Volume 2

UROPATHOLOGY

Edited by

Gary S. Hill, M.D.

Associate Professor
Department of Pathology
Johns Hopkins University School of Medicine
Chief
Department of Pathology
Francis Scott Key Medical Center
Baltimore, Maryland

CHURCHILL LIVINGSTONE
New York, Edinburgh, London, Melbourne
1989

Library of Congress Cataloging in Publication Data

Uropathology / edited by Gary S. Hill.
    p.   cm.
    Includes bibliographies and index.
    ISBN 0-443-08194-8 (set)
    1. Genitourinary organs — Diseases. 2. Genitourinary organs — Pathophysiology.
I. Hill, Gary S.
    [DNLM: 1. Genitalia, Male — pathology. 2. Urinary tract — pathology. 3. Urologic
Diseases — pathology. WJ 100 U798]
RC873.9.U76 1989
616.6′07 — dc19
DNLM/DLC
for Library of Congress
                                     88-22940
                                           CIP

© **Churchill Livingstone Inc. 1989**

Distributed in the United Kingdom by Churchill Livingstone, Robert Stevenson House, 1–3 Baxter's Place, Leith Walk, Edinburgh EH1 3AF, and by associated companies, branches, and representatives throughout the world.

Accurate indications, adverse reactions, and dosage schedules for drugs are provided in this book, but it is possible that they may change. The reader is urged to review the package information data of the manufacturers of the medications mentioned.

The Publishers have made every effort to trace the copyright holders for borrowed material. If they have inadvertently overlooked any, they will be pleased to make the necessary arrangements at the first opportunity.

Acquisitions Editor: *Robert A. Hurley*
Copy Editor: *Ann Ruzycka*
Production Designer: *Jill Little*
Production Supervisor: *Jocelyn Eckstein*

Printed in the United States of America

First published in 1989

To **R. H. Heptinstall, M.D.,**
a friend and mentor for
a quarter of a century,

and **Martha,**
whose patience
and understanding
have sustained me
throughout this long effort

CONTRIBUTORS

Claire Billey-Kijner, M.D.

Staff Pathologist, Hôpital de la Maison Nanterre, Nanterre; Attachée, Department of Pathology, Hôpital de Saint Germain-en-Laye, Saint Germain-en-Laye, France

David Brandes, M.D.

Associate Professor Emeritus, Department of Pathology, Johns Hopkins University School of Medicine; Staff Pathologist, Francis Scott Key Medical Center, Baltimore, Maryland

James W. Eagan, Jr., M.D.

Assistant Professor, Department of Pathology, Johns Hopkins University School of Medicine; Associate Pathologist, St. Joseph's Hospital, Baltimore, Maryland

Gary S. Hill, M.D.

Associate Professor, Department of Pathology, Johns Hopkins University School of Medicine; Chief, Department of Pathology, Francis Scott Key Medical Center, Baltimore, Maryland

Robert S. Katz, M.D.

Assistant Clinical Professor, Department of Pathology, College of Physicians and Surgeons of Columbia University, New York, New York; Director, Blood Bank, Department of Pathology, Morristown Memorial Hospital, Morristown, New Jersey

Juan C. Millan, M.D.

Associate Professor, Department of Pathology, Division of Laboratory Medicine, John Hopkins University School of Medicine; Chief of Laboratory Medicine, Department of Pathology, Francis Scott Key Medical Center, Baltimore, Maryland

Frank Rudy, M.D.

Clinical Assistant Professor, Department of Pathology, Pennsylvania State University College of Medicine, Hershey, Pennsylvania; Associate Pathologist, Department of Pathology, Polyclinic Medical Center, Harrisburg, Pennsylvania

John E. Tomaszewski, M.D.

Assistant Professor, Department of Pathology and Laboratory Medicine, University of Pennsylvania School of Medicine, Philadelphia, Pennsylvania

James E. Wheeler, M.D.

Professor, Department of Pathology and Laboratory Medicine, University of Pennsylvania School of Medicine, Philadelphia, Pennsylvania

PREFACE

Knowledge in all areas of pathology is expanding at a rapid rate. Nowhere is this explosion more dramatic than in urologic pathology. It has become difficult for the pathologist or the urologist to keep up to date with every advance. This expansion also has made it more important than ever to have available a uropathology text which attempts to tie together what has become a broad field. With this goal in mind, we have written a book which covers the entire urinary tract and the male reproductive system.

We have also tried to put together a book which represents a more faithful reflection of urologic practice than is available in any other text. We have placed strong emphasis on congenital anomalies, infectious and inflammatory processes, and obstructive uropathy rather than on neoplastic lesions.

When we began to write the book, we realized that simply describing the morphology of the various lesions was not enough. There are a number of problem areas in urologic pathology in which the morphology is reasonably straightforward but the underlying pathogenesis is poorly understood or controversial, or both. Notable among these topics are the various renal cystic and dysplastic lesions and their relation to intrauterine obstruction, reflux nephropathy, interstitial cystitis, the mechanisms of obstructive nephropathy, bladder cancer, the interrelations of the various types of testicular malignancies, the testicular substrate of infertility, and the relation of human papillomaviruses to penile neoplasms. In these areas and others we have included extended discussions of etiology and pathogenesis in an attempt to fully lay out opposing views and, where possible, give a synthesis of current thinking. By contrast, we have limited our discussion of therapy and prognosis, with the primary goal of putting the lesion into the appropriate clinical context.

I would like to acknowledge a number of individuals who have contributed to the production of this book, starting with three without whose help it literally could not have been completed. Janet Zirckel provided untold hours of superb secretarial assistance, not only typing manuscripts and checking references for Drs. Katz, Brandes, and Millan, as well as a portion of my own manuscript, but catching and correcting innumerable grammatical, numerical, and factual errors and inconsistencies. Milton Tudahl, Sr., did almost all of the beautiful photomicrographs which enrich this volume, taking great pains to be sure that the lighting and focus were perfect for each. Over the years he had also taken many of the gross photographs. William Klosicki was responsible for the remaining excellent gross photographs and the conversion of many gross photographs from lantern slides and 35-mm photographs to black and white prints suitable for publication, as well as charts and photographs from other authors and publications.

Other persons who made significant contributions were Sandra Harris and Laura Klein, who helped with manuscript and library research; Medical Media of Baltimore, particularly Kristine

Rasmussen, who provided numerous handsome line drawings; Barbara White, who did most of the remaining drawings; Robert Bone and Bob Philips, who did library research; and the histology lab at Francis Scott Key Medical Center, under Ruby Slusser, which cut many sections and performed numerous special stains so that cases might be photographed to best advantage. In Philadelphia, Linda Paul and Lisa DiLemmo provided excellent secretarial assistance to Drs. Wheeler and Tomaszewski.

I would also like to thank Dr. Joseph C. Eggleston for making available abundant surgical pathology material from the Johns Hopkins Hospital and Dr. Robert H. Heptinstall for allowing me to mine the rich lode of material in the autopsy files at Johns Hopkins. My appreciation also goes to those with whom I have worked at Churchill Livingstone, particularly to Robert Hurley, Editor-in-Chief, who has been so incredibly patient during the protracted gestation of this book, and to Ann Ruzycka, our copy editor, and Jill Little, our book designer, who presided so well over its actual delivery. If the book succeeds, it will be in substantial measure because of their efforts.

Lastly, I would like to thank my wife, Martha, for all of her understanding and support during this very long period, and for taking on much of my share of responsibility to our sons, Paul and Justin, despite her own heavy commitments. I am sure that my fellow authors join me in expressing my gratitude to their families for their forbearance during the writing of their chapters as well. In a very real way, it was they who made the book possible.

Gary S. Hill, M.D.

CONTENTS

Volume 1

URINARY TRACT OBSTRUCTION

Volume 2

NEOPLASIA IN THE URINARY TRACT

LESIONS OF THE TESTIS

15

Tumors of the Kidney

Juan C. Millan

Primary malignant tumors of the kidney include Wilms' tumor (nephroblastoma), renal cell carcinomas, and various types of sarcoma. In 1987 renal malignant tumors represented 2 to 3 percent of all cancers, with 21,900 estimated new cases of genitourinary carcinoma (excluding the bladder).[248] These epidemiologic data fail to distinguish tumors that arise in the renal pelvis from those in the renal parenchyma and do not highlight the marked age difference between renal cell adenocarcinoma and Wilms' tumor. Important etiologic and epidemiologic characteristics distinguish these tumors.

Wilms' tumor (nephroblastoma), accounting for 2 to 4 percent of all kidney cancers, usually appears during the first 5 years of life; and in 95 percent of cases it presents before the age of 15 years.[259] Rarely, it appears in adults, with fewer than 200 cases reported in the literature.[236]

Renal cell adenocarcinoma constitutes 85 to 95 percent of all kidney tumors.[259] It occurs almost exclusively in adults, although cases in children and adolescents have been described.[2,82,269] Sarcomas, representing 1 percent of all kidney tumors,[259] also occur mainly in persons more than 15 years of age.

Benign tumors are represented by oncocytomas, juxtaglomerular cell tumors, angiomyolipomas, renomedullary interstitial tumors, and the usual benign mesenchymal tumors: lipomas, leiomyomas, hemangiomas, and lymphangiomas.

RENAL TUMORS OF CHILDHOOD

Primary tumors of the kidney during childhood present numerous unresolved points concerning their nomenclature, histogenesis, and prognosis. In 1969 the National Wilms' Tumor Study (NWTS) was created to increase the understanding of renal tumors of childhood and to develop improved therapeutic approaches; it has published three major reports of its observations since then.[22,52,79,80] During that period there has been a dramatic increase in survival with the use of multimodal treatment. Characterization of these relatively rare tumors has also been achieved.[20,80]

The principal primary kidney tumors of childhood are the following:

Wilms' tumor (nephroblastoma)
Nephroblastomatosis
Cystic partially differentiated nephroblastoma
Congenital mesoblastic nephroma
Clear cell sarcoma of the kidney (bone-metastasizing renal tumor of childhood)
Malignant rhabdoid tumor

Wilms' Tumor (Nephroblastoma)

INCIDENCE AND EPIDEMIOLOGY

Approximately 450 cases of Wilms' tumor are diagnosed annually in the United States.[296] In Great Britain a rate of 0.5 case per 100,000 children per year has been documented,[203] and the incidence has been reported to be remarkably constant among various populations in the world.[144] This statement has been challenged, however, in view of the remarkable racial difference in incidence reported from the Greater Delaware Valley tumor registry. Wilms' tumor comprises 5.3 percent of all cancers among white children compared to 11.3 percent among nonwhite children.[165] This higher proportion in black children was also associated with a higher incidence of congenital anomalies.

The peak incidence of nephroblastoma occurs during the second to fourth year of life, with 50 percent of the cases being diagnosed at approximately 3 years of age.[51] However, some cases have been detected in fetuses, and the tumor has also been reported in adults.[57,69]

Wilms' tumors that are bilateral, familial, and generally associated with congenital anomalies appear in younger patients; the median age of the children at diagnosis being 25.5 months. The median age at diagnosis of nephroblastomas that are unilateral and presumably sporadic is 36.1 months.[51] Age at presentation is also related to sex. The male incidence peaks during the second to third year of life, whereas for girls it remains high into the fourth year.[51] Although it has been reported in the past that there are no sex differences, the National Wilms' Study II (NWTS-II) reported a slightly higher proportion of the tumor in girls (male/female ratio of 0.896 : 1.000).[51] Nonwhite girls have the highest incidence rate, 14.6 per 1,000,000 children age 0 to 14 years, compared with 9.4 for nonwhite boys, and 6.0 and 6.3 for white girls and white boys, respectively.[165]

ETIOLOGY

Numerous factors have been implicated in the etiology of nephroblastoma-like tumors in experimental animals, including chemicals, (N-nitroso compounds, methane, cycasin, dimethylbenzatracene), radiation, and infectious agents.[29] A rat Wilms' tumor model morphologically identical to the human tumor has been used to study tumor biology and therapeutic modalities.[205]

In humans the associations with congenital anomalies,[76,77,219] heredity, and chromosomal disorders[160] are of definite etiologic significance, whereas gestational factors and occupational exposure of parents have not been conclusively demonstrated.

Congenital Anomalies

Aniridia, or absence of the iris, occurs in a sporadic and a familial form. The sporadic form has been present in about 1 percent of the cases of Wilms' tumors reviewed by the NWTS group, and it is esti-

mated that 30 percent of children with aniridia develop Wilms' tumor. Nephroblastomas have also been reported in the familial form of aniridia.[298]

Genitourinary anomalies[51] ranging from double collecting systems (1.52 percent of all cases of Wilms' tumor), horseshoe kidneys (0.43 percent),[195] cryptorchidism (2.78 percent), hypospadias (1.78 percent), to pseudohermaphroditism have been described. This last association has been referred to as the Drash syndrome.[92] It is also associated with chronic glomerulonephritis in which electron-dense deposits have been demonstrated.[188,254]

Hemihypertrophy, in which one side of the body is significantly larger than the other, was first reported with Wilms' tumor by Miller et al.[198] and was found in 2.47 percent of the 1,905 cases reported by the NWTS group between 1969 and 1981.

Other conditions associated with somatic overgrowth have been related to a higher incidence of Wilms' tumor. They include the *Beckwith-Weidemann syndrome* (macroglossia, gigantism, umbilical hernia, and kidney and pancreatic hyperplasia) and the *Klippel-Trenaunay syndrome* (multiple nevi, hemangiomas, mental retardation, and seizures).

Associations between various congenital anomalies occur, especially between aniridia and genitourinary malformations. Other congenital anomalies have also been described,[51] as have entities such as neurofibromatosis.[261]

Heredity and Familial Cases

The NWTS included 20 patients (1 percent) who had one or more relatives with Wilms' tumor.[51] Larger numbers of bilateral tumors were found in these family members. Wilms' tumor has also occurred in monozygous twins,[187] with at least four twin pairs demonstrating tumors in both twins.

In 1972 Knudson and Strong[161] analyzed familial an sporadic cases. Familial cases have an earlier average age of diagnosis, a higher incidence of bilaterality (21 percent), and a pattern of inheritance consistent with autosomal dominant transmission. Nonhereditary cases are diagnosed later, and only 5 to 10 percent are bilateral. Knudson and Strong suggested a two-mutational model in which two mutations are required for tumor development. In this model familial cases would represent one inherited germinal mutation plus a subsequent somatic mutation. Nonhereditary cases would be the result of two successive somatic mutations. It was estimated that 62 percent of the Wilms' tumor cases were of the nonhereditary form. Hemihypertrophy-associated Wilms' tumor was thought to result from two somatic mutations. Lately, it has been suggested that some of the associations with congential anomalies, especially dysgenesis, can also be explained by two postzygotic events. They must occur early enough in embryogenesis to affect developing renal and genital tissue on both sides of the midline.[51] The presence of tumor in one of a pair of monozygous twins but not in the other lends support to the two-mutation requirement for development of the tumor.[187]

Chromosome Abnormalities

It has been reported that mutant forms of one or more loci contained within the 11p 13 band on chromosome 11 predispose to the formation of this tumor.[298] Deletion of this region has been seen in tumor cells, without occurring in the normal somatic cells of patients. It may be due to an abnormal segregation with loss of a homologous chromosome and reduplication of the remaining homologue.[162]

Gestational factors may also be implicated in the development of this tumor but have not been conclusively demonstrated. The possibility that occupational exposures among fathers of children with Wilms' tumor influence its development has been suggested. It has been reported the proportionally more nephroblastoma patients have fathers that work in either lead- or hydrocarbon-related occupations.[152] However, another study did not find a statistical difference in the frequency of occupational exposure to lead, lead alkyls, and lead salts for fathers of children with Wilms' tumor. In this study, case fathers were found more likely to have been exposed to boron.[291] Maternal use of hair-coloring products, hypertension and fluid retention during pregnancy, tea drinking, and vaginal infections have also been associated with increased risk of Wilms' tumor.[55a] Additional studies are required to clarify these associations.

PATHOGENESIS

The origin of Wilms' tumor from metanephric blastema is widely accepted.[20,29] Controversy exists whether this tumor develops from persistent renal blastema or from differentiated cells that regain embryonic potential.

The presence of persistent renal blastema has been demonstrated in systematic reviews of pediatric autopsies. Bennington and Beckwith[29] reported an incidence of blastemal rests in pediatric autopsies of 1 per 204. The incidence was 1 per 115 in infants less than 3 months old. Lesions were multiple, associated with congenital malformations, and situated in the periphery of renal lobules. Independent foci of renal blastema are also present in 17 to 27 percent[29] of nephroblastomas. The cell rests apparently result from developmental disturbances of the kidneys.[19] Aspirin has been implicated in a case where a maturation defect was observed followed by a diffuse nephroblastic proliferation.[46]

Another type of dysgenetic lesion seems to be important in a subgroup of Wilms' tumors. These lesions are nephroblastic proliferations in the deep cortical areas and in the midzones of the lobules (intralobular). The stromal component of the proliferations may show heterotopic tissue, and it has been related to nephroblastomas that show minimal epithelial differentiation. They remain blastemal or differentiate toward a stroma with immature skeletal muscle.[20,182]

The possibility of the development of nephroblastomas from differentiated cells that regain embryonic potential is raised by the occasional appearance of the tumor in adults and by the presence of embryonal hyperplasia of Bowman's capsule in end-stage dialysis kidneys.[143] In a review of 108 pairs of end-stage kidneys obtained prior to transplantation, we saw small foci of renal blastema in six cases (5.45 percent). The mean age of the patients was 36 years, with no cases under 10 years of age (unpublished data). Most renal tumors that develop in end-stage renal failure have renal cell differentiation rather than blastemal differentiation. It appears, then, that some if not all adult Wilms' tumors are explained by persistence into adulthood of the nephroblastomatosis complex and subsequent malignant transformation.[242]

The ability of blastemal cells to differentiate into tubular and stromal elements forming the triphasic component of Wilms' tumor has been described.[243] Cells of Wilms' tumor resemble blastemal cells of the intermediate cell mass that derives from primary mesenchyme. Both have epithelial features, being closely apposed and demonstrating intercellular junctions.

The plasma membrane of the cells is also occasionally lined by a thick layer of flocculent, moderately electron-dense material with a basement membranelike appearance. There is immunohistochemical evidence that it actually corresponds to a basement membrane antigen.[105] This material is characteristic of Wilms' tumor and when present can be used in the differential diagnosis from other pediatric neoplasms such as neuroblastomas and rhabdomyosarcomas.

Tubular areas are formed by a greater degree of organization of the diffuse blastemal epithelium. Open spaces become central lumens, and the flocculent material develops into discrete basal lamina. The tubular elements, however, do not differentiate completely into the normal segments of the renal tubules.

Transitions between blastema cells and loosely arranged stroma, with flocculent basement membranelike material lying against stromal cells, have also been shown. The differentiation of the stroma into heterotopic tissue is thought to occur by way of anomalous differentiation.[243]

Attention has also been given to the presence of intermediate filament proteins that indicate the embryonic differentiation of cells.[214] In a study of nine nephroblastomas, blastemal cells demonstrated the presence of vimentin and cytokeratin, the tubules showed cytokeratin positivity, and stroma cells were positive for vimentin only. In immature nephroblastomas only vimentin was shown — in a pattern analogous to that of primitive mesodermal cells. It has been postulated that primitive blastemal cells can differentiate into two pathways: (1) *epithelial,* with first co-expression of vimentin and cytokeratin (blastema) and later with only cytokeratin (tubules); and (2) *mesenchymal,* with maintenance of vimentin (stroma, fibrocytes, chondrocytes, osteocytes). In smooth and skeletal muscle there is first co-expression of vimentin and desmin, and later the vimentin system is turned off.[4]

Cell membrane glycosylation, determined by lectin histochemistry, demonstrates a similar pattern of differentiation for fetal, adult, and Wilms' tumor nodules. An increased complexity in glycosubstances is present with progressive epithelial differentiation.[295a]

PATHOLOGY

The NWTS-I and NWTS-II results have made it evident that predicting the prognosis of Wilms' tumor depends on an accurate description of tumor extension and on the microscopic characteristics, favorable or unfavorable, of the tumor.[22,52,79]

Grossly, the tumor appears as a large, well circumscribed mass that replaces most of the kidney (Fig. 15-1). On cut section it bulges over the cut surface. It is soft to firm and gray or white, in contrast with neuroblastomas, which are reddish purple. Nephroblastomas may also have a variegated appearance with foci of hemorrhage and gelatinous areas or cysts. A pseudocapsule is commonly present with compression of the surrounding kidney parenchyma, but often the tumor has infiltrative margins. Calcifications may be present.

Size is not a prognostic factor. NWTS-I had shown that combined kidney and tumor weights under 250 g gave a favorable prognosis.[53] NWTS-II has now demonstrated that neither tumor size nor age at diagnosis are independent prognostic features.[52] This difference in findings likely reflects the advances in therapy that have occurred during the period between the two studies. *Multifocal* masses are found in about 7 percent of cases, and 5 percent of cases are bilateral.[51] The tumor occurs somewhat more frequently in the left kidney (51.4 percent), but laterality does not influence prognosis.[52]

Local spread occurs by direct invasion of the tumor through the renal capsule into the perirenal soft tissue. Renal vessels may also be invaded, with propagation as a tumor thrombus into the renal vein (10 percent) and inferior vena cava (4 percent). It is accompanied by an increase in the rate of distant metastasis. NWTS-II patients with negative renal vein invasion had a 15 percent relapse rate compared with 22.2 percent for patients with renal vein thrombus and 36.4 percent for those with a thrombus in the inferior vena cava.[52]

Lymph node metastases in the regional lymph nodes comprise one of the more important prognostic factors in both NWTS groups and the European experience.[147] Approximately 18 percent of patients had lymph node metastases. The 2-year relapse-free survival rate was 54 percent for patients with metastases and 82 percent for those with no evidence of node involvement.[79] Lymph node metastases must be evaluated microscopically. It has been reported that half of the patients considered by surgeons to have positive lymph nodes failed to have microscopic confirmation of this finding.[52]

Abdominal spread and *operative spillage* are two im-

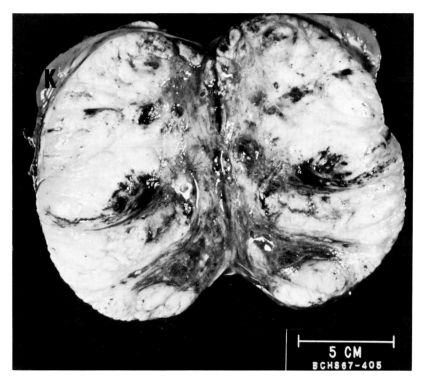

Fig. 15-1 Wilms' tumor. Gross appearance shows a minute area of residual kidney (K). Note the large, whitish solid tumor with hemorrhagic foci.

portant characteristics that must be evaluated by the surgeon. The surgeon's indication of regional spread or spillage during operation are strongly associated with abdominal recurrence, relapse, and mortality. Abdominal spread was demonstrated in 17 percent of cases; local operative spillage was seen in 10 percent of cases, and diffuse operative spread to the general peritoneal cavity was present in 2.4 percent of NWTS-II patients.[52] The degree of spill is currently under review as a prognostic factor. Preoperative radiation therapy decreases the frequency of tumor rupture but may complicate the microscopic evaluation of the tumor for detection of unfavorable microscopic features.[42]

Staging

The current staging system used in NWTS-III has been refined by the knowledge acquired through the first two cooperative studies.

Stage I: tumor limited to the kidney and completely excised

Stage II: tumor extending beyond the kidney but completely excised

Stage III: residual nonhematogenous tumor confined to the abdomen

Stage IV: hematogenous metastases

Stage V: bilateral renal involvement at diagnosis

Staging[24] is based on both gross and microscopic identification of tumor and metastases. Favorable or unfavorable histologic patterns do not modify the stage. In a stage I tumor the surface of the renal capsule is intact. The tumor has not been ruptured before or during removal, and there is no residual tumor beyond the margins of resection. A report from the NWTS-III has highlighted the importance of capsular invasion, presence of pseudocapsule, renal sinus penetration (hilar structures and soft tissue), and intrarenal vein invasion. All the Stage I cases with favorable histology that relapsed had one or more of these features.[284a] Stage II is characterized by penetration through the renal capsule into the perirenal soft tissues. Vessels outside the kidney substance are infiltrated or contain tumor thrombus. The tumor may have been biopsied, or there has been local spillage of tumor confined to the flank. There is no residual tumor at the margins of excision.

Stage III may have (1) lymph node involvement at the hilus, periaortic chain, or beyond; (2) diffuse peritoneal contamination of tumor by either operative tumor spillage beyond the flank or penetration of tumor growth through the peritoneal surface; (3) peritoneal implants; (4) tumor extending beyond the surgical margins grossly or microscopically; (5) tumor that is not completely resectable because of local infiltration of vital structures.

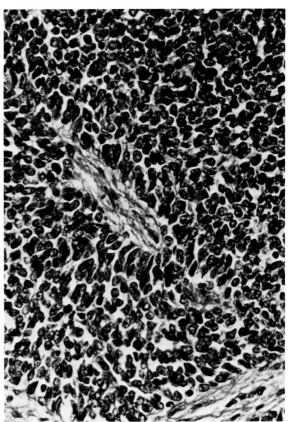

Fig. 15-3 Wilms' tumor. In this high-power view of blastemal cells, the nuclei are oval or elongated, and the cytoplasm is scarce. ×378.

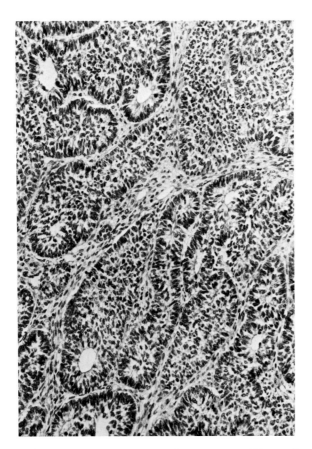

Fig. 15-2 Wilms' tumor. Note the aggregates of blastemal cells, with some tubular differentiation separated by stroma. ×152.

With stage IV, distant hematogenous metastases are present. Eleven percent of the cases are in this stage at diagnosis, with 95 percent of these cases showing metastases in the lungs. Another, less common site is the liver. With stage V disease each side should be staged according to the above criteria. Subsequent bilateral involvement does not seem to alter prognosis.

Microscopic Appearance

Classically, the tumor appears as a triphasic renal neoplasm in which blastemal, epithelial, and stromal cells are seen (Fig. 15-2), with each cell type having a variety of patterns and lines of differentiation. Transitions are observed between these cell lines, and some tumors exhibit a biphasic or monotopic pattern.[29]

Blastema cells are oval or slightly elongated cells

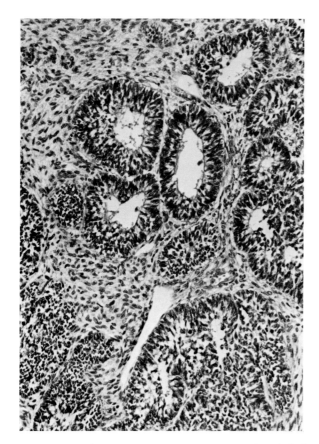

Fig. 15-4 Wilms' tumor. Low-power view of epithelial differentiation with recognizable tubular formation. There is nuclear polarization to a central lumen and a clearly defined luminal border. ×152.

with scanty cytoplasm (Fig. 15-3); they are closely packed together and generally separated by stroma into nodules or trabecula. Tubular differentiation may be apparent either centrally or at the periphery (Fig. 15-2).

Epithelial differentiation may be barely apparent, or there may be well developed tubules (Figs. 15-4 and 15-5). Papillary patterns, glomeruloid bodies with no vascularization, and heterotopic cells and tissues may be encountered. Less differentiated epithelial cells can assume a basaloid or cordlike pattern. Transitional, squamous, mucinous, and ciliated columnar epithelium have been described. Argentaffin and argyrophil cells, neuroblasts, and ganglion cells (Fig. 15-6) have also been seen.[20]

Stromal cells are predominantly fibroblastic or myxoid, sharp contrast to the dark blastemal cells (Fig. 15-7). Smooth muscle (Fig. 15-8) and skeletal muscle may be present, as well as cartilage (Fig. 15-9), fat cells, and bone. Uncommonly, anaplastic elements are found.

Monomorphous variants of Wilms' tumor represent a gray zone between Wilms' tumor and other renal neoplasms. Degeneration of blastema with oncocytoid features[29] as well as cases that closely resemble adenocarcinoma have been described.[20] Because nearly all parenchymal renal neoplasms originate from metanephric blastema or its differentiated derivatives, it may be argued that all are related to Wilms' tumor.[19] However, it is better to consider them separate entities for diagnostic and therapeutic purposes. Two other tumors have been distinguished from nephroblastomas as a result of conclusions from the first NWTS collaborative study[22]: *clear cell sarcoma* of

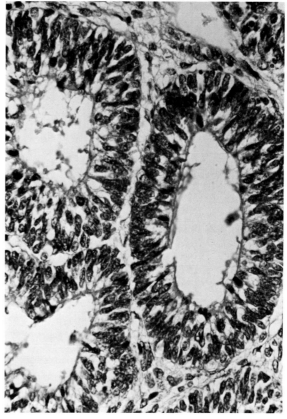

Fig. 15-5 Wilms' tumor. High-power view of Fig. 15-4. ×378.

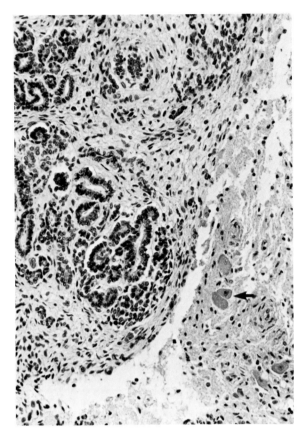

Fig. 15-6 Wilms' tumor. Ganglion cell differentiation (arrows). ×165.

the kidney and *malignant rhabdoid tumor* (see below). They do not represent Wilms' tumor variants.

Monotopic tubular tumors are said to have a better prognosis,[63] as do nephroblastomas with fibroadenomatouslike structures.[88] The criterion for this diagnosis is the finding of coarse infolded lobular formations of blastema, forming slitlike lumens similar to those seen with fibroadenomas of the breast and ovary.

The randomly assorted heterotopic tissues occasionally seen in Wilms' tumor raise the possibility of a renal teratoma.[279] This diagnosis is reserved for tumors that definitely exhibit organogenesis, with attempts to form organs other than kidney. Among 2,600 cases in the NWTS, Beckwith described only one such case.[20]

The most important microscopic features for establishing the prognosis of nephroblastoma are the cri-

teria for *anaplasia* developed as a consequence of the analysis of NWTS-I.[22] As stated by Beckwith, it is a major responsibility of the pathologist to ascertain if anaplastic cells are present. A combined series from NWTS-I and NWTS-II found 7.3 percent of tumors with anaplasia.[42] Anaplasia may involve blastemal, epithelial, or stromal elements or any combination of them. Its incidence increases with age, appearing mainly in children 1 to 2 years older than the average age of 3 years. A higher percentage of nonwhite children are seen in the anaplastic tumor group (31 percent versus 11 percent in the nonanaplastic tumor group). Almost 50 percent of the 84 children with anaplastic Wilms' tumor suffered a relapse, and 42 percent died from tumor after at least a 4-year follow-up.[42] Initially the monotopic sarcomatous elements represented by clear cell sarcoma and malignant rhabdoid tumor were included in the unfavorable prog-

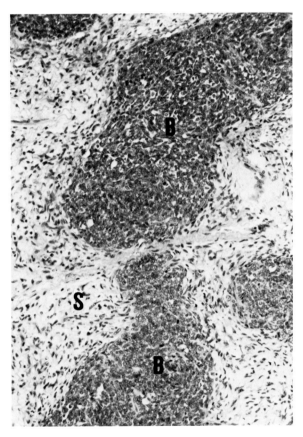

Fig. 15-7 Wilms' tumor. Note the contrasting appearance of stromal (S) and blastemal (B) cells. ×152.

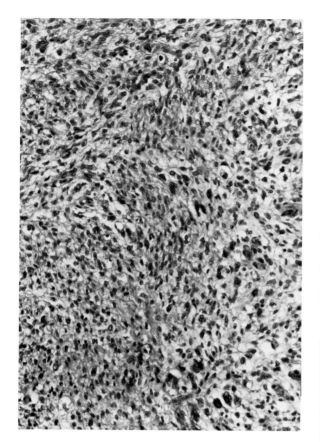

Fig. 15-8 Wilms' tumor. Note the areas with smooth muscle differentiation. ×152.

nostic group. They are currently separated as distinct entities.

The minimal definition of anaplasia requires that all *three* of the following criteria[20] be met.

1. Marked enlargement of some nuclei within blastemal, epithelial, or stromal cells to at least three times the diameter of adjacent nuclei of the same cell type (Fig. 15-10). Skeletal muscle is excluded, as anaplasia limited to skeletal muscle has not been associated with a worse prognosis.
2. Marked hyperchromatism of the enlarged nuclei (Fig. 15-10).
3. Multipolar mitotic figures (Fig. 15-11).

Anaplasia has been characterized as *focal* if 10 percent or less of the submitted tumor sections meet the outlined criteria, or *diffuse* if more than 10 percent of the tissue submitted meets the criteria. The NWTS-II

experience has shown an improved survival with aggressive chemotherapy in anaplastic tumors. Importantly, there is no difference in relapse and survival between focal and diffuse anaplasia.[42] Even in those cases with focal anaplasia involving only one microscopic slide, the prognosis is worsened. Thorough sampling is necessary, then, to evaluate these tumors. The NWTS recommendation is one section of tumor for each centimeter of largest tumor diameter. It has also been stated by some of the principal investigators that they take two to three times this number of sections when anaplasia is suspected, and that lymph nodes are carefully examined because of the high association between anaplasia and lymph node metastases. If the tumor is multicentric, each nodule should be analyzed.

Reliable identification of anaplasia requires well fixed tissue free of compression artifact, sectioned

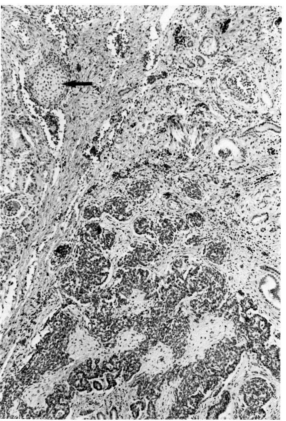

Fig. 15-9 Wilms' tumor. Note the cartilagenous structures (arrow) as part of mesenchymal differentiation. ×74.

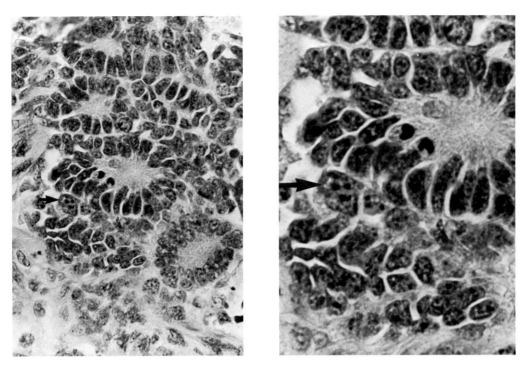

Fig. 15-10 Wilms' tumor. Nuclear anaplasia is evident. **(B)** Enlarged pleomorphic nuclei with abnormal chromatin aggregates (arrows) are shown at higher magnification. **A,** ×500; **B,** ×1,000.

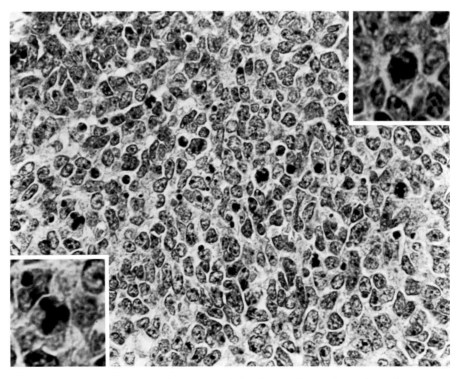

Fig. 15-11 Wilms' tumor. Note the atypia and the abnormal irregular and tripolar mitoses in blastemal cells. The latter appear enlarged in the insets in the right upper and left lower corners. ×640; **insets,** ×1,280.

Table 15-1 Wilms' Tumor Survival at 2 Years According to Stage, Lymph Nodes, and Histology

Parameter		%
Stage		
I:	Tumor limited to kidney	95
II:	Tumor extends beyond kidney	90
III:	Residual nonhematogenous tumor	84
IV:	Hematogenous metastases	54
Lymph node		
Negative		82
Positive		54
Histology		
Favorable		90
Unfavorable		54

(Modified From D'Angio et al.,[79] with permission.)

thin, and well stained. False identification of anaplasia can be made if care is not taken to differentiate it from megakaryocytes, either circulating or in areas of extramedullary hematopoiesis. Crush artifact with fusion of nuclear material, overlapping cells in thick sections, overstaining with inadequate removal of excess nuclear stain, foreign material, tissue calcification, and psammoma bodies must all be carefully distinguished from true anaplasia.[20] Use of preoperative irradiation should be carefully evaluated. It diminishes the risk of operative spillage with large tumors but creates difficulty for evaluating the unfavorable histology of anaplasia. Cytomorphology of anaplastic cells indicates an abnormal DNA content, and evaluation with flow cytometry has recently been performed.[244a]

When reviewing the pathology of Wilms' tumor, both staging with the crucial feature of metastasis to lymph nodes and favorable or unfavorable (anaplasia) histologic features must be carefully evaluated. Table 15-1 shows 2-year survival rates of NWTS-II.[79] Note that NWTS-II results included periaortic lymph node involvement as a stage II lesion. It is considered in NWTS-III as stage III disease. Also, in NWTS-III peritoneal contamination limited to the local flank has been down-graded to stage II.

"NATURAL" HISTORY AND EVOLUTION

The natural history of this tumor has been dramatically altered as a result of the cooperative studies during the early 1970s in the United States (NWTS) and Europe (International Society for Pediatric Oncology; SIOP). It is believed that during the early 1900s most children with Wilms' tumor died; in 1920 the mortality rate was more than 90 percent; during the 1940s, survival approached 50 percent with the advent of postoperative radiotherapy and improved surgical methods; and during the mid-1970s a 90 percent survival rate had been achieved with the addition of combination chemotherapy.[24] This change in the natural history of Wilms' tumor after intensive therapy,[71] however, has resulted in a series of complications and sequelae of therapy, including second malignant tumors.

CLINICAL PRESENTATION

Most children appear healthy when first seen. In most cases the tumor is found incidentally during a well-baby examination or is noted by the parents. An enlarging mass is easily palpable. The tumor generally protrudes forward, and the mass is hard and sometimes lobulated. Associated signs and symptoms are often nonspecific.[292]

1. Pain is seldom severe until there is local infiltration.
2. Hematuria is seen in one-third of cases, generally the result of thrombosis in obstructed veins.
3. Mild fever occurs in 30 percent of cases and may be associated with hemorrhage into the tumor.
4. Elevations of systolic pressure with or without diastolic elevations have been found in 63 percent of cases.[266] Though it is possible that secretion of renin by the tumor cells may be responsible for the observed hypertension,[255] local ischemia in the adjacent kidney is a more likely explanation.
5. Trauma to the flank may lead to rupture of a Wilms' tumor, with pain and signs of blood loss. It must be differentiated from traumatic rupture of the spleen or liver. Confined hemorrhage within the capsule may account for some of the peripheral calcifications seen with some nephroblastomas.

DIAGNOSIS

Detection of a flank mass is the usual presentation. Excretory urography (intravenous pyelogram, IVP) and chest films are generally the only additional tests required. In this age range, pulmonary nodules found in association with an intrarenal mass are virtually always due to the presence of a Wilms' tumor. On

IVP the mass is intrarenal and displaces and distorts the renal collecting system. Sonography, computed tomography (CT), and angiography, though they may identify the tumor more precisely, are seldom necessary, particularly as any child with a flank mass must be surgically explored. Additional studies are used only when there is doubt that the mass is intrarenal and when there is suspicion of bilateral involvement.[78,164]

Inferior venacavography seems to be particularly indicated when tumor thrombus is suspected, e.g., for a nonvisualized kidney on routine IVP or a prominent collateral venous pattern in the anterior abdominal wall. Bilateral involvement is sometimes inconspicuous, and the entire surface of the contralateral kidney should be examined at operation, especially in cases of nephroblastomatosis or Beckwith-Weidemann syndrome. Careful clinical examination with IVP and CT is the most valuable means of following patients at risk of disease or for contralateral involvement.

The lungs are the most frequent site of metastasis. In NWTS-II 95 percent of stage IV tumors had lung metastases, either alone or associated with other sites. The liver is also involved in metastatic spread, with a 15 percent incidence for stage IV tumors (alone or in combination with other sites). Follow-up with chest x-ray films is advocated every 6 months for the first 3 years after operation and yearly thereafter. This regimen is especially relevant as treatment of metastases has been associated with a 50 percent 2-year survival.[79] Liver metastases indicate an apparently worse prognosis.[52a]

DIFFERENTIAL DIAGNOSIS

The differential diagnosis includes benign conditions such as cystic lesions, abscesses, hemorrhage, dysplastic kidney and mesoblastic nephroma, and malignant tumors such as neuroblastoma, sarcoma, and renal cell carcinoma.[96]

Cystic lesions can produce x-ray findings similar to those of Wilms' tumor. They may be differentiated by sonography, but the possibility of the presence of a cystic nephroblastoma should also be considered.

Mesoblastic nephroma has a radiologic appearance similar to that of nephroblastoma even with the newer supplementary studies. The differential diagnosis is made by the characteristic gross and microscopic morphology (see below).

Intrarenal neuroblastoma is the most common source of misdiagnosis. Neuroblastomas have stippled or flaky calcifications instead of the infrequent (5 percent of cases) spotlike or ringlike calcification of nephroblastoma. Neuroblastic rosettes are sometimes confused with the embryonic tubular pattern of Wilms' tumors. Beckwith[20] stressed that neuroblastic rosettes lack lumens and have multilayered, nonpalisading cells surrounding fibrillary centers without a peripheral basal lamina. In contrast, tubules of Wilms' tumor have lumens and a single layer of well aligned cells (Fig. 15-12) surrounded by a basal lamina (Fig. 15-13). The stroma is also different. Neuroblastomas have a fibrovascular and neurofibrillar stroma,

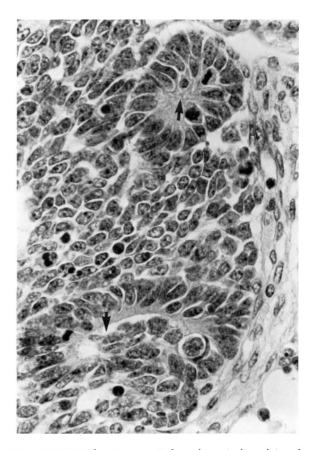

Fig. 15-12 Wilms' tumor. Enlarged atypical nuclei and atypical mitosis in structures with tubular differentiation. The tubule at the top resembles a rosette seen with neuroblastoma. The presence of a primitive lumen (arrows) and basement membrane material seen by electron microscopy (Fig. 15-13) facilitates the differential diagnosis. ×621.

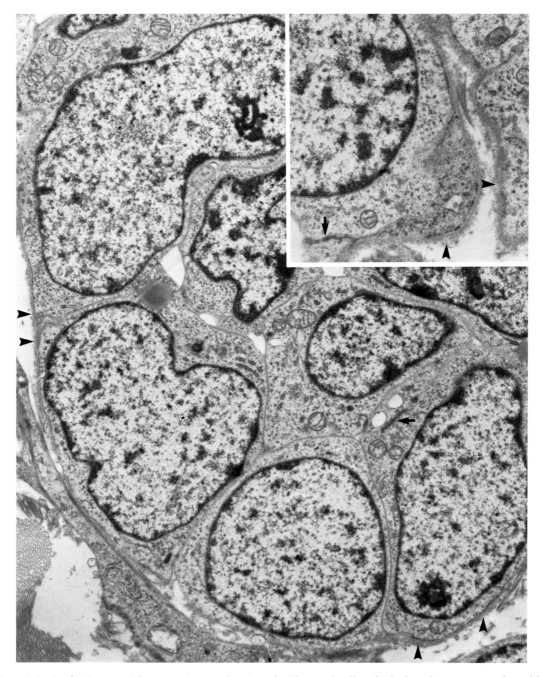

Fig. 15-13 Wilms' tumor. Electron micrograph. Note the blastemal cells, which show basement membranelike material (arrowheads) and tight junctions (arrow). **(Inset)** Basement membrane material (arrowheads). Tight junctions (arrow) are evident at this higher magnification. ×7,438. **Inset,** ×10,625.

whereas with nephroblastomas the stroma is fibro-myxoid, with mesenchymal cells exhibiting other types of heterotopic differentiation such as smooth and skeletal muscle, and cartilage. Wilms' tumors are also more variegated in appearance than neuroblastomas.

Biochemical studies such as vanillylmandelic acid and homovanillic acid in the urine are also helpful in differentiating neuroblastoma from Wilms' tumor. Inactive renin has been proposed as a tumor marker in nephroblastoma.[61a] Electron microscopy of neuroblastomas demonstrates the presence of neurosecretory granules, and studies for neuron-specific enolase are positive.[125] Wilms' tumors have a characteristic thick layer of flocculent, moderately electron-dense material surrounding the blastemal cells (Fig. 15-13).[20]

TREATMENT

The marked success achieved with the multimodal treatment currently used in both the NWTS[79] and the European experience (SIOP)[170] underscores three fundamental considerations in the treatment of Wilms' tumor. First, when treating these young children, the risk of the acute and long-term sequelae of treatment must be considered. Second, treatment has achieved a high degree of survival, and some of the initial prognostic factors (age, size) are no longer valid. Patients with more unfavorable prognostic variables stand out more clearly, and those at low risk begin to merge into a single group.[20] Evaluation of a subgroup who require less treatment becomes more difficult but perhaps more imperative as the risk/benefit ratio of the various therapies must be defined.[24] Third, 2-year survival in Wilms' tumor without recurrence, as for most childhood embryonal tumors, is equivalent to cure.[170] The results of treatment protocols can then be rapidly assessed.

Surgery

Surgery remains the cornerstone of therapy. Total nephrectomy with a transabdominal approach is indicated. The abdomen and the opposite kidney are thoroughly explored. The renal fossa is dissected, and the involved kidney and associated lymph nodes are removed. The renal vein and inferior vena cava are handled carefully so as not to dislodge tumor emboli.

Initially, SIOP employed preoperative radiotherapy, but it was later changed to preoperative chemotherapy — vincristine (VCR) and actinomycin D (AMD) — for 3 weeks.[170] The benefits of this approach seem to be a reduction in tumor spillage at the time of operation and an "improved" surgical pathology stage (because more stage I tumors that do not require radiation therapy are created).[87] The American investigators of the NWTS take strong exception to preoperative treatment; they believe that the important prognostic clues of tissue histology and extent of disease, especially lymph node metastasis, may be missed, which may cause a less precise treatment to be used. NWTS-III is also studying if radiation therapy is necessary for stage II (local extension) tumors. A preliminary report indicates that more than 70 percent of children with tumors of favorable histology and who are free of distant metastases at diagnosis do not require irradiation.[75]

Radiation Therapy

Initially routine postoperative irradiation to the flank was used. It has been shown that stage I patients who have received adjuvant chemotherapy do not need irradiation, and that VCR added to AMD substitutes for postoperative irradiation.[79] Currently, NWTS-III is testing actinomycin D and intensive vincristine therapy in comparison with triple-agent chemotherapy [VCR + AMD + adriamycin (ADR)], with or without postoperative radiotherapy in stage II disease. Radiotherapy is also the standard therapy for lung metastases. The role of surgery and intensive chemotherapy needs to be evaluated in relation to pulmonary metastases.

Chemotherapy

Actinomycin D and VCR used for 15 months comprise the standard therapy. NWTS-III is trying to determine if a shorter period of treatment, 10 weeks to 6 months, can be used for stage I disease. Also, intensive VCR plus AMD is being evaluated against triple-drug therapy (VCR + AMD + ADR). Patients with unfavorable histology of any stage and stage IV patients undergo postoperative irradiation and triple-agent (VCR + AMD + ADR) or quadruple-agent (VCR + AMD + ADR + cyclophosphamide) therapy.

For bilateral tumors of synchronous or metachronous appearance, treatment must be individualized. Partial nephrectomy has been attempted in order to remove all tumor in both kidneys. Postoperative radiotherapy is used if there is residual tumor. Renal transplantation has been done in patients with severely impaired or absent renal function. Waiting for at least a year after treatment of the tumor, if possible, significantly reduces the incidence of recurrence or metastases.[220]

TREATMENT COMPLICATIONS

Acute complications include surgical rupture of the tumor during nephrectomy which heightens the risk of peritoneal seeding.[169] This situation requires irradiation to the whole abdomen, which in turn may cause subsequent intestinal disorders and impaired ovarian function.

Other acute complications are related to the use of chemotherapeutic drugs.[169] Low blood counts, risk of infections, nausea, vomiting, and alopecia frequently develop. The combination of VCR + AMD + ADR after radiotherapy was the most toxic regimen in NWTS-II, with 17.1 percent of patients showing leukocyte counts of less than $1,000/mm^3$, 7.6 percent of patients with platelets under $50,000/mm^3$, and 30.9 percent with hemoglobin levels under 8 g/dl.[79]

A total of 122 deaths among 803 children occurred in NWTS-II. Of them, 17 were attributed to causes other than tumor progression. Seven were due to infection during periods of drug-induced leukopenia, and four were related to liver failure with hemorrhagic necrosis. Other causes were radiation pneumonitis, intestinal obstruction secondary to adhesions, renal failure, myocardial disease, and encephalopathy. The report stressed the additive toxic effect of irradiation and chemotherapy. Children under 1 year of age initially had an inordinate amount of toxicity, requiring a 50 percent reduction of chemotherapeutic doses in this group. Efforts to reduce toxicity are perhaps among the more important goals of the cooperative studies. In NWTS-II, of 44 deaths in groups III and IV, 10 were due to toxicity (23 percent toxic deaths).[148]

Sequela and *delayed complications* seem to be related to late effects of radiation therapy on growing children, possibly enhanced by intensive chemotherapy.[169] Spinal deformities with kyphosis and scoliosis and under-development of the flank soft tissue become obvious at the growth spurt that occurs at puberty. Radiotherapy to both lungs, used for metastatic disease, impairs the growth of the lungs and thoracic wall. Vital capacity and dynamic compliance have been reduced by 20 to 50 percent of the predicted values.[33]

Second malignant neoplasms have begun to be recognized as the success of multiple modality therapy prolongs survival.[174] A report from the Late Effect Study Group (LESG), which involved 12 leading centers in the United States, Canada, and western Europe, included 36 children with Wilms' tumor and a second neoplasm. Almost 30 percent of these cases had characteristics compatible with a prezygotic or genetic form of the tumor, suggesting that second malignant neoplasms occur excessively in the familial form of Wilms' tumor. The most frequent second malignancies found were soft tissue sarcomas (nine cases), leukemia/lymphomas (seven), bone sarcomas (six), thyroid carcinoma (four), and brain tumor (three).[194] It has been reported that children who develop one malignancy have a tenfold increased risk of developing a new cancer and that 3 to 12 percent do so within 20 years of the first diagnosis. It is clear from the LESG study that genetic predisposition, radiation therapy, and chemotherapy, especially with alkylating agents, are the important factors in the development of second malignancies. The lifetime incidence of additional malignancies cannot be estimated at present. The latent period for the development of solid tumors after irradiation is more than 15 years, as reported from the Japanese atomic survival data.[194]

The aim of the present studies (NWTS-III, SIOP-6) is to reduce the long-term sequelae and risk of late effects by reducing the intensiveness of the treatment while retaining the progress achieved. A preliminary report on NWTS-III appears to indicate that stages I, II, and III favorable-histology patients can be treated successfully with less intensive regimens. No improvement seems to have been achieved for stage IV or unfavorable-histology patients.[52a,80] (Table 15-1)

Nephroblastomatosis Complex

In 1961 Hou and Holman[140] described a 32 weeks' premature infant who died soon after delivery. She presented bilateral symmetrical enlargement of the kidneys due to massive proliferation of renal blastema.

In view of the presence of transitional zones from the areas of blastema to normal developing kidney and the universal involvement with the blastematous process, they postulated that this lesion was different from bilateral nephroblastoma and used the term nephroblastomatosis. The term was subsequently expanded to include nodular proliferations of renal blastema present in infants with trisomy 18, congenital anomalies, and proliferations associated with Wilms' tumors.[47] Some form of aberrant metanephric differentiation has been demonstrated in 30 percent of Wilms' tumors, including nodular renal blastema, metanephric hamartomas (admixtures of epithelial and collagenized stroma), and Wilms' tumorlets (monomorphic epithelial lesions 1.0 to 3.5 cm in diameter). These lesions are also members of the nephroblastomatosis complex.[48]

Nephroblastomasis is defined as the persistence of metanephric blastema past the stage when nephrogenesis is usually complete (36 weeks' gestation). Various morphologic patterns have been described, with the hyperplastic blastema appearing as discrete superficial multifocal masses or as a diffuse cap surrounding the entire kidney (Fig. 15-14). The latter produces diffuse renal enlargement with preservation of the normal fetal lobulation and contour. The incidence of blastemal rests in autopsies of children varies from 1 per 204 to 1 per 115 for infants less than 3 months.[29] Etiologic factors considered relevant in the familial cases of Wilms' tumor are also related to nephroblastomatosis. The association of the superficial or subcapsular form with trisomy 18/13, congenital anomalies, and bilateral nephroblastomas is well documented.[48] It has been postulated that aniridia is probably related to the deep intralobular type of nephroblastomatosis.[182] Deletion of the short arm of chromosome 11 (11p-), an abnormality associated with Wilms' tumor, has also been demonstrated in a case of nodular renal blastema.[133a]

Microscopically, two types of nephroblastomatosis have been described. *Superficial nephroblastomatosis* is characterized by a diffuse subcapsular proliferation or nodules of embryonal cells with minor degrees of tubular differentiation (Fig. 15-15). No embryonal stromal proliferation is seen in this form, although collagenized stroma can be present in the "sclerosing metanephric hamartomas." Immature fetal glomeruli, sclerosis of some glomeruli, focal dysplasia, and cystic change are associated findings.[48] With *intralo-*

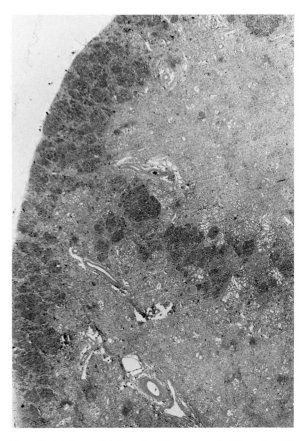

Fig. 15-14 Superficial nephroblastomatosis. Note the diffuse subcapsular proliferation of embryonal cells and the intraparenchymal extension through the normal fetal lobulations. ×15.

bar nephroblastomatosis, as described by Machin and McCaugley,[182] the nephroblastic proliferation is present at the junction between cortex and medulla and has well differentiated tubules, usually with a layer of stroma between the epithelium and the blastema, and glomeruloid forms with hyperchromatic parietal epithelium. Cysts and a stromal component with heterotopic tissue are also seen.[20,182] This form has been related to nephroblastomas that show minimal epithelial differentiation and that remain in a blastema stage or differentiate to rhabdomyomatous stroma (or both).[20,182,290] The presence of cysts and polypoid growth in the pelvicalyceal septum has also led some investigators to propose an association of intralobular nephroblastomatosis with cystic partially differentiated nephroblastoma.[182] It has been postu-

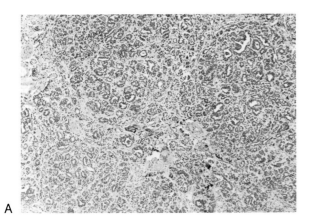

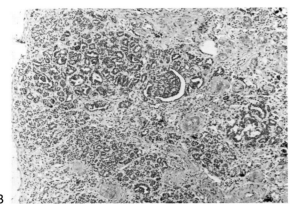

Fig. 15-15 Superficial nephroblastomatosis. Tubular differentiation and glomeruloid structures are seen in the blastemal elements. **A,** ×47; **B,** ×58.

lated that the early renal blastema is principally stromatogenic, and that its persistence can give rise to the deep cortical intralobular nephroblastomatosis.

The imprecise boundaries between what is called nephroblastomatosis and nephroblastoma have been stressed by Beckwith.[19] There is a gradual multistep progression from precursor lesion to frank tumor. The ends of the spectrum are clearly distinguished, but the dividing line is difficult to define. The entire clinical picture must be taken into account. Bilaterality, extension, and focality must be carefully evaluated. Young age at presentation, long-standing flank mass, and a family history of renal anomalies or renal tumors suggest the diagnosis of nephroblastomatosis. It must be considered a bilateral process but not necessarily with symmetrical and equal involvement of both kidneys. Sometimes only examination of both kidneys at surgery permits the diagnosis to be established.

Careful radiographic and ultrasound examination in suspected cases is necessary, as the potential of a contralateral tumor dictates a conservative approach, with emphasis on partial, small wedge resections instead of total nephrectomy.[133] Ultrasound is also recommended for follow-up because of the unknown risk imposed by the multiple low-level radiation exposures with conventional radiographic methods. These patients are followed by image examination every 3 to 6 months.

Nephroblastomas associated with nephroblastomatosis have similar rates of recurrence to unilateral tumors when stratified for stage and histologic grade. Only five patients in NWTS-III have developed metachronous Wilms' tumor, suggesting that the risk is low, even when nephroblastomatosis is present, provided that therapy as in NWTS-II is used.[19]

The therapy used in cases of nephroblastomatosis should take into consideration that it is a precursor lesion and not a malignancy per se. Therapy should be no more deleterious to the patient than the lesion itself. The maximum amount of renal tissue is preserved in order to delay the age when dialysis or renal transplantation must be considered. The good results with imaging techniques for detecting the development of tumors at an early stage, when current therapy is highly successful, permit a conservative approach to treatment. The use of chemotherapy has reduced the size of the lesions of nephroblastomatosis, but it is questionable if it reduces the occurrence of Wilms' tumor in this condition.[133]

Cystic Partially Differentiated Nephroblastoma

Cystic partially differentiated nephroblastoma (CPDN)[149] has been variously designated *benign multilocular cystic nephroma, polycystic nephroma, benign cystic differentiated nephroblastoma,* and *well differentiated polycystic nephroblastoma.* It has also been confused with solitary multilocular renal cyst of the kidney, so strict criteria have been proposed for diagnosis of the latter condition.[29] The different terms that have been used clearly indicate that morphologically there is a continuum between (1) a nephroblastoma with a few cysts at one end and (2) a mass with multiple cysts and a thin wall with well differentiated mesenchyme (multilocular renal cyst) at the other.

The lesion is defined as a predominantly or almost totally multicystic mass, with cysts lined by epithelium and septa that show a combination of blastemal, epithelial, and mesenchymal elements with varying degrees of differentiation and organization.

The incidence of the cystic partially differentiated nephroblastoma is not known, although it was reported to represent 2.6 percent of renal tumors in one center.[109] The pathogenesis of CPDN is controversial, particularly as to whether it represents a congenital malformation or true neoplasia. Some investigators believe that there is initial maldevelopment of the ureteric bud, giving rise to a multilocular cyst. Poor induction of the metanephric blastema in the cyst would then give rise to the immature epithelium and stroma of CPDN.[270] Others have postulated that the cysts form as an expression of tubular differentiation of the metanephric blastema that becomes cystically dilated. A lesion similar to CPDN has been induced experimentally in the opossum with ethylnitrosourea,[149] and a case associated with multiple congenital anomalies and trisomy 8 mosaicism has been reported.[208]

A relation between deep cortical intralobular nephroblastomatosis and CPDN has also been proposed as constituting a form of early dysfunction in the metanephric blastema[182] (Fig. 15-16).

Grossly, a predominant or totally multicystic mass, frequently encapsulated and measuring 6 to 18 cm, is present. The cysts vary in size from a few millimeters to several centimeters and contain thin, yellowish, clear fluid. They do not communicate with each other or with the renal pelvis. The septa of the cysts are usually thin but in some areas may be up to 3 cm thick. The surrounding parenchyma is compressed but not invaded. Neither metastasis nor vascular or capsular involvement are seen.

Microscopically, the cysts are lined by cuboidal or flattened epithelium. The septa show varying degrees of cellularity and thickness, with nodular prolifera-

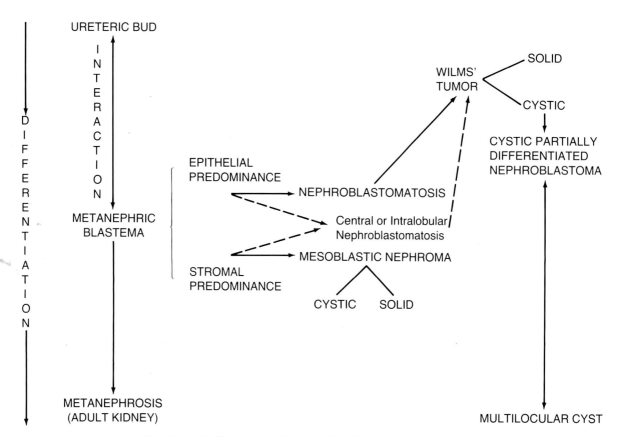

Fig. 15-16 Differentiation of metanephric blastema: proposed stages.

tion of blastemal cells, tubular structures, glomeruloid structures, undifferentiated mesenchymal myxoid areas, rhabdomyoblasts, and striated muscle. The degree of differentiation varies from area to area in the tumor.

The age range of those affected is 3 weeks to 24 months, with a preponderance of girls (11:6, girls/boys). The clinical behavior has been invariably benign. No recurrence or metastasis has been reported.

Clinically, the differential diagnosis is that of a renal mass. Because of advances in ultrasound imaging techniques it is possible to characterize the mass as cystic. In the pediatric age group, predominantly cystic renal masses fall mostly into the category of multilocular renal cysts, but Wilms' tumors, mesoblastic nephromas, and clear cell sarcomas may also be cystic.[21]

Multilocular renal cysts (MRC), the principal lesion to be distinguished from CPDN, must be unilateral and solitary, with noncommunicating, multilocular cystic cavities lined by epithelial cells. The septa between cysts must not contain metanephric blastemal cells, immature tubules, glomeruli, or fully mature nephrons. The residual kidney is normal on gross and microscopic examination in MRC (see Ch. 4).

Some have advocated conservative treatment,[12] but it has been suggested that this approach can be used only in cases where imaging techniques reveal an overwhelming preponderance of cystic spaces separated by thin, delicate septa and no evidence of solid regions.[19] In most cases the clinical diagnosis has been Wilms' tumor, and treatment was total nephrectomy. No additional therapy is presently indicated.[117]

Congenital Mesoblastic Nephroma

In 1967 Bolande et al. delineated clinically and pathologically a benign renal mesenchymal tumor of infancy that had been called variously *fetal renal hamartoma, leiomyomatous hamartoma, fibroma,* or *leiomyoma.*[41] These authors used the term congenital mesoblastic nephroma (CMN) to emphasize the congenital nature of the tumor, the preponderance of mesenchymal elements, and its existence as an entity separate from Wilms' tumor.[40]

The tumor is defined as a benign fibroblastic or leiomyomatous proliferation usually present during the first 3 months of life. CMN is rare with a reported incidence of 2.8 percent[141] to 3.2 percent[240] among

renal tumors of children. The pathogenesis is controversial, with some investigators favoring the development of the tumor from the more central stromatogenic mesenchyme associated with the early divisions of the ureteric bud[110] (Fig. 15-16). In a study of four nonmetastatic mesoblastic nephromas, fibronectin, but not laminin, was demonstrated, suggesting an origin from primitive mesenchymal cells. Laminin is present in metanephric blastema but absent in the more primitive nephrogenic mesenchyme.[167]

Grossly, a unilateral mass measuring 5 to 10 cm in diameter, replacing 50 to 90 percent of the kidney parenchyma, is present (Fig. 15-17). On section, it has a firm, rubbery consistency and a whitish-yellowish, trabeculated appearance. It resembles a uterine fibroid but is not encapsulated; it extends into the normal kidney parenchyma and perirenal connective tissue,

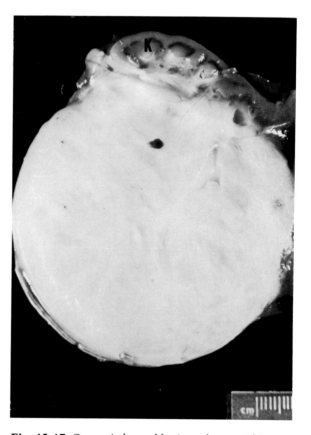

Fig. 15-17 Congenital mesoblastic nephroma. This gross specimen shows the residual kidney (K), as well as the rubbery, "fibroid", whitish yellow, trabeculated appearance of the tumor.

especially at the hilus. The tumor can be cystic or show areas of necrosis and hemorrhage.

Microscopically, the predominant histologic feature is of tightly interlaced sheets and bundles of benign fibroblasts and smooth muscle cells. Myxoid and angiomatoid areas may be present, and rhabdomyocytes and cartilage have been described occasionally; renal blastema is not seen in this tumor. Interspersed throughout the connective tissue and at the periphery of the tumor are discrete collections of tubules and glomeruli (Fig. 15-18) that may be dysplastic[40a] or mature. Cysts lined by cuboidal epithelium may be present. The tumor extends via fingerlike projections that merge imperceptibly with the renal stroma or adjacent perirenal fat.[40]

Areas with dense cellularity, a high mitotic rate, necrosis, and hemorrhage may be present. This find-

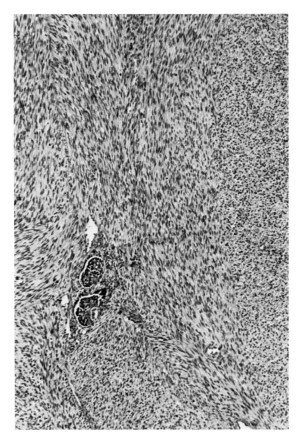

Fig. 15-18 Congenital mesoblastic nephroma. Note the interlacing bundles of smooth muscle cells and fibroblasts, with occasional trapped tubular and glomerular structures. ×136.

ing led Joshi et al. to propose the term *atypical mesoblastic nephroma* for tumors where these features are prominent to indicate a potentially aggressive behavior.[150] Beckwith and Weeks commented that at least 25 to 30 percent of congenital mesoblastic nephromas in patients less than 3 months old contain such areas. Though such findings in these infants may not be worrisome, their possible biologic behavior in children older than 3 months should be a matter of concern.[23] Cytogenetic analysis of a cellular and pleomorphic area in one case demonstrated an aneuploid clone with 54 chromosomes.[162b]

Ultrastructurally (Fig. 15-19), the cells contain sparse organelles with rough endoplasmic reticulum forming dilated and anastomotic cisternae. Microfilaments and dense bodies are seen. The consensus is that the cells represent myofibroblasts with variable expression of these characteristics.[101,107,110,111,289]

The mean age at diagnosis is 3.4 months (newborn to 9 years),[141] although the lesion has been reported in rare adults.[37,173] NWTS figures show a male/female ratio of 1.8 : 1.0[141] but in the European experience (SIOP) girls predominate (male/female 0.6 : 1.0).[240] A palpable abdominal mass is the most common sign at presentation, with some patients showing hematuria. Maternal polyhydramnios has been sometimes associated with the tumor,[40] but in the NWTS experience this association was not present.[141] IVPs demonstrate an intrarenal mass in practically all cases.

Prognosis in the typical lesions is excellent after nephrectomy. No additional treatment is required even if there has been intraoperative rupture.[141]

Controversy exists concerning the more aggressive atypical variants of this tumor, with recurrence being reported in 11 cases. The age at diagnosis and adequacy of the resection are extremely important factors in the relapse of the tumor.[23,62a] Congenital mesoblastic nephromas have a tendency to infiltrate into the perirenal soft tissue by way of irregular filamentous extensions. Adequate margins are necessary; although when resection of adjacent organs appears necessary, a second-look operation has been advocated.[141] According to Beckwith and Weeks,[23] the only infant under 3 months with recurrence had a positive ureteral margin. In children older than 3 months with atypical features, administration of actinomycin D and vincristine has been recommended.[62a,141] Pulmonary metastases have been successfully treated with chemotherapy, radiotherapy, and resection.[119]

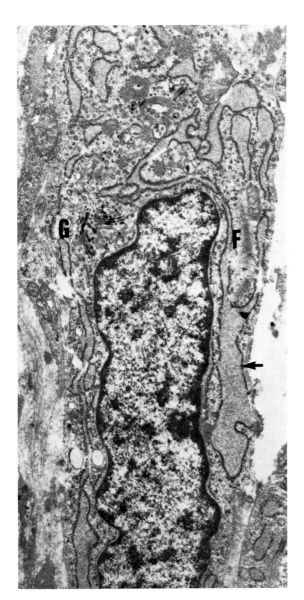

Fig. 15-19 Congenital mesoblastic nephroma. Well developed rough endoplasmic reticulum, with dilated anastomosing cisternae (arrow), Golgi (G), and filaments (F) can be observed. ×7,000.

Clear Cell Sarcoma of the Kidney

In 1970 Kidd[158] called attention to renal sarcomas with a predisposition to metastasize to bone rather than to lung and suggested that these tumors were different from the classic Wilms' tumor. More or less simultaneously, but with different names for the tumors, three groups described the lesions' clinical and pathologic features.[22,186,202] The European literature favors the term proposed by Marsden et al.,[186] *bone metastasizing renal tumor of childhood,* emphasizing this distinct pattern of metastasis. In the United States the preferred term appears to be *clear cell sarcoma of kidney,* emphasizing the predominant histopathologic pattern described by Beckwith and Palmer.[22] Still others prefer the term *undifferentiated sarcomas*[115] with the addition of a metastatic pattern or histologic appearance. They point out that not all specimens of clear cell sarcoma of kidney have cells with optically clear cytoplasm, and that in the combined experience of NWTSI-III (75 cases) only 17 percent developed bone metastasis.[125] A more constant or characteristic morphological pattern appears to be an alveolar or arborizing vascular network pattern.[226a,239a] The cell of origin is unknown; and the descriptive term *clear cell sarcoma* will be used in this chapter.

Clear cell sarcoma of kidney (CCSK) is defined as a highly malignant tumor of childhood with predilection for bone metastasis and a characteristic sarcomatous pattern of polygonal, generally clear cells with a prominent capillary pattern.[19]

Ultrastructural studies have attempted to define the histogenesis of the tumor. A blastemal origin has been denied because of the absence of frank epithelial or stromal differentiation, the lack of basal lamina, the presence of intermediate cytoplasmic filaments, and the demonstration of only poorly developed cell junctions. The cells appear as primitive mesenchymal cells, and a relation with malignant congenital mesoblastic nephroma has been proposed.[125] An association with epithelioid elements has been reported, although vimentin, a type of intermediate filament present in mesenchymal cells, was also said to be present in some CCSK.[244]

Clear cell sarcoma of kidney comprises about 4 percent of childhood renal tumors in the NWTS. The mean age at presentation is 3 years, and the tumor rarely occurs in children under 1 year of age. The male/female ratio in the United States is 1.7:1.0,[125] remarkably different from the 7.6:1.0 male sex predominance reported from Great Britain.[186]

Grossly, the tumor appears as a large tan renal mass, often with cystic areas that may be large and multiloculated. The tumor is firm, with a rubbery consistency, and appears to be demarcated from the adjacent parenchyma. Only about 40 percent are confined to the kidney, 5 percent have distant metastasis, and 55 percent have penetration of the capsule, vessels, or lymph nodes. In some specimens the tumor appears to originate centrally in relation to the renal medulla.[125]

The light microscopic appearance[20] is usually that of polygonal to stellate cells of uniform size, with poorly outlined pale cytoplasm that often appears vacuolated. Nuclei are oval to round, with finely granular chromatin and inconspicuous nucleoli. Mitotic figures are rare, giving a deceptively bland appearance to the tumor. A prominent arborizing network of small blood vessels is present (Fig. 15-20),[20] and Marsden et al. stressed this capillary pattern as one of the main diagnostic features.[186] It is present in 73 percent of the tumors in NWTS-III[226a] and is the constant microscopic feature of the 33 cases in the SIOP experience.[239a] An epithelioid trabecular pattern, with cells aligned in parallel fashion in relation to vascular septa and having a columnar appearance with a dark cytoplasm, has been described in some tumors. Other sections in these same tumors demonstrate the "classic" pattern of CCSK. This pattern was previously called osteosarcomatoid,[22] but it is now recognized that both CCSK and malignant rhabdoid tumors may contain extracellular hyaline material. Cysts may also be prominent. Tubules may be trapped, especially at the periphery. Neurolemmomalike nuclear palisading and an angiectatic pattern have also been demonstrated.

Ultrastructurally, the cells contain little glycogen and only rarely cytoplasmic fat. The clear appearance is given by the mosaic arrangement of the cells that may include pools of abundant pale extracellular matrix (Fig. 15-21). Condensation of microfilaments following formalin fixation may also be responsible for this light microscopic appearance.[125]

The great predilection of this tumor for bone metastasis is intriguing. It has been proposed that this property may be related to the capacity of CCSK to migrate into native collagen gels as well as to the lack

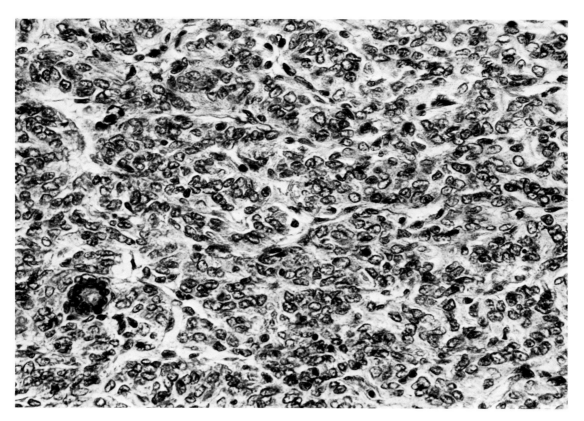

Fig. 15-20 Clear cell sarcoma. Cords and columns of tumor cells with oval or round nuclei are defined by vascular septa. An entrapped tubule is present at lower left. ×427. (From Haas et al.,[125] with permission.)

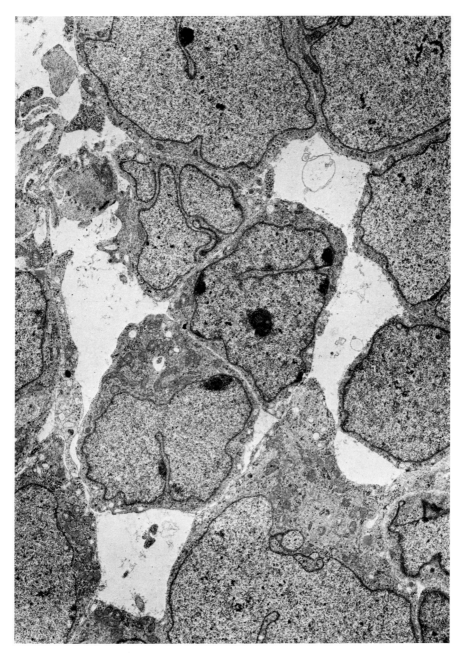

Fig. 15-21 Clear cell sarcoma. Prominent, pale extracellular matrix surrounds clusters of tumor cells. Some nuclei are deeply cleaved and appear to be pleomorphic. ×5,148. (From Hass et al.,[125] with permission.)

of fibronectin in the tumor cells. Addition of fibronectin to cultures of these cells markedly reduced the ability of the cells to migrate into native collagen gels.[166]

The prognosis is much worse than that of Wilms' tumor. Of 31 cases in NWTS-I and NWTS-II, 65 percent relapsed and 48 percent died of tumor.[20] The introduction of adriamycin in NWTS-III trials has changed survival to 80 percent.[226a] Tumors with hyalinizing pattern appear to have a worse prognosis with five year recurrence free survival of only 20 percent in the SIOP experience.[239a]

Malignant Rhabdoid Tumor of the Kidney

In 1978 Beckwith and Palmer[22] identified a monomorphic rhabdosarcomatoid variant of Wilms' tumor with an unfavorable prognosis. Subsequently, it became clear that it was a separate and distinct neoplasm unrelated to rhabdomyosarcoma or Wilms' tumor.[126] The rhabdoid tumor has also been described at other sites, such as thymus,[171] soft tissue, and liver.[116]

Malignant rhabdoid tumor is distinguished clinically by its poor prognosis and its tendency to early metastatic spread. Histopathologically it is characterized by the presence of cells with abundant acidophilic cytoplasm (Fig. 15-22) resembling skeletal rhabdomyoblasts.

The origin of this tumor is highly controversial. The neoplasm is generally monophasic and, unlike Wilms' tumor, does not recapitulate nephrogenesis. Recently a possible origin from cells of the infantile renal medulla has been suggested.[284b] Although light microscopy has suggested a rhabdomyoblastic origin, immunoperoxidase has failed to demonstrate myoglobin.[238] Ultrastructurally, features of carcinoma such as nexus-type cellular junctions and cytoplasmic tonofilaments have been demonstrated. The presence of arrays of thin filaments (6 to 9 mm in diameter) packed in nonmembrane-bound, whorled inclusions is characteristic (Figs. 15-23 and 15-24). They are different from the parallel bundles of alternating thin and thick filaments with primitive Z bands of condensation seen in true myogenous tumors.[126] A histiocytic origin has been proposed for this tumor on the basis of some of the ultrastructural features, the pres-

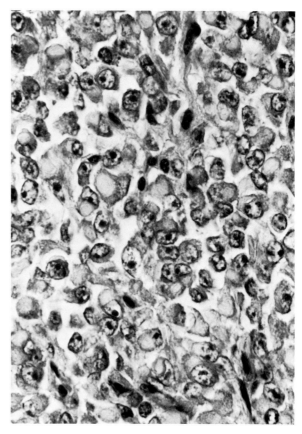

Fig. 15-22 Malignant rhabdoid tumor. Note the cells with abundant eosinophilic cytoplasm with rounded hyaline inclusions, as well as the eccentric vesicular nuclei with prominent nucleoli ("owl-eye"). ×614.

ence of muramidase and complement receptors, and its ability to phagocytose.[116] It has also been suggested that rhabdoid tumors are of neuroectodermal origin, though neurosecretory granules have not been detected. Ultrastructurally, the filamentous aggregates in this tumor appear similar to those seen in some APUD (amine precursor uptake and decarboxylation cell) tumors.[126] It has been proposed that these filamentous cytoplasmic inclusions may be seen in APUD cells of endodermal, rather than neural crest, origin.[247] Microfilaments are believed to have a role in the migration of endocrine secretory granules,[18] and a decreased number of membrane-bound granules and an increase in filamentous inclusions may represent an anomaly of differentiation of APUD cells.[126] Sparse

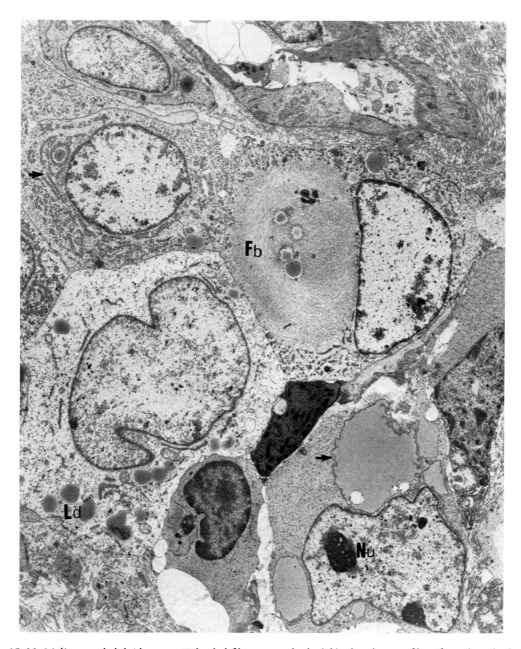

Fig. 15-23 Malignant rhabdoid tumor. Whorled filamentous body (Fb), abundant profiles of rough endoplasmic reticulum (arrows) in different stages of distension, lipid droplets (Ld), and vesicular nuclei with knotted, ropy nucleoli (Nu) are characteristic of these tumors. ×6,720. Survey electron micrograph.

lipid droplets and rough endoplasmic reticulum is also seen. Sometimes the endoplasmic reticulum shows remarkably dilated cisterna. The nucleolus has a characteristic reticular configuration (Figs. 15-23 and 15-24).

An association with embryonal primary tumors in the central nervous system has also been described. Most of these additional primary malignancies have been cerebellar medulloblastomas, but it has been concluded that there is no morphologic evidence that

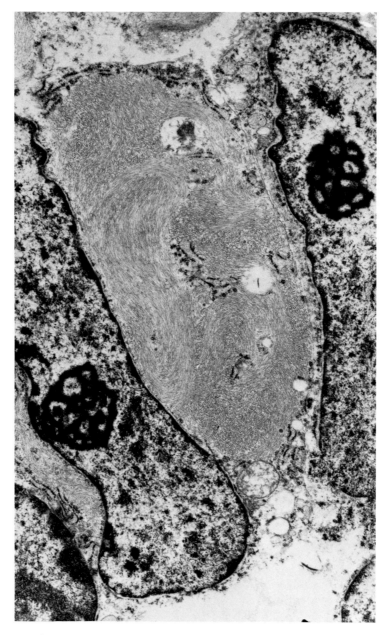

Fig. 15-24 Malignant rhabdoid tumor. A cytoplasmic rounded mass of tightly packed, 6- to 9-nm filaments is referred to as a whorled filamentous body. A few profiles of ergastoplasm are present in the inclusion. ×12,800. Electron micrograph. (From Haas et al.,[126] with permission.)

the malignant transformations in the kidney and brain occur in histogenetically related cells.[43] Studies have also been performed to characterize the intermediate filaments of the malignant rhabdoid tumor in order to determine its cell of origin. It has been shown that the tumors contain vimentin, a mesenchymal protein, and a 54-kilodalton cytokeratin, present in nonsquamous epithelium.[281] This dual mesenchymal and epithelial differentiation has also been described in renal cell carcinomas, where 57 percent of the cytokeratin-positive tumors were also vimentin-positive.[139] The coexpression of these intermediate filament proteins is also present in the blastemal cells of Wilms' tumor.[4]

In summary, evidence for the origin of this tumor is inconclusive. It is clear that it is not of rhabdomyoblastic origin, and the possibilities include renal cell, renal medulla, renal blastema, a histiocytic or neuroepithelial origin, or a mixed epithelial/mesenchymal origin.

Malignant rhabdoid tumor of the kidney is a rare neoplasm. Of the patients entered in NWTS between 1969 and 1978, this tumor was seen in only 21 cases (2 percent).[216] The tumor does not have any distinctive gross features. Histopathologically,[20,216] the borders tend to be infiltrative rather than expansile. The growth pattern is usually diffuse, with a monotonous population of cells with prominent eosinophilic cytoplasm and a large eccentric nucleus with a single large (owl's eye) nucleolus (Figs. 15-22 to 15-25). The hallmark of malignant rhabdoid tumor is the presence of hyaline, globular, generally single cytoplasmic inclusions of a size similar to that of the nucleus of the cell. The inclusion corresponds to the array of intermediate filaments described by electron microscopy (Fig. 15-25). The tumors may also have a trabecular or alveolar pattern. Occasionally, intercellular collagenous stroma condenses into hyaline bands, and sometimes the tumor presents focal spindle cell areas that may simulate the interwoven fasicles of mesoblastic nephroma or leiomyosarcoma (Fig. 15-26).

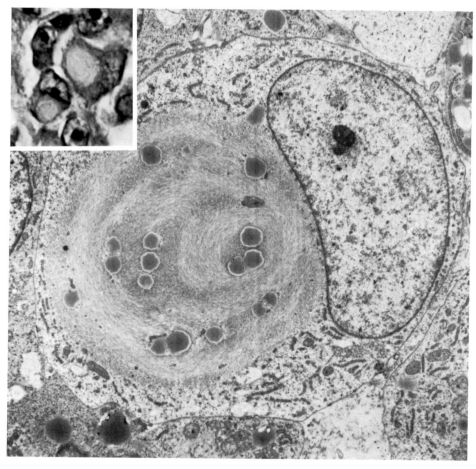

Fig. 15-25 Malignant rhabdoid tumor. Electron micrograph shows the details of a whorled filamentous body with lipid droplets. This structure correlates with the PAS-positive globular cytoplasmic hyaline inclusion seen by light microscopy **(inset).** ×6,972. **Inset,** ×1,062.

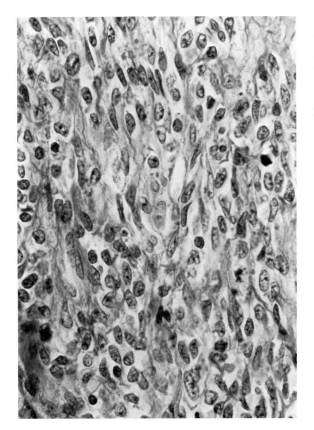

Fig. 15-26 Malignant rhabdoid tumor. Note the area of tumor with sarcomatoid appearance. ×460.

Malignant rhabdoid tumor of the kidney has a male/female ratio of 1.8 : 1. Seventy-eight percent of the cases are diagnosed before 25 months of age with a median age at diagnosis of 18 months.[284b]

The differential diagnosis on morphologic grounds includes epithelioid sarcomas that may contain cells with eosinophilic cytoplasm and intracellular filamentous eosinophilic inclusions that are indistinguishable from those of MRT. Immunohistochemically, both lesions are vimentin-positive. The distinction is currently based on clinical features, such as presentation of an epithelioid sarcoma in the distal extremities of young adults, a tendency to multiple recurrences, and a protracted clinical course. Epithelioid sarcomas tend to grow in nodular or pseudonodular patterns. The presence of these characteristic intermediate filamentous inclusions in epithelioid sarcomas and malignant rhabdoid tumor is intriguing.[106]

The prognosis is dismal. Death occurred in 51 of the 67 cases in the NWTS. Stage and gender are the most useful predictor factors with 60 percent survival for stage I, 33 percent for stage II, 26 percent for stage III, and 0 percent for stage IV. Girls survived in 37 percent of cases in contrast with only 14 percent survival for boys.[284b] Metastasis may occur at multiple sites, especially lungs and liver. Recurrences in the tumor bed as well as brain and heart metastases have also been reported. Relapses generally occur within 1 year, and all deaths have occurred within 2 years of diagnosis.[216]

Mesonephroid Blastoma

A single case of a large multicystic and hemorrhagic renal tumor presenting in a 4.5-year-old child with clear or pale epithelial tubules and a myxoid stroma has been reported. The authors proposed that it represents a mesonephroid blastoma in view of its similarity with tubuloalveolar prostatic glands, ducts, and vas deferens. However, a scrotal metastasis had a histologic appearance indistinguishable from that of blastemal cells of Wilms' tumor.[118]

RENAL TUMORS IN ADULTS

Renal Cell Adenocarcinoma

INCIDENCE AND EPIDEMIOLOGY

Renal cancer represents 2 to 3 percent of all cancers, placing it 13th in frequency. The American Cancer Society estimates that there were 21,900 new cases of urinary carcinomas (excluding bladder) in 1987 with an annual estimate of 9,400 deaths; 85 percent of these new cases were renal cell adenocarcinomas.[248]

The tumor affects men 1.6 times more frequently than women and its frequency increases with advancing age, occurring generally during the fifth or sixth decade of life. It rarely arises in children and adolescents.[2,82,269] Mortality rates for renal cell carcinoma are low in Asia, Africa, South and Central America, and southern Europe. High rates are seen in Iceland, Sweden, and Denmark, with intermediate rates in most European countries, North America, and Australia. Mortality rates since 1958 have shown an increase especially in Japan, Finland, France, Ireland,

and Italy. The incidence of kidney cancer has also increased in Sweden, Norway, Finland, and centers with a high population density in the United States.[259] Clustering of cases of renal cell carcinoma in the north central area of the United States has been related to an elevated risk for the development of this tumor in individuals of German and Scandinavian origin.[191]

Studies suggest that smoking doubles the risk of developing renal cell adenocarcinoma, especially smokers of cigars and pipes.[30,31,191,296a] It may be related to dimethylnitrosamine, a known inducer of renal cell adenocarcinoma in rodents.[129] It has been suggested that occupational hazards may be important[176]; coke, coal-gas, and petrochemical workers appear to be especially at risk.[191,229,272] A positive correlation has been established with animal protein and more importantly total fat consumption.[7,294] Coffee consumption, especially decaffeinated coffee, and diuretic use have been associated with increased risk of developing renal cell carcinoma.[119a,296a] The exact relation of these associations with carcinogenesis are not known.

Obesity,[119a,191,296a] hypercholesterolemia, atherosclerosis, and diabetes mellitus are also common in patients with renal cell carcinoma.[287]

ETIOLOGY

Numerous factors have been implicated in the development of renal cell adenocarcinomas, including chemicals, drugs, natural products, irradiation, hormones, and viruses.[211a,215,218] Genetic factors, congenital abnormalities, and chronic renal failure have also been considered to be of possible etiologic significance.

Chemicals, Drugs, and Natural Products

The association between chemicals, drugs, and natural products with renal cell carcinoma is not strong. Although compounds such as nitrosoamines, hydrazines, alkylating agents, and chloroform have been implicated in the development of tumors in experimental animals, their etiologic significance in man has not been proved. Cadmium and lead have been associated in some studies with a higher incidence of renal cancer,[29,34] but studies specifically examining occupational exposure to these metals have failed to

show an excess of renal cancers in the exposed workers.[81] An interesting association between renal adenoma and carcinomas and cycasin has been described in the rat.[253] Cycasin can be extracted from nuts used as a source of starch by the indigenous populations in Guam and East Africa, but there is not yet evidence of an increase in renal cell carcinoma in these populations.[215]

Irradiation

Whole-body irradiation and radioactive compounds such as polonium 210 and strontium 90 have been related to renal carcinogenesis in experimental animals.[218] There have been no reports of increased risk for renal cell carcinoma among individuals exposed to radiation. Although Thorotrast has been related to kidney tumors, the evidence for a cause-and-effect relation is weak.[81]

Hormones

Renal adenocarcinomas can be induced with prolonged administration of natural and synthetic estrogens in the male Syrian and European hamster. This induction of tumors and its control by cortisone, progestational agents, adrenalectomy, or orchiectomy in experimental animals have led to attempts to treat human renal adenocarcinomas with hormones, particularly in view of the presence of hormone receptors in the tumors and the striking male/female ratio.[153,154] The relation between hormones and renal cancer remains controversial, and the hamster model cannot be readily extrapolated.[211a]

Viruses

The spontaneous renal carcinoma (Lucke's tumor) that occurs in the North American leopard frog (*Rana pipiens*) is due to a herpes simplex virus.[123] Herpes simplex virus antigens have been identified in human renal adenocarcinoma[72] as well as in other human tumors, however, rendering this association uncertain. In one study antigenic material related to the main structural protein of the mammalian retrovirus p30 was demonstrated in all 27 cases of renal cell carcinoma examined as well as in the three cases of oncocytoma studied,[282] suggesting that it may play a role in the pathogenesis of this tumor. Other viruses that produce a sarcomatous pattern in hamsters and other rodents are polyoma virus, simian virus SV40, and adenovirus 7.

Genetic Factors and Congenital Abnormalities

A familial incidence of renal adenocarcinoma has been described.[73,228] It has been associated with a chromosomal translocation[73] apparently due to a deletion in the proximal end of 3p.[217] As with other familial cancers that can be ascribed to genetic factors, these patients are young, the tumor is often multifocal, and the probability of bilaterality increases with age. Study of tumor tissue in sporadic renal cell cancer has demonstrated abnormalities in the short arm of chromosome 3 with a DNA sequence deletion at 3p 14–21 region.[299a] It suggests the association between fragile chromosome sites and oncogenes in the development or evolution of renal cell carcinoma. A higher incidence has also been noted in patients of blood group A, certain HLA types, and those with color blindness.[124] It is interesting that no differences in incidence have been noted in the United States among caucasian, black, or Mexican groups. An association with horseshoe kidney and von Hippel-Lindau disease has also been described, with a reported renal cell carcinoma incidence of 10 to 35 percent in the latter.[183a]

Acquired Renal Cystic Disease and Chronic Renal Failure

In 1977[93] Dunnill described the presence of multiple renal cysts in patients on renal dialysis and the association with renal neoplasms. Numerous other reports have documented this association. The incidence has been estimated to be 2.1 to 3.5 percent, a 1,000-fold increase over renal cell carcinoma in a regular population.[145]

In our experience, tumors have been small and multifocal,[50] although clinically significant masses and metastatic tumors have been reported[50,145,227] with an overall metastatic rate of 6 to 27 percent.[54,142a] The importance of these potentially bilateral lesions in patients with chronic renal failure who are known to have an increased risk of malignancy,[201] the need for periodic examination by either ultrasound or CT scanning, and the indication of nephrectomy in radiologically uncertain or equivocal lesions must be stressed[50] (see also Ch. 4).

SMALL RENAL CELL TUMORS OR ADENOMAS

A discussion of the etiology of renal cell carcinoma must take into account the concept of renal cell adenoma. Largely based on the original paper of Bell,[25] it was assumed that renal cell tumors less than 3 cm in diameter were benign and that the potential for metastasis correlated with a tumor larger than 3 cm. In Bell's study the frequency of metastasis was as follows: 1 of 24 tumors measuring 1 to 2 cm; 0 of 12 tumors measuring 2 to 3 cm; and 4 of 12 tumors 3 to 4 cm in size. He stated that, "In general the large tumors are more apt to form metastases," but he also said, "We may conclude that the small tumors (so called adenomas) are early stages of large growths, and that no certain distinctions can be made between adenoma and carcinomas."[25] Bennington and Beckwith[29] recommended that all cortical glandular neoplasms of the kidney regardless of size must be considered renal adenocarcinomas, stating, however, that if the tumor is less than 3 cm in diameter the risk of metastasis is slight.

Bannayan and Lamm[13] recommended avoidance of the term renal cell adenoma, especially for surgically removed specimens. They suggested that tumors less than 3 cm be referred to as borderline renal cell tumors.

A remarkable study done by Hellsten et al.[135] defined malignancy as "all tumors measuring 2 cm or more" and other smaller tumors "when local infiltration, vascular growth or metastasis were revealed or when the cellular picture agreed with renal cell carcinoma." This series is from the city of Malmö, where the hospital's autopsy rate was 99 percent (16,294 autopsies in 12 years), corresponding to 62.2 percent of all persons succumbing in this city. A total of 350 renal tumors were detected, 115 recognized clinically and 235 (two-thirds of cases) clinically unrecognized, with 56 of the latter already metastatic (24 percent). In this series, 82 (34 percent) of the clinically unrecognized tumors were less than 3 cm, 3 of them with metastasis at autopsy and 26 with vascular or pericapsular growth. Thus of a total of 82 tumors less than 3 cm, 29 (35 percent) had undisputable malignant characteristics (Figs. 15-27 and 15-28) despite the fact that they would have been called adenomas if judged only on size.

It is evident that small lesions that are largely papillary, cystic, or tubular with no atypia or capsular inva-

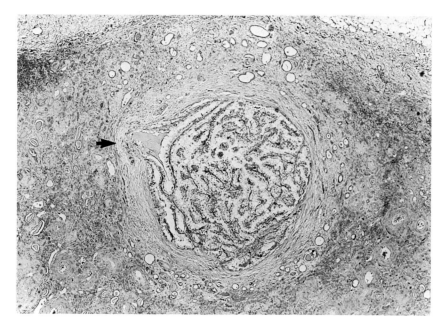

Fig. 15-27 Small renal cell adenocarcinoma. Note the focal infiltration into the surrounding stroma (arrow). ×31.

sion behave in a benign fashion and have a low, if any, metastatic potential (Fig. 15-29) and that size should not be the sole malignant criterion.[281a]

PATHOGENESIS

Studies with proximal tubular brush border antigens have demonstrated their presence in a high proportion of renal cell carcinomas.[284] Conversely, Tamm-Horsfall glycoprotein, a distal tubule marker, has been absent. It has been shown that most renal cell carcinomas express cytokeratin antigens as a sign of epithelial origin and characteristics of proximal convoluted cells (80 percent positive for brush border antigen and negative for Tamm-Horsfall protein).[139] Lectin-binding sites that are typical for normal tubular cells are markedly modified in carcinoma.[139]

Electron microscopy has also demonstrated similarities with proximal tubular cells, brush border with tightly packed microvilli, pinocytosis, glycocalyx, infoldings of plasma membrane, and abundant elongated and tortuous mitochondria.[28] Infolding of the basal plasma membrane and abundant mitochondria are also present in distal convoluted tubules; and when the apical cytoplasmic specialization is not demonstrated, a distal convoluted tubule contribution to the tumor has been suggested.[94]

Scarring might be implicated in the development of cysts, epithelial hyperplasia, regeneration and renal

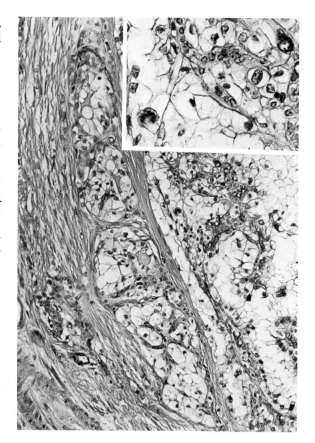

Fig. 15-28 Small renal cell adenocarcinoma. Note the detail of stromal invasion and the presence of atypia (inset). ×131. Inset, ×326.

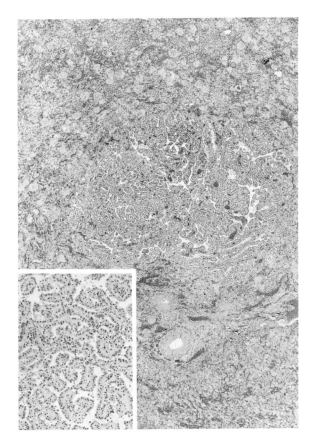

Fig. 15-29 Small, benign renal tumor. Note the papillary appearance and lack of atypia **(inset).** ✕ 30. **Inset,** ✕ 60.

tumors.[55] It may be related to the tumors that develop with acquired renal cystic disease. Both regenerative and neoplastic epithelium demonstrate the presence of brush border antigen (proximal tubule) and epithelial membrane antigen (distal tubule) raising the possibility that renal cell carcinoma develops from regenerating cells.[102a]

HORMONE RECEPTORS

Estrogen, progesterone, and androgen receptors have been demonstrated in normal kidney and approximately 20 percent of renal cell adenocarcinomas.[113,154,209] The steroid receptors can undergo nuclear translocation; and in some experimental animals estrogen is able to induce transformation of the proximal convoluted tubular cells. Hormonal treatment initially was reported to produce a tumor response in 7 to 25 percent of cases.[38] Lately, with more

rigorous objective measures of tumor response parameters, it seems that the response is a disappointing 2 percent.[142,224] Receptor data have not been helpful for selecting patients who will respond to therapy,[153] and no correlation has been found between histopathologic findings and receptor studies.[209] It has been proposed that the low content of the receptor in tumor tissue may explain the poor treatment response.[204]

PATHOLOGY

The overall prognosis of renal cell adenocarcinoma depends on a comprehensive and accurate description of size, extent, and microscopic characteristics of the tumor.

Grossly,[28,29,271] the tumor is a bosselated, pale yellow, sometimes variegated mass with occasional grayish septa and focal cystic, necrotic, or hemorrhagic zones (Fig. 15-30). Viable areas where there is

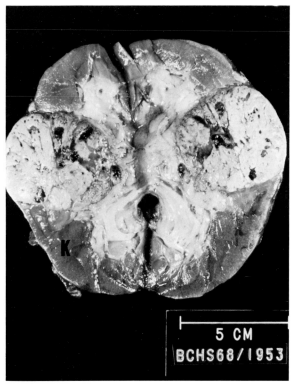

Fig. 15-30 Renal cell carcinoma. This gross specimen shows portions of remaining kidney parenchyma (K) and tumor with a variegated appearance. Areas of hemorrhage and necrosis are visible. A pseudocapsule is also seen.

significant intracellular lipid are yellow to orange, whereas lipid-poor zones appear grayish white. The tumor is generally soft and bulges over the cut surface. It has a pseudocapsule even when it has extended through the renal capsule (Fig. 15-31).

Size, although overrated as the defining factor of adenoma, is still an important feature. The tumor can attain a remarkable size, which has led to the general belief that it is a relatively slow-growing tumor. Prognosis worsens with a larger tumor, and the possibility of associated vascular invasion, local extension, or metastasis increases with size.[8,156] It has been estimated that the percentage of patients who have metastasis with a tumor 2 cm in diameter is practically zero but increases to 80 percent when the tumor measures 10 cm (Table 15-2).

Local extension is one of the important prognostic factors. A tumor confined to the kidney (Fig. 15-30) is associated with a 5-year survival rate of 60 to 80 percent and a 10-year survival rate of 56 percent. Exten-

Table 15-2 Tumor Size and Percentage of Metastasis

Tumor Diameter (cm)	% Patients with Metastasis
2	0
4	20
6	40
8	60
10	80

(Modified from Bennington et al.,[29] with permission.)

sion to the perinephric fat (Fig. 15-31) drops the survival rate at 5 years to 45 to 51 percent to 28 percent at 10 years.[155,192,250] Direct extension to the adrenal occurs within Gerota's fascia in 6 to 10 percent of patients and is considered prognostically in the same group as perinephric fat extension.[235] Renal pelvis involvement has not been evaluated as a single variable because it generally occurs associated with capsular, venous, or nodal involvement.[192] Pelvic involvement has not been found to affect survival in patients who also have lymph node or renal vein invasion (10-year survival is 21 percent versus 19 percent in the absence of renal pelvis involvement).[192]

Renal vein invasion has generated some controversy as a prognostic factor. According to Robson et al.,[235] tumors with renal vein invasion or lymph node metastasis are considered stage III carcinomas. Bennington and Beckwith[29] supported the view that survival at 10 years is significantly worse with renal vein invasion and closely approaches that of tumors with lymph node metastasis.[235] However, others have claimed that perinephric fat involvement is more important.[8] Yet other studies have found distant metastases, as frequently as 40 percent, in patients with tumors strictly confined to the kidney, as well as in those with tumors confined to the kidney but with renal vein invasion.[108] McNichols et al.[192] showed a slightly worse prognosis for patients who have tumors with renal vein invasion than in those with tumors exclusively confined to the kidney or with only perinephric involvement. They cautioned that some of the patients with venous involvement alone may have had microscopic metastasis because lymph node dissections were not performed. It appears, then, that renal vein invasion should be analyzed as a separate parameter and carefully evaluated in the surgical pathology specimens.

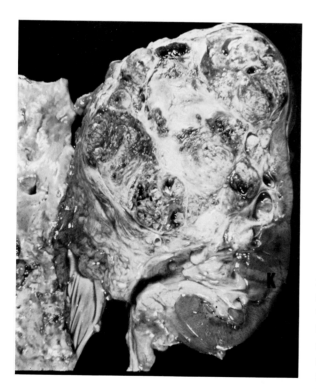

Fig. 15-31 Renal cell carcinoma. This gross specimen shows the remaining kidney parenchyma (K) and tumor with areas of necrosis and hemorrhage. There is extension to the perinephric fat and formation of a pseudocapsule.

Inferior vena cava extension of tumor may represent a significant surgical challenge, but in patients with no distant metastasis cumulative data show that 50 percent (33 of 66) of patients were alive after aggressive surgery with follow-up of 3 to 199 months.[251] Inferior vena cava involvement seems to markedly worsen the prognosis in comparison with extension only to the renal vein.[249] In one series the 5-year survival rate was 29 percent when inferior vena cava was involved, compared with a 56 percent 5-year survival rate when the involvement was limited to the renal vein.[17] There is also a suggestion that the level of extension of the tumor thrombi in the inferior vena cava is important. Extension to the level of hepatic veins or beyond worsens the prognosis (Fig. 15-32).[252]

Regional lymph node metastasis has been reported to be present in 23 percent of patients who underwent extensive lymphadenectomy with radical nephrectomy.[235] Spread to lymph nodes carries a poor prognosis with a 5-year survival rate of 33.5 percent and of 20 percent at 10 years.[192]

Other factors such as number of tumors, location in the kidney, and calcification appear to be of little prognostic significance.

Staging

Robson et al. in 1969[235] modified the system proposed by Flocks and Kadesky.[103] It considers all the basic features discussed in relation to tumor extension.

Stage I: Confined to the kidney

Stage II: Invasion of perinephric fat but confined to Gerota's fascia; adrenal involvement considered to be stage II

Stage III: A. Invasion of renal vein or vena cava

             B. Metastasis to regional lymph nodes

             C. Invasion to renal vein or vena cava and metastasis to regional lymph nodes

Stage IV: A. Invasion to adjacent organs other than adrenal gland

             B. Distant metastasis

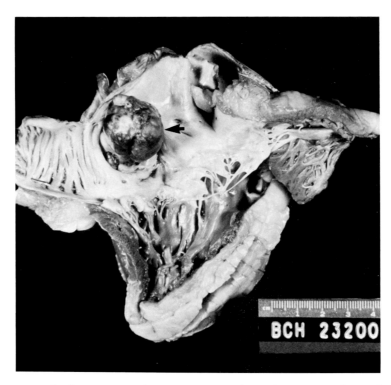

Fig. 15-32 Renal cell carcinoma. This gross specimen shows the invasion of the inferior vena cava with tumor protrusion into the right atrium (arrow).

An alternative subgrouping has been defined by the American Joint Committee for Cancer Staging and End Results Reporting.[6] However, it has not gained wide acceptance, and most statistics are reported in only four stages (Table 15-3). It may change, though, as more information on the prognostic significance of separating renal vein, vena cava, and lymph node involvement becomes available. This staging considers separately the characteristics of the primary tumor, lymph nodes, and metastasis.

Primary tumor (T)

Tx: Minimum requirement cannot be met

T0: No evidence of primary tumor

T1: Small tumor, minimal renal and caliceal distortion or deformity, circumscribed neovasculature surrounded by parenchyma

T2: Large tumor with deformity and/or enlargement of kidney and/or collecting system

T3a: Tumor involving perinephric tissue

T3b: Tumor involving renal vein

T3c: Tumor involving renal vein and infradiaphragmatic vena cava

T3d: Tumor involving renal vein and infradiaphragmatic and supradiaphragmatic vena cava

T4a: Tumor extending into neighboring organs or abdominal wall

T4b: Intracardiac extension

Nodal involvement (N): regional lymph nodes = paraaortic and paracaval nodes

Nx: Minimal requirements not met

N0: No evidence of involvement of regional nodes

N1: Single, homolateral regional nodal involvement

N2: Involvement of multiple regional or contralateral or bilateral nodes

N3: Fixed regional nodes (assessable only at surgical exploration)

Distant metastases (M)

Mx: Not assessed

M0: No (known) metastases

M1: Distant metastasis present; specify

The pretreatment clinical classification is designated cTNM; the postoperative classification is done

Table 15-3 Renal Cell Carcinoma in 499 Patients: Survival According to Stage

Stage	Survival (%)			
	5 years	10 years	15 years	20 years
I	67.0	56.0	44.0	33.0
II	51.0	28.0	18.5	10.5
III	33.5	20.0	10.5	5.0
IV	13.5	3.0	4.0	3.5

(Modified from McNichols et al.,[192] with permission.)

after evaluation of operative findings and pathologic analysis and is designated pTNM. The shortcoming of this system is the great number of subgroups that are identified. The benefit is that it can more precisely address the prognosis of individual patients. It has been shown that patients with only perinephric fat involvement (T3a) have a 72 percent chance of 5-year survival versus a 56 percent chance of survival for patients with only renal vein involvement, and a 29 percent chance for patients with only inferior vena cava involvement. If there is extension into the inferior vena cava and the perinephric fat (pT3a–c), the mean survival is 18 months, compared with 40 months when only the inferior vena cava is involved (pT3c).[17]

It is thus important to provide a careful and accurate pathologic description of the tumor, especially if new therapeutic modalities are to be evaluated for such an unreliable tumor as renal cell cancer.

Microscopic Appearance

Markedly varied histologic and cellular patterns can be found in these tumors. Some tumors are composed of clear cells (Fig. 15-33), rich in lipid and glycogen and containing few cytoplasmic organelles. Others have granular cells (Fig. 15-34) with little lipid or glycogen but filled with mitochondria and organelles, giving a granular and eosinophilic cytoplasm. At the end of the spectrum of granular tumors there are some that have cells so tightly packed with organelles as to have glassy, homogeneous, dark red cytoplasm. These cells used to be called "dark cells" but currently are referred to as oncocytic or oncocytoid cells. Most of the tumors have a heterogeneous cell pattern with an admixture of all cells and frequent

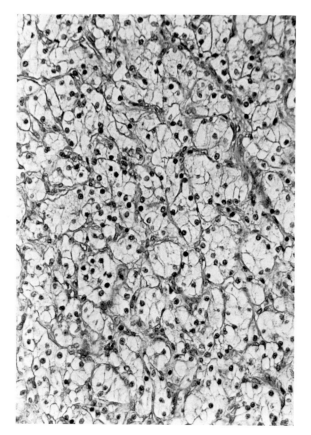

Fig. 15-33 Renal cell carcinoma. It is of the clear cell variety with solid appearance. ×236.

transitions between the various cell types present (Fig. 15-35).

Architecturally, solid (Fig. 15-33), tubular (Fig. 15-36), papillary (Figs. 15-37 and 15-38), or cystic (Fig. 15-39) configurations may be seen. Solid patterns have islands of cells separated by myxoid stroma or only occasionally interrupted by delicate fibrovascular septa (Fig. 15-33).

The tubular pattern is characterized by small tubules in an orderly arrangement with a rather inconspicuous lumen (Fig. 15-36) or by large, irregular, dilated tubules. Intervening stroma might be represented only by thin-walled capillaries or more abundant collagen and macrophages.

The papillary pattern is formed by proliferation of

frondlike structures into the tubular lumens (Fig. 15-38). The stroma of the papillary structures is generally delicate and may contain foamy macrophages (Fig. 15-37) and laminated, calcified psammoma bodies.

Cystic lesions generally have a papillary epithelial proliferation in a rather large lumen (Fig. 15-39). They appear well defined, although areas of infiltration are present.

A sarcomatoid appearance is present in approximately 0.5 to 4.8 percent of renal cell carcinomas (Fig. 15-40),[232b,245a,274] with elongated and sometimes bizarre spindle-shaped cells.

Different histologic patterns may be present in the same tumor with most renal cell carcinomas showing

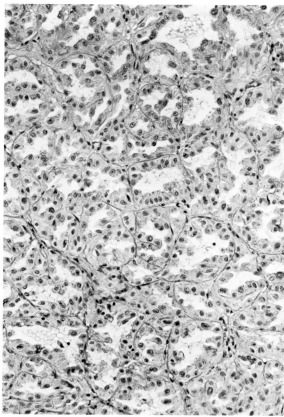

Fig. 15-34 Renal cell carcinoma. It is of the granular cell variety. ×144.

a bimorphic pattern as well as the previously described admixture of clear and granular cells (Fig. 15-35) and even apparent transitions from clear cells to spindle sarcomatoid elements (Fig. 15-41).

It has been reported that papillary tumors, including their cystic variant, have a better prognosis than tumor with other patterns.[184] However, no definitive statistical correlation has been found between survival and histologic configuration,[231,267] with the exception of the sarcomatoid pattern, where the dismal prognosis is well recognized (median survival 6.3 months to 13.0 months with newer therapeutic modalities).[245a,274]

In contrast to the situation with histologic pattern, controversy surrounds the importance of cell type in

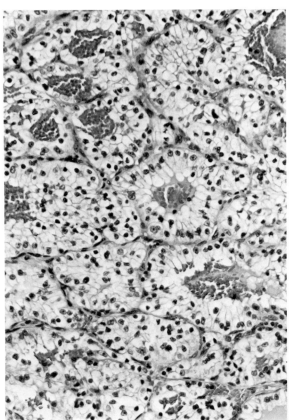

Fig. 15-36 Renal cell carcinoma. It is of the tubular architectural configuration. Red blood cells are present in the lumen. ×233.

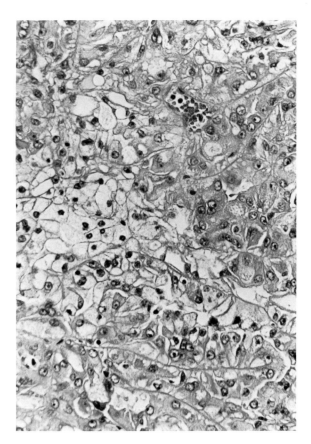

Fig. 15-35 Renal cell carcinoma. It is an admixture of the clear cell and granular cell varieties. ×142.

predicting behavior. Murphy and Mostofi[206] observed that patients with granular cells have the worst survival rate. This finding has been correlated with a greater incidence of the more undifferentiated tumors in this group,[13,108] whereas clear-cell-type tumors are more differentiated. It is perhaps important to note that at least one-third of cases are classified as mixed cell type, and that the well differentiated (low grade) granular cell tumors correspond to the "oncocytomas"[159] or to the granular cell tumors with oncocytic features.[159,175] Oncocytomas, defined restrictively, are invariably benign in contradistinction to the well differentiated clear cell carcinomas, which are true malignancies.[275]

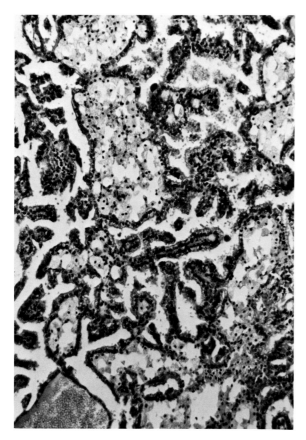

Fig. 15-37 Renal cell carcinoma. It is a papillary tumor with abundant foamy macrophages (F). ×144.

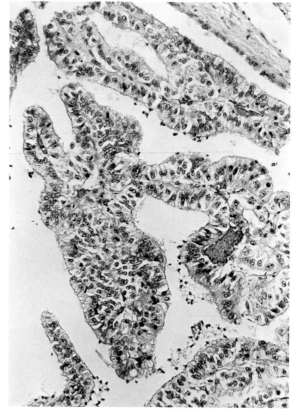

Fig. 15-38 Renal cell carcinoma. This detail of the tumor shows its papillary configuration. ×178.

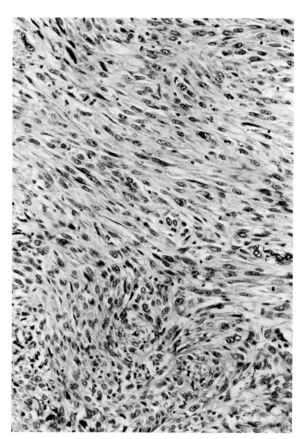

Fig. 15-40 Renal cell carcinoma. Note the areas of sarcomatoid configuration of tumor cells. ×144.

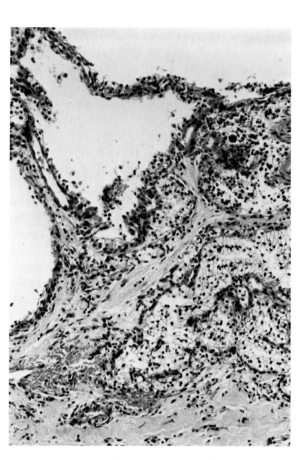

Fig. 15-39 Renal cell carcinoma. Note the cystic configuration with papillary proliferations. A clear cell component infiltrates the wall of the cyst. ×144.

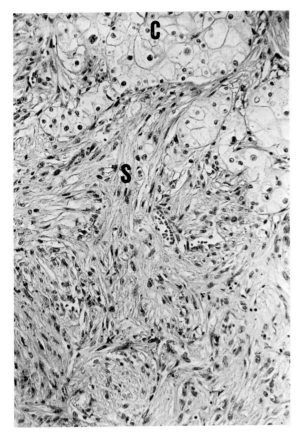

Fig. 15-41 Renal cell carcinoma. There is an admixture of clear cell (C) and sarcomatoid (S) elements. ×144.

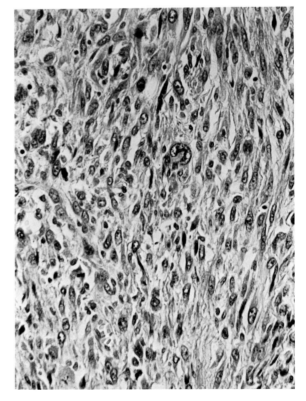

Fig. 15-42 Renal cell carcinoma, nuclear grade 4. In an area that has sarcomatoid features. ×236.

It appears that the independent histologic feature that best predicts behavior is *nuclear grade.* A system of evaluating differentiation on the basis of the nuclear structure has been proposed.[108,250,267] Size, presence of nucleoli, anisonucleosis, irregularity of nuclear outline, chromatin distribution, and number of mitoses are analyzed. Using these characteristics, tumors have been divided into four grades (Table 15-4; Figs. 15-42 to 15-47). The system correlates well with survival, although grades 2 and 3 are sometimes difficult to separate. Some encouraging preliminary results have been obtained with image analyzers and nuclear morphometry.[276] Skinner et al.[250] stated that if more than one high power field shows grade 3 nuclei the tumor should be called grade 3. Fuhrman et al.[108] also ana-

lyzed development of metastasis in 45 tumors confined to the kidney and its relation to nuclear grade. No patient with nuclear grade 1 had subsequent metastases. For grades 2 and 3 the percentage with metastasis was 44 and 67 percent, respectively.

Studies of DNA content in renal cell carcinoma have shown that patients with diploid/near-diploid tumors have a better prognosis than patients with aneuploid tumors.[32,159a] A positive correlation also exists between nuclear grade and DNA content.[159a] Practically all tumors of nuclear grades 1 and 2 are diploid/near-diploid, whereas in grade 3 and 4 tumors aneuploidy is present in 32 and 58 percent, respectively.[178] There is a better correlation between DNA content and survival time when the analysis is performed on

Table 15-4 Renal Cell Carcinoma Survival According to Nuclear Grade

Skinner et al.[250]		Syrjanen & Hjelt[267]		Fuhrman et al.[108]	
Grade & Description	5-Year Survival (%)	Grade & Description	5-Year Survival (%)	Grade & Description	5-Year Survival (%)
Grade 1: nuclei indistinguishable from normal tubular cells	75.0	Grade 1: spherical nuclei, equal size; delicate chromatin strands; rare mitosis	86.7	Grade 1: small (10 μm) round uniform nuclei; inconspicuous or absent nucleoli	65.0
Grade 2: nuclei pyknotic, slightly irregular and slightly enlarged; no abnormal nucleoli	65.0	Grade 2: spherical nuclei of approximately same size; distinct chromatin as bands; nucleoli; scattered mitosis	69.0	Grade 2: larger nuclei (15 μm) with irregularities in outline; nucleoli present	31.0
Grade 3: nuclei moderately enlarged irregular, pleomorphic; nucleoli large but no abnormal forms	56.0	Grade 3: anisonucleosis; clumped chromatin; prominent nucleoli; frequent mitosis	44.5	Grade 3: large, irregular (20 μm) nuclei; prominent nucleoli	35.0
Grade 4: numerous bizarre giant nuclei	26.0	Grade 4: profound anisonucleosis with large nuclei; coarse clumped chromatin; large irregular nucleoli; frequent mitoses with frequent pathologic figures	28.5	Grade 4: similar to grade 3 plus bizarre multilobed nuclei; heavy chromatin clumps; frequent spindle-shaped cells	10.0

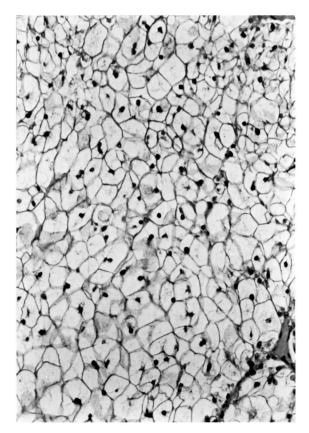

Fig. 15-43 Renal cell carcinoma, nuclear grade 1. Note the small, uniform nuclei with densely packed chromatin and the absence of nucleoli in most cells. ×236.

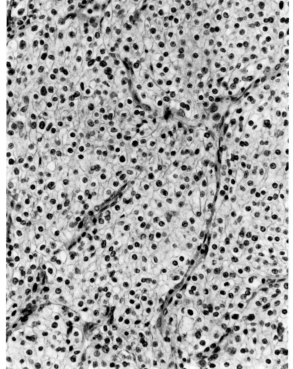

Fig. 15-44 Renal cell carcinoma, nuclear grade 2. There is mild nuclear pleomorphism, and the chromatin pattern is less compact. The nucleoli, although present in many cells, are rather inconspicuous. ×236.

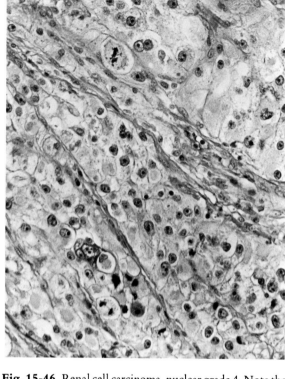

Fig. 15-46 Renal cell carcinoma, nuclear grade 4. Note the marked nuclear pleomorphism. The nuclei are large and irregular in size and shape. The chromatin is "open" with a vesicular appearance. Nucleoli are frequent, prominent, and irregular. Mitoses are frequent, with many atypical figures. ×236.

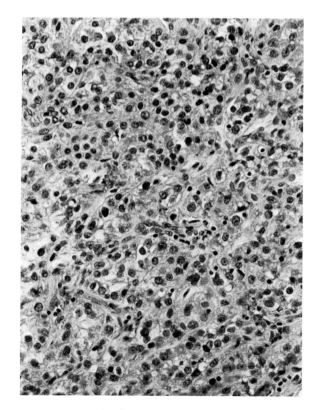

Fig. 15-45 Renal cell carcinoma, nuclear grade 3. Nuclear pleomorphism is conspicuous, with many "open" and distinct chromatin aggregates. Nucleoli are frequent and distinct. ×236.

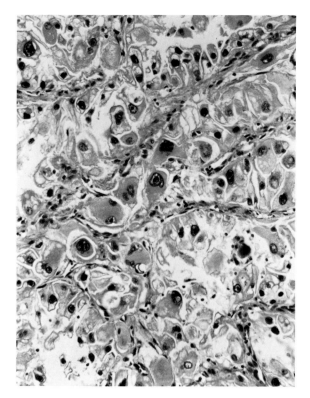

Fig. 15-47 Renal cell carcinoma, nuclear grade 4. A granular cell tumor with high nuclear grade. ×236.

Colloidal iron is positive at cell surfaces, glycocalyx, and in the cytoplasm of some of the tumor cells; but the reaction is not prevented by preincubation with hyaluronidase. This finding indicates that the substances responsible for the colloidal iron stain contain sialomucins but not hyaluronic acid.

The glycocalyx present in this tumor stains strongly with Alcian blue below pH 3.0, with toluidine blue at low pH, and with the PAS stain, suggesting sulfated but weakly acidic acid mucopolysaccharide composition.[146] It is located extracellularly on the cell membrane. True epithelial mucins are not present, and mucicarmine stains are negative.

Intermediate filaments are present in the cytoskeleton of epithelial cells (7 to 11 mm in diameter), and antibodies to intermediate filaments have been used to study normal and neoplastic renal tissue.[139,277] With cryostat sections, practically all renal adenocarcinomas stain for low-molecular-weight cytokeratin,

the metastatic lesion, probably because of the greater cell population homogeneity.[177] Static as well as flow cytometry have been used in the evaluation of paraffin embedded tumors.[235a]

Histochemistry and Immunohistochemistry

Glycogen, neutral lipid, and phospholipid can be demonstrated in the clear cells of renal adenocarcinomas. Glycogen is shown with the periodic acid-Schiff (PAS) reaction and verified by removal by prior diastase digestion (Figs. 15-48 and 15-49). Neutral lipid stains with oil red O (Fig. 15-50), Sudan IV, or perchloric acid naphthoquinone on frozen sections. The staining is completely removed by xylene or chloroform with methyl alcohol. Phospholipids are not removed by these compounds and can be shown by Sudan black.

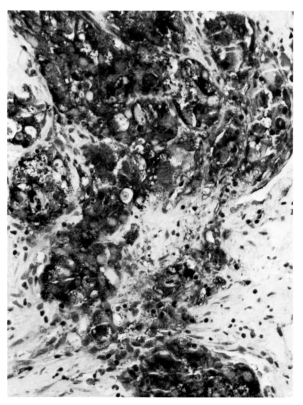

Fig. 15-48 Renal cell carcinoma. Positive cytoplasmic staining for glycogen (PAS reaction). PAS stain; ×236.

and approximately 50 percent also show positive staining for vimentin.[139,283] The latter is present in blastemal cells, and this pattern of reaction suggests a derepression of the genome, as seen during nephrogenesis. The dual expression of cytokeratin of low molecular weight and vimentin is potentially useful for distinguishing sarcomatoid renal cell carcinoma from a true sarcoma or in the differential diagnosis of a metastatic lesion of unknown primary site. Only a limited number of carcinomas exhibit this pattern of reaction (endometrium, ovary, salivary gland, lung, and thyroid).[10a,193]

Although there is no good explanation, leukocyte differentiation antigens also have a distinctive pattern of reaction in the normal segments of the nephron, and this reactivity is preserved in renal neoplasia.[44] Common ALL antigen, DU-HL60-4 and p24, have been used. DU-HL60-4 stained all renal cell carcinomas regardless of tumor grade or cell type, and p24 stained all nephroblastomas.[44]

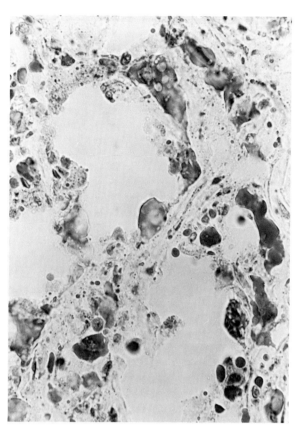

Fig. 15-50 Renal cell carcinoma. Oil red O stain demonstrates lipid granules in the cytoplasm of tumor cells. ×614.

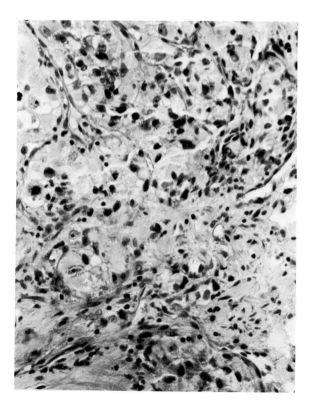

Fig. 15-49 Renal cell carcinoma. Pretreatment of sections with diastase has removed the glycogen. The PAS stain is now negative for cytoplasmic glycogen. PAS stain; ×236.

Antibodies to epithelial membrane antigens and to rat brush border antigen are positive in a high percentage of renal cell carcinomas.[102,139] Regretfully, staining is generally not seen in poorly differentiated tumors.

Currently great efforts are being made to develop antibodies to renal cell carcinoma cells that will provide a more definitive and specific immunocytochemical diagnosis.

Electron Microscopy

Electron microscopy demonstrates particulate glycogen and fat in the *clear cells,* with little endoplasmic reticulum, few Golgi apparatus, and few mitochondria (Figs. 15-51 and 15-52). *Granular cells* have numerous mitochondria and dense bodies (Fig. 15-53), a developed Golgi apparatus, and endoplasmic reticu-

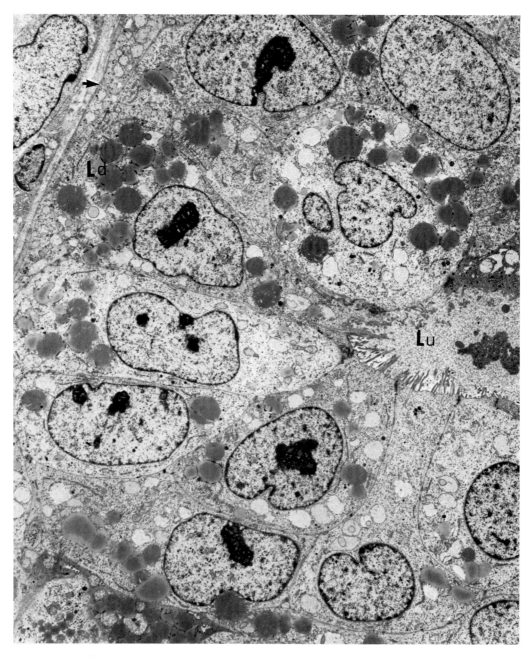

Fig. 15-51 Renal cell carcinoma. Electron micrograph of an area with tubular differentiation, a central lumen (Lu) and microvilli, and basement lamina (arrow). There are abundant lipid droplets (Ld) and glycogen in the cytoplasm. Note also the nuclear atypia with prominent nucleoli. ×3,591.

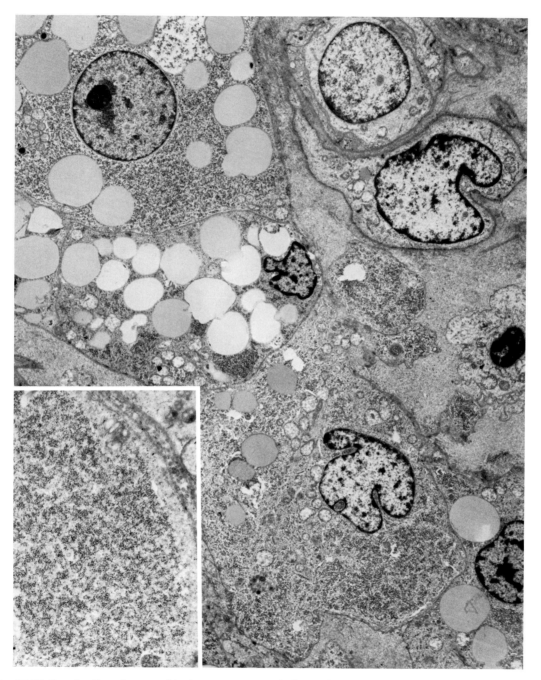

Fig. 15-52 Renal cell carcinoma. This electron micrograph shows clear cells with abundant particulate glycogen and lipid droplets. Particulate glycogen is seen in the inset. ×3,591. **Inset,** ×10,838.

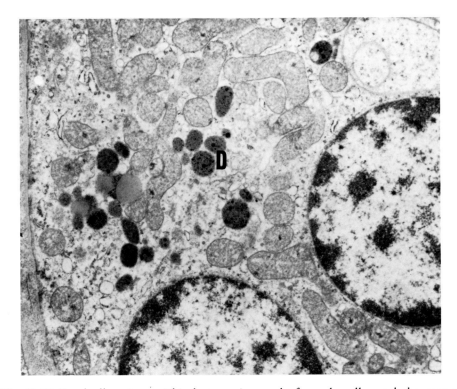

Fig. 15-53 Renal cell carcinoma. This electron micrograph of granular cells reveals the presence of abundant mitochondria and dense bodies (D). ×12,000.

lum. Some of the mitochondria are atypical, with bizarre arrangement of the cristae.[29] Both types of cell show multiple similarities to the proximal convoluted tubules, with tightly packed microvilli in a brush border, membrane-associated vesicles that may be involved in pinocytosis, and a membrane coating of extracellular material (glycocalyx). Also present are intercellular junctions, basal infoldings of the plasma membrane, and abundant mitochondria. The last three elements cited are also found in distal convoluted tubules.[271] Ultrastructural studies in sarcomatoid renal cell tumors have demonstrated desmosomal junctions.[43a,83]

NATURAL HISTORY AND CLINICAL PRESENTATION

Renal adenocarcinoma presents with subtle symptoms and misleading physical and laboratory findings. It has been said that it rivals tuberculosis and syphilis as the great masquerader or mimic in clinical medicine. Symptoms of presentation are vague, and 30 to 45 percent of patients have no presenting symptoms directly related to the tumor.[137] Ectopic hormone production and other paraneoplastic syndromes occur in approximately 30 percent of patients. They may appear early in the natural history of the tumor, and they do not necessarily imply the presence of metastasis.[232,232a] There are enough reports about spontaneous regression, including metastases, to raise questions about host–tumor relations. All of these facts make it difficult to precisely define the natural history of this tumor. Moreover, no agreement exists about the definition of renal cell adenoma and adenocarcinoma in the literature. The deep-seated nature of this tumor has precluded the sequential analysis that has been performed with carcinoma of the cervix, where the preinvasive phase has a duration of 13 to 20 years. It is believed that the latent period of renal cell carcinoma may be of similar duration.[137]

Renal cell carcinoma has a variety of presentations, frequently with significant delay in diagnosis. Early manifestations are nonspecific, e.g., cachexia, malaise, fever, and anemia. The classic triad of hematuria, flank pain, and abdominal mass occurs in only 5 to 15 percent of patients.[232,234] It is generally present in advanced disease, and 47 percent of these patients already have metastasis.[207] Any one of the classic symptoms and signs (hematuria, flank pain, abdominal mass) is present in only 65 percent of cases[234] (Table 15-5).

Hematuria is usually intermittent and painless, unless it is brisk enough to produce clots. It occurs in 60 percent of patients[137] and should prompt a thorough investigation of the urologic tract. It indicates invasion into the calyceal system, pelvis, or intrarenal circulation and is generally a late event.

Flank pain, described as a dull ache in 38 percent of combined series,[232] is a late and inconstant finding. Unfortunately, it has also been reported as not helpful for establishing the diagnosis.[127] A palpable mass is present in one-third of cases and is also a late manifestation.

Acute varicocele is found in 2 percent of cases[127] and is due to obstruction of the left internal spermatic vein. It can also occur on the right side owing to involvement of the right vein by tumor; on the right side it is even more suggestive of tumor, as most idiopathic varicoceles are left-sided.

Cardiac failure of the high-output type may be caused by massive arteriovenous fistulas within the tumor.[137] Presentation with metastatic disease has been described in 5 to 20 percent of cases.[29,127] A solitary metastasis leading to pathologic fracture in a long bone or to visual defects, priapism, etc. may call attention to this tumor.

Approximately 30 percent of patients with renal adenocarcinomas have paraneoplastic signs or syndromes at presentation. These signs may be nonspecific or may be characteristic paraneoplastic endocrinopathies.[232,168a] The nonspecific paraneoplastic signs and syndromes include: normochromic, normocytic anemia of chronic disease (33 percent); elevated erythrocyte sedimentation rate (60 percent); fever (16 percent); weight loss (27 percent); fatigue (20 percent); anorexia; cachexia; abnormalities of liver function (40 percent), with elevated alkaline phosphatase, haptoglobin, and bilirubin, and a prolonged prothrombin time; amyloidosis (3 to 5 percent); neuromyopathy (4 percent); leukemoid reaction; disorders of coagulation; and a variety of vague gastrointestinal symptoms.

The anemia observed in renal cell carcinoma may

Table 15-5 Symptoms and Signs of Renal Cell Carcinoma

Symptoms/Signs	Incidence (%)	At Presentation (%)
Local carcinoma		
Hematuria	60	
Flank pain	38	5 – 15
Palpable mass	36	
Varicocele	2	
Metastasis		5 – 20
Paraneoplasm		30
Nonspecific		
Anemia	33	
Elevated ESR	60	
Fever	16	
Weight loss	27	
Fatigue	20	
Liver dysfunction	0 – 40	
Amyloidosis	3 – 5	
Neuropathy	4	
Hypertension		30
Erythrocytosis		1.8 – 6.0
Hypercalemia		10
Incidental findings		8

(Data from Ritchie and Chisholm,[232] Haertig and Kuss,[127] and Bennington and Beckwith.[29])

be related to an ectopic production of lactoferrin by the tumor. Lactoferrin is a glycoprotein that binds free iron and shunts it into the reticuloendothelial system.[176a]

Hepatic dysfunction associated with nonmetastatic renal cell carcinoma has been called the Stauffer syndrome.[260] It is associated not only with renal malignancy but also with other gastrointestinal tumors and xanthogranulomatous pyelonephritis.[234] Histologically, the liver manifests a nonspecific triaditis and Kupffer cell hyperplasia.[131,278]

Paraneoplastic endocrinopathies are associated with hypersecretion by the tumor of a substance indistinguishable from a hormone. The substance secreted may be associated normally with the kidney (e.g., renin, erythropoietin, or prostaglandins A and E) or be ectopically produced in the tumor. Hypertension is present in more than one-third of the patients. Although an elevated renin level is found in one-third of the patients, it may not be related to hypertension.[66] It has been reported that a high proportion of tumors contain renin in the inactive form.[275a] Erythrocytosis has been described in 1.8 to 6.0 percent of cases,[29] and in one study erythropoietin was increased in 36 of 51 patients.[265] An erythropoietinlike substance has been isolated from clones of a human renal carcinoma cell line.[268] Prostaglandin E has been associated with hypercalcemia and prostaglandin A with hypotension. Ectopic hormones such as parathormone are associated with hypercalcemia, gonadotropins with feminization or hirsutism and amenorrhea, and ACTH with Cushing's syndrome; prolactin and insulinlike activity have also been described.[66,239] Hypercalcemia has been reported in 10 percent of cases of renal cell carcinoma. It may be due to skeletal metastases, which are typically osteolytic, or to the secretion of parathyroid hormonelike substances or prostaglandins.[65]

Paraneoplastic syndromes are of important clinical significance as they generally represent early manifestations of the disease. Disappearance after nephrectomy confirms that the tumor is indeed responsible for the abnormality.

The tumor may also appear as an incidental finding during the investigation of other conditions (8 percent incidence). A high index of suspicion is mandatory to make the diagnosis of a tumor that presents with such varied symptomatology.

METASTATIC SPREAD

Renal cell carcinoma grows by expansion, producing a pseudocapsule. It spreads by direct extension or by invasion of lymphatics or intrarenal veins (Table 15-6). *Local spread* includes extension to perinephric fat, pelvic tissue, adrenal gland, or other adjacent organs (liver, colon). In 6 to 10 percent of cases, direct extension to the adrenal gland occurs within Gerota's fascia.[234] Also, veins in the perirenal fat communicate with adrenal veins,[137] forming an expedited route of spread. The incidence of adrenal involvement has been reported to be 19 percent in an autopsy series[29] and was present in 29 percent of the clinically unrecognized renal cell carcinomas in the Malmö series. Ninety-four percent of these cases also had lymph node metastasis.[134]

The *lymphatic drainage* of the kidney is to adjacent lateral, aortic, or caval lymph nodes. The lymphatics from the perinephric fat empty in a more cranial position. Lymphatic metastases are present in 23 percent of patients undergoing extensive lymphadenectomy with radical nephrectomy.[234] Lymph node metastases were present in 34 percent of an autopsy series,[29] and retroperitoneal lymph nodes were positive in 44 percent of the clinically unrecognized renal cell carcinomas of Hellsten et al.[134] The first lymph nodes involved are those of the renal hilum. Progression continues to the midline group of retroperitoneal lymph nodes and to the mediastinum. Disorderly progression has also been noted.[84] Lymph nodes can also drain to the cisterna chyli and from there to supraclavicular lymph nodes. Caudal extension has been noted when retroperitoneal lymph nodes are extensively involved.

Malignant cells may gain access to the thoracic duct and thence to the superior vena cava, right heart, and pulmonary circulation with a lymphohematogenous route of spread.[29] The thoracic duct occasionally divides into two branches, with the right emptying into the subclavian vein. Both supraclavicular areas can then have metastastic foci.[137] The difficulty of predicting the pattern of metastasis is also explained by

Table 15-6 Renal Cell Carcinoma: Site and Frequency of Metastasis

Site of Metastasis	Autopsy series[29] (%)	Clinically recognized[134] (103 cases) (%)	Unrecognized tumors[135] (56 cases) (%)
Lung	55	72	82
Lymph nodes	34	65[a]	64[a]
Bone	32	49	48
Adrenals	19	32	29
Liver	33	48	23

[a] Includes supraclavicular and tracheobranchial lymph nodes.

the marked neovascularity of this tumor. The new vessels are accompanied by lymphatics that may give rise to metastasis to any point between the diaphragm and the pelvis. This unpredictability of behavior makes difficult exicision of all tumor-bearing lymphatic tissue.[84]

Invasion of renal veins or *hematogenous spread* of the tumor is probably the most important route of spread. Thirty percent of patients at operation have renal vein invasion,[234] and 55 percent of the patients with metastasis showed growth into a vein, in contrast to only 6 percent of patients without metastatic growths.[134]

Four vascular routes of spread have been postulated: (1) up through the vena cava to the right heart and into the lungs; (2) down to the pelvic structures via the left spermatic or ovarian vein; (3) along the axial skeleton by the Batson's plexus (paravertebral); and (4) from the pulmonary circulation to the arterial circulation.[29]

Invasion of the inferior vena cava has been found in 7 percent of tumors,[134] but reviews of patients with inferior vena cava extension and no distant metastasis has shown a 5-year survival of approximately 50 percent.[64,251] The frequency of vein invasion and its relative lack of negative influence on survival, especially in contrast with lymph node metastasis, has led to studies of host resistance. Tumor cells are shed from aggregates of tumor cells growing in intravascular spaces, but some mechanism of elimination of these cells and prevention of implantation must be active. A significant increase in natural killer cells has been found in patients with tumors at stage III of Robson. Also, a drop in the helper/suppressor ratio due to a decrease in helper cells has been noted as the stage of the tumor progresses.[232]

Metastasis to the pelvic and genitourinary organs has been explained through retrograde embolization via the left gonadal vein.[1] Although renal adenocarcinoma cells have been observed in the urine, there are no substantial data to support implantation of malignant cells as a significant mechanism for bladder and ureter metastasis.[237] It has been suggested that minor trauma to the urothelium may allow exfoliated renal tumor cells to implant and grow.[246]

Tumor cells may enter the vertebral veins from the vena cava during periods of increased abdominal pressure. This route explains the frequent metastasis in the axial skeleton (pelvis, spine, skull) and adjacent organs such as brain and thyroid. Skeletal metastases are seen in 32 percent of patients dying of renal cell carcinoma. Typically they are osteolytic.[29]

The lungs are involved in about one-half of patients with metastasis in autopsy series. Passage of malignant cells through the pulmonary circulation has been demonstrated. Passage to the arterial circulation probably explains the unusual sites of metastasis, a well recognized peculiarity of this tumor.

The incidence of metastasis in patients at presentation is 24 to 28 percent,[232] and metastases were found in 24 percent of patients with a clinically unrecognized renal cell carcinoma.[134] The common sites of metastasis are lung, lymph nodes, bone, adrenals, and liver.

Hepatic metastasis may be explained by direct extension to mesenteric veins or by direct passage through systemic portal shunts.[137] Not unexpectedly, liver metastases were twice as common in the clinically recognized cases of renal tumor as in those unrecognized clinically.[135] Apparently solitary metastases are present in 1 to 3 percent of cases. Aggressive surgical management has been advocated,[273] but others believe it is of little value.[197]

Involvement of both kidneys has been found in 2.0 to 5.5 percent. The difficulty of defining a simultaneously occurring primary bilateral renal cell carcinoma from metastatic disease has been discussed by several authors.[135,232] Renal cell adenocarcinoma is somewhat unusual in that patients may live many years with metastasis, or metastases may occur at a late date. Among patients surviving 10 years, 11 percent had late recurrence.[192] Late metastases, occurring as long as 15 to 20 years after the appearance of the primary, have also been described. Idiopathic or spontaneous regression of primary tumors and metastases have been reported.[137] Pronounced histologic regression of the primary tumor, with lymphocytic infiltration and fibrosis, was shown in 8 of 235 (3.4 percent) cases of unrecognized carcinoma in the series of Hellsten et al.[135] Regression of metastasis after nephrectomy is also relatively rare. In combined series it is reported to occur in 0.3 to 0.8 percent,[273] which is much lower than the current mortality rate for nephrectomy alone.

Although this tumor is associated with a high mortality rate, only 21 percent of the patients with clinically unrecognized renal cell carcinoma died of the tumor. Cardiovascular disease (44 percent) and other malignant tumors (20 percent) were the other main causes of death.[134] These findings must be kept in mind when treating elderly patients with coexistent cardiovascular disease.

DIAGNOSIS

A renal mass with central and mottled calcifications seen on plain abdominal film is usually a renal cell carcinoma. Unfortunately, calcifications are not common, with 80 percent of renal cell carcinomas not showing them.[112]

Intravenous urography is the initial examination performed for detection of a renal mass. IVP demonstrates enlargement of the kidney in 88 percent of patients with renal cell carcinoma but in only 16 percent of those with a renal cyst. Other findings that are less specific for renal malignancy include calyceal deformities, pelvis displacement, and irregular renal outlines. Cystic hypernephromas occur in approximately 4 percent of patients, although most of them have only minor cystic changes.[97]

Tomography helps in the distinction between cysts and tumors. Cysts appear radiolucent with homogeneous density, have a thin and well defined wall, and demonstrate an acute crescentic angle at the junction with the cortex. Carcinomas show irregular densities, calcifications, and irregular and thick walls. Margins at the interface between tumor and the normal renal parenchyma are poorly defined. If the renal anatomic landmarks are well defined, a 95 percent accuracy rate has been reported with these studies; regretfully, it is achieved with confidence in only 70 to 80 percent of cases.

Sonography is particularly helpful for demonstrating internal echoes and little if any acoustic enhancement if the mass is a renal cell carcinoma. Computed tomography can produce kidney images with a slice thickness of as little as 2 mm. This technique is not only accurate but also sensitive, as it can detect previously unrecognized renal masses. With renal cell carcinoma, a thick wall, irregular contrast enhancement, parenchymal calcification, central necrosis, and densities near those of renal parenchyma are usually demonstrable.

Angiography has been relegated to the study of renal vein or inferior vena cava tumor extension. Digital subtraction angiography with injection of the contrast medium through an intravenous route has been used for renal artery visualization, although computed tomography appears superior for tumor diagnosis and staging.[98]

Fluid aspiration from cysts followed by examination of gross characteristics, cytology, and chemical analysis might also be helpful for distinguishing benign cysts from tumors. Benign cysts have a clear, straw-colored fluid with a low content of protein, lactic dehydrogenase (LDH), and lipids (cholesterol and total lipids)[221,262]; tumors, on the other hand, generally contain murky or hemorrhagic fluid and a high content of protein, LDH, and lipids.

Cytology does not appear to be helpful for diagnosing renal cell adenocarcinoma. Urine cytology is not an adequate screening procedure as it fails to detect early carcinomas in adequate numbers. Even with multiple specimens only approximately 50 percent of patients with known renal cell carcinoma had malignant cells in the urine.[222] Fine-needle aspiration has also been used, but its usefulness is controversial. The combination of fine-needle aspiration and immunoperoxidase staining with a tumor specific monoclonal antibody has been reported to reduce the number of false-positive cases.[241b]

DIFFERENTIAL DIAGNOSIS

The differential diagnosis includes cystic and histiocytic lesions, clear cell tumors, and spindle, poorly differentiated malignancies. In general, multiple sections should be taken in problem cases, where the demonstration of a characteristic differentiated pattern may establish the correct diagnosis. Histochemistry and electron microscopy are sometimes fundamental to the diagnosis of difficult tumors.

Unilateral multilocular cyst may be considered in the differential diagnosis of a largely cystic renal cell carcinoma. The presence of small tubules lined by large cuboidal cells with a large vesicular nucleus, hobnail cells lining large septal spaces, and immature mesenchyme favors the diagnosis of a unilateral multilocular cyst over cystic renal cell carcinoma.

Histiocytic lesions such as xanthogranulomatous pyelonephritis and malakoplakia should be ruled out. They appear grossly as tan to orange bulging nodules with central necrosis or as tan to yellow mucosal plaques. Although generally confined to the medulla, they may replace the whole kidney. Histologically, they are composed of histiocytes with clear, foamy or granular eosinophilic cytoplasm. Pseudoacinar or pseudotubular structures may be present. The differential diagnosis is established by the absence of the fibrovascular stroma and the glandular and acinar pattern present in renal cell carcinoma as well as the prominence of an acute and chronic inflammatory component in xanthogranulomatous pyelonephritis and malakoplakia. Cholesterol clefts and multinucleated cells are prominent in xanthogranulomatous lesions, whereas the diagnosis of malakoplakia is made by demonstrating Michaelis-Gutmann bodies. It must be remembered that xanthogranulomatous pyelonephritis has been described in kidneys with renal cell carcinoma.[120]

With clear cell lesions the possibility of ectopic adrenal tissue is worth considering. Generally, it appears as a subcapsular nodule of up to 2 cm in diameter in the upper pole. Microscopically, it resembles adrenal zona fasciculata.

Clear cell tumors have been described as arising in multiple organs. The demonstration of mucin in such a tumor rules out a renal cell origin. Glycogen-rich clear cell carcinomas have been described in the thyroid[62,70] and breast,[27] joining other tumors (female genital tract, parotid gland, and lung) in which the clear cell appearance is due to glycogen accumulation. Although in hematoxylin-eosin preparations these tumors may initially be confused with renal cell tumors, they do not contain fat as do renal cell carcinomas. Thyroglobulin has been demonstrated in thyroid clear cells[62] and clear cell thyroid carcinomas[70] by immunocytochemistry. This technique might be of value when assessing the presence of a metastatic lesion without an obvious primary tumor. Perhaps the most difficult differential diagnosis occurs in a metastatic clear cell tumor to the skin. Sebaceous carcinoma is a rare tumor that contains both glycogen and lipid. The differential diagnosis rests in the presence of a lobular arrangement, poorly differentiated cells at the margin of the lobules, and foci of keratinization in sebaceous carcinoma.[29]

A clear cell carcinoma can also be metastatic to the kidney. The presence of multiple nodules and mucin and the absence of fat establish the diagnosis of metastatic malignancy.

Spindle cell malignancies in the kidney may represent sarcomatoid renal cell carcinomas, spindle cell transitional cell carcinoma, nephroblastomas with only a mesenchymal component, or true sarcomas. An exhaustive search for typical areas, the demonstration of fat by special stains, and searching for desmosomes, brush borders, and basement membranes by electron microscopy are some of the approaches to the diagnosis of sarcomatoid renal cell carcinoma. The diagnosis of spindle or sarcomatoid transitional cell carcinoma is based on finding areas that are recognizable as invasive or in situ transitional cell carcinoma. Sarcomatoid renal cell carcinomas stain positively for low-molecular-weight cytokeratin and vimentin. Vimentin has not been demonstrated in transitional cell carcinoma, but blood group antigens' immunoreactivity is present in the sarcomatoid variant of this carcinoma.[288] Rarely, transitional cell carcinoma coexists with renal cell carcinoma.[179] In an adult, a nephroblastoma composed almost exclusively of immature spindle mesenchymal cells is a difficult, but fortunately rare, diagnostic problem. The presence of blastemal immature epithelial cells, high-molecular-weight keratin, and leukocyte differentiation antigen are helpful for establishing this diagnosis.[44]

True sarcomas of the kidney are rare. Most spindle cell malignancies of the kidney are sarcomatoid renal cell carcinomas.[43a,232b,274] All sarcomatous histologic patterns may be present. The carcinoma may appear with areas of malignant fibrous histiocytoma, hemangiopericytoma, fibrosarcoma, leiomyosarcoma, rhabdomyosarcoma, liposarcoma, osteosarcoma, or chondrosarcoma. A true sarcoma should stain negatively for low-molecular-weight keratin and positively for vimentin. An absence of epithelial differentiation after generous sampling in electron microscopy is consistent with a mesenchymal tumor. Leiomyosarcomas and rhabdomyosarcomas should also be desmin-positive.

Malignant melanoma, another pleomorphic tumor, must also be considered in the differential diagnosis of renal cell carcinoma. Demonstration of melanin and melanosomes as well as staining for S-100 protein are used to establish this diagnosis. Malignant melanoma does stain with vimentin.[10a,121]

TREATMENT

Complete surgical excision of the tumor is the only effective treatment for renal cell carcinoma.[85a] Regrettably, 50 percent of the patients either present with metastasis at diagnosis or metastases develop after the operation.[85] Patients with tumors that do not invade the perinephric fat but extend to the inferior vena cava have a similar cure rate from early-stage renal carcinoma if treated with complete removal of the thrombus and nephrectomy.

Surgical enucleation has been used with good results in patients with bilateral renal cell carcinomas or carcinoma in a solitary kidney. Most patients had a low-grade stage I carcinoma.[213] Partial nephrectomy is thought to offer better quality of life in these cases than complete nephrectomy and dialysis.

The role of nephrectomy in patients with distant metastases is controversial. No improvement in survival has been shown, and tumor regression appears insignificant. It may be indicated in patients with solitary metastases where improved survival has been seen and in those who undergo experimental therapy with debulking or immunotherapy.[85]

Irradiation pre- or postoperatively does not appear to play a significant role in the treatment of renal cell carcinoma.[49] The use of transcatheter embolization with radioactive infarct particles has been used[168] in patients with advanced disease, achieving some palliation and treatment response.

Hormonal therapy also does not appear to make a significant contribution.[142,224] It produces a small proportion of incomplete responses of short duration. Treatment with the progestational agent medroxyprogesterone acetate has been advocated because of the lack of a more effective therapy and the absence of side effects[132]; it does not, however, appear to be of therapeutic benefit in patients who have undergone radical nephrectomy.[224]

Chemotherapy has not been of help with this tumor. Vinblastine appears to be the most effective drug, and combination chemotherapy produces a higher rate of response. Tumor response is rare, however, and the appropriateness of the course of chemotherapy has been questioned.[85,132]

Immunologic therapies initially raised significant expectations. Renal cell carcinoma is known for undergoing spontaneous regression on rare occasion, and it has been postulated that this response is due to an immunologic phenomenon. Bacillus Calmette Guérin (BCG) has been used as a nonspecific immunotherapy with little effect,[190] and adjuvant immunotherapy has been tried with little success.[104] Immune RNA and autologous tumor cells have also been used. Interferon therapy appears promising for inducing partial tumor response.[86,207a] Additional data are needed on its long-term effectiveness, dose schedule, or combination with chemotherapy.[211,241a]

Adoptive immunotherapy with lymphokine activated killer cells or with tumor infiltrating cytotoxic lymphocytes and interleukin two (IL-2) are newer approaches that may prove to be of value.[235b,235c]

In summary, surgical excision is still the basic treatment for a contained renal cell carcinoma and the search for systemic therapy for metastatic disease continues with new and challenging approaches.

Oncocytoma

Klein and Valensi[159] first called attention to the benign behavior of a kidney tumor composed purely of oncocytic cells. Oncocytes are altered epithelial cells of multiple origins that have an abundant homogeneous eosinophilic cytoplasm and a small, round nucleus. Characteristically, the cells contain strikingly abundant mitochondria, a paucity of other organelles, and high ATPase and oxidative enzyme activity. Oncocytes have been described as appearing in cells of salivary glands, thyroid, parathyroid, lacrimal glands, adenohypophysis, bronchial mucous glands, pancreas, and kidneys.[130]

The origin of renal oncocytomas is somewhat controversial. Initially it was suggested that they were proximal tubular adenomas in view of the similarities with the staining characteristics and mitochondrial content of proximal tubules.[159] It has also been suggested that they represent a senescent or degenerative change. Oncocytes increase with advancing age and are seen in cachectic individuals.[67] The absence of true brush borders, the presence of round to oval mitochondrial profiles, and protrusion of basal membrane into concavities in the plasmalemma have lent support to a distal convoluted tubule origin.[94,241] The controversial origin of oncocytes supports the use of the descriptive term oncocytoma for this tumor and not the designation proximal tubular adenoma, as initially proposed by Klein and Valensi.[159]

The incidence of the tumor among renal cell carcinomas has been reported to be between 3 percent[175] and 7 percent.[67] An analysis of 44 cases in the literature showed that most cases are asymptomatic (89 percent) and are discovered incidentally on IVP for nonspecific symptoms. The male/female ratio is

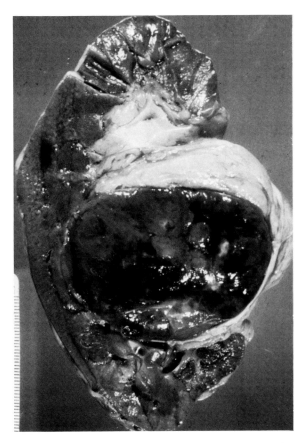

Fig. 15-54 Renal oncocytoma. This gross specimen shows a circumscribed, encapsulated tumor. The color is uniformly tan-brown.

homogeneous nephrogram, and a sharp, smooth rim have been described.[5] There is no evidence of puddling of the contrast medium, arteriovenous shunting, or renal vein invasion, as is seen with renal cell carcinoma.

Microscopically, renal oncocytomas are composed exclusively of brightly eosinophilic epithelial cells with fine, uniform, compactly arranged cytoplasmic granules. The nuclei are usually round and uniform without mitotic activity (Fig. 15-56). A minimal degree of focal nuclear pleomorphism resembling that seen in endocrine adenomas is accepted. The cells are arranged in an alveolar tubular or trabecular pattern (Fig. 15-57). A few cases with a focal minor papillary pattern have been described.[16] In contrast, renal cell carcinomas contain an admixture of clear and granular cells with basophilic or eosinophilic cytoplasm; they

2.4 : 1.0, and most patients are elderly with a mean age of 63.8 years.[67]

Grossly, the tumors are well circumscribed, encapsulated, and without extension to pericapsular, pelvicalyceal system or renal vein (Fig. 15-54). Unlike renal cell carcinomas, which are golden yellow or gray with areas of hemorrhage and necrosis, oncocytomas are tan-brown and uniform in color. In larger tumors a central fibrous scar with radiating bands (stellate scar) may be present (Fig. 15-55). The tumors range from 0.3 to 20.0 cm in diameter (average 7.4 cm). Multicentricity and bilaterality seem to be increasingly described.[180]

Angiographic findings are distinctive in renal oncocytomas. A spoke-wheel pattern with peripheral vessels radiating toward the center of the lesion, a

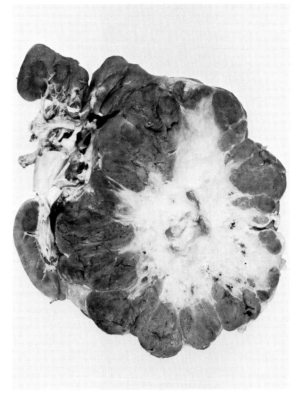

Fig. 15-55 Renal oncocytoma. This gross specimen, with a section through the tumor, reveals a stellate fibrous scar. Residual kidney tissue is seen at left. (From Eble et al.,[94] with permission.)

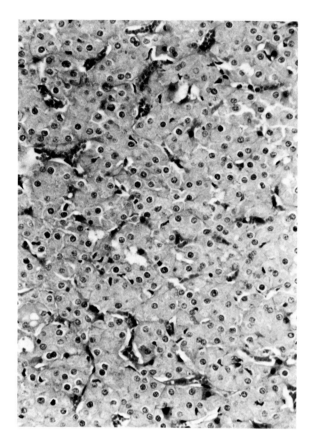

Fig. 15-56 Renal oncocytoma. Note the eosinophilic cytoplasm with compact granularity. Nuclei are round and uniform. ×233.

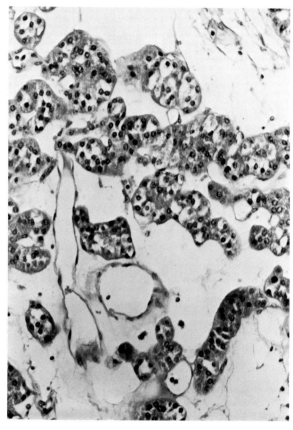

Fig. 15-57 Renal oncocytoma. Note the trabecular arrangement of the tumor cells. ×233.

reveal a multiplicity of patterns, including a sarcomatous component. Mitotic activity and nuclear pleomorphism are also prominent in renal cell carcinoma and absent in oncocytomas (Table 15-7).

Ultrastructurally, oncocytomas are composed totally of cells that have compactly arranged mitochondria, a paucity of other organelles, and an absence of fat vacuoles (Fig. 15-58). Renal cell carcinomas of the granular type contain a variable number of mitochondria, Golgi apparatus, rough endoplasmic reticulum, lipid droplets, and glycogen (see Table 15-7, below).

Prognostically, oncocytomas are nonaggressive, benign tumors. Restriction of this term to tumors composed of purely oncocytic and well differentiated cells (grade 1) reveals definitive clinicopathologic correlation. In the Mayo Clinic study[175] none of the 62 patients with grade 1 tumor developed metastases,

demonstrating that oncocytic neoplasms have a sluggish local growth potential and an excellent prognosis. This benign tumor should not be included within the classification of renal cell carcinoma, as it will artificially improve the prognosis or therapeutic response.[175]

Some authors have used the term "congeners of renal oncocytomas" to describe some renal cell carcinomas that have morphologic features that pose potential difficulty in the diagnosis, and they have cautioned against a frozen section or needle aspiration diagnosis.[16,297] Others have argued against the stringency of some of the morphologic criteria, including in this entity small cells with less cytoplasm, more nuclear pleomorphism, and microfocal capsular penetration.[94] It is well recognized that in some individual fields or sections of renal cell carcinoma an onco-

Table 15-7 Pathologic and Clinical Comparison of Oncocytoma and Renal Cell Carcinoma

Parameter	Oncocytoma	Renal Cell Carcinoma
Gross appearance	Tan-brown	Golden yellow-orange
	Uniform; no hemorrhage or necrosis, large tumors with central stellate scar	Hemorrhage and necrosis
	Well circumscribed	Infiltrative with spread to pericapsule and metastasis
Microscopic appearance	Uniform eosinophilic epithelial cells	Admixture of clear granular cells with eosinophilic or basophilic cytoplasm
	Alveolar or tubular pattern	All patterns, including sarcomatous
	No mitosis	Mitosis sometimes present
Electron microscopic appearance	Enlarged and swollen mitochondria	Lipid droplet, glycogen, organelles
Presentation	Incidental; no symptoms or weight loss	Flank pain, hematuria

cytic pattern may be present, but the diagnosis of oncocytoma should be reserved for those tumors that have exclusively characteristic, well differentiated oncocytic cells with abundant eosinophilic cytoplasm. A purely eosinophilic tumor that exhibits nu-

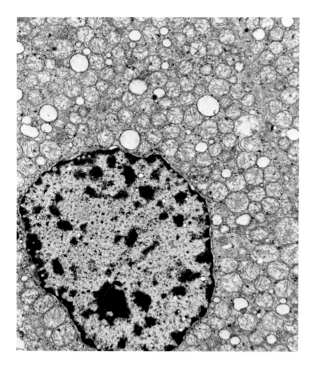

Fig. 15-58 Renal oncocytoma. This electron micrograph demonstrates the cytoplasm of an oncocytoma cell with its characteristic overload of mitochondria. ×9,800 (From Eble et al.,[94] with permission.)

clear pleomorphism must be excluded from a diagnosis of oncocytoma, as it cannot be ascertained that it would have a benign behavior. It is preferable to err on the safe side in nuclear irregularity. The Mayo Clinic study shows that of 28 patients with grade 2 lesions (larger, more irregular nuclei, and variation in cell size and configuration) 4 died of metastatic disease (14 percent).[175] Until a larger study is able to evaluate the potential of some of the lesions with less stringent diagnostic criteria, the diagnosis of oncocytoma should include only tumors that are universally accepted as benign (grade 1 and exclusively oncocytic). DNA analysis has given conflicting results with both normal diploid[95] and aneuploid nuclear patterns.[32] Cytogenetic analysis and study of intermediate filament proteins appear to demonstrate a distinct pattern for renal oncocytomas that could help in its differentiation from renal cell carcinomas.[162a,233a]

The possibility of treating this benign tumor with only partial renal resection has been raised,[175,297] although caution must be exercised in frozen sections and needle aspiration where adequate sampling cannot be ascertained.

Juxtaglomerular Cell Tumor (Angioreninoma)

In 1967 Robertson et al.[233] reported a renal cortical lesion in a young man with severe diastolic hypertension and hypokalemia. Histologically, the lesion resembled an hemangiopericytoma and contained large quantities of renin. Twenty cases have since been reported,[58,89,256] establishing the association of a cortical renal tumor with the clinical syndrome of hypertension, hyperreninemia, and secondary hyperaldosteronism due to the release of excessive amounts of renin.

This tumor presumably originates from the juxtaglomerular cells that arise from metaplasia of smooth muscle of the arterial vasculature.[14,60] The metaplasia to endocrine functioning cells has been induced by experimental manipulation even at considerable distance from the afferent arteriole.[60] The presence in this tumor of cells containing renin secretory granules and myofilaments with attachment bodies also supports a smooth muscle origin.[58] Admixture with neural elements has raised the possibility of a hamartomatous lesion, although juxtaglomerular cells are normally innervated by nonmyelinated fibers of sympathetic origin.[15]

Juxtaglomerular cell tumors are primarily lesions of the second decade (seven cases) and third decade (six cases). The oldest reported patient was a 69-year-old woman.[58] Twelve cases in women and seven in men have been reported. Symptomatology at presentation includes headaches, polyuria or nocturia, or both. Hypertension is severe (mean blood pressue 216/141 mmHg), the mean serum potassium is 2.9 mEq/liter, and plasma renin assays have ranged from two- to seven-fold the upper limits of normal. Postoperative blood pressure was shown to be significantly decreased (mean 132/89 mmHg) in cases where pertinent data were available. The tumors are small, 3 to 5 cm in diameter, cortical, well circumscribed or encapsulated, and gray-white. Light microscopy demonstrates a thin capsule separating the tumor from the adjacent compressed renal tissue. Small epithelioid, fairly uniform cells with slightly granular cytoplasm in an organoid or trabecular arrangement are seen to be admixed (Fig. 15-59), with areas of spindle-shaped cells merging into muscular vessel walls. In all cases the tumors are richly vascularized with capillaries arranged in an endocrinelike pattern, veins, and small muscular arteries. The tumor cells form poorly developed swirling patterns around vessels accentuated by stromal reticulin. Mast cells have also been described to be irregularly distributed between tumor cells. Occasional nuclear pleomorphism of the type present in endocrine tumors is seen (Fig. 15-60). Mitoses are absent.

The granules in the tumor cells stain deep blue to purple with Bowie stain in Zenker formalin-fixed material. PAS stain is positive and resistant to both diastase and trypsin digestion. Fluorescein-labeled anti-renin antibodies and immunoperoxidase staining with and without prior renin absorption have been used to demonstrate the presence of renin.[58,90] Electron microscopy demonstrates a discontinuous basal lamina, micropinocytotic vesicles and submembranous plaques, myofilaments, rare desmosomes, and abundantly developed rough endoplasmic reticulum and mitochondria[256] (Fig. 15-61). Various numbers of intracytoplasmic granules are present. The most characteristic are rhomboid protogranules with a fairly organized, crystalloid substructure (Fig. 15-61, inset), such as described in the human juxtaglomerular complex.[36] Electron probe microanalysis has demonstrated the presence of zinc,[90,256] which appears to play some role in the storage and secretion of endocrine cells.

Prognostically, it is a benign tumor. No case has been shown to have a recurrence or metastasis, with follow-up from 0.5 to 15.0 years (average 6.6 years) in one series.[256] Nevertheless, the tumor is potentially lethal owing to complications of extreme hypertension or the subsequent development of sustained benign hypertension probably as a result of hypertensive vascular damage (27 percent of patients).

The differential diagnosis of a juxtaglomerular cell tumor includes renal cell carcinoma, interstitial cell tumor, Wilms' tumor variants, and renal leiomyoma. The differentiation is made by the characteristic clinical presentation, the distinctive endocrine pattern with admixture of spindle cells, the demonstration of renin by histochemistry, and the characteristic electron microscopy features. Renin alone does not define this tumor, as the production of renin and hypertension has been described in at least one clear cell carcinoma of the kidney.[138]

Alveolar soft part sarcomas (ASPSs) have been proposed as malignant angioreninomas[90] because of the demonstration of renin in a series of four tumors and the suggested origin from modified smooth muscle cell for both juxtaglomerular tumors and ASPSs. Juxtaglomerularlike cells have been documented outside the kidney at sites related to the vasculature. No association with hypertension is present in such slowly progressing (10 to 15 years) malignant tumors of soft tissue, probably because of the presence of an inactive reninlike product or the inability of the tumor cell to secrete it.

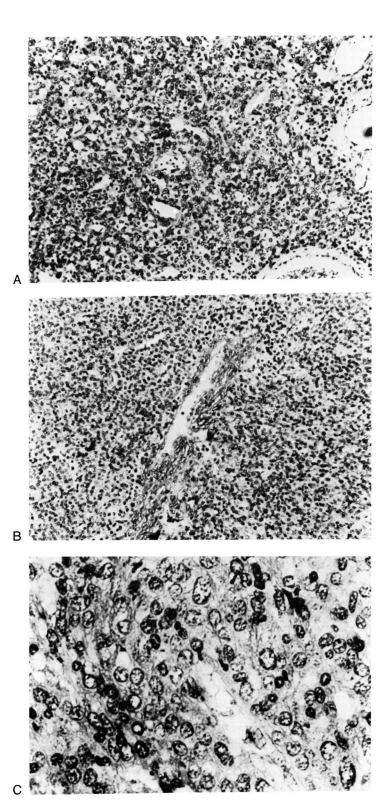

Fig. 15-59 Renin-screting renal tumor. **(A)** Tumor cells are arranged between endothelium-lined blood spaces. **(B)** Fine basement membrane surrounds the cells and condenses around the arterioles. **(C)** Tumor cells appear to merge with smooth muscle cells of a blood vessel wall. **A&B,** ×83; **C;** ×323. (From Robertson et al.,[233] with permission.)

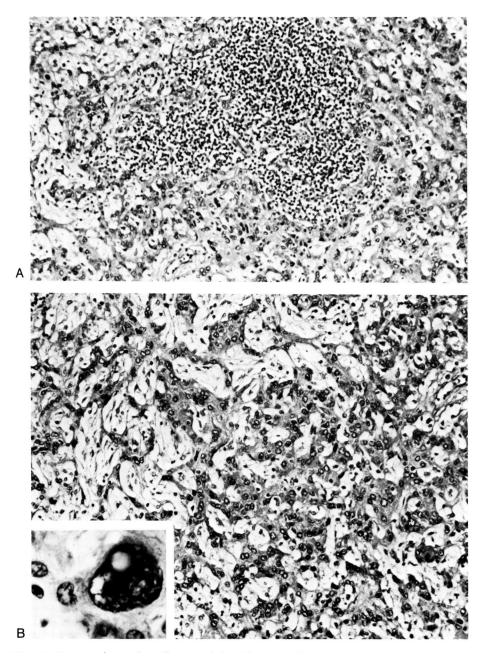

Fig. 15-60 Juxtaglomerular cell tumor. **(A)** Collections of lymphocytes are seen in the tumor. **(B)** Acidophilic cells set in a myxoid stroma are mostly uniform with occasional enlarged, hyperchromatic cells **(inset). A,** ×119; **B,** ×214; **inset,** ×741. (From Squires et al.,[256] with permission.)

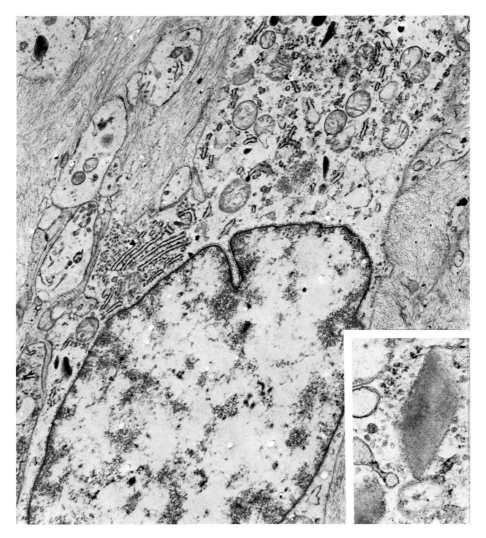

Fig. 15-61 Juxtaglomerular cell tumor. The tumor cell is surrounded by collagen. Small processes of unmyelinated nerve fibers are next to the cell border. Stacks of rough endoplasmic reticulum, angulated electron-dense crystals, and round mitochondria are visible. **(Inset)** Note the characteristic rhomboid granules with crystalline substructure. $\times 12,000$; **inset,** $\times 39,450$. (From Squires et al.,[256] with permission.)

Juxtaglomerular cell tumors must also be distinguished from hemangiopericytoma, though all juxtaglomerular cell tumors can be considered, in a sense, "differentiated" hemangiopericytomas because they are derived from pericytes (smooth muscle cells). A distinction must be made from ordinary hemangiopericytomas, which arise in the renal fossa in older patients; the latter spread to the retroperitoneum and cause death from local tumor growth or metastasis in 50 percent of cases.[256] Gross appearance here is also helpful, as juxtoglomerular cell tumors are solitary, well circumscribed cortical lesions.

Distinctions must also be made clinically, as any tumor may cause hypertension by a Goldblatt clamp mechanism; and malignant hyperreninemic hypertension unassociated with a renal tumor may mimic the clinical picture of juxtaglomerular cell tumor.

Once the diagnosis has been established, the treatment, if technically possible, should be partial nephrectomy. In practice, however, only lateralization is possible, and the treatment ends by being a total nephrectomy.

Angiomyolipomas

Angiomyolipomas are benign tumorlike lesions in the kidney formed by heterotopic tissue. They are most properly considered hamartomas containing tissue normally present in the kidney — smooth muscle, blood vessels, fat — but abnormal in arrangement, quantity, and degree of maturation. Thus they are not true neoplasms.[29,293] Angiomyolipomas can be found in approximately 0.3 percent of autopsies.[126a]

Traditionally, angiomyolipomas of the kidney have been categorized into two clinical variants: those associated with the tuberous sclerosis complex[68] and sporadic cases without this association.

TUBEROUS SCLEROSIS-ASSOCIATED ANGIOMYOLIPOMAS

Bourneville's[45] classic case of tuberous sclerosis-associated angiomyolipoma was a mentally retarded child with widespread adenoma sebaceum and uncontrolled epilepsy. On autopsy, large potatolike sclerotic plaques were demonstrated in the cerebral cortex and primitive cell tumors of the kidney. Moolten[200] proposed the term tuberous sclerosis complex, defining it as "a congenital developmental anomaly characterized by the occurrence of tumor-like malformations in various organs" representing widespread hamartomatosis. Cutaneous tumors such as angiofibromas on the face (adenoma sebaceum), paraungual fibromas, and shagreen patches (thickened plaques generally in the lumbosacral area) are associated with hamartomas of the brain, eyes (glial tissue plaques, or phacomas), bone (cysts), heart (rhabdomyomas), lungs (cysts), and kidneys (angiomyolipomas). As many as 80 percent of the patients with the severe form of tuberous sclerosis have renal angiomyolipomas, which are usually bilateral, multiple, small, and asymptomatic.[74] Fifty percent of the patients have a family history of mental retardation, epilepsy, characteristic skin lesion, or other mental conditions. Inheritance is thought to be on the basis of an autosomal dominant gene with incomplete penetrance, with another modifying gene affecting the severity of expression. The disease affects females more than males and occurs in approximately 1 of every 150,000 births.[26]

SPORADIC ANGIOMYOLIPOMAS

The second type, sporadic angiomyolipoma, occurs rarely among the general population, with slightly more than 200 cases described. They appear sporadically as large unilateral, symptomatic masses. The female/male ratio is 4:1. No overt symptoms of tuberous sclerosis are present,[293] although it has been postulated that the solitary angiomyolipomas may represent a *forme fruste* of the disease.[225] In 2 of the 32 cases of angiomyolipoma described by Farrow et al., there was no other evidence of the tuberous sclerosis complex; nevertheless each of these two women had a child with severe disease of the central nervous system believed to be tuberous sclerosis.[99]

A large proportion of the benign mixed mesenchymal tumors of the kidney are myolipomas, whereas the others have a prominent angiomatous component or are pure leiomyomas or lipomas. All have been considered probably to be hamartomas in the same group as angiomyolipomas. They may or may not be associated with the tuberous sclerosis complex.[29] Angiomyolipomas (predominantly of the solitary variety) can be found in approximately 0.3 percent of autopsies.[126a]

Grossly, the tumor appears as a smooth or bosselated mass that is gray, yellow, or hemorrhagic de-

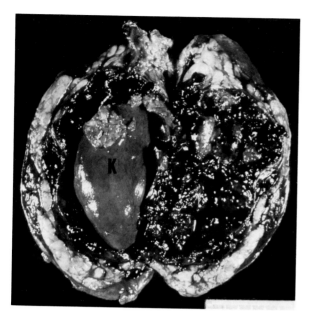

Fig. 15-62 Angiomyolipoma. This gross specimen shows a yellowish tumor that has ruptured and produced massive hemorrhage in the pericapsular tissue. K=kidney.

pending on the predominance of smooth muscle or fat tissue and if there is disruption of the angiomatous component. The growth is generally circumscribed and expansile, with distension of the renal capsule and in some cases extension into the perirenal tissue. Rarely, it involves the pelvicalyceal system. The tumor may appear as a multicentric growth and have focal areas of adipose tissue with an oily texture that can be clearly differentiated from the golden yellow appearance of a renal cell carcinoma. Massive hemorrhage may also be present (Fig. 15-62).

The histopathology is characterized by an admixture of adipose tissue, blood vessels, and smooth muscle in inconstant proportions (Figs. 15-63 and 15-64). The fat is of the adult type with an eccentric pyknotic nucleus. Occasional lipoblasts with prominent centrally placed nuclei and finely vacuolated cytoplasm are present. Fat necrosis and giant cell reaction are common. The vacular component is represented by small and medium-size muscular vessels with tortuous appearance, imperfect walls, and incomplete or only occasional fragmented elastic lamellae. The defective vessel walls may account for the frequent hemorrhagic complications. Elongated spindle smooth muscle cells form collarettes (Fig. 15-63 inset) around

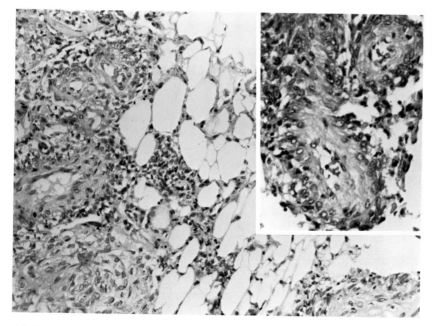

Fig. 15-63 Angiomyolipoma. Note the admixture of fat cells and vessels with a streaming collarette of smooth muscle cells. ×148; **inset,** ×296.

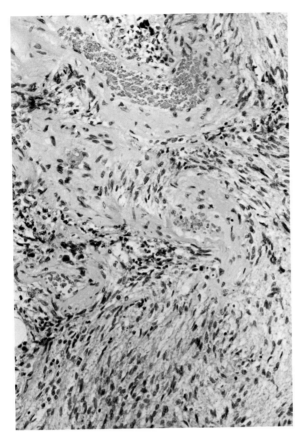

Fig. 15-64 Angiomyolipoma. Elongated, spindle smooth muscle cells stream from an abnormal vessel and form interlacing fascicles throughout the tumor. ×144.

The clinical presentation in symptomatic cases is usually due to hemorrhage with hypovolemia, an enlarging palpable mass (47 percent), hematuria (40 percent), and mild to acute abdominal pain (87 percent) generally in the flank.

Radiologically, the lesions appear radiolucent because of the fat content, but hemorrhage may obscure the lucency. IVP reveals distortion of the calyceal system by a mass. Multiple angiomyolipomas must be differentiated from polycystic disease, which may also have lucent areas. On angiography, hypervascularity with abnormal, tortuous, branching ectatic vessels is present, in contrast to polycystic kidneys, which are generally relatively avascular. Discrete inter- and intralobular arterial aneurysms have been described as a characteristic radiologic feature.[189,280] The combination of this vascular pattern with the radiolucent fat aids in the differentiation between renal cell carcinoma and angiomyolipoma.

Treatment has been complete nephrectomy. The other kidney should first be examined to determine if bilateral or multicentric angiomyolipoma (tuberous sclerosis-associated) is present, in which case conservative treatment with preservation of a maximum amount of renal parenchyma for as long as possible is desirable. An occasional extensive tumor, especially if there is extrarenal extension, may recur locally if inadequately excised.[163] Conservative management with observation, elective exploration and renal preserving operation is currently being advocated.[39a,213a]

the vessels and stream out from them or form interlacing fascicles throughout the tumor (Fig. 15-64). The smooth muscle cells may show considerable pleomorphism, hyperchromatism, and scattered mitotic figures. Occasionally, these cells have a clear cytoplasm, as seen in epithelioid leiomyomas or leiomyoblastomas.

The tumors appear to extend to the adjacent tissue, vascular extension has been documented, and in a small proportion of cases deposits have been present in regional lymph nodes.[56] The addition of multicentricity, bizarre cells, and mitoses has led to the diagnosis of malignancy, but distant metastasis have not been substantiated. The consensus is that regional lymph node involvement represents another expression of the multicentric origin of these hamartomatous lesions.[293]

Renomedullary Interstitial Tumor (Medullary Fibroma, Medullary Fibrous Nodule)

In 1972 Lerman et al.[172] established the relation between so-called medullary fibromas and the interstitial cells of the renal medulla. Small, multiple, poorly circumscribed, gray-tan nodules measuring 0.1 to 0.3 cm in diameter are commonly present in the midportion of the renal medulla in older individuals (Fig. 15-65). They had been considered hamartomas or benign fibroblastic tumors. In autopsy series the incidence has varied between 26 and 41 percent,[29] with Lerman et al.'s series of 103 unselected consecutive autopsies showing a 30 percent incidence.[172] They are present in equal numbers in men and women and are seen in those over age 50.

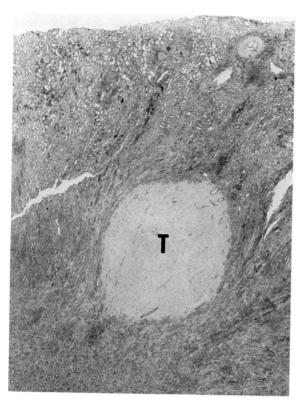

Fig. 15-65 Renomedullary interstitial tumor. The tumor (T) is in the midportion of the medulla. ×15.

Microscopically, these tumors are unencapsulated, with margins compressing the adjacent parenchyma. Trapped tubules are seen particularly at the periphery (Fig. 15-66). The tumors tend to be sparsely cellular with a loose basophilic or dense eosinophilic, hyalinized matrix and occasional ovoid to spindle cells with indistinct cytoplasmic borders. Special stains reveal the presence of neutral lipid (oil red O), phospholipid (Sudan black), and acid mucopolysaccharides (colloidal iron and alcian blue). Collagen is present in abundance, but no reticulin or elastic fibers are seen. Electron microscopy demonstrates cells similar to renomedullary interstitial cells, with elongated processes closely adherent to capillaries and electron-dense osmophilic droplets.

Interstitial cells of the medulla are known to have an antihypertensive effect and to contain prostaglandins.[185] A similar function was postulated for renomedullary interstitial tumors. Lerman et al.[172] proposed that the stimulatory effect of the hypertensive

state in patients would cause either hyperplasia or adenomatous transformation of the interstitial cells. However, a study comparing heart weight, the heart weight/body weight ratio, and blood pressure in patients with renomedullary interstitial tumors at autopsy and matched controls has failed to support the idea that renomedullary interstitial tumors arise in response to hypertension.[264]

These tumors are incidental findings at autopsy and do not require treatment.

A relation has been suggested between a rare tumor described in the renal pelvis[114] and renomedullary interstitial tumor. The former presents generally with hematuria and with a lucent filling defect of the renal pelvis on IVP. It appears to represent a large (approximately 3 cm in diameter) renomedullary interstitial tumor with a stalk that protrudes into the calyceal system and arises from a renal papilla. Seven of the eight cases reported have been in women. Histologically, these lesions are similar to renomedullary inter-

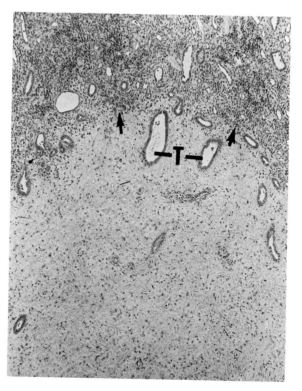

Fig. 15-66 Renomedullary interstitial tumor. Note the compressing margins (arrows) and entrapped tubules (T). ×51.

stitial tumors. Nephrectomy has been the most common treatment. In some cases the diagnosis of benign tumor by frozen section has resulted in conservative treatment.[114]

Benign Mesenchymal Tumors

Benign neoplasms are generally incidental findings at autopsy, being found in 8 to 11 percent of autopsied patients (Table 15-8).[29,230,295]

LEIOMYOMA AND LIPOMA

Leiomyomas and lipomas are the most common mesenchymal tumors. They are found frequently in patients over 40 years of age and occur more frequently in women than men. A large number of the tumors contain both smooth muscle and fat. It has been postulated that most are hamartomas, although an origin from multipotential mesenchymal cells of the renal cortex or capsule cannot be ruled out.[29] Typically, leiomyomas or lipomas appear as subcapsular lesions, well circumscribed with a gray-white, firm cut surface. Tumors found at autopsy are usually silent, with an average size of 0.5 cm in diameter. Larger tumors are rare. Microscopically, the tumor has interlacing bundles of smooth muscle tissue or fat tissue or an admixture of both. Thick-walled vessels are also seen.[29] Pure lipomas, intrarenal or capsular, have also been reported.[91,263]

HEMANGIOMA

Hemangiomas are relatively uncommon, with men and women affected equally. The presenting symptom is hematuria. They may be multiple, appearing as

Table 15-8 Benign Tumors in Two Autopsy Series

Tumor	250 Autopsies[295] (No.)	212 Autopsies[230] (No.)
Leiomyomas	13	12
Lipomas	2	7
Myolipomas	5	13
Fibromas (medullary)	67	68

small (0.3 to 0.4 cm) hemorrhagic nodules. Microscopically, they are generally of the capillary type, sometimes with dilated cavernous vessels.

LYMPHANGIOMA

Lymphangiomas are rare lesions generally appearing in children. They are large, unencapsulated multicystic nodules that replace the kidney. Microscopically, they have widely dilated thin-walled vessels lined by flattened endothelial cells. There have been no cases of metastasis or recurrence. The lesion must be differentiated from multilocular cystic disease in which the cystic spaces are lined by epithelium sometimes with a hobnail appearance.

FIBROMAS

Fibromas of the renal cortex are rare. The so-called medullary fibromas must be considered renomedullary interstitial cell tumors.

Sarcomas

Sarcomas are rare malignant mesenchymal tumors of the kidney with a variety of histologic types (Table 15-9). The incidence of sarcomas is difficult to estimate. Two large series, one from the Mayo Clinic and the other from Memorial Sloan–Kettering (MSK) Cancer Center, indicated that sarcomas constitute about 1 percent of all malignant renal tumors.[100,257]

The age range is from 16 to 75 years, with most patients being over age 40. There seems to be a slightly increased incidence in men (male/female ratio 1.25 : 1.00). The most common symptoms and signs at presentation in the MSK series were flank pain (55.5 percent) and a palpable mass (33.3 percent).[257] In the Mayo Clinic series a palpable mass was present in 20 of 26 cases, and the tumors were large, weighing from 190 g to 9.5 kg.[100] The tumor was found incidentally in four patients in the MSK series (22 percent).[257]

The clinical differential diagnosis with renal cell carcinoma may be impossible, and the x-ray findings may not be helpful. IVP generally shows a large mass in a nonfunctional or poorly functioning kidney. A diagnosis of sarcoma may be suspected on angiography if there is a relatively hypovascular tumor with prominent capsular vascular formation.[122]

Table 15-9 Sarcomas: Distribution by Type

Sarcoma	Mayo Clinic 1906–1966[100] (2,386 Malignant Kidney Tumors)	Memorial Sloan-Kettering 1950–1980[257] (1,699 Malignant Kidney Tumors)
	26	16
Leiomyosarcoma	15	8
Liposarcoma	5	—
Rhabdomyosarcoma	1	3
Fibrosarcoma	—	2
Fibrous histiocytoma	—	1
Hemangiopericytoma	5	1
Undifferentiated spindle cell sarcoma	—	1

All types of sarcoma have been described in the kidney. Some are infrequent, and others such as osteogenic sarcoma are exceedingly rare and are not seen even in series as large as those from the Mayo Clinic and Memorial Sloan–Kettering Cancer Center.

LEIOMYOSARCOMA

Leiomyosarcoma is the most common sarcoma, with more than 85 cases reported. They may appear near the cortical surface (in relation to the capsule),[212] in the hilus (renal pelvis), or in the kidney parenchyma (one-third of the cases show extensive renal parenchymal involvement).[100] The gross appearance is of a glistening tan to light gray mass, whorled and lobulated, that protrudes from the cortical surface or pushes into the calyceal system and pelvis. Areas of hemorrhage, cystic change, and calcification may be present.[29] On microscopic examination the characteristic appearance of leiomyosarcoma is present, with interlacing fascicles of plump to spindle-shaped cells with a rodlike or oval nucleus and eosinophilic or fibrillary cytoplasm. Moderate pleomorphism and mitotic figures are present. Electron microscopy demonstrates myofilaments. The overall prognosis is poor, with survival dependent on the tumor's being well encapsulated and localized to the kidney[257] and with a low mitotic count.[29] Metastases appear generally in the lungs, associated with local recurrence.

Leiomyosarcomas, as a primary tumor in the kidneys, must be differentiated from retroperitoneal leiomyosarcomas with extension and metastasis to the kidneys and from leiomyosarcomas of the renal vein.[136]

LIPOSARCOMA

Liposarcomas are generally believed to arise in nondifferentiated mesenchymal tissue.[100] There are few reliable data on their incidence. They represented 5 of 26 cases in Farrow et al.'s series and none in the MSK series. Angiomyolipomas may have pleomorphic areas, and some earlier cases of renal liposarcomas have been associated with tuberous sclerosis. Involvement of the kidney by a retroperitoneal liposarcoma also must be excluded. Liposarcomas generally show a mucoid, yellow cut surface. Microscopically, they may have any of the histologic patterns of liposarcomas with lipoblasts (fat-forming cells) at various stages of differentiation (see Ch. 29). Myxoid liposarcomas with little fat, abundant intercellular substance, and prominent plexiform vascular patterns are also seen.[59,100]

RHABDOMYOSARCOMA

Rhabdomyosarcoma has been reported in other organs with no intrinsic striated muscle, e.g., gallbladder and bile duct. There is no convincing evidence to support the arguments that rhabdomyosarcoma in the kidney represents an overgrowth of nephroblastoma, and it is generally believed that the tumor arises from undifferentiated mesenchyme.[29,257] On gross examination, it appears as a large, pale, nodular tumor with extensive infiltration and areas of necrosis. Microscopically, the tumors are pleomorphic with undifferentiated mesenchymal and strap-shaped cells with occasional cross striations (see Ch.

29). This tumor behaves poorly despite the multiple modalities of treatment that have been attempted (nephrectomy, irradiation, chemotherapy).[257]

FIBROSARCOMA

Fibrosarcoma has virtually disappeared as a diagnosis with the advent of histochemistry, electron microscopy, and the realization that leiomyosarcoma is a relatively common malignant mesenchymal tumor in the kidney. The rare fibrosarcomas that do occur develop usually from the capsule of the kidney and grow rapidly.[151] The tumors are large, pale, fibrous masses, sometimes circumscribed. On cut section they are hard and homogeneous. Histologically, they show spindle-shaped cells, often with substantial fibrosis. The prognosis is poor.[257] It should be emphasized that this diagnosis is one of exclusion, and lesions must be carefully scrutinized for other types of differentiation before being diagnosed as fibrosarcoma.

FIBROUS HISTIOCYTOMA (FIBROXANTHOSARCOMA)

Fibrous histiocytoma (fibroxanthosarcoma) occurs in the abdomen or retroperitoneum in 16 percent of all cases[286] but rarely as a primary tumor of the kidney. Only ten cases have been described.[181,245,257] The tumors are generally bulky with a mottled, red-white to yellow appearance with areas of necrosis and hemorrhage. Microscopically, the tumor is generally of the pleomorphic variety with bizarre mono- or multinucleated tumor cells and a malignant stroma of spindle cells arranged in interdigitating bands and whorls (storiform pattern). Pleomorphism, hyperchromatism, lipid droplets, and plump histiocytes are also present. The inflammatory variant may have a prominent inflammatory reaction with numerous segmented granulocytes and interspersed eosinophils, lymphocytes, and plasma cells.[157] This inflammatory variant must be distinguished from xanthogranulomatous pyelonephritis. The differential diagnosis between the two is based on the atypical, large, sometimes foamy histiocytic cells seen with malignant fibrous histiocytoma and the absence of an atypical spindle component in xanthogranulomatous pyelonephritis. Local recurrence and metastasis to the lung have been reported.

HEMANGIOPERICYTOMA

Hemangiopericytomas[29] generally arise from the renal capsule; and although they may appear encapsulated, some invade the kidney superficially. Microscopically, they have vascular channels lined by endothelial cells surrounded by plump spindle cells with pale cytoplasm and indistinct borders. On reticulin stain the cells appear in perivascular whorls or collarettes. The tumor has been associated with hypoglycemia.[9] The largest number of cases has been described by Farrow et al.,[100] only with a few cases reported by others.[199,257,285] The outcome is difficult to predict, with a certain number of patients dying of generalized metastasis.

ANGIOSARCOMA

Angiosarcomas (malignant hemangioendotheliomas) are rare tumors. Malignant cells line the inside of vascular channels or grow in packed cell groups. Mitoses are prominent. The tumors are highly malignant.[3,226]

OSTEOGENIC SARCOMA

Only eight cases of osteogenic sarcoma have been reported.[196] Radiography demonstrates the presence of calcifications in a tumor mass. The presence of bone formation must be differentiated from osseous metaplasia or dystrophic calcification within a tumor of other histologic type by thoroughly sampling the specimen and ruling out metastatic involvement. Microscopically, pleomorphic spindle cells with focal osteoid and bone formation are present. The tumor grows rapidly and is fatal. It is believed that it originates from indifferent or metaplastic mesenchyme.[10]

CHONDROSARCOMA

Chondrosarcoma is another rare sarcoma.[210,223] It has a characteristic morphologic appearance of cartilaginous matrix and chondrocytes within lacuna.

SUMMARY

It can be said that the overall prognosis of renal sarcomas is abysmal. The tumors are bulky, infiltrating adjacent structures at the time of diagnosis.

Treated with nephrectomy, they recur locally and give rise to distant metastases. The only two long-term survivors in the MSK series had well encapsulated tumors localized to the kidney (one leiomyosarcoma and one fibrosarcoma). Chemotherapy followed by surgery has been suggested if a preoperative diagnosis can be established.[257]

Rare Tumors of the Kidney

PRIMARY OAT CELL CARCINOMA

Primary oat cell carcinoma of the kidney has been described,[61] in which calcitonin has been demonstrated in 10 percent of tumor cells; sparsely endocrine-granulated cells are also seen by electron microscopy. The tumor replaced most of the kidney parenchyma, violated the capsule, destroyed the pelvis, and produced extensive metastasis to periaortic lymph nodes. No other organs were involved by the tumor.

CARCINOID TUMORS

Carcinoid tumors of the kidneys have also been reported,[258,299] as have an enteroglucagon-producing tumor[39] and a vipoma[128] producing vasoactive intestinal peptide.

INTRARENAL PHEOCHROMOCYTOMA

Intrarenal pheochromocytoma is a rare cause of hypertension. Eight of the ten cases described have been associated with ipsilateral renal artery stenosis.[35] Heterotopic adrenal tissue can be found in the kidney; and although it is generally cortical adrenal tissue, large masses also contain medullary tissue.[29]

TRANSITIONAL CELL CARCINOMA OF THE RENAL COLLECTING TUBULES

Transitional cell carcinoma of the renal collecting tubules has been demonstrated with or without carcinoma of the renal pelvis. Papillary structures, umbrella cells, keratohyaline, and parakeratosis have been shown in these cases, suggesting urothelial origin. It is not surprising, as the collecting tubules, pelvis, and ureter are derived from the ureteric bud.[11,101a,183]

REFERENCES

1. Abeshouse BS: Metastasis to the ureters and urinary bladder from renal carcinoma: report of two cases. J Int Coll Surg 25:117, 1956
2. Abrams HJ, Buchbinder MI, Sutton AP: Renal carcinoma in adolescents. J Urol 121:92, 1979
3. Allred CD, Cathey WJ, McDivitt RW: Primary renal angiosarcoma: a case report. Hum Pathol 12:665, 1981
4. Altmannsberger M, Osborn M, Schaefer H, et al: Distinction of nephroblastomas from other childhood tumors using antibodies to intermediate filaments. Virchows Arch [Cell Pathol] 45:113, 1984
5. Ambos MA, Bosniak MA, Valensi QJ, et al: Angiographic pattern of renal oncocytomas. Radiology 129:633, 1977
6. American Joint Committee for Cancer Staging and End-Results Reporting of the American College of Surgeons: Manual for Staging of Cancer 1977. American Joint Committee, Chicago, 1980
7. Armstrong B, Doll R: Environmental factors and cancer incidence and mortality in different countries, with special reference to dietary practices. Int J Cancer 15:617, 1975
8. Arner O, Blanck C, Von Schreeb T: Renal adenocarcinoma: morphology—grading of malignancy—prognosis: a study of 197 cases. Acta Chir Scand [Suppl] 346:1, 1965
9. Asa SL, Bedard YC, Buckspan MB, et al: Spontaneous hypoglycemia associated with hemangiopericytoma of the kidney. J Urol 125:864, 1981
10. Axelrod R, Naidech HJ, Myers J, Steinberg A: Primary osteosarcoma of the kidney. Cancer 41:724, 1978
10a. Azumi N, Battifora H: The distribution of vimentin and keratin in epithelial and non epithelial neoplasms: A comprehensive immunohistochemical study on formalin and alcohol fixed tumors. Am J Clin Pathol 88:286, 1987
11. Balsev E, Fischer S: Transitional cell carcinoma of the renal collecting tubules ("renal urothelioma"). Acta Pathol Microbiol Scand [A] 91:419, 1983
12. Bamier MP, Pollack HM, Chatten J Witzleben C: Multilocular renal cysts: radiologic-patologic correlation. AJR 136:239, 1981
13. Bannayan G, Lamm D: Renal cell tumors. Pathol Annu 271:308, 1980
14. Barajas L: The development and ultrastructure of the juxtaglomerular cell granule. J Ultrastruct Res 15:400, 1966
15. Barajas L: The innervation of the juxtaglomerular apparatus: an electron microscopic study of the innerva-

tion of the glomerular arterioles. Lab Invest 13:916, 1964

16. Barnes CA, Beckman EN: Renal oncocytomas and its congeneres. Am J Clin Pathol 79:312, 1983

17. Bassil B, Dosoretz DE, Prout GR Jr: Validation of the tumor, nodes, and metastasis classification of renal cell carcinoma. J Urol 134:450, 1985

18. Battifora HA: Ultrastructure of endocrine neoplasms. Am Clin Lab Sci 9:164, 1979

19. Beckwith JB: Histopathological aspects of renal tumors in children. p. 1. In Kuss R, Murphy GP, Khoury S, Karr JP (eds): Renal Tumors. Proceedings of the First International Symposium on Kidney Tumors. Alan R. Liss, New York, 1982

20. Beckwith JB: Wilms' tumor and other renal tumors of childhood: a selective review from the National Wilms' Tumor Study Pathology Center. Hum Pathol 14:481, 1983

21. Beckwith JB, Kiviat NB: Multilocular renal cysts and cystic renal tumors. AJR 136:435, 1981

22. Beckwith JB, Palmer NF: Histopathology and prognosis of Wilms' tumor: results from the First National Wilms' Tumor Study. Cancer 41:1937, 1978

23. Beckwith JB, Weeks DA: Congenital mesoblastic nephroma: when should we worry? (editorial). Arch Pathol Lab Med 110:98, 1986

24. Belasco J, D'Angio GJ: Wilms' tumor. CA 31:258, 1981

25. Bell ET: Classification of renal tumors. J Urol 39:238, 1938

26. Bender BL, Yunis EJ: The pathology of tuberous sclerosis. Pathol Annu 17:339, 1982

27. Benisch B, Peison B, Newman R, et al: Solid glycogen-rich clear cell carcinoma of breast: a light and ultrastructural study. Am J Clin Pathol 79:243, 1983

28. Bennington JL: Cancer of the kidney, etiology, epidemiology and pathology. Cancer 32:1017, 1973

29. Bennington JL, Beckwith JB: Atlas of Tumor Pathology, Second Series 2, Fascicle 12: Tumors of the Kidney, Renal Pelvis, and Ureter. p. 12. Armed Forces Institute of Pathology, Washington, DC, 1975

30. Bennington JL, Ferguson BR, Campbell PB: Epidemiologic studies of carcinoma of the kidney. II. Association of renal adenoma with smoking. Cancer 22:821, 1968

31. Bennington JL, Laubscher FA: Epidemiologic studies on carcinoma of the kidney: association of renal adenocarcinoma with smoking. Cancer 21:1069, 1968

32. Bennington JL, Mayall BH: DNA-cytometry on four micrometer sections of paraffin-embedded human renal adenocarcinomas and adenomas. Cytometry 4:31, 1983

33. Benoist MF, Lemerle J, Jean R, et al: Effect of pulmonary function of whole lung irradiation for Wilms' tumor in children. Thorax 37:175, 1982

34. Berg JW, Burbank F: Correlations between carcinogenic trace metals in water supplies and cancer mortality. Ann NY Acad Sci 199:249, 1972

35. Bezirdjian DR, Tegtmeyer CJ, Johnsey LL: Intrarenal pheochromocytoma and renal artery stenosis. Urol Radiol 3:121, 1981

36. Biava CG, West M: Fine structure of normal human juxtaglomerular cells. II. Specific and nonspecific cytoplasmic granules. Pathology 49:955, 1966

37. Block NL, Grabstald AG, Melamed MR: Congenital mesoblastic nephroma (leiomyomatous hamartoma): first adult case. J Urol 110:380, 1973

38. Bloom HJG: Hormone induced and spontaneous regression of metastatic renal cell cancer. Cancer 32:1006, 1973

39. Bloom SR: An enteroglucagon tumor. Gut 13:520, 1972

39a. Blutze ML, Malek RS, Segura J: Angiomyolipoma: clinical metamorphosis and concepts for management. J Urol 139:20, 1988

40. Bolande RP: Congenital mesoblastic nephroma of infancy. Perspect Pediatr Pathol 1:227, 1973

40a. Bolande RP, Bernstein J, Libcke J: Tubulogenesis in mesoblastic nephroma. Lab Invest 58:2P, 1988

41. Bolande RP, Bough AJ, Izant RJ Jr: Congenital mesoblastic nephroma of infancy: a report of eight cases and the relationship to Wilms' tumor. Pediatrics 40:272, 1967

42. Bonadio JF, Storer B, Norkool P, et al: Anaplastic Wilms' tumor: clinical and pathological studies. J Clin Oncol 3:513, 1985

43. Bonnin JM, Rubinstein LJ, Palmer NF, Beckwith JB: The association of embryonal tumors originating in the kidney and in the brain: a report of seven cases. Cancer 54:2137, 1984

43a. Bonsib SM, Fisher J, Plattner S, Fallon B: Sarcomatoid renal tumors: clinicopathologic correlation of three cases. Cancer 59: 527, 1987

44. Borowitz MJ, Weiss MA, Bossen EH, et al: Characterization of renal neoplasm with monoclonal antibodies to leukocyte differentiation antigens. Cancer 57:251, 1986

45. Bourneville DM: Contribution a l'etude de l'idiotic, sclerose tubereuse des circonvolutions cerebrales, idiotic et hemiplegique. Arch Neurol 1:69, 1880

46. Bove KE, Bhathena D, Wyatt RJ, et al: Diffuse metanephric adenoma after in utero aspirin intoxication: a

unique case of progressive renal failure. Arch Pathol Lab Med 103:187, 1979

47. Bove KE, Koffler H, McAdams J: Nodular renal blastema: definition and possible significance. Cancer 24:323, 1969

48. Bove KE, McAdams J: The nephroblastomatosis complex and its relationship to Wilms' tumor: a clinicopathologic treatise. Perspect Pediatr Pathol 3:185, 1976

49. Brady LW: Carcinoma of the kidney: the role for radiation. Semin Oncol 10:417, 1983

50. Brendler CB, Albertsen PC, Goldman SM, et al: Acquired cystic disease in endstage kidney: urologic implications. J Urol 132:548, 1984

51. Breslow NE, Beckwith JB: Epidemiological features of Wilms' tumor: results of the National Wilms' Tumor Study. J Natl Cancer Inst 68:429, 1982

52. Breslow NE, Churchill G, Beckwith JB, et al: Prognosis for Wilms' tumor patients with non-metastatic disease at diagnosis — results of the Second National Wilms' Tumor Study. J Clin Oncol 3:521, 1985

52a. Breslow NE, Churchill G, Nesmith B, et al: Clinicopathologic features and prognosis for Wilms' tumor patients with metastases at diagnosis. Cancer 58:2501, 1986

53. Breslow NE, Palmer NF, Hill LR, et al: Prognostic factors for patients without metastasis at diagnosis. Cancer 41:1577, 1978

54. Bretan PN, Busch MP, Hricack H, Williams RD: Chronic renal failure: a significant risk factor in the development of acquired renal cysts and renal carcinoma. Cancer 57:1871, 1986

55. Budin R, McDonnell PJ: Renal cell neoplasias: their relationship with arteriosclerosis. Arch Pathol Lab Med 108:138, 1984

55a. Bunin GR, Kramer S, Marrero O, Meadows AT: Gestational risk factors for Wilms' tumor: results of a case control study. Cancer Res 47:2972, 1987

56. Busch FM, Bark CJ, Clyde HR: Benign renal angiomyolipoma with regional lymph node involvement. J Urol 116:715, 1976

57. Byrd RL, Evans AE, D'Angio GD: Adult Wilms' tumor: effect of combined therapy on survival. J Urol 127:648, 1982

58. Camilleri JP, Hinglais N, Bruneval P, et al: Renin storage and cell differentiation in juxtaglomerular cell tumors: an immunohistochemical and ultrastructural study of three cases. Hum Pathol 15:1069, 1984

59. Cano Y, D'Atorio RA: Renal liposarcoma: case report. J Urol 115:747, 1976

60. Cantin M, Araujo-Nascimento MdeF, Benchimol S, Desormeaux Y: Metaplasia of smooth muscle cells into juxtaglomerular cells in the juxtaglomerular apparatus, arteries, and arterioles of the ischemic (endocrine) kidney. Am J Pathol 87:581, 1977

61. Capella C, Eusebi V, Rosai J: Primary oat cell carcinoma of the kidney. Am J Surg Pathol 8:855, 1984

61a. Carachi R, Lindop BM, Leckie BJ: Inactive renin: a tumor marker in nephroblastoma. J Pediatr Surg 22:278, 1987

62. Carcangiu ML, Sibley RK, Rosai J: Clear cell change in primary thyroid tumors. Am J Surg Pathol 9:705, 1985

62a. Chan HSL, Cheng M-Y, Mancer K, et al: Congenital mesoblastic nephroma: a clinicopathologic study of 17 cases representing the pathologic spectrum of the disease. J Pediatr 111:64, 1987

63. Chatten J: Epithelial differentiation in Wilms' tumor: a clinicopathologic appraisal. Perspect Pediatr Pathol 3:225, 1976

64. Cherrie RJ, Goldmann DG, Linder A, et al: Prognostic implications of vena cava extension of renal cell carcinoma. J Urol 128:910, 1982

65. Chisholm GD: Hypercalcemia. p. 293. In Kuss R, Murphy GP, Khoury S, Karr JP (eds): Renal Tumors. Proceedings of the First International Symposium on Kidney Tumors. Alan R. Liss, New York, 1982

66. Chisholm GD: Paraneoplastic syndromes: introduction. p. 277. In Kuss R, Murphy GP, Khoury S, Karr JP (eds): Renal Tumors. Proceedings of the First International Symposium on Kidney Tumors. Alan R. Liss, New York, 1982

67. Choi H, Almagro UA, McManus JT, et al: Renal oncocytoma: a clinicopathologic study. Cancer 51:1887, 1983

68. Chonko AM, Weiss SM, Stein JH, Ferris TF: Renal involvement in tuberous sclerosis. Am J Med 56:124, 1974

69. Chung TS, Reyes CV, Stefani SS: Wilms' tumor in adults. Urology 24:275, 1984

70. Civantos F, Albores-Saavedra J, Nadji M, Morales AR: Clear cell variant of thyroid carcinoma. Am J Surg Pathol 8:187, 1984

71. Clouse JW, Thomas PRM, Griffith RC, et al: The changing management of Wilms' tumor over a thirty year period 1949–1978. Cancer 56:1484, 1985

72. Cocchiara R, Tarro G, Flaminio G, et al: Purification of herpes simplex virus tumor associated antigen from human kidney carcinoma. Cancer 46:1594, 1980

73. Cohen AJ, Li FP, Berg S, et al: Hereditary renal-cell carcinoma associated with a chromosomal translocation. N Engl J Med 301:592, 1979

74. Cutchley M, Earl CJC: Tuberous sclerosis and allied conditions. Brain 55:311, 1932

75. D'Angio GJ: SIOP and the management of Wilms' tumor (editorial). J Clin Oncol 1:595, 1983

76. D'Angio GJ, Beckwith JB, Breslow NE, et al: Wilms' tumor: an update. Cancer 45:1798, 1980

77. D'Angio GJ, Evans AE: Wilms' tumor: genetic aspects and etiology. p. 43. In Kuss R, Murphy GP, Khoury S, Karr JP (eds): Renal Tumors. Proceedings of the First International Symposium on Kidney Tumors. Alan R. Liss, New York, 1982

78. D'Angio GJ, Evans AE: Wilms' tumor updated: evolution of ideas and trends. p. 123. In Kuss R, Murphy GP, Khoury S, Karr JP (eds): Renal Tumors. Proceedings of the First International Symposium on Kidney Tumors. Alan R. Liss, New York, 1982

79. D'Angio GJ, Evans A, Breslow NE, et al: The treatment of Wilms' tumor: results of the Second National Wilms' Tumor Study. Cancer 47:2302, 1981

80. D'Angio GJ, Evans AE, Breslow NE, et al: Results of the Third National Wilms' Tumor Study (NTWS-3): a preliminary report. Proc Am Assoc Cancer Res 25:183, 1984

81. Dayal H, Kinman J: Epidemiology of kidney cancer. Semin Oncol 10:366, 1983

82. Dehner LP, Liestma JE, Price EBJ: Renal cell carcinoma in children: a clinicopathologic study of 15 cases and review of literature. J Pediatr 76:358, 1970

83. Deitchman B, Sidhie GS: Ultrastructural study of sarcomatoid variant of renal cell carcinoma. Cancer 46:1152, 1980

84. DeKernion J: Lymphadenectomy for renal cell carcinoma: therapeutic implications. Urol Clin North Am 7:697, 1980

85. DeKernion JB: Treatment of advanced renal cell carcinoma—traditional methods and innovative approaches. J Urol 130:2, 1983

85a. DeKernion JB, Mukamel E: Selection of initial therapy for renal cell carcinoma. Cancer 60:539, 1987

86. DeKernion JB, Sarna G, Figlin R, et al: The treatment of renal cell carcinoma with human leukocyte alpha interferon. J Urol 130:1063, 1983

87. DeKraker J, Voute PA, Lemerle J, et al: Preoperative chemotherapy in Wilms' tumor: results of clinical trials and studies on nephroblastomas conducted by the international society of paediatric oncology (SIOP). p. 131. In Kuss R, Murphy GP, Khoury S, Karr JP (eds): Renal Tumors. Proceedings of the First International Symposium on Kidney Tumors. Alan R. Liss, New York, 1982

88. Delemarre JFM, Sandstedt B, Tournade MF: Nephroblastoma with fibroadenomatous-like structures. Histopathology 8:55, 1984

89. Dennis RL, McDougal WS, Glick AD, MacDonell RC: Juxtaglomerular cell tumor of the kidney. J Urol 134:334, 1985

90. DeSchryver-Kecskemeti K, Kraus FT, Engleman W, Lacy PE: Alveolar soft-part sarcoma: a malignant angioreninoma: histochemical, immunochemical, and electron-microscopic study of four cases. Am J Surg Pathol 6:5, 1982

91. Dineen MR, Venable DD, Misra RP: Pure intrarenal lipoma: report of a case and review of the literature. J Urol 132:104, 1984

92. Drash A, Sherman F, Hartman WH, Blizzard RM: A syndrome of pseudohermaphroditism, Wilms' tumor, hypertension and degenerative renal disease. J Pediatr 76:585, 1970

93. Dunnill MS, Millard PR, Oliver D: Acquired cystic disease of the kidneys: a hazard of long-term intermittent maintenance haemodialysis. J Clin Pathol 30:868, 1977

94. Eble JN, Hull MT: Morphological features of renal oncocytoma: a light and electron microscopic study. Hum Pathol 15:1054, 1984

95. Eble JN, Sledge G: Euploidy of renal oncocytomas: analysis of cellular DNA content using flow cytometry. Lab Invest 52:20A, 1985

96. Ehrlich RM, Bloomberg SD, Gyepes MT, et al: Wilms' tumor, misdiagnosed preoperatively: a review of 19 National Wilms' Tumor Study I cases. J Urol 122:790, 1979

97. Emmett JL, Levine SR, Woolner LB: Co-existence of renal cyst and tumor: incidence in 1,007 cases. Br J Urol 35:403, 1963

98. Engelmann U, Schaub T, Schweden F, et al: Digital subtraction angiography in staging renal cell carcinoma: comparison with computerized tomography and histopathology. J Urol 132:1093, 1984

99. Farrow GM, Harrison EG Jr, Utz DC, Jones DR: Renal angiomyolipoma: a clinicopathologic study of 32 cases. Cancer 22:564, 1968

100. Farrow GM, Harrison EG Jr, Utz DC, ReMine WH: Sarcomas and sarcomatoid and mixed malignant tumors of the kidney in adults—part I. Cancer 22:545, 1968

101. Favara BE, Johnson W, Ito J: Renal tumors in the neonatal period. Cancer 22:845, 1968

101a. Fleming S, Lewi HJE: Collecting duct carcinoma of the kidney. Histopathology 10:1131, 1986

102. Fleming S, Lindo GBM, Gibson AAM: The distribution of epithelial membrane antigen in the kidney and its tumors. Histopathology 9:729, 1985

102a. Fleming S, Matthews TJ: Renal tubular antigens in regenerative epithelium and renal carcinoma. Br J Urol 60:103, 1987

103. Flocks RH, Kadesky MC: Malignant neoplasm of the

kidney: an analysis of 353 patients followed five years or more. J Urol 79:196, 1958

104. Fowler JE: Failure of immunotherapy for metastatic renal cell carcinoma. J Urol 135:22, 1986

105. Franklin WA, Ringus JC: Basement membrane antigen in Wilms' tumor. Lab Invest 44:375, 1981

106. Frierson HF, Mills SE, Innes DJ Jr: Malignant rhabdoid tumor of the pelvis. Cancer 55:1963, 1985

107. Fu Y, Kay S: Congenital mesoblastic nephroma and its recurrence. Arch Pathol 96:66, 1973

108. Fuhrman SA, Lasky LC, Limas C: Prognostic significance of morphologic parameters in renal cell carcinoma. Am J Surg Pathol 6:655, 1982

109. Gallo GE, Penchansky L: Cystic nephroma. Cancer 39:1322, 1977

110. Ganick DJ, Gilbert EF, Beckwith JB, Kiviat N: Congenital cystic mesoblastic nephroma. Hum Pathol 12:1039, 1981

111. Garcia-Bunuel R, Brandes D: Fetal hamartoma of the kidney: case report with ultrastructural and cytochemical observations. Johns Hopkins Med J 127:213, 1970

112. Gatenby RA: Diagnostic evaluation of a renal mass. Semin Oncol 10:401, 1983

113. Ghanadian R, Williams G, Coleman AP: Steroid receptors in kidney tumors. Prog Clin Biol Res 100:245, 1982

114. Glover SD, Buck AC: Renal medullary fibroma: a case report. J Urol 127:758, 1982

115. Gonzalez-Crussi F, Baum ES: Renal sarcomas of childhood: a clinicopathologic and ultrastructural study. Cancer 51:898, 1983

116. Gonzalez-Crussi F, Goldschmidt R, Hsueh W, Trujillo YP: Infantile sarcoma with intracytoplasmic filamentous inclusions: distinctive tumor of possible histiocytic origin. Cancer 49:2365, 1982

117. Gonzalez-Crussi F, Kidd JM, Hernandez RJ: Cystic nephroma: morphologic spectrum and implications. Urology 20:88, 1982

118. Gonzalez-Crussi F, Lin J-N, Hsueh S, et al: Mesonephroid blastoma: a previously undescribed renal tumor of childhood. Am J Surg Pathol 7:707, 1983

119. Gonzalez-Crussi F, Sotelo-Avila C, Kidd JM: Malignant mesenchymal nephroma of infancy: report of a case with pulmonary metastasis. Am J Surg 4:85, 1980

119a. Goodman MT, Morgenstern H, Wynder EL: A case control study of factors affecting the development of renal cell cancer. Am J Epidemiol 124:926, 1986

120. Goulding FJ, Miser A: Xanthogranulomatous pyelonephritis associated with renal cell carcinoma. Urology 23:385, 1984

121. Gown AM, Vogel AM: Monoclonal antibodies to intermediate filament protein. III. Analysis of tumors. Am J Clin Pathol 84:413, 1985

122. Granmayeh W, Wallace S, Barret AF, et al: Sarcoma of the kidney: angiographic features. AJR 129:107, 1977

123. Granoff A: Herpesvirus and the Lucké tumor. Cancer Res 33:1431, 1973

124. Griffin JP, Hughes CV, Peeling WB: A survey of the familial incidence of adenocarcinoma of the kidney. Br J Urol 39:63, 1967

125. Haas JE, Bonadio JF, Beckwith JB: Clear cell sarcoma of the kidney with emphasis on ultrastructural studies. Cancer 54:2978, 1984

126. Haas JE, Palmer NF, Weinberg AG, Beckwith JB: Ultrastructure of malignant rhabdoid tumor of the kidney: a distinctive renal tumor of children. Hum Pathol 12:646, 1981

126a. Hadju SI, Foote FW: Angiomyolipoma of the kidney: report of 27 cases and review of the literature. J Urol 102:396, 1969

127. Haertig A, Kuss R: Clinical signs in renal neoplasia: a comparison of two series of three hundred cases. p. 337. In Kuss R, Murphy GP, Khoury S, Karr JP (eds): Renal Tumors. Proceedings of the First International Symposium on Kidney Tumors. Alan R. Liss, New York, 1982

128. Hamilton I, Reis L, Bilimoria S, Long RG: A renal vipoma. Br Med J 281:1323, 1980

129. Hamilton JM: Renal carcinogenesis. Adv Cancer Res 22:1, 1975

130. Hamperl H: Benign and malignant oncocytoma. Cancer 15:1019, 1962

131. Hanash KA: The nonmetastatic hepatic dysfunction syndrome associated with renal cell carcinoma (hypernephroma): Stauffer's syndrome. p. 301. In Kuss R, Murphy GP, Khoury S, Karr JP (eds): Renal Tumors. Proceedings of the First International Symposium on Kidney Tumors. Alan R. Liss, New York, 1982

132. Harris PT: Hormonal therapy and chemotherapy of renal cell carcinoma. Semin Oncol 10:422, 1983

133. Heideman RL, Haase GM, Foley CL, et al: Nephroblastomatosis and Wilms' tumor: clinical experience and management of seven patients. Cancer 55:1446, 1985

133a. Heideman RL, McGavran L, Waldstein G: Nephroblastomatosis and deletion of 11p: the potential etiologic relationship to subsequent Wilms' tumor. Am J Pediatr Hematol Oncol 8:231–234, 1986

134. Hellsten S, Berge TH, Linell F, Wehlin L: Clinically unrecognized renal cell carcinoma: an autopsy study. p. 273. In Kuss R, Murphy GP, Khoury S, Karr JP (eds): Renal Tumors. Proceedings of the First Interna-

tional Symposium on Kidney Tumors. Alan R. Liss, New York, 1982

135. Hellsten S, Berge TH, Wehlin L: Unrecognized renal cell carcinoma: clinical and pathological aspects. Scand J Urol Nephrol 15:273, 1981

136. Herman C, Morales P: Leiomyosarcoma of renal vein. Urology 18:395, 1981

137. Holland JM: Proceedings: cancer of the kidney—natural history and staging. Cancer 32:1030, 1973

138. Hollifield JW, Page DL, Smith C, et al: Renin-secreting clear cell carcinoma of the kidney. Arch Intern Med 135:859, 1975

139. Holthofer H, Miettinen A, Paasivuo R, et al: Cellular origin and differentiation of renal carcinomas: a fluorescence microscopic study with kidney specific antibodies, anti-intermediate filament antibodies and lectins. Lab Invest 49:317, 1983

140. Hou LT, Holman RL: Bilateral nephroblastomatosis in a premature infant. J Pathol Bacteriol 82:249, 1961

141. Howell GG, Othersen HB, Kiviat NE, et al: Therapy and outcome in 51 children with mesoblastic nephroma: a report of the National Wilms' Tumor Study. J Pediatr Surg 17:826, 1982

142. Hruschesky WJ, Murphy GP: Current status of the therapy of advanced renal cell carcinoma. J Surg Oncol 9:277, 1977

142a. Hughson MD, Buchwold D, Fox M: Renal neoplasia and acquired cystic kidney disease in patients receiving long term dialysis. Arch Pathol Lab Med 110:592, 1986

143. Hughson MD, McManus JF, Hennigar GR: Studies on 'end-stage' kidneys. II. Embryonal hyperplasia of Bowman's capsular epithelium. Am J Pathol 91:71, 1978

144. Innis MD: Nephroblastoma: possible index of cancer of childhood. Med J Aust 1:18, 1972

145. Ishikawa I, Shinoda A: Renal adenocarcinoma with or without acquired cysts in chronic hemodialysis patients. Clin Nephrol 20:321, 1983

146. Ito S: The enteric surface coat on intestinal microvilli. J Cell Biol 27:475, 1965

147. Jereb B, Tournade MF, Lemerle J, et al: Lymph node invasion and prognosis in nephroblastoma. Cancer 45:1632, 1980

148. Jones B, Breslow NE, Takashiwa J: Toxic deaths in the Second National Wilms' Tumor Study. J Clin Oncol 2:1028, 1984

149. Joshi VV: Cystic partially differentiated nephroblastoma: an entity in the spectrum of infantile renal neoplasia. Perspect Pediatr Pathol 5:217, 1979

150. Joshi VV, Kaznica J, Walters TR: Atypical mesoblastic nephroma. Arch Pathol Lab Med 110:100, 1986

151. Kansara V, Powell I: Fibrosarcoma of the kidney. Urology 16:419, 1980

152. Kantor AF, Curnen MG, Meigs JW, et al: Occupations of fathers of patients with Wilms' tumor. J Epidemiol Community Health 33:253, 1979

153. Karr JP, Pontes JE, Schneider S, et al: Clinical aspects of steroid hormone receptors in human renal cell carcinoma. J Surg Oncol 23:117, 1983

154. Karr JP, Schneider S, Rosenthal H, et al: Receptor profiles in renal cell carcinoma. p. 211. In Kuss R, Murphy GP, Khoury S, Karr JP (eds): Renal Tumors. Proceedings of First International Symposium on Kidney Tumors. Alan R. Liss, New York, 1982

155. Kaufman JJ: Reasons for nephrectomy. JAMA 204;607, 1968

156. Kay S: Renal carcinoma: a 10-year study. Am J Clin Pathol 50:428, 1968

157. Kempson RL, Kyriakas M: Fibroxanthosarcoma of the soft tissues: a type of malignant fibrous histiocytoma. Cancer 29:961, 1972

158. Kidd JM: Exclusion of certain renal neoplasms from the category of Wilms' tumor. Am J Pathol 58:16a, 1970

159. Klein MJ, Valensi QJ: Proximal tubular adenomas of the kidney with so-called oncocytic features: a clinicopathologic study of 13 cases of a rarely reported neoplasm. Cancer 38:906, 1976

159a. Klöppel G, Knöfel WT, Baisch H, Otto U: Prognosis of renal cell carcinoma related to nuclear grade, DNA content and Robson stage. Eur Urol 12:426, 1986

160. Knudson AG Jr: Cancer genes in man. Curr Probl Cancer 7:4, 1983

161. Knudson AG Jr, Strong LC: Mutation and cancer: a model for Wilms' tumor of the kidney. J Natl Cancer Inst 48:313, 1972

162. Koufos A, Hansen MF, Lampkin BC, et al: Loss of alleles at loci on human chromosome 11 during genesis of Wilms' tumor. Nature 309:170, 1984

162a. Kovacs G, Szücs S, Eichner W, et al: Renal oncocytoma: a cytogenetic and morphologic study. Cancer 59:2071, 1987

162b. Kovacs G, Szücs S, Maschek H: Two chromosomally different cell populations in a partly cellular congenital mesoblastic nephroma. Arch Pathol Lab Med 111:383, 1987

163. Kragel PJ, Toker C: Infiltrating recurrent renal angiomyolipoma with fatal outcome. J Urol 133:90, 1985

164. Kramer SA: Pediatric urologic oncology: symposium on advances in pediatric urology. Urol Clin North Am 12:31, 1985

165. Kramer SA, Meadows AT, Jarrett P: Racial variation

in incidence of Wilms' tumor: relationship to congenital anomalies. Med Pediatr Oncol 12:401, 1984

166. Kumar S, Marsden HB, Calabing MC: Childhood kidney tumors: in vitro studies and natural history. Virchows Arch [Pathol Anat] 405:95, 1984

167. Kumar S, Marsden HB, Carr T, Kodet R: Mesoblastic nephroma contains fibronectin but lacks laminin. J Clin Pathol 38:507, 1985

168. Lang EK, Sullivan J, deKernion JB: Work in progress: transcatheter embolization of renal cell carcinoma with radioactive infarct particles. Radiology 147:413, 1983

168a. Laski ME, Vugrin D: Paraneoplastic syndromes in hypernephroma. Semin Nephrol 7:123, 1987

169. Lemerle J: Complications and sequelae of the treatment of Wilms' tumor. p. 119. In Kuss R, Murphy GP, Khoury S, Karr JP (eds): Renal Tumors. Proceedings of the First International Symposium on Kidney Tumors. Alan R. Liss, New York, 1982

170. Lemerle J: The treatment of Wilms' tumor in 1982: the status of the art. p. 167. In Kuss R, Murphy GP, Khoury S, Karr JP (eds): Renal Tumors. Proceedings of the First International Symposium on Kidney Tumors. Alan R. Liss, New York, 1982

171. Lemor LB, Hamrondi AB: Malignant thymic tumor in an infant: malignant histiocytoma. Arch Pathol Lab Med 102:84, 1978

172. Lerman RJ, Pitcock JA, Stephenson P, Muirhead EE: Renomedullary interstitial cell tumor (formerly fibroma of renal medulla). Hum Pathol 3:559, 1972

173. Levin NP, Damajnow I, Depillis UJ: Mesoblastic nephroma in an adult patient. Cancer 49:573, 1982

174. Li FP, Yan JC-J, Sallan S, et al: Second neoplasms after Wilms' tumor in childhood. J Natl Cancer Inst 71:1205, 1983

175. Lieber MM, Tomera KM, Farrow GM: Renal oncocytoma. J Urol 125:481, 1981

176. Lilis R: Long term occupational lead exposure, chronic nephropathy and renal cancer: a case report. Am J Industr Med 2:293, 1981

176a. Loughlin KR, Grittes RF, Partridge D, Stelos P: The relationship of lactoferrin to the anemia of renal cell carcinoma. Cancer 59:566, 1987

177. Ljunberg B, Stenling R, Roos G: DNA content and prognosis in renal cell carcinoma: a comparison between primary tumors and metastasis. Cancer 57:2346, 1986

178. Ljunberg B, Stenling R, Roos G: DNA content in renal cell carcinoma with reference to tumor heterogeneity. Cancer 56:503, 1986

179. Lundell C, Kadir S, Engel R, Nyberg LM: Concurrent renal cell and transitional cell carcinoma in a single kidney: a case report. J Urol 127:761, 1982

180. Maatman TJ, Novick AC, Tancinco BJ, et al: Renal oncocytoma: a diagnostic and therapeutic dilemma. J Urol 132:878, 1984

181. MacEachern NH, Anderson KR, Wright WC: Fibroxanthosarcoma of the kidney: report of a case. J Urol 126:684, 1981

182. Machin GA, McCaugley WTE: A new precursor lesion of Wilms' tumor (nephroblastoma): intralobular multifocal nephroblastomatosis. Histopathology 8:35, 1984

183. Madadevia PS, Karwa GL, Koss LG: Mapping of urothelium in carcinomas of the renal pelvis and ureter. Cancer 51:890, 1983

183a. Malek RS, Omess PJ, Benson RC, Zincke H: Renal cell carcinoma in von Hippel-Lindau syndrome. Am J Med 82:236, 1987

184. Mancilla-Jimenez R, Stanley R, Blatz R: Papillary renal cell carcinoma: a clinical, radiologic and pathologic study of 34 cases. Cancer 38:2469, 1976

185. Mandal AK: The renal papilla and hypertension: an up-to-date review. Pathol Annu 16:295, 1981

186. Marsden HB, Lawler W, Kumar PM: Bone metastasizing renal tumor of childhood: morphological and clinical features, and differences from Wilms' tumor. Cancer 42:1922, 1978

187. Maurer HS, Pendergrass TW, Borges W, Honig GR: The role of genetic factors in the etiology of Wilms' tumor: two pairs of monozygous twins with congenital abnormalities (aniridia; hemihypertrophy) and discordance for Wilms' tumor. Cancer 43:205, 1979

188. McCoy FE, Franklin WA, Aronson AJ, Spargo BH: Glomerulonephritis associated with male pseudohermaphroditism and nephroblastoma. Am J Surg Pathol 7:388, 1983

189. McCullough DL, Scott R Jr, Seybold HM: Renal angiomyolipoma (hamartoma): review of the literature and report of 7 cases. J Urol 105:32, 1971

190. McCure C: Immunologic therapies of kidney cancer. Semin Oncol 10:431, 1983

191. McLaughlin JK, Mandel JS, Blot WJ, et al: A population-based case-control study of renal cell carcinoma. J Natl Cancer Inst 72:275, 1984

192. McNichols DW, Segura JW, DeWeend JH: Renal cell carcinoma: long-term survival and late recurrence. J Urol 126:17, 1981

193. McNutt MA, Bolen JW, Gown AM, et al: Co-expression of intermediate filaments in human epithelial neoplasms. Ultrastruct Pathol 9:31, 1985

194. Meadows AT, Baum E, Fossati-Bellani F, et al: Second malignant neoplasms in children: an update from the Late Effect Study Group. J Clin Oncol 3:532, 1985

195. Mesrobian H-GJ, Kelalis PP, Hrabovsky E, et al:

Wilms' tumor in horseshoe kidneys: a report from the National Wilms' Tumor Study. J Urol 133:1002, 1985

196. Micolonghi TS, Liang D, Schwartz S: Primary osteogenic sarcoma of the kidney. J Urol 131:1164, 1984

197. Middleton AW Jr: Indications for and results of nephrectomy for metastatic renal cell carcinoma. Urol Clin North Am 7:711, 1980

198. Miller RW, Fraumeni JF, Manning MD: Association of Wilms' tumor with aniridia hemihypertrophy and other congenital malformations. N Engl J Med 270:922, 1964

199. Mondal A, Choridhung S, Mukheyce PK: Primary malignant haemangio-pericytoma of kidney. J Postgrad Med 29:120, 1983

200. Moolten SE: Hamartial nature of tuberous sclerosis complex and its bearing on the tumor problem: report of a case with tumor anomaly of the kidney and adenoma sebaceum. Arch Intern Med 69:589, 1942

201. Moorthy AV, Beirne GJ: Acquired cystic disease of kidney. Lancet 1:663, 1978

202. Morgan E, Kidd JM: Undifferentiated sarcoma of the kidney: a tumor of childhood with histopathologic and clinical characteristics distinct from Wilms' tumor. Cancer 42:1916, 1978

203. Morris-Jones PM: MRC nephroblastoma trial results. Arch Dis Child 53:112, 1978

204. Mukamel E, Bruhis S, Nissenkorn I, Servadio C: Steroid receptors in renal cell carcinoma: relevance to hormonal therapy. J Urol 131:227, 1984

205. Murphy GP: An experimental Wilms' tumor. p. 15. In Kuss R, Murphy GP, Khoury S, Karr JP (eds): Renal Tumors. Proceedings of the First International Symposium on Kidney Tumors. Alan R. Liss, New York, 1982

206. Murphy GP, Mostofi KK: The significance of cytoplasmic granularity in the prognosis of renal cell carcinoma. J Urol 94:48, 1965

207. Murphy GP, Schirmer HKH: The diagnosis and treatment of hypernephroma. Geriatrics 18:354, 1963

207a. Muss HB: Interferon therapy for renal cell carcinoma. Semin Oncol 14:36, 1987

208. Nakamura Y, Nakashima H, Fukuda S, et al: Bilateral cystic nephroblastomas and multiple malformations with trisomy 8 mosaicism. Hum Pathol 16:754, 1985

209. Nakano E, Tada Y, Fujioka H, et al: Hormone receptors in renal cell carcinoma and correlation with clinical response to endocrine therapy. J Urol 132:240, 1984

210. Nativ O, Horowitz A, Lindner A, Many M: Primary chondrosarcoma of the kidney. J Urol 134:120, 1985

211. Neidhart JA: Interferon therapy for the treatment of renal cancer. Cancer 57:1696, 1986

211a. Newsom GD, Vugrin D: Etiologic factors in renal cell adenocarcinoma. Semin Nephrol 7:109, 1987

212. Ng WD, Chan KW, Chan YT: Primary leiomyosarcoma of renal capsule. J Urol 133:834, 1985

213. Novick AC, Zinck H, Neves RJ, Topley HM: Surgical enucleation for renal cell carcinoma. J Urol 135:235, 1986

213a. Oesterling JE, Fishman EK, Goodman SM, Marshall FF: The management of renal angiomyolipoma. J Urol 135:1121, 1986

214. Osborn M, Weber K: Tumor diagnosis by intermediate filament typing: a novel tool for surgical pathology. Lab Invest 48:372, 1983

215. Outzen HC, Maguire HC Jr: The etiology of renal cell carcinoma. Semin Oncol 10:378, 1983

216. Palmer NF, Sutow W: Clinical aspects of the rhabdoid tumor of the kidney: a report of the National Wilms' Tumor Study Group. Med Pediatr Oncol 11:242, 1983

217. Pathak S, Strong LC, Ferrell RE, Trindade A: Familial renal cell carcinoma with a 3;11 chromosomal translocation limited to tumor cells. Science 217:939, 1982

218. Pavone-Macaluso M, Ingargiola GB, Lamartina M: Aetiology of renal cancer. p. 255. In Kuss R, Murphy GP, Khoury S, Karr JP (eds): Renal Tumors. Proceedings of the First International Symposium on Kidney Tumors. Alan R. Liss, New York, 1982

219. Pendergrass TW: Congenital anomalies in children with Wilms' tumor: a new survey. Cancer 37:403, 1976

220. Penn I: Renal transplantation for Wilms' tumor: report of 20 cases. J Urol 122:793, 1979

221. Pettersson S, Kleist H, Jonsson O, et al: Diagnostic value of lipid content in cyst fluid. In Kuss R, Murphy GP, Khoury S, Karr JP (eds): Renal Tumors. Proceedings of the First International Symposium on Kidney Tumors. Alan R. Liss, New York, 1982

222. Piscioli F, Pusiol T, Scappine P, Luciani L: Urine cytology in the detection of renal adenocarcinoma. Cancer 51:2251, 1985

223. Pitfield J, Preston BJ, Smith PG: A calcified renal mass: chondrosarcoma of kidney. Br J Radiol 54:262, 1981

223a. Pitz S, Moll R, Störkel S, Thoener W: Expression of intermediate filament proteins in subtypes of renal cell carcinomas and in renal oncocytomas: distinction of two classes of renal cell tumors. Lab Invest 56:642, 1987

224. Pizzocaro G, Piva L, Salvioni R, et al: Adjuvant medroxyprogesterone acetate and steroid hormone receptors in category M0 renal cell carcinoma: an interim

report of a prospective randomized study. J Urol 135:18, 1986

225. Price EG Jr, Mostofi K: Symptomatic angiomyolipoma of the kidney. Cancer 18:761, 1965

226. Prince CL: Primary angioendothelioma of the kidney: report of a case and brief review. J Urol 47:787, 1942

226a. Pysher TJ, Beckwith JB: Clear cell sarcoma of the kidney (CCSK): analysis of 82 cases from the Second and Third National Wilms' Tumor studies (NWTS-2 and NWTS-3). Lab Invest 58:73A, 1988

227. Ratcliff PJ, Dunnill MS, Oliver DO: Clinical-importance of acquired cystic disease of the kidney in patients undergoing dialysis. Br Med J 287:1855, 1983

228. Reddy ER: Bilateral renal cell carcinoma—unusual occurrence in three members of one family. Br J Radiol 54:8, 1981

229. Redmond CK, Ciocco A, Lloyd JW, et al: Long-term mortality study of steelworkers. VI. Mortality from malignant neoplasms among coke over wokers. J Occup Med 14:621, 1972

230. Reese AJ, Winstanley DP: The small tumour-like lesions of the kidney. Br J Cancer 12:507, 1958

231. Reznicek SB, Narayana AS, Culp DA: Cystoadeno-carcinoma of the kidney: a profile of 13 cases. J Urol 134:256, 1985

232. Ritchie AWS, Chisholm GD: The natural history of renal carcinoma. Semin Oncol 10:390, 1983

232a. Ritchie AWS, DeKernion JB: The natural history and clinical features of renal carcinoma. Semin Nephrol 7:131, 1987

232b. Ro JY, Ayala AG, Sella A, et al: Sarcomatoid renal cell carcinoma: clinicopathologic: a study of 42 cases. Cancer 60:516, 1987

233. Robertson PW, Klidjian A, Harding IK, et al: Hypertension due to renin-secreting renal tumor. Am J Med 43:963, 1967

234. Robson CJ: The natural history of renal cell carcinoma. p. 447. In Kuss R, Murphy GP, Khoury S, Karr JP (eds): Renal Tumors. Proceedings of the First International Symposium on Kidney Tumors. Alan R. Liss, New York, 1982

235. Robson CJ, Churchill BM, Anderson W: The results of radical nephrectomy for renal cell carcinoma. J Urol 101:297, 1969

235a. Roos G, Stenling R, Ljungberg B: DNA content in renal cell carcinoma: a comparison between flow and static cytometric methods. Scand J Urol Nephrol 20:295, 1986

235b. Rosenberg SA, Lotze MT, Mull LM, et al: A progress report on the treatment of 157 patients with advanced cancer using lymphokine-activated killer cells and interleukin-2 or high dose interleukin-2 alone. New Engl J Med 316:889, 1987

235c. Rosenberg SA, Speis P, Lafreniere R: A new approach to the adoptive immunotherapy of cancer with tumor infiltrating lymphocytes. Science 233:1318, 1986

236. Roth DR, Wright J, Cawood CD Jr, Pranke DW: Nephroblastoma in adults. J Urol 132:108, 1984

237. Russo P, McClennan B, Bauer W, Fair W: Hematuria 5 months after left radical nephrectomy. J Urol 130:319, 1982

238. Rutledge J, Beckwith JB, Benjamin D, Haas JE: Absence of immunoperoxidase staining for myoglobin in the malignant rhabdoid tumor of the kidney. Pediatr Pathol 1:93, 1983

239. Samaan N: Paraneoplastic syndromes associated with renal carcinoma. p. 73. In Johnson DE, Samuels ML (eds): Cancer of the Genitourinary Tract. Raven Press, New York, 1979

239a. Sandstedt BE, Delemarre JFM, Harms D, Tournade MF: Sarcomatous Wilms' tumour with clear cells and hyalinization: a study of 38 tumours in children from SIOP nephroblastoma file. Histopathology 11:273, 1987

240. Sandstedt B, Delemarre JFM, Kuell EJ, Tournade MF: Mesoblastic nephromas: a study of 29 tumours from SIOP nephroblastoma file. Histopathology 9:741, 1985

241. Sarkar K, Ejeckam GC, McCaughy WTE, Tolnai G: Oncoytic tumors of the kidney (so-called "renal oncocytomas"). Lab Invest 40:282, 1979

241a. Sarna G, Figlin R, DeKernion JB: Interferon in renal cell carcinoma: the UCLA experience. Cancer 59:610, 1987

241b. Schärfe T, Yokoyama M, Alken P, et al: Immunoperoxidase staining of fine needle aspiration biopsies of renal cell carcinoma using tumor-specific monoclonal antibody. Eur Urol 13:331, 1987

242. Scharfenberg JC, Beckman EN: Persistent renal blastema in an adult. Hum Pathol 15:791, 1984

243. Schmidt D, Dickersin GR, Vawter GF, et al: Wilms' tumor: review of ultrastructure and histogenesis. Pathobiol Annu 12:281, 1982

244. Schmidt D, Harms D, Evers KG, et al: Bone metastasizing renal tumor (clear cell sarcoma) of childhood with epithelioid elements. Cancer 56:609, 1985

244a. Schmidt D, Wiedemann B, Keil W, et al: Flow cytometric analysis of nephroblastomas and related neoplasm. Cancer 58:2494, 1986

245. Scriven RR, Thrasher TV, Smith DC, Stewart SC: Primary renal malignant fibrous histiocytoma: a case report and literature review. J Urol 131:948, 1984

245a. Sella A, Logothetis CJ, Ro JY, et al: Sarcomatoid

renal cell carcinoma: treatable entity. Cancer 60:1313, 1987

246. Seppanen J, Williams R: Implant metastasis to the ureteral stump from hypernephroma: report of a case. Scand J Urol Nephrol 4:81, 1970

247. Sidher GS: The endodermal origin of digestive and respiratory tract APUD cells: histopathologic evidence and review of the literature. Am J Pathol 96:5, 1979

248. Silverberg BS, Lubera J: Cancer statistics, 1987. CA 37:2, 1987

249. Siminovitch JMP, Montie JE, Straffon R: Prognostic indicators in renal adenocarcinoma. J Urol 130:20, 1983

250. Skinner DG, Colvin RB, Vermillion CD, et al: Diagnosis and management of renal cell carcinoma: a clinical and pathologic study of 309 cases. Cancer 28:1165, 1971

251. Sogani P, Herr H, Bain M, Whitmore W Jr: Renal cell carcinoma extending into inferior vena cava. J Urol 130:660, 1983

252. Sosa RE, Muecke EC, Vaughan ED Jr, McCarron JP Jr: Renal cell carcinoma extending into the inferior vena cava: the prognosis significance of the level of vena caval involvement. J Urol 132:1097, 1984

253. Spatz M: Toxic and carcinogenic alkylating agents from cycads. Ann NY Acad Sci 163:848, 1969

254. Spear GS, Hyde TP, Gripps RA, Slusser R: Pseudohermaphroditism, glomerulonephritis with nephrotic syndrome and Wilms' tumor in infancy. J Pediatr 79:677, 1971

255. Sphar J, Demers LM, Schochat SJ: Renin producing Wilms' tumor. J Pediatr Surg 16:32, 1981

256. Squires J, Ulbright TM, DeSchryver-Kecskemeti K, Engleman W: Juxtaglomerular cell tumor of the kidney. Cancer 53:516, 1984

257. Srinivas V, Sogani PC, Hajdu SS, Whitmore WF Jr: Sarcomas of the kidney. J Urol 132:13, 1984

258. Stahl RE, Sidher GS: Primary carcinoid of the kidney: light and electron microscopic study. Cancer 44:1345, 1979

259. Staszewski J: Cancer of the kidney: international mortality patterns and trends. WHO Statist Q 33:42, 1980

260. Stauffer MH: Nephrogenic hepatosplenomegaly. Gastroenterology 40:694, 1969

261. Stay EJ, Vawter G: The relationship between nephroblastoma and neurofibromatosis (Von Recklinghausen's disease). Cancer 39:2250, 1977

262. Steg A: Does percutaneous puncture still have a role to play in the diagnosis of renal tumors? p. 417. In Kuss R, Murphy GP, Khoury S, Karr JP (eds): Renal Tumors. Proceedings of the First International Symposium on Kidney Tumors. Alan R. Liss, New York, 1982

263. Stone NN, Cherry J: Renal capsular lipoma. J Urol 134:118, 1985

264. Stuart R, Salyer WR, Salyer DC, Heptinstall RH: Renomedullary interstitial cell lesions and hypertension. Hum Pathol 7:327, 1976

265. Sufrin G, Mirand EA, Moore RH, et al: Hormones in renal cancer. J Urol 117:433, 1977

266. Sukawchana J, Folentino W, Kieseweitter WB: Wilms' tumor and hypertension. J Pediatr Surg 7:573, 1972

267. Syrjanen J, Hjelt L: Grading of human renal adenocarcinoma. Scand J Urol 12:49, 1978

268. Sytkowski A, Bicknell K, Smith G, Garcia J: Secretion of erythropoietin-like activity by clones of human renal carcinoma cell line GKA. Cancer Res 44:51, 1984

269. Talerman A, Knjestedt WF: Testicular tumor as the first manifestation of renal carcinoma. J Urol 111:584, 1974

270. Tang TT, Harb JM, Oechler HW, Camitta BM: Multilocular renal cyst: electronmicroscopic evidence of pathogenesis. Am J Pediatr Hematol Oncol 6:27, 1985

271. Tannenbaum M: Surgical and histopathology of renal tumors. Semin Oncol 10:385, 1983

272. Thomas TL, Decoufle P, Moure-Eraso R: Mortality among workers employed in petroleum refining and petrochemical plants. J Occup Med 22:97, 1980

273. Tolia BM, Whitmore WF Jr: Solitary metastases from renal cell carcinoma. J Urol 114:836, 1975

274. Tomera KM, Farrow GM, Leiber MM: Sarcomatoid renal carcinoma. J Urol 130:657, 1983

275. Tomera KM, Farrow GM, Lieber MM: Well differentiated (grade 1) clear cell renal carcinoma. J Urol 129:933, 1983

275a. Tomita T, Poisner A, Inagami T: Immunohistochemical localization of renin in renal tumors. Am J Pathol 126:73, 1987

276. Tosi P, Luzi P, Baak JPA, et al: Nuclear morphometry as an important prognostic factor in stage I renal cell carcinoma. Cancer 58:2512, 1986

277. Ulrich W, Horvart R, Krisch K: Lectin histochemistry of kidney tumors and its pathomorphologic relevance. Histopathology 9:1037, 1985

278. Utz DC, Warren MM, Gregg JA, et al: Reversible hepatic dysfunction associated with hypernephroma. Mayo Clin Proc 45:161, 1970

279. Variend S, Spicer RD, Mackinnon AE: Teratoid Wilms' tumor. Cancer 53:1936, 1984

280. Viamonti M Jr, Ravel R, Politano V, Bridges B: Angiographic findings in a patient with tuberous sclerosis. AJR 98:723, 1966

281. Vogel AM, Gown AM, Caughlan J, et al: Rhabdoid tumors of the kidney contain mesenchymal specific and epithelial specific intermediate filament proteins. Lab Invest 50:232, 1984

281a. Vugrin D: Biological aspects of renal cell carcinoma. Semin Nephrol 7:117, 1987

282. Wahlstrom T, Suni J, Nieminen P, et al: Renal cell adenocarcinoma and retrovirus p 30-related antigen excreted to urine. Lab Invest 53:464, 1985

283. Waldherr R, Schwechheimer R: Co-expression of cytokeratin and vimetin intermediate-sized filaments in renal cell adenocarcinomas. Virchows Arch [Pathol Anat] 108:15, 1985

284. Wallace AC, Narrn RC: Renal tubular antigens in kidney tumors. Cancer 29:977, 1972

284a. Weeks DA, Beckwith JB, Luckey DW: Relapse associated variables in Stage I favorable histology Wilms' tumor: report of the National Wilms' Tumor Study. Cancer 60:1204, 1987

284b. Weeks DA, Beckwith JB, Mierau GA: Rhabdoid tumor of kidney, the National Wilms' Tumor Study experience. Lab Invest 58:101A, 1988

285. Weiss JP, Pollack HM, McCormick JF et al: Renal hemangiopericytoma: surgical, radiological and pathological implications. J Urol 132:337, 1984

286. Weiss SW, Enzinger FM: Malignant fibrous histiocytoma: an analysis of 200 cases. Cancer 41:2250, 1978

287. Whisenand JM, Kostas D, Sommers SC: Some host factors in the development of renal cell carcinoma. West J Surg 70:284, 1962

288. Wick MR, Perrone TL, Burke BA: Sarcomatoid transitional cell carcinoma: An ultrastructural and immunocytochemical study. Arch Pathol Lab Med 109:55, 1985

289. Wigger HJ: Fetal hamartoma of kidney: a benign, symptomatic, congenital tumor, not a form of Wilms' tumor. Am J Clin Pathol 51:323, 1969

290. Wigger HJ: Fetal rhabdomyomatous nephroblastoma—a variant of Wilms' tumor. Hum Pathol 7:613, 1976

291. Wilkins JR, Sinks TH Jr: Occupational exposure among fathers of children with Wilms' tumor. J Occup Med 26:427, 1984

292. Williams DI, Martin J: Renal tumors. p. 381. In Williams DI, Johnston JH (eds): Paediatric Urology. 2nd Ed. Butterworth, London, 1982

293. Wong AL, McGeorge A, Clark AH: Renal angiomyolipoma: a review of the literature and report of 4 cases. Br J Urol 53:406, 1981

294. Wynder EL, Mabuchi K, Whitmore WF: Epidemiology of adenocarcinoma of the kidney. J Natl Cancer Inst 53:1619, 1974

295. Xipell JM: The incidence of benign renal nodules (a clinicopathologic study). J Urol 106:503, 1971

295a. Yeger H, Baumal R, Harason P, Phillips MJ: Lectin histochemistry of Wilms' tumor: comparison with normal adult and fetal kidney. Am J Clin Pathol 88:278, 1987

296. Young JL Jr, Miller RW: Incidence of malignant tumors in United States. J Pediatr 86:254, 1978

296a. Yu MC, Mack TM, Hanisch R, et al: Cigarette smoking, obesity, diuretic use and coffee consumption as risk factors for renal cell carcinoma. J Natl Cancer Inst 77:351, 1986

297. Yu GSM, Rendler S, Herskowitz A, Molnar JJ: Renal oncocytoma: report of five cases and review of literature. Cancer 45:1010, 1980

298. Yunis JJ, Ramsay NKC: Familial occurrence of aniridia—Wilms' tumor syndrome with deletion 11p 13-14.1. J Pediatr 96:1027, 1980

299. Zak FG, Jindrak K, Capozzi F: Carcinoidal tumor of the kidney. Ultrastruct Pathol 4:51, 1983

299a. Zbar B, Branch H, Talmadge C, Linehan M: Loss of alleles of loci on the short arm of chromosome 3 in renal cell carcinoma. Nature 327:721, 1987

16

Urothelial Neoplasms: Etiologic Considerations

James W. Eagan, Jr.

Numerous environmental agents have been implicated in the development of urothelial neoplasms, most at least by association if not in a direct cause-and-effect relation. The relations appear relatively firm in at least a few areas, e.g., aromatic amines in the development of bladder carcinoma and phenacetin abuse in the development of upper tract carcinomas. The role of cigarette smoking, perhaps the most commonly cited factor, is still not completely defined. The influence of other agents, e.g., coffee and artificial sweeteners, continues to be debated. Still other factors, e.g., ionizing radiation, that may play significant roles in the development of neoplasia in other organ systems appear to have little overall effect in the development of urothelial tumors in a numerical sense. Although the "risk ratio" might be higher for radiation exposure than for cigarette smoking, for example, the contribution of the latter to urothelial carcinogenesis would be much more significant simply because the "denominator" is so much larger; that is, smokers outnumber those exposed to radiation by many orders of magnitude. This element must be kept in mind when assessing all such risk factors.

Suspected agents are briefly outlined. Other factors and clinical situations of possible etiologic importance, e.g., lithiasis and paraplegia, are also discussed.

INDUSTRIAL CARCINOGENS

The observations of Rehn[113] in 1895 concerning the presence of bladder complications in workers involved in the production of fuchsin in an analine dye factory are cited among the earliest perceptions of chemicals as possible carcinogens. The author noted the occurrence of bladder carcinomas in 3 of 45 workers studied, all with long-term exposure, varying from 15 to 20 years. He also observed that the tumors occurred in the trigonal area and near the ureteral orifices, which he thought was a reflection of the concentration of urine, and thus the chemical irritant, in this area. Two lesions were described as "fibroma papillare" and the third a sarcoma. A camera lucida drawing of a representative area of the former seems to correspond to our present-day impression of a grade III papillary transitional cell carcinoma. The author also noted five cases of fuchsin-related bladder toxicity resulting in hematuria, urgency, dysuria, and darkly colored urine, with subsequent oliguria. Analine was found in the urine of the affected workers.

Similar observations in American dye workers were made by Heuper[62] in 1934, with subsequent laboratory confirmation of at least one of the active agents as β-naphthylamine (2-aminonaphthalene, or 2-

naphthylamine). The same author and co-workers[63] administered this agent to dogs both subcutaneously and orally over a period of 20 to 26 months. What were termed "preneoplastic" and neoplastic formations (papillomas and carcinomas) were found in 13 of the 16 animals treated. The pathologic changes were described in detail by the authors and ran the gamut of urothelial neoplasia seen in humans. Also described were associated hyperplastic changes and areas of "pretumorous" epithelium, essentially carcinoma in situ, surrounding areas of infiltrative tumor.

Since these observations were made, various chemical carcinogens have been identified in association with bladder carcinoma. Most belong to the family of aromatic amines (arylamines),[78] including β-naphthylamine, the compound studied by Hueper. Examples of other members of this family implicated in urothelial carcinogenesis in humans include benzidine (4,4'-diaminobiphenyl),[13,61] xenylamine (4-aminodiphenyl),[87] and α-naphthylamine.[13] Initial efforts were concentrated on workers exposed to such chemicals, which were predominantly used as dyestuff intermediates. However, as pointed out by Morrison,[95] far less than 1 percent of men have such exposure, and they account for a small fraction of the total bladder cancer experience. Nonetheless, the strength of the association made the dye industry a prime target for early efforts at preventive medicine, and fortunately so for those directly involved in such industries. Huben et al.,[61] for example, reported results from an ongoing study of 360 workers previously involved in the manufacture of benzidine, with initial exposures from 1916 to 1946. As of 1985, 111 of the 360 had died, with an astounding 40 of the 111 dead of bladder cancer.

Despite the initially grudging removal of some of the more notorious offensive agents from the work place, however, Lower[78] noted the still widespread presence of arylamines as reagents used in the preparation of textile dyes, hair dyes, and paint pigments, and also as antioxidants used in the preparation of rubber for manufacture of tires and cables. Of perhaps even more concern in our present "plastic society" is their use as curing agents to prepare epoxy resins and polyurethanes. The potential effects of the persisting exposure are reflected in modern-day epidemiologic studies, such as that reported by Cole and colleagues.[19] These investigators surveyed industrial concerns in eastern Massachusetts, including the Boston metropolitan area, examining the incidence of carcinoma of the lower urinary tract among workers in various occupations. Excess risk of tumor development was found in five of the eight occupation categories examined, including statistically significant increases in the rubber industry and in leather workers as well as similar trends among workers in the dyestuff, paint, and other organic chemical industries. Patients with a history of exposure were found to be younger than tumor patients without such a history. Overall, for males, it was thought that approximately 18 percent of the bladder carcinomas encountered in the area of study could be attributed to occupational exposure. Upon review of the literature, however, the authors stated: "Yet, even among men in industrialized societies, probably not more than one-fourth of the disease can be attributed to occupational exposures."

One senses that such studies of the more blatant examples of urothelial carcinogenesis in the work place are little more than views of the tip of an iceberg, the remainder of which may be difficult, if not impossible, to see. Indeed, the ill effects of such industrial exposure are still being discovered.[21] As we are finding with asbestos, low level exposure to various known carcinogens, not to mention as yet undetected elements, may be an almost ubiquitous phenomenon in today's society. Yet in studies ranging from that reported by Rehn[113] in 1895 to those of recent times, the fact remains that, although risks may be markedly increased, even in the setting of prolonged exposure to the most potent of known human urothelial carcinogens most workers do not develop urothelial carcinoma. Unfortunately, this "negative" population and the reasons for the seeming resistance are most often ignored in studies of industrial carcinogenesis.

CIGARETTE SMOKING

Cigarette smoking has been implicated in the development of malignant neoplasms at various body sites, most notably the lung, and appears to play an important role in the development of bladder carcinoma. With the complex mixture of potentially noxious agents found in cigarette smoke, it has been difficult to assign guilt to a particular chemical, but a number of candidates are obvious. It is known that smoke contains arylamines[58] as well as other carcinogens such as nitrosamines, which have been implicated in the development of urothelial tumors as well as other cancers in animal studies[79] (see "N-Nitroso Compounds" below).

The possibility of a relationship between cigarette smoking and bladder cancer was raised by Holsti and Ermala[59] who noted the occurrence of bladder neoplasms in mice in association with intraoral application of tobacco tar. Following this report, Lilienfeld and co-workers[76] examined the history of tobacco usage among various groups of patients at the Roswell Park Memorial Institute. Patients with bladder cancer were compared to patients with other cancers as well as noncancerous conditions, and the authors found a significantly larger proportion of cigarette smokers among men with bladder carcinoma than in patients in the other groups. The association appeared to be limited to those who had smoked for 30 years or more and was noted to be of a lower degree than that found in smokers with lung carcinoma.

Since the appearance of these original observations, numerous reports have contributed evidence to substantiate a relation between cigarette smoking and bladder cancer. In a review of epidemiologic studies of bladder cancer by Ross et al.,[115] the relative risk of developing bladder carcinoma for male cigarette smokers ranged from 0.8 to a high of 7.3, with most values in the neighborhood of 2.0. Most but not all studies also noted an increasing risk with increasing amounts of tobacco usage. Whatever the risk ratios, the importance of the "denominator" is again emphasized because of the still widespread prevalence of the smoking habit; from a public health standpoint, even well-known occupational risks appear substantially less important than cigarette smoking.[96] When all of the various major risk factors are compared, cigarette smoking is cited as accounting for 39 to 61 percent of bladder cancers in men and 26 to 31 percent in women.[56]

Of perhaps even greater concern is the possibility that cigarette smoking may potentiate the effects of other hazards, notably industrial carcinogens.[48,49] Glashan and Cartwright,[48] who studied the occurrence of bladder carcinoma in the West Yorkshire area in England, found an increased risk of bladder carcinoma in association with cigarette smoking for both men and women in general, with risk ratios of 1.8 and 1.6, respectively. Chemical industry workers overall had a relative risk of 2.9, with a figure of 3.5 noted for that subset of workers involved in dye man-ufacturing. When subclassified into smokers and nonsmokers, however, dye workers who smoked had a relative risk of 4.6, whereas nonsmokers in the same occupation had a relative risk of only 1.9 of developing bladder carcinoma. It should be noted, however, that in some more recent studies of industrial carcinogenesis,[8,97] including further examination of the dye industry in the West Yorkshire area,[8] the potentiating role of cigarette smoking has been much less clear.

It should also be noted that even in studies commonly cited in support of the general association between urothelial carcinoma and cigarette smoking, such as that of Cole et al.,[20] the linkage is not clear-cut. These authors indicated that the association, if causal, appeared to be "rather indirect," and also noted the considerably lower magnitude of risk increase among smokers for developing bladder cancer versus lung cancer. In this regard, Weinberg and associates,[121] in a study of bladder and lung carcinoma in Los Angeles County, found that the epidemiologic patterns of bladder carcinoma differed markedly from those of lung carcinoma, and only the patterns of the latter tumor closely paralleled the known epidemiology of cigarette smoking. The authors also pointed out that nationally, comparing survey data from 1947–48 to 1969–71, there was only a modest rise in the incidence rate for bladder cancer in white men, and the incidence rates for white women actually decreased during this period, by approximately 20 percent. In contrast, however, during the same time period incidence rates for lung cancer rose markedly, with increases of 131 and 122 percent for white men and white women, respectively. Such observations suggested to the authors that factors other than cigarette smoking and occupational exposure may be of significant etiologic importance in the development of bladder carcinoma. Coffee consumption in particular was indicated to be a suspected element.

COFFEE DRINKING

Coffee drinking has been cited as another of the "life style" factors potentially influencing the development of urothelial carcinoma. As noted above, the study of Weinberg et al.[121] actually demonstrated a much better "fit" of epidemiologic data when matching the pattern of coffee drinking in the Los Angeles area to the occurrence of bladder carcinoma compared to the pattern of cigarette smoking. As the study was primarily one of descriptive rather than analytic epidemiology, however, risk ratios for the two factors were not given.

Cole[18] originally reported an apparent independent association of coffee drinking and urothelial carcinoma in a population-based study in eastern Massachusetts. When controlled for age, cigarette smoking, and (for men) occupation, the relative risk of developing bladder carcinoma in coffee drinkers was 1.24 for men and 2.58 for women. The author found, however, that there was an inconsistent dose–response relation and that the association in men was low, with "the conclusion reached only that the relationship between coffee drinking and bladder cancer warrants investigation."

Fraumeni et al.,[41] using the approach of Cole, reexamined data from a case–control study in the New Orleans area. Statistics were analyzed for the occurrence of bladder carcinoma relative to coffee drinking in four race/sex groups, with figures again adjusted for age and cigarette smoking. White male coffee drinkers showed a relative risk of 1.78, black males 2.10, and black females 5.65. White female coffee drinkers, however, showed a negative correlation, with a relative risk of 0.51. Again, no dose–response relation was noted. This finding and the inconsistencies when examined by race and sex were cited as indicators of either an indirect or perhaps a noncausal relation. Similar conclusions have been reached in other studies,[90,117] and still others have not been able to confirm any correlation at all between coffee consumption and the development of urothelial carcinoma.[49,67,93,118] The question of a relation therefore is unsettled at present.

ARTIFICIAL SWEETENERS

Evidence that saccharin, one of the most commonly used artificial sweeteners, could produce bladder tumors in mice was presented by Allen and coworkers[2] in 1957. These authors studied the effects of a large number of known carcinogens and other compounds, including saccharin, by direct pellet implantation into the bladders of the experimental animals. Although saccharin led to an increased number of tumors by the implantation technique, parenteral administration of the compound did not result in tumor induction. As the pellet implantation technique was not thought suitable for evaluating the hazards of orally ingested compounds, oral administration was employed in rats by Price et al.[108] They used a saccharin/cyclamate mixture, with or without supplemental cyclohexylamine (a metabolite of cyclamate) added toward the latter part of the experiment. Among 240 rats receiving the saccharin/cyclamate mixture at various dose levels, bladder neoplasms were found in 8 of the surviving animals in the highest dosage group, 3 of which had received supplemental cyclohexylamine and 5 of which had not. It was of interest that in all but one instance the tumors developed in rats that could convert cyclamate to cyclohexylamine. The induction of bladder tumors in rats by cyclamate alone, without added saccharin, was also noted by Friedman et al.[43]

Because of the widespread and increasing usage of such compounds, these reports resulted in obvious concern regarding the compounds' possible role in human urothelial carcinogenesis. From an epidemiologic viewpoint, however, their influence in the development of human tumors remained questionable. For example, in diabetics, who have a considerably higher-than-usual use of artificial sweeteners,[60] Kessler[70] found a *decreased* incidence of bladder tumors in a review of general cancer mortality figures in the population seen at the Joslin Clinic. Howe et al.,[60] in a case–control study in three provinces in Canada, showed a positive association between the use of artificial sweeteners and the risk of developing bladder carcinoma among men in the population at large, with a risk ratio of 1.6 and a significant dose–response relation noted. Female users, however, showed a risk ratio of only 0.6. Diabetic patients were analyzed separately in this study, and as in Kessler's study,[70] there appeared to be a slightly decreased risk overall for the development of bladder carcinoma. On further analysis, however, the authors found that a number of the diabetics had no history of artificial sweetener usage, and when this fact was taken into account, diabetic users were found to have a slightly increased risk of bladder carcinoma, comparable to that of male nondiabetic users. In contrast to these findings, however, numerous other epidemiologic studies have shown little or no risk attributable to the usage of these sugar substitutes.[67,93,98,121]

Although they do not appear to play a significant role as primary agents in tumorigenesis, the potential hazard of artificial sweeteners as synergistic agents, acting in concert with more potent urothelial carcinogens, has also been questioned. Such an additive effect was noted by Hicks and Chowaniec[53] in an experimental rat model using the potent bladder carcinogen N-methyl-N-nitrosourea (MNU) with diets containing saccharin and cyclamate. The authors pointed out the epidemiologic problems encountered when a "weak carcinogen" reaches a wide cross section of the population and listed an astounding array of products that contained sodium cyclamate in England prior to its withdrawal, ranging from the expected soft drinks and ice cream to the rather unexpected pickles, toothpaste, lipstick, etc. Prior to its withdrawal from the "generally regarded as safe" list in the United States in 1969, the authors noted that: "It would appear that cyclamate must have been consumed unwittingly by almost the entire population (not only those on a low-calorie diet for obesity or other health problems). The same is probably still true for saccharin."

Despite the concerns, it appears at the present time that the wheel on artificial sweeteners is coming full circle. In an update on food additives and contaminants, Newberne and Conner[102] reviewed the opinions on saccharin and cyclamates, as well as the increasingly popular artificial sweetener aspartame. With regard to human carcinogenesis, these substances appear to have received a relatively "clean bill of health," at least for the moment.

DRUGS

Phenacetin

In 1965 Hultengren and colleagues[64] reported six cases of transitional cell carcinoma of the renal pelvis in a group of over 100 patients with renal papillary necrosis. Five of the six patients had a history of excessive use of phenacetin-containing analgesics. Approximately a decade later, Rathert et al.[112] reported an additional two cases and in a literature review were able to find 119 published cases of renal pelvic carcinoma associated with phenacetin abuse. All patients had ingested drugs containing phenacetin for prolonged periods of time, ranging from 5 to 40 years, with at least 2-year periods where excessive ("1 g daily") usage was noted. Three-fourths of the cases

reported had associated renal papillary necrosis, which, although commonly present in such cases, may in fact itself be an independent risk factor for carcinoma of the upper tract.[84] Phenacetin-associated cases of renal pelvic carcinoma have shown a much higher incidence among women than expected, with male/female ratios generally on the order of 1:1, in contrast to the male preponderance in cases not associated with analgesic abuse.[112]

Although less prominent in the literature, the development of both bladder[65,107,112] and ureteral[65,105,112] tumors has also been observed in the setting of analgesic abuse, often associated with a history of recurrent urinary tract infections and, to a lesser degree, renal papillary necrosis.[65] As with renal pelvic tumors, these tumors tend to occur at a somewhat younger age and show a higher than expected occurrence in women compared to those in patients without a history of analgesic abuse.[65,107] It has been noted that such bladder and ureteral tumors tend to be lower grade, by and large, than the more frequently high grade renal pelvic tumors seen in patients with a history of phenacetin abuse, possibly indicative of lower carcinogenic activity of the compound in the bladder and ureters.[65]

Phenacetin structurally belongs to the group of aromatic amides, and the development of active carcinogens from the compound[101] presumably proceeds along pathways similar to those suggested for the general group of aromatic amines and amides by Miller and Miller.[91] Although the occurrence of carcinogenesis in the setting of phenacetin abuse may thus possibly be explained biochemically, it is disturbing to note that the risk of renal pelvic carcinoma may also be increased in patients using non-phenacetin-containing analgesics. McCredie et al.[83] examined the histories of analgesic consumption of 67 patients with carcinoma of the renal pelvis, and it was found that regular consumption of phenacetin *and* non-phenacetin-containing analgesics resulted in an increased risk of renal pelvic carcinoma in both men and women. The authors noted the difficulty of sorting out the exact role of phenacetin, however. The study was conducted in Australia, where, as in many countries in which phenacetin has enjoyed popularity as an analgesic (e.g., Darvon compound in the United States[107]), the drug is generally available only in compound form, most commonly mixed with aspirin and caffeine. Similar difficulties were encountered when assigning specific risk ratios to nonphenacetin analgesics such as aspirin, paracetamol, and salicylamide, again because of routine usage in multidrug compounds. In the final analysis, comparing patients exposed primarily to phenacetin-containing analgesics to those taking nonphenacetin compounds, *each* type of preparation showed an increased risk for development of renal pelvic carcinoma. Moderate total consumption (0.1 to 4.9 kg) of either preparation doubled the risk ratio, and heavy consumption (5 kg or more) conferred a risk of 6 to 16 times that seen in nonconsumers. Thus as with the artificial sweeteners, what intially appeared to be a straightforward situation with an equally straightforward solution, i.e., withdrawal of the agent from the market, may not be as simple as it seems. The last word on analgesics and urothelial carcinoma does not appear to have been written.

Alkylating Agents

The family of cytotoxic drugs called alkylating agents has enjoyed widespread use for the treatment of systemic malignancies over the past 20 to 30 years and, more recently, for the induction of immunosuppression to treat nonneoplastic disorders. Two agents in particular, cyclophosphamide (Cytoxan) and busulfan (Myleran), are of particular importance with regard to the urinary tract.

Cyclophosphamide is the cyclic phosphamide of nitrogen mustard, inactive in its native form, converted to an active cytotoxic agent primarily in the liver,[37] and eventually excreted via the urinary tract. It may be administered either intravenously or orally. A primary complication and limiting factor in use of the drug is the development of hemorrhagic cystitis, reported to occur in 4 to 36 percent of patients treated,[6] with a dose–response relation generally noted with both modes of administration. Symptoms may appear long after the drug has been discontinued; and according to Bennett,[6] it is difficult to predict who will suffer from the disorder and when symptoms will occur. More severe complications, e.g., bladder fibrosis[66] and mural necrosis with sloughing,[82] have been noted.

Busulfan is an alkylating agent with antineoplastic and immunosuppressive properties similar to those of cyclophosphamide. It also has multiple side effects that sometimes curtail the use of the drug, perhaps the

most widely publicized being the "busulfan lung."[77] In contrast to cyclophosphamide, however, urinary complications are generally limited to epithelial alterations, with only a single case of hemorrhagic cystitis having been reported in association with its use.[89]

Of particular interest to the urologist and pathologist is the ability of both drugs to induce severe epithelial abnormalities in the urinary tract[38,73,100] and, particularly in the case of busulfan, in many other anatomic sites as well.[73,100] Following treatment with these drugs, urothelial cytologic abnormalities may develop that are so marked that distinction from carcinoma may be impossible on morphologic grounds alone.[38] The practicing cytologist is well advised to proceed with caution in the diagnosis of urothelial malignancy in this situation. In fact, at least for cyclophosphamide, the morphologic similarities to carcinoma have proved to be more than just "mimetic" at times, and urinary tract malignancies, primarily epithelial[9,45] but occasionally stromal,[116] have been reported in association with use of the drug.

Fuchs et al.[45] culled from the literature 15 cases of urothelial carcinoma associated with a history of cyclophosphamide treatment and noted that most of the tumors were high grade transitional cell or squamous carcinomas resulting in the death of the patient. The authors added an additional six patients of their own, two with renal pelvic and four with bladder carcinoma. These six patients had been treated with cyclophosphamide over the course of 4 to 12 years for various lymphomas and leukemia. All developed intermediate or high grade transitional cell malignancies that resulted in death for two of the six.

Of perhaps even more concern is the increasing use of cyclophosphamide for immunosuppression in patients with nonneoplastic disorders, many of whom will enjoy a considerably longer life-span in which to develop carcinoma of the bladder and the upper tract, both situations having now been reported.[46,86]

Most patients who have developed urinary tract malignancies following treatment with cyclophosphamide have received doses of more than 150 g total,[86] although some cases have been noted after considerably smaller amounts.[9] The average time lapse from treatment to discovery of urothelial malignancy has been approximately 7 years.[86] It has been suggested that patients so treated be followed closely for the development of urothelial carcinoma by the use of scheduled cystoscopy, excretory urography, and urinary cytology.[45] As noted, cytologic studies may be difficult to interpret, and particular emphasis should be placed on the use of directed biopsies to obtain histologic correlation as well.

N-NITROSO COMPOUNDS

N-Nitroso compounds, including nitrosamines and nitrosamides, are carcinogenic in experimental animals and may also demonstrate varying toxic, mutagenic, and teratogenic effects.[79] In fact, members of this class of chemicals, e.g., BBN (*N*-butyl-*N*-butanol (4)-nitrosamine)[27] and MNU[54] have served as reliable inducers of bladder cancer in various animal models.[79]

As noted by Hicks et al.,[55] nitrate is always present in urine, derived from dietary sources, as are small amounts of secondary amines formed by intestinal bacterial action on ingested material with reabsorption into the bloodstream and subsequent excretion into the urine. With the addition of certain strains of nitrate-reducing bacteria, the setting is ripe for the local production of nitrosamines.[55] In fact, such compounds have been detected in the urine of patients with both *Proteus mirabilis* and *Escherichia coli* infections,[111] and thus the question of a possible role for these compounds in human urothelial neoplasia has been raised.

Radomski and colleagues[111] examined this question in patients with urinary tract infections involving nitrate-reducing bacteria. They also examined the possibility that certain commonly used drugs, e.g., tetracycline, might actually serve as chemical substrates that react with nitrates present in the infected urine to even further increase nitrosamine production. Contrary to what was expected, the nitrosamine levels fell promptly after the administration of tetracycline, with the antibacterial activity of the drug apparently offsetting its function as a source of dimethylamine groups. Therefore the actual time during which *N*-nitroso compounds may be present in the setting of typically treated urinary tract infections in Western countries may be small.

Long-term infections, on the other hand, may present a different story. To examine this situation, Hicks and co-workers[51,55] analyzed urine specimens for *N*-nitroso compounds in a population of adolescents and young adults in an area of Egypt where bilharziasis is endemic and bladder cancer prevalent.

Chronic secondary bacterial infection of the bilharzial bladder is frequent, posing some difficulty when sorting out the various factors involved. In this particular population, however, urinary tract bacterial infections in young males are also frequent even in the absence of bilharziasis. Subjects in this group in fact showed significantly higher levels of detectable *N*-nitroso compounds in their urine than did controls without bacterial infection, and these levels were comparable to those found in individuals with either combined bacterial-schistosomal infections or schistosomal infections alone. Therefore significant long-term exposure to urinary nitrosamines may, at least in this population, predate the almost inevitable chronic bilharzial infection and perhaps figure into laying the groundwork for subsequent bladder carcinoma.

Indication that *chronicity* may be a necessary component in this scenario has also been noted in animal studies. Davis et al.,[26] for example, showed that apparently neoplastic as well as hyperplastic and dysplastic changes of the urinary bladder could be induced in rats by the use of repeated injections of nitrate-reducing bacteria over a long course of time, thereby maintaining a state of chronic urinary tract infection. Single intravesical bacterial injections produced no such changes, but introduction of a foreign body into the murine bladder, followed by a single bacterial injection, appeared to serve the same function as repeated injections, with resultant long-term infections. In a subsequent analysis[25] these investigators noted that in the rats with long-term infections by either method, dimethylnitrosamine was detected in the urine of most of the infected animals by 12 weeks, and in some it was detected as early as 2 weeks. The chemical was not detected, however, in those with only transient urinary tract infections resulting from a single intravesical injection of bacteria.

Numerous questions regarding the effects of these chemicals in the development of human urothelial malignancies have yet to be answered.[51,111] Perhaps the major loose end is the fact that nitrosamines must still be activated to a locally reactive moiety. It may take place in the liver but has thus far not been shown to take place in the bladder.[57,111] According to Hicks,[51] at present there is no *direct* evidence that any of the *N*-nitroso compounds may be linked with urothelial carcinogenesis either via urinary tract infections or otherwise. The data thus far, particularly those derived from the Egyptian population studied by Hicks and colleagues as well as others,[1] certainly raises suspicion, however.

INFECTIOUS AGENTS

Bilharziasis (Schistosomiasis)

The possible relation between infestation with *Schistosoma hematobium* and the development of bladder carcinoma was first noted by Ferguson in 1911.[35] As with Ferguson's report, most epidemiologic data regarding the association have emanated from Egypt, where schistosomal infection is endemic and the incidence of bladder carcinoma remarkably high. In fact, the most common malignancy among males in Egypt is carcinoma of the bilharzial bladder, accounting for fully 27 percent of all new cancers seen each year at the Cairo Cancer Institute.[33,34] In contrast to bladder carcinoma in Western countries, the tumor occurs in a younger population, peaking during the fifth decade, and the predominant tissue type is squamous carcinoma.[33,34] Lesions are generally at a high stage at the time of diagnosis although with relatively more limited nodal metastases than would be expected of comparable stage tumors in a Western population.[31,34] Because of the advanced stages as well as the relatively larger sizes of these tumors, endoscopic resection has not proved of value.[34,47] Adding to the dismal picture is the lack of response to standard chemotherapeutic agents that have been found to be of use for disseminated transitional cell carcinoma.[122]

The nature of the association between bilharziasis and bladder cancer has yet to be elucidated. The number of patients from the Egyptian studies is striking, and certain ancillary findings (e.g., a selectively increased schistosomal egg burden in areas of tumorous bladder tissue[16]) add strength to the plausibility of a relation. Experimental studies, however, have thus far failed to show a direct cause-and-effect situation.[33] It is also of note that outside of Egypt the clinical data are not nearly so impressive. Although other areas where schistosomal infection is endemic, particularly the Middle East, have shown an increased incidence of bladder carcinoma,[30,34,99] this not universal. For example, Kaye and Isaacson,[68] in a study of urban black males in South Africa, found bladder cancer to be rare despite widespread bilharziasis.

It appears that chronic schistosomal infestation more likely plays a propagating role than one of initiation,[33,52] with the production of an intractable cystitis resulting in fertile soil for tumor growth following exposure to potentially carcinogenic agents such as urinary nitrosamines as outlined above. Again, however, the role of these *N*-nitroso compounds remains unclear.

Bacterial Infection

It is likely that in Western populations urinary tract infections play little if any role in urothelial carcinogenesis. In support of this statement is the much lower incidence of urothelial neoplasms in women versus men, despite the higher incidence of urinary tract infections in women. The predominant organism in Western population urinary tract infections is *Escherichia coli*, with *Proteus* species also common offenders. Both, as noted, are capable of promoting nitrosamine formation, perhaps the only *potential* link thus far with urothelial carcinogenesis. Once tumor growth has been established by other means, however, particularly in the urethra and bladder neck region as well as in the upper tract, obstruction often results in secondary bacterial infection. This in turn perhaps serves in a propagating role similar to that suggested for schistosomal infestation.

Viral Infection

The possibility of viruses having a role in the production of human urothelial tumors was suggested by the isolation of RNA virus from three renal pelvic transitional cell carcinomas by Fraley et al.[40] The same group of investigators subsequently recovered an RNA virus from bladder tumors that was morphologically and biochemically similar to known RNA oncogenic viruses.[32] Subsequent to these discoveries, increasingly sophisticated techniques have been used to demonstrate viruslike cores containing RNA-directed DNA polymerase and high-molecular-weight RNA in the urine of patients with prostate, bladder, and urethral cancer.[22] Molecular evidence of viruslike biochemical activities has also been found in assays of tumor tissue proper from patients with bladder and urethral carcinomas as well as prostate carcinoma and hypernephroma.[23]

The meaning of such findings remains open to speculation at present, although advances in tumor virology continue at a rapid pace. It was not long ago that human neoplasms seemed somehow outside the realm of viral oncogenesis that obtained elsewhere in the animal kingdom. Yet recent discoveries, notably the relations between papillomaviruses and cervical cancer[123] and retroviruses and adult T-cell leukemia,[120] suggest that light may be shed on the above discoveries in urothelial neoplasia in the near future.

TRYPTOPHAN

Metabolism of the amino acid tryptophan results in a number of intermediates (e.g., kynurenine, 3-hydroxyanthranilic acid, and 2-amino-3-hydroxyacetophenone) that are aromatic amines structurally similar to industrial bladder carcinogens discussed above. The studies of Dunning and co-workers[29] indicated a potential role for tryptophan metabolites in chemically induced bladder tumors in rats, raising the possibility of "endogenous carcinogenesis." The finding of elevated levels of these metabolites in the urine of patients with bladder carcinoma following administration of ingested tryptophan suggested that an individual's biochemical peculiarities might result in excess exposure to such metabolites,[109] with possible carcinogenic effects. Thus far, however, there has been no direct evidence that tryptophan or its metabolites, in and of themselves, produce bladder cancer in humans.[15] Subsequent studies by Teulings et al.[119] indicated that abnormally high excretion of tryptophan metabolites was generally seen in patients with tumors associated with obstruction to urinary outflow. In contrast, patients with carcinoma but no evidence of obstruction and patients "cured" of bladder cancer (average follow-up of 5.2 years) showed urinary tryptophan metabolite levels comparable to those of controls. Thus the possibility that tryptophan metabolite elevation may result from the effects, rather than serve as a cause, of urothelial carcinoma was raised. The question of such metabolites acting as promoting agents in neoplasms induced by other means, as suggested by animal experiments,[15] remains open at the present time. In at least one study of bladder cancer patients who were identified as hypersecretors of tryptophan metabolites, however, correc-

tion of the hypersecretion by oral pyridoxine (vitamin B_6) did not affect the rate of tumor recurrence compared to that in similar patients not so treated.[75]

BALKAN NEPHRITIS

There is a high incidence of a peculiar interstitial nephritis among inhabitants along certain rivers in Yugoslavia, Bulgaria, and Romania, as well as an impressive associated incidence of both renal pelvic and ureteral tumors in affected patients.[81,106] The renal parenchymal lesions are not unlike those of analgesic nephropathy. Morbidity and mortality are striking, and the largest percentage of deaths in these patients occurs during the third to fifth decades.[81] Associated renal pelvic and ureteral tumors may be seen in as many as one-third of autopsied cases, with approximately 32 percent of cases showing multiple ipsilateral tumors and 10 percent bilateral tumors.[106] These lesions are generally low grade papillary ones, however, and patients usually die as the result of chronic renal failure rather than malignancy.[106] The nephritis has been attributed to the high level of silicates in the drinking water, with conversion to silicic acid leading to renal toxicity.[81] The relation, if any, of the silicates to tumor development is not clear, however.

BLADDER EXSTROPHY

Bladder exstrophy, a relatively uncommon condition with an estimated incidence of approximately 1 per 50,000 births,[104] has been associated with the subsequent development of bladder carcinoma in approximately 4 percent of afflicted patients.[50] O'Kane and Megaw,[104] in a review of the literature, noted 56 cases of carcinoma developing in exstrophied bladders, seen as early as the third decade, with the bulk of cases reported in patients aged 30 to 59. A subsequent update review by Nielsen and Nielsen,[103] adding 25 more cases, showed similar statistics, with one of the additional cases noted in the 0 to 19 years age bracket.

In contrast to routine bladder carcinoma, the predominant tumor type has been adenocarcinoma, found in 87 percent of O'Kane and Megaw's collected cases. This finding may relate to the almost universal epithelial alterations seen in exstrophied bladder mucosa, with glandular metaplasia observed in the considerable majority of such bladders examined.[24] The nature of the relation is uncertain, however, as an even larger percentage of exstrophied bladders examined show squamous metaplasia,[24] yet squamous carcinoma accounted for less than 4 percent in the series collected by O'Kane and Megaw.[104] A report by Bullock et al.,[12] wherein widespread intestinal metaplasia in nonexstrophic bladders was found to have seemingly ominous connotations, suggests the possibility that the malignant potential may somehow relate to the glandular metaplasia per se, or at least the circumstances giving rise to the intestinal metaplasia.

Despite the increased incidence of carcinoma in the exstrophic bladder, the prognosis with such neoplasms appears to be relatively good, as only 2 of 56 patients in O'Kane and Megaw's series died as a result of metastatic disease.[104] It may reflect earlier detection in these patients as well as perhaps a tendency to more aggressive surgery at an earlier stage, particularly as the bladder is already nonfunctional. As surgical methods of early bladder reconstruction improve,[92] it will be of interest to note whether the incidence of bladder carcinoma in these patients in fact decreases, as the benign epithelial alterations, including glandular metaplasia, have been noted as early as age 2 weeks.[24]

HEREDITARY FACTORS

Fraumeni and Thomas[42] first suggested the possibility of hereditary factors in the development of urothelial neoplasia in a 1967 case report of malignant bladder tumors in a man and his three sons. Since that time, a handful of reports documenting similar familial occurrences have appeared. McCullough et al.[85] presented a case study wherein six family members from two generations were found to have bladder carcinoma, with two patients having upper tract lesions as well. The pattern of inheritance suggested an autosomal dominant trait. There was no history of common carcinogenic exposure, and studies of immunologic competence and tryptophan metabolism were unrevealing. Of note was the occurrence of the lesions at a younger than expected age, with a median age at onset of 48 years, as well as the fact that five of

the six patients had associated nonurothelial malignancies.

Despite these sometimes striking occurrences, such reports have appeared only sporadically. One epidemiologic study, conducted by Purtilo and colleagues,[110] noted a surprising 11 cases of transitional cell carcinoma of the bladder in five unrelated families from a total study population of 162 patients with bladder carcinoma. Again, patients were younger than expected, and familial occurence of other malignancies was noted. All but three patients had a history of cigarette smoking and possible industrial carcinogen exposure, however, which might have explained the phenomenon, as other epidemiologic studies have not found a significant incidence of familial occurrence.[94,118] The common theme of multiple nonurothelial as well as urothelial malignancies in these occasional reports suggests the possibility that many of these patients may suffer from the "cancer family syndrome," as noted in a more recent report by Frischer et al.[44]

RADIATION

There appears to be some increase in the development of urothelial malignancies following radiation exposure, with, for example, data accumulated on long-term survivors of the atomic bomb explosions in Hiroshima and Nagasaki indicative of a two- to threefold risk increase for all urinary tract neoplasms.[72] On a more practical level, patients who have undergone therapeutic pelvic irradiation show increased risk as well.

Duncan et al.[28] examined the long-term incidence of bladder malignancies in more than 2,000 women from the Cincinnati Tumor Registry who had been previously irradiated for cervical cancer. They found eight cases of bladder carcinoma among 2,674 women. A similar study from Rotterdam revealed five cases among 2,772 women irradiated for cervical carcinoma.[36] These figures suggest an increased risk on the order of eight times that expected, with figures of similar magnitude noted elsewhere.[69]

Even with such direct exposure, however, the numbers still indicate the development of bladder tumors in only a relative handful among the thousands of women so treated, and it is reasonable to conclude that radiation exposure plays little role in the development of urothelial neoplasia in the general population, a point borne out in more general epidemiologic studies.[118]

LITHIASIS

That calculi may serve in the induction of urothelial tumors has been suggested by animal experiments.[14,17] However, as Hicks indicated,[52] stones more likely act as a nonspecific irritant serving as a propagating stimulus to growth initiated by other factors. Calculi are found not infrequently in association with urothelial neoplasms, particularly upper tract lesions, which are often aggressive squamous carcinomas.[74] Some no doubt are formed secondarily following obstruction and the onset of chronic infection, but in other cases lithiasis has been presumed to predate tumor formation by virtue of prior clinical and radiologic information.[80] The increased incidence of urothelial neoplasms in certain groups of patients prone to lithiasis, e.g., paraplegics (see below), adds to the suspicion of some etiologic relation.

In this regard, it is important to be aware that urinary cytology preparations may show disturbing abnormalities in the presence of calculi, mimicking those seen with carcinoma,[7] even when no such lesion is present. Lithiasis is among the most common clinical situations wherein false-positive cytologic diagnoses are made.[39,114] These alterations may clear completely following removal of the calculi,[7] but in the event they do not, further careful evaluation is indicated.

PARAPLEGIA

An increased incidence of bladder carcinoma has been noted in paraplegics, with estimates of the eventual development of malignancy in long-term survivors in the range of 0.28 to 1.0 percent.[10,88] Of particular interest is the disproportionate number of squamous carcinomas compared to the more common transitional cell carcinomas in the general population.

Broecker et al.[10] noted that of the 24 patients with spinal cord injury and bladder carcinoma reported in three studies, 29 percent had pure squamous carcinomas, and an aggregate of 67 percent showed at least some squamous elements in their tumors. Preexisting squamous metaplasia is exceedingly common in this group of patients, particularly among those with indwelling catheters. However, its relation to subsequent squamous malignancies remains speculative.

The underlying etiology also remains uncertain. Such lesions usually occur years after the initial insult, with a range of 10 to 42 years between spinal cord injury and eventual tumor development.[10,88] Although a definite inciting agent or agents may not be identifiable, it seems that recurrent bouts of cystitis, indwelling catheters, and frequent calculus formation would at the very least serve as an effective set of promoting agents in the development of carcinoma. It has been emphasized[5,10] that the onset of hematuria in a patient with spinal cord injury, often ascribed to chronic bladder infection or irritation, must result in careful scrutiny of not only the bladder but also the upper tract, particularly in patients whose injuries occurred in the distant past.

SUMMARY OF ETIOLOGIC FACTORS

Of necessity, this chapter has been little more than a brief sketch of the most commonly cited factors associated with the development of urothelial malignancies. As the reader will have noted, there remain many more questions than answers in this area, and it is hoped that continued examination of the questions will result in the discovery of additional basic information concerning urothelial carcinogenesis. At the present time, exciting advances in oncology appear to be taking place at an even more basic level, that of molecular biology. The discovery of the importance of oncogenes in human neoplasia,[11,71] for example, has rightly been noted by Baltimore[4] to have led to a "revolution in our thinking about the underlying changes that distinguish a cancer cell from a normal cell." From these advances may come eventual revolutionary changes in the ability to categorize human neoplasms as well as to treat them.

Yet as Baltimore also pointed out, it does not yet appear that the "magic bullet" is on the horizon, and at least for the time being it behooves both clinician and pathologist to be aware of some of the more pedestrian relations that have been examined in this chapter, as such awareness may prove to be of practical value for the diagnosis and treatment of urothelial neoplasms.

REFERENCES

1. Abdel-Tawab GA, Aboul-Azm T, Ebied SA, et al : The correlation between certain tryptophan metabolites and the N-nitrosamine content in the urine of bilharzial bladder cancer patients. J Urol 135:826, 1986
2. Allen MJ, Boyland E, Dukes CE, et al: Cancer of the urinary bladder induced in mice with metabolites of aromatic amines and tryptophan. Br J Cancer 11:212, 1957
3. Al-Shukri S, Alwan MH, Nayef M, Rahman AA: Bilharziasis in malignant tumors of the urinary bladder. Br J Urol 59:59, 1987
4. Baltimore D: The impact of the discovery of oncogenes on cancer mortality rates will come slowly. Cancer 59:1985, 1987
5. Belldegrun A, Loughlin K, Fam B, et al: Squamous cell carcinoma of bladder in spinal cord injury patients. J Urol 133:302-A, 1985
6. Bennett AH: Cyclophosphamide and hemorrhagic cystitis. J Urol 111:603, 1974
7. Beyer-Boon ME, Cuypers LHRI, deVoogt HJ, Brussee JAM: Cytological changes due to urinary calculi. Br J Urol 50:81, 1978
8. Boyko RW, Cartwright RA, Glashan RW: Bladder cancer in dye manufacturing workers. J Occup Med 27:799, 1985
9. Brenner DW, Schellhammer PF: Upper tract urothelial malignancy after cyclophosphamide therapy: a case report and literature review. J Urol 137:1226, 1987
10. Broecker BH, Klein FA, Hackler RH: Cancer of the bladder in spinal cord injury patients. J Urol 125:196, 1981
11. Brosman SA, Liu BCS: Oncogenes: their role in neoplasia. Urology 30:1, 1987
12. Bullock PS, Thoni DE, Murphy WM: The significance of colonic mucosa (intestinal metaplasia) involving the urinary tract. Cancer 59:2086, 1987
13. Case RAM, Hosker ME, McDonald DB, Pearson JT: Tumors of the urinary bladder in workmen engaged in the manufacture and use of certain dyestuff intermediates in the British chemical industry. I. The role of aniline, benzidine, alpha-naphthylamine, and beta-naphthylamine. Br J Industr Med 11:75, 1954
14. Chapman WH, Kirchheim D, McRoberts JW: Impact of the urine and calculus formation on the incidence of bladder tumors in rats implanted with paraffin wax pellets. Cancer Res 33:1225, 1973
15. Chowaniec J: Aetiology: epidemiological and experimental considerations. p. 118. In Skrabanek P, Walsh A (eds): Bladder Cancer: A Series of Workshops on the Biology of Human Cancer. Report No. 13. International Union Against Cancer, Geneva, 1981
16. Christie JD, Crouse D, Kelada AS, et al: Patterns of Schistosoma haematobium egg distribution in the human lower urinary tract. III. Cancerous lower urinary tracts. Am J Trop Med Hyg 35:759, 1986
17. Clayson DB: Bladder carcinogenesis in rats and mice: possibility of artifacts (editorial). J Natl Cancer Inst 52:1685, 1974
18. Cole P: Coffee-drinking and cancer of the lower urinary tract. Lancet 1:1335, 1971
19. Cole P, Hoover R, Friedell GH: Occupation and cancer of the lower urinary tract. Cancer 29:1250, 1972
20. Cole P, Monson RR, Haning H, Friedell GH: Smoking and cancer of the lower urinary tract. N Engl J Med 284:129, 1971
21. Connolly JG, Gospodarowicz MK, Rawlings GA, Lopatin WB: Bladder cancer in rubber workers. J Urol 133:303-A, 1985
22. Cuatico W, Cheung CH, Sy F: Detection of viral-like cores from the urine of patients with genito-urinary malignancies. Cancer 41:706, 1978
23. Cuatico W, Cheung CH, Sy F: Molecular evidence of viral-like biochemical activities in human genitourinary malignancies. J Urol 123:895, 1980
24. Culp DA: The histology of the exstrophied bladder. J Urol 91:538, 1964
25. Davis CP, Cohen MS, Anderson MD, et al: Urothelial hyperplasia and neoplasia. II. Detection of nitrosamines and interferon in chronic urinary tract infections in rats. J Urol 134:1002, 1985
26. Davis CP, Cohen MS, Gruber MB, et al: Urothelial hyperplasia and neoplasia: a response to chronic urinary tract infections in rats. J Urol 132:1025, 1984
27. Druckrey H, Preussmann R, Ivankovic S, et al: Selektive erzeugung von Blasenkrebs an ratten durch Dibutyl-und N-butanol (4)-nitrosamin. Z Krebsforsch 66:280, 1964
28. Duncan RE, Bennett DW, Evans AT, et al: Radiation-induced bladder tumors. J Urol 118:43, 1977
29. Dunning WF, Curtis MR, Maun ME: The effect of

added dietary tryptophane on the occurrence of 2-ace-tylaminofluorene-induced liver and bladder cancer in rats. Cancer Res 10:454, 1950

30. El-Akkad SM, Amer MH, Lin GS, et al: Pattern of cancer in Saudi Arabs referred to King Faisal Specialist Hospital. Cancer 58:1172, 1986
31. El-Bolkainy MN, Mokhtar NM, Ghoneim MA, Hussein MH: The impact of schistosomiasis on the pathology of bladder carcinoma. Cancer 48:2643, 1981
32. Elliott AY, Fraley EE, Castro AE, et al: Isolation of an RNA virus from transitional cell tumors of the human urinary bladder. Surgery 74:46, 1973
33. Elsebai I: Parasites in the etiology of cancer—bilharziasis and bladder cancer. CA 27:100, 1977
34. Elsebai I: Cancer of the bilharzial bladder. Urol Res 6:233, 1978
35. Ferguson AR: Associated bilharziosis and primary malignant disease of the urinary bladder, with observations on a series of forty cases. J Pathol Bacteriol 16:76, 1911
36. Fokkens W, Hop WCJ: Re: radiation-induced bladder tumors. J Urol 121:690, 1979
37. Foley GE, Friedman OM, Drolet BP: Studies of the mechanism of action of Cytoxan: evidence of activation in vivo and in vitro. Cancer Res 21:57, 1961
38. Forni AM, Koss LG, Geller W: Cytological study of the effect of cyclophosphamide on the epithelium of the urinary bladder in man. Cancer 17:1348, 1964
39. Frable WJ, Paxson L, Barksdale JA, Koontz WW Jr: Current practice of urinary bladder cytology. Cancer Res 37:2800, 1977
40. Fraley EE, Elliott AY, Hakala TR, et al: RNA virus isolation from papillary tumors of renal pelvis. Surg Forum 23:529, 1972
41. Fraumeni JF Jr, Scotto J, Dunham LJ: Coffee drinking and bladder cancer. Lancet 2:1204, 1971
42. Fraumeni JF Jr, Thomas LB: Malignant bladder tumors in a man and his three sons. JAMA 201:97, 1967
43. Friedman L, Richardson HL, Richardson ME, et al: Toxic response of rats to cyclamates in chow and semisynthetic diets. J Natl Cancer Inst 49:751, 1972
44. Frischer Z, Waltzer WC, Gonder MJ: Bilateral transitional cell carcinoma of the renal pelvis in the cancer family syndrome. J Urol 134:1197, 1985
45. Fuchs EF, Kay R, Poole R, et al: Uroepithelial carcinoma in association with cyclophosphamide ingestion. J Urol 126:544, 1981
46. Garvin DD, Ball TP: Bladder malignancy in patient receiving cyclophosphamide for benign disease. Urology 18:80, 1981
47. Ghoneim MA, Awaad HK: Results of treatment in

carcinoma of the bilharzial bladder. J Urol 123:850, 1980
48. Glashan RW, Cartwright RA: Occupational bladder cancer and cigarette smoking in West Yorkshire. Br J Urol 53:602, 1981
49. Gonzalez CA, Lopez-Abente G, Errezola M, et al: Occupation, tobacco use, coffee, and bladder cancer in the county of Mataro (Spain). Cancer 55:2031, 1985
50. Goyanna R, Emmett JL, McDonald JR: Exstrophy of the bladder complicated by adenocarcinoma. J Urol 65:391, 1951
51. Hicks RM: Nitrosamines as possible etiologic agents in bilharzial bladder cancer. p. 455. In Magee PN (ed): Nitrosamines and Human Cancer. Banbury Report 12. Cold Spring Harbor Laboratory, New York, 1982
52. Hicks RM: Multistage carcinogenesis in the urinary bladder. Br Med Bull 36:39, 1980
53. Hicks RM, Chowaniec J: The importance of synergy between weak carcinogens in the induction of bladder cancer in experimental animals and humans. Cancer Res 37:2943, 1977
54. Hicks RM, Wakefield JStJ: Rapid induction of bladder cancer in rats with N-methyl-N-nitrosourea. I. Histology. Chem Biol Interact 5:139, 1972
55. Hicks RM, Walters CL, Elsebai I, et al: Demonstration of nitrosamines in human urine: preliminary observations on a possible etiology for bladder cancer in association with chronic urinary tract infections. Proc R Soc Med 70:413, 1977
56. Hill GB: Epidemiologic considerations. p. 5. In Javadpour N (ed): Bladder Cancer. International Perspectives in Urology, Vol. 12. Williams & Wilkins, Baltimore, 1984
57. Hill MJ: Bacterial metabolism and human carcinogenesis. Br Med Bull 36:89, 1980
58. Hoffmann D, Masuda Y, Wynder EL: Alpha-naphthylamine and beta-naphthylamine in cigarette smoke. Nature 221:254, 1969
59. Holsti LR, Ermala P: Papillary carcinoma of the bladder in mice, obtained after peroral administration of tobacco. Cancer 8:679, 1955
60. Howe GR, Burch JD, Miller AB, et al: Artificial sweeteners and human bladder cancer. Lancet 2:578, 1977
61. Huben RP, Tomasello E, Gamarra M, et al: Benzidine and human bladder cancer. J Urol 133:253-A, 1985
62. Hueper WC: Cancer of the urinary bladder in workers of chemical dye factories and dyeing establishments: a review. J Indust Hyg Toxicol 16:255, 1934
63. Hueper WC, Wiley FH, Wolfe HD, et al: Experimental production of bladder tumors in dogs by ad-

ministration of beta-naphthylamine. J Industr Hyg Toxicol 20:46, 1938

64. Hultengren N, Lagergren C, Ljungqvist A: Carcinoma of the renal pelvis in renal papillary necrosis. Acta Chir Scand 130:314, 1965

65. Johansson S, Wahlqvist L: Tumors of urinary bladder and ureter associated with abuse of phenacetin-containing analgesics. Acta Pathol Microbiol Scand [A] 85:768, 1977

66. Johnson WW, Meadows DC: Urinary-bladder fibrosis and telangiectasia associated with long-term cyclophosphamide therapy. N Engl J Med 284:290, 1971

67. Kabat GC, Dieck GS, Wynder EL: Bladder cancer in nonsmokers. Cancer 57:362, 1986

68. Kaye V, Isaacson C: Genitourinary pathology in urban male blacks of South Africa. J Urol 123:51, 1980

69. Kennedy DRH: Radiation-induced bladder cancer. Br J Urol 53:74, 1981

70. Kessler II: Cancer mortality among diabetics. J Natl Cancer Inst 44:673, 1970

71. Kirschenbaum A, Droller MJ: Update on oncogenes and relevance in urology. Urology 29:121, 1987

72. Kohn HI, Fry RJM: Radiation carcinogenesis. N Engl J Med 310:504, 1984

73. Koss LG, Melamed MR, Mayer K: The effect of busulfan on human epithelia. Am J Clin Pathol 44:385, 1965

74. Li MK, Cheung WL: Squamous cell carcinoma of the renal pelvis. J Urol 138:269, 1987

75. Lieman SJ, Newman AJ, Carlton CE Jr, et al: Tryptophan metabolism and bladder cancer: a double-blind study with pyridoxine (vitamin B$_6$) versus placebo. J Urol 133:211A, 1985

76. Lilienfeld AM, Levin ML, Moore GE: The association of smoking with cancer of the urinary bladder in humans. Arch Intern Med 98:129, 1956

77. Littler WA, Kay JM, Hasleton TS, Heath D: Busulphan lung. Thorax 24:639, 1969

78. Lower GM, Jr: Concepts in causality: chemically induced human urinary bladder cancer. Cancer 49:1056, 1982

79. Magee PN, Montesano R, Preussmann R: N-Nitroso compounds and related carcinogens. p. 491. In Searle CE (ed): Chemical Carcinogens. ACS Monograph 173. American Chemical Society, Washington, DC, 1976

80. Mahadevia PS, Karwa GL, Koss LG: Mapping of urothelium in carcinomas of the renal pelvis and ureter. Cancer 51:890, 1983

81. Markovic B: Endemic nephritis and urinary tract cancer in Yugoslavia, Bulgaria, and Rumania. J Urol 107:212, 1972

82. Marsh FP, Vince FP, Pollock DJ, Blandy JP: Cyclophosphamide necrosis of bladder causing calcification, contracture and reflux; treated by colocystoplasty. Br J Urol 43:324, 1971

83. McCredie M, Ford JM, Taylor JS, Stewart JH: Analgesics and cancer of the renal pelvis in New South Wales. Cancer 49:2617, 1982

84. McCredie M, Stewart JH, Carter JJ, et al: Phenacetin and papillary necrosis: independent risk factors for renal pelvic cancer. Kidney Int 30:81, 1986

85. McCullough DL, Lamm DL, McLaughlin AP, Gittes RF: Familial transitional cell carcinoma of the bladder. J Urol 113:629, 1975

86. McDougal WS, Cramer SF, Miller R: Invasive carcinoma of the renal pelvis following cyclophosphamide therapy for nonmalignant disease. Cancer 48:691, 1981

87. Melick WF, Escue HM, Naryka JJ, et al: The first reported cases of human bladder tumors due to a new carcinogen — xenylamine. J Urol 74:760, 1955

88. Melzak J: The incidence of bladder cancer in paraplegia. Paraplegia 4:85, 1966

89. Millard RJ: Busulfan-induced hemorrhagic cystitis. Urology 18:143, 1981

90. Miller AB: The etiology of bladder cancer from the epidemiological viewpoint. Cancer Res 37:2939, 1977

91. Miller JA, Miller EC: The metabolic activation of carcinogenic aromatic amines and amides. Prog Exp Tumor Res 11:273, 1969

92. Mollard P: Bladder reconstruction in exstrophy. J Urol 124:525, 1980

93. Morgan RW, Jain MG: Bladder cancer: smoking, beverages and artificial sweeteners. Can Med Assoc J 111:1067, 1974

94. Morganti G, Gianferrari L, Cresseri A, et al: Recherches clinico-statistiques et génétiques sur les néoplasies de la vessie. Acta Genet (Basel) 6:306, 1956

95. Morrison AS: Public health value of using epidemiologic information to identify high-risk groups for bladder cancer screening. Semin Oncol 6:184, 1979

96. Morrison AS: Epidemiology and environmental factors in urologic cancer. Cancer 60:632, 1987

97. Morrison AS, Ahlbom A, Verhoek WG, et al: Occupation and bladder cancer in Boston, USA, Manchester, UK, and Nagoya, Japan. J Epidemiol Community Health 39:294, 1985

98. Morrison AS, Buring JE: Artificial sweeteners and cancer of the lower urinary tract. N Engl J Med 302:537, 1980

99. Mustacchi P, Shimkin MB: Cancer of the bladder and infestation with Schistosoma hematobium. J Natl Cancer Inst 20:825, 1958

100. Nelson BM, Andrews GA: Breast cancer and cytologic dysplasia in many organs after busulfan (Myleran). Am J Clin Pathol 42:37, 1964

101. Nery R: The binding of radioactive label from labelled phenacetin and related compounds to rat tissues in vivo and to nucleic acids and bovine plasma albumin in vitro. Biochem J 122:311, 1971

102. Newberne PM, Conner MW: Food additives and contaminants: an update. Cancer 58:1851, 1986

103. Nielsen K, Nielsen KK: Adenocarcinoma in exstrophy of the bladder — the last case in Scandinavia? A case report and review of literature. J Urol 130:1180, 1983

104. O'Kane HOJ, Megaw JM: Carcinoma in the exstrophic bladder. Br J Surg 55:631, 1968

105. Palvio DHB, Andersen JC, Falk E: Transitional cell tumors of the renal pelvis and ureter associated with capillarosclerosis indicating analgesic abuse. Cancer 59:972, 1987

106. Petković SD: Epidemiology and treatment of renal pelvic and ureteral tumors. J Urol 114:858, 1975

107. Piper JM, Tonascia J, Matanoski GM: Heavy phenacetin use and bladder cancer in women aged 20 to 49 years. N Engl J Med 313:292, 1985

108. Price JM, Biava CG, Oser BL, et al: Bladder tumors in rats fed cyclohexylamine or high doses of a mixture of cyclamate and saccharin. Science 167:1131, 1970

109. Price JM, Wear JB, Brown RR, et al: Studies on etiology of carcinoma of urinary bladder. J Urol 83:376, 1960

110. Purtilo DT, McCarthy B, Yang JPS, et al: Familial urinary bladder cancer. Semin Oncol 6:254, 1979

111. Radomski JL, Greenwald D, Hearn WL, et al: Nitrosamine formation in bladder infections and its role in the etiology of bladder cancer. J Urol 120:48, 1978

112. Rathert P, Melchior H, Lutzeyer W: Phenacetin: a carcinogen for the urinary tract? J Urol 113:653, 1975

113. Rehn L: Blasengeschwülste bei Fuchsin-arbeitern. Arch Klin Chir 50:588, 1895

114. Rife CC, Farrow GM, Utz DC: Urine cytology of transitional cell neoplasms. Urol Clin North Am 6:599, 1979

115. Ross RK, Paganini-Hill A, Henderson BE: Epidemiology of bladder cancer. p. 113. In Skinner DG (ed): Urological Cancer. Grune & Stratton, New York, 1983

116. Seo IS, Clark SA, McGovern FD, et al: Leiomyosarcoma of the urinary bladder — 13 years after cyclophosphamide therapy for Hodgkin's disease. Cancer 55:1597, 1985

117. Simon D, Yen S, Cole P: Coffee drinking and cancer of the lower urinary tract. J Natl Cancer Inst 54:587, 1975

118. Sullivan JW: Epidemiologic survey of bladder cancer in greater New Orleans. J Urol 128:281, 1982

119. Teulings FAG, Peters HA, Hop WCJ, et al: A new aspect of the urinary excretion of tryptophan metabolites in patients with cancer of the bladder. Int J Cancer 21:140, 1978

120. Wachsman W, Golde DW, Chen ISY: HTLV and human leukemia: perspectives 1986. Semin Hematol 23:245, 1986

121. Weinberg DM, Ross RK, Mack TM, et al: Bladder cancer etiology — a different perspective. Cancer 51:675, 1983

122. Yagoda A: Chemotherapy of metastatic bladder cancer. Cancer 45:1879, 1980

123. Zur Hausen H: Papillomaviruses in human cancer. Cancer 59:1692, 1987

17

Urothelial Neoplasms: Pathologic Anatomy

James W. Eagan, Jr.

This chapter is devoted to a general discussion of the morphology of urothelial neoplasms and associated epithelial changes throughout the urinary tract. First, however, normal urothelial morphology as well as certain nonneoplastic alterations and their possible relations to neoplasia are briefly considered. Certain problem areas are also addressed, such as the classification of low grade papillary tumors.

Although urothelial neoplasms of the upper tract, bladder, and proximal urethra are often considered separately, the common threads, at least from the pathologic point of view, are such that they may be discussed collectively at the outset for the following reasons.

1. Throughout the urothelium, the most common tumors are of the transitional cell or "urothelial" type, with pure squamous lesions accounting for only a small minority at all sites and pure adenocarcinomas an even lesser number.

2. The histologic types encountered at one site are encountered at all sites, in roughly similar proportions.

3. Among the transitional cell neoplasms at all sites, most have a papillary configuration, at least at the time of initial diagnosis.

4. For reasons that are not entirely clear, multiplicity of involvement is commonplace, both at an individual site, e.g., multiple bladder tumors, or at various sites, e.g., concomitant or sequential bladder, ureteral, and renal pelvic neoplasms.

5. Benign neoplasms, admittedly hazily defined (a problem that is examined here), are in a distinct minority at all sites.

Individual tumor sites and their attendant peculiarities are considered in depth in Chapters 18 and 19, with interrelations among the various sites also discussed.

NORMAL HISTOLOGIC ANATOMY

Recognition of neoplastic alterations at any body site obviously presupposes a knowledge of normal histologic anatomy. With the sometimes subtle variations found in lesions designated as low grade carcinomas in the urinary tract, a solid knowledge of the normal urothelial appearance and common nonneoplastic variations is of utmost importance.

Normal urothelium, or transitional epithelium (Figs. 17-1 and 17-2), consists of multiple tiers of cells that vary from rounded to cuboidal, elongated in a direction perpendicular to the basement membrane. The surface is covered by specialized cells, at times multinucleated, termed "umbrella cells" by Koss.[111] As the name implies, these cells extend to cover a

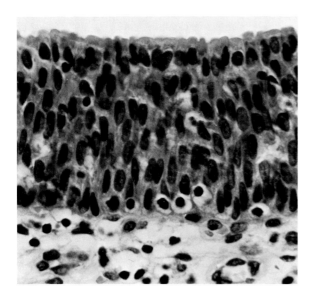

Fig. 17-1 Normal urothelium, contracted. ×570.

number of the smaller underlying cells. These underlying cells have been divided, as with other epithelia, into intermediate and basal cell layers on the basis of electron microscopic differences.[214] It is difficult to distinguish the basal and intermediate cells by light microscopy, however, and for practical purposes urothelial cells are generally divided into two categories: deep and superficial.

Both cytoplasmic configuration and the number of nuclear layers or tiers vary with the area examined. Renal pelvic mucosa is generally more attenuated in appearance than bladder mucosa, and both are gener-

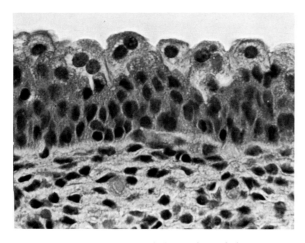

Fig. 17-2 Normal urothelium, distended. ×570.

ally less thick than normal ureteral mucosa. The apparent thickness of the latter presumably relates in part to the normally tightly contracted state of the ureter, with the ureteral epithelium often thrown into "pseudopapillary" folds.

Artifactual distension of the urinary bladder, during either cystoscopy with the use of distilled water or saline or inflation with formalin in the routine handling of cystectomy specimens, may result in an apparent decrease in cell layer number. Contrasting appearances in normal urothelium are noted in Figures 17-1 and 17-2. Figure 17-1 demonstrates the normal appearance of contracted urothelium. Note in particular the vertical orientation of the nuclei and that the superficial or umbrella cells as distinct entities are relatively inapparent. The outermost cytoplasmic border is sometimes smooth but at other times is thrown into a corrugated or "picket fence" appearance. In contrast, distended urothelium (Fig. 17-2) shows an apparent decrease in cell layer number, with vertical orientation of the nuclei less well maintained. The superficial cells are more readily discerned, and their cytoplasmic borders can be seen to extend over a number of the underlying cells. Note also the now apparent multinucleation of some of the superficial cells, as well as their occasional enlarged nuclei and recognizable nucleoli. These features may be cause for undue concern in both histologic and cytologic preparations. The presence or absence of the superficial cell layer has been found to be useful for the determination of pathologic tumor grade, with the disappearance of these cells most commonly associated with higher grade neoplasms.

Another finding seen to a variable degree is that of cytoplasmic "clearing." At least some of this appearance may be attributed to the normal presence of intracytoplasmic vesicles and/or intracellular glycogen, and the absence of such clearing is thought by some to be associated with neoplastic and preneoplastic change.[153] We have not found this alteration to be reliable in this context, however, having seen many biopsy specimens of otherwise normal urothelium with little or no cytoplasmic clearing and others with persistent clearing despite noticeable nuclear atypia (Fig. 17-3). At least in part, such cytoplasmic alteration may relate to either fixation artifact or to specimens having been obtained from a bladder distended with distilled water or solutions of low osmolarity, with imbibition of hypotonic fluid during the proce-

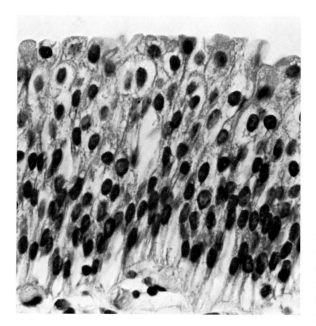

Fig. 17-3 Cytoplasmic "clearing" in atypical urothelium. ×570.

dure. In the latter situation, Tannenbaum et al.[214] noted marked ultrastructural alterations of the cytoplasm of the basilar cells in particular.

According to Koss,[111] the number of nuclear layers or tiers in normal human urothelium should range between five and seven, but this number may vary considerably depending on the factors noted above. Although it should not be considered a hard and fast rule, numbers exceeding seven to ten layers are generally considered abnormal in histologic sections of human urothelium. Among the chief reasons for not adhering strictly to the practice of "layer counting" is the difficulty in being sure for any given microscopic area, particularly with small irregular biopsy specimens, that one is dealing with a true perpendicular section. Even a minor bias may lead to an apparent increase in what is in fact no more than seven-layer epithelium. Conversely, in many instances where nuclear features warrant a diagnosis of carcinoma in situ, the epithelium may be less than seven tiers thick and yet be obviously malignant. As with all other histologic alterations, the number of nuclear layers must be taken in context.

The urinary tract, unlike the gastrointestinal tract, only rarely contains a distinct, continuous muscularis mucosa[182a]. Therefore neither "lamina propria" nor "submucosa" seems correct to describe the soft tissue layer between the mucosa and muscularis.[74] In practice, however, the terms are used interchangeably, correctly or not, particularly with reference to the level of tumor invasion.

NONNEOPLASTIC UROTHELIAL ALTERATIONS

A variety of mucosal alterations are commonly found throughout the urothelium, often associated with chronic irritation, but at other times as seemingly normal variants or at least without obvious explanation. Under certain circumstances these alterations have been found in association with urothelial neoplasms. However, at the present time the associations have not been translated into cause and effect; and, with a few possible exceptions, which are discussed later, a label of "premalignant" for any of the following conditions does not appear warranted.

Squamous Metaplasia

Transformation of the normal bladder mucosa into an epidermoid-type lining may be seen at cystoscopy or on gross examination of a resection specimen as an irregular whitish area, more or less apparent depending on the presence or absence and degree of keratinization. It is most commonly found in the female bladder and much less often in the male bladder.

Histologically, the appearance closely simulates that of normal squamous epithelium when fully developed (Fig. 17-4). The altered areas most commonly do not show evidence of surface keratinization, but it may be prominent in certain clinical situations (see below). The individual cells may show cytoplasmic clearing, presumably secondary to the presence of glycogen, and this may be prominent in the squamous epithelium that is often found in the area of the female trigone and proximal urethra. The inferior border may be flat or thrown into folds similar to that of the normal rete ridge pattern found in skin, as noted in Figure 17-4.

In the renal pelvis squamous metaplasia is unusual, and it is most commonly seen with chronic pyelitis, particularly in the presence of stones. The ureter is rarely the site of noticeable squamous metaplasia,

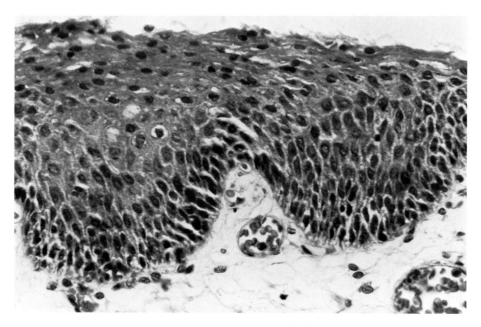

Fig. 17-4 Squamous metaplasia, bladder. ×360.

with the exception of the distalmost ureter in association with schistosomiasis, as noted below.

In the bladder the most common pathologic setting for squamous metaplasia in Western populations is chronic cystitis, in some cases with associated chronic urethritis. It is seen far more commonly in women than in men[112] with an approximate 9 : 1 female/male ratio in one series of cystoscopy patients.[232] The preponderance of women may partially result from the inclusion of a subcategory that Koss noted separately as that of "vaginal-type epithelium in the area of the bladder trigone in women."[111] As the name implies, the metaplasia is generally confined to the trigone and adjacent urethra, and it is of the nonkeratinizing type normally found in the menstrual era vagina. In an autopsy series Tyler[218] found no trigonal squamous epithelium in newborns or children, although occasional patches were noted in the proximal urethra. Squamous epithelium in the trigone was found in 86 percent of premenopausal women, however, and in 50 percent of postmenopausal women. Interestingly, the morphology of the squamous epithelium appeared to correspond to the hormonal pattern seen in the vaginal epithelium in a given patient. Thus the incidence of squamous metaplasia found at cystoscopy in association with chronic recurrent cystitis in

women, which has been found in excess of 80 percent,[166] is difficult to interpret without comparative figures for women during the reproductive years without cystitis, a group unlikely to undergo cystoscopic examination.

Four clinical situations merit special mention with regard to squamous metaplasia. The first is schistosomiasis, previously discussed in Chapter 16, which is associated in certain countries such as Egypt with a high incidence of bladder carcinoma.[59] Although squamous metaplasia is common in urinary bladders infested with *Schistosoma hematobium,* the absence of a high incidence of associated bladder malignancies in other countries where the disease is endemic casts doubts on the possibility of a cause-and-effect relation between the metaplasia and subsequent neoplasia.

The second clinical situation, also discussed in Chapter 16, is that of squamous carcinoma in paraplegics, who are often victims of chronic urinary tract infections and lithiasis. Again, the relation between the relatively frequent (compared to adult men) squamous metaplasia and the increased incidence of both bladder carcinoma in general and squamous carcinoma in particular is not clear. Although a direct relation between the two cannot be excluded, it can be argued that a common stimulus may result in the occurrence of squamous metaplasia as well as the induction of such differentiation in neoplasms caused by other factors.

A third clinical situation in which squamous metaplasia is commonly found, most often with associated glandular metaplasia, is bladder exstrophy. Despite the association of both types of metaplasia, most carcinomas of the bladder found in patients with this disorder are adenocarcinomas. Squamous carcinomas, conversely, account for no higher a percentage of tumors in this group than in the general population.

A fourth situation, that of squamous metaplasia with prominent keratinization, is not clearly defined, particularly with regard to premalignant potential. Various labels have been used for the entity, including "leukoplakia,"[21,176] "cholesteatoma,"[109] and "keratinizing desquamative squamous metaplasia."[90] The lesion is seen most commonly in the bladder, less often in the upper tract, and least commonly in the urethra.[21] It may occur in conjunction with other disease processes, e.g., chronic infection, lithiasis, and tuberculosis, but a significant number of cases have no clear-cut association with other disorders.[21] The most distinctive feature is the formation of often large amounts of keratin, occasionally sufficient to occlude the urinary passages when occurring in the upper tract.[109] Some authors, e.g., Benson et al.,[21] have observed a distinct association with malignancy, most commonly squamous carcinoma, whereas others have not found such an association.[90] It is of importance in

this regard to note that Benson et al.[21] recorded *dysplastic* epithelial changes as well as squamous metaplasia and hyperkeratosis; the former finding in particular is certainly cause for concern in biopsy material.

Perhaps the most compelling argument against a direct relation between squamous metaplasia, at least of the nonkeratinizing variety, and subsequent squamous carcinoma is the very fact that squamous metaplasia is so much more common in the female population — perhaps the rule rather than the exception in the adult premenopausal woman. Yet the overall incidence of bladder carcinoma, including squamous carcinoma, is quite low in women. Therefore the finding of squamous epithelium in urothelial biopsy material should not in itself be cause for alarm. Distinct keratinization, however, should arouse some suspicion, and again, if there are *dysplastic* as well as metaplastic features, the possibility of associated malignancy should be considered, similar to the situation at other body sites such as cervix, bronchus, etc.

Glandular Metaplasia

Although submucosal alterations with a glandlike configuration are common, true surface glandular metaplasia is unusual, with the most readily available examples found in exstrophic bladders. Mucinous metaplasia has also been induced experimentally by *Escherichia coli* infection.[91] Alterations may range from a simple one-layered cuboidal or columnar con-

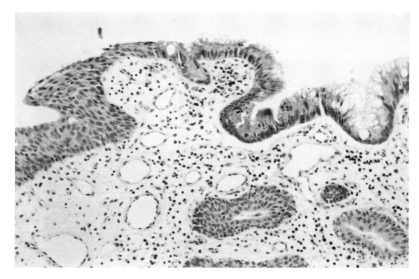

Fig. 17-5 Surface glandular metaplasia, bladder. Note the abrupt change from transitional epithelium at left to mucin-secreting glandular epithelium with goblet cell formation. Cystitis cystica is also present. ×144.

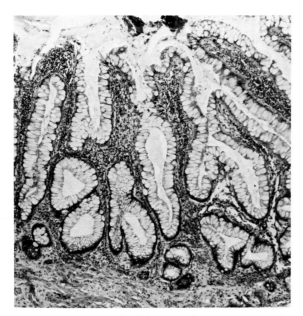

Fig. 17-6 Complex glandular metaplasia in an exstrophic bladder. ✕58.

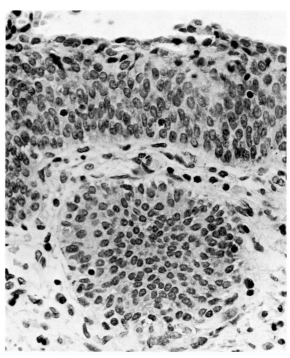

Fig. 17-7 Brunn's nest formation. ✕360.

figuration (Fig. 17-5) to a more complex arrangement, again typically found in the exstrophic bladder, which may faithfully mimic the appearance of large or small intestinal mucosa, at times even complete with Paneth and argentaffin cells (Fig. 17-6). Occasionally this more elaborate type of intestinal mucosa occurs in the upper tract.[77,184]

As with squamous metaplasia, the mere finding in biopsy material of *isolated* foci of glandular metaplasia that are not histologically atypical should not, in and of itself, be cause for alarm.[113] *Extensive* replacement of urothelium by complex glandular metaplasia simulating intestinal mucosa (as illustrated above) is another matter. It has been reported rarely in the nonexstrophic bladder as well as the upper tract, generally in the setting of chronic irritation or infection, and may be associated with a significant risk of malignancy.[31]

Brunn's Nests

Throughout its distribution, urothelium has a propensity to proliferate focally into the soft tissue immediately subjacent to the mucosa, leading to the formation of discrete epithelial aggregates termed "the nests of von Brunn" or, simply, Brunn's nests (Fig. 17-7). They are frequently found in the bladder and are common in the supramontanal prostatic urethra,[107] and may also be seen in the renal pelvis and ureter. The nests often show a point of attachment to the overlying mucosa, at times demonstrable only in serial sections, but may appear truly isolated from the mucosa in a given section. In fact, although many of these nests are true downward proliferations, others are probably not much more than exaggerated folds in a contracted mucosa.

Melicow[140] noted that these epithelial nests are frequently seen in association with bladder carcinoma, but to date no convincing evidence has linked them with carcinoma in a causal fashion. In fact, in a series of thoroughly examined bladders from 100 consecutive autopsies without grossly apparent vesical abnormalities, Koss found Brunn's nests in 89 of the 100 cases studied.[112] There was no significant difference in distribution in men versus women. Koss was able to find no relation between Brunn's nests and inflammatory states. This view is in contrast to that of earlier pathologists, such as Morse,[144] and it is also in conflict with experimental evidence that Brunn's nests, as well as mucinous metaplasia, may be induced by *E. coli* infection.[91] One potential explanation for the disparity of opinions might be that Brunn's nests persist long after the inflammation abates. In any event, it appears that the presence of Brunn's nests, at least in adult bladders, is the rule rather than the exception. In 58 pairs of ureters examined in Koss' study, Brunn's nests were also found in 10 to 20 percent of the specimens sectioned.

Perhaps the most important aspect of recognizing this type of proliferative activity is in the interpretation of small biopsy specimens from patients with carcinoma. One must be cautious of overinterpreting what appears to be extension of tumor into the submucosa, particularly if the extension is well circumscribed. The individual cytologic features must be noted as well, as the apparent "invasion" may be nothing more than a preexisting Brunn's nest or, if

cytologically atypical features are present, merely an extension of the neoplastic process to involve these epithelial nests rather than true invasion (Fig. 17-8).

Cystitis (Pyelitis, Ureteritis) Cystica

Also seen throughout the urothelium-lined areas, cystitis (pyelitis, ureteritis) cystica appears to be an alteration of a Brunn's nest type of structure.[144,145] It is characterized by the appearance of a lumen within the solid aggregate of cells, which may or may not be filled with an eosinophilic, periodic acid-Schiff (PAS)- and mucin-positive material (Fig. 17-9). In contrast to normal urothelium, ultrastructural and immunofluorescence microscopic evaluations indicate a now active secretory state,[224] and in the early

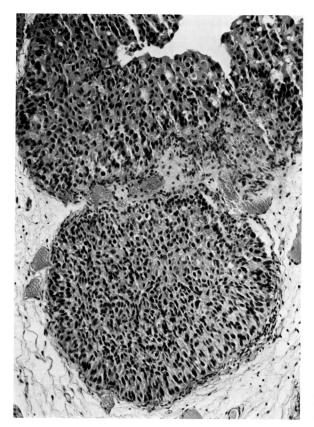

Fig. 17-8 Transitional cell carcinoma involving Brunn's nest. ×110.

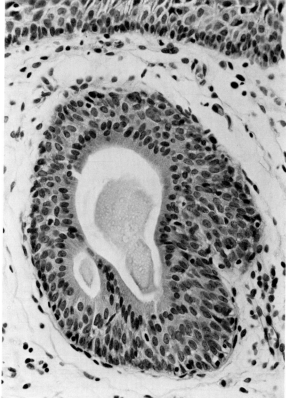

Fig. 17-9 Cystitis cystica. Note the eosinophilic material in the lumen. ×273.

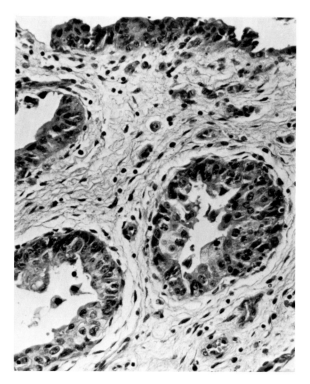

Fig. 17-10 Carcinoma in situ, with involvement of underlying areas of cystitis cystica. ×230.

Cystitis (Pyelitis, Ureteritis) Glandularis

Cystitis glandularis is a histologic alteration which also appears as nests in the submucosa but, at least in its completely developed form, is much less common than either Brunn's nests or cystitis cystica. The hallmark is that of mucin-producing glandular epithelium similar, and at times virtually identical, to intestinal mucosa (Fig. 17-11), not only morphologically but also histochemically.[229] Cystitis glandularis apparently evolves along a continuum that includes Brunn's nests and cystitis cystica.[91,145] In fact, spotty mucin production may be seen in individual cells in otherwise typical examples of cystitis cystica, and urothelial cell remnants may be seen surrounding the mucin-producing cells in otherwise typical examples of cystitis glandularis.

Although on occasion, similar to surface glandular metaplasia, this alteration is seen in association with adenocarcinoma,[160] as with the other "mucosal variants" there is no convincing evidence linking the glandularis abnormalities in a more than incidental fashion, and some studies have shown no association at all.[5]

stages the inner layer of cells about the lumen is overtly columnar. In older cysts the luminal border cells may be flattened or cuboidal, and eventually the cystic portions may enlarge enormously, leaving only an attenuated epithelial border.

Cystitis cystica was noted in most normal bladders studied by Koss,[112] although less frequently than Brunn's nests, with only 60 of 100 bladders demonstrating these structures. In 57 of the 60 cases they were found in direct association with Brunn's nests, supporting the concept of the relation of these two entities. Similar to Brunn's nests, the lesions were most commonly seen, but not confined to, the trigonal area.

The admonition regarding interpretation of Brunn's nests in tumor-containing biopsy material also applies to cystitis cystica (Fig. 17-10). In the case of atypical changes in association with an overlying tumor, both the recognizable lumen and the well-defined border should alert the investigator that the area in question is a preexisting structure involved by the neoplastic process rather than an area of true invasion.

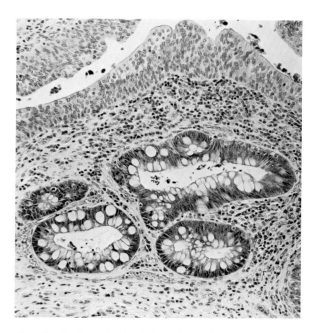

Fig. 17-11 Cystitis glandularis. Note the resemblance to intestinal mucosa. ×130.

At least for the present, it appears that cystitis glandularis and adenocarcinoma are merely two reflections of the facility of urothelium to be transformed into other types of epithelium, some neoplastic and some nonneoplastic.

UROTHELIAL HYPERPLASIA

Urothelial hyperplasia occupies the "gray zone" between nonneoplastic and neoplastic transformation of urothelium, at least from the morphologic point of view. It is the major example of alterations that must be taken in context when dealing with urothelial pathology.

Generally speaking, the phenomenon of hyperplasia, or an increase in cell number, is seen not uncommonly throughout the body in various sites, both epithelial and stromal. It may represent a physiologic process (e.g., the increase in acinar cells in the lactating breast), or a pathologic process or reaction thereto

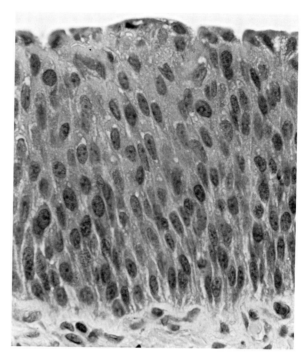

Fig. 17-13 Urothelial hyperplasia. There is a less prominent increase in number of nuclear tiers than in Figure 17-12, but note the minor degree of anisonucleosis, the increase in nuclear chromaticity, and the occasional small nucleoli. ×470.

(e.g., the thickening of the esophageal mucosa seen with chronic reflux esophagitis).

Similar changes occur in the transitional epithelium of the urinary tract. The histologic evidence of hyperplasia is similar to that seen in the esophagus, for example (i.e., an increase in the apparent number of epithelial cell layers, estimated by counting the nuclear tiers from the basilar area to the surface). With more pronounced examples, often seen in inflammatory settings, there may be some loss of nuclear polarity (Fig. 17-12), and occasional abnormal nuclei may be seen (Fig. 17-13), usually demonstrating relatively minor increases in nuclear size, nuclear hyperchromaticity, and small nucleolar formations. The superficial cell layer is generally intact, at times attenuated, but at other times even more prominent than usual.

Urothelial hyperplasia often occurs as a "reactive process," most commonly in the setting of chronic or recurrent inflammation. In a prospective study of urothelial changes in spinal cord injury patients, for example, Broecker et al.[30] found mucosal hyperplasia

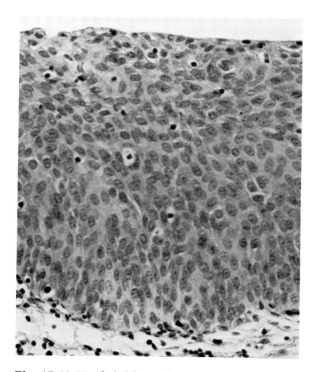

Fig. 17-12 Urothelial hyperplasia. Note the marked increase in the number of nuclear tiers, with some loss of nuclear polarity. Note also the otherwise bland nuclear features and attenuated superficial layer. ×300.

relatively common, occurring in approximately 30 percent of patients, both in a group with indwelling catheters and in one without. All patients in both groups showed chronic inflammation, and squamous metaplasia was also noted in 22 and 13 percent of the catheterized and noncatheterized patients, respectively.

Frequent settings for at times striking urothelial hyperplasia are benign prostatic hyperplasia (BPH) and chronic prostatitis. As illustrated in Figure 17-14, hyperplastic transitional mucosa may be seen in the periurethral segments of transurethral resection specimens, often accompanied by submucosal chronic inflammation, at times extending deep into the periurethral prostatic ducts. This phenomenon should be kept in mind when examining prostatic specimens for possible extension of transitional cell carcinoma of the bladder, generally from a patient population most likely to have unrelated BPH. Although benign uro-

thelial proliferation may be alarming at low power, occasionally almost filling the periurethral ducts, higher power examination reveals the hyperplastic cells to be cytologically bland and not part of a neoplastic process.

With urothelial hyperplasia in a noninflammatory setting, however, care must be taken when interpreting these changes because essentially the same epithelial appearance, *when present in a papillary configuration,* constitutes sufficient evidence to warrant a diagnosis of low grade carcinoma. In fact, whereas high grade urothelial malignancies are not frequently associated with hyperplastic changes in the remaining bladder, low grade lesions commonly show hyperplastic foci in the remaining mucosa.[190] If present in a flat configuration, they cannot be reliably distinguished from hyperplasia found in nonneoplastic conditions. One type of hyperplasia with a more distinctive appearance, however, may also be seen in association with

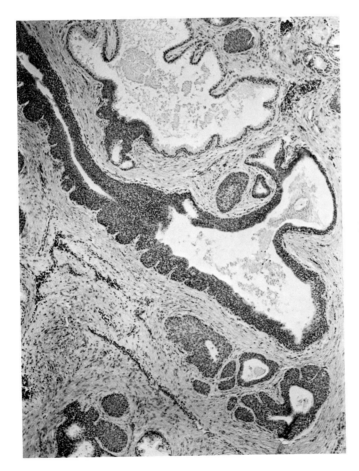

Fig. 17-14 Urothelial hyperplasia in periurethral prostatic ducts. ×66.

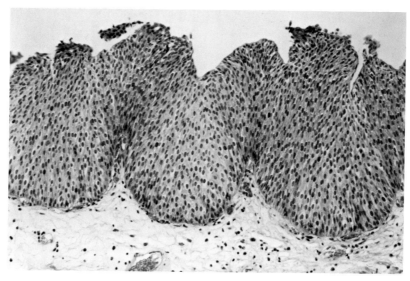

Fig. 17-15 Urothelial hyperplasia with "accordian pleat" appearance. It is a presumed early recognizable stage of papillary neoplasia. ×230.

low grade papillary carcinoma (Fig. 17-15), demonstrating a corrugated or "accordion-pleat" appearance. This alteration represents perhaps the earliest stage that is definitely recognizable in the development of a papillary neoplasm.

Therefore when presented microscopically with simple hyperplasia (increase in cell layer number, no significant cytologic atypia, and *flat* configuration), one must look to the setting to determine its significance. If associated with low grade papillary neoplasms or a history of such, it may well be part of the neoplastic process. Outside this setting, it might still represent the "dawn of neoplasia" but may just as well be part of a nonneoplastic, reactive process despite the fact that it appears identical to hyperplasia associated with low grade papillary carcinomas. So-called atypical hyperplasia is discussed later.

UROTHELIAL NEOPLASMS

Most urothelial neoplasms encountered throughout the urinary tract are of the transitional cell type, a morphologically distinct group of tumors. Considerable controversy still surrounds the nomenclature of these lesions, and certain "problem areas" (for want of a better term) are considered here prior to a general discussion of their histologic appearance.

Problem Areas

For various reasons, at least some of which seem unnecessarily self-inflicted, designation and terminology of urothelial neoplasms is a source of confusion to many urologists and pathologists. Part of the confusion stems from well-meaning attempts to "clear up the confusion" by the ongoing introduction of new systems of tumor classification, grading, and staging, a practice better left to those in the lymphoma field, in my opinion.

If the changing systems present difficulty to those directly involved in the field, they must surely be almost impossible sources of irritation for the practicing clinician or pathologist who is only occasionally faced with the problem of urothelial neoplasia. In few areas of medicine is the interaction of clinician and pathologist more important than when dealing with urothelial neoplasms; there is a particular need for precise exchange of information between the two to rationally determine therapy and prognosis for a given patient.[68] A significant area of potential confusion, and therefore one of great importance to both patient and physician, is the classification of low grade papillary lesions, particularly with regard to what morphologic features constitute sufficient evidence to warrant a diagnosis of "carcinoma." As the controversy is unlikely to be settled one way or another in the forseeable future, it is important that clinicians and pathologists be aware of the issues involved.

"Flat" Versus "Papillary" Lesions

Papillary change, or the formation of fingerlike projections of epithelium surrounding a usually delicate fibrovascular core, is common to many lesions in pathology. The lesions are often recognizable as such on examination of the gross material, appearing as arborescent structures with a filiform texture to the surface, as illustrated in Figure 17-16. The origin of the papillary configuration is presumed to be an increase in epithelial cell number, or epithelial "hyperplasia" in the broadest sense of that word, vis-à-vis the underlying stroma. Eventually, there is "pleating" of the epithelium into the adjacent lumen or surrounding tissue, and, growing with it, a sustaining fibrovascular stromal core.

The mere presence of a growth with a papillary configuration is regarded as evidence in certain sites, e.g., colon, of at least possible benign neoplastic transformation. In other sites, e.g., thyroid, the presence of the papillary configuration, *when accompanied by appropriate cytologic alterations,* is regarded de facto evi-

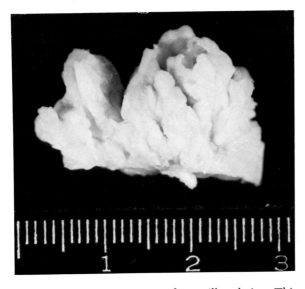

Fig. 17-16 Gross appearance of a papillary lesion. This segment was taken from a papillary transitional cell carcinoma of bladder.

dence of neoplastic alteration with a potential for malignant behavior.

So too with the urothelium. At any site — renal pelvis, ureter, bladder, or proximal urethra — the presence of an epithelial lesion with a papillary configuration must arouse concern, as under present systems of classification it is generally considered an indication of neoplastic transformation despite the fact that other histologic aspects may not be at all alarming. Presuming that such papillary lesions are neoplastic, we then turn to the major area of controversy, the pathologic designation "low grade papillary tumors."

Benign Papilloma Versus Papillary Carcinoma, Grade I

In virtually all areas of tumor pathology, the fundamental question remains: "Is this lesion benign or malignant?" The pathologist is often able to readily settle the issue on a purely morphologic basis, and the addition of clinical information, laboratory and radiologic data, etc. allows this judgment to be made accurately in most cases. In some diagnostic areas (e.g., smooth muscle tumors of the uterus and certain types of ovarian epithelial lesions), subsets of tumors with indeterminate malignant capabilities, at least by routine analysis, have been segregated. The usual situation is that most such lesions behave in a benign fashion if adequately treated, but a relative handful of lesions with identical appearance pursue a malignant course. Criteria for inclusion in these subsets have been defined, and terms such as "borderline malignancy" and "tumors of low malignant potential" are applied. Finally, there seems always to be the occasional lesion that defies classification by other than the test of time. As one wise pathologist advised, such lesions are best sent off to a trusted expert, "not so much to be diagnosed, but pronounced!"

In no other area in pathology has the distinction between "benign" and "malignant" been so blurred as with the diagnosis of papillary transitional cell neoplasms, in particular transitional cell papilloma versus grade I papillary transitional cell carcinoma. If we consider general tumor pathology, some of the reasons for the lack of clarity are apparent.

When assessing neoplasms in any body site, many aspects of the process are taken into account before arriving at an opinion concerning a lesion's "biologic potential." Such factors include the patient's age, sex, and race; the location of the lesion; symptoms; chronicity of the lesion; and clinical evidence of possible invasion and metastasis. Although some consider possession of such information by the pathologist as possibly deleterious to objective assessment of a lesion,[197] an opinion with which I strongly disagree, it may at least serve as a guideline to keep the pathologist on the right track. An example of the usefulness of such information is the occasional worrisome but "not quite malignant" melanocytic lesion seen in day-to-day practice. In an adult the pathologist might consider a given lesion potentially malignant or at least "premalignant," whereas a similar lesion in a 5-year-old child should elicit a much more circumspect approach. It is imperative for the clinician to recognize that the clinical information supplied with the specimen may be of pivotal importance. As Lattes[123] observed: ". . . surgical pathology is not a guessing game; sur-

gical pathologists should not operate in a vacuum but should have all available clinical information, *and they should be influenced by it.* This will protect them and the patients from serious mistakes of interpretation, with all of the related side effects and complications."

It is also true with the pathologic information, where all of the facts should be gathered before arriving at a diagnosis. Here one takes into account the gross appearance of the lesion, information often of necessity supplied by the clinician when only a small biopsy specimen is submitted. Microscopically, many features are noted, including the "low power" configuration, evidence of possible invasion, and so on. "High power" observations concentrate on epithelial structural organization (how closely the lesion appears to progress through the normal maturation sequence expected for epithelium of its type) and on cytologic alterations (how closely the individual cells resemble those of normal epithelium of the same type). Significant cytologic deviations would include anisocytosis, anisonucleosis, nuclear membrane irreg-

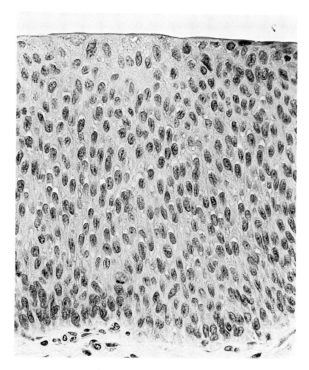

Fig. 17-17 Urothelial hyperplasia. Note the mild degree of loss of nuclear polarity but otherwise bland nuclear features. Changes such as those seen here and those depicted in Figure 17-18 are seen in association with low grade papillary neoplasms but may also be seen in nonneoplastic reactive situations. ×300.

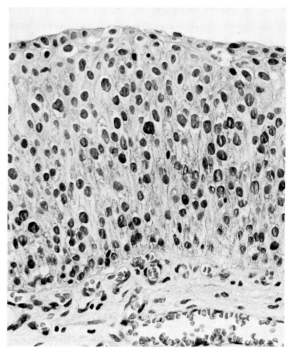

Fig. 17-18 Urothelial hyperplasia with atypical features. Nuclear polarity is less well maintained than in the lesion in Figure 17-17, and occasional, enlarged, hyperchromatic nuclei, some with small nucleoli, are seen. ×300.

ularities, increased nuclear chromaticity, increased nuclear/cytoplasmic ratio, numerous nucleoli, macronucleoli, increased number of mitotic figures, and abnormal mitotic figures. Particularly when the lesion is still confined to its site of origin and invasion is not demonstrable, such cytologic alterations have proved to be the best predictors of malignancy or, more accurately, of the potential for malignant behavior, in standard pathology practice at such sites as lung, cervix, and gastrointestinal tract.

A significant deviation from the above concepts has occurred in the diagnosis of urothelial neoplasms. When considering alterations in "flat" or planar urothelium, traditional concepts of hyperplasia, dysplasia or atypia, and malignant neoplasia still apply. For example, the epithelium in Figure 17-17 shows, first, a flat configuration. The only alteration of note is an increase in the epithelial cell layers to almost twice the expected seven to ten. This lesion, in flat epithelium, would be diagnosed as showing "hyperplasia." Figure 17-18 shows, again, flat epithelium exhibiting not only an increase in number of cell layers but low power structural alterations, in particular some loss of nuclear polarity. There are significant cytologic alterations as well, including anisonucleosis and nuclear

hyperchromaticity. Overall, the epithelium shows some, but not all, of the classic features associated with malignancy, and these intermediate lesions would be classified as showing "dysplasia," "atypia," or "atypical hyperplasia." (See Nonpapillary Transitional Cell Carcinoma, below, for further discussion.) Such lesions are apparent in patients with overt urothelial carcinomas when the grossly uninvolved urothelium is biopsied or sectioned,[112] as was the case with the specimen in Figure 17-18. However, similar, and at times even more striking alterations are occasionally found in apparently "reactive" situations. Figure 17-19, for example, shows an area from the renal pelvis in a kidney removed from a young woman with chronic obstructive pyelonephritis. Aside from such foci of atypia, which were generally seen in areas of severe inflammation, there was no evidence of urothelial malignancy here or elesewhere in the urinary tract. Again, all such alterations must be taken in context. Figure 17-20, a specimen taken from the ureter

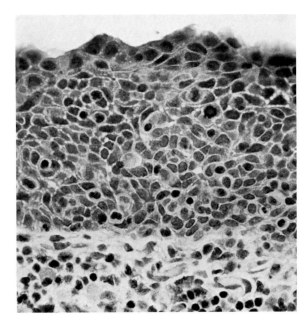

Fig. 17-19 Severely atypical "reactive" hyperplasia. This was found in the renal pelvis of a young woman with obstructive pyelonephritis. ×300.

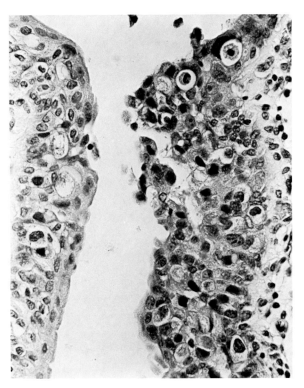

Fig. 17-20 Carcinoma in situ (right side) located in the ureter in a section adjacent to an area of invasive carcinoma. Compare to Figure 17-19. Note also the lesser degree of atypia of apposing mucosa. ×435.

of a patient with invasive high grade transitional cell carcinoma distal to this site, shows epithelium in a flat configuration exhibiting total disarray along one luminal face, with many of the traditional features of malignancy listed above. This appearance in an epithelial biopsy would be sufficient to warrant a diagnosis of carcinoma in situ. Note the focal nuclear alterations in the apposing ureteral mucosa, lesser in degree but sufficient to be diagnosed as atypical or dysplastic.

Most urothelial neoplasms, however, do not have a "flat" configuration. According to Koss,[112] about 90 percent of bladder tumors are found to have a papillary configuration when first seen by the urologist. When presented with such lesions, the pathologist must be aware that, because of the papillary configuration, all other features that are required for a diagnosis of carcinoma in flat epithelium are down-scaled. The epithelium in Figure 17-21, for example, shows a

papillary configuration but otherwise has structural and cytologic features that would be indicative of, at most, atypical hyperplasia if found in flat mucosa. This type of lesion, however, would be regarded at present by most pathologists as at least a low grade papillary transitional cell carcinoma. In contrast, the epithelium in Figure 17-22, also from a papillary lesion, shows structural and cytologic alterations that would be sufficient in and of themelves to warrant a diagnosis of carcinoma in flat epithelium. In the papillary configuration this lesion would be regarded as a high grade papillary transitional cell carcinoma.

The above philosophy regarding diagnosis of malignancy in urothelial papillary lesions is generally held as majority opinion at present. In particular, it is reflected in such standard pathologic references as the Armed Forces Institute of Pathology (AFIP) fasicles on both urinary bladder[111,113] and upper urinary tract

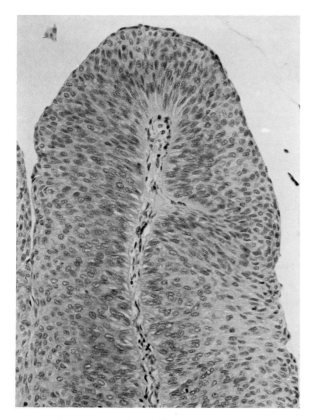

Fig. 17-21 Low grade papillary transitional cell carcinoma. Note the minimal degree of atypical features. ×179.

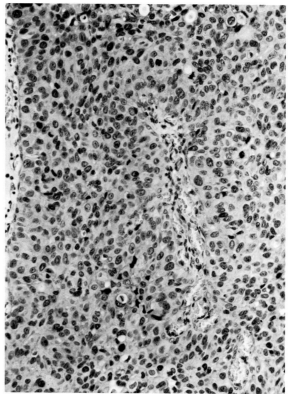

Fig. 17-22 High grade papillary transitional cell carcinoma. Compare its architectural and cytologic features with those in Figure 17-21. ×208.

tumors[20] as well as the World Health Organization (WHO) monograph on the histologic typing of urinary bladder tumors.[147] Under this system, the preponderance of all papillary urothelial tumors are diagnosed as at least low grade carcinomas, with lesions acceptable as "transitional cell papillomas" (i.e., "a papillary tumor with a delicate fibrovascular stroma covered by regular transitional epithelium indistinguishable from that of the normal bladder and not more than six layers thick" — WHO classification[147]) virtually legislated out of existence.

It must be noted, however, that there is a prominent minority opinion that maintains that papillary lesions showing increased epithelial thickness but only minor cytologic and architectural alterations should be diagnosed as papillomas rather than low grade papillary carcinomas. The fact that the cited incidence of "papillomas" in the literature ranges from as low as 3 percent to as high as 30 to 40 percent serves as witness that not everyone is giving the same lesion the same name.[140] Perhaps the most important proponent of this line of thinking is the Memorial Hospital (of the Memorial Sloan-Kettering Cancer Center), an institution from which has emanated so much of value and influence in the literature on genitourinary malignancies. In simple terms, a lesion that would be classified as papillary transitional cell carcinoma, grade I, in many institutions would be relegated to the "histologically benign papilloma" category at Memorial Hospital and at other centers as well. Further adding to the confusion is the fact that still other institutions are even more stringent in their requirements for a diagnosis of "carcinoma," with only lesions showing histologic evidence of actual invasion accepted as carcinoma, and noninvasive papillary lesions designated as such and graded according to their degree of atypicality.[177]

Arguments can be marshaled for both the "liberal" and the "conservative" approach to the diagnosis of carcinoma in papillary urothelial lesions. There are two principal reasons for the former approach, i.e., designating virtually all papillary lesions as carcinomas, as is done by most popular classification systems. The first is the fact that for many patients presenting with such lesions it is merely the first episode in a lengthy, recurrent, often multifocal disease process, and at least some of these patients eventually die from bladder cancer. Exact figures for such progression are difficult to come by, as most large series are published by referral centers or groups of centers with a possible selection bias toward difficult cases. One study of interest in this regard was reported by Gilbert and colleagues[76]; they recorded 365 patients evaluated and treated for papillary bladder tumors in the Southern California Kaiser Permanente group. As the study followed the course of an unselected, nonreferral center group of prepaid health plan patients, it was thought to be more reflective of the natural history of such lesions in the general population. Most patients were treated conservatively, with total cystectomy used only for advanced primary or recurrent lesions. Radiation therapy was seldom used except for medically inoperable patients, for patients with unresectable cancers, or in conjunction with vesical resection — and then as a postoperative measure. No patients were lost to follow-up, and all were followed at least 5 years.

In this study, 155 patients were classified at initial presentation as having papillary transitional cell carcinoma, grade I. Approximately 60 percent (92/155) suffered recurrent tumors, and 21 of these 92, or approximately 13 percent of the original group, had advances in tumor grade with recurrence. Of the 21 patients, 12 advanced to grade II lesions and 9 to grade III lesions. These final 9 patients all progressed to grade III disease in less than 2 years, and all went on to die of their disease.

In a study of referral patients seen with grade I papillary transitional cell carcinoma at the Mayo Clinic,[80] recurrence rates were even higher: 73 percent overall. Patients initially presenting with multiple tumors who were amenable to treatment by transurethral resection showed the highest recurrence rate: 88 percent. Although the higher recurrence rates noted in the Mayo Clinic series probably are in part reflective of the referral-based population, part of the increase relates to a longer follow-up period. The 5-year recurrence rate, 58 percent, was virtually identical to the Kaiser group figure. As an aside, this finding underscores another important aspect of the disease, i.e., its chronicity; and it is emphasized that a 5-year disease-free interval is not synonomous with cure. In the Mayo Clinic series, the time of first recurrence ranged from 3 months or less *to longer than 10 years in 8 percent of the patients.* Overall, 22 percent of the Mayo Clinic patients had recurrence at a higher grade, and mural invasion was detected in 10 percent, all of whom died of their disease.

A second major reason for the liberal approach to the diagnosis of bladder carcinoma is the basic unpredictability of the disease, i.e., the problem of deciding which patients among the many presenting with "bladder cancer" will go on to die of their disease. As Cummings noted,[42] the inability to predict the biologic behavior of malignant bladder epithelium *for an individual patient* is a dilemma. In no area is it more apparent than in predicting from day 1 which patients with low grade tumors will suffer recurrent disease, how soon and how often the disease will recur, and in particular which patients in this group will be in the 6 to 10 percent who go on to higher-grade disease, invasion, and death. Numerous factors have been cited as possibly predictive of the latter course, such as multiplicity of the lesions, number of recurrences, and time to first recurrence. Various adjunctive studies may also help differentiate which patients will develop more aggressive disease, including cell surface antigen assays, chromosome analysis, and electron microscopic examination. (Each of these topics is covered in detail subsequently.) Even when all possible predictors are taken into account, however, no one has yet been able to state with unfailing accuracy which patient presenting with low grade/low stage disease will go on to eventually die of urothelial cancer unless major therapeutic intervention is undertaken. For this reason in particular, many clinicians and pathologists advocate labeling virtually all papillary lesions as carcinoma, with rare exceptions (illustrated later).

There are a number of arguments in favor of a more conservative diagnostic approach to urothelial papillary lesions, however. One is the fact that convincing evidence of true invasion, particularly into the musculature, by tumors that maintain the appearance of grade I papillary transitional cell carcinoma is scarce and evidence of metastatic capability even more so. If we concentrate on bladder carcinoma, where initial conservative treatment is the rule and the natural history is therefore more accurately assessed, deaths related to metastases of grade I papillary transitional cell carcinomas are most unusual.[156]

A second reason for a conservative diagnostic approach is that, for patients with low grade bladder lesions treated by transurethral resection, life expect-ancy approaches that of a comparable population without bladder carcinoma, provided progression to higher grade disease does not occur.[156] Similar survival rates have been found in upper tract lesions as well.[150] These figures are, if anything, conservative, as many of the smaller lesions may be treated by simple fulguration without submission of pathologic material.

Another fact of note in this regard is that only a minority of patients with bladder carcinoma die as a result of their *original* disease, and these lesions are uniformly high grade tumors at presentation, according to Cummings.[42] Furthermore, when one speaks of death from "recurrences," it should be noted that this word has been used loosely with reference to urothelial carcinoma in general and low grade papillary lesions in particular. In fact, aside from inadequate resection in certain situations, e.g., tumors involving the ureteral orifices, most such "recurrences" are thought not to be reappearances of the original tumor. It is much more likely that they are new tumors, reflective of widespread but not yet clinically apparent abnormalities throughout much of the remaining urothelium.[171] Finally, there is good reason to believe that in studies noting the increased rate of subsequent invasive disease from low grade papillary lesions *with associated mucosal atypias or carcinoma in situ*, we are in fact looking at the hole rather than the doughnut; that is, the important facet is not the papillary tumor but the associated flat mucosal abnormalities. Koss,[112] commenting on mapping studies of the urinary bladder in neoplasia, suggested that these low grade papillary lesions may be considered focal indicators of the proliferative activity in the urothelium, "per se, quite harmless, but which may be followed by other manifestations of neoplasia." Furthermore, the associated nonpapillary lesions, which would be diagnosed as atypical hyperplasia and carcinoma in situ in biopsy material, are much more likely the principal sources of invasive and eventually metastatic bladder carcinoma in these patients.

A final reason for a conservative approach to the diagnosis of low grade papillary lesions is a more general concern that is often lost in the welter of statistical data: that is, the implication of the diagnosis of "cancer" for the patient presenting with such a lesion. This fact is too often given small play, particularly in this era of sweeping schemas regarding the spectrum of neoplasia, a notable example being that of the "CIN" system in gynecologic pathology.[179] In fact, anyone who has given more than a passing thought to the development of malignant neoplasms must presume that the lesions we finally accept in most body sites as diagnostic of "cancer" represent but a late stage in the developmental process, and that recognition by whatever means of earlier stages may improve prevention or treatment and thereby prognosis. However, it must be borne in mind that wherever in the spectrum of development we as clinicians and pathologists choose to call lesions "malignant," the word, warranted or not, has obvious dire implications for the patient and family. Here the simple converse of one of the major arguments for diagnosing low grade papillary lesions as "grade I carcinomas" may be noted: Although it is obviously a matter of concern that some of the patients initially presenting with low grade papillary lesions eventually die of urothelial carcinoma (approximately 6 percent in the Kaiser Permanente series[76]), the fact remains that most, despite multiple recurrences of low grade lesions, do not. The only thing of which one can be assured is that many of the effects, both practical and emotional, of the word "carcinoma" may be the same for those in the 94 percent group and those in the less fortunate 6 percent group.

Although the conservative rather than the liberal approach to classification of papillary lesions is personally preferable, the importance of uniformity in nomenclature may supersede the above considerations, and the liberal approach seems to be the more firmly entrenched at present. Therefore that approach is reflected in this chapter. It is important to be aware, however, that not everyone subscribes to the same system of classification. This disagreement has obvious implications at the individual case level, and clear communication between clinician and pathologist regarding the system used is imperative. Here a fundamental working knowledge of the basic pathology of urothelial neoplasms is invaluable to the practicing urologist. On a larger scale, particularly when trying to assess the efficacy of published treatment methods, care must be taken to ascertain the pathologic criteria used when assigning patients to the various categories. For the pathologist, it is imperative that diagnostic terms be used with clarity and the system of nomenclature made known to the clinician. There is no room for confusion, as it can only undermine the confidence the clinician places in the pathology report, witness a respected urologist who once advised his clinical colleagues, in print, that: "All pathology specimens should be examined microscopically by the urologist, or in lieu of this, by a pathologist"![14]

UROTHELIAL NEOPLASMS: HISTOLOGIC CLASSIFICATION

The classification of urothelial neoplasms by light microscopy remains the cornerstone on which prognosis and therapy are based. Because of the difficulty of predicting the long-term course of lower-grade papillary neoplasms in particular, a number of adjunctive studies have evolved, including cell surface isoantigen evaluation, chromosome analysis, and diagnostic electron microscopic examination (see below). At the present time, however, the microscopic appearance of a given lesion is the single best predictor of tumor behavior. The standard classifications of urothelial neoplasms may be applied to lesions throughout the extent of the urothelium,[147] and, as noted, virtually all types of tumors cited are found throughout, from renal pelvis to proximal urethra. With the standard practice of assigning all papillary transitional cell lesions showing even mild histologic deviations to the low grade carcinoma category, the group of urothelial neoplasms designated benign is small, with only a few subsets. The bulk of the discussion is therefore devoted to malignant neoplasms and their classification, with the following features considered here as well as in more detail in subsequent chapters.

Epithelial Type

Tumors are segregated into the usual tissue types including transitional cell, squamous, glandular, mixed histologic, and undifferentiated carcinomas. At all sites most lesions are transitional cell in type, generally accounting for approximately 75 to 90 percent of all lesions.[69,104,140] In typical Western population studies, squamous carcinoma accounts for approximately 6 to 15 percent of lesions at all sites. Pure adenocarcinoma and undifferentiated epithelial lesions that cannot be further subclassified constitute most of the small number of remaining cases. Tumors listed as "mixed histologic type" vary from 5 to 10 percent of the total number in some studies[69] to none in other series.[140] They are generally lesions showing primarily transitional cell differentiation, with some squamous or glandular features, and the variable numbers presumably reflect the authors' particular requirements for differentiation of the subtypes.

Growth Pattern

As noted in the WHO classification of bladder tumors,[147] growth pattern, particularly the presence or absence of a papillary configuration, is an important prognostic indicator in urothelial neoplasms. With low grade carcinomas, the papillary configuration itself, when coupled with minor histologic alterations, is the feature on which the diagnosis of malignancy rests. Most of the noninvasive or only superficially invasive lesions encountered show this papillary pattern. Conversely, the presence of a "solid" or "sessile," or more simply "nonpapillary" configuration is most often associated with higher-grade lesions, usually more aggressive from inception. It should be emphasized that some high grade, deeply invasive carcinomas that are seemingly nonpapillary may still show some remnants of a papillary configuration, particularly along the superficial aspects of the tumor; this characteristic should be noted in the diagnosis. Such lesions, despite their invasiveness, may be associated with a better prognosis than their solid counterparts, as they appear less likely to involve lymphatics than solid tumors, and seem more likely to be destroyed by preoperative or definitive irradiation.[172,202]

Pathologic Grade

Despite all attempts at objectivity, grading of urothelial tumors remains in part a subjective exercise.[164] Although a four-tiered grading system is still used in some centers, the recommendation of the WHO[147] and the AFIP[20,111] that grading be limited to three levels — I, II, and III, corresponding to the traditional pathologic assessment of well, moderately, and poorly differentiated carcinoma, respectively — seems preferable. These grades may be applied to all of the epithelial subtypes seen. A drawback is found when grading transitional cell lesions, however, as

grade I carcinomas are by definition papillary, with histologic abnormalities otherwise so slight as to be unrecognizable as carcinoma in flat urothelium. Therefore all nonpapillary or solid lesions are by definition at least grade II or III histologically.

Pathologic Stage

Similar to other body sites, one prognostic dividing line in urothelial tumors is the presence or absence of invasion. If a lesion is clearly confined to its epithelial site of origin, however high the pathologic grade, that lesion per se is curable with adequate resection. The occasional reports of subsequent metastases from such lesions may be a reflection of inadequate histologic sampling of the particular tumor, with invasive areas overlooked. More often, such occurrences probably are reflective of abnormalities elsewhere in the urothelium, as areas of occult invasive disease are found not infrequently when resection specimens are examined in their entirety.[112]

In lesions still confined to the epithelial site of origin, a dichotomy in nomenclature has developed. Lesions with a flat or nonpapillary configuration, which are recognizable only by a severe degree of cytologic abnormality and architectural alteration, are designated the traditional "carcinoma in situ." Papillary lesions with no evidence of extension through the basement membrane, on the other hand, are referred to as "noninvasive" rather than "papillary carcinoma in situ." The reason for this escapes me.

If invasion has taken place, the level to which the tumor has extended is assessed, again with prognostic implication. Details of staging systems for bladder and upper tract lesions are discussed in their respective sections.

Another feature that should be noted is the manner of invasion. Lower-grade papillary lesions generally extend into the underlying tissue in a "broad front" pattern[203] (Fig. 17-23), the equivalent of en bloc extension or "pushy border" invasion referred to by Koss.[112] Tissue reaction is usually correspondingly minimal. Higher-grade lesions, conversely, more often show evidence of "tentacular" invasion, with individual cells and cell groups spreading in a disorganized fashion, most often with a surrounding fibroinflammatory response (Fig. 17-24). An additional facet that should be noted is the presence or

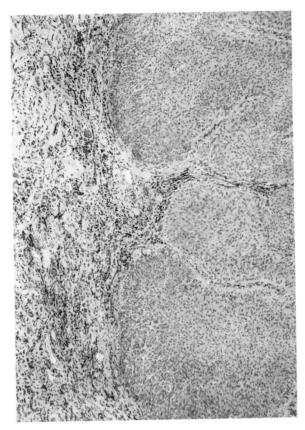

Fig. 17-23 Low grade transitional cell carcinoma of the renal pelvis invading the renal parenchyma in a "broad front" pattern. ×60.

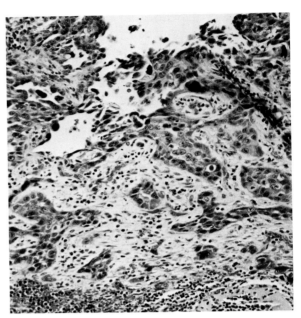

Fig. 17-24 High grade transitional cell carcinoma of the bladder invading the submucosa in a "tentacular" pattern. Note the residual in situ disease. ×126.

absence of lymphatic or vascular invasion,[147] which is discussed in more detail in subsequent chapters.

At least three major nomenclature systems for classification of urothelial neoplasms of the bladder have been proposed (Table 17-1), and these classifications may be extended to all areas of urothelium. The first is that of the WHO.[147] The second was proposed by Koss in an AFIP fascicle.[111] The third is a modification of these two by Friedell et al.,[69] used by the National Bladder Cancer Group (NBCG), formerly the National Bladder Cancer Collaborative Group A,[154] a cooperative study group responsible for many of the more rational comments on urothelial neoplasia. The latter classification has been further modified[71] to correspond more closely with the other two classifications, primarily by deleting the term "carcinoma in situ" in favor of "noninvasive" when referring to papillary lesions confined to the surface.

Some differences are immediately apparent. For example, in contrast to the AFIP classification, both the WHO and NBCG classifications retain the prefix "transitional cell" for carcinomas, and this prefix is still used almost universally in the clinical literature. The WHO classification is the most compact. However, it makes no provision for such entities as truly "mixed" tumors. Although the "mixed" tumors may behave similarly to transitional cell carcinomas with only occasional foci of squamous or glandular differentiation, this is a point that has not been adequately studied. Neither the WHO nor the NBCG classification separately categorizes "spindle and giant cell" (pleomorphic) carcinomas, and so they are presumably placed in the undifferentiated category with tumors that may be quite dissimilar.

Each system has its advantages and disadvantages. To capitalize on the former, Table 17-2 is presented as an adaptation of these three standard classifications of urothelial tumors. Each lesion is illustrated and discussed below. Benign neoplasms and certain other "tumorlike" lesions such as nephrogenic adenomas and prostatic polyps are presented, and concepts of "premalignant" states, e.g., dysplasia and atypical hyperplasia, are discussed.

Table 17-1 Urothelial Neoplasms: Morphologic Classification

WHO[147]	AFIP[111]	NBCG[71]
Transitional cell papilloma	Papilloma	Papilloma
Transitional cell papilloma, inverted type	Inverted papilloma	—
Squamous cell papilloma	—	—
Transitional cell carcinoma (grades 1, 2, 3)	Papillary carcinoma (grades I, II, III)	Papillary transitional cell carcinoma, noninvasive (grades 1, 2, 3)
	Invasive urothelial carcinoma (nonpapillary)	Transitional cell carcinoma, invasive (grades 1, 2, 3)
	Nonpapillary carcinoma in situ	Transitional cell carcinoma in situ (grade 3)
Variants of transitional cell carcinoma With squamous carcinoma With glandular metaplasia With squamous & glandular metaplasia	Mixed carcinoma	Mixed carcinoma
Squamous cell carcinoma	Squamous cell carcinoma	Squamous carcinoma
Adenocarcinoma	Adenocarcinoma	Adenocarcinoma
Undifferentiated carcinoma	—	Undifferentiated carcinoma
—	Spindle & giant cell carcinoma	—

Modified from Mostofi et al,[147] Koss,[111] and Friedell et al.[71]

Table 17-2 Urothelial Neoplasms

Benign
  Transitional cell papilloma
  Transitional cell papilloma, inverted type
  Other rare lesions (e.g., villous adenoma)
Malignant
  Transitional cell ("urothelial") carcinoma
    Papillary transitional cell carcinoma, noninvasive, invasive (grades I, II, III)
    Nonpapillary ("flat") transitional cell carcinoma in situ (grades II, III)
    Nonpapillary ("solid," "sessile") transitional cell carcinoma, invasive (grades II, III)
  Squamous carcinoma
    Squamous carcinoma in situ
    Squamous carcinoma, invasive (grades I, II, III)
  Adenocarcinoma, invasive (grades I, II, III)
  Mixed carcinoma (transitional cell–squamous, transitional cell–adeno, etc.)
  Undifferentiated carcinoma
    Small cell type
    Large cell type
  Pleomorphic carcinoma ("spindle and giant cell carcinoma")
  Carcinosarcoma ("malignant mesodermal mixed tumor")

Modified from Koss,[111] Mostofi et al.,[147] and Friedell et al.[71]

BENIGN UROTHELIAL TUMORS AND TUMORLIKE LESIONS

Transitional Cell Papilloma

As defined by such popular classifications as those of the WHO[147] and the AFIP,[111] transitional cell papillomas are distinctly uncommon tumors. (Again, it is emphasized that some institutions still use the term "papilloma" for lesions that would be clearly placed in the "papillary transitional cell carcinoma, grade I" category of the major classifications.[79,230])

These lesions are only rarely seen intact by the pathologist; more often they are incidental findings in resection specimens removed for more obvious tumors. As isolated lesions they usually measure no more than a few millimeters in diameter and, if detected cystoscopically, are often fulgurated rather than resected. Microscopically, the tumors are composed of delicate, fingerlike projections of urothelium arising from the surface mucosa and surrounding thin fibrovascular cores (Fig. 17-25). The epithelium should closely resemble normal urothelium (Fig. 17-26), with no more than seven layers of cells, according to Koss,[111] and with no cytologic abnormalities such as nuclear enlargement or hyperchromatism.

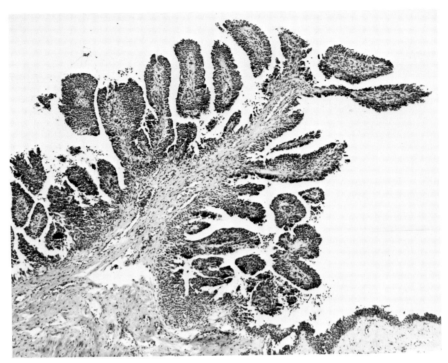

Fig. 17-25 Transitional cell papilloma. This was an incidental finding in a bladder removed because of carcinoma. ×60.

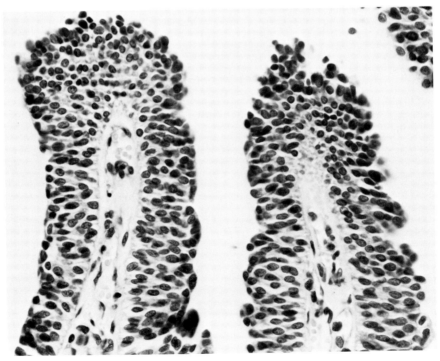

Fig. 17-26 Transitional cell papilloma. Note the virtually normal mucosal appearance aside from the papillary configuration. ×370.

These lesions are subject to surface damage with resultant hemorrhage,[20] and the pathologic findings should be interpreted cautiously in the presence of such damage.

Transitional Cell Papilloma, Inverted Type

The transitional cell papilloma, inverted type, is an unusual tumor, and is also referred to as "inverted papilloma" and "Brunnian adenoma."[108] According to DeMeester et al.,[48] it was first reported in the German literature by Paschkis[168] in 1927. In a literature review, Kunze and colleagues[117] noted that a total of 110 patients had been reported through 1980, among whom the average age was 57.3, with a male/female ratio of approximately 9:1. Approximately 80 per-

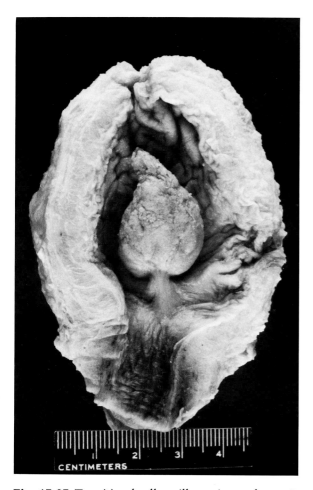

Fig. 17-27 Transitional cell papilloma, inverted type. It arises in the typical trigonal location in the bladder. (From Kim et al.,[108] with permission.)

cent of the lesions were localized in the bladder neck and trigone area, with only four cases involving the prostatic urethra and one the renal pelvis. Other cases have been reported involving the ureter[75] and the ureteropelvic junction[51]; according to Schulze et al.,[196] 24 cases of upper tract disease have now been reported. The most common presenting complaints are hematuria and symptoms related to obstruction.[48]

These inverted papillomas may be sessile or pedunculated, with the surface having a generally smooth or somewhat lobulated appearance, and they may reach considerable size (Fig. 17-27). Microscopically, the lesions are composed primarily of anastomosing epithelial cords and nests focally connected to the overlying transitional epithelium, the latter appearing hyperplastic to attenuated (Fig. 17-28). The individual cords are composed of bland cells, with peripheral perpendicular orientation and a central spindled appearance. They may have areas of squamous metaplasia and also cystic structures that may contain PAS-positive material. In some cases the latter finding is prominent, with some authors suggesting subdivision into "trabecular" and "glandular" types.[117]

At times these tumors bear morphologic similarity to very proliferative areas of cystitis cystica and glandularis. In their classic form, however, the lesions are generally considered benign neoplasms,[48] and Friedell et al.[70] considered that they may in fact be the endophytic counterpart of transitional cell papilloma. They are usually treated with local resection and fulguration. DeMeester et al.[48] noted only one recurrence in 18 patients with adequate follow-up and in only 1 in 28 cases reported in the literature to that time. It should be mentioned, however, that isolated case reports[124,231] have described lesions consistent with inverted papillomas in association with low grade transitional cell carcinoma, and a number of authorities are of the opinion that differentiation of these neoplasms from low grade carcinomas is not always clear-cut.[70,113] Therefore the overall morphologic appearance must be taken into account, with generous histologic sampling of lesions thought to be inverted papillomas before they are diagnosed as such.

Other Benign Epithelial Tumors and Tumorlike Lesions

Epithelial lesions other than the above that are considered true benign neoplasms are most uncommon, generally noted in isolated case reports. Rare exam-

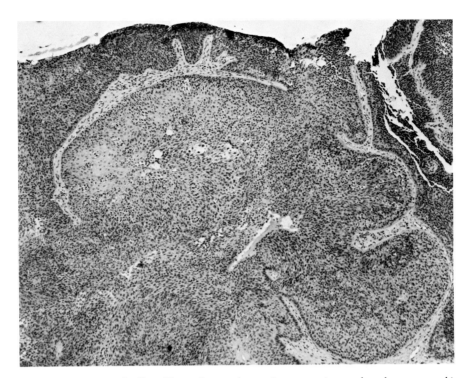

Fig. 17-28 Transitional cell papilloma, inverted type. Anastomosing cords and nests extend into the mural area, with a focal connection to the overlying mucosa. Note the perpendicular orientation of peripheral cells, with central areas varying from spindled to squamoid (upper left) in appearance. ×60.

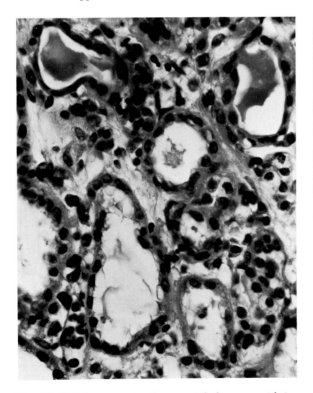

Fig. 17-29 Nephrogenic adenoma, tubular area, with intraluminal material that may be PAS-positive. ×420.

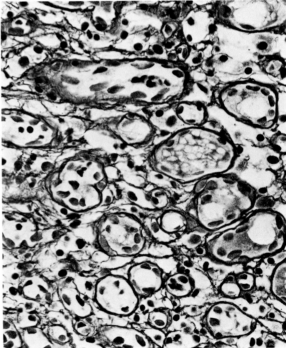

Fig. 17-30 Nephrogenic adenoma, with the silver stain demonstrating basement membranes. Reticulin stain. ×370.

ples of tumors virtually identical to villous adenomas of the intestine have been noted in the bladder[13] and urethra[174] as well as the urachus.[54] Squamous cell papillomas, presumably the squamous counterpart of transitional cell papillomas,[70] are probably rarer still. Others, such as "nephrogenic adenomas," have been considered in times past to be neoplastic in origin but are now thought more likely to represent tumorlike metaplasias. Still other lesions encountered, e.g., prostatic urethral polyps, condyloma acuminatum, and endometriosis, although nonneoplastic, may be confused with true neoplasms, particularly in biopsy material.

NEPHROGENIC ADENOMA

The nephrogenic adenoma is a "tumor" that has been described in the urinary bladder and urethra from the first through the ninth decades[199]; it is also seen, but less commonly, in the ureter and renal pelvis.[137,237] Its status as a true neoplasm has been questioned,[142,165] with more noncommittal names such as "adenomatoid polyp"[223] and "adenosis"[113] applied. At present it is thought to represent a metaplastic phenomenon occurring in the urothelium[137,199] and rarely in nonurothelial sites.[207] The cases share a common historical theme of infection, chronic irritation, previous surgical trauma, etc. Two cases have been reported following topical bacillus Calmette Guèrin (BCG) therapy for superficial carcinoma.[206] The trigonal localization of most early cases led to the hypothesis that the lesion might be related to the small portion of bladder epithelium derived from the caudal ends of the mesonephric ducts. (This anatomic area indeed been shown to share properties with nephrogenic adenomas.[49]) O'Shea et al.[165] noted, however, that as more cases have been recognized it has become evident that any portion of the urothelium may be involved.

Bhagavan et al.,[23] in a series of eight cases, indicated that nephrogenic adenoma may be mistaken at cystoscopy for papillary carcinoma or urothelial carcinoma in situ. The gross appearance in their cases ranged from granular to polypoid nodules, usually multifocal, up to 5 mm in diameter, with one lesion showing a condylomatous appearance. Most lesions are small, as in this series, but sizes up to 7 cm have been described by others.[237] Nodular or polypoid aspects may not be apparent in some cases, with 20 percent show-

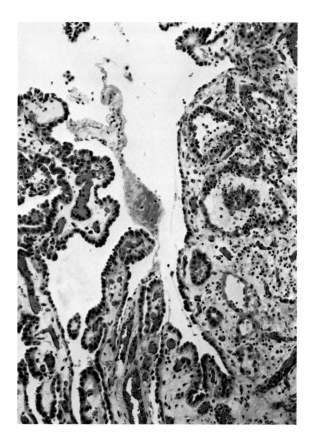

Fig. 17-31 Nephrogenic adenoma, papillary area. ×126.

ing only a flat, reddened appearance,[137] which may mimic carcinoma in situ. Microscopically, the lesions are composed of aggregates of tubular structures generally confined to the lamina propria but rarely extending into the muscularis.[237] They are lined by cuboidal to columnar cells having eosinophilic to partially cleared cytoplasm, with PAS-positive, diastase-resistant material noted in occasional lumens (Fig. 17-29). Cystic dilatation of occasional tubules is often present. Tubules are surrounded by distinct basement membranes, more readily seen by silver stain (Fig. 17-30). Similar epithelium often extends onto the surface of the lesions, with formation of delicate papillary projections (Fig. 17-31), which predominate in some cases.[237] Inflammatory infiltrate is common. Disturbing cytologic and architectural features have been noted in some cases,[23,165] but the few reported cases of presumably malignant change in these lesions are disputed.[23] At least some authors believe that they may rarely serve as precursors of adenocarcinoma, however, and some reports still suggest an association between the two.[95] In the AFIP experience, 18 of 86 patients had recurrent disease following conservative therapy, but in no case was it associated with unequivocal malignant change.[199] Certain features, e.g., large lesion size, patient age more than 35, widespread "clear cell" changes, and significant pleomorphism and mitotic activity, should suggest the possibility that one is not dealing with a nephrogenic adenoma at all but, rather, a clear cell adenocarcinoma, as emphasized by Young and Scully[236,237] (see Adenocarcinoma, below).

PROSTATIC POLYP

According to Butterick et al.,[33] prostatic polyps are found most often in young adult men who usually present with intermittent painless hematuria, or, less frequently, symptoms of obstruction or hemospermia. Other studies[178] have shown a somewhat higher average age, however, with a lesser incidence of he-

maturia. The typical location is in the prostatic urethra in the area of the verumontanum, but virtually identical masses have been reported in the membranous urethra[178] as well as the bladder proper, involving primarily the trigonal area.[178,183]

Histologically (Figs. 17-32 and 17-33) prostatic polyps usually have a papillary surface that may be covered in part by often attenuated transitional epithelium and in part by columnar epithelium that is typically prostatic in appearance. Varying numbers of glandular structures are seen within the body of the lesion. They are morphologically identical to prostatic glands, typically lined by tall columnar epithelium having basally located nuclei with a surrounding layer of flattened nuclei and even containing occasional corpora amylacea. Although there is usually no doubt as to the prostatic origin of such processes, in questionable cases it may be confirmed by immunoperoxidase demonstration of prostatic acid phosphatase and prostate-specific antigen.[178] The lesions are not considered to be neoplastic, and metaplasia, ecto-

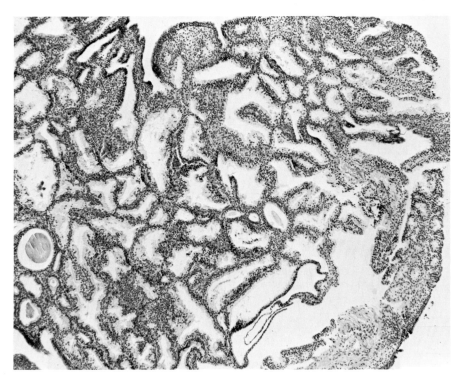

Fig. 17-32 Prostatic polyp in the prostatic urethra. Note the transitional epithelium focally along the surface with the remainder of the lesion composed of typical prostatic-type mucosa. ×60.

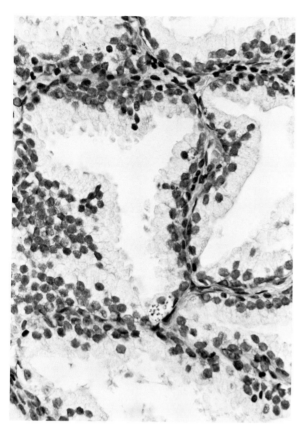

Fig. 17-33 Prostatic polyp. Prostatic-type mucosa is readily apparent. ×370.

pia, and extension from the prostatic tissue immediately underlying the urethra[183] have been considered as likely explanations for these occurrences. In most cases simple evagination of hyperplastic prostatic tissue into the prostatic urethra appears plausible,[183] but it does not explain the few cases recorded outside the area of the prostate. Simple transurethral resection or fulguration is again the treatment of choice.

CONDYLOMA ACUMINATUM

Condyloma acuminatum, a growth caused by members of the papovavirus group, has been seen with increasing frequency in clinical practice. The lesions occur chiefly in young adults but may be found in individuals of any age. Although they generally present on the external genitalia and perineal area, involvement of the vagina and cervix is not uncommon, and there may be extension of the disease to involve the urinary tract in either sex. Typical urinary involvement consists of distal urethral lesions associated with present or prior external lesions.[45,185] Involvement of the entire urethra with bladder extension has been noted, however,[24,45] which may present difficult problems from a management standpoint.

As with external lesions, those involving the urinary tract are soft, verrucous nodules that may coalesce into larger aggregates. The microscopic appearance is also typical, with mucosal features including acanthosis, varying degrees of papillomatosis, and irregular extension downward in a rete ridge pattern. Cells in the equivalent of the stratum malpighii show enlarged hyperchromatic nuclei with variable perinuclear clearing (Fig. 17-34). As with external lesions, caution against overinterpreting atypical features is in order, particularly if there has been recent topical therapy.

Most cases may be treated conservatively with excision and fulguration, cryotherapy,[185] or laser therapy.[191,204] More proximal or multiple lesions may require the addition of topical chemotherapy with agents such as 5-fluorouracil (5-FU).[45] As noted by Debenedictis and colleagues,[45] therapy must be carefully planned because of the possibility of spreading the disease proximally during instrumentation.

One other word of caution was also sounded by Walther et al.[225]: underinterpretation of "condylomatous changes" in biopsy specimens that are actually from superficial aspects of the rare verrucous carcinomas. Particularly in large lesions, biopsies from the base as well as superficial areas may help in differentiation.

OTHER LESIONS

Fibroepithelial polyps may be seen in both children and adults, most commonly involving the ureter and ureteropelvic junction[135,152,208,221] and less frequently the renal pelvis.[25,234] Essentially identical lesions may be seen in the posterior urethra in children,[64,152] and rarely in the bladder as well.[152] They are considered by most authors to be benign neoplasms of mesodermal origin but are not of consequence with regard to malignant potential. Of greater concern is the possibility of mistaking them for malignancies from a clinical or radiologic viewpoint, with needless radical surgery ensuing. They generally present no difficulties in pathologic diagnosis, as the epithelial surface lining is

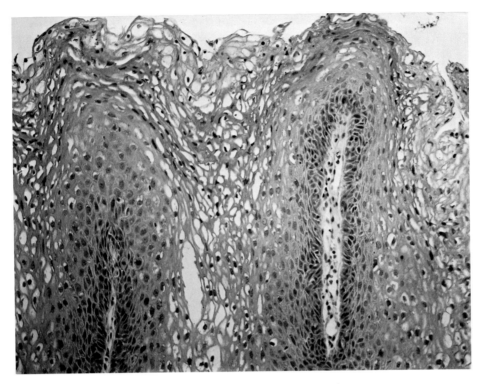

Fig. 17-34 Condyloma acuminatum of the urethra. ×148.

normal or attenuated in appearance, and the bulk of the lesion consists of the underlying fibrovascular stromal core.

Another unusual lesion sometimes noted in cystoscopic biopsy material is *endometriosis* (Fig. 17-35), as vesical involvement may be seen in 1 to 2 percent of patients with this disorder and may in fact result in a filling defect or even a palpable bladder mass.[4] Although the glands are at times somewhat disturbing, the presence of the associated endometrial stroma allows easy diagnosis. This disease is not confined to the bladder, and numerous cases of upper tract involvement, notably ureteral,[149,205] are also on record. The disease is seen most commonly during the menstrual era, but the diagnosis cannot be excluded merely because a woman is postmenopausal.[169] Nor is the disease confined to female patients: Rare cases of endometriosis have occurred in elderly men on estrogen therapy for prostatic cancer,[194] the lesions presumably arising from müllerian remnants.

Other processes that may appear clinically as possible epithelial tumors, e.g., papillary cystitis or urethri-

tis,[147] catheter-associated polypoid cystitis,[55] malakoplakia, and amyloidosis,[147] generally are readily recognized microscopically as nonneoplastic conditions.

MALIGNANT UROTHELIAL TUMORS

Papillary Transitional Cell Carcinoma

PAPILLARY TRANSITIONAL CELL CARCINOMA, GRADE I

The grade I papillary transitional cell carcinoma, generally larger than the transitional cell papilloma, may present as an isolated lesion or as one of many lesions at various sites throughout the urothelium. Grossly, the lesion appears as an irregularly lobulated mass, at times with a prominent filiform texture, raised from the surface, with minimal if any gross

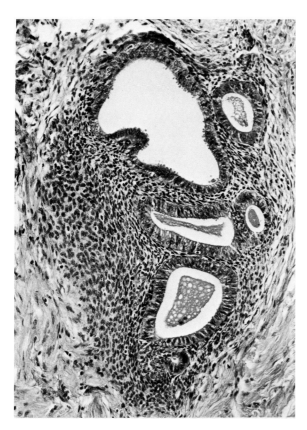

Fig. 17-35 Endometriosis involving the bladder wall. ×148.

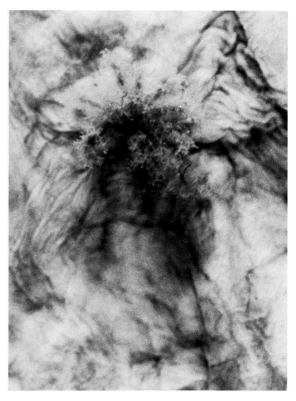

Fig. 17-36 Bladder segment with papillary transitional cell carcinoma, submerged in water to simulate its appearance at cystoscopy.

evidence of necrosis. The arborescent nature may be even more apparent at cystoscopy, as illustrated in Figure 17-36, which shows a low grade papillary carcinoma discovered at autopsy that has been photographed while submerged in water. Mural changes suggestive of invasive disease are unusual and, if present, suggest higher grade disease.

Microscopically, the appearance of individual papillae may vary from relatively short to elongated and villiform (Fig. 17-37). In contrast to the epithelium of the transitional cell papilloma, there is now a mild deviation structurally and cytologically from normal urothelium. The number of cell layers is generally increased, to more than ten, according to Koss,[111] or to more than six, according to Friedell et al.[71] Such "layer counting" may present difficulties in any given histologic section, and often considerable variation is found from one frond to the next. If reliance is placed

on this feature, one should choose areas for evaluation that appear to be perpendicularly cut, with the fibrovascular core evident centrally, as tangential cuts may artifactually increase the layer count.

At higher power (Fig. 17-38), there should be no more than a mild degree of cytologic alteration compared to normal urothelium. Abnormal features may include some loss of nuclear polarity, mild degrees of nuclear hyperchromaticity in occasional cells, and mild nuclear enlargement. Nucleoli, if present, are small and usually limited to one per nucleus. Nuclear chromatin dispersion is uniform and finely granular, and mitotic figures should be rare to absent. In many areas the superficial cell layer is still recognizable, although often attenuated. Less often these "umbrella cells" are prominent, with enlarged nuclei containing sizable nucleoli; such abnormalities are disregarded, however, provided they are *confined* to a recognizable

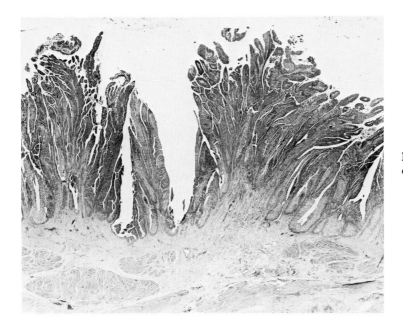

Fig. 17-37 Papillary transitional cell carcinoma, grade I, of the bladder. ×9.

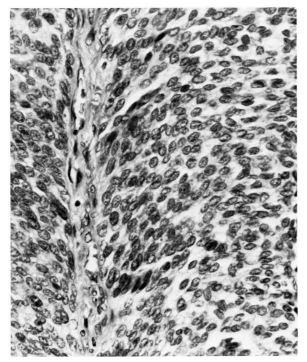

Fig. 17-38 Papillary transitional cell carcinoma, grade I. ×310.

superficial cell layer. Invasion is unusual in lesions with only the above abnormalities and, if present, almost invariably occurs with a "pushing border" (Fig. 17-23).

PAPILLARY TRANSITIONAL CELL CARCINOMA, GRADE II

Grade II papillary transitional cell carcinoma typically shows a lobulated appearance (Fig. 17-39), grossly similar to grade I papillary transitional cell carcinoma, although hemorrhage and focal necrosis may be more readily apparent. Only a minority are deeply invasive, and in these cases mural thickening may be seen in definitive resection specimens.

Microscopically, the tumor shows a still recognizable fronded appearance (Fig. 17-40) with easily discernible fibrovascular cores. There are often more than six to ten cell layers, but this feature is variable owing to loss of portions of the papillary surfaces. Compared to grade I lesions, normal maturation is disturbed, with increasingly haphazard arrangement of nuclei throughout the thickness of the epithelium. Variation in nuclear size is more apparent, as is overall nuclear enlargement, with concomitant increase in the nuclear/cytoplasmic (N/C) ratio (Fig. 17-41).

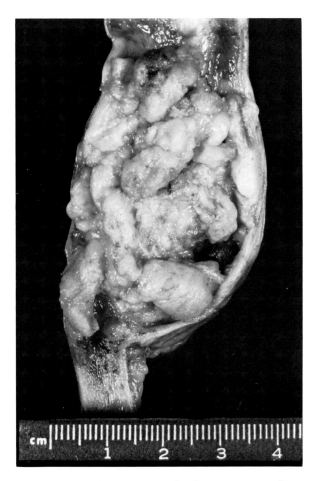

Fig. 17-39 Papillary transitional cell carcinoma, grade II, of the ureter. Note the proximal ureteral dilatation.

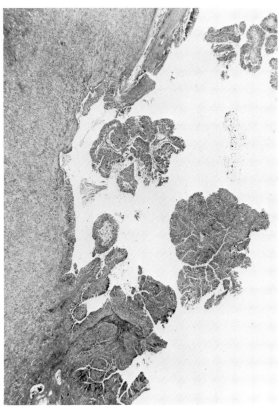

Fig. 17-40 Papillary transitional cell carcinoma, grade II, of the renal pelvis. ×11.

Nuclei appear more hyperchromatic than in grade I lesions, with a more coarsely granular texture the chromatin pattern. Nucleoli may now be seen in some cells, and mitotic figures may be identified. Scattered nuclei may show even more disturbing features, but they are in the minority; most nuclei, in contrast to grade III lesions, still have a rounded or ovoid contour. The superficial cell layer is usually retained in some areas but is often no longer recognizable in others; and focal necrosis, particularly along the surface, may be noted.

Koss[111] described a number of morphologic variants, including small cell, columnar–spindle cell, and clear cell types. Prognostic implications of the various appearances are not given, however, and such subdivision is not commonly practiced.

PAPILLARY TRANSITIONAL CELL CARCINOMA, GRADE III

Grade III papillary transitional cell carcinomas are generally the most clinically aggressive of the papillary lesions. Although the surface may still be lobulated and velvety focally (Fig. 17-42), this may be less apparent because of extensive necrosis and hemorrhage. These lesions, even at initial presentation, are often accompanied by an invasive component, with associated mural changes readily discerned on examination of resection specimens.

Histologically, the papillary nature of the lesion may be seen only in some areas (Fig. 17-43), but in others, where there is a great deal of necrosis, it may be no longer recognizable. For reasons noted above, these lesions should still be placed into the papillary category despite their paucity of papillary areas.

At the microscopic level, we have finally arrived at a stage where virtually all pathologists would agree on

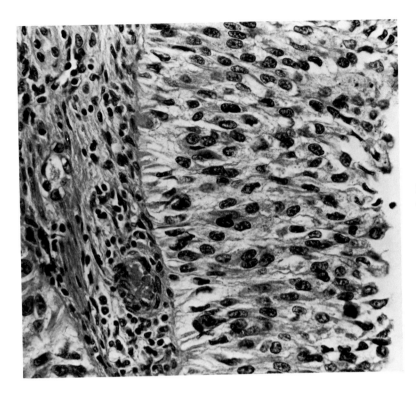

Fig. 17-41 Papillary transitional cell carcinoma, grade II. ×310.

a diagnosis of "carcinoma" by morphologic standards applied to other organ sites. Architecturally, the epithelium shows considerable variation in cell layer number, and all vestiges of organization from base to surface of the papillary fronds may be lost (Fig. 17-44). Recognizable superficial cells are generally absent. There is marked anisonucleosis, with prominent nuclear enlargement, a high N/C ratio in many cells, nuclear membrane irregularities, and a prominent increase in chromaticity in many nuclei. The chromatin pattern is coarse, with abnormal parachromatin clearing. Nucleoli are often prominent in these high grade tumors and are frequently multiple; macronucleoli may also be seen. However, some high grade tumors show all of the other nuclear features of malignancy but have few recognizable nucleoli. Mitotic figures are found without difficulty, and abnormal mitoses may also be present.

An interesting paradox has been found in the evaluation of high grade lesions by immunohistochemical methods. Ramaekers and colleagues[175] noted that although both normal and neoplastic urothelium express keratin positivity, studies of a subtype of intermediate filament protein—cytokeratin 18—showed

somewhat unexpected results. In normal urothelium, this protein is expressed only in superficial cells, presumably the most differentiated cells of the mucosa. Low grade papillary tumors give a similar pattern, i.e., staining of only superficial cells, with deeper cells negative. Intermediate grade tumors, however, were noted to show single cells and clusters in the deeper layers now positive for cytokeratin 18, with cases of high grade papillary carcinoma, carcinoma in situ, and invasive carcinoma showing positive staining throughout. The implications of these unexpected findings are not known.

Nonpapillary Transitional Cell Carcinoma

NONPAPILLARY ("FLAT") TRANSITIONAL CELL CARCINOMA IN SITU

Nonpapillary ("flat") transitional cell carcinoma in situ may be found throughout the urothelium, either as an isolated entity or in association with solid or papillary carcinomas. The natural history of the le-

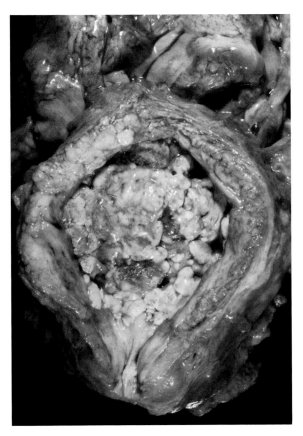

Fig. 17-42 Papillary transitional cell carcinoma, grade III, of the bladder. Note the mural involvement.

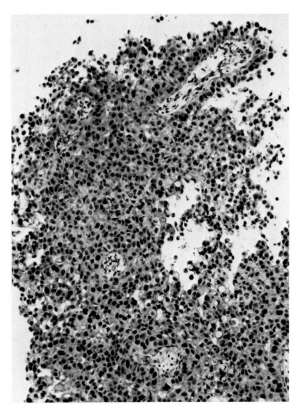

Fig. 17-43 Papillary transitional cell carcinoma, grade III, of the bladder. ×110.

sion, when found without accompanying tumors in the bladder, is not well defined (a subject covered in depth in Chapter 18). Even less is known about its behavior in the renal pelvis and ureter, as it is rarely discovered in the absence of clinically recognizable upper tract or vesical malignancies. Whatever the clinical setting, however, it must be considered a potential precursor lesion to overt high grade invasive transitional cell neoplasms, an association first suggested by Melicow[139] during the early 1950s.

If detectable at all, the gross appearance may be subtle during cytoscopic examination and even more so in resection specimens. In patients with extensive bladder involvement (those most often symptomatic), cystoscopy may reveal an appearance similar to that seen with cystitis. In fact, a significant percentage of patients initially thought to have "interstitial cystitis" in particular on clinical and cystoscopic grounds may

actually have carcinoma in situ.[239] Areas of mottled reddish discoloration may be found, slightly raised or granular in appearance, with poorly defined borders.[220] In patients with more focal disease, often asymptomatic and picked up incidentally by urinary cytology, attempts at cystoscopic definition of the lesion may be disappointing.[88]

Microscopically, these lesions are, by definition, confined to their site of origin. Various subtypes have been noted,[111] including large cell and small cell varieties, but the value of such subcategorization, if any, is not clear. A two-grade system for "flat" transitional cell carcinoma has been utilized, corresponding to those changes seen in grades II and III papillary lesions.[69] The former is best seen in flat areas associated with intermediate grade papillary neoplasms (Fig. 17-45); it is characterized by moderate anisonucleosis, nuclear enlargement, occasional mitotic figures, and in particular a haphazard nuclear arrangement with

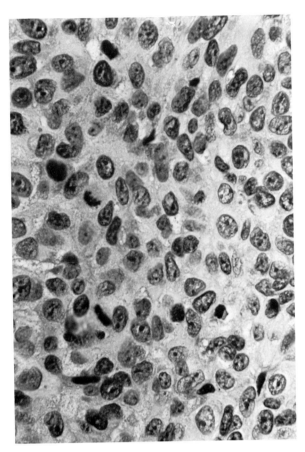

Fig. 17-44 Papillary transitional cell carcinoma, grade III. ×310.

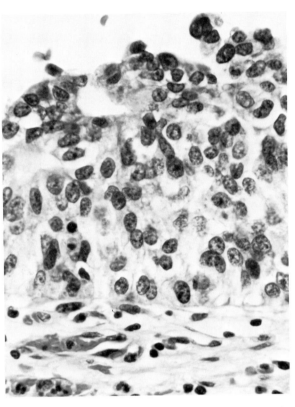

Fig. 17-45 Nonpapillary transitional cell carcinoma in situ, grade II. ×500.

loss of polarity. The number of cell layers may be increased but this is not necessary for diagnosis.

The prognostic significance of such division has not been clarified, and in fact most major classifications at present recognize only a single grade of flat transitional cell carcinoma in situ.[71,111,147] I would favor retention of a two-tiered system, however, with the designation of "grade III" carcinoma in situ reserved for those cases with an appearance generally corresponding to that of grade III papillary and invasive nonpapillary neoplasms (Fig. 17-46). One would think intuitively that patients with in situ lesions as depicted in Fig. 17-46 might fare worse than those with lesions similar to that seen in Figure 17-45.

Nuclear pleomorphism is the most striking feature in grade III lesions. There is usually complete loss of normal architectural arrangement, with mitotic figures frequently detectable, and nucleoli, particularly macronucleoli, often evident. Again, however, in contrast to prostatic carcinomas, for example, nucleoli may be inapparent even in lesions that otherwise show all of the nuclear features of high grade malignancy. As noted by Murphy,[151] mucosa from areas of carcinoma in situ is readily detached, either at cystoscopy or during processing; and biopsy specimens from these areas often show mucosa partially denuded of epithelium, leaving nothing more than an inflamed base, usually with a prominent vascular pattern. Diligent search, occasionally necessitating multiple-step sections through the biopsy blocks, often eventually reveals at least a few adherent cells. These cells, if adequately preserved, may show sufficient pleomorphism to warrant a diagnosis of carcinoma in situ (Fig. 17-47). The yield in these cases may also be increased by separate cytologic processing of the fluid in which the biopsy specimens are submitted, as it may contain residual grossly inapparent yet diagnostically helpful material.[44]

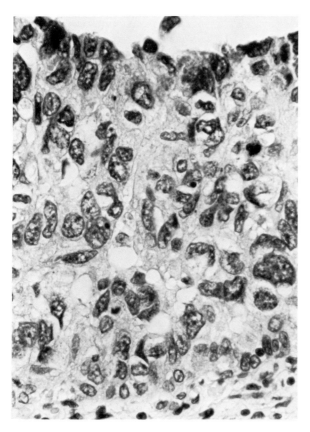

Fig. 17-46 Nonpapillary transitional cell carcinoma in situ, grade III. ×450.

DYSPLASIA, ATYPIA, AND ATYPICAL HYPERPLASIA

As a corollary to the topic of carcinoma in situ, dysplasia, atypia, and atypical hyperplasia are briefly considered as it is obvious that urothelial changes of carcinoma in situ do not result from instantaneous morphologic transformation. Thorough examination of a cystectomy specimen with carcinoma in situ reveals a number of areas showing some but not all of the changes described above. The changes vary from one site to another, with some foci showing occasional atypical nuclei with otherwise normal maturation, others a disorderly nuclear arrangement yet with little in the way of individual cell atypia, etc. Categorization of these abnormalities is controversial,[70,72,228] but conventional terms applied to other areas, such as dysplasia,[70,151,228] atypia, and atypical hyperplasia[115] (dysplastic nuclear features with an in-creased epithelial thickness), are used in practice. Dysplasia and atypia are used synonymously by some but not by others,[228] and the former appears to have gained the greater popularity with reference to changes in the neoplastic spectrum. Whatever the term used, these alterations are considered to be at least potentially representative of "premalignant lesions,"[70] and morphologic criteria for their recognition have been proposed by authorities in the field.[70,153]

In the early portion of this morphologic spectrum, the significance of mild changes is difficult to define. Focal abnormalities (e.g., increased mucosal thickness, mild anisonucleosis, some loss of nuclear polarity, occasional hyperchromatic nuclei, and mitotic figures) are certainly seen on occasion as isolated entities, particularly in inflammatory situations (Fig. 17-48), at times to a striking degree (Fig. 17-19). (As an aside, it is emphasized that the pathologist should take every opportunity to become familiar with the surprisingly wide range of urothelial abnormalities seen in "reactive settings." The alterations in nephrectomy specimens in cases of lithiasis and transurethral prostatic resection specimens, particularly those from recently instrumented patients, can be instructive in this regard.) In other cases, such alterations may in fact be the first morphologic evidence of neoplastic change, but at the present time there is no completely reliable way to sort out which is which. Diagnostically, such changes must be taken in context by both pathologist and urologist.

Figure 17-49, from a renal pelvic section, illustrates such a case. The atypical features are similar in magnitude to those seen in Figure 17-48. This section, however, was taken immediately adjacent to the base of a grade II papillary transitional cell carcinoma, which showed essentially identical cytologic features. Therefore, *in this setting,* this picture would qualify for the diagnosis of a "precursor lesion" of neoplasia. Certainly, if the setting is not clear, the possibility that such changes represent preneoplastic lesions should be noted, with careful clinical follow-up advised.

At the far end of the spectrum, areas of urothelium may be seen that show most of the features of carcinoma in situ but still fall short of typical carcinoma in situ in one respect or another. The finding of even a few *nonsuperficial* cells with markedly atypical nuclei, particularly along the basilar layer, should arouse suspicion, as this may reflect "pagetoid spread" (Fig.

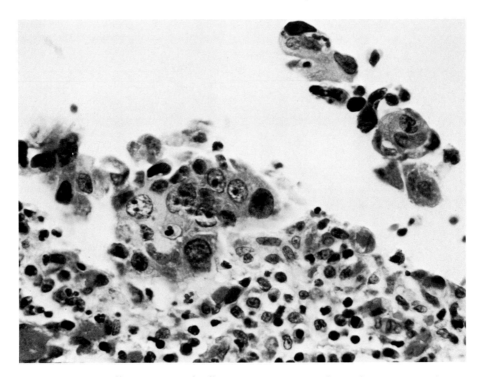

Fig. 17-47 Nonpapillary transitional cell carcinoma in situ, grade III, demonstrating the common phenomenon of partial mucosal denudation. ×500.

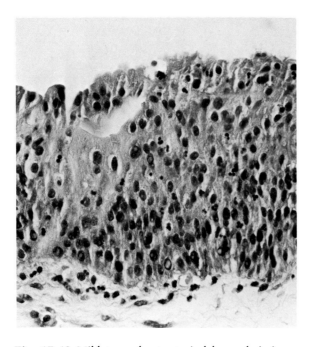

Fig. 17-48 Mild to moderate atypical hyperplasia in an inflammatory setting. ×300.

17-50) from adjacent areas of overt in situ or invasive disease. Simple perusal of the edges of histologic foci of carcinoma in situ demonstrate how common this phenomenon is. Finding such cells in a biopsy section should lead to further cuts, which may reveal a fully developed picture of carcinoma in situ. The reader is again cautioned against "overinterpretation" for both histologic and cytologic preparations when such abnormalities are limited to apparently superficial cells (Fig. 17-51). As Murphy[151] indicated, these cells often react to various noxious stimuli and may develop large nuclei with many of the features of malignancy, yet be of no apparent prognostic importance. Even the more strikingly altered cells usually have generous amounts of cytoplasm, with normal or low N/C ratios; moreover, particularly when they are multinucleated, they are easily recognized by both appearance and position over subjacent normal mucosa. This differentiation is not always clear-cut, however. On occasion, bizarre cells with many of the features of superficial cells, particularly a low N/C ratio, may also be seen focally along the surface of high grade malignancies (Fig.

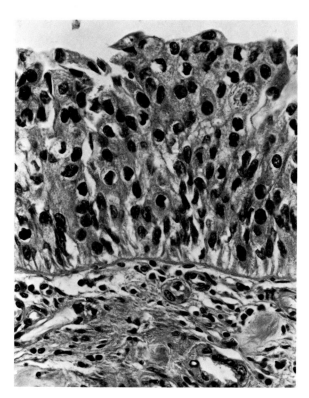

Fig. 17-49 Mild to moderate atypical hyperplasia found adjacent to grade II papillary transitional cell carcinoma. ×310.

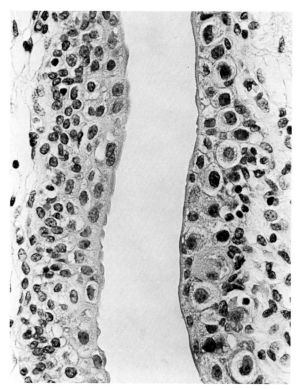

Fig. 17-50 "Pagetoid spread" of high grade malignancy. In this ureteral section the right side shows scattered cells identical to those which were seen in adjacent mucosa with overt carcinoma in situ. ×391.

17-52), and they are obviously part of the malignant process. Perhaps the safest course of action for the pathologist is to avoid making firm judgments regarding "preneoplastic" alterations when nuclear abnormalities are *confined* to apparent superficial cells. This point is most important when assessing follow-up biopsy material in patients being treated with topical chemotherapy, where superficial cells overlying otherwise normal urothelium seem particularly prone to rather bizarre changes in appearance.[157]

The unpredictability of disease progression in patients with dysplasia and atypical hyperplasia is emphasized. Some may go for years with no evidence of deterioration, whereas others seem to progress rapidly to invasive disease and death. This may be a reflection of more serious alterations outside the available biopsy material, but it must also be noted that direct invasion from areas showing a morphologic appearance of no more than dysplasia or atypical hyperplasia has been documented,[112] and such diagnoses must be viewed with concern by the clinician.

NONPAPILLARY TRANSITIONAL CELL CARCINOMA, INVASIVE

It is difficult to state with certainty what percentage of urothelial malignancies are purely "solid" (i.e., nonpapillary) lesions from their inception. Melicow,[140] surveying more than 900 bladder malignancies seen over a 10-year period, observed that approximately 80 percent of the lesions were papillary and approximately 20 percent nonpapillary. A somewhat higher percentage of nonpapillary lesions may be seen in the upper tract.[85,159] One factor tending to obscure the true number of solid tumors is that they may be found in association with papillary neoplasms,[203] and thus a given patient may fall into either category. A second is that high grade, invasive papillary lesions may lose all vestiges of their papillary configuration as a result of surface necrosis, ulceration, etc., and there is evidence that many solid tumors have probably evolved from preexisting papillary ones.[155] Even in far

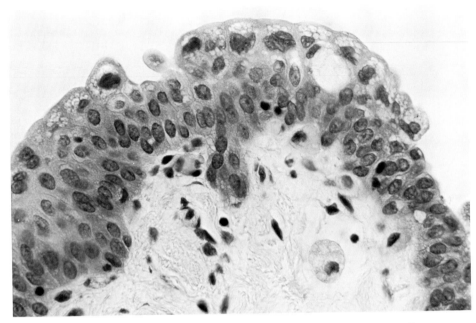

Fig. 17-51 Marked nuclear abnormalities are present, confined to superficial cells. Note the multinucleation, low nuclear/cytoplasmic (N/C) ratio, and comparatively normal underlying cells in the intermediate and basilar layers. ×500.

advanced tumors, however, any remnants of papillary growth should be mentioned in the diagnosis because of the possibility of a greater degree of radiosensitivity and the lesser likelihood of lymphatic or vascular invasion in these tumors.

Although the true percentages are difficult to define, there remains a subgroup of patients who present *ab initio* with nonpapillary invasive malignancies, presumably originating directly from areas of carcinoma in situ or atypical hyperplasia.[112] These lesions usually

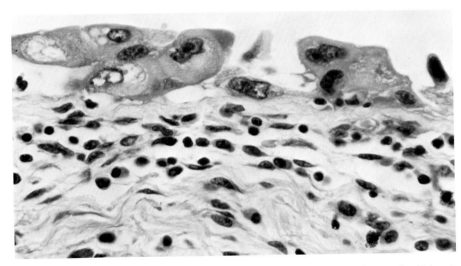

Fig. 17-52 High grade transitional cell carcinoma in situ, with markedly abnormal cells bearing a resemblance to superficial cells (see text). ×510.

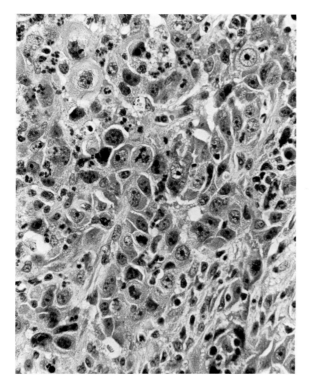

Fig. 17-53 Nonpapillary ("solid") transitional cell carcinoma, grade III. ×310.

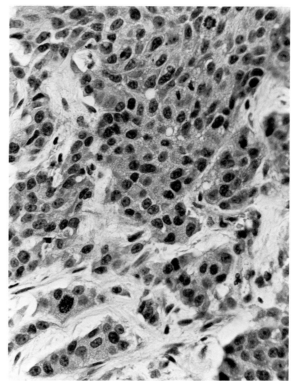

Fig. 17-54 Nonpapillary ("solid") transitional cell carcinoma, grade II. ×310.

show an irregularly nodular appearance grossly, with variable coloration ranging from white-tan to dark red-brown. Focal hemorrhage, ulceration, and necrosis are often apparent. Cut section usually readily reveals gross evidence of invasion, with firm, whitish areas of mural distortion and occasionally necrosis.

Microscopically, such lesions are most often high grade malignancies, (Fig. 17-53) with nuclear pleomorphism obvious, mitotic figures easily identified, and abnormal mitoses often present. Cytologically, these tumors correspond to grade III papillary neoplasms. Occasional tumors that appear as otherwise typical nonpapillary neoplasms may show a lesser degree of cytologic atypia (Fig. 17-54), and they may be classified as grade II carcinomas. In fact, there may be considerable variation from one area to another in a given tumor, and prognosis with these lesions is much more dependent on stage than grade. These lesions typically infiltrate in a tentacular pattern (Fig. 17-54), with varying degrees of surrounding fibroinflammatory response. Compared to papillary lesions of similar grade, they are more likely to exhibit lymphatic or

vascular invasion (Fig. 17-55), although diligent search may be necessary to identify this feature.

Squamous Carcinoma (In Situ and Invasive)

The incidence of squamous carcinoma of the bladder and upper urinary tract varies from series to series, with figures ranging from approximately 3 to 13 percent,[69,79,102] presumably due to variation in histologic criteria for establishing the diagnosis. One reason for the variability is the fact that the morphologic hallmarks of squamous differentiation (keratin pearl formation, individual cell keratinization, and prominent intercellular bridge formation) may become less and less apparent in more poorly differentiated tumors. Lesions that would be classified as high grade squamous carcinomas in other sites such as lung, where squamous lesions are typically seen, merge imperceptibly with poorly differentiated transitional cell lesions in the urothelium.

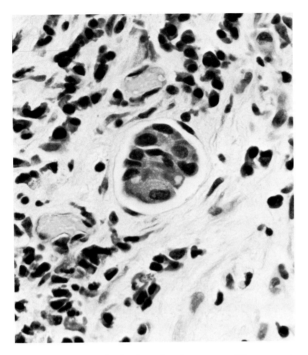

Fig. 17-55 Lymphatic invasion by nonpapillary transitional cell carcinoma. Note the identifiable endothelial lining cells. ×500.

Moreover, various systems of classification demand more or less in the way of such overt squamous differentiation for the diagnosis of squamous carcinoma. One pathologist's squamous carcinoma may be another's mixed transitional cell–squamous carcinoma or poorly differentiated transitional cell carcinoma with focal squamous differentiation.

Our practice has been to classify lesions as squamous carcinoma if they are purely squamous *or* if they show focal squamous differentiation in an otherwise obviously high grade tumor with little in the way of other differentiation. If a distinct pattern of transitional cell or adenocarcinomatous differentiation is seen elsewhere, they are then classified as mixed carcinomas (see below).

Grossly, squamous carcinomas tend much more often to be solitary than their transitional cell counterparts, at least in Western populations.[102] In certain Eastern populations where squamous carcinoma is the predominant lesion, most often in association with schistosomiasis,[57,59] multiple lesions are present in up to 25 percent of cases.[59] Again, in contrast to transitional cell lesions, the typical picture is that of an ulcerated, infiltrating tumor (Fig. 17-56), rarely exo-

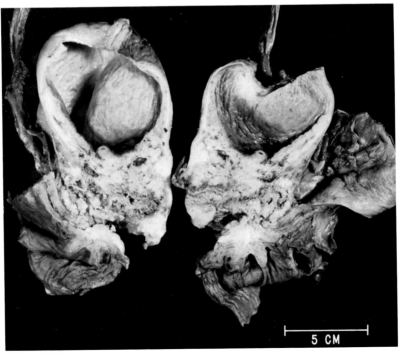

5 CM

Fig. 17-56 Squamous carcinoma of the bladder, with extension into surrounding soft tissue and invasion of the rectum.

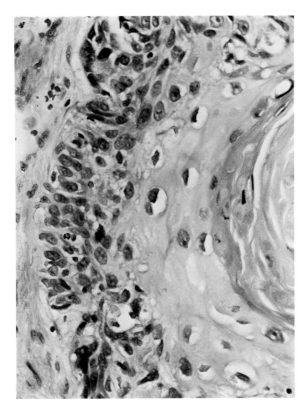

Fig. 17-57 Squamous carcinoma, grade I. Maturation is seen from the periphery (left) of the tumor nest, with increasing keratinization and central "pearl" formation (right). Compare the nuclear features with those seen in Figure 17-58. ×270.

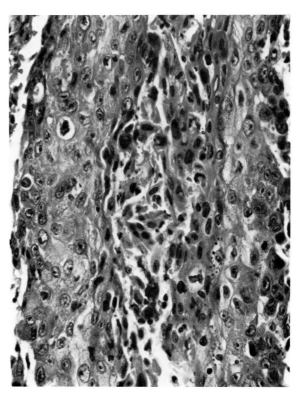

Fig. 17-58 Squamous carcinoma, grade II. Nuclear features are more disturbing than those in a low grade lesion (Fig. 17-57); but maturation, with central keratinization, is still easily recognized. ×285.

phytic or fungating, often deeply invasive at the time of initial presentation.[102] They are usually whitish, at times with a somewhat grumous appearance in tumors with prominent keratinization.

Histologically, grade I, or well differentiated tumors (Fig. 17-57) generally infiltrate in a sheetlike pattern. Basaloid cells rim the aggregates, and cells with progressively increasing amounts of eosinophilic cytoplasm are found centrally, with varying degrees of individual cell keratinization and keratin pearl formation.

Although the degree of cytoplasmic differentiation tends to decrease with increasing nuclear grade, it should be kept in mind that it is not always the case. When grading squamous lesions, therefore, particular attention must be paid to the nuclear features, which in grade I lesions tend to be bland, with only mild degrees of pleomorphism and mitotic activity. Grade II squamous carcinomas exhibit more disturbing nu-

clear features (Fig. 17-58), and a grade III designation is generally reserved for tumors with pronounced nuclear pleomorphism and mitotic activity. These tumors often show only focal cytoplasmic differentiation, such as poorly developed keratin pearls (Fig. 17-59), or just foci of cells with eosinophilic cytoplasm and prominent intercellular bridge formation (Fig. 17-60).

Histologic grade is of less help prognostically in patients with squamous carcinoma of the urothelium compared to those with transitional cell carcinoma.[57,102] One of the reasons may be overemphasis on the cytoplasmic aspects of the cells. When assigning grade to these tumors, again the pathologist is urged to pay more attention to nuclear details and less to the degree of cytoplasmic differentiation. Also, these tumors may be less apt to show uniformity throughout than their transitional cell counterparts, and tumors showing considerable variation in grade

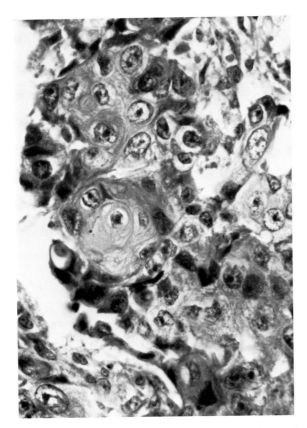

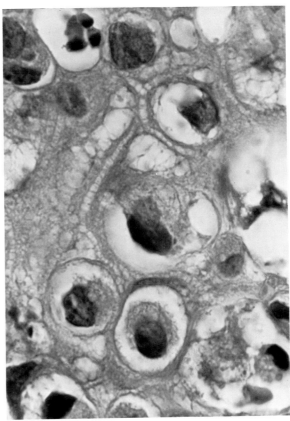

Fig. 17-59 Squamous carcinoma, grade III. A small area of "pearl" formation is seen to the left of center. The tumor otherwise showed little recognizable cytoplasmic differentiation, with typical nuclear features of a high grade lesion. ×500.

Fig. 17-60 Squamous carcinoma, grade III, with intercellular bridge formation. ×1080.

from one microscopic focus to the next are not uncommon. In such cases, as with tumors at other body sites, grade is assigned on the basis of the most poorly differentiated areas.

In situ squamous carcinoma may be seen focally in association with invasive carcinoma. As an isolated entity, it is rare in the urinary tract in Western populations, and the prognostic implications, although assumed to be similar to those of transitional cell carcinoma, are essentially unknown.[70] Figure 17-61 illustrates residual in situ disease adjacent to a deeply invasive carcinoma. The epithelium exhibits obviously malignant nuclear features as well as typical cytoplasmic features of squamous differentiation.

Rare examples of verrucous carcinoma may also be seen in the urothelium.[225] Although unusual in Western populations, El-Bolkainy et al.[57] noted a 3 to 4 percent incidence of verrucous carcinoma in tumors associated with schistosomiasis. The lesion illustrated in Figure 17-62 was classified as a carcinoma primarily on the basis of its large size and noticeable cytologic atypia, with some extension into the lamina propria in a "broad front" pattern. The morphologic similarities to condyloma acuminatum are obvious, and it is again emphasized that adequate biopsy specimens of such lesions be taken from the base as well as the superficial areas, particularly when dealing with large lesions.[225]

Adenocarcinoma

Primary adenocarcinomas of urothelial origin are uncommon lesions, accounting for only a small percentage of cases in any major series of bladder malignancies; they are equally uncommon in the upper tract. The single exception to this rule occurs in patients with bladder exstrophy, where adenocarcinomas comprise more than 80 percent of bladder

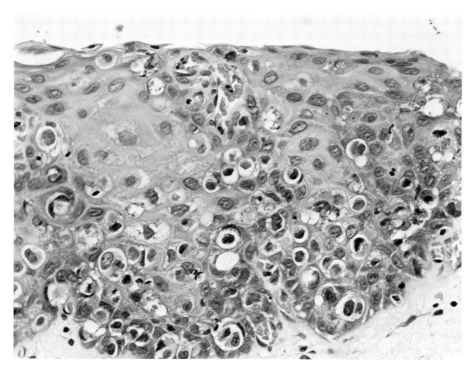

Fig. 17-61 Area of residual squamous carcinoma in situ in a patient with a deeply invasive squamous carcinoma. ×310.

malignancies.[163] Among cases of bladder adenocarcinoma not associated with exstrophy, those occurring in urachal remnants constitute a sizable number, estimates varying from approximately 10 percent[53] to more than one-third[148,216] of all cases. The mere presence of urachal remnants, however, in contrast to the exstrophy situation, does not appear to predispose to adenocarcinoma or other malignancies. Careful examination of unselected autopsy cases reveals such remnants to be present in 30 to 70 percent of all bladders examined,[27,195] with approximately two-thirds of the remnants showing transitional epithelial lining and the remainder columnar epithelium.

In contrast to transitional cell lesions, approximately 75 percent[148] to 90 percent[10] of adenocarcinomas are solitary tumors, predominantly sessile but at times papillated, often with a glary mucoid surface. Glandular metaplasia[1] and significant dysplastic lesions[158] may be seen in adjacent mucosa on occasion, but we are not aware of any reported cases of in situ adenocarcinoma without an associated invasive component. These tumors may be found throughout the urothelium, with a disproportionate number of bladder primaries found in the region of the dome,[10] pre-

sumably reflective of urachal origin in this location. Mostofi et al.[148] established criteria for delineation of urachal primaries (see Ch. 18), although these tumors may be so extensive at the time of diagnosis that origin from surface epithelium cannot be definitely excluded.

Histologically, virtually all of the standard types of adenocarcinoma found elsewhere have been described in the urothelium,[1,10] including gland-forming (Fig. 17-63), papillary (Fig. 17-64), mucinous (Fig. 17-65), and signet ring cell.[29,38,47] "Clear cell" tumors (Fig. 17-66), may also be seen, a subject reviewed by Young and Scully.[236] These tumors resemble clear cell or mesonephric carcinomas of the female genital tract, with a typical clear cell and "hobnail cell" appearance; they may occur in the urethra[36,236] and the bladder.[236] They show glycogen as well as focal mucin positivity.[236] Of greatest importance, they are occasionally confused with nephrogenic adenomas,[237] particularly in biopsy material, but features such as large size, abundant cytoplasmic clearing, prominent glycogen content, nuclear pleomorphism, and mitotic activity are helpful for defining the lesion as a clear cell adenocarcinoma. "Endometrial adenocarcinoma" arising in

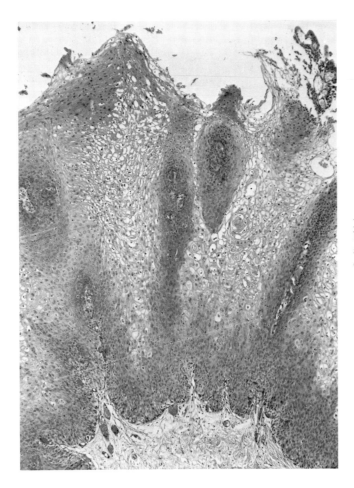

Fig. 17-62 Verrucous carcinoma of the bladder. Note the "condylomatous" appearance and the broad front extension into underlying stroma. ×51.

the prostatic ducts may also present as a gland-forming lesion in the urethra, similar in appearance to routine endometrial carcinomas, but this lesion may be defined as such by the demonstration of acid phosphatase.[238]

Urothelial adenocarcinomas are usually morphologically identical to adenocarcinomas found elsewhere, often with a striking resemblance to intestinal primaries by light microscopy as well as by histochemical, immunochemical, and ultrastructural analyses.[1,7] Because of their rarity, it is incumbent on the clinician to exclude the possibility of metastasis from a covert primary elsewhere. The finding of residual in situ transformation, often of help in establishing tumor origin at other body sites, is unusual in primary urothelial adenocarcinomas, so its absence does not exclude a urothelial origin. The conclusion regarding the primary site is more often a clinical than a pathologic one.

Prognostically, tumor grade for adenocarcinoma is assigned in the usual fashion for the sake of uniformity, with poorly differentiated, signet ring cell tumors apparently the most aggressive of the lot.[47] However, whatever the grade assigned, many of these tumors are far advanced at the time of presentation; and, as with squamous carcinomas, tumor stage appears to be the most important factor.[10] Even in series where well differentiated tumors predominate,[101] high-stage disease appears to be the rule rather than the exception.

Mixed Carcinoma

Mixed patterns of epithelial differentiation are seen in urothelial malignancies at all sites. The typical situation is that of transitional cell carcinoma with focal squamous or glandular differentiation (Fig. 17-67), at times with all three patterns noted in the same tumor. Such squamous or glandular foci may be seen in as

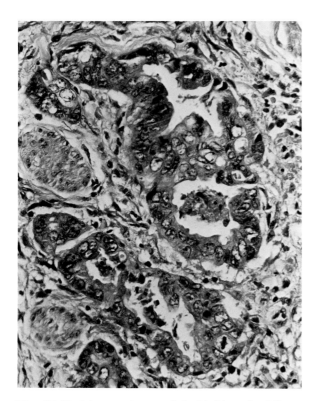

Fig. 17-63 Adenocarcinoma of the bladder, gland-forming type. ×276.

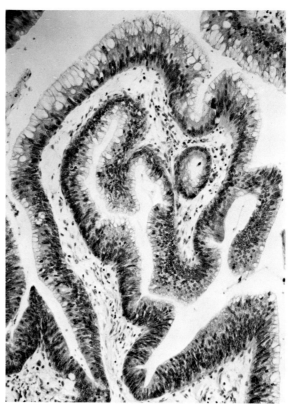

Fig. 17-64 Adenocarcinoma of the bladder, papillary type. ×113.

many as 65 percent of high grade transitional cell tumors,[155] but it is unusual to see areas of squamous or glandular alteration in low grade papillary transitional cell carcinomas. Other, much less common alterations, such as trophoblastic metaplasia, complete with human chorionic gonadotropin (hCG) production,[32] are encountered occasionally.

The exact frequency of "mixed" tumors is difficult to assess from the literature. One large series of bladder tumors[69] revealed that approximately 6 percent had a mixed pattern. Richie[180] noted that approximately 20 percent of ureteral tumors may demonstrate some evidence of squamous or glandular differentiation. Fraley[67] indicated that transitional cell tumors account for approximately 90 percent of all renal pelvic carcinomas, "often accompanied by either squamous or glandular metaplasia or both." He pointed out that electron microscopic examination of many cancers that appear to be pure transitional cell neoplasms by light microscopy reveals ultrastructural features consistent with squamous carcinoma in particular. Focal evidence of secretory activity is also not

uncommon in high grade transitional cell lesions. This evidence ranges from prominent glandular structures, strongly mucicarminophilic, to more subtle individual cell vacuolation, mucin-variable, presumably corresponding to intracytoplasmic lumen formation, with ultrastructural characteristics as described by Alroy et al.[6] We have found the latter feature to be particularly common in high grade transitional cell tumors; however, it is of unknown significance, as we have occasionally seen it in more bland low grade tumors as well.

The WHO classification[147] suggests that such mixed lesions should be classified as "variants of transitional cell carcinoma," noting the usual predominance of the transitional cell pattern. We classify lesions that are predominantly transitional cell in type as such, with a notation of minor squamous or glandular elements. However, we also believe that lesions exhibiting a truly "mixed" appearance, with more than one type of differentiation prominent, should be

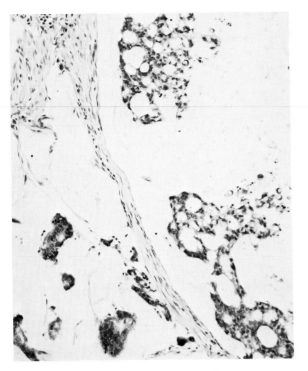

Fig. 17-65 Adenocarcinoma of the bladder, mucinous or "colloid" type. ×124.

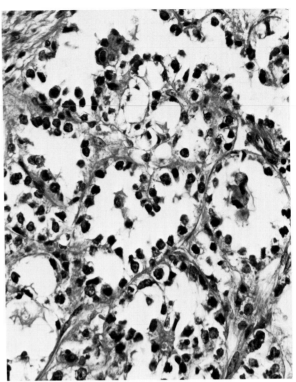

Fig. 17-66 Clear cell adenocarcinoma of the urethra. ×280.

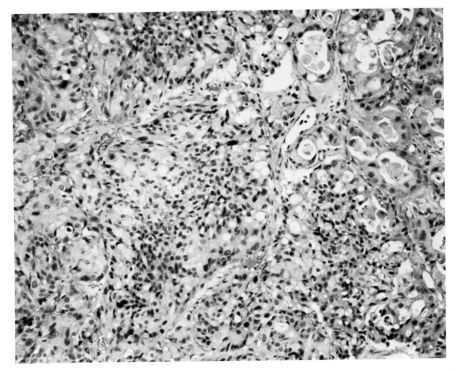

Fig. 17-67 Mixed carcinoma. Note the poorly differentiated transitional cell carcinoma (left), with gland-forming adenocarcinoma (right). ×124.

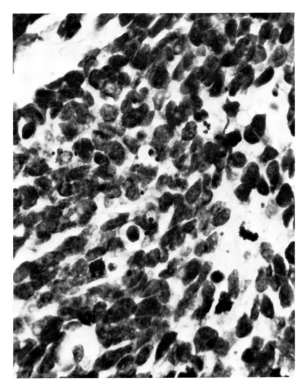

Fig. 17-68 Undifferentiated carcinoma, small cell type. Note the typical hyperchromatic nuclei, with some degree of nuclear molding, and a virtually indiscernible cytoplasmic component to the individual cells. ×512.

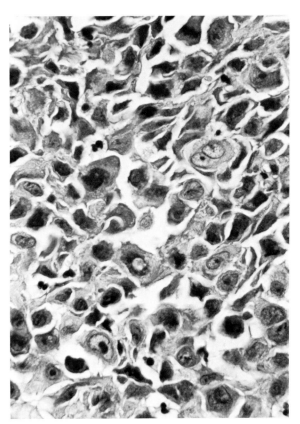

Fig. 17-69 Undifferentiated carcinoma, large cell type. ×500.

separately classified in order to gain more meaningful data on their behavior. From the limited information available, however, the behavior of tumors with mixed differentiation appears to be similar to that of tumors with a single pattern of differentiation, and outcome generally depends on the stage and grade of the disease.[111]

Undifferentiated Carcinoma

Sometimes urothelial malignancies are encountered that defy classification because of lack of any discernible differentiation along the lines outlined above. Such lesions are distinctly unusual, accounting for only 0.2 percent of more than 450 bladder primaries examined by Friedell et al.[69] As noted by these authors, the diagnosis is one of exclusion.

The WHO classification[147] indicates that the word "undifferentiated" should be used in a histologic

sense to denote "primitive tissue" and not as a synonym for anaplasia. Lesions with varying appearance have been included in this category.[147] Tumor cells are often loosely cohesive and may infiltrate in patterns that suggest nonepithelial derivation. Individual cells show varying amounts of cytoplasm, usually with a high N/C ratio. Nuclear pleomorphism varies from a small degree, with an appearance virtually identical to that of small cell undifferentiated lung primaries (Fig. 17-68), to prominent pleomorphism (Fig. 17-69), analogous to large cell undifferentiated lung primaries. The former in particular may be found in pure form or coexistent with areas of recognizable transitional cell, squamous, or glandular malignancy[233]; it may also be found to have arisen elsewhere in the area, notably the prostate.[215] The similarities of this small cell variant of undifferentiated bladder carcinoma to its pulmonary counterpart may be more than just morphologic, as ectopic hor-

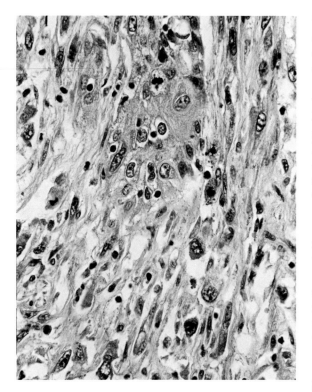

Fig. 17-70 Pleomorphic carcinoma. Most of the lesion has a sarcomatoid appearance, with only focal areas (top, center) of recognizable epithelial differentiation. ×310.

"pseudosarcoma."[111] Evidence of epithelial origin can often be ascertained by light microscopy, provided adequate material is available, with at least focal areas of discernible epithelial differentiation noted (Fig. 17-70). Immunochemical and ultrastructural evaluation may also be of value for differentiating these lesions from true sarcomas.[217] The epithelial component may be of the transitional, squamous, or glandular type; thus this subgroup of tumors is actually not a distinct class. It is designated as such in the AFIP classification[111] but is lumped in the "undifferentiated" category in the WHO classification.[147]

As the name implies, pleomorphic carcinomas are generally bizarre in appearance, often with a predominant "sarcomatoid" element of spindle cells, with variable numbers of large, frequently multinucleated giant cells interspersed. The nuclei are generally a showcase for all of the cytologic features of malignancy, mitotic figures are abundant, and abnormal mitoses are easily found (Fig. 17-71). In the case illustrated, a renal pelvic primary tumor, transition be-

mone production has been noted with these tumors.[167]

Use of the term "poorly differentiated carcinoma," without modifiers, is inappropriate, as this diagnosis implies that one has been able to discern at least some degree of differentiation. This situation is often the case if numerous areas of the tumor are examined; and if focal differentiation is identifiable, the lesion should be so classified.

Because of their infrequent occurrence, the biologic behavior of these lesions is difficult to state with certainty; but as with similar lesions elsewhere, they generally behave in a highly aggressive fashion.[233]

Pleomorphic Carcinoma

Pleomorphic carcinomas, also referred to as "spindle and giant cell carcinoma,"[111] may be confused with the rare sarcomas found throughout the genitourinary tract—hence the use of another synonym,

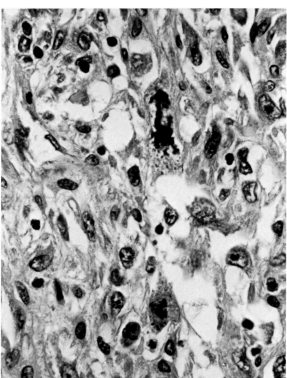

Fig. 17-71 Pleomorphic carcinoma. Note the abnormal mitotic figures. ×512.

tween the poorly differentiated epithelial component and the "sarcomatoid" component could be discerned in a number of areas. The case also illustrates the fact that renal primaries in particular must be viewed in the overall gross and histologic context. Foci of sarcomatoid differentiation may also be seen in primary renal cell carcinomas that extend secondarily to involve the pelvis. Delineation of the epithelial component usually settles the issue in questionable cases, with a typical "clear cell" pattern in other areas indicative of renal parenchymal origin, and transitional cell and squamous patterns indicative of pelvic origin.

The significance of the giant cells in pleomorphic carcinomas has been a subject of some debate.[126] In the past they have been viewed as "end stage cells," but tissue culture studies of bladder carcinomas by Leighton et al.[126] suggested that they may actually play an intrinsic role in subsequent tumor propagation. Although some of the morphologic issues concerning these tumors remain open to question, the clinical behavior does not: These tumors are highly aggressive neoplasms associated with a poor prognosis.[111]

One entity to keep in mind when confronted with such morphology is that of "postoperative spindle cell nodules of the genitourinary tract resembling sarcomas" described in the bladder and elsewhere in the lower genitourinary tract by Proppe et al.[170] These lesions, generally nodular in appearance, may range up to 4 cm in size; and as the name implies, they occur within weeks to a few months following various surgical procedures. The histologic appearance can be alarming, showing pronounced spindle cell proliferation with numerous mitotic figures. Such lesions have been mistaken for sarcomas[170] but may obviously also bear some resemblance to spindled pleomorphic carcinomas. The clinical setting, relative uniformity of nuclear appearance, absence of abnormal mitotic figures, and lack of a tendency to epithelial differentiation should allow the distinction between these and truly neoplastic lesions.

Carcinosarcoma

True carcinosarcomas of urothelial origin, also referred to as "malignant mesodermal mixed tumors,"[105,111] are distinct rarities, with, according to Young,[235] only 35 acceptable cases of primary bladder lesions reported through 1987. Upper tract lesions are even more rare.[34,182] For bladder tumors, the reported age range of the patients is 33 to 82,[235] with a male/female ratio similar to that for urothelial carcinoma in general.[193,235] Grossly the lesions are polypoid or pedunculated in 89 percent and sessile in 11 percent, without an apparent predilection for any particular site.[235] Microscopically, as the name implies, there is an admixture of epithelial elements, which may show transitional cell, squamous, or glandular differentiation, as well as malignant stromal elements. These tumors are generally classified into those exhibiting homologous-type stroma, with leiomyomatous differentiation the only recognizable tissue type qualifying, and those with heterologous differentiation, which may assume various appearances, cartilaginous in close to one-half of all cases.[235] Figures 17-72 and 17-73 illustrate rhabdomyosarcomatous and chondrosarcomatous differentiation in the renal pelvis and bladder, respectively, each associated with high grade epithelial components. As Ridolfi and Eggleston[182]

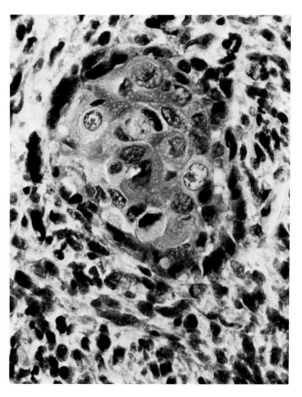

Fig. 17-72 Carcinosarcoma. Rhabdomyoblasts surround an island of poorly differentiated squamous carcinoma. ×446.

advised, the designation "carcinosarcoma" should be reserved for those lesions having both epithelial and one of the definitely recognizable sarcoma subtypes. When such an appearance is seen by light microscopy, electron microscopic and immunohistochemical studies support a genuine mesenchymal nature to the sarcomatous components.[94] The mere finding of a prominent "spindle cell" component in a given epithelial lesion, however, is insufficient evidence for this designation. Such tumors are better termed pleomorphic carcinomas, as described above.

The origin of the sarcomatous elements in these tumors remains uncertain. One may postulate that both the carcinomatous and sarcomatous elements arise from a single malignant cell line, with the soft tissue elements generally viewed as "metaplastic." Equally likely, however, is simultaneous malignant transformation of both epithelial and mesenchymal elements in a given region. Similar to pleomorphic carcinomas, prognosis with these tumors is relatively grim. Death usually occurs within 1 year following diagnosis and therapy,[193] although prolonged survivals have been noted.[235]

OTHER MORPHOLOGIC CONSIDERATIONS

The practicing pathologist is sometimes faced with two not uncommon questions. The first arises when biopsy material is submitted from another body site such as lung or lymph node, with the question: "Could it be a metastasis from a urothelial primary?" Fortunately, most urothelial malignancies are of the transitional cell type, a relatively distinctive tumor. The clinical setting is a great deal of help, for it is most unusual to be faced with an "occult primary" of urothelial origin presenting initially as a distant metastasis. As Marshall noted,[136] totally unsuspected or asymptomatic bladder tumors are rare. Upper tract lesions may remain clinically silent somewhat more frequently, but again occult disease presenting first

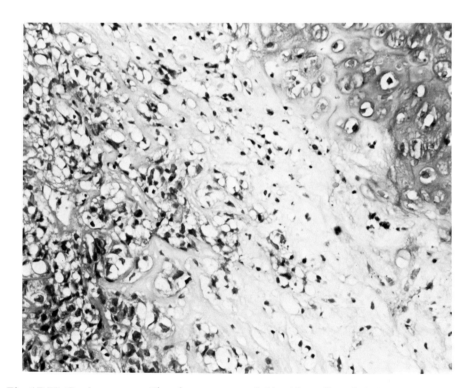

Fig. 17-73 Carcinosarcoma. Chondrosarcomatous field, with small epithelial nests at lower left. ×198.

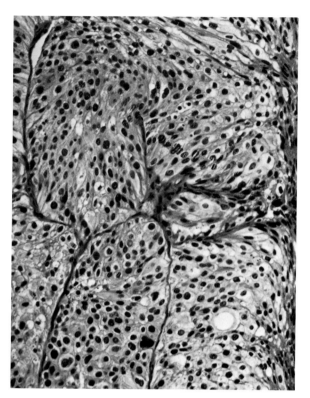

Fig. 17-74 Metastatic transitional cell carcinoma, lung biopsy. ×198.

with extraurinary tract signs or symptoms is infrequent. Given the clinical setting of preexisting urothelial malignancy therefore, particularly with prior resection material in hand, assurance that such lesions as the one illustrated in Figure 17-74 (a biopsy from a lung lesion in a patient with previously diagnosed transitional cell carcinoma of the bladder) are of urothelial origin is not difficult. In addition to lung, other common sites for metastases include liver, bone, adrenals, and kidneys (renal parenchyma).[140]

It should be noted, however, that other carcinomas sometimes show differentiation similar to that of transitional cell neoplasms. In the pelvis in particular, we have seen lesions bearing at times strong resemblance to transitional cell carcinoma of the urinary tract in the anorectal area, another body site containing "transitional epithelium," in "cloacogenic carcinomas." We have also seen focal differentiation along these lines in clinically typical cervical and colorectal carcinomas (Fig. 17-75). Perhaps the lesion bearing

the most striking resemblance and occasionally identical appearance to papillary transitional cell carcinoma in this area is the borderline ("proliferative") Brenner tumor of ovarian origin, as illustrated in Figure 17-76. As Scully noted,[198] however, it is an unusual lesion, with a benign clinical course in almost all instances. One case report[211] described a patient with low grade papillary transitional cell carcinomas of the bladder as well as what appeared to be bilateral proliferative Brenner tumors of the ovaries. The possibility of the bladder primaries having metastasized to the ovaries could not be excluded, but it would have been distinctly unusual behavior for such low grade urothelial lesions.

The second question deals with the converse situation: "Is this kidney, ureteral, bladder, or urethral lesion a primary urothelial tumor or a secondary deposit from elsewhere?" Again, because of the distinctive appearance of the transitional cell lesion, this question is usually easily settled. Tumors arising elsewhere with secondary involvement of the urothelium that are both aggressive enough to have done so and yet morphologically similar enough to be mistaken for transitional cell carcinoma are distinctly unusual. Carcinomas with squamous and glandular features are another matter, however. As the bladder may be secondarily involved by tumors from virtually any site,[111] careful clinical evaluation is often necessary to settle this issue. Figure 17-77 is from a case of an elderly woman who presented with gross hematuria and who was found to have a large, polypoid bladder mass on cystoscopy. As illustrated, it proved to be a moderately to poorly differentiated gland-forming adenocarcinoma, and subsequent evaluation revealed an unsuspected primary in the cecum.

Another such case, where tumor was found at the bladder neck, is illustrated in Figure 17-78. This lesion appeared as a poorly differentiated tumor with some suggestion of gland formation. Immunoperoxidase stain for prostatic acid phosphatase was positive, however, and the lesion was thought therefore to most likely be a prostatic primary (see below). This situation is perhaps the most common one wherein secondary involvement of the bladder by extrinsic adenocarcinoma is found. Considering the rarity of primary adenocarcinomas of the bladder, the mere finding of a glandular tumor in transurethral resection material should immediately arouse suspicion of a possible prostatic primary. As noted by Mostofi and

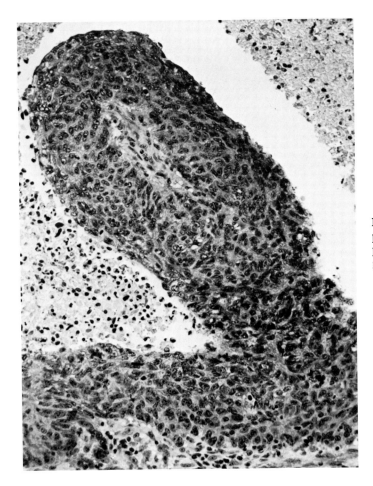

Fig. 17-75 Transitional cell appearance in a poorly differentiated colonic primary neoplasm. The tumor showed a more typical glandular appearance in other areas. ×198.

Price,[146] involvement of the prostatic urethra and bladder neck by prostatic carcinoma may be observed in as many as 50 percent of cases. A good differential point emphasized by the authors is that although the submucosal soft tissue is commonly involved, the urothelium lining the posterior urethra and bladder seems resistant to the spread of carcinoma. Hence mucosal ulcerations secondary to extension of prostatic carcinoma are unusual.

To return briefly to the use of immunoperoxidase methods in the differential diagnosis of bladder versus prostatic adenocarcinoma, a study by Epstein et al.[60] is of interest. These authors studied both pure adenocarcinomas as well as mixed transitional cell adenocarcinomas in cystoprostatectomy specimens, wherein prostatic tumors could be excluded. Among the pure adenocarcinomas, 3 of 11 were positive for prostatic acid phosphatase (PSAP) in male patients, and two of four in female patients. Mixed tumors showed one of five and two of four positive for PSAP in male and female patients, respectively. Conversely, none of the tumors in either sex was positive for prostate-specific antigen (PSA). The latter marker therefore seems to be the more reliable in this particular differential diagnosis.

ADJUNCTIVE DIAGNOSTIC STUDIES

At least for the present, pathologic diagnosis of urothelial neoplasms, as with neoplasms elsewhere, remains the purview of the light microscopist. This is so for a number of reasons, perhaps the most important of which is the considerable weight of experience accumulated over years of examining these and other pathologic lesions almost solely at the gross and light microscopic level. Other factors include the rapidity

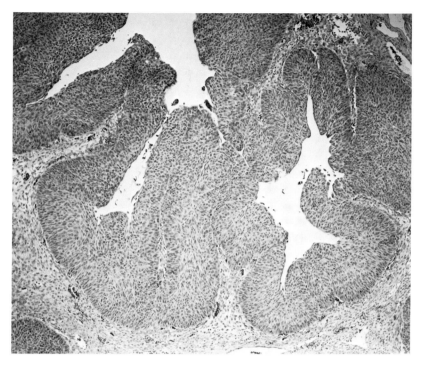

Fig. 17-76 Transitional cell appearance of "proliferative Brenner tumor" of the ovary. ×54.

of the analysis, its relative inexpensiveness, and the attainability of an acceptable level of competence for tissue processing and diagnostic acumen in even the smallest pathology laboratories. For the occasional "difficult case," the portability of diagnostic material for consultation is also useful, and the retrievability of such material for further examination and retrospective study has proved of great value.

Nevertheless, pathologists are among the first to admit the limitations of routine histologic analysis, not only for the diagnosis and classification of these lesions, but particularly for predicting the "biologic potential" of such neoplasms and of the remainder of the urothelial field in any given patient.

By light microscopic analysis, the ends of the spectrum of urothelial neoplasia, as with most spectra, are relatively straightforward. Patients presenting with isolated transitional cell papillomas by the most stringent criteria may be expected to do well following resection. Conversely, most patients with high-grade bladder or upper tract carcinomas, of corresponding high stage, may be expected to die of their disease whatever mode of therapy is employed. Between these two ends of the spectrum, however, exists a large collection of variants on the theme of urothelial

neoplasia, wherein the degree of unpredictability rivals or surpasses that of virtually any other site in the body.

In view of the commonly widespread involvement of the urothelial field by neoplastic alteration, part of the unpredictability results from simple limitations of sampling. Observing the changes in a small bladder biopsy, for example, tells one nothing with certainty about the state of the remaining bladder urothelium. Even when the entirety of the bladder and proximal urethral mucosa are examined in a cystectomy specimen, the remaining urothelium in the ureters and the renal pelves is still uncharted. Moreover, even if we could somehow view the entirety of the urothelium under the light microscope, one may presume that there are numerous features of predictive value that are simply not detected by the method.

The problem of sampling error has been addressed in part by cytologic examination of the urothelium, although this area remains fraught with controversy. Acknowledgement of the simple limitations of light microscopy has engendered a number of other valuable adjunctive tests in recent years. In the course of time they may be perfected to a point where they greatly supplement and perhaps even surpass evalua-

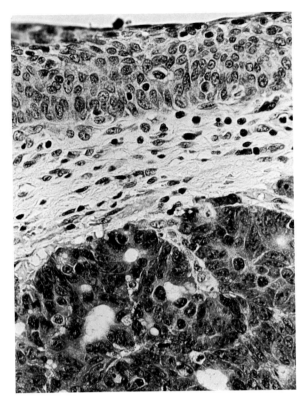

Fig. 17-77 Unsuspected cecal adenocarcinoma that had invaded the bladder. The patient presented with hematuria and a polypoid bladder mass. Note the reactive-appearing transitional epithelium overlying a moderately to poorly differentiated adenocarcinoma. ×310.

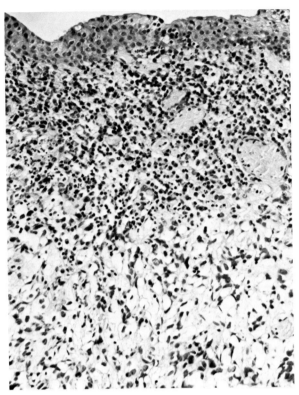

Fig. 17-78 Poorly differentiated prostatic carcinoma in a deep submucosal area of a biopsy from the bladder neck. ×159.

tion by light microscopy, with regard to both diagnosis and prognosis. These tests, including electron microscopy, cell membrane antigen analysis, and chromosome examination, have been developed principally during the study of bladder neoplasia because of the greater availability of patients compared to those with upper tract neoplasms, as well as the accessibility of diagnostic material. It might be predicted, however, that such methods will be applied with equal success to the extravesical urothelium in the future.

Urinary Tract Cytology

Despite a number of problems, urinary tract cytology has proved to be a valuable aid not only in the primary diagnosis of urothelial malignancies, but es-

pecially in the further evaluation and follow-up of the remaining urothelium in patients who have undergone conservative therapy for primary tumors.[35,173] Although this topic is covered in depth in Chapter 21, a few brief comments, particularly with regard to limitations of the method, are made here.

First, cytologic evaluation is of optimal use when dealing with higher grade neoplasms, for the obvious reason that the higher the grade of the tumor the more likely it is to shed cells into the urine that are recognizable as malignant. The diagnosis of low grade lesions, conversely, has been particularly disappointing.[56] This should come as no surprise, for as Friedell et al.[73] noted: "Grade 1 in situ papillary carcinomas simply do not possess the cytologic characteristics — and more particularly the nuclear characteristics — of malignancy which would permit the diagnosis to be made with any appreciable degree of frequency."

Second, although cytology may help solve the problem of direct biopsy sampling error, as cells shed from everywhere in the urothelial field may be detected in urinary cytology preparations, this facility is a two-edged sword. That is, the malignant cells may have arisen anywhere from the renal pelvis through to the proximal urethra, with no indication of origin.

Third, cytology suffers from greater "technical" limitations than does histology. Obviously, not all tumors necessarily shed diagnostic cells into any given specimen, particularly a single voided urine. Presuming that cells are shed, there is the potential for degeneration of cells residing for any length of time in urine, a medium that can be somewhat inhospitable. If in fact the cells shed are well preserved at the time of collection, the ability to process and stain the cells may vary considerably from one laboratory to another, much more so than with histologic processing, in my opinion.

Fourth, perhaps most important, are basic "diagnostic" limitations. A cytology preparation puts the pathologist at an immediate disadvantage compared to a histologic preparation because structural abnormalities, e.g., number of cell layers and loss of nuclear orientation, cannot be assessed. In the absence of well-preserved tissue fragments, reliance is placed almost solely on the presence or absence of nuclear features of malignancy, which obviously increases the element of subjectivity in diagnosis.

Despite these limitations, cytopathology remains by far the most valuable adjunctive study in the management of patients with urothelial neoplasms. The field continues to evolve, and advances such as the employment of automated methods[114,138] (see Ch. 21) may lead to improved diagnostic accuracy. Accuracy, as with all areas of diagnostic pathology, remains the key word. For the clinician, it obtains provided unrealistic expectations of the methods are not held, e.g., the unfailing diagnosis of low grade papillary lesions. It also applies to the pathologist, as "positive diagnoses" should be reserved for those cases demonstrating a sufficient number of the classic cytologic features of malignancy. These cases also happen to be, not by coincidence, those posing the greatest threat to the health and life of the patient. Forced attempts to overextend oneself in order to "look sharp" in diagnosing low grade neoplasms do little more in the end than destroy the pathologist's most valuable asset — his credibility.

Electron Microscopy

Electron microscopy has been used predominantly as a research tool for urothelial neoplasia, but recent advances have suggested its possible value as a diagnostic aid. The ultrastructural details of both normal human urothelium[17,214] and urothelial neoplasms[18,214] have been well characterized by standard transmission electron microscopy (TEM), and observations of the ultrastructural deviations in neoplastic cells have proved to be of great interest. Of particular importance has been the development of scanning electron microscopy (SEM), which has made available remarkably detailed studies of urothelial topography, ranging from isolated cell morphology to that of the intact mucosa, in both animal models[97] and human material.[52,99,192,214]

The superficial cells of normal urothelium, as viewed by SEM (Fig. 17-79) have an irregularly corrugated surface membrane system with an anastomosing system of microridges. The underlying basal and intermediate cells demonstrate surface microvilli, but they are short and regular in appearance.[99] In contrast, in experimental systems[97] the earliest recognizable morphologic change in the neoplastic progression of bladder tumors induced by chemical carcinogens has been considered to be the appearance of "pleomorphic microvilli," which involve not only the surface cells but the underlying intermediate and basal cells as well.

Studies of human material[96,99,214] have shown similar alterations, particularly in lower grade papillary neoplasms (Fig. 17-80). Cells covered by such pleomorphic microvilli may be found in approximately 40 percent of cells from grade I transitional cell neoplasms, 20 to 25 percent of grade II lesions, and a similar number of cells from grade III lesions.[99] However, in the highest grade lesions, although some cells retain surface pleomorphic microvilli (Fig. 17-81) a number of cells have lost this characteristic feature, perhaps secondary to fusion of microvilli (Fig. 17-82), whereas other cells have entirely smooth surfaces, presumably reflective of degenerative changes.[99]

One potentially valuable aspect of SEM is that it may also be applied to cytologic material.[98,210] Schmidt et al.[192] examined bladder washings from 61 patients with grades 1 to 3 urothelial tumors, with analysis by SEM, TEM, morphometry, and carcinoembryonic antigen assay. In their experience, even

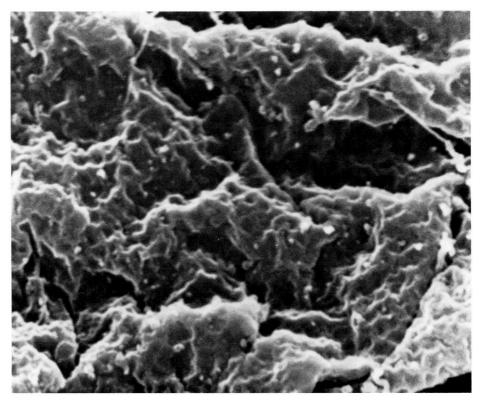

Fig. 17-79 SEM demonstrating the normal anastomosing microridge system of bladder superficial ("umbrella") cells. ×14,000. (From Jacobs et al.,[99] with permission.)

though SEM surface features were examined blindly, there were no false-positive or false-negative diagnoses of malignancy. The tumors were correctly graded in 77 percent of cases and within one grade in the remaining 23 percent of cases.

It should be noted, however, that enthusiasm for the technique is not universally shared[52]; and other studies, such as that of Suzuki et al.,[210] have shown not only a high false-negative rate in patients with known tumors but also a significant false-positive rate among patients with lithiasis and urinary tract infections. Although the appearance of pleomorphic microvilli in apparently neoplastic cells is a striking alteration, it has been emphasized that it is not necessarily a sign of irreversible neoplastic transformation,[99] as underscored by the findings of Suzuki et al.[210] as well as others.[9]

Electron microscopy may also offer the possibility of increasingly early detection of invasive disease. Tannenbaum and Romas[213] found that TEM, in con-

junction with careful histologic examination, revealed that many lesions at first considered confined to the mucosa were actually beginning to extend into the underlying lamina propria. Interestingly, the areas that had undergone transformation to carcinoma in situ were no longer producing basement membrane material but, rather, abutted directly onto the lamina propria. The authors contended that this fact may be the cause for the phenomenon known to any pathologist of experience, the "nude biopsy," where epithelium has disappeared somewhere between the patient and the slide, with nothing more than vesical wall left to examine. Although it is certainly seen in nonneoplastic disorders, it is distressingly common in biopsy specimens obtained to evaluate other areas of mucosa in patients with high grade neoplasms.

Unfortunately, at the present time, even if electron microscopic techniques were 100 percent reliable, the limitations of the method are obvious: The equipment is expensive, and few pathologists have suffi-

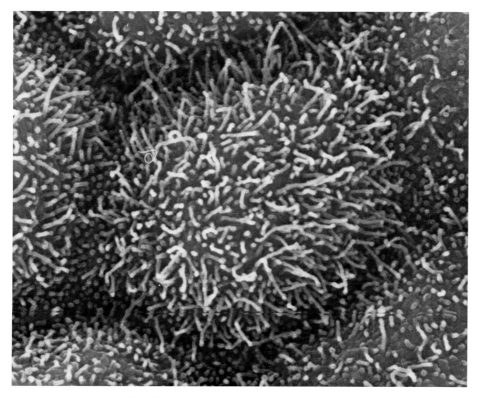

Fig. 17-80 SEM of surface pleomorphic microvilli in human bladder cancer. These structures may be particularly prominent in low grade tumors. ×8,600. (From Jacobs et al.,[99] with permission.)

cient diagnostic expertise in this area. The former may be partially obviated by the development of preliminary methods for fixation,[22] affording the possibility of processing at established electron microscopy laboratories. The latter is of obvious importance, particularly if the method is to give a true indication of what may be among the earliest recognizable signs of neoplastic transformation and invasion, unable to be corroborated by other standard methods. For the moment, the practical value of electron microscopy in human urothelial neoplasia remains speculative.

Cell Surface Antigen Studies

Evaluation of cell surface antigens of normal and neoplastic tissue has received considerable attention in recent years. In urologic oncology, a particular goal has been improvement of prognostication for patients with low and intermediate grade transitional cell neoplasms of low stage. Much of the work, reviewed by Lloyd,[133] has involved the ABH(O) blood group–related antigens, although more recently other blood group-related antigens have been studied, such as those of the Lewis system[129] as well as precursor antigens such as the Thomsen-Friedenreich antigen (TAg).[40,125,130] (For discussion of other tumor-associated antigen studies, see Immunologic Evaluation below.)

Although the ABH(O) isoantigen system was first described in studies of red blood cells, these and other "blood group antigens" are also expressed on the cell surfaces of numerous tissues.[92] Altered expression of these surface antigens has been described in urothelial neoplasms as well as malignancies at other body sites.[116,127,131] Methods for detecting the presence or absence of the antigens include the specific red blood cell adherence test (SRCA) (Fig. 17-83), originally described by Kovarik et al.,[116] and immunohistochemical analysis.[26,41,227] Both methods may be used with fixed tissues, although the SRCA technique appears

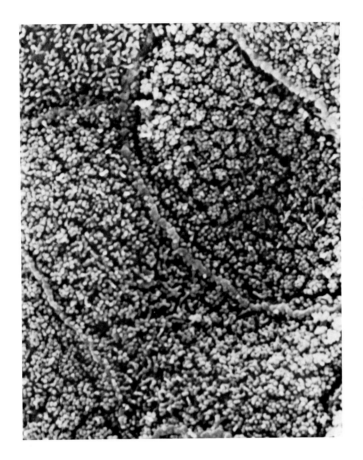

Fig. 17-81 SEM of clustered surface pleomorphic microvilli, with thickened intercellular seams, characteristic of higher grade tumors. ×5,740. (From Jacobs et al.,[99] with permission.)

to give less reliable results on paraffin embedded material than on frozen section material,[128] perhaps because of the vulnerability of the H antigen (blood group O patients) to processing techniques as well as its comparatively weak antigenicity. In this group of patients in particular, testing by immunoperoxidase methods is thought to be preferable.[26,41,100]

Kay and Wallace,[106] in an early study of urothelial malignancies in patients of blood groups A, B, and AB, noted instances of tumor cell surface antigen deletion, particularly among the more pleomorphic, infiltrating, and rapidly fatal tumors. The authors also observed, however, that "exceptions were numerous"; in particular, surface antigens were still detectable in some of the invasive tumors examined. A study by Decenzo et al.[46] indicated a potentially useful predictive value in assessment of superficial bladder tumors. In their report the tumors of 22 patients with stage A disease were evaluated by the SRCA technique; and of these patients, 13 showed retention of

cell surface antigens. None of the 13 patients progressed to the stage of invasive malignancy during follow-up ranging from 5 to 14 years. Of the nine patients whose initial tumors were surface antigen-negative, however, five progressed to stage B disease within 5 years, with three of the remaining four proceeding to invasion at 7, 8, and 11 years, respectively. The fourth patient had only a brief period of follow-up. The authors discussed the findings of Kay and Wallace,[106] and questioned the possibility that at least some of the tumors in that study may have been squamous rather than transitional cell. They noted that superficial squamous cell lesions destined to become deeply invasive may, in contrast to transitional cell lesions, retain their antigenicity, although studies of bilharziasis-associated squamous carcinomas indicate that a significant number do not.[81]

The results of Decenzo et al.[46] were met with great enthusiasm, as one of the major problems in urothelial neoplasia has been the inability to predict by routine

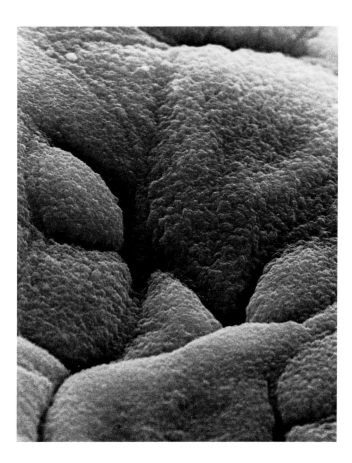

Fig. 17-82 SEM of cell type also characteristically seen in higher grade tumors, with pleomorphic villi not apparent. ×4,350. (From Jacobs et al.,[99] with permission.)

histologic methods which of the patients presenting with lower grade, noninvasive tumors will develop aggressive disease. In a review of the literature, Catalona[37] found that the aggregate results of surface antigen studies indicated that subsequent invasive disease developed within 5 years in 66 percent of patients initially presenting with superficial antigen-negative tumors, whereas only 4 percent with antigen-positive tumors went on to invasive disease during the same time period. For the antigen-negative group, the figures are even more impressive in view of the fact that invasion may occur considerably past the 5-year point of follow-up.[46] Other findings stressed by Catalona[37] included the general correlation between grade of tumor and antigenic expression and the correlation between loss of antigen expression and subsequent tumor recurrences. Ninety percent of patients whose initial tumors were antigen-negative suffered recurrences, whereas only 46 percent of those who were initially antigen-positive developed subsequent

tumors. Also, approximately 95 percent of recurrent tumors maintained the antigenic expression pattern of the original tumor. Of further interest in this regard is the fact that antigenicity of biopsy specimens of "uninvolved" mucosa taken at the time of tumor resection may prove to be of value for predicting tumor recurrence.[43]

Enthusiasm for the technique has not been found in all quarters, however, particularly with regard to long-term prognosis. Askari et al.,[12] in a controlled blind study of 73 bladder cancer patients, did not find definite statistical evidence that loss of antigen expression could be independently equated with poor prognosis. In particular, when patients were examined according to blood group, those in group A whose tumors were initially antigen-positive showed no statistical difference in 5-year survival compared to those whose tumors were antigen-negative. All but 4 of 35 patients in blood group O were antigen negative, so survival comparison in this group was unin-

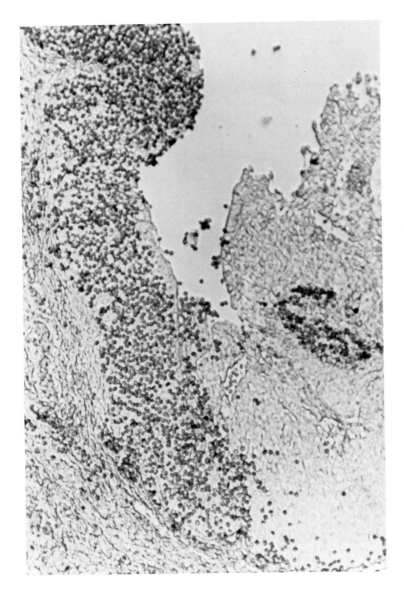

Fig. 17-83 ABH(O) surface isoantigen analysis by the specific red blood cell (RBC) adherence assay. Intermediate-grade transitional cell carcinoma (right) shows no RBC adherence, indicating a loss of surface antigens. Note the adherence of RBCs to adjacent normal mucosa (left) and vascular endothelium. ×88. (From Limas et al.,[131] with permission.)

formative. When grouped according to grade, they found that antigen negativity did not indicate a poor prognosis in grade 1 and 2 lesions, although patients with grade 3 lesions that were antigen-negative fared less well than those whose tumors were antigen-positive.

A number of significant problems remain with the technique. One is the aforementioned difficulty of detecting blood group H substance (type O) compared to A and B substance.[12] The immunoperoxidase method, among its other advantages, appears to have alleviated this problem[26,41,100]; and monoclonal anti-

body technology, allowing for production of essentially unlimited quantities of highly specific reagents, will no doubt further improve the situation.[133] Another source of difficulty is the tendency to decreased expression of surface antigens in general with increasing age.[12] A third is the potential reappearance of antigen expression in patients treated with radiotherapy, a finding recorded in some studies[8] but not in others.[181] A fourth, alluded to above and cited as a possible explanation of the variable results noted in the original work by Kay and Wallace,[106] is the lack of similar correlation in lesions demonstrating squamous

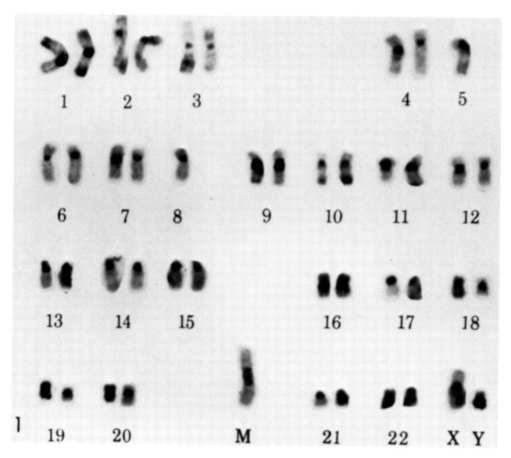

Fig. 17-84 Karyotype from noninvasive papillary transitional cell carcinoma of the bladder with 45 chromosomes. Note the missing chromosomes in groups 5 and 8, and the marker chromosome (M). (From Sandberg,[186] with permission.)

differentiation.[46] They may be antigen-positive in 40 percent of cases[37] despite their commonly high stage presentation. Similar lack of correlation between antigen expression and stage has also been found with adenocarcinomas.[7] As emphasized by Limas and Lange,[127,128] some of the difficulties encountered may be due to the fact that loss of expression is a *quantitative* phenomenon that may be affected by numerous factors. In some, loss of reactivity is in fact a true indicator of potentially aggressive behavior. In others it may merely reflect variations from one type of tumor to the next, modifying therapeutic factors, or methodologic differences in tissue processing, titer of antisera, etc.

For the present, the available data seem to be most helpful for evaluating behavior of urothelial neo-

plasms as a whole. As noted by Cummings,[42] however, the results are not now applicable as accurate predictors in an individual case. For patients with low grade/low stage neoplasms, retention of surface antigen expression may be reassuring, as it appears that only a small number of such patients develop invasive disease. The converse situation is much more unsettled, however, particularly with regard to major "early" therapeutic intervention, as a significant number of patients presenting with low grade/low stage disease whose tumors are surface antigen-negative do *not* go on to develop invasive disease, at least within the first 5 years of follow-up. With regard to upper tract lesions, the application of the method to cytologic specimens may possibly prove to be of value. Cytologic indication of low grade disease, combined

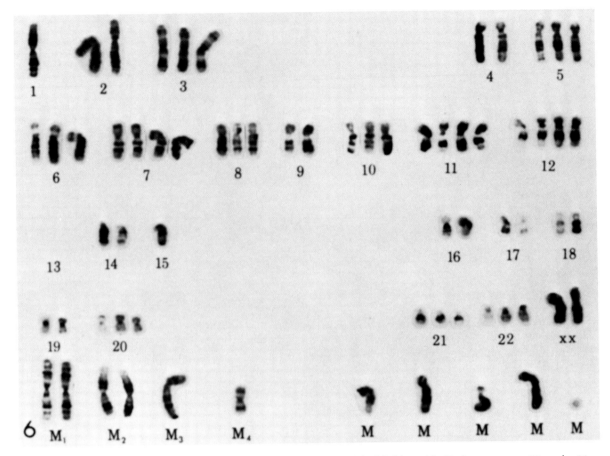

Fig. 17-85 Karyotype from invasive transitional cell carcinoma of the bladder with 67 chromosomes. Note the 11 marker chromosomes, only six of which (M1 to M4) could be further characterized by banding techniques. (From Sandberg,[186] with permission.)

with antigen positivity, may prove valuable when deciding which upper tract lesions might be dealt with in a more conservative fashion than the standard nephroureterectomy.[82]

Chromosome Analysis

Increasingly refined analysis of chromosome abnormalities in urothelial neoplasms has been performed over the last two decades.[188] As with ultrastructural evaluation and cell surface antigen studies, results have been largely from examination of bladder tumors.

Aspects suitable for analysis include modal chromosome number, derived from a survey of multiple karyotypes performed from an individual tumor sample, and morphology of the individual chromosomes. (Determination of DNA content by flow cytometric analysis is discussed in Chapter 21.)

Early studies concentrated on evaluation of chromosome number,[118,201] with particular attention to the contrast between noninvasive and invasive tumors. The former most commonly showed numerical correspondence with the normal diploid complement of 46 chromosomes, whereas the latter showed significant aneuploidy (i.e., deviation from the normal 46, or two sets of 23 homologous chromosomes). There was a tendency to polyploidy (i.e., more than the normal two sets of chromosomes), a finding that may have been predicted by mere inspection of the enlarged, hyperchromatic nuclei in high grade invasive tumors. As these two groups of tumors could often be easily distinguished by routine microscopy, with prognostic differences equally obvious, such studies added little predictive value.

With examination of chromosome morphology, one initial hope was that some specific, recognizable chromosome anomaly might be identified as an earmark of malignant transformation in urothelium, as with the Philadelphia chromosome in chronic myelogenous leukemia. However, such a single abnormality, common to most or all urothelial neoplasms, has not been found, although certain subgroups of abnormalities now appear to be emerging.[188] Significant advances in technique, in particular the introduction of chromosome banding,[103] have resulted in much more precise karyotype analysis and more discerning evaluation of individual chromosome alterations, with increased facility in recognizing abnormal, or "marker," chromosomes.[63] With this technique, much more subtle abnormalities, e.g., reciprocal translocations and deletions of small bands of chromosome material, can be detected.[187] Other advances, e.g., enzymatic disaggregation of tumor cells,[222] have been of use particularly for the evaluation of low grade lesions, where previous techniques had resulted in a relatively small number of mitotic figures for analysis.[187] With the help of such methodologic improvements, a detectable pattern seems to have been discerned that may help sort out which patients with low grade tumors may eventually suffer recurrence or invasive disease.

In a study from Sandberg's laboratory[186] at Roswell Park, for example, 62 noninvasive papillary tumors and 75 invasive transitional cell carcinomas were examined, as were 75 specimens from normal bladder mucosa. In the normal specimens, more than 90 percent of the karyotypes in each case examined had a normal diploid complement of 46 chromosomes, with a small percentage in each case showing what was thought to be consistent with random chromosome loss. In particular, no evidence of polyploidy was noted in more than 700 metaphases examined.

Of the 62 noninvasive papillary tumors, 12 were diagnosed as benign lesions, although the histologic criteria used for diagnosis were not noted in the report. Of these 12 lesions, 10 showed a predominantly diploid arrangement, and no evidence of recurrence was noted in these patients, with follow-up from 8 months to 3 years. Of the remaining two, one showed only 45 chromosomes in one-fourth of the meta-

phases examined. This patient suffered recurrent tumor, with invasion, within 11 months, interestingly with aneuploidy similar to that originally observed. The other patient also had recurrence 1.5 years after analysis but without evidence of invasion.

The remaining 50 papillary, yet noninvasive tumors were malignant as assessed by light microscopy, and they also had modal chromosome numbers in the diploid range. However, all were noted to show some detectable abnormality, in either chromosome number, appearance of marker chromosomes, or both (Fig. 17-84). Thirty-two of the 50 cases contained markers, no more than two per cell, appearing in 5 to 100 percent of the cells examined in a given case. The most common markers originated from chromosome 1 or involved a translocation of chromosomes 14, 17, and some of those in the C group. Other than these findings, no common thread was apparent.

Of these 50 patients with noninvasive papillary tumors, 11 suffered recurrent disease, most within 6 months. Of the 11 recurring tumors, 10 were invasive, and all 10 demonstrated at least one identifiable marker chromosome. The only tumor without a marker that recurred did not become invasive.

Sandberg[186] examined 75 cases of invasive transitional cell carcinoma for comparison. The more well differentiated, locally invasive tumors remained in the near-diploid range, whereas high grade tumors showed a noticeable tendency to polyploidy in the near-triploid and tetraploid range. More striking was a significant increase in the number of marker chromosomes with progression of the cancer. Most common were two large markers of metacentric morphology, possibly originating from chromosome 1, present in most of the cases examined. Some cases demonstrated even more blatant abnormalities (Fig. 17-85). An interesting observation was a possible increase in radiosensitivity of tumors with the higher relative number of markers. This may merely be a reflection of a phenomenon seen with other tumors — small cell carcinoma of the lung, for example — where the more poorly differentiated tumors may respond most rapidly to radiotherapy, which unfortunately seems to have little influence on the eventual outcome.

Similar results have been noted in other studies. Summers et al.[209] evaluated 65 patients with low grade neoplasms (grade 1 or 2) at initial biopsy. Of these 65 patients, 20 demonstrated no marker chromosomes, and only 2 of the 20 suffered recurrences, again superficial and noninvasive. With follow-up ranging from 9 months to 10 years, only one of these 20 patients died, of unrelated causes. Another 20 patients had noninvasive tumors "histologically and visually identical" to those in the first group but did exhibit marker chromosomes. In this group recurrent disease was found in 18 of the 20 patients, with one patient dying of tumor-related disease. The last group comprised 25 patients with similar low grade tumors, all with marker chromosomes, differing from the other two groups in that their tumors showed submucosal invasion. Recurrences in this group were noted in 20 of the 25 patients; but, most strikingly, the patients averaged three recurrences per year, and within 6 years half of the patients were dead of their disease. Other findings of interest included examination of patients with cystitis cystica or cystitis glandularis, which the authors found to "never evoke chromosomal aberrations," and the fact that over the more than 10 years of analyzing chromosome material from more than 600 specimens only three instances of invasive tumors, stage B1 or deeper, did *not* show marker chromosomes or fragments and marker aneuploidy. This dogma does not hold for all situations, however. Among 34 patients with bilharziasis-associated bladder carcinoma, which is virtually always invasive, Abu Farha et al.[2] found markers in *none* of the tumors.

The figures for chromosome analysis are encouraging, particularly with regard to prognosis in patients with lower grade tumors. As with all other techniques, however, certain drawbacks should be noted. One is that in the situation where predictiveness is most needed, i.e., in patients with low grade papillary lesions, difficulties with analysis are greatest. An adequate number of cells in metaphase must be obtained in order to ensure detection of significant deviations from diploidy and, most important, to optimize chances for detection of marker chromosomes. Hopefully, improved techniques will circumvent this problem. Another difficulty, which was essentially unmasked with the advent of banding techniques, is the sometimes subtle variations that indicate the presence of "marker" chromosomes. The method in general is time-consuming, requires the use of fresh tissue, and necessitates expertise not only technologically but particularly for interpretation. A final criticism is the degree of predictability afforded by the presence of marker chromosomes. For example, despite the high number of patients with recurrent disease in the marker group reported by Summers et al.,[209] it should be noted that in Sandberg's series[186] 21 of the 32 cases with a marker chromosome (from a total of 50 noninvasive papillary carcinomas) did *not* recur, at least over the stated period of observation.

Despite these drawbacks, the data support the potential usefulness of cytogenetic analysis for predicting biologic behavior, particularly of lower grade papillary lesions. Moreover, with advances in technique, information on cytogenetic abnormalities of urothelial neoplasms,[188] as well as other solid tumors,[189] continues to expand. In one report[188] Sandberg detailed subgroups of chromosome abnormalities in urothelial tumors that now appear to be coming into focus, including formation of an isochromosome for the short arm of chromosome 5, monosomy of chromosome 9, and trisomy of chromosome 7. The implications of these findings, particularly with regard to possible oncogene activation, are discussed by the author, and it remains an exciting area of development, not only in urologic oncology but in basic tumor biology as a whole.

Immunologic Evaluation

Because of the complexity and rapid evolution of the subject of "tumor immunology" it is difficult to present anything but a brief sketch of certain aspects of the field, much of which will no doubt be outdated in the near future. The reader is referred to more general reviews of the subject,[162] as well as specific reviews dealing with urothelial neoplasia.[120,141] Two aspects of potential importance with regard to prognosis are discussed here. The first is evaluation of tumor-associated antigen production as a measure of tumor occurrence or recurrence. The second is assessment of basic immunologic competence of the individual patient.

TUMOR-ASSOCIATED ANTIGEN PRODUCTION

The cells of urothelial neoplasms are similar to all other cells, normal and neoplastic, in that they are capable of elaborating antigenic substances. Lange[120] divided them into three groups: normal antigens, tumor-specific (transplantation) antigens, and onco-developmental antigens.

The first set, normal antigens, includes cell surface antigens usually associated with normal adult cells. Examples include the histocompatibility antigens and the ABH(O) blood group-related antigens described above, as well as normal antigenic substances found in blood and other body fluids, which may be elevated in patients with urothelial neoplasms. Although the histocompatibility antigen content of tumors has not been directly characterized, there is indirect evidence that expression of histocompatibility antigens may be decreased with increasing degrees of malignancy, similar to the situation with the blood group-related antigens.[226] Efforts have also been directed toward characterization of patient histocompatibility antigen profiles, but the results reported in the literature have been variable.

Herring et al.,[89] for example, reported 101 patients with transitional cell carcinoma of the bladder and noted that the antigenic frequencies of HLA B5 and Cw4 in these patients were higher than in the general population. Other studies have failed to support this association, however. Lytton et al.[134] examined 70 patients with transitional cell carcinoma of the bladder and found no significant differences at the A, B, C, or DR loci between their patients and a comparable normal population. DR4 was the most common antigen expressed in bladder cancer patients, yet allelic frequency was only 39 percent compared to 28 percent in the normal population. The presence or absence of the DR4 antigen was not related to the stage or the grade of the tumor.

Other studies have examined normal antigenic substances that may be elevated in the plasma or urine of patients with urothelial neoplasms, e.g., haptoglobin, transferrin, albumin, immunoglobulins, and fibrin/fibrin degradation products. Increased amounts of such substances have been found in urine from tumor patients, particularly those with higher grade transitional cell carcinomas[84] as well as higher stage lesions.[61] Some may be traced to the tumor itself, and some may be of extratumoral origin, resulting from glomerular deposition of tumor-derived antigen–antibody complexes.[84] Gozzo et al.[78] found that panel analysis of such urinary proteins allowed the diagnosis of 64 percent of bladder papillomas and 77 percent of bladder carcinomas, with only a 7 percent false-positive rate for urine specimens from normal controls.

Such elevations may be nonspecific, however. The same research group[161] found increased urinary levels of IgG, IgA, transferrin, orosomucoid, haptoglobin, fibrinogen, and α_1-antitrypsin in patients with urinary tract infection. Because large, invasive tumors often show necrosis, inflammation, and secondary infection, results of such urinary screening must be interpreted with caution.

The second set of tumor-associated antigenic substances is that of tumor-specific (transplantation) antigens (TSA). Defined in animal studies by evaluating immune responses in syngeneic hosts,[120] they include antigenic substances that are not found in normal cells and that are unique to a given tumor in the case of chemically induced lesions or to group of tumors in the case of virus-induced lesions. Identification and characterization of such antigens have been hampered in the past by methodologic problems, in particular the difficulties encountered in the production of "pure" antibodies by classic techniques. The advent of hybridoma technology[110] has resulted in the ability to produce highly specific antibody preparations (monoclonal antibodies, or MABS) in quantity,[15,16,143] and with this advance a whole new avenue of investigation has been made available. Numerous previously uncharacterized antigens have now been discovered that may be expressed by urothelial neoplasms and detected in various ways.[11,15,28,39,65,66,93,132,212]

Although it was initially hoped that such markers might be truly "tumor-specific," it now appears that they more likely represent normal and developmental antigens of restricted expression[11,66,132] and that they are not limited to neoplasms. Nonetheless, the degree of restricted expression is such that evaluation for such antigens, particularly when panels of multiple antibodies are used, may eventually allow better definition of tumor subsets and their biologic potentials[66] and perhaps serve also in eventual attempts at directed immunotherapy.[15]

The third set, oncodevelopmental antigens, includes those elaborated by normal cells, usually early in development, but that at times persist to later stages. Again, such substances may be attached to the cell surface, be released by the cells, or both. As noted above, many of the "tumor-associated antigens" may well belong to this category. Among these antigens, perhaps the three most commonly mentioned in the literature with regard to human neoplasms are the carcinoembryonic antigen (CEA), α-fetoprotein (AFP), and human chorionic gonadotropin (hCG).

Carcinoembryonic antigen, best characterized in association with colorectal neoplasms, belongs to a group of cross-reacting isoantigens,[219] some variants of which are preferentially expressed during normal ontogenic development. CEA levels may also be increased in patients with noncolorectal tumors, and elevated CEA levels in both serum and urine have been detected in patients with transitional cell carcinoma.[50,83,120] As noted by Hall,[83] however, measurement of urinary CEA level in particular is associated with a high false-negative rate in the face of demonstrable tumor. Conversely, a high number of false-positive results may be found with urinary tract infection, with specimens contaminated by vaginal secretions, and in patients who have had cystectomy with the establishment of an ileal conduit. An interesting paradox was found by Shevchuk et al.[200] in direct immunoperoxidase studies of benign and neoplastic urothelium. They noted that CEA was detectable in normal transitional epithelium, yet its level often appeared to decrease in malignant transitional epithelium. This finding was in direct contrast to the elevated urinary levels of CEA in patients with tumors compared to normals. The authors thought this paradox to be explainable on the basis of increased cell mass and turnover rate in bladder neoplasms compared to normal bladder. They cautioned that CEA should not be used as a biomarker in direct studies of urothelium, and Hall[83] thought that for the present CEA measurement is not reliable in either the diagnosis or the management of urologic cancer.

The value of hCG analysis has been suggested by some investigators[50] but denied by others.[120] Measurement of other oncodevelopmental antigens, e.g., AFP, of interest in other areas of genitourinary neoplasia, notably testicular tumors, has not been found useful thus far in the diagnosis and management of urothelial tumors.[120]

HOST IMMUNOCOMPETENCE

As noted above, at least in animal studies it is apparent that some tumors elaborate antigens that serve to distinguish them from normal host cells, with tumor transplantation experiments indicative of the potential for inducing at least partial resistance to neoplasms in previously sensitized host animals.[120]

Initially it was thought that such resistance was primarily the result of activation of cell-mediated immunity mechanisms, with little part, if any, played by humoral mechanisms. As noted in excellent reviews by Lange and co-workers,[120,122] early concepts contrasting cell-mediated immunity versus humoral immunity were oversimplified. With the further subdivision of the lymphocyte population into cytotoxic T lymphocytes, suppressor and helper lymphocytes, natural killer cells, etc., and the recognition of the interactive roles played by both T and B cells as well as nonlymphocyte effector cells, it has become much more difficult to assign specific roles in the immune response in an individual situation. However, despite these difficulties, the generalization may be made that patients with deficient cell-mediated immune responsiveness seem to have a poorer prognosis than those with normal responsiveness.[62]

Immunologic tests of patients with genitourinary malignancies may be considered in two categories: tests of general immunologic status and tests of antitumor immunity.[119] The first category includes in vivo testing of skin reactivity both to recall antigens (e.g., PPD and *Candida*) and, more informative, to such primary antigens as dinitrochlorobenzene (DNCB) and dinitrofluorobenzene (DNFB).[3,58,62] Fahey et al.[62] examined DNCB reactivity in patients with transitional cell carcinoma and found increasing impairment of reactivity with increasing tumor burden. In those with localized tumors, 45 percent showed no reactivity to DNCB. A second group, with invasive disease still localized regionally, showed 60 percent negative reactivity. A third group, with proven metastatic disease, showed 75 percent negative reactivity. Surgical removal of tumor led to restoration of reactivity in a number of patients. Interestingly, patients who were originally thought to have localized disease but who later developed clinically apparent metastatic disease had had poor reactivities initially. Furthermore, responsiveness appeared to be predictive even within stage. All five patients with stage D disease who retained reactivity were alive at 20 months, yet only approximately 20 percent of patients in stage D with negative reactivity survived for a similar length of time. The authors discussed the problem of decreased reactivity following radiotherapy, a phenomenon that has been noted after such other insults as surgery and anesthesia,[19] that is obviously of some potential concern in therapeutic considerations.

Numerous other methods have been used to assess the general immunologic status of patients, including counts of lymphocyte types and subtypes, measurement of lymphoproliferative response to mitogens, and observation of mixed lymphocyte culture reactivity to allogeneic cells.[86,87] Again, possible predictive value has been noted, but data remain limited at present.

The second category of tests (antitumor immunity) has been used in an attempt to measure possible tumor-specific immune response in a given patient, primarily via in vitro tests such as the lymphocyte-mediated microcytotoxicity assay,[121] although in vivo skin testing with either crude or refined tumor extracts has also been tried.[119] As noted by Lange et al.,[121] the lymphocyte-mediated microcytotoxicity assay has been the most popular method used for attempts to assess specific antitumor immunity, although initial optimism has diminished somewhat as a greater understanding of the mechanisms affecting the assay has evolved. In particular, sorting-out changes in specific antitumor activity from the welter of non-tumor-related immunologic changes effected by therapy and other events poses considerable difficulty.

Overall, the field of "tumor immunology" must at present be considered to be in a state of flux. Certain tests, such as blood group-related antigen assay and assessing reactivity to primary antigens such as DNCB, have proved to be of some predictive value in *groups* of patients, although they have not been definitively applicable for *individual* patients independent of other factors such as tumor grade or stage. The field nonetheless remains perhaps the most exciting in the study of neoplasia in the genitourinary tract as well as elsewhere, particularly with regard to the possibility of discovering distinct tumor-specific antigens and, hopefully, developing directed immunotherapy.

REFERENCES

1. Abenoza P, Manivel C, Fraley EE: Primary adenocarcinoma of urinary bladder: clinicopathologic study of 16 cases. Urology 29:9, 1987
2. Abu Farha OM, Hamoud F, El-Garbawy M, et al: Cytogenetic study of carcinoma of bilharzial bladder. J Urol 133:300A, 1985
3. Adolphs HD, Steffens L: Evaluation of the immuno-competence of patients with transitional cell carcinoma of the bladder. Urol Res 5:29, 1977
4. Aldridge KW, Burns JR, Singh B: Vesical endometriosis: a review and 2 case reports. J Urol 134:539, 1985
5. Allen TD, Henderson BW: Adenocarcinoma of the bladder. J Urol 93:50, 1965
6. Alroy J, Pauli BU, Hayden JE, Gould VE: Intracytoplasmic lumina in bladder carcinomas. Hum Pathol 10:549, 1979
7. Alroy J, Roganovic D, Banner BF, et al: Primary adenocarcinomas of the human urinary bladder: histochemical, immunological and ultrastructural studies. Virchows Arch [Pathol Anat] 393:165, 1981
8. Alroy J, Teramura K, Miller A W III, et al: Isoantigens A, B, and H in urinary bladder carcinomas following radiotherapy. Cancer 41:1739, 1978
9. Anderström C, Ekelund P, Hansson HA, Johansson SL: Scanning electron microscopy of polypoid cystitis —a reversible lesion of the human bladder. J Urol 131:242, 1984
10. Anderström C, Johansson SL, von Schultz L: Primary adenocarcinoma of the urinary bladder: a clinicopathologic and prognostic study. Cancer 52:1273, 1983
11. Arndt R, Dürkopf H, Huland H, et al: Monoclonal antibodies for characterization of the heterogeneity of normal and malignant transitional cells. J Urol 137:758, 1987
12. Askari A, Colmenares E, Saberi A, Jarman WD: Red cell surface antigen and its relationship to survival of patients with transitional cell carcinoma of the bladder. J Urol 125:182, 1981
13. Assor D: A villous tumor of the bladder. J Urol 119:287, 1978
14. Baker R: Correlation of circumferential lymphatic spread of vesical cancer with depth of infiltration: relation to present methods of treatment. J Urol 73:681, 1955
15. Bander NH: Monoclonal antibodies in urologic oncology. Cancer 60:658, 1987
16. Bander NH: Monoclonal antibodies: state of the art. J Urol 137:603, 1987
17. Battifora H, Eisenstein R, McDonald JH: The human urinary bladder mucosa: an electron microscopic study. Invest Urol 1:354, 1964
18. Battifora H, Eisenstein R, Sky-Peck HH, McDonald JH: Electron microscopy and tritiated thymidine in gradation of malignancy of human bladder carcinomas. J Urol 93:217, 1965
19. Bean MA: Some immunological considerations relevant to the study of human bladder cancer. Cancer Res 37:2879, 1977
20. Bennington JL, Beckwith JB: Tumors of the kidney,

renal pelvis, and ureter. Fasicle 12, 2nd Series. Atlas of Tumor Pathology, Washington, DC, 1975

21. Benson RC Jr, Swanson SK, Farrow GM: Relationship of leukoplakia to urothelial malignancy. J Urol 131:507, 1984

22. Bertrand B, Mason A, Jacobs JB: A simple apparatus and a novel method of cell collection for combined light microscopic and scanning electron microscopic exfoliative cytology. Acta Cytol (Baltimore) 23:427, 1979

23. Bhagavan BS, Tiamson EM, Wenk RE, et al: Nephrogenic adenoma of the urinary bladder and urethra. Hum Pathol 12:907, 1981

24. Bissada NK, Cole AT, Fried FA: Extensive condylomas acuminata of the entire male urethra and the bladder. J Urol 112:201, 1974

25. Blank C, Lissmer L, Kaneti J, et al: Fibroepithelial polyp of the renal pelvis. J Urol 137:962, 1987

26. Boileau MA, Cowles RS, Schmidt KL, Schmidt WA: Comparison of specific red-cell adherence and immunoperoxidase staining techniques for ABO(H) blood-group cell-surface antigens on superficial transitional cell carcinoma of the bladder. J Surg Oncol 30:72, 1985

27. Bourne CW, May JE: Urachal remnants: benign or malignant? J Urol 118:743, 1977

28. Braesch-Andersen S, Paulie S, Koho H, Perlmann P: Isolation and characterization of two bladder carcinoma-associated antigens. J Immunol Methods 94:145, 1986

29. Braun EV, Ali M, Fayemi AO, Beaugard E: Primary signet-ring cell carcinoma of the urinary bladder: review of the literature and report of a case. Cancer 47:1430, 1981

30. Broecker BH, Klein FA, Hackler RH: Cancer of the bladder in spinal cord injury patients. J Urol 125:196, 1981

31. Bullock PS, Thoni DE, Murphy WM: The significance of colonic mucosa (intestinal metaplasia) involving the urinary tract. Cancer 59:2086, 1987

32. Burry AF, Munn SR, Arnold EP, McRae CU: Trophoblastic metaplasia in urothelial carcinoma of the bladder. Br J Urol 58:143, 1986

33. Butterick JD, Schnitzer B, Abell MR: Ectopic prostatic tissue in urethra: a clinico-pathological entity and a significant cause of hematuria. J Urol 105:97, 1971

34. Byard RW, Bell MEA, Alkan MK: Primary carcinosarcoma: a rare cause of unilateral ureteral obstruction. J Urol 137:732, 1987

35. Cant JD, Murphy WM, Soloway MS: Prognostic significance of urine cytology on initial follow-up after intravesical mitomycin C for superficial bladder cancer. Cancer 57:2119, 1986

36. Cantrell BB, Leifer G, DeKlerk DP, Eggleston JC: Papillary adenocarcinoma of the prostatic urethra with clear-cell appearance. Cancer 48:2661, 1981

37. Catalona WJ: Practical utility of specific red cell adherence test in bladder cancer. Urology 18:113, 1981

38. Choi H, Lamb S, Pintar K, Jacobs SC: Primary signet-ring cell carcinoma of the urinary bladder. Cancer 53:1985, 1984

39. Chopin DK, deKernion JB, Rosenthal DL, Fahey JL: Monoclonal antibodies against transitional cell carcinoma for detection of malignant urothelial cells in bladder washing. J Urol 134:260, 1985

40. Coon JS, McCall A, Miller AW III, et al: Expression of blood-group-related antigens in carcinoma in situ of the urinary bladder. Cancer 56:797, 1985

41. Coon JS, Weinstein RS: Detection of ABH tissue isoantigens by immunoperoxidase methods in normal and neoplastic urothelium: comparison with the erythrocyte adherence method. Am J Clin Pathol 76:163, 1981

42. Cummings KB: Carcinoma of the bladder: predictors. Cancer 45:1849, 1980

43. Das G, Buxton NJC, Stewart PA, Glashan RW: Prognostic significance of ABH antigenicity of mucosal biopsies in superficial bladder cancer. J Urol 136:1194, 1986

44. DeBellis CC, Schumann GB: Cystoscopic biopsy supernate: a new cytologic approach for diagnosing urothelial carcinoma in situ. Acta Cytol (Baltimore) 30:356, 1986

45. Debenedictis TJ, Marmar JL, Praiss DE: Intraurethral condylomas acuminata: management and review of the literature. J Urol 118:767, 1977

46. Decenzo JM, Howard P, Irish CE: Antigenic deletion and prognosis of patients with stage A transitional cell bladder carcinoma. J Urol 114:874, 1975

47. DeFillipo N, Blute R, Klein LA: Signet-ring cell carcinoma of bladder: evaluation of three cases with review of literature. Urology 29:479, 1987

48. DeMeester LJ, Farrow GM, Utz DC: Inverted papillomas of the urinary bladder. Cancer 36:505, 1975

49. Devine P, Ueci AA, Gavris VE, et al: Nephrogenic adenoma, mesonephric, and metanephric tubules share Arachis hypogea receptor sites. Lab Invest 50:16A, 1984

50. Dexeus F, Logothetis C, Hossan E, Samuels ML: Carcinoembryonic antigen and beta-human chorionic gonadotropin as serum markers for advanced urothelial malignancies. J Urol 136:403, 1986

51. Di Cello V, Brischi G, Durval A, Mincione GP: Inverted papilloma of the ureteropelvic junction. J Urol 123:110, 1980

52. Domagala W, Kahan AV, Koss LG: The ultrastructure of surfaces of positively identified cells in the

human urinary sediment: a correlative light and scanning electron microscopic study. Acta Cytol (Baltimore) 23:147, 1979

53. Dowd JB: Case records of the Massachusetts General Hospital: case 8-1981. N Engl J Med 304:469, 1981

54. Eble JN, Hull MT, Rowland RG, Hostetter M: Villous adenoma of the urachus with mucusuria: a light and electron microscopic study. J Urol 135:1240, 1986

55. Ekelund P, Johansson S: Polypoid cystitis: a catheter associated lesion of the human bladder. Acta Pathol Microbiol Scand 87A:179, 1979

56. El-Bolkainy MN: Cytology of bladder carcinoma. J Urol 124:20, 1980

57. El-Bolkainy MN, Mokhtar NM, Ghoneim MA, Hussein MH: The impact of schistosomiasis on the pathology of bladder carcinoma. Cancer 48:2643, 1981

58. El-Mahrouky AS, Dawson DV, Paulson DF, Sanfilippo F: The predictive value of 2,4-dinitrochlorobenzene skin testing in patients with bilharzial bladder cancer. J Urol 129:499, 1983

59. Elsebai I: Parasites in the etiology of cancer — bilharziasis and bladder cancer. CA 27:100, 1977

60. Epstein JI, Kuhajda FP, Lieberman PH: Prostate specific acid phosphatase immunoreactivity in adenocarcinomas of the urinary bladder. Hum Pathol 17:939, 1986

61. Ewing R, Tate GM, Hetherington JW: Urinary fibrin/fibrinogen degradation products in transitional cell carcinoma of the bladder. Br J Urol 59:53, 1987

62. Fahey JL, Brosman S, Dorey F: Immunological responsiveness in patients with bladder cancer. Cancer Res 37:2875, 1977

63. Falor WH, Ward RM: DNA banding patterns in carcinoma of the bladder. JAMA 226:1322, 1973

64. Foster RS, Garrett RA: Congenital posterior urethral polyps. J Urol 136:670, 1986

65. Fradet Y, Cordon-Cardo C, Thomson T, et al: Cell surface antigens of human bladder cancer defined by mouse monoclonal antibodies. Proc Natl Acad Sci 81:224, 1984

66. Fradet Y, Cordon-Cardo C, Whitmore WF, Jr., et al: Cell surface antigens of human bladder tumors: definition of tumor subsets by monoclonal antibodies and correlation with growth characteristics. Cancer Res 46:5183, 1986

67. Fraley EE: Cancer of the renal pelvis. p. 134. In Skinner DG, DeKernion JB (eds): Genitourinary Cancer. Saunders, Philadelphia, 1978

68. Friedell GH: Urinary bladder cancer: selecting initial therapy. Cancer 60:496, 1987

69. Friedell GH, Bell JR, Burney SW, et al: Histopathology and classification of urinary bladder carcinoma. Urol Clin North Am 3:53, 1976

70. Friedell GH, Hawkins IR, Nagy GK: Urinary bladder. p. 295. In Henson DE, Albores-Saavedra J (eds): The Pathology of Incipient Neoplasia. Saunders, Philadelphia, 1986

71. Friedell GH, Parija GC, Nagy GK, Soto EA: The pathology of human bladder cancer. Cancer 45:1823, 1980

72. Friedell GH, Soloway MS, Hilgar AG, Farrow GM: Summary of workshop on carcinoma in situ of the bladder. J Urol 136:1047, 1986

73. Friedell GH, Soto EA, Nagy GK: Cytologic and histopathologic study of bladder cancer patients. Urol Clin North Am 3:71, 1976

74. Friedell GH, Soto EA, Parija GC, Nagy GK: The renal pelvis, ureter, urinary bladder, and urethra. p. 1125. In Silverberg SG (ed): Principles and Practice of Surgical Pathology. Wiley, New York, 1983

75. Geisler CH, Mori K, Leiter E: Lobulated inverted papilloma of the ureter. J Urol 123:270, 1980

76. Gilbert HA, Logan JL, Kagan AR et al: The natural history of papillary transitional cell carcinoma of the bladder and its treatment in an unselected population on the basis of histologic grading. J Urol 119:488, 1978

77. Gordon A: Intestinal metaplasia of the urinary tract epithelium. J Pathol Bacteriol 85:441, 1963

78. Gozzo JJ, Gottschalk R, O'Brien P, et al: Use of heterogenous and monospecific anterisera for the diagnosis of bladder cancer. J Urol 118:748, 1977

79. Grabstald H, Whitmore WF, Melamed MR: Renal pelvic tumors. JAMA 218:845, 1971

80. Greene LF, Hanash KA, Farrow GM: Benign papilloma or papillary carcinoma of the bladder? J Urol 110:205, 1973

81. Halim A, Javadpour N, Kasraeian A, Young JD: Cell surface antigen in bilharzial bladder tumours. Br J Urol 58:523, 1986

82. Hall L, Faddoul A, Saberi A, Edson M: The use of red cell surface antigen to predict the malignant potential of transitional cell carcinoma of the ureter and renal pelvis. J Urol 127:23, 1982

83. Hall RR: Carcinoembryonic antigen and urological carcinoma: a review after 7 years. Br J Urol 52:166, 1980

84. Hemmingsen L, Rasmussen F, Skaarup P, Wolf H: Urinary protein profiles in patients with urothelial bladder tumors. Br J Urol 53:324, 1981

85. Heney NM, Nocks BN, Daly JJ, et al: Prognostic factors in carcinoma of the ureter. J Urol 125:632, 1981

86. Herr HW: Suppressor cells in immunodepressed bladder and prostate cancer patients. J Urol 123:635, 1980

87. Herr HW: Association of depressed mixed lympho-

cyte reactivity with the development of bladder carcinoma in patients with papillomas. Cancer 51:344, 1983

88. Herr HW: Carcinoma in situ of the bladder. Semin Urol 1:15, 1983

89. Herring DW, Cartwright RA, Williams DDR: Genetic associations of transitional cell carcinoma. Br J Urol 51:73, 1979

90. Hertle L, Androulakakis P: Keratinizing desquamative squamous metaplasia of the upper urinary tract: leukoplakia-cholesteatoma. J Urol 127:631, 1982

91. Hill GS: Experimental production of pyeloureteritis cystica and glandularis. Invest Urol 9:1, 1971

92. Holborow EJ, Brown PC, Glynn LE, et al: The distribution of the blood group A antigen in human tissues. Br J Exp Pathol 41:430, 1960

93. Huland H, Arndt R, Huland E, et al: Monoclonal antibody 486 P3/12: a valuable bladder carcinoma marker for immunocytology. J Urol 137:654, 1987

94. Huszar M, Herczeg E, Lieberman Y, Geiger B: Distinctive immunofluorescent labeling of epithelial and mesenchymal elements of carcinosarcoma with antibodies specific for different intermediate filaments. Hum Pathol 15:532, 1984

95. Ingram EA, De Pauw P: Adenocarcinoma of the male urethra, with associated nephrogenic metaplasia: case report and review of the literature. Cancer 55:160, 1985

96. Jacobs JB: The potential of scanning electron microscopic (SEM) exfoliative cytology in the clinical management of human bladder cancer. p. 95. In Bonney WW, Prout GR Jr (eds): Bladder Cancer. AUA Monographs, Vol. 1. Williams & Wilkins, Baltimore, 1982

97. Jacobs JB, Arai M, Cohen SM, Friedell GH: A long-term study of reversible and progressive urinary bladder cancer lesions in rats fed N-[4-(5-nitro-2-furyl)-2-thiazolyl]formamide. Cancer Res 37:2817, 1977

98. Jacobs JB, Cohen SM, Arai M, Friedell GH: SEM on bladder cells. Acta Cytol (Baltimore) 21:3, 1977

99. Jacobs JB, Cohen SM, Farrow GM, Friedell GH: Scanning electron microscopic features of human urinary bladder cancer. Cancer 48:1399, 1981

100. Javadpour N, Vafrier J, Worsham GF, O'Connel K: Peroxidase antiperoxidase versus specific red cell adherence in detection of O (H) antigen in bladder cancer: a blind study. J Surg Oncol 27:112, 1984

101. Johnson DE, Hogan JM, Ayala AG: Primary adenocarcinoma of the urinary bladder. South Med J 65:527, 1972

102. Johnson DE, Schoenwald MB, Ayala AG, Miller LS: Squamous cell carcinoma of the bladder. J Urol 115:542, 1976

103. Jones KW: Chromosomal and nuclear location of mouse satellite DNA in individual cells. Nature 225:912, 1970

104. Kakizoe T, Fujita J, Murase T, et al: Transitional cell carcinoma of the bladder in patients with renal pelvic and ureteral cancer. J Urol 124:17, 1980

105. Kanno J, Sakamoto A, Washizuka M, et al: Malignant mixed mesodermal tumor of bladder occurring after radiotherapy for cervical cancer: report of a case. J Urol 133:854, 1985

106. Kay HEM, Wallace DM: A and B antigens of tumors arising from urinary epithelium. J Natl Cancer Inst 26:1349, 1961

107. Kiernan M, Gaffney EF: Brunn's nests and glandular metaplasia: normal urothelial variants in the supramontanal prostatic urethra. J Urol 137:877, 1987

108. Kim YH, Reiner L: Brunnian adenoma (inverted papilloma) of the urinary bladder: report of a case. Hum Pathol 9:229, 1978

109. Kirschenbaum AM, Cohen EL, Goldman HJ, et al: Ureteroscopic management of ureteral cholesteatoma. Urology 28:397, 1986

110. Köhler G, Milstein C: Continuous cultures of fused cells secreting antibody of predefined specificity. Nature 256:495, 1975

111. Koss LG: Tumors of the urinary bladder. Fascicle 11, 2nd Series. Atlas of Tumor Pathology. Armed Forces Institute of Pathology, Washington, DC, 1975

112. Koss LG: Mapping of the urinary bladder: its impact on the concepts of bladder cancer. Hum Pathol 10:533, 1979

113. Koss LG: Tumors of the urinary bladder. Supplement, Fascicle 11, 2nd Series. Atlas of Tumor Pathology. Armed Forces Institute of Pathology, Washington, DC, 1985

114. Koss LG, Bartels PH, Sychra JJ, Wied GL: Diagnostic cytologic sample profiles in patients with bladder cancer using the TICAS system. Acta Cytol (Baltimore) 22:392, 1978

115. Koss LG, Tiamson EM, Robbins MA: Mapping cancerous and precancerous bladder changes. JAMA 227:281, 1974

116. Kovarik S, Davidsohn I, Stejskal R: ABO antigens in cancer: detection with the mixed cell agglutination reaction. Arch Pathol 86:12, 1968

117. Kunze E, Schauer A, Schmitt M: Histology and histogenesis of two different types of inverted urothelial papillomas. Cancer 51:348, 1983

118. Lamb D: Correlation of chromosome counts with histological appearances and prognosis of transitional cell carcinoma of bladder. Br Med J 1:273, 1967

119. Lange PH: Immunologic testing of patients with genitourinary malignancies. Urol Clin North Am 6:587, 1979

120. Lange PH: Tumor immunology: a review of basic concepts with special reference to bladder cancer. p. 119. In Bonney WW, Prout GR Jr (eds): Bladder Cancer. AUA Monographs, Vol. 1. Williams & Wilkins, Baltimore, 1982

121. Lange PH, Hakala TR, Fraley EE: Classification of the bladder cancer patient based on in vitro measurements of the immune response. Cancer Res 37:2885, 1977

122. Lange PH, Hakala TR, Fraley EE: Current concepts in immunobiology of genitourinary tumors. p. 607. In Devine CJ Jr, Stecker JF Jr (eds): Urology in Practice. Little, Brown, Boston, 1978

123. Lattes R: Surgical pathology reports. Hum Pathol 15:598, 1984

124. Lazarevic B, Garret R: Inverted papilloma and papillary transitional cell carcinoma of urinary bladder: report of four cases of inverted papilloma, one showing papillary malignant transformation, and review of the literature. Cancer 42:1904, 1978

125. Lehman TP, Cooper HS, Mulholland SG: Peanut lectin binding sites in transitional cell carcinoma of the urinary bladder. Cancer 53:272, 1984

126. Leighton J, Abasa N, Tchao R, et al: Development of tissue culture procedures for predicting the individual risk of recurrence in bladder cancer. Cancer Res 37:2854, 1977

127. Limas C, Lange P: Altered reactivity for A, B, H antigens in transitional cell carcinomas of the urinary bladder: a study of the mechanisms involved. Cancer 46:1366, 1980

128. Limas C, Lange P: A, B, H antigen detectability in normal and neoplastic urothelium: influence of methodological factors. Cancer 49:2476, 1982

129. Limas C, Lange PH: Lewis antigens in normal and neoplastic urothelium. Am J Pathol 121:176, 1985

130. Limas C, Lange P: T-antigen in normal and neoplastic urothelium. Cancer 58:1236, 1986

131. Limas C, Lange P, Fraley EE, Vessella RL: A, B, H antigens in transitional cell tumors of the urinary bladder: correlation with the clinical course. Cancer 44:2099, 1979

132. Liu BC-S, Neuwirth H, Zhu LW, et al: Detection of oncofetal bladder antigen in urine of patients with transitional cell carcinoma. J Urol 137:1258, 1987

133. Lloyd KO: Blood group antigens as markers for normal differentiation and malignant change in human tissues. Am J Clin Pathol 87:129, 1987

134. Lytton B, O'Toole C, Tiptaft R, et al: Histocompatibility testing in patients with carcinoma of the bladder. Cancer 52:645, 1983

135. Macksood MJ, Roth DR, Chang CH, Perlmutter AD: Benign fibroepithelial polyps as a cause of intermittent ureteropelvic junction obstruction in a child: a case report and review of the literature. J Urol 134:951, 1985

136. Marshall VF: Current clinical problems regarding bladder tumors. Cancer 9:543, 1956

137. McIntire TL, Soloway MS, Murphy WM: Nephrogenic adenoma. Urology 29:237, 1987

138. Melamed MR, Klein FA: Flow cytometry of urinary bladder irrigation specimens. Hum Pathol 15:302, 1984

139. Melicow MM: Histological study of vesical urothelium intervening between gross neoplasms in total cystectomy. J Urol 68:261, 1952

140. Melicow MM: Tumors of the bladder: a multifaceted problem. J Urol 112:467, 1974

141. Mitchell MS: Tumor immunology and immunotherapy: principles and studies in genitourinary cancers. p. 349. In Skinner DG (ed): Urological Cancer. Grune & Stratton, New York, 1983

142. Molland EA, Trott PA, Paris AMI, Blandy JP: Nephrogenic adenoma: a form of adenomatous metaplasia of the bladder: a clinical and electron microscopical study. Br J Urol 48:453, 1976

143. Moon TD, Vessella RL, Lange PH: Monoclonal antibodies in urology. J Urol 130:584, 1983

144. Morse HD: The etiology and pathology of pyelitis cystica, ureteritis cystica, and cystitis cystica. Am J Pathol 4:33, 1928

145. Mostofi FK: Potentialities of bladder epithelium. J Urol 71:705, 1954

146. Mostofi FK, Price EB Jr: Tumors of the male genital system. Fascicle 8, 2nd Series, Atlas of Tumor Pathology. Armed Forces Institute of Pathology, Washington, DC, 1973

147. Mostofi FK, Sobin LH, Torloni H (eds): International Histological Classification of Tumours, No. 10: Histological Typing of Urinary Bladder Tumours. World Health Organization, Geneva, 1973

148. Mostofi FK, Thomson RV, Dean AL Jr: Mucous adenocarcinoma of the urinary bladder. Cancer 8:741, 1955

149. Mourin-Jouret A, Squifflet JP, Cosyns JP, et al: Bilateral ureteral endometriosis with end-stage renal failure. Urology 29:302, 1987

150. Murphy DM, Zincke H, Furlow WL: Primary grade I transitional cell carcinoma of the renal pelvis and ureter. J Urol 123:629, 1980

151. Murphy WM: Current topics in the pathology of bladder cancer. Pathol Annu 18:1, 1983

152. Musselman P, Kay R: The spectrum of urinary tract fibroepithelial polyps in children. J Urol 136:476, 1986

153. Nagy GK, Frable WJ, Murphy WM: Classification of

premalignant urothelial abnormalities: a Delphi study of the National Bladder Cancer Collaborative Group A. Pathol Annu 17:219, 1982

154. National Bladder Cancer Collaborative Group A (NBCCGA): Development of a strategy for a longitudinal study of patients with bladder cancer. Cancer Res 37:2898, 1977

155. Neumann MP, Limas C: Transitional cell carcinomas of the urinary bladder: effects of preoperative irradiation on morphology. Cancer 58:2758, 1986

156. Nichols JA, Marshall VF: Treatment of histologically benign papilloma of the urinary bladder by local excision and fulguration. Cancer 9:566, 1956

157. Nieh PT, Daly JJ, Heaney JA, et al: The effect of intravesical thio-tepa on normal and tumor urothelium. J Urol 119:59, 1978

158. Nielsen K, Nielsen KK: Adenocarcinoma in exstrophy of the bladder — the last case in Scandinavia? A case report and review of literature. J Urol 130:1180, 1983

159. Nocks BN, Heney NM, Daly JJ, et al: Transitional cell carcinoma of the renal pelvis. Urology 19:472, 1982

160. O'Brien AME, Urbanski SJ: Papillary adenocarcinoma in situ of bladder. J Urol 134:544, 1985

161. O'Brien P, Gozzo JJ, Monaco AP: Urinary proteins as biological markers: bladder cancer diagnosis versus urinary tract infection. J Urol 124:802, 1980

162. Oettgen HF, Hellstrom KE: Tumor immunology. p. 1029. In Holland JF, Frei E III (eds): Cancer Medicine. Lea & Febiger, Philadelphia, 1982

163. O'Kane HOJ, Megaw JM: Carcinoma in the exstrophic bladder. Br J Surg 55:631, 1968

164. Ooms ECM, Anderson WAD, Alons CL, et al: Analysis of the performance of pathologists in the grading of bladder tumors. Hum Pathol 14:140, 1983

165. O'Shea PA, Callaghan JF, Lawlor JB, Reddy VC: "Nephrogenic adenoma": an unusual metaplastic change of urothelium. J Urol 125:249, 1981

166. Packham DA: The epithelial lining of the female trigone and urethra. Br J Urol 43:201, 1971

167. Partanen S, Asikainen U: Oat cell carcinoma of the urinary bladder with ectopic adrenocorticotropic hormone production. Hum Pathol 16:313, 1985

168. Paschkis R: Über adenome der harnblase. Z Urol Chir 21:315, 1927

169. Plous RH, Sunshine R, Goldman H, Schwartz IS: Ureteral endometriosis in post-menopausal women. Urology 26:408, 1985

170. Proppe KH, Scully RE, Rosai J: Postoperative spindle cell nodules of genitourinary tract resembling sarcomas: a report of eight cases. Am J Surg Pathol 8:101, 1984

171. Prout GR Jr: Introduction: management (control) of early bladder lesions. Cancer Res 37:2891, 1977

172. Prout GR Jr: Classification and staging of bladder carcinoma. Cancer 45:1832, 1980

173. Prout GR Jr, Bassil B, Griffin P: The treated histories of patients with Ta grade 1 transitional-cell carcinoma of the bladder. Arch Surg 121:1463, 1986

174. Raju GC, Roopnarinesingh A, Woo J: Villous adenoma of female urethra. Urology 29:446, 1987

175. Ramaekers FCS, Moesker O, Huysmans A, et al: Intermediate filament proteins in the study of tumor heterogeneity: an in-depth study of tumors of the urinary and respiratory tracts. Ann NY Acad Sci 455:614, 1985

176. Reece RW, Koontz WW Jr: Leukoplakia of the urinary tract: a review. J Urol 114:165, 1975

177. Reichborn-Kjennerud S, Hoeg K: The value of urine cytology in the diagnosis of recurrent bladder tumors: a preliminary report. Acta Cytol (Baltimore) 16:269, 1972

178. Remick DG Jr, Kumar NB: Benign polyps with prostatic-type epithelium of the urethra and the urinary bladder. Am J Surg Pathol 8:833, 1984

179. Richart RM: Cervical intraepithelial neoplasia. p. 301. In Sommers SC (ed): Pathology Annual. Appleton-Century-Crofts, New York, 1973

180. Richie JP: Management of ureteral tumors. p. 150. In Skinner, DG, DeKernion JB (eds): Genitourinary Cancer. Saunders, Philadelphia, 1978

181. Richie JP, Yap WT: Further observations on the specific red cell adherence test: effects of radiation therapy. J Urol 125:493, 1981

182. Ridolfi RL, Eggleston JC: Carcinosarcoma of the renal pelvis. J Urol 119:569, 1978

182a. Ro JY, Ayala AG, El-Naggar A: Muscularis mucosa of urinary bladder. Importance for staging and treatment. Am J Surg Pathol 11:668, 1987

183. Rubin J, Khanna OP, Damjanov I: Adenomatous polyp of the bladder: a rare cause of hematuria in young men. J Urol 126:549, 1981

184. Salm R: Combined intestinal and squamous metaplasia of the renal pelvis. J Clin Pathol 22:187, 1969

185. Sand PK, Shen W, Bowen LW, Ostergard DR: Cryotherapy for the treatment of proximal urethral condyloma acuminatum. J Urol 137:874, 1987

186. Sandberg AA: Chromosome markers and progression in bladder cancer. Cancer Res 37:2950, 1977

187. Sandberg AA: Chromosomes in bladder cancer. p. 81. In Bonney WW, Prout GR Jr (eds): Bladder Cancer. AUA Monographs, Vol. 1. Williams & Wilkins, Baltimore, 1982

188. Sandberg AA: Chromosome changes in bladder

cancer: clinical and other correlations. Cancer Genet Cytogenet 19:163, 1986

189. Sandberg AA, Turc-Carel C: The cytogenetics of solid tumors: relation to diagnosis, classification and pathology. Cancer 59:387, 1987

190. Sarma KP: Genesis of papillary tumours: histological and microangiographic study. Br J Urol 53:228, 1981

191. Schilling A, Böwering R, Keiditsch E: Use of the neodymium-YAG laser in the treatment of ureteral tumors and urethral condylomata acuminata. Eur Urol 12, Suppl 1:30, 1986

192. Schmidt KL, Riddouch MD, Hilburn PJ, et al: Scanning and transmission electron microscopy, morphometry, and carcinoembryonic antigen of bladder washings. Lab Invest 48:75A, 1983

193. Schoborg TW, Saffos RO, Rodriquez AP, Scott C Jr: Carcinosarcoma of the bladder. J Urol 124:724, 1980

194. Schrodt GR, Alcorn MO, Ibanez J: Endometriosis of the male urinary system: a case report. J Urol 124:722, 1980

195. Schubert GE, Pavkovic MB, Bethke-Bedürftig BA: Tubular urachal remnants in adult bladders. J Urol 127:40, 1982

196. Schulze S, Holm-Nielsen A, Ravn V: Inverted papilloma of upper urinary tract. Urology 28:58, 1986

197. Schwartz WB, Wolfe HJ, Pauker SG: Pathology and probabilities: a new approach to interpreting and reporting biopsies. N Engl J Med 305:917, 1981

198. Scully RE: Tumors of the ovary and maldeveloped gonads. Fascicle 16, 2nd Series, Atlas of Tumor Pathology. Armed Forces Institute of Pathology, Washington, DC, 1979

199. Sesterhenn IA, Davis CJ, Mostofi FK: Nephrogenic adenomas of bladder and urethra. Lab Invest 50:53A, 1984

200. Shevchuk MM, Fenoglio CM, Richart RM: Carcinoembryonic antigen localization in benign and malignant transitional epithelium. Cancer 47:899, 1981

201. Shigematsu S: Significance of the chromosome in vesical cancer. In: Proceedings, XIII Cong. Soc. Inter. Urologie, London, 1965, p. 111

202. Shipley WU, Prout GR, Jr., Kaufman D, Perrone TL: Invasive bladder carcinoma: the importance of initial transurethral surgery and other significant prognostic factors for improved survival with full-dose irradiation. Cancer 60:514, 1987

203. Soto EA, Friedell GH, Tiltman AJ: Bladder cancer as seen in giant histologic sections. Cancer 39:447, 1977

204. Stein BS: Laser treatment of condylomata acuminata. J Urol 136:593, 1986

205. Stillwell TJ, Kramer SA, Lee RA: Endometriosis of ureter. Urology 28:81, 1986

206. Stilmant MM, Siroky MB: Nephrogenic adenoma associated with intravesical bacillus Calmette-Guérin treatment: a report of 2 cases. J Urol 135:359, 1986

207. Strand WR, Alfert HJ: Nephrogenic adenoma occurring in an ileal conduit. J Urol 137:491, 1987

208. Stuppler SA, Kandzari SJ: Fibroepithelial polyps of ureter. Urology 5:553, 1975

209. Summers JL, Falor WH, Ward R: A 10-year analysis of chromosomes in non-invasive papillary carcinoma of the bladder. J Urol 125:177, 1981

210. Suzuki T, Cano M, Cohen SM: Scanning electron microscopic exfoliative urinary cytology in patients with malignant and nonmalignant diseases of lower urinary tract. Urology 28:62, 1986

211. Svenes KB, Eide J: Proliferative Brenner tumor or ovarian metastases? Cancer 53:2692, 1984

212. Takahashi N, Takahashi S, Takahashi K, et al: A monoclonal antibody to human transitional cell carcinoma of the bladder: production and characterization. J Urol 138:207, 1987

213. Tannenbaum M, Romas NA: The pathobiology of early urothelial cancers. p. 232. In Skinner DG, deKernion JB (eds): Genitourinary Cancer. Saunders, Philadelphia, 1978

214. Tannenbaum M, Tannenbaum S, Carter HW: SEM, BEI, and TEM ultrastructural characteristics of normal, preneoplastic, and neoplastic human transitional epithelia. Scan Electron Microsc 2:949, 1978.

215. Têtu B, Ro JY, Ayala AG, et al: Small cell carcinoma of the prostate. I. A clinicopathologic study of 20 cases. Cancer 59:1803, 1987

216. Thomas DG, Ward AM, Williams JL: A study of 52 cases of adenocarcinoma of the bladder. Br J Urol 43:4, 1971

217. Tungekar MF, Al Adnani MS: Sarcomas of the bladder and prostate: the role of immunohistochemistry and ultrastructure in diagnosis. Eur Urol 12:180, 1986

218. Tyler DE: Stratified squamous epithelium in the vesical trigone and urethra: findings correlated with the menstrual cycle and age. Am J Anat 111:319, 1962

219. Uriel J: Retrodifferentiation and the fetal patterns of gene expression in cancer. Adv Cancer Res 29:127, 1979

220. Utz DC, Hanash KA, Farrow GM: The plight of the patient with carcinoma in situ of the bladder. J Urol 103:160, 1970

221. Van Poppel H, Nuttin B, Oyen R, et al: Fibroepithelial polyps of the ureter: etiology, diagnosis, treatment and pathology. Eur Urol 12:174, 1986

222. Wake N, Slocum HK, Rustum YM, et al: Chromosomes and causation of human cancer and leukemia. XLIV. A method for chromosome analysis of solid tumors. Cancer Genet Cytogenet 3:1, 1981

223. Walker AN, Mills SE, Fechner RE, Perry JM: Epithelial polyps of the prostatic urethra. Am J Surg Pathol 7:351, 1983

224. Walther MM, Campbell WG, Jr., O'Brien DP III, et al: Cystitis cystica: an electron and immunofluorescence microscopic study. J Urol 137:764, 1987

225. Walther M, O'Brien DP III, Birch HW: Condylomata acuminata and verrucous carcinoma of the bladder: case report and literature review. J Urol 135:362, 1986

226. Walton GR, McCue PA, Graham SD Jr.: Beta-2-microglobulins as a differentiation marker in bladder cancer. J Urol 136:1197, 1986

227. Weinstein RS, Coon JS, Alroy J, Davidsohn I: Tissue-associated blood group antigens in human tumors. p. 239. In DeLelis RA (ed): Diagnostic Immunohistochemistry. Masson, New York, 1981

228. Weinstein RS, Coon JS, Schwartz D, et al: Pathology of superficial bladder cancer with emphasis on carcinoma in situ. Urology, suppl. 4, 26:2, 1985

229. Wells M, Anderson K: Mucin histochemistry of cystitis glandularis and primary adenocarcinoma of the urinary bladder. Arch Pathol Lab Med 109:59, 1985

230. Whitmore WF, Jr.: Bladder cancer. CA 28:170, 1978

231. Whitesel JA: Inverted papilloma of the urinary tract: malignant potential. J Urol 127:539, 1982

232. Widran J, Sanchez R, Gruhn J: Squamous metaplasia of the bladder: a study of 450 patients. J Urol 112:479, 1974

233. Wolfe JT III, Mills SE, Weiss MA, Fowler JE: Small cell undifferentiated carcinoma of the urinary tract. Lab Invest 54:71A, 1986

234. Wolgel CD, Parris AC, Mitty HA, Schapira HE: Fibroepithelial polyp of renal pelvis. Urology 19:436, 1982

235. Young RH: Carcinosarcoma of the urinary bladder. Cancer 59:1333, 1987

236. Young RH, Scully RE: Clear cell adenocarcinoma of the bladder and urethra: a report of three cases and a review of the literature. Am J Surg Pathol 9:816, 1985

237. Young RH, Scully RE: Nephrogenic adenoma: report of 15 cases, review of the literature, and comparison with clear cell adenocarcinoma of the urinary tract. Am J Surg Pathol 10:268, 1986

238. Zaloudek C, Williams JW, Kempson RL: "Endometrioid" adenocarcinoma of the prostate: a distinctive tumor of probable prostatic duct origin. Cancer 37:2255, 1976

239. Zincke H, Utz DC, Farrow GM: Review of Mayo Clinic experience with carcinoma in situ. Urology, suppl. 4, 26:39, 1985

18

Urothelial Neoplasms: Urinary Bladder

James W. Eagan, Jr.

In this chapter we consider epithelial neoplasia of the urinary bladder, with attention given also to the proximal urethra. Because the clinical aspects of the disease are so closely intertwined with the pathologic aspects, particularly in key areas such as tumor staging, an overview of both is given. In all areas of pathology, a sound grasp of the clinical situation may be an invaluable aid to the pathologist at the microscope. Indeed, one who chooses to ignore the clinical circumstances resulting in the advent of the specimen at hand does so at his or her own peril.

Epithelial tumors account for the vast majority of all neoplasms encountered in the urinary bladder. Among all epithelial neoplasms, greater than 99 percent are considered malignant,[53] at least according to the criteria established in conventional classifications such as those of the World Health Organization (WHO)[126] and the Armed Forces Institute of Pathology (AFIP).[94] Thus, for practical purposes, urothelial bladder neoplasia and "bladder cancer" are essentially synonymous.

As the reader will note, however, there is a decided lack of homogeneity among patients and their "bladder cancers," with obvious implications regarding diagnosis, therapy, and prognosis. Much of the chapter, therefore, will focus upon how these patients and their disease processes may best be subclassified.

INCIDENCE

As noted, incidence figures for urothelial neoplasms of the bladder are essentially those for bladder cancer; benign tumors, as defined in the preceding chapter, are seen so infrequently that meaningful figures are difficult to assemble. Only two types of benign lesion that are thought definitely to be of neoplastic nature—transitional cell papilloma and transitional cell papilloma, inverted type—are seen with any degree of frequency, but even they are uncommon in day-to-day practice. The former lesion, transitional cell papilloma, as defined by the WHO,[126] is not frequently encountered by itself. When it occurs as an isolated lesion, it is generally small and more likely to be fulgurated than resected. Most examples of this entity are discovered as incidental findings in patients being followed for papillary transitional cell carcinoma. Inverted transitional cell papillomas are even more unusual, generally the subject of isolated case reports and compendia of previous case reports. Other benign tumors and tumor-like lesions, which rarely may present major surgical problems,[32] have been discussed in Chapter 17.

For malignant epithelial neoplasms, or "bladder cancers," the estimated incidence of new cases in the United States in 1987 is 45,400, with men predominating over women in a ratio of approximately 2.7 : 1.[168] The estimated number of deaths due to bladder cancer during the same time period is 10,600, with a somewhat lower male/female ratio, approximately 2.1 : 1, indicating that, overall, women seem to fare less well with this disease.

The lifetime risks of developing bladder cancer are on the order of approximately 2.8 and 1.0 percent for white men and women, respectively, with blacks showing lower risks: 0.9 percent for men and 0.6 percent for women.[161,167] For men, the risk of bladder cancer increases at a nearly constant rate throughout adult life, with an annual incidence of less than 2 per 100,000 population among males in their third decade, rising to more than 200 per 100,000 during the eighth and ninth decades.[124] A bimodal incidence curve has been found for women, however, rising sharply during the fifth decade, falling somewhat, and then rising again during the seventh to ninth decades, possibly reflective of increased cigarette smoking in the younger female population.[124]

Melicow,[119] in a series of more than 900 cases of vesical tumors, found that 97 percent of primary bladder malignancies in both men and women were seen after age 40, with the greatest incidence in both sexes from ages 60 to 69. The mean age for the subgroup with only low grade papillary lesions is somewhat lower, in the mid fifties range according to Nichols and Marshall.[136] The disease is seen essentially throughout life, however, although Benson et al.,[12] in a review of transitional cell carcinoma of the bladder in children and adolescents, found only 100 patients in the literature with bladder cancer occurring before age 21, and only 14 documented cases in children during the first decade of life. Prognosis for patients under age 40 has been noted as better than that usually cited for the over-40 group, perhaps the result of a generally low grade/low stage presentation,[193] but it should be noted that aggressive disease is seen in younger patients on occasion and must be treated accordingly.[98]

There appears to be a minor trend toward an increasing overall incidence in men, but opinions are somewhat divergent on changes in female incidence.[124] The various factors associated with an increased risk of developing bladder cancer, including industrial exposure, cigarette smoking, etc. are discussed at length in Chapter 16.

The above "standard data" are generally descriptive of the situation that obtains in patients with transitional cell carcinoma. The data for patients with less common tumors show many similarities and a few dissimilarities.

Pure squamous carcinoma in Western populations, for example, is also a disease seen primarily in patients in their sixties, with a broad range from the thirties through the eighties.[48,85] Significant male predominance is not the case, however, with the male/female ratio approaching 1 : 1.[48,85]

Blacks appear more likely to develop squamous carcinoma than whites,[159] although such tumors still account for only a minority of bladder cancers in both races. Bilharziasis-associated carcinoma, on the other hand, is a strikingly different matter, with squamous carcinomas clearly predominating over other types. According to Elsebai,[43] cancer of the bilharzial bladder is the most common cancer in Egyptian men, accounting for more than one-fourth of *all* tumor cases admitted to the Cairo Cancer Institute each year, with somewhat lesser incidences noted in other Middle Eastern countries. Here the male/female ratio is approximately 5:1, and the usual presentation is during the forties, with patients in their twenties seen not infrequently.

Adenocarcinoma of the bladder, outside the setting of bladder exstrophy, has been seen from the third to the ninth decades[1,2,76,84,127] but is predominantly seen in patients in their fifties and sixties.[76,84] Similar to transitional cell carcinoma, the male/female ratio is approximately 3 : 1.[1,127] Figures on racial distribution are not available. Both adenocarcinomas and squamous carcinomas are seen with increased frequency in the setting of lithiasis.

Patients presenting with carcinoma in situ alone, without associated or prior neoplasms, are generally elderly men.[47,117] Farrow et al.[47] detailed 69 such cases seen over a 6-year period at the Mayo Clinic, discovered as part of a prospective urinary cytology study. Of the 69 patients, 63 were men, but the age span of 31 to 87 years and mean age of 63.1 years were similar to statistics cited for transitional cell carcinoma of the bladder in general.

CLINICAL PRESENTATION

Hematuria is the presenting manifestation in most patients with bladder carcinoma. Massey et al.,[113] in a study of more than 300 patients with bladder cancer, all grades considered, found that 80 percent presented with gross hematuria, with an additional 5 percent having had only microscopic hematuria. Although 60 percent of the patients were seen within 3 months of their first symptoms, 9 percent were not seen until 2 years or more following the onset of symptoms. Greene and colleagues[61] noted similar figures among patients with low grade papillary lesions in a referral population at the Mayo Clinic, with 73 percent of patients demonstrating gross hematuria and an additional 12 percent at least microscopic hematuria. Of interest in this series was a delay in presentation of up to 20 years following the onset of symptoms, a magnitude of delay noted in another large series of patients with low grade tumors reported by Lerman et al.[103]

Hematuria is also the most common complaint among patients with adenocarcinoma[1,76,127] and squamous carcinoma,[48,85] although irritative symptoms of urgency, frequency, and dysuria may be the presenting complaints in both situations as well.[84,85] If irritative symptoms are the dominant complaint, however, one should be alerted to the possibility of carcinoma in situ, as approximately 90 percent of patients having only carcinoma in situ present in this fashion, at first frequently suggestive of cystitis or prostatitis.[197,198] Accompanying gross hematuria will often be present, however, and, as noted by Farrow and co-workers,[47] virtually all of these patients are found to have at least microscopic hematuria. The reason for the disparity in presenting symptoms between patients with carcinoma in situ and most of the patients with other forms of bladder cancer is not clear; it may relate to the fact that there is no mass lesion prone to focal hemorrhage in patients with only carcinoma in situ. (It would be of interest to know how many patients with nonpapillary invasive carcinomas had suffered from irritative symptoms, possibly during an in situ phase of their disease, prior to the onset of hematuria, an event more likely to prompt a visit to the doctor.)

Much less frequently, patients with bladder cancer present with obstructive symptoms at the outset, an event more commonly seen with adenocarcinoma[76] and squamous carcinoma[85] than transitional cell carcinoma. Few patients with any tumor type present with metastatic disease as the initial manifestation, with absolutely no signs or symptoms to suggest an occult bladder primary.

Although most patients with bladder cancer manifest gross or at least microscopic hematuria, the converse is not the case; that is, the majority of adult patients presenting because of hematuria do *not* have bladder or other cancers, although the percentage that do is still rather striking. In a series of 110 consecutive adults presenting with *gross hematuria*, Carter and Rous[19] found somewhat fewer than one-fourth to have genitourinary neoplasms, including 9 percent bladder, 6 percent renal, 6 percent prostate, and 1 percent urethral primaries. In patients with only asymptomatic *microscopic hematuria*, the incidence is less, with only approximately 10 percent of adult patients found to have genitourinary neoplasms[31,59]; in one large series,[59] 51 percent had no demonstrable urologic lesion whatever, either at presentation or after follow-up for at least 2 years. Hematuria in an adult patient must always be viewed with suspicion, however; and even though other possible explanations may be found, a thorough evaluation is indicated. Patients with gross hematuria[19] are commonly found initially to have urinary tract infection, another obvious cause of hematuria. If evaluation is terminated following the finding of pyuria and bacteriuria, however, a significant number of patients with underlying neoplasms will be missed. Pyuria is frequently seen with bladder tumors,[61,198] and in patients with partial obstruction bacteriuria is also common. In the series of patients with squamous carcinomas reported by Johnson et al.,[85] urethral obstruction was frequent, and urinary tract infection was present at the time of diagnosis in 93 percent of patients.

In summary, hematuria, with or without associated symptoms, must be viewed as a "red flag." Particularly in patients in their fifties and sixties, a full workup must be pursued despite such immediately apparent explanations as urinary tract infection or calculi.

PATIENT EVALUATION

A thorough history and complete physical examination are the primary steps of evaluation. In addition to documenting the patient's symptoms, the history covers possible predisposing factors such as occupational exposure, usage of analgesics and tobacco products, travel history, previous infections, and lithiasis. Prior or concurrent diseases, particularly a history of neoplasia elsewhere in the body, and a record of treatment, should also be noted. Physical examination should be equally thorough, including complete abdominal and pelvic examination in the female patient and rectal examination in the male patient.

Cytologic examination of at least one voided urine specimen (preferably prior to prostatic examination) may prove a relatively inexpensive first clue to the presence or absence of urothelial malignancy, particularly with high grade disease. Although less sensitive than specimens obtained during cystoscopy, artifactual changes related to instrumentation are circumvented.

Preoperative radiologic evaluation should include at least a routine chest film and intravenous urography. Bladder filling defects suggestive of tumor may be seen with low grade disease[61] and in more than two-thirds of patients presenting with low stage disease with all grades represented.[210] Hydroureteronephrosis and/or nonfunction of a renal unit associated with ipsilateral bladder tumor are generally associated with deep tumor extension,[27,63] although such findings were also noted at presentation in 6 percent of patients with low grade noninvasive disease by Greene et al.[61] Transabdominal ultrasonography may also be of value in answering the basic question of presence versus absence of a mass lesion,[34] although evolving methods of transurethral sonography seem to offer better results for both initial diagnosis and subsequent staging.[35,70]

Cystoscopic examination with bimanual palpation of the abdomen remains the cornerstone of the primary evaluation of patients with suspected urothelial neoplasms and is done following the initial workup.[27,184] At the outset of the procedure, a cystoscopically obtained urine specimen for cytology should be collected, after which many clinicians obtain a bladder washing specimen.[184] Although the former has been viewed as possibly superfluous if the latter is obtained, Murphy et al.[129] demonstrated that the two techniques may be complementary; diagnostic cells were usually present in both specimens but were found *only* in the cystoscopic urine specimen in 13.1 percent of their patients. One situation where this test may be of particular use is that in which biopsy specimens and bladder washings are indicative of low grade disease, but an admixture of high grade cells in the cystoscopy urine specimen indicates the possibility of a more serious lesion elsewhere in the urothelial tract.

After obtaining the cytology specimens, thorough

cystoscopic and urethroscopic examinations are performed. According to Persky et al.,[139] approximately 45 percent of all bladder tumors are located on the lateral walls, 20 percent in the trigone region, 15 percent on the posterior wall, 5 percent in the bladder neck area, and 6 to 8 percent each on the anterior wall and in the vault. The location, appearance, and estimated size of the lesion or lesions are carefully recorded, with graphic charting of the findings as recommended by Prout and the National Bladder Cancer Group (NBCG)[140] (Fig. 18-1). Photography of the lesions may also be of value.[182] All apparent lesions are subject to at least biopsy if not primary transurethral resection. Although simple fulguration of small lesions is usually performed during subsequent cystoscopy, resection for microscopic evaluation should be considered for all visible lesions during the initial evaluation. The preferred method to obtain a tumor biopsy specimen is with a resectoscope; underlying muscle, necessary for proper pathologic staging, is obtained as well.[139] The remaining "normal mucosa" may have as much and at times more bearing on the patient's prognosis as the tumor itself,[45,95] particularly with lower grade tumors. For this reason, selected-site biopsies of the mucosa adjacent to the tumor, lateral to each ureteral orifice, and in the posterior midline are obtained.[140] They are best performed using the "cold cup" biopsy technique, aimed at obtaining superficial specimens where mucosal evaluation is the primary purpose.

There has been some controversy concerning possible secondary implantation of tumor related both to resection and biopsy. Soloway,[178] who has done considerable research on this important issue, noted that although iatrogenic tumor implantation in man has not been definitely proved, laboratory studies in animals and circumstantial evidence in man have suggested that this phenomenon may account for at least some of the recurrences common to bladder carcinoma. The clinician is well advised to give serious consideration to the use of topical chemotherapeutic agents following cystoscopic resection of the tumorous urothelium,[60,72] an idea actually proposed many years back by Dr. Melicow[118] in his original work regarding the importance of the "remaining urothelium" in the prognosis of patients with bladder carcinoma.

The above evaluation permits initial classification

CYSTOSCOPY REPORT FORM

Pt. Name _ Unit Number _

Date of Cystoscopy _ _ _ _ / _ _ _ / _ _ _ Surgeon _

Number of visible tumors seen: 0 _ _ _ _ _

1 _ _ _ _ _

2 _ _ _ _ _

3 _ _ _ _ _

≥ 4 _ _ _ _ _

Susp. areas only _ _ _ _ _

Size of largest tumor: < 1cm _ _ _ _ _

1 − 1.9 _ _ _ _ _

2 − 2.9 _ _ _ _ _

3 − 3.9 _ _ _ _ _

4 − 4.9 _ _ _ _ _

5+ _ _ _ _ _

unable to estimate _ _ _ _ _ _

Shapes of tumor present: papillary _ _ _ _ _

sessile _ _ _ _ _

nodular _ _ _ _ _

flat _ _ _ _ _

other _ _ _ _ _

Biman. exam: Not done _ _ _ _ _

Normal _ _ _ _ _

Induration of bl. wall _ _ _ _ _

Palp. mobile mass _ _ _ _ _

Tumor invading prost/

vagina _ _ _ _ _

Tumor fixed _ _ _ _ _

Check which of the following procedures were done:

Bladder wash for cytology _ _ _ _ _

Cold cup tumor biopsy _ _ _ _ _

Selected mucosal biopsy _ _ _ _ _

Transurethral resection _ _ _ _ _

▶ ▶ ▶ PLEASE USE PRE−PRINTED BIOPSY

▶ ▶ ▶ LABEL SPECIMENS FOR ALL PATHOLOGY

MATERIAL!!

PLEASE COMPLETE DIAGRAM: MARK LOCATION OF TUMORS AND BIOPSY SITES.
IF TUMOR REMAINS AT THE END OF THE PROCEDURE PLEASE INDICATE ITS LOCATION
BY MARKING AS INDEX ON DIAGRAM.

LUO = Left Ureteral Orifice
RUO = Right Ureteral Orifice
PW = Posterior Wall
RW = Right Wall
LW = Left Wall
TR = Trigone
PN = Posterior Neck
AN = Anterior Neck
D = Dome
RAW = Right Anterior Wall
LAW = Left Anterior Wall
PU = Prostatic Urethra
FEM U = Female Urethra
PS = Prostatic Substance
(ab = Air Bubble

} Biopsy Site

CC−T = Cold cup biopsy of tumor
TUR = transurethral resection of tumor
ADJ = Cold cup biopsy adjacent to tumor
SUSP = Cold cup biopsy of suspicious area
SMB = Cold cup selected mucosal biopsy
POOL = Pooled resection specimens

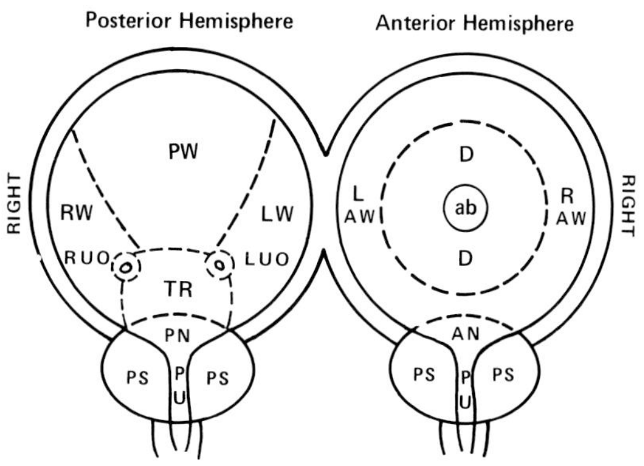

} Type of Biopsy

Fig. 18-1 Cystoscopy report form, detailing all pertinent elements of the procedure, including "mapping" diagrams for tumor localization. (Courtesy of Dr. G. R. Prout, Jr., Chairman, National Bladder Cancer Group, Massachusetts General Hospital, 1985.)

of the patient and the disease process. It may be done according to a number of schemas, but all are generally a combination of clinical and pathologic assessments that should include the following.

1. Tumor location, size, and number
2. Pathologic type and configuration
3. Pathologic grade
4. Clinical and pathologic stage
5. Mode of infiltration, if present, and the presence or absence of vascular or lymphatic invasion
6. Presence or absence of other urothelial abnormalities in areas away from the primary site
7. Results of adjunctive studies, including cytology, and other studies, e.g., cell surface antigen and chromosome analysis, if they are performed

The prognostic implications of each category are considered in detail in the following sections. Most of the data cited derive from the study of transitional cell carcinoma or from general studies of "bladder cancer," where such lesions account for most of the cases. Information for the less common tumor types, such as it is, is also given.

TUMOR LOCATION, SIZE, AND NUMBER

As noted above,[139] approximately 80 percent of all bladder tumors occur on the lateral walls, trigone, or posterior wall and are readily viewed through the cystoscope. Other less apparent sites are obviously not infrequent, however. Melicow's review of more than 800 cases of primary lesions, for example,[119] revealed a 10 percent tumor occurrence in the bladder dome; such lesions tend to be clinically "silent" and are often discovered late in their course. Also noted were tumors occurring in diverticula in 7 percent of all cases, another area where tumors may be difficult or impossible to detect. Primary carcinoma in situ, which comprised only 3 percent of Melicow's cases, is most commonly seen at the bladder base, trigone, and around the ureteral orifices,[197] although exact location and extent is obviously difficult to delineate at cystoscopy. In a series of squamous carcinomas,[85] tumors were located on the lateral walls in 38 of 90 cases, with the remaining tumors distributed elsewhere throughout the bladder. Adenocarcinomas are

also distributed generally but with a propensity toward occurrence in the dome area, presumably reflective of the fact that 20 to 50 percent[76,127,195] may be of urachal origin.

Although many of the subsequent tumors appearing during the patient's course may in fact be "new occurrences" rather than "recurrences,"[135,202] one area prone to true recurrence as the result of incomplete excision and regrowth is the ureteral orifice and region immediately adjacent. Here the risks of ureteral injury following attempts at deep or extensive resection, including resulting obstruction, urinary extravasation, etc. may be such that complete removal transurethrally is impossible.

The size of the patient's tumor may have some bearing on initial success at complete removal, particularly for the largest lesions, for obvious technical reasons (Table 18-1). However, maintenance of "disease-free status" over the long term is not so dependent on the size of the initial lesion.[28] If one looks only at patients presenting with low and intermediate grade, noninvasive lesions, however, initial tumor size may have a direct bearing on the ability to achieve and maintain disease-free status.[51] Still other studies, such as that reported by Narayana et al.,[132] have found tumor size to be independently predictive of long-term outcome, with large tumors in general associated with poor survival.

As the above discussion suggests, a comparison of predictive value of tumor size should probably be confined to given grades. For example, many of the bulkiest tumors may be low grade superficial papillary lesions with an expected good prognosis, whereas often smaller but higher grade lesions may already be deeply invasive at the time of presentation.

Table 18-1 Tumor Size Versus Achievement of Disease-Free Status

Tumor Size (cm)	Percent of Patients	Percent Achieved Disease-Free Status	Percent Remained Disease-Free at 36 Months
<1	18	98	53
1–2	38	89	45
3–4	25	92	43
≥5	19	68	44

(Data modified from Cutler et al.,[28] for the NBCG.)

As Prout noted,[140] bladder carcinoma is a "po-lychronotopical neoplastic diathesis" in many patients, with multiplicity of lesions both at initial presentation and over the course of time characteristic of the disease. A significant minority of patients have multiple tumors when first seen,[28,61,91,103,135] with definite implications regarding their subsequent course.[28,51,61,91,135] Among patients with grade I transitional cell carcinomas, Greene et al.[61] found that disease recurred in 88 percent of patients initially presenting with multiple tumors compared to only 68 percent of those with single tumors. In the NBCG study,[28,135] where newly diagnosed patients with all grades and stages of disease were evaluated, approximately 40 percent had multiple lesions at presentation, and of these only an average of 43 percent were disease-free at 24 months compared to 56 percent of those presenting with single tumors.

This proclivity for recurrence in patients with initial multifocal disease is not necessarily reflected in overall survival statistics, however. In a review of 167 patients presenting with T 1 bladder tumors (submucosal invasion), Williams et al.[210] noted virtually identical survival at 3 and 5 years' follow-up when comparing patients presenting with single versus multiple tumors. Nor did multiple tumors have predictive value with regard to survival in the group reported by Narayana et al.[132]

When coupled with other factors, however, multifocality may be of importance. Cummings[26] noted in a review that initial noninvasive multifocal disease that recurred was not more lethal than unifocal disease; both had an approximately 9 percent mortality rate. However, when disease was initially multifocal *and* showed any degree of invasiveness, there was a 45 percent incidence of death from recurrent disease.

Squamous carcinomas, conversely, presented as solitary masses in 81 of 90 cases reported by Johnson et al.[85] More patients with bilharziasis-associated carcinoma present with multiple lesions, though still less than one-fourth of all cases, and the majority of these are transitional cell rather than squamous lesions.[89] Figures for *adenocarcinoma* are quite variable, ranging from as low as 10 to as high as 50 percent[76] of patients with multiple lesions. By far the most common tumor type to present as multifocal disease is primary *transitional cell carcinoma in situ,* with approximately 70 percent of patients demonstrating such involvement in the Mayo Clinic series.[198] This is somewhat difficult

to characterize as such, however, because of problems in grossly identifying the extent of disease, but at the microscopic level, widespread involvement is often noted.

Overall, for transitional cell carcinomas, including carcinoma in situ, multiplicity may have obvious implications for the ability to control the disease. For squamous carcinomas and adenocarcinomas, typically more aggressive than transitional cell carcinomas as a group, the prognosis is much more likely to depend on initial stage than on multiplicity.

TUMOR TYPE AND CONFIGURATION

Primary bladder neoplasms exhibit transitional cell-type differentiation in approximately 76 to 90 percent of cases, with squamous cell carcinomas accounting for 3 to 15 percent, mixed types (primarily transitional cell plus squamous) 6 to 8 percent, and adenocarcinoma, undifferentiated carcinoma, etc. accounting for the small number of remaining cases.[28,53,85,119] The type of epithelial differentiation has a distinct bearing on prognosis, although there is an obvious strong interrelation with other prognostic factors such as stage and grade. For example, patients with transitional cell carcinoma enjoy a far better prognosis as a group than those with pure squamous or adenocarcinomas, but it is because of a large number of patients included in the group who have low grade tumors, which are either noninvasive or only superficially invasive at the time of initial diagnosis. By contrast, patients with squamous and adenocarcinomas rarely present with noninvasive disease. Although prognosis is said to be poorer for patients with squamous and adenocarcinoma, survival is probably similar to that with transitional cell carcinoma if disease is compared stage for stage.[84,85]

Among patients with transitional cell carcinomas, tumor configuration is also important prognostically. Papillary lesions account for approximately 80 percent[119] to 86 percent[28] of cases; and as a group, patients with papillary lesions fare better than those with solid tumors. In a retrospective analysis of 500 patients, Cummings[26] found that only 28 percent of patients with papillary lesions died of bladder carcinoma versus 75 percent of the group with tumors originally classified as solid or sessile.

Although papillary tumors usually present as low grade/low stage disease, this tumor configuration has some predictive value even when other factors are held constant.[132] For tumors of comparable high grade, Kern[88] found only 22 percent of papillary lesions to penetrate to the outer muscularis or beyond compared to 79 percent of nonpapillary tumors of the same grade. Two other factors, cited by Slack and Prout,[173] may account for some of the difference in survival: When invasive tumors are compared, those with a papillary configuration seem less likely to involve lymphatics than their solid counterparts; also they appear to be more radiosensitive, and this fact should be taken into account particularly if contemplating definitive radiotherapy for patients with invasive disease.[165,166]

Clear-cut estimates of the importance of tumor configuration are difficult to make, however, because patients with high grade/high stage disease at cystectomy often have varying combinations of papillary tumors, solid tumors, and carcinoma in situ.[190] It may be impossible to state with certainty if the final invasive tumor or tumors arose directly from a papillary lesion, despite a long history of papillary neoplasia. In fact, such a history may be much less common than is usually thought. Brawn,[17] for example, examined what he termed the "widely held idea that the majority of invasive carcinomas of the bladder occur in patients with a history of papillary neoplasms of the bladder." In actuality, he found that only 20 of a series of 104 consecutive cases of invasive bladder carcinoma had any history of papillary neoplasia, whereas the remaining 84 cases had no such history. Morphologically, only 26 of the 104 cases had gross or microscopic features suggestive of a papillary growth pattern. Whether accompanied or preceded by papillary tumors, or presenting as solitary lesions de novo, it is safe to say that the bottom line is as follows: Solid or nonpapillary tumors should generally be viewed with greater alarm than papillary tumors.

Lesions with pure *squamous* differentiation portend a dismal outlook. Faysal[48] reported 2- and 5-year survival figures of approximately 28 and 20 percent, respectively. Johnson et al.[85] reviewed a group of 90 patients with squamous carcinoma seen at the M. D. Anderson Hospital who had even more disheartening results. There was only a 13.3 percent 5-year survival rate, and this decreased to 5.3 percent at 10 years among the 73 patients who were treated. The remaining 17 patients were apparently beyond treatment, with 15 of 17 dead within a year and the remaining 2 following shortly thereafter.

The overall prognosis for patients with *adenocarcinoma* may be clouded by the fact that most series contain a number of tumors of probable urachal origin (see below), a clinical situation that, according to Mostofi et al.,[127] has a 5-year "success rate" (i.e., freedom from disease) of only about 6 percent. Their series of adenocarcinomas in general, including those of probable urachal origin (reported in 1955), showed only 11 of 44 alive without tumor, although only 8 of these patients had been followed for at least 5 years. Anderström et al.,[6] in a more recent review of 64 patients with primary adenocarcinoma, noted that in their series location did not appear to affect prognosis. Tumors occurring in the anterior wall and dome, the usual location for urachal lesions, had essentially the same prognosis found for the group as a whole. Overall 5-year survival was only 18 percent, a somewhat discouraging figure with regard to therapy for this disease, as all of their cases were seen between 1958 and 1973, whereas the cases reported by Mostofi et al.,[127] with a similar or better survival rate, were all received at the Armed Forces Institute of Pathology prior to 1951.

The natural history of *transitional cell carcinoma in situ* of the urinary bladder is more difficult to define.[217] In earlier reports[198] progression to invasive cancer occurred in a high percentage of patients. However, Farrow et al.,[47] subsequently noted that some patients followed for the disease, including a number who had also been treated for prior bladder neoplasms, were perhaps being seen late in their course. A more accurate chronology of events was accomplished when 106 patients at the Mayo Clinic were found to have cytologic evidence of carcinoma *without* a cystoscopically visible bladder tumor or previous history of malignancy.[47] Sixty-nine of these patients were proved to have in situ transitional cell carcinoma of the bladder by biopsy. The age range of the patients and the mean age were similar to figures for transitional cell carcinoma in general (range 31 to 87 years, average 63.1 years). Most patients had symptoms of bladder irritation, and all had at least microhematuria. The average duration of symptoms prior to the first detected cytologic abnormality was more than 32 months but ranged to surprising lengths in some patients, the longest recorded being 12 years.

The patients were treated in various ways. Only eight of 58 patients with follow-up data developed overt invasive disease, with three of the eight having cystectomy early on. In the remaining five the period from first positive cytologic examination to discovery of invasive disease ranged from 20 to 58 months, with an average of 41.2 months. There were no reported deaths among the patients with invasive disease. Subsequent data from the same institution,[196,217] however, indicated a relatively small number of deaths in an expanded group of patients treated with cystectomy. Most presumably were related to the presence of occult invasive disease at the time of surgery, which was found in a surprising 34 percent of the cystectomy specimens examined. The projected 5-year survival for those with no evidence of invasion was 91 percent, but this figure dropped to 70 percent when invasion was present. Thus "the plight of the patient with carcinoma in situ of the bladder," as originally reported by the Mayo Clinic Group[198] was found to be not so bad as it first seemed, and it appears that most of these patients can be dealt with effectively, particularly with the advent of newer treatment regimens. On the opposite side of the coin, however, the fact remains that a small percentage of the Mayo Clinic patients developed significant invasion and died of their disease under what seems to have been as close scrutiny as possible.

TUMOR GRADE

The morphologic assessment that determines tumor grade is based on the degree of differentiation of the tumor when compared subjectively to that normal tissue which it most closely resembles. Departures from normal appearance include overall architectural rearrangement as well as individual cellular abnormalities. At the "low power" architectural level, numerous alterations may be noted, e.g., increased cellularity, nuclear crowding, disturbances of nuclear polarity, and failure of normal differentiation from base to surface. At the individual cell level one sees varying degrees of change in nuclear size and shape, abnormal nuclear chromatin patterns, increased nuclear/cytoplasmic ratio, irregular nuclear membrane configurations, an increase in mitotic figures, abnormal mitoses, etc.

One factor that may contribute to the subjective variation that seems inherent in most grading systems is sampling bias. Although most bladder tumors show a relatively uniform grade throughout,[45] occasional lesions are relatively well differentiated in one area but much more poorly differentiated in another area, as illustrated in Figures 18-2 and 18-3. This factor may be partially overcome by generous histologic sampling of surgical specimens, but it obviously cannot be circumvented in small biopsies.

Another factor that contributes to the problem is the inevitable inter- and intraobserver variations among pathologists. In an interesting study reported by Ooms et al.,[137] both variations were found to be distressingly high, even among a group that included experienced observers.

Despite the limitations, however, grading of transitional cell lesions in particular provides useful prognostic information. In fact, it is here that grading is most crucial, as the simple diagnosis of "transitional cell carcinoma," without modifiers, tells little prog-

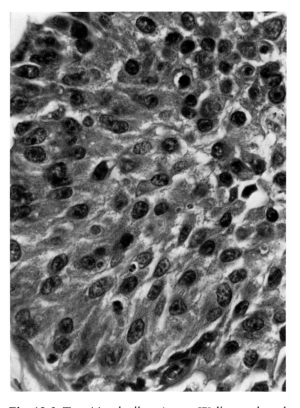

Fig. 18-2 Transitional cell carcinoma. Well to moderately differentiated area of tumor. Compare to Fig. 18-3. ×500.

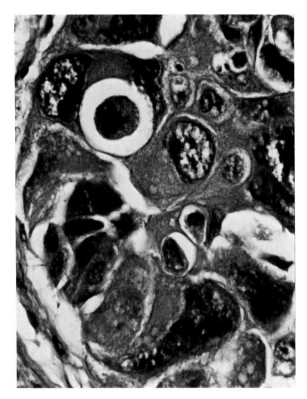

Fig. 18-3 Transitional cell carcinoma. Poorly differentiated area in the same lesion depicted in Figure 18-2. ×485.

nostically. Indeed, Broders' original observations on the grading of tumors in general might well be applied by substituting "transitional cell carcinoma" for "cancer"[18]:

> The term cancer is used loosely, but it is very important to know the type of cancer in a given case. No one would think of putting the ordinary garter snake and the death-dealing cobra in the same class, but they are both snakes!

What is the percentage distribution expected among the various grades of transitional cell carcinomas? In a number of large series[28,53,113,119] grade I lesions have accounted for 23 to 35 percent, grade II lesions for 34 to 50 percent, and grade III (as well as grade IV lesions where this grading system is used) for 27 to 40 percent of all cases.

Of note for transitional cell tumors is the fact that, as a general rule, stage and grade tend to run parallel,[111,112] with high stage disease in most of the cases

found also to be high grade disease. Of the approximately 10 percent of all patients with bladder carcinoma who die as a result of their *original* tumor, virtually all have high grade neoplasms.[26]

Although grade and stage often go hand in hand, tumor grade has beeen shown to be of independent predictive value with regard to overall survival.[132] Marshall,[112] for example, found a 69 percent 5-year survival among 142 patients presenting with low grade/low stage disease but only a 47 percent 5-year survival among 74 patients with high grade but similar low stage disease. In a survey of patients with T1 bladder tumors, all treated similarly, Williams et al.[210] noted 5-year survivals of 73 percent for grade I lesions, 71.2 percent for grade II lesions, and 58.8 percent for grade III lesions. A high or moderate degree of pleomorphism was noted as a "particularly unfavourable" prognostic element, despite the early stage at presentation. Lutzeyer and co-workers,[109] in an analysis of more than 300 cases of superficial bladder cancer, found even more striking differences in survival among their T1 cases, with 3-year survival rates of 92, 72, and 57 percent for patients with grade I, II, and III tumors, respectively. Jakse et al.[79] indicated that superficially invasive grade III lesions were associated with a noticeably poorer prognosis among all cases of low stage tumors, accounting for 11 of 13 cancer-related deaths among 172 patients presenting with Ta, T1 lesions.

When only low and intermediate grade tumors are considered, differences in disease progression are also striking. Althausen and colleagues,[3] in a review of 129 patients with low stage transitional cell carcinomas, found that subsequent muscle-invasive tumors developed in only 15 percent of patients presenting with grade I lesions compared to 50 percent with grade II lesions.

The literature, however, shows a number of somewhat confusing observations with regard to the significance of grade. For example, England et al.[44] studied 332 patients with T1 bladder cancer and came to the conclusion that "neither grade nor stage had any effect on the liability to grow new tumours." Conversely, Cutler et al.,[28] based on the NBCG data, observed that "the relationship of grade to prognosis is clear—the higher the grade, the sooner the disease is likely to recur." Moreover, even if some of the conclusions regarding the prognostic importance of grade are firm, the therapeutic implications are not, at least for standard surgical approaches. As Whitmore[203] noted:

High grade tumors are more aggressive than low grade ones. For each method of treatment, data exist that clearly demonstrate that patients with low grade, low stage tumors survive better than patients with high grade, low stage tumors. What is not clearly known is to what extent (if any) the method of surgical treatment favorably alters the adverse impact of tumor grade on survival. Within the constraints of the treatment selection criteria previously enumerated, does radical treatment of a high grade, low stage cancer offer a better prospect of controlling that lesion than does conservative treatment? This question is not resolvable from existing data.

Fortunately, the addition of topical forms of adjuvant therapy (discussed later) appears to favorably alter the course of at least some patients with superficial high grade disease, without resorting to radical surgery at the outset.

The influence of tumor grade on prognosis in patients with squamous and adenocarcinomas is virtually impossible to assess as an independent variable. Even at large university centers and primary oncology centers, the subsets of patients with pure squamous or adenocarcinoma remain relatively small, and literature series have correspondingly small numbers of patients for analysis.[48,85] These data are usually collected over long periods of time, and treatment is generally not systematized. Division into even smaller subgroups, e.g., variable grade-comparable stage, results in numbers of essentially anecdotal significance.

For *squamous carcinomas,* reports of tumor grade in the literature vary from one series to the next. Faysal,[48] in a series of 46 patients with pure squamous cell carcinoma seen at Stanford, noted 22 percent of the cases to be well differentiated, 41 percent moderately differentiated, and 37 percent poorly differentiated. In an overall review of 457 cases of bladder tumors seen at the New England Deaconess and New England Baptist Hospitals, Friedell et al.[53] noted a subgroup of 68 patients with squamous cell carcinoma, with tumor grades not so evenly distributed as in the Stanford series. They found only 3 percent of their patients to have well differentiated lesions and 19 percent moderately differentiated lesions, with most (71 percent) of the patients presenting with poorly differentiated tumors. An additional 7 percent showed only in situ carcinoma. This preponderance

of higher-grade lesions was also noted in Melicow's report from Columbia Presbyterian Hospital[199] where close to one-half of 54 patients with squamous lesions showed poorly differentiated tumors.

In Faysal's series,[48] with all stages grouped together, there were 30 and 27 percent 5-year survivals in the well and moderately differentiated categories respectively, but only 5 percent in the poorly differentiated category. In contrast, Johnson et al.,[85] reporting 90 patients with squamous carcinoma, found that the histologic grade of the tumor "offered little aid in regard to prognosis." They observed that high grade tumors were most often found with advanced disease, but the four patients in their series with grade I lesions were all dead within a year of diagnosis. This apparent lack of correlation between stage and grade also seems to obtain in the bilharziasis-associated squamous carcinomas reported from Egypt, where 80 percent of lesions are well differentiated yet advanced stage disease is the rule, with deep muscle invasion almost always present and extravesical extension common at the time of diagnosis.[43]

In various series of patients with *adenocarcinoma,* incidence rates by grade are again variable. Anderström et al.[6] noted that in their series of 64 patients only 9 percent presented with well differentiated tumors, 27 percent had moderately differentiated tumors, and 64 percent poorly differentiated tumors. Yet Johnson and colleagues,[84] in a smaller series from the M.D. Anderson Hospital, found that most of their patients had well differentiated lesions. Although grade appeared to be of some prognostic importance in the report of Anderström et al.,[6] higher grade lesions were generally of a higher stage as well, although this is relative, as five of their six patients with well differentiated tumors showed at least muscle invasion. Despite the preponderance of well differentiated lesions in the M.D. Anderson series,[84] again these lesions tended to be advanced, with approximately two-thirds showing at least deep muscle invasion at the time of diagnosis.

Although reference to variations in grade of urothelium diagnosed as showing *carcinoma in situ* has been made in the literature,[47,53,198] the implications, if any, of such differentiation are not given.[47,198] Present standard classifications, such as those of the AFIP[94] and the NBCG[54] do not subdivide carcinoma in situ by grade; and if this diagnosis is made, it is presumed to show morphologic features equal to those seen in high grade invasive neoplasms. As noted in Chapter 17, however, it seems reasonable to separate these lesions into grades II and III, with cellular morphologies corresponding to their respective invasive counterparts. Additional study will be obviously necessary, however, to examine the prognostic utility of such subdivision.

TUMOR STAGE

The stage of a tumor, i.e., the extent to which the lesion has spread either locally or distantly, remains the single most reliable prognostic factor at present and generally is the primary basis on which therapeutic decisions are made. Thus the need for accuracy demands a systematic combined clinical-pathological approach.

During the mid-1940s, having noted the disappointing results of treatment for bladder carcinoma, Jewett and Strong[83] reviewed 107 cases that had come to autopsy, a study that was to form the groundwork for present-day staging systems. The authors examined the relation of depth of penetration of the bladder wall by tumor to the incidence of three factors: metastases, lymphatic capillary invasion (termed "incipient metastasis"), and perivesical fixation. The cases were divided into three groups: group A, in which tumor cells were confined to the submucosa; group B, in which tumor had infiltrated into, but not through, the muscularis; and group C, where tumor had extended completely through the bladder wall with perivesical infiltration. The study was obviously a theoretical attempt to determine which patients might have been cured by surgery based on the presence or absence of the above three factors in relation to depth of invasion. In a subsequent study,[80] published in 1952, Jewett suggested further division of stage B, the muscle-invasive category, into superficial (B1) and deep (B2) extension, noting the greater likelihood of successful therapy in the former group.

That same year the "Marshall modification" of the Jewett–Strong system appeared.[111] It lumped noninfiltrating papillary tumors, in situ carcinomas, and biopsy-proved tumors no longer present in the definitive resection specimen into a separate group, stage 0. Furthermore, stage D, a category for neoplasms that had spread beyond the limits of the bladder and perivesical fat, was divided into stage D1 and D2. The

former group included cases with widespread disease still confined to the pelvis, and the latter contained cases with "distant metastases, metastases in lymph nodes external to the inguinal ligament, and in nodes above the sacral promontory."

Marshall compared the clinical preoperative estimate of tumor extent to that found in the definitive pathologic specimen from 104 consecutive radical cystectomies. The clinical staging correlated correctly with the pathologic findings in 81 percent of the group as a whole. However, there was a significant underestimation in patients with clinical stage 0, A, and B1 disease, where 10 of 29 patients so categorized were found to have stage B2 or greater disease at definitive resection. Conversely, for patients thought clinically to be in stage B2 or greater, only 10 of 75 cases (13 percent) were found to be understaged. A general correlation of increasing stage with increasing grade was noted, and it was pointed out in particular that most clinical understaging occurred with high grade neoplasms. Three-fourths of such lesions thought clinically to be stage A or B1 were found to be in a higher stage at surgery. The estimate of A or B1 disease with low grade tumors was surprisingly good, however, with only 1 of 17 such tumors found to be in a higher stage at surgery.

During the same era the European community witnessed the evolution of the TNM system for the general classification of malignancies, under the auspices of the Union Internationale Contre le Cancer (UICC or IUAC).[74] Tumors were classified according to the extent of the primary tumor (T), as well as the presence or absence of lymph node involvement (N) and/or metastases (M). This method of classification was adopted by the American Joint Committee for Cancer Staging and End-Results Reporting of the American College of Surgeons (AJC) for the staging of bladder carcinoma, with a number of modifications. The system, as described in the AJC *Manual for Staging of Cancer,*[8] is a comprehensive staging classification that incorporates not only the initial extent of the tumor (clinical-diagnostic staging) but also subsequent restaging at the time of definitive surgery and pathologic examination as well as at the time of eventual retreatment, if necessary. It also documents histopathologic aspects including tumor type, tumor grade, and the additional factor of "performance status" of the patient.

Corresponding stages in the Jewett–Strong–

Marshall system and the AJC–UICC "TNM" systems are as listed in Table 18-2. Note that the AJC section is in outline form for comparative purposes, and the reader is referred to both the *Manual*[8] as well as thorough discussions of the system by Prout[140,141] for further details.

The AJC system offers a number of advantages over the Jewett–Strong–Marshall system, in particular a more comprehensive evaluation of the patient's situation, a clear indication of at which point in the course, and by what means, the data were collected, as well as a short-hand method of data recording that lends itself well to statistical analysis. As Prout[141] noted, however, the AJC classification has not been embraced with enthusiasm. The Jewett–Strong–Marshall system is still perhaps the most widely used method of staging in the United States and appears frequently in

the literature. It is somewhat ironic that Dr. Jewett, who was instrumental in the formulation of both classifications, does not use the "Jewett system," and bladder specimens at Johns Hopkins are routinely classified according the AJC recommendations.

In a review of the two staging systems, Skinner[169] cited various advantages of the TNM system, one of which is the distinction between staging based on clinical evaluation versus that based on histopathologic evaluation. As the system is used, however, there are some facets that lend themselves to confusion. In the literature, for example, T stages are referred to as "clinical stages" and P stages as "pathologically determined stages." In fact, T stages are not derived from clinical assessment alone but from both clinical evaluation *and* pathologic evaluation of biopsy or transurethral resection specimens, or both. Con-

Table 18-2 Bladder Cancer Staging

Jewett–Strong–Marshall System		American Joint Committee for Cancer Staging and International Union Against Cancer Systems	
Stage	Primary Tumor/Lymph Nodes/Metastases	Stage	Primary Tumor/Lymph Nodes/Metastases
		Primary tumor	
		Tis	Carcinoma in situ (nonpapillary)
O	Intraepithelial	Ta	Papillary noninvasive carcinoma
A	Invasion of lamina propria	T1	Invasion of lamina propria
B_1	Invasion of superficial muscle	T2	Invasion of superficial muscle
B_2	Invasion of deep muscle	T3a	Invasion of deep muscle
C	Invasion of perivesical fat	T3b	Invasion of perivesical fat
D_1	Lymph node metastases below the level of the sacral promontory	T4	Tumor fixed or invades neighboring structures
D_2	Lymph node metastases above the level of the sacral promontory, external to the inguinal ligament, and/or distant metastases	T4a	Tumor invading substance of prostate (microscopically proved), uterus, or vagina
		T4b	Tumor fixed to pelvic wall or infiltrating abdominal wall
		Lymph nodes	
		N0	No involvement of regional lymph nodes
		N1	Involvement of a single homolateral regional lymph node
		N2	Involvement of contralateral, bilateral, or multiple regional lymph nodes
		N3	A fixed mass on the pelvic wall with a free space between it and the tumor
		Distant metastases	
		M0	No (known) distant metastases
		MI	Distant metastases present (specify site)

(Data from Refs. 8, 74, 80, 83, 111, 112.)

versely, P stages are derived from pathologic findings in a definitive resection specimen, either cystectomy or segmental resection. For practical purposes, references in this chapter to TNM stages are generally listed as T stages in order to correspond to the usual method of reference in case series in the literature.

A second advantage of the TNM system that Skinner[169] noted is the addition of a separate category for carcinoma in situ (Tis). Since the time of that review, a further category (Ta) has been added, used in reference to noninvasive papillary carcinomas. In the Jewett–Strong–Marshall classification, these two lesions had been lumped together in a category that originally also included all cases where no tumor was found in the definitive resection specimen. Clearly the prognosis would be expected to differ for one patient with a low grade noninvasive papillary tumor compared to that of a second with extensive carcinoma in situ and to a third with a deeply invasive tumor that is no longer detectable at cystectomy following preoperative transurethral resection, irradiation, or both. All of these patients, however, would be classified as "stage 0" under the Jewett–Strong–Marshall system.

In contrast to these advantages, Skinner[169] also voiced a number of criticisms of the TNM system. One is that the addition of "N" and "M" groupings may be of little practical therapeutic importance because of serious limitations in our ability to detect early metastases, as well as a relative inability to influence prognosis once clinically apparent metastases have occurred. A second deficiency is the perpetuation of the long-criticized segregation of muscle-invasive tumors into those confined to the superficial half of the musculature (B1–T2) and those extending more than half-way into the musculature (B2–T3a). It is important to emphasize here that, *in theory,* the prognostic distinction between superficially and deeply invasive muscle tumors is a useful concept. As discussed in an editorial by Jewett[81] (aptly titled "Two B's or Not Two B's: That Is the Question"), there have been no indisputable data published to disprove the original observation that the incidence of dissemination was directly proportional to the depth of penetration of the bladder wall. This concept has certainly gained support in other areas of oncology, such as treatment of melanomas and cervical carcinomas. Dr. Jewett's statement that "It is unlikely that most cancers, deep in the muscularis, extending to its outer-most fibers, are as easy to cure as those that have barely begun to invade it . . ."[81] makes eminent good sense. Obviously, there are exceptions to the rule, such as occasional superficial tumors that already have progressed to lymphatic and/or vascular invasion with dissemination, but these exceptions must be viewed in statistical context.

The primary criticism leveled against the segregation of tumors into "superficial" and "deeply invasive" categories has centered around the gross inaccuracy of clinical compared to pathologic staging in the midportion of the invasive spectrum. As noted originally by Marshall and also by Prout,[140] when estimating tumor stage in the B1, B2, and C range by clinical means the cumulative error approaches 40 percent. A great deal is made of this inaccuracy in the literature, appropriately so, because of the possible differences in treatment of superficial versus deep lesions. Unfortunately, in this midportion of the invasive spectrum, the inaccuracy is inherent to the situation, with no improvement offered by merely changing designations from one staging system to the next.

Arguments concerning the two systems will no doubt persist in the literature. Opponents of the Jewett–Strong–Marshall system continue to argue that it is too simplistic, with insufficient subclassification, and with certain groups containing patients who may have quite disparate prognoses. Opponents of the AJC TNM classification argue that it, on the other hand, is too complex, with some of the subcategorization based on rather "soft" information.[169] For better or for worse, the issue of changing systems for many clinicians boils down to a matter of inertia, and both systems will no doubt continue to be used for the forseeable future.

For the practicing pathologist, perhaps the best advice is to stand clear of the problem by spelling out, as completely and succinctly as possible, the pathologic diagnoses one is able to make from the specimen submitted. The primary goal is to note all of the information available, including the anatomic location, the designated procedure, and the descriptive findings; for example:

Right periureteral area (transurethral resection specimen): Papillary transitional cell carcinoma, grade III, with invasion of lamina propria. Numerous segments of muscle show no evidence of tumor infiltration. No evidence of lymphatic and/or vascular invasion.

This description may be followed by a notation of stage according to either of the above systems, but the most important part of the diagnosis is the former. If certain important features cannot be accurately diagnosed, it is important to say so as well. "Unreadable" tissue, such as a specimen with severe cautery artifact (Fig. 18-4), is just that—inadequate for diagnosis—and should be reported as such.

With regard to muscle invasion, the first order of business in a transurethral resection specimen is to note if muscle is present.[52] If it is and it has been invaded by tumor, it is difficult to estimate the extent of invasion in both biopsy and transurethral resection specimens. Section planes exactly perpendicular to the surface mucosa are found only fortuitously. When faced with fragments containing both muscle and tumor, about all one can say is that muscle involvement is present,[52] and assessments of the depth of invasion are only speculative (Fig. 18-5). About the

only situation in which one may make a relatively educated guess is in the completely resected transurethral specimen that shows focal extension into muscle in fragments where the submucosa and mucosa are clearly identified, with all other muscular fragments showing no evidence of tumor. In this particular situation, it might reasonably be concluded that there is only superficial muscle invasion, but this cannot be guaranteed with complete certainty. Occasionally one may be tempted to speculate on the possibility of deep muscle invasion when there is extensive muscle involvement in a sizable fragment of tissue without other landmarks, but tangential sections through fragments of superficial muscle may give an appearance of equally "extensive" muscle involvement. With regard to true deep muscle invasion, the presence of immediately adjacent perivesical fat in an area of invasion of muscle by tumor may be an indication that the neoplasm has spread to the B2 or T3a level;

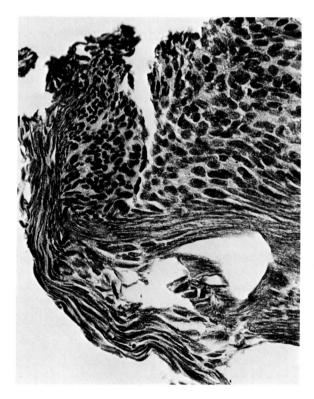

Fig. 18-4 Marked "cautery artifact." Morphologic details, nuclear features in particular, are not sufficiently preserved for accurate diagnosis. ×273.

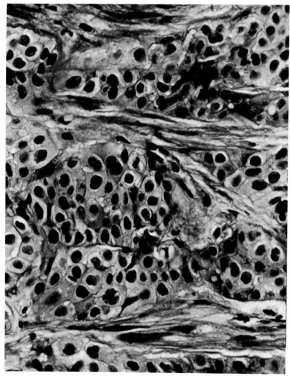

Fig. 18-5 Muscle invasion. Transitional cell carcinoma is penetrating between the smooth muscle fibers in a fragment from a transurethral resection. ×300.

but fortunately for the patient, such inadvertant "through and through" transurethral resection specimens are seen only infrequently.

In the final analysis, inherent difficulties of clinical staging by present methods preclude an accurate categorization of every patient with newly diagnosed bladder cancer. The overall estimate of error in clinical staging may range up to 50 percent according to Schmidt and Weinstein,[158] with sources of error including: (1) a variable assortment of diagnostic studies performed; (2) inaccuracies inherent in the diagnostic measures utilized; (3) insufficient corroboration by surgical and pathologic staging; (4) lack of a satisfactory means of detecting micrometastasis; and (5) confusion and controversy regarding the various classification systems available for clinical staging. The clinician formulating therapeutic decisions based on studies reported in the literature should always bear these limitations in mind.

Transitional Cell Carcinoma

At what stages do patients with transitional cell carcinoma generally present? Among the more reliable figures are those of the National Bladder Cancer Group (formerly the National Bladder Cancer Cooperative Group A), which took a relatively rigid systematic approach to patient classification. This group reported on 850 patients registered over a 2-year period.[28]

As noted in Table 18-3, among the subgroup of newly diagnosed patients with transitional cell carcinoma, approximately two-thirds presented with "su-

Table 18-3 Transitional Cell Carcinoma: Stage at Presentation

Stage	National Bladder Cancer Group[28] (Percent)	Lutzeyer et al.[109] (Percent)
Ta–O	40	30
T1–A	27	28
T2–B$_1$	20	16
T3–B$_2$		13
T4–D	10	6
	(Additional 3 percent unevaluable)	(Additional 7 percent: papilloma, dysplasia, etc.)

Table 18-4 Transitional Cell Carcinoma: Stage/Grade Correlation

Stage (Percent)	Grade (Percent)		
	I	II	III
Ta–0	25	4	1
T1–A	11	15	2
T2–B$_1$	3	8	5
T3–B$_2$,C	—	5	8
T4–D	—	2	4

(Data from Lutzeyer et al.[109])

perficial" disease (Ta to T1); similar figures were found in a large series from West Germany reported by Lutzeyer et al.[109] The latter study also cross-tabulated stage and tumor grade (Table 18-4) and showed the expected strong correlation between the two.

The prognosis, stage by stage, for transitional cell carcinoma is somewhat difficult to state with certainty from the available published data. One troublesome point is the tendency in the literature to lump categories together for various reasons, therapeutic in particular. A common approach has been to group patients into categories of "superficial disease" and "deeply invasive disease." Earlier publications tended to set this dividing line at the midmuscularis. Of late, however, the "superficial disease" category has more often been limited to disease invading at most the lamina propria (Ta/T1-0/A), with further extension relegated to the "deeply invasive" category. Although such groupings may be appropriate with regard to therapy, there appear to be distinctly different prognoses for the various stages in the two groups, as can be seen in Tables 18-5 and 18-6.

For example, although the prognosis for "superficial" disease is generally good, in fact noninvasive (Ta–0) disease should be distinguished from disease showing invasion of lamina propria (T1–A). Such distinction seems logical, as the former tumor has not, by definition, had a chance for distant spread. Theoretically, therefore, if such lesions can be completely resected, *barring recurrent disease* either at this site or elsewhere, such lesions should be universally cured.

A second problem associated with attempts to correlate stage with prognosis is this propensity for new and often distinctly separate tumors to arise within the urothelium. If a patient dies as a result of her cervical carcinoma, for example, we may trace it back to the

Table 18-5 Transitional Cell Carcinoma—"Superficial Disease": Prognosis by Stage

Parameter	Noninvasive (Ta–O) (Percent)	Lamina Propria Invasion (T1–A) (Percent)
"Disease-free" status achieved	98	90
Recurrent disease		
12 months	31	39
24 months	45	52
36 months	54	56
Progression to muscle invasive disease at 2 years	3 (all cases)	25 (all grades) 40 (grade III)
Overall 3-year survival	97 (grade I) 90 (grade II)	92 (grade I) 72 (grade II) 57 (grade III)

(Data modified from Cutler, et al.[28] for the NBCG, and Lutzeyer, et al.[109])

stage of her original tumor. If she dies of bladder carcinoma, however, where recurrence or "new occurrence" is the rule, which tumor should be put in our staging figures? Her first? Her second or third? All three?

As an illustration of this phenomenon, in the NBCG study[28] (Table 18-5) 98 percent of Ta patients achieved "disease-free status" and thereby were presumed to have had all of their initial tumor removed, yet 31 percent of these patients had evidence of new or recurrent tumors at 12 months, 45 percent at 24 months, and 54 percent at 36 months. Among these patients some will have had more aggressive subsequent tumors, and some of these tumors may have little relation to the original Ta lesion, yet they affect the prognostic data if the original tumor stage is that which enters the statistics.

In view of the fact that more than one-half of the patients with initial Ta lesions eventually have recurrent disease, it is obviously important to know how many such recurrences are of a potentially more serious nature than the original lesion. Using muscle invasion as the hallmark, it was noted in the NBCG study[28] that only 3 percent of patients with initial Ta lesions showed eventual "disease progression" to this point. So despite the propensity for recurrent disease, the overall prognosis for patients with noninvasive tumors, particularly grade I tumors, is excellent; Lutzeyer et al.[109] reported 97 and 90 percent 3-year survivals in stage Ta patients with grades I and II tumors, respectively. Williams and colleagues[210] also found only a 3 percent death rate from subsequent tumor in this group; and among 160 patients with Ta–grade I lesions Prout et al.[144] noted only one tumor-related death. In general, even with multiple recurrences, most of these patients can be managed by conservative means.

Patients with tumors that have invaded the lamina propria (T1–A) do *not* fare so well as those with noninvasive lesions. There is an obvious interdependence on grade, with increasing numbers of patients in this category with grade II and higher disease compared to those with noninvasive disease. Again, it seems logical that the prognosis should be worse with *any* degree of invasion, for it is at this point that the tumor first gains access to vascular and lymphatic channels which may serve as avenues for metastasis; and the first such avenues, however sparse, sit immediately beneath the basement membrane (Fig. 18-6).

As noted in Table 18-5 "disease-free status" may also be achieved by conservative means in most patients with lamina propria invasion, and disease recurrence rates are comparable to those for noninvasive disease. Progression to muscle-invasive disease is considerably higher, however, particularly for those with grade III lesions, and overall prognosis is correspondingly poorer.

In patients with muscle-invasive tumors (T2, T3a–B1, B2), most (72 percent) may also be rendered "disease-free" at the time of initial therapy by conserva-

Table 18-6 Transitional Cell Carcinoma—"Deeply Invasive Disease": Prognosis by Stage

	Superficial Muscle Invasion (T2–B1)	Deep Muscle Invasion (T3a–B2)	Perivesical Extension (T3b–C)
5-yr survival (%)	38	35	16

(Modified from Skinner.[169])

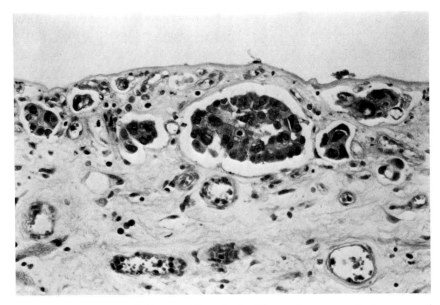

Fig. 18-6 Tumor invasion of submucosal lymphatics. The surface mucosa is almost completely denuded in this area. ×198.

tive means, according to the NBCG study.[28] Moreover, the percentages of patients who *remain* disease-free at 12, 24, and 36 months are also impressive: 60, 51, and 51 percent, respectively. Despite these findings, however, the overall prognosis for these patients is considerably worse than for those with no evidence of muscle invasion (Table 18-6). This fact presumably relates to a greater likelihood of "silent" metastases, more dire consequences of recurrent disease, or a combination of the two, with many of the deaths occurring past the 3-year mark.

Within the group of patients with muscle-invasive tumors, despite the former separation of superficial versus deep muscular invasive disease prognostically, more recent studies indicate that survival statistics for these two subgroups may be similar.[152] In a review of a number of studies in the literature comparing survival among patients in these two subgroups, most of whom were treated by cystectomy, Skinner[169] (Table 18-6) noted an aggregate 5-year survival of 38 percent for patients with superficial muscular-invasive disease (T2–B1) versus 35 percent for those with deep muscle invasion (T3a–B2). Particularly for the group with superficial muscular invasion, this represents a marked decrease in survivability compared to those with only lamina propria invasion.

Once tumor has spread beyond the confines of the bladder wall, prognosis becomes dismal. Skinner[169] cited combined study figures that averaged a 16 percent 5-year survival in patients whose tumors had penetrated into the perivesical soft tissue (stage T3b–C). With more advanced regional disease, few patients are curable, and the presence of distant metastases essentially reduces the prognostic discussion to one of complete versus partial response with intensive chemotherapy, both usually of temporary duration.

Squamous Carcinoma

For patients with pure squamous carcinoma, the average initial stage is distinctly higher than for those with transitional cell carcinoma, in both Western countries and areas with endemic bilharziasis (Table 18-7). As representative of the disease in Western countries, data were combined from two major series —those of Johnson et al. from the M. D. Anderson Hospital[85] and those of Faysal from the Stanford University Medical Center[48]—giving a total of 136 patients. As noted in Table 18-7, not a single patient in either series presented with noninvasive disease, and in only 3 percent was invasion limited to the lamina propria. Even at this stage, only one of four patients survived for 5 years. The largest subgroup (37 per-

Table 18-7 Squamous Carcinoma: Stage at Presentation

Stage	Nonbilharzial[a] (Percent)	Bilharzial (Percent)
Ta–O	—	0.2
T1–A	3	2.7
T2–B$_1$	24	11.7
T3a–B$_2$		61.5
T3b–C	29	
T4–D	37	23.9

[a] Remaining cases were not able to be accurately staged. (Data from El-Bolkainy, et al.,[42] Faysal,[48] and Johnson, et al.[85])

cent) had either advanced regional disease or metastases. Treatment by various modalities produced disappointing results overall, in part because of the high number of patients with advanced disease at the outset. The Stanford study,[48] in which all patients with muscle-invasive lesions were grouped together, showed a 50 percent survival rate at 5 years. The M. D. Anderson study[85] distinguished superficial from deep muscle-invasive disease, with some difference in survival noted at the 3-year mark: "B1" patients had a better than 50 percent survival; "B2" patients had an approximately 25 percent survival rate. This difference became less apparent at 5 years, with the "B1" survival curve approaching the "B2" curve. Stage T3b–C cases showed a survival of approximately 13 to 20 percent at 5 years. All 41 patients with T4–D1,D2 disease were dead within 3 years, most of them within a year or less from the time of diagnosis.

With bilharziasis-related bladder carcinoma, most commonly squamous, high stage disease is also the rule rather than the exception. El-Bolkainy and colleagues[42] reported 1,095 patients, all treated by radical cystectomy, which allowed accurate pathologic staging. As noted in Table 18-7, their data indicated that the largest number of patients had deep muscle or perivesical invasion. Despite the generally advanced local stage of the disease, however, the frequency of lymph node metastases was limited, generally comparable to that reported in Western countries. The overall 5-year survival figure from another group of 1,007 patients with bilharziasis-associated disease, reported by Elsebai,[43] was 27.3 percent. When pelvic lymph nodes were involved, localized to the obturator and/or external iliac nodes on one side, the 5-year

survival rate was 18 percent; when other groups were involved, no long-term survivals were recorded.

Adenocarcinoma

Certain parallels between adenocarcinoma and squamous carcinoma are found: Noninvasive lesions are rarely encountered[6,84]; tumors invading muscle or beyond are the rule (Table 18-8); almost one-third of patients are found to have either regional or distant metastases.

Survival figures are equally dismal. In one of the larger series available, that of Anderström et al.,[6] which documented 64 cases of primary adenocarcinoma of the bladder and urachus, 13 of 24 patients with tumor infiltrating the lamina propria or muscularis died from their tumor, 7 died from intercurrent disease, and only 4 patients were alive and tumor-free by the conclusion of the study. Of the 21 patients with tumors that had penetrated the bladder wall, 18 died from advanced local recurrence or distant metastases, 2 died of intercurrent disease, and another died of unrelated causes with tumor detected only at autopsy. Of 18 patients with advanced regional disease, 17 died of tumor and the remaining patient died of congestive heart failure, with tumor discovered incidentally at autopsy.

MODE OF TUMOR SPREAD

In Mostofi's opinion,[125] mode and location of tumor spread are two pathologic features that have not been given sufficient attention. He noted two patterns of invasion: (1) a "broad front," or en bloc, pattern (Fig. 18-7), where the infiltrating tumor

Table 18-8 Adenocarcinoma: Stage at Presentation

Stage	Percent of Patients
Ta–O	—
T1–A	9.9
T2–B$_1$	
T3a–B$_2$	29.6
T3b–C	29.6
T4–D	30.9

(Data from Anderström, et al.,[6] and Johnson, et al.[84])

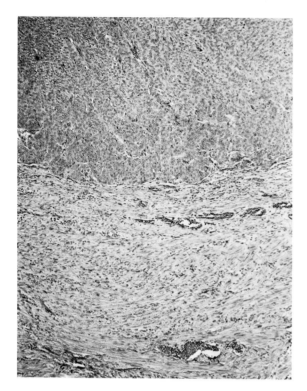

Fig. 18-7 "Broad front" invasion pattern. Note the circumscribed invasive border. ×56.

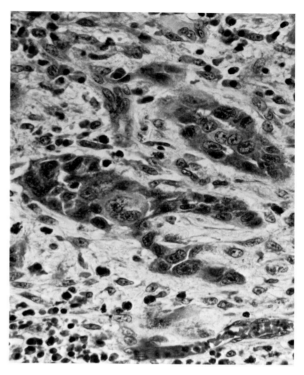

Fig. 18-8 Tentacular invasion. Note the irregular tumor borders and typical stromal response. ×320.

maintains a relatively circumscribed border; and (2) a "tentacular" pattern (Fig. 18-8), where the tumor spreads in an irregular, fingerlike fashion through the adjacent structures and has poorly circumscribed borders.

It is generally acknowledged that a tentacular mode of invasion is associated with a poorer prognosis, although this feature is not an independent variable. That is, tumors with a tentacular pattern of invasion are often nonpapillary, high grade lesions with a greater tendency to vascular and lymphatic invasion, and this pattern is most often associated with higher stage disease. In their study of giant sections from cystectomy specimens, Soto et al.[190] found a predominant tentacular pattern of invasion in 20 of 27 specimens with deeply invasive disease (T3a–B2,C), whereas the broad front invasion pattern predominated in 11 of 16 specimens with superficial disease (T1,T2–A,B1). As the authors indicated, however, both patterns may be seen in different areas of a single tumor.

Despite its lack of independence as a variable, this feature should be recorded. There is certainly precedent in other areas of pathology for prognostic differences between the two patterns, such as the poorer prognosis of infiltrating duct carcinoma of the breast (tentacular pattern) versus typical medullary carcinoma of the breast (broad front pattern).

Mostofi also advised noting any tendency to "lateral spread," wherein tumor extends to involve and undermine adjacent normal-appearing mucosa, with the potential for misleading the urologist who is attempting to remove an adequate uninvolved margin via the transurethral route.[125] Such change is most often confined to the immediate region of the grossly apparent tumor. However, occasional cases are encountered where intramucosal extension is much more extensive, both within the bladder and involving adjacent areas such as the distal ureters and prostate (see below). Subtle "pagetoid" spread may also be noted (Fig. 18-9); here malignant-appearing nests of tumor cells are found not only adjacent to the primary tumor but sometimes far removed from the grossly apparent tumor.

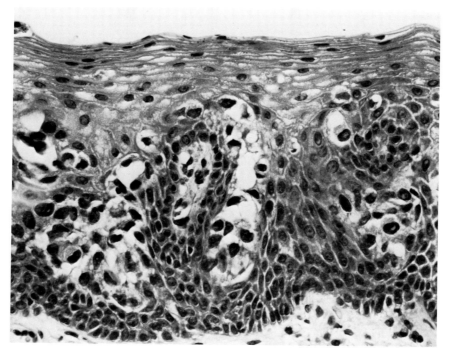

Fig. 18-9 "Pagetoid spread" involving the distal urethral mucosa in a patient with bladder carcinoma. Note the tumor nests along the mid and deep aspects of mucosa. ×320.

LYMPHATIC AND VASCULAR INVASION

Transitional Cell Carcinoma

Jewett and Strong[83] first emphasized the importance of lymphatic capillary invasion in the spread of bladder carcinoma in their landmark paper on the relation of local spread of carcinoma to the occurrence of metastases. They found an increasing incidence of this phenomenon with greater depth of tumor penetration and presumed that its presence would have an adverse effect on prognosis. That they were correct was shown within the next few years by McDonald and Thompson,[115] who noted a reduction in the 5-year survival rate, despite what appeared to be adequate surgery, when lymphatic invasion was present. These authors also called attention to the importance of blood vessel invasion.

Again, the degree of independence of this variable is difficult to sort out. Its incidence rises not only with increasing depth of invasion but also with high grade versus low grade tumors as well as solid versus papil-

lary tumors. Nonetheless, there appears to be a definite trend toward poorer survivability among patients with lymphatic and vascular invasion when other factors are held constant. For example, Jewett et al.[82] found that 19 of 48 patients treated for superficial disease eventually died of bladder cancer, and 7 of the 19 demonstrated lymphatic invasion by their initial tumors. Conversely, among the remaining 29 patients with superficial disease who were cured, not a single tumor showed lymphatic invasion. Most strikingly, for the group as a whole, 87 percent of patients who had lymphatic permeation demonstrated in their original material, *whatever the stage,* died of their disease. Therefore particular concern should be aroused when dealing with patients with low stage disease who demonstrate this feature, where conservative therapy using transurethral resection is contemplated. In the study of Anderström et al.,[5] 99 patients with tumors infiltrating the lamina propria had overall 5- and 10-year survivals of 71 and 64 percent, respectively. However, in a subgroup of 10 patients whose tumors had invaded lymphatics, all 10 patients died within 6 years of diagnosis, 7 as a result of their bladder carcinoma. The authors suggested that a more radical approach to therapy should be considered when this feature is present.

Because of the prognostic and possible therapeutic implications, care must be taken in the diagnosis of this feature. Invasion of blood vessels with muscular walls is the easiest type of invasion to recognize microscopically (Fig. 18-10) but also, unfortunately, the least frequent. A distinct point of attachment of the tumor to the vessel wall or associated thrombus formation, (Fig. 18-11) should be sought. This is sometimes apparent only after serial sections are performed. In some tumors fixation results in artifactual contraction of tumor nests, particularly those invading in a tentacular fashion. An endothelial lining (Fig. 18-12) should therefore be identified prior to accepting a focus as definitely showing lymphatic or small blood vessel permeation.

In cases where vascular or lymphatic invasion is suspected, but definitive identification of the potential spaces involved as truly vascular cannot be made on routine hematoxylin and eosin (H & E) sections, immunoperoxidase techniques that can be applied to

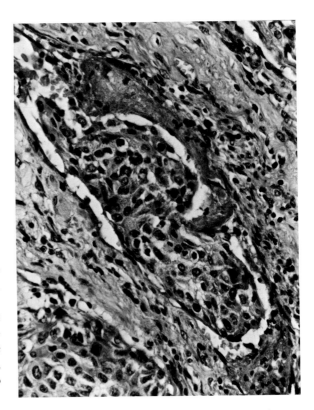

Fig. 18-11 Tumor invasion of a small blood vessel. Note the adjacent thrombus. ×282.

paraffin-embedded tissue may be helpful. Various antigen markers of vascular endothelial cells may be identified by this technique, e.g., factor VIII-related antigen,[128] as well as the factor or factors which bind the lectin *Ulex europaeus* agglutinin I.[56] With the latter technique, as noted by Fujime et al.,[56] capillaries and small vessels, both blood and lymphatic, stain with great intensity compared to larger vessels; this finding is of particular importance, as these vessels are the most difficult to identify with certainty on routine H & E sections.

It is not always possible to distinguish small blood vessels from lymphatics, as the muscular coats surrounding the former may not be apparent, even with special stains. This may not be crucial, however. In their study of giant sections from cystectomy specimens, Soto et al.[190] noted that when lymphatic invasion was present there was almost invariably concomitant invasion of venules. They also found that the frequency of blood vessel invasion paralleled tumor

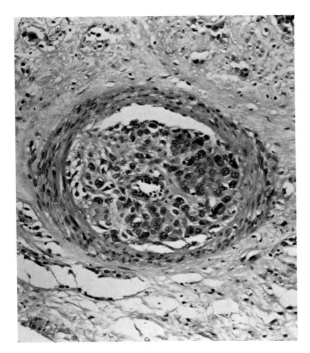

Fig. 18-10 Tumor invasion of medium-sized blood vessel. The muscular wall of the vessel is readily apparent. ×159.

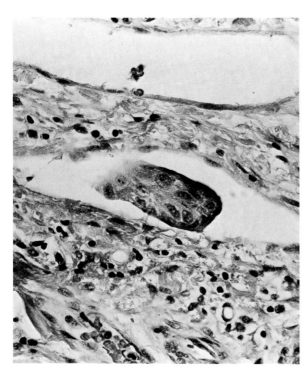

Fig. 18-12 Tumor nest in a small vessel, probably a dilated lymphatic channel. Note the endothelial lining cells. ×320.

stage, present in only 3 of 16 cases with stage A–B1 disease but noted in 21 of 27 cases with stage B2–C disease. It is also of interest, in contrast to previous published findings,[7] that the authors found involved vessels to lie generally within the tumor masses themselves or in the immediate vicinity, with little evidence of distant vascular or lymphatic spread. True "tumor emboli" within the surgical specimen were rarely seen, and in only two cases (of 45) was tumor found in vessels more than 4 cm from the main tumor mass. A further finding, corroborating earlier impressions, was that tumors demonstrating tentacular invasion were more likely to show vascular involvement than those invading with a broad front pattern, with this feature noted in 68 percent of the former tumors versus 33 percent of the latter.

Other Carcinomas

There is little information available on the propensity for lymphatic and blood vessel invasion by the less common tumor types. Jewett et al.[82] found a high percentage of lymphatic invasion in the subgroup of patients with high grade squamous cell carcinoma. Soto et al.,[190] noted that all seven of their cases of squamous carcinoma were deeply invasive tumors, and all showed blood vessel invasion. The incidence of lymphatic and blood vessel invasion by adenocarcinomas is not known, but the implications of such a finding would presumably be similar to those for transitional cell carcinoma.

ASSOCIATED UROTHELIAL ABNORMALITIES

In his classic article, published in 1952, Melicow[118] addressed the issue of the distressingly high recurrence rate in patients treated for bladder carcinoma. To study this phenomenon, he evaluated ten tumor-bearing bladders obtained at surgery, as well as five control bladders from the autopsy service. He carefully examined not only the tumors but also the grossly uninvolved mucosa. On microscopic examination Melicow found ". . . in the *grossly normal-looking mucosa* of tumor-bearing bladders varying numbers of *microscopic foci* of cellular activity, some of which were definitely malignant, and others, which in the course of time, would probably have blossomed into grossly obvious growths." His report is richly illustrated (fortunately having been written during an era when editors would accept 25 illustrations for an 18-page article), and the author demonstrated a number of microscopic lesions including hyperplasia, atypical hyperplasia, and carcinoma in situ. It is presumably from such altered epithelium that many of the "recurrences" arise in patients with bladder cancer.

A number of other thorough studies of cystectomy specimens have shown the widespread existence of such changes in grossly nontumorous areas of bladder epithelium.[96,97,190] Koss et al.[96] summarized the experience with histologic mapping of 20 cystectomy specimens and noted the presence of widespread abnormalities in all cases, including atypical hyperplasia and nonpapillary carcinoma in situ, at times far afield from the grossly visible lesions for which the bladders were removed. Moreover, they found areas of grossly inapparent *invasive* carcinoma extending not only from foci of carcinoma in situ but also from areas that would be classified as no more than atypical hyperplasia. The lateral and posterior walls were the areas most frequently involved by these "precancerous" lesions. Of greatest importance is the fact that these studies draw attention to the potential severity of lesions, up to and including early invasive carcinoma, in seemingly innocuous-appearing bladder mucosa.

For this reason multiple-site mucosal biopsies have become an integral part of patient evaluation, along with biopsy or resection of the more obvious tumor mass or masses. As recommended by the NBCG,[134] cold-cup biopsy specimens are taken from selected sites, including mucosa adjacent to the cystoscopically apparent tumor, lateral to each ureteral orifice, and in the posterior midline. Directed biopsy specimens should also be taken from areas with noticeable but at times subtle abnormalities when viewed cystoscopically. Wallace et al.,[200] for example, called attention to two mucosal appearances at cystoscopy which they found to give a particularly good yield on biopsy. The first was flat mucosa with a reddened appearance, suggesting increased vascularity, wherein 51 percent of biopsies showed abnormalities including hyperplasia, dysplasia, and carcinoma, either in situ or with some invasion, with 14 percent in the latter two categories. The second appearance was described as granular, edematous, or "red mossy." Here abnormalities were found in 81.5 percent, with 42 percent classifiable as carcinoma. Newer techniques, such as selective surface staining of abnormal mucosa using methylene blue, as described by Gill and colleagues,[58] similar to Schiller's iodine staining of cervical abnormalities, may result in an even greater yield of significantly abnormal biopsies at endoscopy, although others have had less success with the method, particularly in patients with prior topical therapy.[217]

Frequency of Biopsy Abnormalities

In the study of Wallace et al.,[200] 154 patients, both new and previously treated, underwent multiple-site biopsies. Among 27 newly diagnosed cases with cystoscopically normal-appearing mucosa away from the tumor, 13 showed microscopic abnormalities in selected-site biopsies (four hyperplasia, seven mild dysplasia, and two severe dysplasia or carcinoma in situ). Of seven newly diagnosed cases with abnormal (flat reddish or granular) appearance to the mucosa, three showed severe dysplasia or carcinoma in situ. In the

series overall, 26 percent of cases were found to have at least carcinoma in situ, if not "frank carcinoma," in biopsy specimens of apparently normal mucosa. Interestingly, as might be expected from the "mapping studies" described above,[96] the abnormalities could be seen far afield, and the mucosa immediately adjacent to apparent tumor did not always give the highest yield. Moreover, such associated abnormalities are not static in patients with bladder carcinoma. For example, in a prospective study with repeated selected-site biopsies, Soloway et al.[187] found 33 percent of patients to have atypicalities in selected-site biopsy material at initial diagnostic evaluation. Biopsies were repeated at 3-month intervals, and by the end of a year, 77 percent had shown at least focal mucosal atypia, and 30 percent had developed severe dysplasia/carcinoma in situ or frank carcinoma.

Prognostic Implications

In perhaps the most frequently cited study, Althausen et al.[3] examined a group of 78 patients with low stage (noninvasive or invasion limited to the lamina propria)/low grade (I to II) disease in whom transurethral resection material contained sufficient adjacent epithelium for adequate evaluation. Slightly more than one-half of the patients showed normal urothelium adjacent to the resected tumor, and of these patients only 7 percent had eventual progression to muscle-invasive disease. Conversely, in the subgroup showing carcinoma in situ associated with their tumor, 83 percent progressed to muscle-invasive disease. Those patients showing associated abnormalities that were atypical but short of carcinoma in situ occupied the intermediate range, with 36 percent progressing to muscle-invasive disease.

In the NBCG study,[28] multiple selected-site biopsies were performed on all patients as part of the initial evaluation. The presence of mucosal abnormalities in conjunction with a cystoscopically apparent tumor was associated with both a significant decrease in the ability to achieve "disease-free status" and an increase in recurrence rate even if a disease-free state were achieved. In a subgroup of patients whose overt tumors showed lamina propria invasion (T1 – A), progression to muscle invasion or beyond by 2 years was seen in 32 percent of patients with associated moderate to severe dysplasia in their selected-site biopsies, compared with only 13 percent with no such abnormalities. It is in just this group, those with low stage disease, that the information may prove of most value with regard to patient management.

Although these figures are alarming, it must be understood that all have been gleaned from studies of such histologic abnormalities *in association with* a clinically apparent neoplasm. Outside this context, the meaning of *histologically identical* abnormalities is less clear. Biopsy-proved carcinoma in situ (Fig. 18-13) must be viewed with concern in any setting. As noted by Herr,[65] however, the natural history of carcinoma in situ shows considerable variation. In particular, it does not necessarily carry the dire prognosis indicated in earlier reports, such as that of Utz et al.,[198] wherein recurrences after treatment were noted in 82 percent of patients, with invasion in 73 percent. Herr[65] discussed three possible settings.

The first is primary carcinoma in situ, in which patients may manifest microhematuria but generally have no significant symptoms and for whom the diagnosis is made incidentally by urinary cytology. Herr noted that the incidence of subsequent invasive cancer in this subgroup, thought to represent the ear-liest portion of the in situ spectrum, is presently unknown, although careful follow-up with conservative therapy is indicated, as the disease will most likely persist (at least) if untreated.

A second setting is that of primary carcinoma in situ, again unassociated with previous or concurrent bladder tumors, but with accompanying overt symptoms, such as urgency, frequency, etc. This group of patients appears much more likely to develop invasive disease and requires a more intensive therapeutic approach.

The final setting—patients presenting with carcinoma in situ in association with prior or concurrent bladder tumors, a more frequent situation than primary carcinoma in situ[55]—is the most worrisome, with the subsequent development of invasive disease noted in 40 to 80 percent of cases. These patients appear to be the most likely to die of invasive bladder cancer.

In passing, it should be noted that although one would think such associated epithelial abnormalities would be more commonly seen with solid, high grade lesions, some studies indicate that this may not be the case. In the study of Soto et al.,[190] carcinoma in situ associated with an overt tumor was in fact more often found with papillary than with nonpapillary tumors, an observation also made by Melicow[118] in his original work on carcinoma in situ. It further underscores the necessity for careful biopsy of the remaining urothelium with even the most innocuous-appearing papillary tumors at the time of first evaluation. Also, particularly for those patients in whom conservative resection followed by intensive topical therapy is contemplated, the possible extension of carcinoma in situ into areas of cystitis cystica or Brunn's nests, and in particular the prostatic ducts, should be kept in mind, as these areas may serve as possible "safe harbors" for tumor during such treatment.[29,45,160,184]

If the course of events with carcinoma in situ is unsettled, the implications of lesser degrees of epithelial abnormalities, criteria for which have been proposed by a panel of experts in the field,[131] are even more difficult to pin down. Lesions showing severe dysplasia are perhaps best categorized as carcinoma in situ.[55,130] Such cases are those wherein full thickness change is not seen but in which many of the features of carcinoma in situ, including marked nuclear pleomorphism, nuclear hyperchromasia, mitotic figures, large nucleoli, etc., are apparent. More difficult, how-

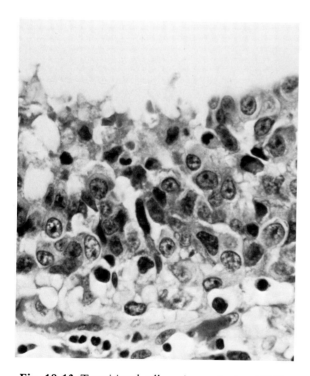

Fig. 18-13 Transitional cell carcinoma in situ. ×500.

ever, are lesser abnormalities, which are lumped in a second category, that of mild to moderate dysplasia. Here such changes as lesser nuclear enlargement, loss of polarization with increasingly rounded nuclei, some degree of nuclear crowding, and increasingly coarsely granular chromatin pattern are seen. Superficial cells are generally still identifiable. Such changes may represent early "precursor lesions" in the development of clinically recognizable neoplastic disease, but here the denominator is somewhat more difficult to define, and in fact morphologically indistinguishable changes may be seen in a number of conditions other than urothelial malignancy.[130] Nonetheless, these findings should at least be noted in patients being evaluated for overt neoplasms; and as more data are accumulated, the meaning of such findings in association with overt tumors might begin to crystallize.

What are the implications of finding simple hyperplasia, i.e., an increase in cell layer number without significant abnormalities of individual nuclei? As noted in Chapter 17, such changes are not infrequently found in nonneoplastic situations, particularly in the setting of chronic inflammation. Hyperplasia may also be seen, however, in association with various vesical tumors. Particularly when a corrugated or "accordian-pleat" appearance is exhibited (see Fig. 17-16), the hyperplasia probably represents the earliest recognizable change in the development of a low grade papillary neoplasm. In a study of the genesis of papillary tumors, Sarma[154] labeled such growths "infant papillary tumors." In a review of 170 cases of papillary tumors of all grades, he found patchy hyperplasia in adjacent mucosa in 79 percent of the cases, with the remaining 21 percent showing no such changes. Sarma graded the extent of the hyperplastic change; and, interestingly, as hyperplasia progressed from slight to moderate to marked, the grade of the primary tumor *decreased,* with the lowest grade tumors showing the most marked areas of associated mucosal hyperplasia. Also of note was the fact that among 13 infiltrating tumors six had no associated hyperplasia, only one had associated marked hyperplasia, and the four tumors with distant metastases all had no apparent adjacent hyperplasia. On examination of recurrence rates, no relation was found between increasing hyperplasia and increasing frequency of recurrence. These findings were reflected in the 2- and 10-year survival rates, with the paradox of increasing degrees of hyperplasia being associated with *increased* survival rates for both periods. Therefore, although simple hyperplasia may be seen in association with urothelial neoplasia, it is generally found with relatively nonaggressive disease and does not appear to bode either an increased propensity for recurrent disease or a poorer prognosis.

Meaningful data on the association and significance of in situ carcinoma or dysplastic epithelial changes with the less common forms of bladder carcinoma are essentially unavailable. With the exception of bilharziasis-associated squamous carcinoma, the finding of dysplastic or in situ lesions with squamous carcinoma is relatively infrequent. In a study of the association of carcinoma in situ with overt carcinoma in cystectomy specimens, Skinner et al.[171] found the expected high incidence of such abnormalities in the transitional cell group but found no evidence of in situ disease in their six cases of squamous carcinoma. Johnson et al.[85] mentioned squamous *metaplasia* of the mucosa adjacent to tumor in 15 of 90 cases of squamous carcinoma but made no mention of dysplastic or in situ lesions. In bilharziasis-associated squamous carcinoma, in contrast, atypical epithelial changes are frequently found in the remainder of the urothelium.[89] In primary adenocarcinoma of the bladder, atypical changes may be noted immediately adjacent to the tumor and at times in Brunn's nests and areas of cystitis cystica,[127] but true in situ surface disease is not commonly seen. In general, however, pure squamous and adenocarcinomas are often advanced tumors at presentation, and the finding of associated in situ changes would have little bearing on either therapy or prognosis. In the unusual event that a tumor in one of these groups is encountered that might be dealt with conservatively, it appears logical to at least sample the remaining urothelium, as one would with transitional cell lesions, with whatever information gleaned applied rationally to management of the case at hand.

INVOLVEMENT OF DISTAL URETERS, URETHRA, AND PROSTATE

It has been clearly documented that patients with widespread mucosal abnormalities of the bladder, particularly carcinoma in situ, may have extension to involve the contiguous distal ureters, prostatic urethra, and prostatic ducts. Various mechanisms are thought to account for this phenomenon.

Farrow et al.,[46] in a study of 21 cystectomies performed for extensive carcinoma in situ, found frequent localization of atypical or dysplastic areas around the borders of in situ carcinoma, with zones of continuous morphologic gradation of change. This suggested a gradual extension of the neoplastic process by a progressive evolution through stages of premalignant atypia. Second, they observed direct intramucosal spread of tumor along the edges of malignant areas, over a range of approximately 1 to 2 mm. The malignant epithelium appeared to extend directly along the basilar regions of the adjacent mucosa, displacing the normal mucosa toward the luminal aspect of the bladder. A third phenomenon, which the authors found as much as 4 mm distant from adjacent in situ carcinoma, was the "pagetoid spread" of tumor described above, wherein small clusters of malignant cells were seen scattered in the normal epithelium, similar to that seen with mammary and extramammary Paget's disease. All three mechanisms could account for involvement of adjacent structures as well as spread within the bladder itself. Obviously, involvement of these adjacent structures is noncontiguous at times, and the "field effect," which is thought to account at least in part for the multifocality of bladder carcinoma, no doubt explains the presence of some of this extravesical spread. Tumor "seeding" of areas in adjacent structures is an additional potential mechanism, and the question of a possible iatrogenic role during the various manipulations and biopsies in these patients remains unsettled.

Whatever the mechanisms, involvement of these structures in mucosal continuity with the bladder may be remarkably widespread and often quite inapparent. Figure 18-14, from a radical cystectomy specimen, illustrates carcinoma in situ of an intramural portion of ureter, which would not have been discovered without cystectomy by any means except directed biopsy or brushing. Figure 18-15, again from a radical cystectomy specimen, shows focal intraprostatic mucosal spread of high grade transitional cell carcinoma, with the blurring of the glandular–stromal interface in one area suggesting early invasion. This mode of intraprostatic spread was emphasized by Seemayer et al.,[160] who found extensive "silent" intraductal prostatic involvement in five of seven patients with carcinoma in situ of the bladder. In three of the five cases,

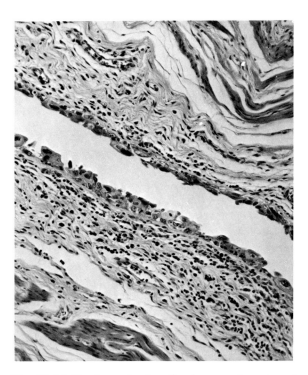

Fig. 18-14 Carcinoma in situ of an intramural portion of the ureter. It was found incidentally in a radical cystectomy specimen containing bladder carcinoma. ×124.

thorough examination revealed microinvasive disease in addition to intraglandular spread. Although inapparent grossly, such involvement was so widespread in some cases as to involve the seminal vesicles (Fig. 18-16) and vas deferens as well.[160] Such findings have also been noted in a number of other detailed studies.[46,110]

Although the highest incidence of involvement of the distal ureters, prostatic urethra, and prostate is seen with high grade disease in the bladder, it is important to note that such extravesical epithelial abnormalities are not confined to this subgroup of lesions. Cooper and colleagues,[23] for example, examined 49 cystectomy specimens in which the gross configuration of the primary neoplasm for which the procedure was performed was papillary in 20 specimens, nonpapillary in 27, and had a combined pattern in 2. Associated "severely atypical abnormalities" (SEAs), essentially the equivalent of carcinoma in situ, were sought. As might be expected, most cases with SEAs in the contiguous ureteral segments were associated with high grade bladder lesions. Yet in one case of ten

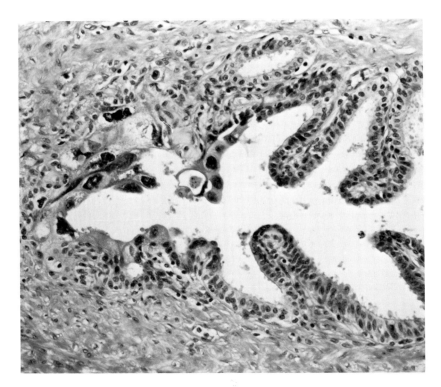

Fig. 18-15 Carcinoma in situ extending into the prostatic glands. There is focal microinvasion of the prostatic stroma at the upper left. ×204.

with intermediate grade primaries, this ureteral change was also noted, and even higher percentages (up to 47 percent in one study[156]) of ureteral abnormalities in association with intermediate or low grade bladder primaries have been recorded at other institutions. The stage of the primary lesion did not appear to have much effect on the presence or absence of ureteral SEAs, as 17 and 19 percent of patients with early and advanced tumors, respectively, showed such ureteral change. Nor was configuration of the bladder primary important; almost equal numbers of patients with papillary and nonpapillary tumors showed ureteral involvement.

In the urethra, SEA was present in 18 percent of cases, either in the membranous or the prostatic portion. Again, most instances were noted in association with high grade bladder primaries, but 2 of 12 patients with intermediate grade primaries showed SEAs in the urethral sections examined. Surprisingly, 20 percent of the patients with early stage bladder primaries showed urethral SEAs versus only 15 percent of those with advanced lesions, and 21 percent with papillary

primaries showed such involvement versus only 15 percent with solid tumors. Four cases contained abnormalities involving both urethra and ureters.

To detect the prostatic changes, Cummings[27] advised biopsy sampling, particularly in men with diffuse carcinoma in situ without frankly invasive tumor. A transurethrally obtained specimen allows evaluation of the prostatic urethral mucosa as well as the immediately subjacent ducts and glands. For the distal ureters, either direct ureteroscopic biopsy or brush biopsy with cytologic evaluation should be considered.

What are the implications of such extravesical spread? Distal ureteral involvement actually appears to affect the clinical situation less than one might expect. In a series of 21 patients undergoing cystectomy for carcinoma in situ reported by Farrow et al.,[46] 12 of the 21 cases showed in situ carcinoma involving one or both ureters. In a later review,[45] after at least 5 years of follow-up, only 1 of the 12 patients had developed an upper tract tumor, and it was in the renal pelvis. Similarly encouraging, Linker and Whit-

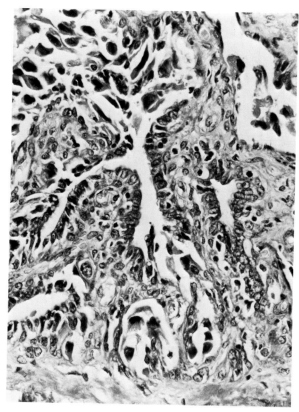

Fig. 18-16 Extension of carcinoma into the seminal vesicle. ×285.

more[104] reported that only 1 of 33 such cases progressed to clinically apparent ureteral tumor. As pointed out by Koss et al.,[96] however, the situation is not clear-cut, as a number of the patients in the latter series died of metastatic bladder cancer. Indeed, this confounding factor in any series of patients with disease aggressive enough to require cystectomy is virtually impossible to surmount. Therefore it seems prudent to continue the common practice of examining ureteral margins by frozen section at the time of cystectomy, with extension of the resections proximally if severe epithelial atypia or carcinoma in situ is detected. Schade and Swinney[156] reported that such disease was most commonly detected in the lower 5 cm of the ureters, and they suggested that resection at the level of the pelvic brim is most often sufficient to encompass the diseased areas.

Data concerning the implications of urethral involvement at the time of cystectomy are also not en-

tirely straightforward, particularly because series vary in terms of the extent of urethral resection. Although the entire urethra is typically removed as part of the cystectomy procedure in women, the extent of resection in male patients is not always stated in the literature.

The occurrence of eventual urethral carcinoma in a series of 174 cystectomies without urethrectomy, reported by Cordonnier and Spjut,[24] was 4.02 percent. Although this overall figure is somewhat comforting, the presence of carcinoma in situ at the urethral margin may pose an important risk. Richie and Skinner[151] reported a series of 12 men who underwent radical cystectomy for bladder cancer, all of whom showed carcinoma in situ at the urethral margin. Six of the seven patients who underwent simultaneous urethrectomy were free of tumor on follow-up, but four of the five patients who did not died of their disease. The authors advised that specimens for routine frozen section examination also be taken from the urethral margin and, for those with carcinoma in situ, that urethrectomy be performed either simultaneously or during the same hospitalization.

One final word with regard to prostatic involvement by transitional cell carcinoma is in order. In a review of cases of transitional cell carcinoma of the prostate, with and without associated bladder tumors, Chibber et al.[21] noted that at times all cases of "prostatic involvement" by urothelial carcinoma are lumped together as high stage disease and placed into the AJC T4a stage. In fact, this category should be reserved for those cases in which "tumor *invades substance of prostate* (microscopically proven), uterus, or vagina."[8] As these authors indicated, actual invasion of the *stroma* of the prostate, either directly from the bladder or via extension from the prostatic duct system, is associated with a dismal prognosis. Even with this finding, though, occasional patients survive for relatively long periods.[172]

Chibber et al.[21] suggested, however, that two other subgroups with "prostatic involvement" should be separately classified. One is *carcinoma in situ* (i.e., high grade, flat, noninvasive disease) involving the prostatic urethra and ducts, with or without similar bladder involvement. In a small group of patients with this type of involvement, three were treated with systemic rather than topical chemotherapy, and a fourth had simple transurethral resection of the prostate; the disease demonstrated no progression in these four patients. Furthermore, according to a report by Montie and co-workers,[121] it appears that such involvement is much more frequent than is usually appreciated. Extensive sampling of the prostate in radical cystectomy specimens showed a 28 percent incidence of tumor involvement, so the investigators prepared whole mount sections of the entire prostate on a series of 62 cases. By this method, prostatic involvement was found in a remarkable 40 percent of cases, but a considerable number (84 percent) showed only intramucosal disease; similar findings have been noted by others.[110] Of particular importance, in agreement with the findings of Chibber et al.,[21] the "prostatic involvement," *if limited to intramucosal disease,* had no adverse effect on survival in the series of Montie and colleagues.[121] Obviously, caution must be exercised when defining the extent of the disease as such on the basis of transurethral sampling. As noted by Seemeyer et al.,[160] areas of microinvasive disease extending out from the ducts may be seen, although it sometimes requires diligent search by the pathologist. In our experience, particularly when there is extensive prostatic duct and gland involvement by tumor, areas of definite stromal invasion are common if sufficient sections are examined.

The other subgroup of prostatic involvement suggested by Chibber and co-workers[21] is that of noninvasive *papillary tumors* of the prostatic urethra and major ducts, occurring with similar bladder tumors. Of 10 such patients, three showed concurrent involvement of the prostate along with the bladder tumor, and the remaining seven developed such prostatic lesions during intervals ranging from 13 months to 10 years following detection of the bladder primary. Most such tumors were well or moderately differentiated at the time of detection, and there was no evidence of extension to involve the prostatic stroma. All patients were managed initially by endoscopic resection and diathermy. Six of the ten were able to be controlled by endoscopic means. In two the tumor in the prostate showed an increase in grade, and in two subsequent tumor with areas of microinvasion of the stroma was encountered. Both such occurrences were considered indications for proceeding to more radical therapy.

Although conservative therapy may be contemplated in patients with prostatic duct extension of low to intermediate grade papillary carcinomas, it is important to realize that even these tumors may at times

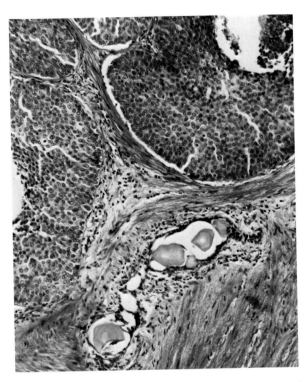

Fig. 18-17 Low to intermediate grade bladder transitional cell carcinoma with invasion of the prostatic stroma. ×108.

invade the substance of the prostate (Fig. 18-17) without an increase in grade. Whatever the grade, conservative therapy in this setting must be contemplated with caution, particularly if reliance is placed on topical chemotherapy or immunotherapy, with the obvious problems of tumor accessibility.

RESULTS OF ADJUNCTIVE STUDIES

The various methods of assessment considered to be "adjunctive studies" are discussed in Chapter 17. Urinary cytology and flow cytometry are discussed separately in Chapter 21. As many of the other studies are of relatively recent origin, or at least of recent application to urothelial neoplasia, the data base at this time must be considered to be in the incipient stage for most such tests, particularly with regard to therapeutic decisions for an individual patient. As noted, most are directed at the problem of determining which patients with superficial lesions will develop more aggressive disease—with the hope that early intervention in this subgroup will lead to improvement in prognosis. Perhaps the only newer studies that may lend themselves in the foreseeable future to application in day-to-day practice are surface isoantigen determination and flow cytometry. The former will have greater applicability as newer immunoperoxidase methods are implemented, as these seem to have circumvented some of the problems associated with the red blood cell adherence method. Flow cytometric analysis shows promise as one of the most accurate method to date of evaluating the malignant potential of transitional cell and other lesions.

SPECIAL SITE CONSIDERATIONS

Although unusual in any series, urothelial neoplasms are occasionally found in urinary diverticula and in areas of urachal remnants. Because of the somewhat differing presentations and prognoses, both situations are briefly considered.

Neoplasms in Vesical Diverticula

In any series of bladder malignancies, the incidence of carcinoma arising in vesical diverticula is small. Faysal and Freiha,[49] for example, found only 12 cases among 850 patients with carcinoma of the bladder seen at Stanford University over a 15-year period, for an incidence of approximately 1.5 percent, with similar figures noted in other series.[90a,119] The reverse figure, i.e., the incidence of neoplastic development in excised diverticula, is somewhat higher in some series, occurring in 4 to 7 percent of such cases.[87,90a] Diverticular carcinoma occurs most often in men,[49,87,90a,119] with the male/female ratio even higher than that cited for routine bladder carcinoma. In the series of Faysal and Freiha,[49] patients were in their forties through eighties with most 50 to 59 years of age. Eight patients presented with gross hematuria, and in the remaining four, the tumors were discovered at cystoscopy performed for obstructive symptoms or cystitis.

Neoplasms in vesical diverticula may be difficult to detect by conventional cystography and cystoscopy, and a significant number of such neoplasms are discovered as incidental findings at operation.[158] Most

such lesions are transitional cell tumors.[49,87,90a,119] In the series of Faysal and Freiha,[49] although nine of the ten transitional cell tumors were papillary, seven were high grade lesions (Figs. 18-18 and 18-19). Two of their 12 patients had squamous carcinomas.

Because of the lack of smooth muscle in the wall of a diverticulum, routine staging is not applicable to these tumors. Generally it is possible to note only whether a tumor is confined to the mucosal layer or has already penetrated the peridiverticular fat.[158] Prognosis for these patients may be poor, related at least in part to the anatomic peculiarities of the situation. Kelalis and McLean[87] reported that 68 percent of their patients were dead less than 1 year after the onset of symptoms, with 84 percent dead at the 3-year mark. Despite the fact that three-fourths of the lesions reported by Faysal and Freiha[49] were papillary, 9 of their 12 patients were dead of disease at 4.5 years, 2 were alive with disease at 2 and 3 years, respectively, and only 1 patient was disease-free at 3.5 years. These authors suggested an aggressive approach, using preoperative radiotherapy and cystectomy. Even this approach may do little to improve the prognosis, however, as what is merely lamina propria invasion in a patient with routine bladder carcinoma is equivalent to perivesical extension in these cases. The importance of tumor grade has been emphasized by Das and Amar,[30] and better differentiated lesions may require less aggressive therapy. (See also Chapter 14.)

Neoplasms of Urachal Origin

The urachus is a vestigial remnant of the early fetal primary excretory organ, the allantois. During fetal development this structure undergoes luminal obliteration and remains as a musculofibrous tube connecting the apex of the bladder to the umbilicus. In the adult the urachus is represented by the median umbilical ligament, bordered by the lateral umbilical ligaments, which represent the obliterated remnants of the umbilical arteries. These structures lie in the space of Retzius, bounded ventrally by the transversalis fascia and dorsally by the peritoneum.[116,164] Epithelial urachal remnants may be found in 30 to 70 percent of all adult patients and thus are extremely common; they are the presumed source of the quite uncommon urachal carcinoma.

According to Mostofi et al.,[127] a tumor is considered to be of urachal origin if it: (1) is situated in the dome

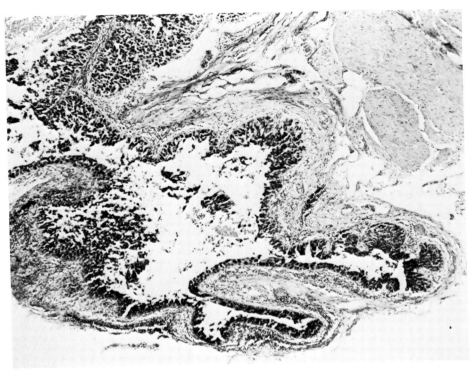

Fig. 18-18 Transitional cell carcinoma involving bladder diverticulum. The disease is still predominantly in situ in this section. ×51.

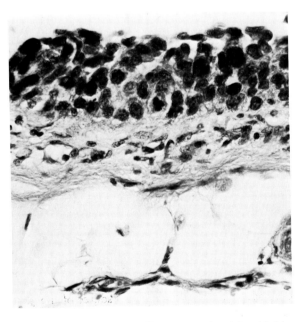

Fig. 18-19 Transitional cell carcinoma involving bladder diverticulum. Higher power view of the diverticular neoplasm seen in Figure 18-19, illustrating an area of high grade carcinoma in situ. ×314.

or anterior wall of the urinary bladder; (2) is mostly intramural; (3) has deep ramifications in the bladder wall; (4) is demonstrated not to be a secondary carcinoma; (5) has an intact or ulcerated surface epithelium overlying the tumor with a sharp demarcation between the tumor and surface epithelium, which should be devoid of glandular and polypoid proliferation; and (6) in addition to ramifications of tumor in the bladder wall, may show extension that involves the space of Retzius, anterior abdominal wall, or umbilicus.

In a report of eight cases and a literature review, Loening and colleagues[105] noted an age span of 15 to 83 years, with most patients between the ages of 40 and 70. The male/female ratio was approximately 4 : 1. Primary presenting symptoms included hematuria, passage of mucoid material, and a palpable mass in the lower abdomen, most commonly in the suprapubic area. Cystoscopic findings were variable; they included ulceration and a sessile mass in the region of the dome. Computerized axial tomography may be of particular diagnostic value.[116]

Nearly all of these tumors are adenocarcinomas, and they may account for a considerable percentage of all adenocarcinomas encountered in the urinary bladder.[9,127,164,195] As noted by Thomas et al.,[195] the tumors may show various types of differentiation, ranging from well differentiated, mucus-secreting papillary adenocarcinomas to poorly differentiated colloid carcinomas with signet ring cell differentiation. These authors, however, found no correlation between the degree of histologic differentiation and survival in their 24 cases. Because of the limited number of such cases, a uniform staging system has not been utilized. In an attempt to examine the prognostic value of staging for these tumors, a system has been proposed by Sheldon et al.,[164] with categories from stage I (no invasion beyond the urachal mucosa) through stage IV (regional nodal or distant metastases). These authors found, however, that most (83 percent) patients presented with high stage disease, extending at least into the bladder proper and/or other regional structures.

Treatment has varied for these patients, ranging from segmental resection to more radical surgery, with or without irradiation. Survival figures have been relatively poor,[36,164] although in occasional reports the results are more encouraging. In the series of Thomas et al.,[195] most patients were treated with partial cystectomy, with approximately one-fourth of them given additional radiotherapy. These authors reported 13 of 24 patients alive, without evidence of disease, at 2 years, with only three additional tumor deaths at the 5-year mark. Loening and colleagues,[105] reporting a smaller series, also noted some encouraging results and suggested early segmental cystectomy or radical cystectomy as the preferred methods of treatment. Others, such as Sheldon et al.,[164] recommended total cystectomy for all patients except those rare cases wherein disease appears confined to the urachal mucosa. In the opinion of Loening et al.,[105] transurethral resection and radiation therapy alone have no place in the management of this disease.

THERAPY

Discussion of therapy of bladder cancer is generally divided into three broad areas: superficial disease, deeply invasive disease, and advanced disease. The subject remains fluid, and only a brief sketch is presented here for the sake of completeness. The reader is urged to consult standard clinical texts as well as current publications for detail.

Therapeutic modalities include those used for treatment of solid tumors at other sites: surgery, radiotherapy, and chemotherapy, either alone or in combination, with "immunotherapy" enjoying success in certain specific situations. As with other areas of oncology, some practices are relatively standard. Fortunately, however, there is more than the usual undertone of controversy in many other areas, so necessary to the evolution of more efficacious means of treatment, and clinical research continues to be vigorously pursued.

Superficial Disease

The category "superficial disease" includes patients with disease confined to the mucosa or invading only the lamina propria. Although superficial muscle invasive disease had been previously considered in this category as well, the inaccuracies of clinical staging in this group and the marked decrease in survival with any degree of muscle invasion noted in some studies[169] suggest that such patients should not be included in this category. Yet even with this group of patients removed, the "superficial disease" category remains anything but homogeneous, as Soloway has noted in thorough reviews of this subject.[177,179,181,182,184] He emphasized the importance of subcategorization of patients with "superficial disease," with both the mode and the intensity of therapy dependent on the likelihood that a given patient will develop muscle-invasive disease and metastases, and eventually die of the disease.

Numerically, one large subcategory includes those with low grade papillary transitional cell carcinomas, accounting for a significant percentage of all bladder carcinomas in the average clinical practice. Most may be handled by transurethral resection, with assessment of additional risk factors for progression both initially and on follow-up.

Initial information should include cytologic evaluation of at least voided urine specimens, and most clinicians also submit cystoscopically obtained urine samples, bladder irrigation specimens, or both for analysis.[182,184] In addition to resection of the primary tumor or tumors at cystoscopy, preselected-site biopsies are also performed. This procedure is most important in this group of patients, as it should be recognized that atypical changes in uninvolved mucosa, although frequently associated with a high grade primary, are also seen in a considerable number of patients with grade I lesions as well.[188] If there is no further indication of higher grade disease elsewhere by cytologic or selected-site biopsy examinations, the patient may generally be followed with repeat cystoscopy and cytologies every 3 to 4 months thereafter, or perhaps even longer,[180,182] with periods lengthened as "disease-free intervals" increase. Although some advocate continuing preselected-site biopsies at repeat cystoscopies even in the absence of visible lesions, I would agree with Soloway[180] that this is not necessary if there is no cytologic evidence of developing high grade lesions. Despite even numerous recurrences over the course of years, many patients may be treated successfully with simple transurethral resection, and various topical agents employed prophylactically may help reduce the number of recurrent tumors that must be resected and increase the intervals between such recurrences.[182]

Certain features indicate the possible need for a more aggressive approach, in particular the use of more intensive adjuvant topical therapy.[177,179,181,182,184] One such feature is that of a *high histologic grade* of the superficial tumor itself. Although recurrences or new occurrences may be seen somewhat less frequently after transurethral resection of superficial higher-grade lesions compared to their low grade counterparts,[28] subsequent disease does occur in many patients with either type of tumor. More important, the propensity for subsequent muscle-invasive disease increases considerably with increasing grade of the initial primary. In the study of superficial lesions reported by Althausen et al.,[3] only 11 percent of patients with grade I lesions developed muscle-invasive disease, whereas 50 percent of patients with grade II primaries did so. *Multiplicity of primary lesions* was another feature of note in that study, with only 1 of 23 patients with single lesions progressing to invasive disease versus 34 of 79 with multiple lesions at presentation. A third alarming feature was *invasion of the lamina propria*, with 42 percent of such patients suffering eventual muscle-invasive disease versus only 28 percent of those with initial noninvasive lesions. A fourth feature was the presence of *associated abnormalities in adjacent mucosa*, which can be extended to include abnormalities in selected-site biopsies, with progression of disease to invasion noted in only 7 percent of those with normal mucosa versus

36 percent for those with atypical mucosa and 83 percent for those with associated carcinoma in situ. To this list should be added a fifth feature, i.e., *persistence of positive cytologies* despite apparent resection of all visible tumor.[40,145,182,184] Each of these factors portends a more pernicious course than usual and if present should lead to a consideration of more aggressive therapy.

If such worrisome factors are encountered during the evaluation of patients with superficial disease, various other methods may be employed either as adjuncts to transurethral resection or, much less commonly, as primary therapy. The most popular at the present time is topical chemotherapy, which is considered in more detail subsequently. Intracavitary or interstitial irradiation has enjoyed success in some hands,[67,199,209] although it has not received wide acceptance in the United States.[142] External radiotherapy, conversely, is thought by some to be of no use as primary treatment for low stage tumors.[149] Although it may destroy superficial lesions, according to Radwin[149] it does so no more effectively than transurethral resection. This author also noted that external radiotherapy is ineffective against carcinoma in situ, that there is no evidence for a protective effect against new tumor formation, that high doses (6,000 to 7,000 rads), with the expected morbidity, may be necessary to achieve tumoricidal range, and that both future surgery and chemotherapy may be compromised by such treatment. Other authors,[148,216] however, have suggested that despite such criticisms it is not unreasonable to consider definitive radiotherapy under certain circumstances.

Immunotherapy has received increasing attention of late, and its use for genitourinary neoplasia has been discussed in excellent reviews by Droller.[37,39] Bacillus Calmette Guérin (BCG) has proved successful in the treatment of superficial bladder neoplasms,[33,38,62,66,101,122,123,157,188] including carcinoma in situ, and has been found to decrease the number of recurrences in patients with superficial disease when compared to controls and to prolong the disease-free interval. Some reports have shown particularly favorable results,[66,157] with encouraging response rates noted among patients who have failed courses of conventional chemotherapy.[188] Topical therapy has been well tolerated in most cases, although occasional potentially serious or even life-threatening situations have been encountered.[100,138] As noted by Droller,[38] enthusiasm for the technique appears merited, but with a number of caveats. One disturbing aspect, for example, reported by Lamm et al.[101] is an apparent balance between enhancement of tumor response under optimum conditions and possible impairment of the immune response, and thus possibly actual tumor growth enhancement, with excess BCG administration. Although many such details still need to be worked out, this area of therapy appears to hold great promise for the treatment of superficial disease.

An additional surgical method which may be of comparable benefit to transurethral resection is segmental resection.[203] As Soloway[177] indicated, however, there are a number of accepted restrictions to its use. First, it should be limited to intermediate and high grade lesions; grade I lesions should be dealt with endoscopically. If a tumor is to be removed by segmental resection, it should be less than 6 to 8 cm in size and located such that a 2-cm margin of normal urothelium can be safely removed along with the tumor. In particular, preoperative selected-site biopsies should have shown no evidence of atypia or carcinoma in situ, as it seems fruitless to perform such a comparatively major procedure with the knowledge that there is an even higher than usual likelihood of recurrent disease in the remaining bladder. Low dose preoperative radiotherapy may also be considered prior to segmental resection, as is commonly done prior to cystectomy (vide infra).

Topical chemotherapy has been employed in various fashions since the concept was introduced in 1948 by Semple,[162] who used podophyllin for the treatment of "bladder papillomata." At present topical chemotherapy is primarily adjunctive, supplementing transurethral resection in the control of superficial disease. With the incidence of recurrent disease as high as it is, it seems logical to supplement standard surgical therapy by some means to either decrease recurrences or new occurrences, as the case may be, or at least prolong the intervals between such events.

The alkylating agent thiotepa (triethylene thiophosphoramide) is still the most commonly used topical drug in the United States. In the multiinstitutional study of the NBCG,[93] the efficacy of topical thiotepa as a therapeutic as well as a prophylactic agent was examined in patients with superficial disease. Patients in the therapeutic category included those with either incompletely resected visible tumor or, in the absence

of visible tumor, carcinoma in situ. After one or, when necessary, two courses of four consecutive weekly instillations of thiotepa, complete remission, i.e., disappearance of disease with no new tumors, was noted in 47 percent of these patients. Adverse factors included (1) tumors that numbered four or more, or (2) primaries that were more than 4 cm in dimension. Of note was the fact that the response did not seem to be affected by either tumor grade or configuration (papillary versus nonpapillary).

In the prophylaxis category, one-third of the patients were from the above group of complete responders to thiotepa in the treatment category. The other two-thirds were disease-free at the time of entry to the study but were considered at high risk because of a history of multiple recurrences, multifocal tumors, etc. These patients were compared to a group of controls with similar risks treated by surgical means alone. At 12 months, 66 percent of patients in the prophylaxis group were free of disease compared to only 40 percent of controls, a trend that continued throughout the 24-month period. The patients who entered the prophylaxis group from the treatment group did significantly better than those who had thiotepa as treatment only, as all of the former were free of disease at the completion of the study versus only 60 percent of the latter. Even the subgroup of patients who underwent only successful treatment (no prophylaxis thereafter) showed a beneficial effect despite discontinuance of therapy, encouraging adjuvant use of the drug even when a prophylactic course is not contemplated. Moreover, in addition to reducing the recurrence rate and increasing the interval between recurrences, more recent data[60] indicate that overall survival appears to be enhanced with the use of such therapy. In general, the NBCG study showed the treatment to be well tolerated, with only 17 percent experiencing complications, including primary urinary tract symptoms as well as the most bothersome of difficulties attributed to thiotepa: bone marrow depression with resultant leukopenia and/or thrombocytopenia. In only a few patients were the complications sufficient to require termination of therapy.

Numerous other drugs have also been used for topical chemotherapy of bladder cancer. Cisplatin (cis-diamminedichloroplatinum), perhaps the most effective single systemic agent for treating advanced disease, has produced disappointing results when used as a topical agent.[14] Another of the drugs with systemic activity, doxorubicin hydrochloride (Adriamycin), has proved efficacious as both a therapeutic and a prophylactic topical agent[13,179] with less systemic absorption than that noted with thiotepa.[108] Epodyl (triethylene glycol diglyceridyl ether), a tumor inhibiting diepoxide, is unavailable in the United States but has been used with benefit for almost two decades in the United Kingdom.[50,153] This drug has been of proved success in difficult-to-manage patients with superficial disease who would otherwise have been treated by cystectomy.[50] It also enjoys the benefit of little systemic toxicity compared with thiotepa, possibly the result of decreased local absorption because of its greater molecular weight.[153] The only other major drug in use in the United States at present is another alkylating agent, mitomycin C. Although it has been used as a systemic agent since the late 1950s,[177] it is only recently that its efficacy as a topical agent for treating bladder carcinoma has begun to be noted in the United States. It may cause severe myelosuppression when administered systemically, but there is apparently little absorption when used topically, again possibly the result of a higher molecular weight than thiotepa,[177,182] and the drug is generally well tolerated when used in this fashion. Reports have indicated not only long-term improvement in recurrence rate, progression rate, and survival,[73] but notable success in patients whose tumors have proved refractory to thiotepa therapy.[75,92] One small series suggested the possibility of even greater efficacy when used in combination with thiotepa at the outset.[71] A significant negative aspect of the drug is its cost, estimated by Hopkins et al.[68] at approximately $5,000 per year, including initiation therapy as well as monthly maintenance. These authors had the rather novel idea of recycling the drug after therapy, as approximately 50 percent of the parent drug can be recovered intact following instillation therapy.

The management of carcinoma in situ, as noted in the above section, requires recognition that not all patients with carcinoma in situ necessarily behave in the same fashion. Herr[65] classified carcinoma in situ into three groups. The first group, patients with *asymptomatic carcinoma in situ* (diagnosed incidentally on cytology examination), may have focal disease that pursues an indolent course. Herr advised endoscopic and cytologic surveillance at 3-month intervals with fulguration and resection of suspicious areas. However, as focal carcinoma in situ may be difficult or impossible to visualize endoscopically, inadequate transurethral resection may be realized only postendoscopically with the return of positive urinary cytology. Furthermore, because all of the above discussed topical therapies have proved to be of some success in at least temporarily eradicating this disease,[50,66,75,78,93] it would seem that this group of patients in particular might be further held in check with the use of these agents. Topical BCG therapy appears to be resulting in an even brighter outlook for the situation.[99]

Herr's[65] second group, patients with *overtly symptomatic carcinoma in situ without associated tumors,* is a more worrisome category, and adjuvant topical chemotherapy is definitely recommended. More recently, Herr et al.[66] reported good results with intravesical BCG therapy, even in patients who had failed courses with conventional topical chemotherapy. A possible exception to this rule, as with superficial tumors in general, is extension of the process into the prostatic urethra and prostatic ducts, areas that may serve as inaccessible repositories for tumors otherwise susceptible to transurethral resection and topical therapy. It is important to have knowledge of this situation at the time of evaluation, and a biopsy of the prostatic urethra should be performed.[65] One might question the risk of tumor implantation in the area as a result of these biopsies, but even more vigorous surgery in the area, i.e., transurethral resection of the prostate simultaneous with transurethral resection of bladder tumors of all grades, does not appear to result in an increase of new tumor occurrences in the prostatic urethra according to a study by Laor et al.[102] Even if some increase in implantation at this site could be proved, the risk of possibly futile treatment of symptomatic bladder carcinoma in situ by topical means in the face of already existing prostatic involvement appears to be the greater evil.

For Herr's third group,[65] patients with *carcinoma in situ associated with prior or concurrent bladder tumors,* he recommended that a brief trial of aggressive topical therapy and transurethral resection be contemplated; but with the later development of infiltrating carcinoma in 50 to 80 percent of these patients, temporizing beyond a reasonable period could prove hazardous, a fact strongly emphasized by Droller and Walsh.[40] Again, more recent work[66,99] has suggested that topical BCG therapy might considerably brighten the picture for these patients. Other methods of dealing with superficial disease, in particular the employment of laser technology, either direct (neodymium-YAG laser therapy[10,163,175,191]) or in conjunction with other modalities (hematoporphyrin derivative photodynamic therapy[11]), are also being explored, again with encouraging results.

For other tumor types, including squamous carcinoma, bilharziasis-associated squamous carcinoma, adenocarcinoma, and undifferentiated carcinoma, the stage of the disease is most often such that conservative management is not an option. One possible exception is the rare verrucous squamous carcinoma, which, if minimally infiltrative at the time of discovery as it often is elsewhere in the body, might be managed conservatively with either transurethral or segmental resection, although delineating the extent of infiltration and the adequacy of resection by the former method may be impossible.

Deeply Invasive Disease

As noted, the category of "deeply invasive disease" should perhaps include *all* tumors aggressive enough to have invaded into the muscularis or beyond, generally requiring an equally aggressive approach therapeutically. However, the question arises with some patients whether tumor that is thought to be invading only the superficial muscularis might be effectively handled by conservative means. Whitmore[205] noted that the greatest proportion of failures in the treatment of such patients is due to distant dissemination, even when treated by radical cystectomy, and that a *selected* group of these patients may be considered for transurethral tumor resection, with expectation of results similar to those achieved by cystectomy. Survival rates of close to 60 percent may be achieved with proper patient selection. According to Whitmore, transurethral resection in this group should be limited to those patients with good bladder function (normal urinary control and capacity of more than 200 cc), who have no more than two tumors present, neither of which should exceed 2 cm at the base. The tumors should be of low grade, with little demonstrable muscle invasion, be unassociated with carcinoma in situ elsewhere, and, in particular, be in areas readily accessible to "safe and sure" transurethral resection. This group remains perhaps one of the most difficult to deal with, as the risks of aggressive disease are high. Considering the alternatives, the temptation to give

conservative therapy a try, even when it may not be the safest procedure, may be equally great for both patient and physician. More recently, the use of neodymium-YAG laser therapy in selected cases of muscle-invasive disease has proved to be of some success.[176] This new approach appears to allow very deep photocoagulation of the bladder wall, yet with maintenance of structural integrity, thus possibly circumventing the major problem of bladder perforation associated with deep transurethral resection by conventional means.

For the remaining and much larger number of patients with deeply invasive disease, there is some disagreement at present regarding standard therapy. Indeed, as Whitmore[206] noted, there may be no "best way" to treat an apparently still localized malignancy ". . . but a series of ways, one of which is best for a particular cancer in a particular patient."

Definitive external beam radiotherapy by itself has been indicated in the past to be of lesser benefit than either surgery or combined radiation and surgery.[149] As Soloway[184] noted, it may be difficult to evaluate the bladder following irradiation for either persistent or new tumor growth, and the latter is not infrequent after full-dose therapy. The patient is then at risk for subsequent cystectomy at an older age, and complication and mortality rates are increased after irradiation. Moreover, there may be considerable morbidity associated with tumoricidal doses given.[149] Not all centers share this negative view of definitive radiotherapy, however; but as emphasized by a number of authors,[165,166,216] proper patient selection may be essential if optimum results are to be achieved.

There remains a group of patients who, for medical or personal reasons, elect definitive radiotherapy; and there has been increasing interest of late in "salvage cystectomy" for the considerable number of these patients who become treatment failures because of recurrent local disease.[25,216] It appears that a certain percentage of patients are indeed salvaged by the procedure. In the report of 37 such cases by Crawford and Skinner,[25] for example, overall survival was a respectable 38 percent, but good results actually seemed limited to those with superficial (stage 0 or A) disease (63 percent) compared to those with stage B or greater disease (19 percent). Moreover, difficulties in clinical staging are even greater in this group of patients as a result of the radiation effects, and the "salvage" surgery appears equally difficult, with an operative mortality rate of 8.1 percent and an early complication rate of 24 percent.[25] At least some of the difficulties encountered are presumably reflective of the nature of the population to begin with, however.

As with superficial disease, there is a place for segmental resection for management of deeply invasive disease *in a small percentage of carefully selected patients,*[143,170,184,205] with the obvious advantages of preservation of bladder function and, in men, potency. Whitmore[205] pointed out that when such patients are appropriately selected survival results are comparable to those achieved with radical cystectomy for lesions of comparable stage. The question of preoperative radiotherapy for the control of local recurrences has not been settled,[143] but it seems not unreasonable in view of the low associated morbidity rate.

At least for the present, the most common mode of treatment for deeply invasive bladder carcinoma is radical cystectomy following preoperative radiotherapy, a combined technique introduced during the 1960s.[57,201] Initially, patients were treated with 4,000 rads followed by delayed cystectomy at 4 to 6 weeks. In a pilot group reported by Whitmore,[201] the 5-year survival rate improved to 37 percent, compared to a 17 percent figure for historical controls treated with surgery alone. In a cooperative study by the NBCG,[173] 475 patients with stage T2 (B1) or greater disease were randomized to undergo similar preoperative radiotherapy with delayed cystectomy versus cystectomy alone. Even in such a large study it was obvious that the heterogeneity of "invasive bladder cancer" resulted in some problematic comparisons in various subgroups, but some conclusions could be reached: (1) Patients treated with preoperative radiotherapy had no apparent residual tumor in the cystectomy specimen in a much larger percentage of cases than those treated by transurethral resection alone followed by cystectomy (34 percent versus 9 percent, respectively). That is, when the effects of transurethral resection were taken into account, tumor appeared to be "down-staged" to P0 (pathologic stage 0: no residual tumor identified in a definitive resection specimen) at the time of cystectomy in at least one-fourth of irradiated patients. (2) Papillary tumors were more likely to be destroyed by preoperative radiotherapy than solid tumors. (3) For the patients whose disease was reduced to P0 in the preoperative radiotherapy group, an improvement in survival was noted compared to the nonirradiated control group.

(4) Those patients with papillary invasive carcinoma, with no evidence of lymphatic invasion, whose tumors had been reduced to P0 by preoperative radiotherapy, had the best 5-year survival rate: in excess of 85 percent.

One major concern from the findings is that for the two large groups directly compared, i.e., preoperative radiotherapy versus no preoperative radiotherapy, there appeared to be no significant *overall* improvement in survival rate for the former group despite the improvement in survival in the subgroup whose disease was reduced to P0 by irradiation. Catalona[20] suggested that this finding may be indicative of irradiation serving merely to identify a subset of patients predetermined to do well even without irradiation. He also noted that, in view of the balance of survival between the two large groups, the preoperative radiotherapy might actually be harming another subset of patients with radiation-resistant tumors, with their poorer survival dragging the overall survival curve downward. In fact, when the study cases were subclassified by Slack and Prout[173] according to the presence or absence of lymphatic invasion, radiotherapy versus no radiotherapy, and P0 versus P+ (residual tumor identified), the best survivorship was enjoyed by the group whose tumors had been irradiated, were reduced to P0, and had no lymphatic invasion. The worst survivorship among all groups, conversely, was found among those whose tumors had also been irradiated but who had residual tumor, with lymphatic invasion (L+), at the time of cystectomy. Patients in this group survived even less well than their nonirradiated P+, L+ counterparts.

There has been a movement in the past decade toward short course, lower dose (2,000 rads) preoperative radiotherapy followed by immediate cystectomy.[150,208] Scanlon and colleagues[155] reported a study comparing patients treated by conventional long course, high dose radiation and delayed cystectomy to those treated with short course, low dose therapy followed by immediate cystectomy. Short course/immediate surgery patients showed reduction of their primaries to P0 in only approximately 2 percent of cases (1 of 49) versus the expected 34 percent in the long course patients. "Down-staging" to less than the preoperative determined stage, but without complete tumor eradication, was also seen in a comparatively smaller number of patients in the short course group (24 percent) versus 56 percent of patients in the long course group. Nonetheless, when the short course and long course groups were compared with each other, overall, regardless of reduction in stage, there was no statistical difference in survival between the two, a phenomenon others have noted as well.[170,208]

The possibility has been raised that irradiation may in fact offer little or no benefit, and that the major improvement in prognosis is the result of improved surgical technique alone.[114,155] Mathur and associates,[114] for example, reported a study of 58 consecutive patients who underwent total cystectomy without preoperative irradiation; pelvic lymphadenectomy was also performed in 70 percent of the patients. The overall 5-year survival rates compared well with those who underwent preoperative irradiation, whether long or short course, with a 62 percent 5-year survival for all patients with transitional cell carcinoma (80 percent for stages 0, A, and B1, and 50 percent for stages B2 and C). As with all studies, however, these seems always to be at least one or more variables that may have significantly influenced results. In this study it was specifically noted that frozen sections were performed on suspicious nodes, with the procedure aborted if the nodes were found to be positive. As lymph node involvement may be high in patients with deeply invasive disease — on the order of 25 percent for P2 lesions and 50 percent for P3 a and b lesions[170] — liberal use of frozen sections at the time of cystectomy may have removed a considerable number of patients with poor prognosis from the study at the outset.

For the present, until more solid data on radical cystectomy alone become available, it appears that the usual therapy for deeply invasive disease will remain low dose (1,500 to 2,000 rads), short course preoperative radiotherapy followed by immediate cystectomy plus total urethrectomy in women and in selected cases in men. The preoperative treatment contributes little in the way of increased morbidity, time, or expense and is generally without serious complications.[205] Moreover, its potential benefits, from decreased local recurrence to improvement in survival for at least some groups of patients,[202] have yet to be disproved. The addition of a meticulous nodal dissection may also improve the lot of some patients, again without adding significantly to the operative morbidity and mortality.[170] For selected patients full course definitive irradiation with salvage cystectomy for tumor persistence or recurrence appears to be a reasonable alternative.[165,205,216] Other avenues, such as the addition of "adjuvant" chemotherapy after radical surgery and/or irradiation, or the use of induction ("neoadjuvant") chemotherapy at the outset of treatment, continue to be explored.[185] It should be emphasized that the treatment of muscle-invasive disease continues to undergo intensive reexamination in the literature,[90] with increasing focus on tailoring therapy to individual patients and their clinical situations.

Advanced Disease

Various chemotherapeutic agents have been used, either singly or in combination, for the treatment of advanced bladder carcinoma, a category that includes patients with locally extensive disease and/or distant metastases. For evaluation of results, the most common categories into which patients undergoing therapy are ordered include the following: (1) complete response or remission (CR), i.e., complete disappearance of all discernible disease by clinical, radiologic, or pathologic examination; (2) partial response or remission (PR), i.e., objective reduction in indicator lesions by clinical or radiologic measurements; and (3) nonresponse (NR). Another category frequently referred to is "disease stabilization." Until recently, most patients in the various studies have been in the PR or NR categories, with few in the CR column. Among these few, *persistent* "complete responders" (i.e., "cures") have been essentially anecdotal.

At present, the most popular single agent for the treatment of advanced bladder cancer is cisplatin. In reviews of the experience with this and other agents, Yagoda[211-213] noted an overall response rate of approximately 30 percent. Most trials have reported few complete responders; but among partial responders and those whose disease appears stabilized, improvement in symptoms may be noted within a week of initiating therapy.[186] Response durations are generally on the order of 5 to 7 months,[212] although occasional complete responders may do so for more than a year.[64] Despite the short duration of response, survival rates compared to those of nonresponders seem to be improved.[186]

Other agents that may be of use in the treatment of advanced disease include doxorubicin (Adriamycin),[185,211,214,215] methotrexate,[133,185,214] and cyclophosphamide (Cytoxan)[185,211,214]; but again, most patient responses are partial and generally of a duration similar to that seen with cisplatin. Vinblastine sulfate, evaluated as a secondary drug following failure on other regimens, has shown some value in inducing further remissions, seen in 18 percent of cases in a study reported by Blumenreich and associates.[16] The drug is well tolerated, something that cannot be said for some of the other drugs in use.

As with other areas of chemotherapy, multiple-drug regimens incorporating the above and other agents have also been evaluated, but in the past they appeared to offer only small or in some instances no major advantages over the single agents in use.[22,174,194,212] Reports on the use of combined regimens such as CISCA (cyclophosphamide, doxorubicin, and cisplatin)[106,107] and M-VAC (methotrexate, vinblastine, doxorubicin, and cisplatin[183,192] have shown much more encouraging results, however.[185,214]

For other, more recent approaches in cases of advanced disease, e.g., "high-dose" therapy with standard agents[15] and combined chemotherapy and radiotherapy,[77] sufficient data are still unavailable for adequate evaluation.

OVERVIEW

By this point, it is hoped that the pathologist will have acquired not only information concerning his or her working area in the field of "bladder cancer" but also a feel for the subject as a whole. There are few areas in oncology where effective interaction between clinician and pathologist is more important,[52] and it behooves the pathologist to be aware of the meaning and relative importance of the various bits of information supplied to the clinician by the laboratory. Careful attention to detail, such as diligently searching for evidence of vascular/lymphatic invasion and reorienting the occasional block to perhaps gain a better perspective on muscle invasion, seems much easier when one realizes the potential importance of such findings.

Despite our best efforts, however, and no doubt because of them as well, many facets of the problem remain enigmatic, and many questions remain unanswered. Perhaps in summation, it is best to concentrate on those aspects that seem relatively certain, with some thought given to those that are not and why they are not.

One certainty is that the umbrella of "bladder cancer" is wide, particularly with regard to the biologic behavior of the disease compared to other lesions such as "lung cancer" or "pancreatic cancer." If one looks at the statistics, for example, simply comparing incidence rates to death rates in a crude fashion,[168] it appears that bladder cancer is a relatively second-rate malignancy with regard to aggressive capability, with only about one of four patients dying as a result of the disease. Compare this figure to the statistics for lung cancer, where approximately five of six patients die of their disease, or pancreatic cancer, where approximately 24 of 25 do so. Unfortunately, the data on bladder cancer are only relatively reassuring compared to those for tumors of other organs, in large part because we choose to call such a widely disparate group of lesions by the same name. The tumors range from those that are little more than a recurring nuisance to patients in their declining years to those that prove every bit as lethal as the most vicious tumors in other body sites.

One of the reasons for the unfortunate width of the umbrella appears to be the misconception briefly alluded to earlier in the chapter that bladder cancer represents a continuous spectrum, with patients most commonly presenting with low stage papillary lesions and subsequently suffering a number of recurrences, with an unfortunate few eventually developing invasive disease progressing to death.

In fact, this sort of course occurs in only a small minority of patients. This is not to say that there is not some degree of continuity among the various groups of patients with "bladder cancer," and the emergence of that first lesion in any patient, however bland it may appear, should always sound the alert that all is not well with the urothelium, setting clinician and pathologist in motion to find out just how "unwell" things are. Nonetheless, particularly in light of recent information, there appears to be not nearly so much continuity between the various subsets of patients with bladder cancer as originally thought. The population of patients might more effectively be divided into three groups, the first and third of which are most easily defined.

The first group consists of those with noninvasive grade I papillary transitional cell carcinomas, which may account for one-fourth[53,109] to one-third[28] of all patients presenting with bladder cancer. Recurrent lesions similar to the primary are the rule rather than the exception. However, *in the absence of associated ur-*

othelial abnormalities (approximately 50 percent of such cases[3]), the chances that these patients will experience subsequent invasive disease are small (only 7 percent in the series reported by Althausen et al.[3]). The chances that they will go on to die of their disease are even smaller.[144] These patients may be managed conservatively, generally with repeated transurethral resections, with or without topical therapy, with an eye to detecting the small number that show evidence of disease progression in grade, stage, or both.

A number of arguments may be put forth for removing these patients from the "malignant" group entirely, some of which were briefly examined earlier: (1) These lesions per se do not behave as carcinomas, and only in the rarest of situations do patients die as the result of invasive or metastatic malignancy that maintains this morphology. (2) Despite the fact that a small number of these patients develop and perhaps die of a malignant lesion, "guilt by association" is rarely accepted as reason for a diagnosis of malignancy elsewhere in pathology. For example, although more than 90 percent of patients with familial polyposis of the colon eventually develop a carcinoma if left untreated, we would not consider calling the great number of polyps in their colon other than what they are—adenomas. When the almost inevitable malignancy occurs, *it* is called a carcinoma. (3) It would considerably narrow the field of patients on which we focus our attention. (4) Perhaps most importantly, it would remove the label "cancer," with all of its connotations, from a large group of patients who have little risk of dying as the result of their disease.

The next group of patients to consider is at the opposite end of the scale, those with deeply invasive disease, most of whom have high grade transitional cell carcinoma, with smaller numbers of patients with squamous carcinoma, adenocarcinoma, etc. Rather than emerging gradually from the ranks of superficial disease, it seems that most of these patients have no such history. Braun,[17] in a study of 104 consecutive cases of invasive disease, found that more than 80 percent had *no* history of preceding papillary lesions. Kaye and Lange[86] found a similar figure of 84 percent in their series of 166 cases of muscle-invasive disease. Hopkins et al.[69] found an even higher number (91 percent) of patients with muscle-invasive disease to have presented as such de novo, with no history of superficial disease. Although it is obvious, at least for lesions arising from the surface mucosa, that all cases

of muscle-invasive disease must have had an in situ and superficially invasive period, for most patients with this most serious form of bladder cancer, the early phase of their disease is either relatively asymptomatic, rapidly progressive, or perhaps both, with no indication of a leisurely advance through the ranks from low-grade, noninvasive disease to their final desperate strait.

Between these two sets is the third group of patients, those with clinically recognized superficial disease who will develop deeply invasive, potentially lethal tumors. Despite the fact that patients with superficial disease in general constitute most of the patients presenting with "bladder cancer,"[69] this group appears to account for no more than 10 to 20 percent of those who may eventually die of their disease. It is precisely these patients whom we are trying to identify early in their course with the hope that appropriate intervention may avert an eventual fatal outcome. With the information gained from the various conventional and adjunctive studies described above, it appears that it may in fact be possible. Hopkins and associates,[69] for example, found that when patients were handled with a combination of aggressive surveillance and intensive intravesical chemotherapy, only 8 of their 215 patients with superficial disease had progression; 4 of the 8 still had disease confined to the bladder at the time of definitive treatment, and 3 of the 4 are still alive without evidence of disease for up to 66 months. These figures are most encouraging.

The intermediate risk group is variously defined but certainly includes those with higher-grade superficial lesions, those with associated significant dysplasia or carcinoma in situ evident on selected-site biopsy specimens, and those with definite invasion of the lamina propria. For these patients much closer surveillance, regular cystoscopy with transurethral resection of new lesions, careful attention to follow-up cytology examination to monitor the development of higher grade disease, and aggressive topical therapy seem in order.

When to intervene with more definitive surgery obviously retains a degree of subjectivity, as there is still no magic earmark to predict with 100 percent accuracy which patient will enter "dangerous waters" or when it will happen. This area remains a difficult one, considering the consequences of a radical cystectomy for the patient; but as Skinner emphasized,[170] avoiding early aggressive therapy may lead to extension beyond the point of curability.

This knowledge must be tempered by a number of facts, however. One is that this group still represents only a minority of patients who die as the result of bladder cancer. Another is that, although many patients who seem to be optimally controlled with aggressive transurethral resection and topical therapy eventually relapse, some do not; and the interval for those who do may be significantly prolonged. Although it may seem to be nothing more than "buying time," and risky time at that, the same may be said for so much else that we do in all areas of medicine when dealing with elderly patients. It must be remembered that we are considering here a population with a mean age of 65, with the considerable majority of patients over age 60, most of whom will die of disease unrelated to their tumors.[147,210]

If aggressive surgery is contemplated for any patient in this group, it is well to recall the words of Dr. Whitmore,[204] who has probably cared for as many of these patients as anyone in the field today.

The diminishing morbidity and mortality of radical cystectomy in treatment of bladder cancer should not blind us to the fact that it is a major procedure with devastating impacts on the quality if not the quantity of life. That patients adjust so well to the procedure is more a tribute to the human spirit than to surgical skill, and continued efforts to diminish the associated urinary and sexual sacrifices involved with the procedure are in order. Progress in the latter area has exceeded that in the former, but efforts to develop a functional, continent, artificial bladder continue.

For patients with deeply invasive disease, inroads appear to have been made, with some improvement in prognosis resulting from better surgical technique, possibly from preoperative radiotherapy, and perhaps from both. Some of the improvement appears to have been the result of better local control of the disease,[146] with most patients who suffer tumor-related deaths now doing so as the result of systemic metastases. Despite the improvements, the dismal fact remains that approximately 50 percent of patients with deeply invasive tumors die with metastases, generally within 2 years.[170] Moreover, a significant number (78 percent in the study by Prout et al.[146]) manifest these metastatic lesions within the first year following surgery, suggesting that the metastases are already present or occur during the perisurgical period.

That this should be the case is not surprising if one looks at some basic principles of cell growth and kinetics. As noted by Anderson,[4] a 5-mm tumor mass, certainly of a size unlikely to be detected by conventional radiologic means, has already undergone approximately 27 doublings since its inception and may contain approximately 10^8 cells. With only three more doublings the tumor will reach 1 cm and contain 10^9 cells. Only five additional doublings, assuming complete survival of all tumor cells, will result in an overall tumor burden of 10^{10} cells, equivalent to widespread metastatic disease. By the time they become clinically apparent, therefore, we are viewing metastases late in their course. The assumption of Prout et al.[146] that these silent metastases are often present at the time of surgery or occur in relation to the surgery is no doubt correct.

There are various approaches to the solution of this problem. The most obvious is earlier detection, as the increasing incidence of systemic disease with increasing stage remains an unchallenged fact. If, as noted, the largest group of patients with muscle-invasive disease presents de novo, new directions for our basic efforts are in order. Preventive measures are obviously the most desirable but often the most difficult to implement. For the present it is perhaps only through the development of cost-effective screening devices, such as urinary flow cytometry in patients with known increased risk (e.g., cigarette smokers and those with exposure to industrial carcinogens), that such patients may be detected at an earlier stage.[69]

A second approach presumes that further refinement in the methods of local control may lead to even further improvement in prognosis, perhaps by a combination of an even greater reduction in pelvic recurrences and perisurgical systemic metastases. One example of potential improvement is found in a study by the Radiation Oncology Study Group, reported by Mohiuddin et al.,[120] wherein patients were given low dose (500 rads) preoperative radiation followed by high dose postoperative radiation. One immediate benefit of this course was the ability to spare those with stage A or lower grade B1 disease at cystectomy from high dose radiation, as this group appears to derive little benefit from adjunctive radiotherapy.[207] For those with high grade B1 lesions, and for all patients with B2 and C disease, a full 4,000 rads was delivered postoperatively, with an overall survival rate of 69 percent at 4 years, which compares well with the usual approximately 50 percent figures cited for this group.

A third approach is that of combined modality therapy, utilizing our best means of local control in conjunction with adjuvant chemotherapy to deal with perisurgical or already established but silent distant metastases. As the chemotherapist's chances for success vary inversely with the "tumor burden,"[4] adjuvant chemotherapy seems most reasonable, for at no point is the patient's tumor burden less than during the immediate postsurgical period. Experience in this area, summarized by Yagoda[213,214] and Soloway,[185] is at present somewhat fragmented, with few available reliable data from well planned, prospectively randomized trials. A number of adjuvant chemotherapy studies are under way,[41,106] but for the present no firm recommendation for adjuvant chemotherapy can be made, except in the context of a prospectively randomized trial. It is hoped that with (1) the development and proper testing of well-thought-out drug regimens, (2) the use of techniques such as rapid in vitro chemosensitivity assays,[189] and (3) the use of newer approaches such as induction or "neoadjuvant" chemotherapy[185] that a chance for survival considerably better than 50 percent will be offered to patients with deeply invasive disease in the future. Barring earlier detection for these patients, this area deserves a concentration of our efforts, as once past this stage the fact remains that at present there is relatively little to offer the patient with bladder cancer in the way of curative therapy.

REFERENCES

1. Abenoza P, Manivel C, Fraley EE: Primary adenocarcinoma of urinary bladder: clinicopathologic study of 16 cases. Urology 29:9, 1987
2. Allen TD, Henderson BW: Adenocarcinoma of the bladder. J Urol 93:50, 1965
3. Althausen AF, Prout GR Jr, Daly JJ: Non-invasive papillary carcinoma of the bladder associated with carcinoma in situ. J Urol 116:575, 1976
4. Anderson T: Developmental concepts: effective chemotherapy for bladder carcinoma. Semin Oncol 6:240, 1979
5. Anderström C, Johansson S, Nilsson S: The significance of lamina propria invasion on the prognosis of patients with bladder tumors. J Urol 124:23, 1980
6. Anderström C, Johansson SL, Von Schultz L: Primary adenocarcinoma of the urinary bladder: a clinicopathologic and prognostic study. Cancer 52:1273, 1983
7. Baker R: Correlation of circumferential lymphatic spread of vesical cancer with depth of infiltration: relation to present methods of treatment. J Urol 73:681, 1955
8. Beahrs OH, Myers MH (eds): Manual for Staging of Cancer. 2nd Ed. American Joint Committee on Cancer. Lippincott, Philadelphia, 1983
9. Begg RC: The colloid adenocarcinomata of the bladder vault arising from the epithelium of the urachal canal: with a critical study of the tumors of the urachus. Br J Surg 18:422, 1931
10. Beisland HO, Seland P: A prospective randomized study of neodymium-YAG laser irradiation versus TUR in the treatment of urinary bladder cancer. Scand J Urol Nephrol 20:209, 1986
11. Benson RC Jr: Treatment of diffuse transitional cell carcinoma in situ by whole bladder hematoporphyrin derivative photodynamic therapy. J Urol 134:675, 1985
12. Benson RC Jr, Tomera KM, Kelalis PP: Transitional cell carcinoma of the bladder in children and adolescents. J Urol 130:54, 1983
13. Blinst Italian Cooperative Group: Intravesical doxorubicin for the prophylaxis of superficial bladder tumors: a mulicenter study. Cancer 54:756, 1984
14. Blumenreich MS, Needles B, Yagoda A, et al: Intravesical cisplatin for superficial bladder tumors. Cancer 50:863, 1982
15. Blumenreich MS, Woodcock TM, Jones M, et al: High-dose cisplatin in patients with advanced malignancies. Cancer 55:1118, 1985
16. Blumenreich MS, Yagoda A, Natale RB, Watson RC: Phase II trial of vinblastine sulfate for metastatic urothelial tract tumors. Cancer 50:435, 1982
17. Brawn PN: The origin of invasive carcinoma of the bladder. Cancer 50:515, 1982
18. Broders AC: Epithelioma of the genito-urinary organs. Ann Surg 75:574, 1922
19. Carter WC III, Rous SN: Gross hematuria in 110 adult urologic hospital patients. Urology 18:342, 1981
20. Catalona WJ: Guest editorial: bladder carcinoma. J Urol 123:35, 1980
21. Chibber PJ, McIntyre MA, Hindmarsh JR, et al: Transitional cell carcinoma involving the prostate. Br J Urol 53:605, 1981
22. Citrin DL, Hogan TF, Davis TE: A study of cyclophosphamide, adriamycin, cis-platinum, and methotrexate in advanced transitional cell carcinoma of the urinary tract. Cancer 51:1, 1983
23. Cooper PH, Waisman J, Johnston WH, Skinner DG:

Severe atypia of transitional epithelium and carcinoma of the urinary bladder. Cancer 31:1055, 1973

24. Cordonnier JJ, Spjut HJ: Urethral occurrence of bladder carcinoma following cystectomy. J Urol 87:398, 1962

25. Crawford ED, Skinner DG: Salvage cystectomy after irradiation failure. J Urol 123:32, 1980

26. Cummings KB: Carcinoma of the bladder: predictors. Cancer 45:1849, 1980

27. Cummings KB: Diagnosis, staging, and classification of bladder tumors. Semin Urol 1:7, 1983

28. Cutler SJ, Heney NM, Friedell GH: Longitudinal study of patients with bladder cancer: factors associated with disease recurrence and progression. p. 35. In Bonney WW, Prout GR Jr (eds): Bladder Cancer. AUA Monographs, Vol. 1. Williams and Wilkins, Baltimore, 1982

29. Daly JJ: Carcinoma-in-situ of the urothelium. Urol Clin North Am 3:87, 1976

30. Das S, Amar AD: Vesical diverticulum associated with bladder carcinoma: therapeutic implications. J Urol 136:1013, 1986

31. Davides KC, King LM, Jacobs D: Management of microscopic hematuria: twenty-year experience with 150 cases in a community hospital. Urology 28:453, 1986

32. Debenedictis TJ, Marmar JL, Praiss DE: Intraurethral condylomas acuminata: management and review of the literature. J Urol 118:767, 1977

33. DeKernion JB, Huang MY, Lindner A, et al: The management of superficial bladder tumors and carcinoma in situ with intravesical bacillus Calmette-Guérin. J Urol 133:598, 1985

34. Dershaw DD, Scher HI: Sonography in evaluation of carcinoma of bladder. Urology 29:454, 1987

35. Devonec M, Chapelon JY, Codas H, et al: Evaluation of bladder cancer with a miniature high frequency transurethral ultrasonography probe. Br J Urol 59:550, 1987

36. Dowd JB: Case records of the Massachusetts General Hospital: case 8-1981. N Engl J Med 304:469, 1981

37. Droller MJ: Immunotherapy in genitourinary neoplasia. Urol Clin North Am 11:643, 1984

38. Droller MJ: Bacillus Calmette-Guérin in the management of bladder cancer. J Urol 135:331, 1986

39. Droller MJ: Biologic response modifiers in genitourinary neoplasia. Cancer 60:635, 1987

40. Droller MJ, Walsh PC: Intensive intravesical chemotherapy in the treatment of flat carcinoma in situ: is it safe? J Urol 134:1115, 1985

41. Einstein AB Jr, Coombs J, Pearse H, et al: Cisplatin (CP) adjuvant therapy following preoperative radiotherapy plus radical cystectomy (RT & RCy) for invasive bladder carcinoma: a randomized trial of the National Bladder Cancer Group (NBCG). J Urol 133:222A, 1985

42. El-Bolkainy MN, Mokhtar NM, Ghoneim MA, Hussein MH: The impact of schistosomiasis on the pathology of bladder cancer. Cancer 48:2643, 1981

43. Elsebai I: Parasites in the etiology of cancer — bilharziasis and bladder cancer. CA 27:100, 1977

44. England HR, Paris AMI, Blandy JP: The correlation of T1 bladder tumour history with prognosis and follow-up requirements. Br J Urol 53:593, 1981

45. Farrow GM: Pathologist's role in bladder cancer. Semin Oncol 6:198, 1979

46. Farrow GM, Utz DC, Rife CC: Morphological and clinical observations of patients with early bladder cancer treated with total cystectomy. Cancer Res 36:2495, 1976

47. Farrow GM, Utz DC, Rife CC, Greene LF: Clinical observations on sixty-nine cases of in situ carcinoma of the urinary bladder. Cancer Res 37:2794, 1977

48. Faysal MH: Squamous cell carcinoma of the bladder. J Urol 126:598, 1981

49. Faysal MH, Freiha FS: Primary neoplasm in vesical diverticula: a report of 12 cases. Br J Urol 53:141, 1981

50. Fitzpatrick JM, Kahn O, Oliver RTD, Riddle PR: Long-term follow-up in patients with superficial bladder tumors treated with intravesical Epodyl. Br J Urol 51:545, 1979

51. Fitzpatrick JM, West AB, Butler MR, et al: Superficial bladder tumors (stage pTa, grades 1 and 2): the importance of recurrence pattern following initial resection. J Urol 135:920, 1986

52. Friedell GH: Urinary bladder cancer: selecting initial therapy. Cancer 60:496, 1987

53. Friedell GH, Bell JR, Burney SW, et al: Histopathology and classification of urinary bladder carcinoma. Urol Clin North Am 3:53, 1976

54. Friedell GH, Parija GC, Nagy GK, Soto EA: The pathology of human bladder cancer. Cancer 45:1823, 1980

55. Friedell GH, Soloway MS, Hilgar AG, Farrow GM: Summary of workshop on carcinoma in situ of the bladder. J Urol 136:1047, 1986

56. Fujime M, Lin CW, Prout GR Jr: Identification of vessels by lectin-immunoperoxidase staining of endothelium: possible applications in urogenital malignancies. J Urol 131:566, 1984

57. Galleher EP Jr, Young JD Jr, Mowad JJ, et al: A follow-up study of supervoltage irradiation followed by cystectomy for bladder cancer. J Urol 99:59, 1968

58. Gill WB, Huffman JL, Lyon ES, et al: Selective surface staining of bladder tumors by intravesical meth-

ylene blue with enhanced endoscopic identification. Cancer 53:2724, 1984

59. Golin AL, Howard RS: Asymptomatic microscopic hematuria. J Urol 124:389, 1980

60. Green DF, Robinson MRG, Glashan R, et al: Does intravesical chemotherapy prevent invasive bladder cancer? J Urol 131:33, 1984

61. Greene LF, Hanash KA, Farrow GM: Benign papilloma or papillary carcinoma of the bladder? J Urol 110:205, 1973

62. Haaff EO, Dresner SM, Ratliff TL, Catalona WJ: Two courses of intravesical bacillus Calmette-Guérin for transitional cell carcinoma of the bladder. J Urol 136:820, 1986

63. Hatch TR, Barry JM: The value of excretory urography in staging bladder cancer. J Urol 135:49, 1986

64. Herr HW: Cis-diamminedichloride platinum II in the treatment of advanced bladder cancer. J Urol 123:853, 1980

65. Herr HW: Carcinoma in situ of the bladder. Semin Urol 1:15, 1983

66. Herr HW, Pinsky CM, Whitmore WF Jr, et al: Long-term effect of intravesical bacillus Calmette-Guérin on flat carcinoma in situ of the bladder. J Urol 135:265, 1986

67. Hewitt CB, Babiszewski JF, Antunez AR: Update on intracavitary radiation in the treatment of bladder tumors. J Urol 126:323, 1981

68. Hopkins SC, Buice RG, Matheny R Jr, Soloway MS: The stability and antitumor activity of recycled (intravesical) mitomycin C. Cancer 53:2063, 1984

69. Hopkins SC, Ford KS, Soloway MS: Invasive bladder cancer: support for screening. J Urol 130:61, 1983

70. Hricak H: Urologic cancer: methods of early detection and future developments. Cancer 60:677, 1987

71. Hu KN, Kim A, Khan AS, et al: Combined thiotepa and mitocycin C instillation therapy for low-grade superficial bladder tumor. Cancer 55:1654, 1985

72. Huland H, Otto U: Use of mitomycin as prophylaxis following endoscopic resection of superficial bladder cancer. Urology, suppl. 4, 26:32, 1985

73. Huland H, Otto U, Droese M, Klöppel G: Long-term mitomycin C instillation after transurethral resection of superficial bladder carcinoma: influence on recurrence, progression, and survival. J Urol 132:27, 1984

74. International Union Against Cancer: TNM Classification of Malignant Tumors. 4th Ed. Springer-Verlag, Berlin, 1987

75. Issell BF, Prout GR Jr, Soloway MS, et al: Mitocycin C intravesical therapy in noninvasive bladder cancer after failure on thiotepa. Cancer 53:1025, 1984

76. Jacobo E, Loening S, Schmidt JD, Culp DA: Primary adenocarcinoma of the bladder: a retrospective study of 20 patients. J Urol 117:54, 1977

77. Jakse G, Frommhold H, Zur Nedden D: Combined radiation and chemotherapy for locally advanced transitional cell carcinoma of the urinary bladder. Cancer 55:1659, 1985

78. Jakse G, Hofstädter F, Marberger H: Intracavitary doxorubicin hydrochloride therapy for carcinoma in situ of the bladder. J Urol 125:185, 1981

79. Jakse G, Loidl W, Seeber G, Hofstädter F: Stage T1, grade 3 transitional cell carcinoma of the bladder: an unfavorable tumor? J Urol 137:39, 1987

80. Jewett HJ: Carcinoma of the bladder: influence of depth of infiltration on the 5-year results following complete extirpation of the primary growth. J Urol 67:672, 1952

81. Jewett HJ: Comments on the staging of invasive bladder cancer: two B's or not two B's: that is the question (editorial). J Urol 119:39, 1978

82. Jewett HJ, King LR, Shelley WM: A study of 365 cases of infiltrating bladder cancer: relation of certain pathological characteristics to prognosis after extirpation. J Urol 92:668, 1964

83. Jewett HJ, Strong GH: Infiltrating carcinoma of the bladder: relation of depth of penetration of the bladder wall to incidence of local extension and metastases. J Urol 55:366, 1946

84. Johnson DE, Hogan JM, Ayala AG: Primary adenocarcinoma of the urinary bladder. South Med J 65:527, 1972

85. Johnson DE, Schoenwald MB, Ayala AG, Miller LS: Squamous cell carcinoma of the bladder. J Urol 115:542, 1976

86. Kaye KW, Lange PH: Mode of presentation of invasive bladder cancer: reassessment of the problem. J Urol 128:31, 1982

87. Kelalis PP, McLean P: The treatment of diverticulum of the bladder. J Urol 98:349, 1967

88. Kern WH: The grade and pathologic stage of bladder cancer. Cancer 53:1185, 1984

89. Khafagy MM, El-Bolkainy MN, Mansour MA: Carcinoma of the bilharzial urinary bladder: a study of the associated mucosal lesions in 86 cases. Cancer 30:150, 1972

90. Klimberg IW, Wajsman Z: Treatment for muscle invasive carcinoma of the bladder. J Urol 136:1169, 1986

90a. Knappenberger ST, Uson AC, Melicow MM: Primary neoplasms occurring in vesical diverticula: a report of 18 cases. J Urol 83:153, 1960

91. Koch M, Hill GB, McPhee MS: Factors affecting recurrence rates in superficial bladder cancer. J Natl Cancer Inst 76:1025, 1986

92. Koontz WW Jr, Heney NM, Soloway MS, et al: Mitomycin for patients who have failed on thiotepa: the National Bladder Cancer Group. Urology, suppl. 4, 26:30, 1985

93. Koontz WW Jr, Prout GR Jr, Smith W, et al: The use of intravesical thio-tepa in the management of non-invasive carcinoma of the bladder. J Urol 125:307, 1981

94. Koss LG: Tumors of the urinary bladder. Fasicle 11, 2nd Series. Atlas of Tumor Pathology. Armed Forces Institute of Pathology, Washington, DC, 1975

95. Koss LG: Formal discussion of "Clinical observations on sixty-nine cases of in situ carcinoma of the urinary bladder." Cancer Res 37:2799, 1977

96. Koss LG, Nakanishi I, Freed SZ: Nonpapillary carcinoma in situ and atypical hyperplasia in cancerous bladders: further studies of surgically removed bladders by mapping. Urology 9:442, 1977

97. Koss LG, Tiamson EM, Robbins MA: Mapping cancerous and precancerous bladder changes: a study of the urothelium in ten surgically removed bladders. JAMA 227:281, 1974

98. Kurz KR, Pitts, WR, Vaughan ED Jr: The natural history of patients less than 40 years old with bladder tumors. J Urol 137:395, 1987

99. Lamm DL: Bacillus Calmette-Guérin immunotherapy: J Urol 138:391, 1987

100. Lamm DL, Stogdill VD, Stogdill BJ, Crispen RG: Complications of bacillus Calmette-Guérin immunotherapy in 1,278 patients with bladder cancer. J Urol 135:272, 1986

101. Lamm DL, Thor DE, Winters WD, et al: BCG immunotherapy of bladder cancer: inhibition of tumor recurrence and associated immune responses. Cancer 48:82, 1981

102. Laor E, Grabstald H, Whitmore WF: The influence of simultaneous resection of bladder tumors and prostate on the occurrence of prostatic urethral tumors. J Urol 126:171, 1981

103. Lerman RI, Hutter RVP, Whitmore WF Jr: Papilloma of the urinary bladder. Cancer 25:333, 1970

104. Linker DG, Whitmore WF: Ureteral carcinoma in situ. J Urol 113:777, 1975

105. Loening SA, Jacobo E, Hawtrey CE, Culp DA: Adenocarcinoma of the urachus. J Urol 119:68, 1978

106. Logothetis CJ, Samuels ML, Johnson DE, et al: Adjuvant (ADJ) CISCA chemotherapy for transitional cell carcinoma of the bladder: a prospective trial. J Urol 135:223A, 1986

107. Logothetis CJ, Samuels ML, Ogden S, et al: Cyclophosphamide, doxorubicin and cisplatin chemotherapy for patients with locally advanced urothelial tumors with or without nodal metastases. J Urol 134:460, 1985

108. Lundbeck F, Pedersen D, Stroyer I, Uldall A: Absorption of doxorubicin hydrochloride during bladder washings in treatment of noninvasive bladder tumors. Urology 18:161, 1981

109. Lutzeyer W, Rübben H, Dahm H: Prognosis parameters in superficial bladder cancer: an analysis of 315 cases. J Urol 127:250, 1982

110. Mahadevia PS, Koss LG, Tar IJ: Prostatic involvement in bladder cancer: prostate mapping in 20 cystoprostatectomy specimens. Cancer 58:2096, 1986

111. Marshall VF: The relation of the preoperative estimate to the pathologic demonstration of the extent of vesical neoplasms. J Urol 68:714, 1952

112. Marshall VF: Current clinical problems regarding bladder tumors. Cancer 9:543, 1956

113. Massey BD, Nation EF, Gallup CA, Hendricks ED: Carcinoma of the bladder: 20-year experience in private practice. J Urol 93:212, 1965

114. Mathur VK, Krahn HP, Ramsey EW: Total cystectomy for bladder cancer. J Urol 125:784, 1981

115. McDonald JR, Thompson GJ: Carcinoma of the urinary bladder: a pathologic study with special reference to invasiveness and vascular invasion. J Urol 61:435, 1948

116. Mekras GD, Block NL, Carrion HM, Ishikoff M: Urachal carcinoma: diagnosis by computerized axial tomography. J Urol 123:275, 1980

117. Melamed MR, Voutsa NG, Grabstald H: Natural history and clinical behavior of in situ carcinoma of the human urinary bladder. Cancer 17:1533, 1964

118. Melicow MM: Histological study of vesical urothelium intervening between gross neoplasms in total cystectomy. J Urol 68:261, 1952

119. Melicow MM: Tumors of the bladder: a multifaceted problem. J Urol 112:467, 1974

120. Mohiuddin M, Kramer S, Newall J, et al: Combined preoperative and postoperative radiation for bladder cancer: results of RTOG/Jefferson study. Cancer 55:963, 1985

121. Montie JE, Mirsky H, Levin, HS: Transitional cell carcinoma of the prostate in a series of cystectomies: incidence and staging problems. J Urol 135:243A, 1986

122. Morales A, Eidinger D, Bruce AW: Intracavitary bacillus Calmette-Guérin in the treatment of superficial bladder tumors. J Urol 116:180, 1976

123. Mori K, Lamm DL, Crawford ED: A trial of bacillus Calmette-Guérin versus adriamycin in superficial bladder cancer: a South-West Oncology Group Study. Urol Int 41:254, 1986

124. Morrison AS, Cole P: Epidemiology of bladder cancer. Urol Clin North Am 3:13, 1976

125. Mostofi FK: Pathology and spread of carcinoma of the urinary bladder. p. 303. In Johnson DE, Samuels ML (eds): Cancer of the Genitourinary Tract. Raven Press, New York, 1979

126. Mostofi FK, Sobin LH, Torloni H (eds): International Histological Classification of Tumours, No. 10: Histological Typing of Urinary Bladder Tumours. World Health Organization, Geneva, 1973

127. Mostofi FK, Thomson RV, Dean AL Jr: Mucous adenocarcinoma of the urinary bladder. Cancer 8:741, 1955

128. Mukai K, Rosai J, Burgdorf WHC: Localization of factor VIII-related antigen in vascular endothelial cells using an immunoperoxidase method. Am J Surg Pathol 4:273, 1980

129. Murphy WM, Crabtree WN, Jukkola AF, Soloway MS: The diagnostic value of urine versus bladder washings in patients with bladder cancer. J Urol 126:320, 1981

130. Murphy WM, Soloway MS: Urothelial dysplasia. J Urol 127:849, 1982

131. Nagy GK, Frable WJ, Murphy WM: Classification of pre-malignant urothelial abnormalities. A Delphi study of the National Bladder Cancer Collaborative Group A. p. 219. In Sommers, SC & Rosen PP, eds.: Pathology Annual. Vol 17. Appleton-Century-Crofts. Norwalk, Connecticut, 1982

132. Narayana AS, Loening SA, Slymen DJ, Culp DA: Bladder cancer: factors affecting survival. J Urol 130:56, 1983

133. Natale RB, Yagoda A, Watson RC, et al: Methotrexate: an active drug in bladder cancer. Cancer 47:1246, 1981

134. National Bladder Cancer Collaborative Group A (NBCCGA): Development of a strategy for a longitudinal study of patients with bladder cancer. Cancer Res 37:2898, 1977

135. National Bladder Cancer Collaborative Group A (NBCCGA): Surveillance, initial assessment, and subsequent progress of patients with superficial bladder cancer in a prospective longitudinal study. Cancer Res 37:2907, 1977

136. Nichols JA, Marshall VF: Treatment of histologically benign papilloma of the urinary bladder by local excision and fulguration. Cancer 9:566, 1956

137. Ooms ECM, Anderson WAD, Alons CL, et al: Analysis of the performance of pathologists in the grading of bladder tumors. Hum Pathol 14:140, 1983

138. Orihuela E, Herr HW, Pinsky CM, Whitmore WF Jr: Toxicity of intravesical BCG and its management in patients with superficial bladder tumors. Cancer 60:326, 1987

139. Persky L, Kursh ED, Soloway M: Uroepithelial tumors. p. 653. In Devine CF Jr, Stecker JF Jr (eds): Urology in Practice. Little, Brown, Boston, 1978

140. Prout GR Jr: Classification and staging of bladder carcinoma. Cancer 45:1832, 1980

141. Prout GR Jr: Classification and staging of bladder carcinoma. p. 133. In Bonney WW, Prout GR Jr (eds): Bladder Cancer. AUA Monographs, Vol. 1. Williams & Wilkins, Baltimore, 1982

142. Prout GR Jr: Commentary: bladder cancer. J Urol 127:607, 1982

143. Prout GR Jr: Surgical therapy for invasive bladder cancer. p. 233. In Bonney WW, Prout GR Jr (eds): Bladder Cancer. AUA Monographs, Vol. 1. Williams & Wilkins, Baltimore, 1982

144. Prout GR Jr, Bassil B, Griffin P: The treated histories of patients with Ta grade 1 transitional-cell carcinoma of the bladder. Arch Surg 121:1463, 1986

145. Prout GR Jr, Coomb LJ, for the National Bladder Cancer Group: a long-term comparison of patients treated with thio-tepa — success versus failure. J Urol 133:212A, 1985

146. Prout GR Jr, Griffin PP, Shipley WU: Bladder carcinoma as a systemic disease. Cancer 43: 2532, 1979

147. Pyrah LN, Raper FP, Thomas GM: Report of a follow-up of papillary tumours of the bladder. Br J Urol 36:14, 1964

148. Quilty PM, Duncan W: Treatment of superficial (T1) tumours of the bladder by radical radiotherapy. Br J Urol 58:147, 1986

149. Radwin HM: Radiotherapy and bladder cancer: a critical review. J Urol 124:43, 1980

150. Reid EC, Oliver JA, Fishman IJ: Preoperative irradiation and cystectomy in 135 cases of bladder cancer. Urology 8:247, 1976

151. Richie JP, Skinner DG: Carcinoma in situ of the urethra associated with bladder carcinoma: the role of urethrectomy. J Urol 119:80, 1978

152. Richie JP, Skinner DG, Kauffman JJ: Radical cystectomy for carcinoma of the bladder: 16 years of experience. J Urol 113:186, 1975

153. Riddle PR, Wallace DM: Intracavitary chemotherapy for multiple non-invasive bladder tumours. Br J Urol 43:181, 1971

154. Sarma KP: Genesis of papillary tumours: histological and microangiographic study. Br J Urol 53:228, 1981

155. Scanlon PW, Scott M, Segura JW: A comparison of short-course, low-dose and long-course, high-dose preoperative radiation for carcinoma of the bladder. Cancer 52:1153, 1983

156. Schade ROK, Swinney J: The association of urothelial atypism with neoplasia: its importance in treatment and prognosis. J Urol 109:619, 1973

157. Schellhammer PF, Ladaga LE, Fillion MB: Bacillus Calmette-Guérin for superficial transitional cell carcinoma of the bladder. J Urol 135:261, 1986

158. Schmidt JD, Weinstein SH: Pitfalls in clinical staging of bladder tumors. Urol Clin North Am 3:107, 1976

159. Schroder LE, Weiss MA, Hughes C: Squamous cell carcinoma of bladder: an increased incidence in blacks. Urology 28:288, 1986

160. Seemayer TA, Knaack J: Thelmo WL, et al: Further observations on carcinoma in situ of the urinary bladder: silent but extensive intraprostatic involvement. Cancer 36:514, 1975

161. Seidman H, Mushinski MH, Gelb SK, Silverberg E: Probabilities of eventually developing or dying of cancer: United States, 1985. CA 35:36, 1985

162. Semple JE: Paillomata of bladder treated with podophyllin: preliminary report. Br Med J 1:1235, 1948

163. Shanberg AM, Baghdassarian R, Tansey LA: Use of Nd:YAG laser in treatment of bladder cancer. Urology 29:26, 1987

164. Sheldon CA, Clayman RV, Gonzalez R, et al: Malignant urachal lesions. J Urol 131:1, 1984

165. Shipley WU, Prout GR Jr, Kaufman SD, Perrone TL: Invasive bladder carcinoma: the importance of initial transurethral surgery and other significant prognostic factors for improved survival with full-dose irradiation. Cancer 60:514, 1987

166. Shipley WU, Rose MA: Bladder cancer: the selection of patients for treatment by full-dose irradiation. Cancer 55:2278, 1985

167. Silverberg E: Statistical and epidemiologic data on urologic cancer. Cancer (suppl. 1) 60:692, 1987

168. Silverberg E, Lubera J: Cancer statistics, 1987. CA 37:2, 1987

169. Skinner DG: Current state of classification and staging of bladder cancer. Cancer Res 37:2838, 1977

170. Skinner DG: Current perspectives in the management of high-grade invasive bladder cancer. Cancer 45:1866, 1980

171. Skinner DG, Richie JP, Cooper PH, et al: The clinical significance of carcinoma in situ of the bladder and its association with overt carcinoma. J Urol 112:68, 1974

172. Skinner DG, Tift JP, Kaufman JJ: High dose, short course preoperative radiation therapy and immediate single stage radical cystectomy with pelvic node dissection in the management of bladder cancer. J Urol 127:671, 1982

173. Slack NH, Prout GR Jr: Heterogeneity of invasive bladder carcinoma and different responses to treatment. p. 213. In Bonney WW, Prout GR Jr (eds): Bladder Cancer. AUA Monographs, Vol. 1. Williams & Wilkins, Baltimore, 1982

174. Smalley RV, Bartolucci AA, Hemstreet G, Hester M: A phase II evaluation of a 3-drug combination of cyclophosphamide, doxorubicin, and 5-fluorouracil and of 5-fluorouracil in patients with advanced bladder carcinoma or stage D prostatic carcinoma. J Urol 125:191, 1981

175. Smith JA Jr: Laser treatment of bladder cancer. Semin Urol 3:2, 1985

176. Smith JA Jr: Treatment of invasive bladder cancer with a neodymium:YAG laser. J Urol 135:55, 1986

177. Soloway MS: The management of superficial bladder cancer. Cancer 45:1856, 1980

178. Soloway MS: Rationale for intensive intravesical chemotherapy for superficial bladder cancer. J Urol 123:461, 1980

179. Soloway MS: Surgery and intravesical chemotherapy in the management of superficial bladder cancer. Semin Urol 1:23, 1983

180. Soloway MS: Superficial bladder cancer: comments on evaluation and management. J Urol 132:91, 1984

181. Soloway MS: Intravesical and systemic chemotherapy in the management of superficial bladder cancer. Urol Clin North Am 11:623, 1984

182. Soloway MS: Overview of treatment of superficial bladder cancer. Urology, suppl. 4, 26:18, 1985

183. Soloway MS: M-VAC for metastatic urothelial cancer. J Urol 135:223A, 1986

184. Soloway MS: Selecting initial therapy for bladder cancer. Cancer 60:502, 1987

185. Soloway MS: Is there a role for induction therapy for locally advanced bladder cancer? Urology 29:577, 1987

186. Soloway MS, Ikard M, Ford K: Cis-diamminedichloroplatinum (II) in locally advanced and metastatic urothelial cancer. Cancer 47:476, 1981

187. Soloway MS, Murphy W, Rao MK, Cox C: Serial multiple-site biopsies in patients with bladder cancer. J Urol 120:57, 1978

188. Soloway MS, Perry A: Bacillus Calmette-Guérin for treatment of superficial transitional cell carcinoma of the bladder in patients who have failed thiotepa and/or mitomycin C. J Urol 137:871, 1987

189. Sondak VK, Bertelsen CA, Kern DH, Morton DL: Evolution and clinical application of a rapid chemosensitivity assay. Cancer 55:1367, 1985

190. Soto EA, Friedell GH, Tiltman AJ: Bladder cancer as seen in giant histologic sections. Cancer 39:447, 1977

191. Staehler G, Chaussy C, Jocham D, Schmiedt E: The use of neodymium-YAG lasers in urology: indica-

tions, technique, and critical assessment. J Urol 134:1155, 1985

192. Sternberg C, Yagoda A, Scher HI, et al: Preliminary results of M-VAC (methotrexate, vinblastine, doxorubicin, and cisplatin) for transitional cell carcinoma of the urothelium. J Urol 133:403, 1985

193. Stokes MA, Kelly DG: Transitional cell carcinoma in patients under forty years of age. Br J Urol 59:536, 1987

194. Tannock IF, Gospodarowicz M, Evans WK: Chemotherapy for metastatic transitional carcinoma of the urinary tract: a prospective trial of methotrexate, adriamycin, and cyclophosphamide (MAC) with cisplatinum for failure. Cancer 51:216, 1983

195. Thomas DG, Ward AM, Williams JL: A study of 52 cases of adenocarcinoma of the bladder. Br J Urol 43:4, 1971

196. Utz DC, Farrow GM: Carcinoma in situ of the urinary tract. Urol Clin North Am 11:735, 1984

197. Utz DC, Farrow GM, Rife CC, et al: Carcinoma in situ of the bladder. Cancer 45:1842, 1980

198. Utz DC, Hanash KA, Farrow GM: The plight of the patient with carcinoma in situ of the bladder. J Urol 103:160, 1970

199. Van der Werf-Messing B, Hop WCJ: Carcinoma of the urinary bladder (category T-1, Nx, Mo) treated either by radium implant or by transurethral resection only. Int J Rad Oncol Biol Phys 7:299, 1981

200. Wallace DMA, Hindmarsh JR, Webb JN, et al: The role of multiple mucosal biopsies in the management of patients with bladder cancer. Br J Urol 51:535, 1979

201. Whitmore WF Jr: The treatment of bladder tumors. Surg Clin North Am 49:349, 1969

202. Whitmore WF Jr: Special article: summary of all phases of bladder carcinoma. J Urol 119:77, 1978

203. Whitmore WF Jr: Surgical management of low stage bladder cancer. Semin Oncol 6:207, 1979

204. Whitmore WF Jr: Urothelial tumor: problems and prospects. Semin Urol 1:2, 1983

205. Whitmore WF Jr: Management of invasive bladder neoplasms. Semin Urol 1:34, 1983

206. Whitmore WF Jr: Long-term effects of initial therapy. Cancer 60:559, 1987

207. Whitmore WF Jr, Batata NA, Ghoneim MA, et al: Radical cystectomy with or without prior irradiation in the treatment of bladder cancer. J Urol 118:184, 1977

208. Whitmore WF Jr, Batata MA, Hilaris BS, et al: A comparative study of two preoperative radiation regimens with cystectomy for bladder cancer. Cancer 40:1077, 1977

209. Williams GB, Trott PA, Bloom HJG: Carcinoma of the bladder treated by interstitial irradiation. Br J Urol 53:221, 1981

210. Williams JL, Hammonds JC, Saunders N: T1 bladder tumors. Br J Urol 49:663, 1977

211. Yagoda A: Future implications of phase 2 chemotherapy trials in ninety-five patients with measurable advanced bladder cancer. Cancer Res 37:2775, 1977

212. Yagoda A: Chemotherapy of metastatic bladder cancer. Cancer 45:1879, 1980

213. Yagoda A: Chemotherapy for advanced urothelial cancer. Semin Urol 1:60, 1983

214. Yagoda A: Chemotherapy of urothelial tract tumors. Cancer 60:574, 1987

215. Yagoda A, Watson RC, Whitmore WF Jr, et al: Adriamycin in advanced urinary tract cancer: experience in 42 patients and review of the literature. Cancer 39:279, 1977

216. Yu WS, Sagerman RH, Chung CT, et al: Bladder carcinoma: experience with radical and preoperative radiotherapy in 421 patients. Cancer 56:1293, 1985

217. Zincke H, Utz DC, Farrow GM: Review of Mayo Clinic experience with carcinoma in situ. Urology, suppl. 4, 26:39, 1985.

19

Urothelial Neoplasms: Renal Pelvis and Ureter

James W. Eagan, Jr.

Compared to primary bladder tumors, the experience with upper tract neoplasms at any given institution is relatively small. In a review of the data from the Memorial Hospital (New York) from 1949 to 1972, Batata and Grabstald[7] reported a total of 3,629 patients registered with primary urothelial tumors. The breakdown included 3,269 bladder tumors and 210 urethral tumors, with only 89 renal pelvic and 77 ureteral tumors registered over the 23-year period, giving a ratio of approximately 19 bladder cases for every upper tract case seen. In other major centers such as the Mayo Clinic, experience is similarly limited, with a few more than 10 patients per year with upper tract disease seen.[41,42] Thus exposure to such cases in day-to-day practice is infrequent. Moreover, because of the limited number of cases, the ability to collect meaningful data on upper tract urothelial malignancies is hampered, particularly with regard to therapy, and it is in this area that well planned collaborative studies would be of greatest use.

BENIGN UROTHELIAL TUMORS OF THE UPPER TRACT

As in the lower tract, most tumors arising in the upper tract are of epithelial origin, and the majority are considered at least low grade malignant neoplasms

by present standards. The benign lesions encountered in the bladder are also seen in the upper tract, although experience with them is essentially anecdotal.

Transitional Cell Papilloma

With strict criteria applied (see Ch. 17), primary transitional cell papillomas of the renal pelvis and ureter are rare lesions (Fig. 19-1). They are generally small excrescences found incidentally in resection specimens removed for other lesions. In and of themselves, these tumors are of no consequence aside from serving as markers of possible proliferative activity elsewhere in the urothelium.

Inverted Transitional Cell Papillomas

Inverted transitional cell papillomas, similar morphologically to those found in the bladder, have also been documented to occur in the renal pelvis,[2] ureter,[21] and ureteropelvic junction.[18] They are even more scarce than their lower tract counterparts, with only 24 cases having been reported in the upper tract according to Schulze et al.[49] Recognizing them as such preoperatively may be difficult or impossible, but the presence of a rounded contour on radiologic studies combined with unremarkable cytologic studies may serve as preoperative clues to their identity

843

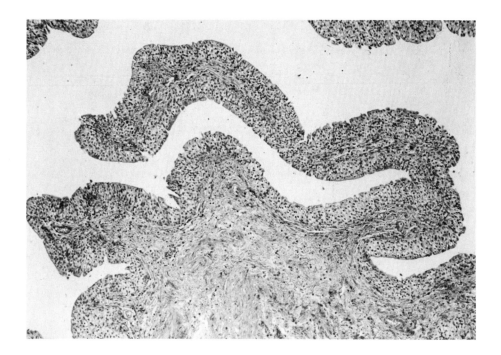

Fig. 19-1 Transitional cell papilloma of the ureter. This lesion was discovered incidentally in a resection specimen for carcinoma. ×82.

and particularly as indicators that they may be treated with conservative surgery if technically possible.

Other Benign Epithelial Tumors and Tumorlike Lesions

Other benign tumors and tumorlike lesions, e.g., nephrogenic adenomas, fibroepithelial polyps, and endometriosis, may rarely be seen in the upper tract. They are described in Chapter 17.

MALIGNANT UROTHELIAL TUMORS OF THE UPPER TRACT

INCIDENCE

Malignant epithelial tumors of the upper tract constitute 5 to 6 percent of all urothelial cancers; therefore, extrapolating from the data for bladder cancer,[51] approximately 2,000 cases per year are seen in the United States. Similarly, of all kidney malignancies, renal pelvic tumors account for only a minority of cases,[56] far overshadowed numerically by renal cell carcinoma. There appears to be no relation between the development of renal pelvic neoplasms and renal cell carcinomas. In fact, in a report of a case of simultaneous renal cell carcinoma and transitional cell carcinoma of the renal pelvis, Lundell et al.[35] could find only 16 such cases previously reported in the literature.

The question of an increasing incidence of upper tract urothelial malignancies has been raised, but the figures are not startling. Although a true increase in incidence is likely, improvement in diagnostic techniques as well as enhancement of the survival of bladder cancer patients may also account for some of the increase noted.[39]

Possible etiologic factors have been discussed in Chapter 16, and it is presumed that some of the same factors cited for bladder carcinoma, e.g., industrial exposure and cigarette smoking, are operative in the upper tract as well.[10] The data are not firm, however, and other large studies have found no definite relation with industrial exposure in particular.[39] The only two situations that appear to be of definite note in the development of upper tract lesions are analgesic abuse and "Balkan nephropathy," and the reader is referred to Chapter 16 for a more complete discussion of these.

The demographic data for upper tract lesions are similar to those for bladder cancer. That is, the tumors are most common in elderly men, with male/female ratios ranging from approximately 2:1 to as high as 4:1, and mean ages ranging from 60 years to 68 years.[4,7,8,17,24,46] These tumors may be seen at any age, however, having been reported even in infants,[32] but they are rare prior to age 30.[10] There is no mention of apparent ethnic or racial predilection in various major series reported.

CLINICAL PRESENTATION

Only rare cases (approximately 2 percent)[39] of upper tract urothelial malignancies are discovered incidentally, and most patients present to the urologist with the disturbing symptom of unexplained hematuria. Gross hematuria, most often painless, the principal manifestation of both renal pelvic and ureteral malignancies, is found in approximately 80 percent of patients.[39] It is the most common symptom regardless of grade, stage, or location (renal pelvis or ureter) of the lesion. At least microscopic hematuria is most often found in the remaining patients.

The close relation between upper and lower tract malignancies is striking. Up to one-fourth of all patients with upper tract malignancies will have already been seen for preceding bladder cancer. Not infrequently, this will have occurred a number of years before.[22] Of even greater concern from a diagnostic standpoint is the fact that *concurrent* bladder lesions may be found in as many as 10 percent of cases (see below), and these lesions may be mistakenly judged as the sole source of urinary bleeding on initial work-up. The upper urinary tract must be evaluated in *all* patients with hematuria, regardless of the presence or absence of overt bladder lesions. Similarly, other ready explanations for hematuria such as calculi[8,42] and infection,[8] as well as associated, possibly misleading phenomena such as pyuria and proteinuria,[11] may be found not infrequently, particularly in association with tumors with squamous and glandular differentiation.[10] In elderly patients especially, they must be viewed as potential "fellow travelers" with malignancy.

Flank pain is noted in roughly one-fourth to one-half of patients,[4,7,17,22] somewhat more commonly in those with renal pelvic versus ureteral lesions[39] and more often in association with invasive tumors and obstructing lesions. A definite palpable mass is another potentially ominous sign; and associated constitutional symptoms, including weight loss, anorexia, and fever, are said to be invariably indicative of far-advanced disease.[39]

PATIENT EVALUATION

As noted, hematuria is the most common symptom in lower tract as well as upper tract disease, and possible differential points in favor of upper tract disease include histories of analgesic abuse, flank pain, and/or renal colic. Physical findings are generally minimal, with palpable masses being the exception rather than the rule. Percussion tenderness at the costovertebral angle may be present in patients with renal pelvic lesions, but this is a rather nonspecific finding.

The initial work-up should include at least one, and preferably three,[20] voided urine cytology specimens, often the first clue to the presence of high grade disease. At the Mayo Clinic, where a four-tiered grading system is used, Murphy et al.[42] found accuracy rates with voided specimens alone of 45, 78, and 83 percent for grade II, III, and IV upper tract tumors, respectively. A confounding factor, however, as with all studies, was the presence of associated bladder lesions in a number of patients. Grade I lesions are considerably more difficult if not impossible to diagnose on cytologic grounds alone (see Ch. 21).

Intravenous pyelography (IVP) provides valuable information concerning the presence or absence of upper tract lesions, regardless of stage or grade. In the Mayo Clinic experience, of 48 patients with grade I disease (47 of whom were also found to have stage I disease), only 3 had normal IVPs.[41] The most common abnormality seen was a filling defect in the renal pelvis or ureter (54 percent), with nonvisualization of the involved upper tract in 19 percent, hydronephrosis without evidence of a filling defect in 17 percent, and evidence of a renal mass in 4 percent. In a review of the Mayo Clinic patients with higher grade tumors,[42] corresponding figures included 45 percent with filling defects, a higher rate of nonvisualization (31 percent), evidence of obstruction in 10 percent, renal mass lesion in 8 percent, and 6 percent with indeterminate abnormalities. Only 1 of the 173 patients examined had an entirely normal IVP. Nonvisualization in particular has been generally associated with higher grade/stage lesions in a number of studies[4,11] but may also, as the above figures indicate, be seen not infrequently in patients with low grade, noninvasive disease.[39,41]

Retrograde pyelography enjoys an even greater success, with all 152 patients showing one or another abnormality in the series of high grade tumors from the Mayo Clinic.[42] It is of particular value for delineating the mass or masses present in the event of a nonvisualizing upper tract on IVP.[39] Other techniques that may prove to be of value are sonography, computerized axial tomography, and, in selected situations, renal arteriography and venography.[39]

A thorough cystoscopic examination is obviously mandatory for all patients with suspected upper tract lesions because of the incidence of concomitant bladder carcinoma. There is often a parallel between grade (and therefore stage) of concomitant upper and lower tract disease, although this is certainly not always the case (see below). Further characterization of the upper tract lesion may be attempted with the use of ureteral catheterized urine cytology,[50] lavage cytology,[33] or brush biopsy with cytologic examination.[12,44]

An encouraging note has been the development of rigid and flexible instruments for evaluation of the upper tract transurethrally.[5,6,25,30,36,37] Rigid instruments have found particular use in upper tract stone manipulation but have also been employed both diagnostically and therapeutically in the management of upper tract tumors. In a report on the use of the ureteropyeloscope, Huffman et al.[25] noted successful completion of the procedure in 28 of 31 patients, 11 of whom were found to have urothelial tumors. Diagnostic biopsies performed under direct visualization allowed distinguishing three patients with high grade, multifocal tumors who needed definitive surgery. Fulguration or resection via the instrument was successfully carried out in the remaining eight patients with apparently localized low grade tumors. Even if attempts at endoscopic therapy do not prove effective, the procedure may at least allow more definitive characterization of upper tract tumors prior to surgery.

CLINICOPATHOLOGIC ASSESSMENT

In contrast to the situation with bladder cancer, local approaches such as ureteropyeloscopic resection are still in the developmental stage. Thus the pathologist is still often presented with a definitive resection specimen in cases of primary renal pelvic or ureteral carcinomas, resulting from either total nephroureterectomy with bladder cuff or lesser, so-called conservative procedures, all of which at present still encompass the entirety of the lesion.

Features of potential prognostic importance, similar to those found in bladder resection specimens, should also be noted. Grade and stage are of prime importance, whereas the significance of the presence or absence of associated urothelial abnormalities, lymphatic or vascular invasion, and the results of adjunctive studies, have not been systematically studied. That which is known about the significance of the various parameters is discussed.

Tumor Location, Size, and Number

The true relative incidence of primary renal pelvic versus primary ureteral malignancies is difficult to glean from the literature, with some studies indicating a preponderance of renal pelvic tumors,[41,42,58] others an almost equal incidence,[7] and still others a preponderance of ureteral primaries.[13] The incidences of concomitant renal pelvic and ureteral primaries, associated bladder lesions, and lesions in the opposite upper tract are discussed later in the chapter under Multiple Urothelial Primaries.

The location of the primary appears to have little bearing on the overall prognosis. In reviews of patients at the Massachusetts General Hospital with ureteral[24] and renal pelvic[43] primaries, survivals were found to be 70 versus 60 percent, respectively, at 2 years, with survival curves approaching each other at 5 years. Others have noted a similar pattern.[4]

Among renal pelvic primaries, Nocks et al.[43] found that 59 percent of the lesions involved the pelvis proper, 23 percent were located in the infundibulocalyceal region, and 18 percent were found to involve both sites. There appeared to be no correlation between the tumor location and stage, grade, or survival.

The predominant location of ureteral primaries in most studies has been the lower one-third of the ureter, ranging from approximately 50 percent[8] to 73 percent,[4] with variable figures for distribution of the remaining tumors in the upper two-thirds. Multiple-site involvement of the ureter may be seen in roughly 10 to 20 percent of patients,[4,8] without apparent effect on survival, although it is an obvious impediment to conservative surgery. The importance, if any, of tumor size is uncertain. In a study of upper tract lesions by Mahadevia et al.,[38] a lesion measuring only 0.5 cm was found to be muscle invasive, yet a number of other lesions of the same grade showed only microinvasion or no invasion at all despite considerably larger size.

Tumor Type and Configuration

Reliable figures for the various tumor types in the upper tract are less readily available than for the bladder, in part because a number of the larger studies are specifically directed at discussion of transitional cell carcinoma, without mention of other types, whereas others may mention only "squamous" or "epidermoid" features, presumably combined with transitional cell features in the same tumor. There may also be some variation in morphologic interpretation from laboratory to laboratory. One pathologist may call a poorly differentiated tumor with occasional keratinized foci a mixed transitional cell–squamous carcinoma, whereas another might sign it out as a squamous carcinoma. As noted in Chapter 17, I prefer to diagnose tumors as having mixed differentiation if two or more definite subtypes are recognized in the same lesion, with the labels of squamous carcinoma and adenocarcinoma reserved for tumors with either complete differentiation along these lines or with predominant squamous or glandular differentiation associated with other areas which show little or no differentiation of any recognizable type.

Bearing this element of subjectivity in mind, it appears that the figures for upper tract primaries are similar to those for bladder neoplasms. Combining the results from a number of studies of both ureteral[4,8,11,57] (total 221 cases) and renal pelvic lesions[22,28,46] (total 248 cases), the figures indicate approximately 90 to 92 percent of tumors to be transitional cell in type, approximately 7 to 8 percent squamous in type or at least with recognizable squamous features, and the remaining 1 percent or so adenocarcinomas, with only rare examples of the other subtypes described in the morphology section (see Ch. 17) reported.

Transitional cell carcinomas as a group enjoy the best prognosis of all tumor types in the upper tract. As with bladder carcinoma, however, this finding is misleading, as the population of lesions included in the transitional cell category shows the same mix of low grade, relatively indolent tumors and higher grade, more aggressive tumors. So to say that a patient has a "transitional cell carcinoma," without modifiers, tells little of the story. Because of the strong dependence of prognosis on grade and stage, these tumors are discussed more fully in following sections.

Tumor configuration (papillary versus nonpapillary, planar, or solid) is also of prognostic significance, but again this feature is closely interrelated with stage and grade.[24,43] The numerical dominance of papillary lesions over nonpapillary lesions appears somewhat less than in the bladder, where approximately 80 percent of tumors are papillary.

In a report on 68 patients with transitional cell carcinoma of the renal pelvis, Nocks et al.[43] found 63 percent to be papillary in configuration and 37 percent nonpapillary. Nonpapillary tumors generally exhibited a significantly higher stage and grade than their papillary counterparts. With regard to stage, 70 percent of papillary lesions were limited to the mucosa and submucosa, whereas only 4 percent of the nonpapillary lesions were so confined. Only 21 percent of papillary tumors had extended beyond the boundaries of the organ and/or metastasized, whereas fully 88 percent of the nonpapillary ones had done so.

Reviewing ureteral tumors from the same institution, Heney et al.[24] found a higher incidence of papillary versus nonpapillary tumors (75 versus 25 percent). Tumor stage figures were similar to those for the renal pelvic primaries, with 64 percent of papillary lesions confined to the mucosa or submucosa, compared to only 14 percent of the nonpapillary lesions. Only 21 percent of the papillary tumors had spread beyond the confines of the organ and/or metastasized, compared to 64 percent of the nonpapillary lesions. Interestingly, among grade III papillary and nonpapillary lesions, in contrast to the situation with bladder carcinoma, survival figures were comparable, although the numbers of patients were small.

Squamous carcinomas in the upper tract appear to merit an even more dismal outlook than their bladder counterparts. The experience with these lesions is small at any given institution, but most studies have noted an almost uniformly poor prognosis.[34,39] In their report of the combined New York Hospital–Memorial Hospital experience, McCarron et al.[39] found that all 11 patients with keratinizing squamous carcinoma of the renal pelvis and 2 patients with similar ureteral lesions had died with metastatic carcinoma within short periods following surgery. As with bladder tumors, the degree of squamous differentiation required to diagnose a lesion as squamous carcinoma varies from one author to the next. Bennington and Beckwith[10] advised that "squamous change," i.e., focal evidence of squamous differentiation in a transitional cell carcinoma, may be found in 18 to 20 percent of upper tract lesions. They thought that these lesions should be separated diagnostically from pure squamous carcinoma. In a series of renal pelvic tumors, however, Grabstald et al.[22] accepted even focal keratinization as evidence of squamous carcinoma, and all five lesions showing such differentiation were high stage tumors at diagnosis.

Adenocarcinomas of the upper tract are generally the subject of isolated case reports and compendiums of previous case reports,[3,14,59] and experience is therefore limited. These lesions, as well as squamous lesions, are commonly associated with inflammation, calculi, and pyelonephritis.[3,14] They often appear relatively well differentiated, but Bennington and Beckwith[10] cautioned against underestimating their aggressive nature on the basis of what is at times a deceptively bland morphology. In general, they are anything but indolent tumors. For example, in a report of a case of ureteral adenocarcinoma and review of 13 other cases from the literature, Brawer and Waisman[14] found that among the six patients with sufficient follow-up mean survival was little more than 2 years.

Carcinoma in situ in the upper tract may be seen in association with overt tumors, but the natural history of this lesion per se, in the absence of associated lesions, is essentially unknown. Such cases are extremely rare in the upper tract, with only five such reports having been found in a literature search by Stragier et al.[53]

Tumor Grade and Stage

For transitional cell carcinomas, it is generally agreed that grade and stage are the two most important prognostic factors in upper tract malignancies, with some studies ascribing more weight to the former[46] and others to the latter.[22] As with bladder cancer, in virtually all studies a strong relation between the two features obtains; that is, low grade lesions are most often low stage, and high grade lesions are most often high stage, with correspondingly excellent and grim prognoses.[17] The interrelation between grade, stage, and prognosis is perhaps even more striking than for bladder cancer. One factor that no doubt contributes to the more uniform parallels among grade, stage, and prognosis is the uniformity of therapeutic approach to these lesions. At least until the recent past, most lesions, whether high grade/stage or low grade/stage, were dealt with in a definitive surgical fashion, i.e., total nephroureterectomy as recommended by Kimball and Ferris in 1934,[31] with lesser procedures usually reserved for special circumstances such as bilateral disease or high operative risk. Because of the conjunctive bearing of grade and stage on prognosis, these two features are discussed together.

Comparison of the data from various reports is somewhat difficult for tumor grade because of the variation in systems used in different institutions. Some centers employ a three-component grading system,[13,17,24,43] whereas others use a four-tiered system.[41,42,46] Still others, such as Memorial Hospital in New York, may totally exclude "histologically benign papillomas," many of which would correspond to grade I transitional cell carcinomas at other centers, from consideration,[8] with an obvious influence on statistics. For the sake of uniformity, as noted in the morphology section, I would recommend adoption of the three-tiered system proposed by the World Health Organization (WHO)[40] and the Armed Forces Insititute of Pathology (AFIP),[10] with grades I, II, and III corresponding to the traditional well, moderately, and poorly differentiated categories, respectively; tumors beyond this level, which show virtually no differentiation, are relegated to the "undifferentiated" category.

So also for tumor staging, which is even more problematic than tumor grading in the literature. Although most systems proposed are similar, everyone seems to add a personal twist. Some authors[13] employ modifications of the TNM system used by the American Joint Committee on Cancer[9] and the International Union Against Cancer (UICC)[27] for bladder lesions. Others[46,57] adapt from the Jewett–Strong–Marshall bladder classification. Still others[22,56] utilize an amalgam of staging and grading, where the relative contributions of either may be difficult to sort out.

Arguments for and against the various systems may be put forth. The most commonly used in the United States appears to be a variation on the Jewett–

Table 19-1 Staging of Upper Tract Urothelial Carcinomas

Primary Tumor Stage	Renal Pelvis	Ureter
Ta	Noninvasive papillary carcinoma	Noninvasive papillary carcinoma
Tis	Nonpapillary carcinoma in situ	Nonpapillary carcinoma in situ
T1	Submucosal invasion and/or microscopic invasion into renal parenchyma	Submucosal invasion
T2	Muscle invasion and/or deep invasion into renal parenchyma	Muscle invasion
T3	Invasion into perirenal soft tissue	Invasion into periureteral soft tissue
T4	Tumor is grossly fixed and/or invades neighboring structures	Tumor is grossly fixed and/or invades neighboring structures

Nodal status

NX	Lymph nodes not assessed
N0	No involvement of regional lymph nodes
NI	Regional lymph nodes involved by tumor

Distant metastases

M0	No known distant metastases
MI	Distant metastases present

Tumor grade

I	Well differentiated
II	Moderately differentiated
III	Poorly differentiated

Strong–Marshall theme, but even it has not been applied uniformly, as one institution's "C" may be another's "D", "O's" may not be separated from "A's", and so on. Therefore, again for the sake of uniformity, I propose that a modification of the current TNM system, presented in Table 19-1, be utilized for upper tract lesions.

There are a number of potential benefits to such a system when compared to the systems now in use. One is that tumor grade, lumped together with extent of involvement in some systems,[22] is clearly distinguished from tumor stage, as is done for bladder tumors. Although the data are limited, there is reason to believe, as with bladder primaries, that higher grade upper tract lesions do worse than lower grade lesions *stage for stage* (see below). Another advantage is that the lumping of "stage IV" patients found in some studies[11,42,56] to include everyone from those with just microscopic extension outside the pelvis or ureter to those with distant metastases is avoided. Whereas prognosis may have been equally poor for all such patients in some studies, other reports have found notable differences in survival comparing those with

only extraorgan invasion to those with metastatic disease.[8,24,43] A third potential benefit is the separation of "low stage" disease into categories similar to those in use for the bladder. At present, noninvasive papillary lesions, superficially invasive papillary lesions, and high grade carcinoma in situ may be grouped together in some schemes. It may have been of no consequence in the past, as, barring associated disease elsewhere, patients with these lesions would be expected to do well following standard definitive resection. As conservative therapy is utilized with increasing frequency, however, clear-cut survival differences may become apparent.

What are the typical grade and stage figures for upper tract malignancies? Combining more than 700 cases from various studies (Table 19-2), for transitional cell carcinomas the distribution of lesions among the three grades in the upper tract is similar to that of bladder cancer but with somewhat fewer low grade lesions encountered. There is variability from series to series, however. In the largest single institution experience in the American literature, that of 224 patients seen at the Mayo Clinic,[41,42] the number of

Table 19-2 Grade and Stage: Transitional Cell Carcinomas
of the Renal Pelvis and Ureter

Incidence	Low (Grade I) (Percent)	Intermediate (Grade II) (Percent)	High (Grades III and IV) (Percent)
Among all cases	16	43	41
By stage			
Ta, Tis	93.4	57.3	13.2
T1	4.4	13.5	4.8
T2	2.2	17.1	13.2
T3/T4/N1/M1	0	12.1	68.8

(Data from Babaian and Johnson,[4] Batata et al.,[8] Bloom et al.,[11] Heney et al.,[24] Murphy et al.,[41,42] Nocks et al.,[43] Rubenstein et al.,[46] and Werth et al.[57])

grade I lesions was somewhat higher (22 percent), and even higher figures have been found in the British literature.[13]

Combining figures from the various studies where grade and stage were specifically cross-tabulated, some rather striking differences from one grade to the next were found (Table 19-2). In particular, in addition to the expected high percentage of grade I lesions still relatively confined, a surprising number (more than 70 percent) of intermediate grade lesions were also either noninvasive or at most superficially invasive. Such stages were distinctly in the minority among high grade lesions, however. In contrast to low grade lesions, close to 70 percent of high grade lesions had already spread beyond the organ confines, with or without metastases, by the time of surgery.

In view of the above, 5-year survival statistics, not unexpectedly, are almost uniformly good for patients with grade I lesions, ranging from 83.3 percent[11] to 100 percent, with a number of studies[4,17,24,43] showing the latter figure. On the other end of the spectrum, grade III lesions, with all stages taken into account, are associated with a poor prognosis, with 5-year survival figures varying from nil[8] to a maximum in the low 30 percent range.[4] Although most series do not contain sufficient patients to stratify survival according to both grade and stage, in the Mayo Clinic series[42] there appeared to be some independent effect of grade alone, as the 5-year survival rate for patients with grade II lesions limited to the mucosa or submucosa was 77 percent, dropping to 54 percent for patients with grade III–IV lesions of identical stage. From examination of their survival curves, there appears to be an independent effect for more advanced

lesions as well, with a 5-year survival rate of 55 percent for patients with grade II lesions that had extended into the muscularis, into the kidney, or beyond, compared into only 13 percent for patients with grade III–IV lesions of similar stages.

For both squamous and adenocarcinomas, the little information available indicates that these tumors are generally high stage lesions at the time of diagnosis, with little apparent effect of grade on the prognosis. Even if well differentiated, with a perhaps more indolent course if found at some other body sites, the aggressive potential of these tumors appears clear when they are found in the renal pelvis or ureter; the outlook is generally poor, whatever the grade assigned.

Mode of Tumor Spread and Vascular/Lymphatic Invasion

Observations of the pattern of invasion are presumed to carry prognostic importance similar to that for bladder cancer. However, there are no systematic studies of these features such as are available for bladder cancer, although documentation of patterns of invasion should be part of the pathology record for upper tract lesions as well.

For invasive lesions, an en bloc or "broad front" pattern of invasion (Fig. 19-2), is generally seen with low to intermediate grade papillary carcinomas. The presence or absence of invasion of this type may be difficult to establish,[10] particularly when the interface between tumor and underlying tissue is partially obscured by inflammatory cells. Conversely, a tentacular pattern of invasion (Fig. 19-3) is more easily recognizable, and it is found almost uniformly with high

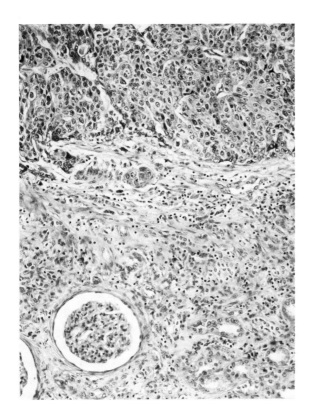

Fig. 19-2 Intermediate grade transitional cell carcinoma of the renal pelvis. The tumor is invading the kidney parenchyma in a predominantly broad front pattern. ×108.

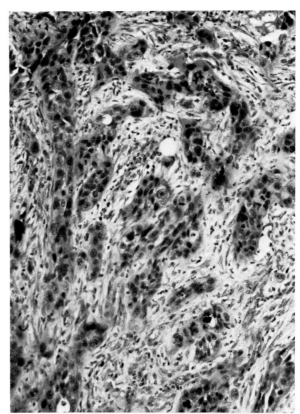

Fig. 19-3 High grade transitional cell carcinoma of the ureter. The tumor is invading in a tentacular pattern. ×262.

grade transitional cell lesions, more commonly solid than papillary. It is also the standard pattern for squamous carcinoma and adenocarcinoma.

Renal pelvic lesions may extend directly into the adjacent renal parenchyma, as illustrated above, but may also show a peculiar manner of parenchymal extension (probably similar to that seen in the prostatic ducts): migration along preexisting collecting ducts (Fig. 19-4). In the "mapping studies" of upper tract lesions reported by Mahadevia et al.,[38] such foci were found in six of the seven renal pelvic tumors examined. The tumor cells appeared to insinuate themselves beneath the collecting duct epithelium, with the surrounding basement membrane still intact. The changes were seen far afield in some instances, involving the entire length of the collecting ducts. At times, we have also seen such spread well removed from the main tumor mass; the potential extent of such changes, without obvious gross alterations,

should be considered if partial nephrectomy is contemplated. As with the prostate, the collecting ducts probably serve as avenues for eventual overt parenchymal and stromal invasion in some cases. The prognostic significance of invasion *limited* to this type is unclear, however. Booth et al.[13] placed such lesions in a separate staging category; and two of three patients whose kidneys showed such involvement, still confined by the collecting duct basement membranes, and who had adequate follow-up, survived for more than 5 years.

The implication of vascular or lymphatic invasion (or both) appears to be similar to that with bladder cancer. Davis et al.,[17] in a study of renal pelvic tumors, found evidence of vascular/lymphatic invasion in 23 patients, 19 of whom had metastases; conversely, among 25 patients without this feature, only 8 suffered metastatic disease. The correlation with tumor grade was as expected, with vascular/lymphatic inva-

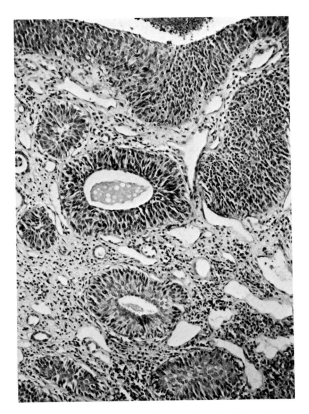

Fig. 19-4 Intermediate grade transitional cell carcinoma. The tumor is extending into the kidney along collecting ducts. ×106.

sion seen in none of the patients with grade I lesions, 25 percent of those with grade II lesions, and 81 percent of those with grade III lesions.

Associated Urothelial Abnormalities

In a study of bladder cancer by Althausen et al.,[1] a correlation was found between the presence of abnormalities in mucosa adjacent to malignancies and the subsequent occurrence of invasive disease. This pathologic feature has also been examined for transitional cell carcinomas of both renal pelvis[43] and ureter[24] in patients seen at the Massachusetts General Hospital. With renal pelvic lesions,[43] only 3 of 66 patients exhibited entirely normal urothelium adjacent to the primary tumor, with a progression in frequency of occurrence of more severe changes with increasing grade of the primary. None of the patients with grade I lesions had more than moderate dysplasia, but 6 of

28 patients with grade II primaries had carcinoma in situ or severe dysplasia in adjacent mucosa, as did 25 of 33 patients with grade III primaries. A similar trend was noted when such associated abnormalities were correlated with the stage of the primary tumors. In a study of ureteral tumors from the same institution,[24] findings were similar, with an even higher percentage of grade III primaries showing associated carcinoma in situ or severe dysplasia (16/19) and with 5 of 25 patients with grade II primaries having associated abnormalities of this degree. All nine patients with grade I lesions, however, showed normal adjacent mucosa. Correlation with increasing stage was also apparent with 100 percent of patients with locally advanced or metastatic disease showing significant associated abnormalities.

In fact, such abnormalities are not limited to the immediately adjacent mucosa, and mapping studies of upper tract specimens have shown that both carcinoma in situ as well as significant dysplasia, with or without associated hyperplasia, may be seen not only immediately adjacent to the grossly apparent primary but also for some distance removed.[16,29,38]

Chasko et al.[16] performed mapping studies on 29 consecutive nephroureterectomy specimens resected for renal pelvic primaries and one partial ureterectomy specimen removed for a ureteral primary. A number of interesting observations were recorded. Similar to the above, all grade I lesions showed, at most, focal minimal atypia in the immediately adjacent urothelium, with only hyperplasia or minimal atypia in areas further removed from the primary. Among the higher grade lesions (II and III), 6 of 23 showed associated unsuspected noninvasive papillary carcinomas. Even more striking, an additional six specimens with associated unsuspected high grade nonpapillary carcinomas were found, one of which was deeply invasive. Six of the nine grade II primaries and all of the grade III primaries showed associated urothelial abnormalities, ranging from atypical hyperplasia to unsuspected areas of carcinoma, with multiple tumors seen in a small but significant number of cases.

Similar widespread associated mucosal abnormalities have been noted in other studies,[29,38] consonant with observations in mapping studies of lower tract disease. As pointed out by Mahadevia et al.,[38] it is of particular interest that, in contrast to the situation with bladder cancer, these upper tract findings are noted in an area that has heretofore been generally inaccessible to manipulation, including biopsy, local resection, and fulguration. They therefore presumably represent basic abnormalities in essentially undisturbed urothelium, lending credence to the "field effect" theory as an explanation for tumor multiplicity and recurrence in urothelial neoplasia.

What is the clinical significance of such associated changes? In the Massachusetts General Hospital study on renal pelvic lesions,[43] 32 of the 68 patients underwent "conservative" procedures (i.e., less than complete nephroureterectomy with bladder cuff). Of these 32 patients, 5 developed tumors in residual ureter segments, 4 of whom had had moderate dysplasia adjacent to the original primary, the other having had associated carcinoma in situ. It is rather striking, however, that the other 27 patients had no recurrence despite the fact that most had associated urothelial abnormalities adjacent to the original primary. It is of even greater interest that the development of tumor in the ureteral stump *did not* appear to have an adverse effect on survival, a fact noted in a number of other series (see below). In the study of ureteral lesions from the Massachusetts General Hospital,[24] the presence of associated abnormalities was also without effect on survival in patients with low stage disease, and patients with high grade lesions appeared to fare equally poorly regardless of whether associated carcinoma in situ was found. One likely explanation for these findings, which again are in contrast to the situation with bladder carcinoma, is that the extirpative nature of the standard therapy for upper tract lesions, and even some of the "conservative" procedures, results in many of these potential sites of further disease being removed along with the original primary.[24]

Adjunctive Studies

Little information concerning the usefulness of adjunctive studies, such as surface antigen evaluation, is available for upper tract lesions, but it is hoped that with systematic application such evaluations may eventually prove to be of some clinical use in the upper tract as well as the bladder.

In one study, Hall et al.[23] retrospectively examined tissue from 29 patients with renal pelvic or ureteral primaries for the presence or absence of surface ABH(O) blood group-related antigens. All patients had been followed for 3 years or longer. Of 13 patients whose tumors were antigen-positive, 9 had noninvasive disease; conversely, 14 of 16 patients with negative tests had invasive lesions, yielding an overall positive correlation of 80 percent. The results were also compared with the grade of the primary and were found to have some independent predictive value for the presence or absence of invasion. As expected, the tumor grade itself was an accurate predictor of invasiveness in low and high grade disease, with neither of the two grade I lesions invasive and, conversely, seven of eight grade III lesions invasive; surface antigen data added little to the picture. With intermediate grade lesions, 11 were invasive and 8 were noninvasive, and thus grade alone gave little indication of whether the lesions were high or low stage. Results of the surface antigen test showed only 2 of 8 with antigen positivity to be invasive, whereas 9 of 11 with antigen negativity were invasive. Thus the test may be of some value for intermediate grade lesions which appear identical by light microscopy.

Obviously, in definitive resection specimens, such retrospective information is of little value at present, as management has already been decided on and carried out. The authors, citing the work of Sadoughi et al.[47] on application of surface antigen assays to cytologic preparations from bladder washings, suggested that such tests might be applied prospectively to upper tract catheter cytology specimens or brush biopsies to help decide on radical versus conservative surgical therapy. Similar to the situation with bladder cancer, however, much more data should be assembled — on the correlation between surface antigen status of upper tract lesions and invasiveness, and particularly on the efficacy of application of the technique to cytologic specimens, as there are numerous potential sources of error to the method.[19] With the advent of ureteropyeloscopy, and thus the ability to obtain adequate preoperative tumor samples, surface antigen analysis may be more effectively utilized in the future.

MULTIPLE UROTHELIAL PRIMARIES

The finding of simultaneous multifocal upper tract lesions is variable in the literature. Fortunately, *concomitant bilateral upper tract tumors* are unusual, seen only once in 224 patients with upper tract disease in the Mayo Clinic series over a 21-year period.[41,42] *Recurrence in the contralateral upper tract* following surgery for the initial lesion was again unusual, found only once in 49 cases of low grade disease[41] and in 3 of 175 cases of high grade disease,[42] for an overall incidence of 1.8 percent.

The incidence of *concomitant ipsilateral upper tract lesions* is variable in the many published studies. The presence of multiple concomitant ureteral primaries shows a wide range in the literature, cited as high as 20 percent of cases in one series[4] but not mentioned at all in others.[41,42,57] In a combined review of 100 patients with renal pelvic primaries, Johansson and Wahlqvist[28] found 11 percent to have multiple tumors in the pelvis proper and 14 percent to have simultaneous ureteral primaries. A large number of patients were found to have a history of phenacetin abuse, however; and in this situation, as well as in others, e.g., "Balkan nephritis" (see Ch. 16), widespread abnormalities might be expected. In a study by Booth et al.,[13] however, a similar percentage of concomitant primary renal pelvic and ureteral lesions (16 percent) was noted among 203 cases of upper tract lesions, although only five patients had a history of long-term analgesic use, with only one judged to be an "analgesic abuser." Still higher figures for concomitant renal pelvic and ureteral primaries have been found in other centers, up to 38 percent in one series.[56]

Bladder tumors, whether preceding, concomitant with, or subsequent to upper tract malignancy, are distressingly common. A significant number of patients with upper tract lesions are in fact diagnosed while being followed for previously resected bladder carcinoma: 23 percent of patients in one series,[13] with similar[8,22] and somewhat smaller figures[4,11,28] in other series. In some studies there appears to be a higher percentage of preceding bladder cancer for ureteral versus renal pelvic primaries, although not so in others. The time interval from the original bladder primary to the subsequent upper tract primary is generally long, with a mean interval of 86 months in the Memorial Hospital experience.[22]

Bladder tumors are found *simultaneously* with upper tract lesions in 7 to 10 percent of cases,[4,11,28,41,42] with similar figures seen whether the upper tract primary is renal pelvic or ureteral. Following surgical treatment of upper tract tumors, the *subsequent* occurrence of bladder carcinoma is again quite high. This is in contrast to the much smaller percentage (approximately 5 percent) of bladder cancer patients who go on to develop upper tract lesions. In the Memorial Hospital experience, 23 percent of patients with renal pelvic primaries developed bladder cancer following therapy,[22] as did 29 percent of patients with ureteral primaries.[8] In contrast to the long latent period between an initial bladder primary and secondary upper tract lesion, the opposite sequence, i.e., upper tract lesion first and bladder lesion subsequently, was relatively rapid, with mean intervals of 21 months (renal pelvic primaries) and 24 months (ureteral primaries). Similar figures were noted from the Mayo Clinic,[41,42] with a slightly higher incidence of subsequent bladder cancer developing in patients with grade II and III upper tract lesions (30 percent) versus patients with grade I lesions (23 percent) and with bladder lesions also seen at a shorter interval in the former group (23 versus 48 months). Experience at both institutions indicates that most bladder lesions (73 to 87 percent) will occur within 3 years from the time of treatment of an upper tract lesion.

Thus the figures for multiple urothelial tumors "in both time and space" in patients with upper tract primaries are impressive. What are the prognostic implications?

Surprisingly, patients with upper tract tumors associated with other urothelial lesions, either in the ipsilateral upper tract, bladder, or both, whether synchronous or asynchronous, appear to fare as well or almost as well as those with isolated upper tract primaries. In the Memorial Hospital data on patients with ureteral primaries,[8] for example, the patients were separated into two general groups: those with associated tumors elsewhere in the urothelium at any time during their course and those without. The authors noted that survival in the two groups was similar "stage for stage, grade for grade, and on combining stage with grade, indicating that survival in both groups was determined mainly by the initial surgicopathologic features of the ureteral cancer rather than by antecedent or concomitant urothelial tumors." This phenomenon has been noted in a number of other major series,[4,24,28,43,46,56] with a smaller number of reports showing somewhat decreased survival for those with upper tract lesions in association with other urothelial tumors versus those presenting with isolated upper tract primaries.[13,22]

The reasons are not clear, as it would appear intuitively that those with multiple lesions should do worse than those with isolated primaries. At least one explanatory factor is that noted above for the apparent lack of influence of associated mucosal atypia; that is, total extirpation of the involved upper tract by nephroureterectomy removes not only multiple upper tract tumors but also potential sites for recurrent tumors from the outset. In fact, in view of the widespread microscopic abnormalities noted on mapping studies of upper tract resection specimens, many of the "isolated" primary cases may have wound up in the "multiple" category had they been dealt with conservatively, with a portion of the upper tract left behind. A second possible factor is the general parallel in grade noted between upper and lower tract tumors. Although not without many exceptions, most low grade upper tract primaries are associated with low grade tumors at other sites,[13,28] and relatively indolent low grade bladder lesions preceding, associated with, or following low grade upper tract lesions would be expected to do little to worsen the patient's prognosis. Conversely, a high stage/high grade upper tract malignancy is quite capable of leading to the patient's rapid demise, with or without the help of an associated bladder tumor of similar aggressive nature. In fact, many studies indicate that those patients with high grade urinary tract lesions are the least likely to develop subsequent bladder tumors, probably in large part due to the fact that they have so little time to do so. Whatever the explanation, it appears that the occurrence of an upper tract urothelial cancer in the setting of "multiple tumors" carries a prognosis that is not much, if at all, worse than that associated with occurrence as an isolated lesion.

THERAPY

In comparison to the therapy for bladder cancer, the treatment of upper tract urothelial carcinoma, as noted, has been relatively standard since the recommendations of Kimball and Ferris[31] in 1934, i.e., total nephroureterectomy with removal of a bladder cuff to include the intramural portion of the ureter. Although lesser procedures of various types have been performed and are noted in virtually every major study, it is difficult to assemble meaningful data on the efficacy of such treatment. The reason is that such procedures have most often been used in special circumstances, notably for patients considered to be poor operative risks for other reasons, patients with bilateral disease, patients with a history of resection of the opposite tract for tumor or other condition, etc. Therefore most studies appear to be inherently biased toward poorer survival in the conservatively managed patients by reason of their selection for such care in the first place, a fact illustrated below.

Arguments for complete extirpation of the involved upper tract are obvious: difficulty in fully characterizing upper tract lesions preoperatively, particularly with regard to stage; the occurrence of multiple simultaneous tumors; the possibility of grossly inapparent mucosal abnormalities either adjacent to or removed from the visible primary; and the potential for recurrence of disease in the portion of the upper tract left behind at surgery. Tumor developing in a ureteral stump left behind, for example, occurs in approximately 5 percent[4] to as high as 40 percent[11] of cases, with most studies showing figures somewhere between, in the range of 10 to 20 percent. For all of these reasons, it appears that total nephroureterectomy with bladder cuff is a reasonable standard approach to upper tract malignancy. Surprisingly, however, despite such arguments, the efficacy of radical versus conservative surgery is not all that clear from the literature.

Booth and associates[13] found a definite difference in survival among their patients with discrete renal pelvic and ureteral tumors according to mode of therapy, with corrected 5-year survival rates of 89.5 percent versus 59.3 percent for those treated by radical versus elective local resection, respectively. Murphy et al.[41] also found lower 5-year survival figures for conservative (75 percent) versus radical (87.5 percent) treatment in patients with low grade upper tract tumors, with even more disparate 10-year survivals (43 percent versus 71 percent). At first glance, the differences are impressive. Yet as the authors noted, of the 47 patients followed, *only two died as a result of urothelial cancer,* and both of these patients had had radical surgery! The figures illustrate the bias introduced by merely stating the comparative survival rates, for, as noted, many of the patients with less than radical procedures had other reasons for the elective surgery, and many of the reasons have obvious influence on survivability. Moreover, numerous studies have noted no differences in survival between radically versus conservatively treated groups.[8,11,22,24,43]

Particularly at the ends of the spectrums of histologic differentiation and extent of disease, it appears at present that the prime determinants of survival in patients with upper tract malignancy are in fact grade, stage, and histologic type of the primary lesion. As McCarron et al.[39] indicated, conservative surgery versus radical surgery may show equally good results for low grade/low stage tumors and equally dismal results for high grade/high stage tumors. The question of conservative versus radical surgery has no simple answer at this point, and the reader is referred to an excellent discussion of the subject by Whitmore[58] for a more in-depth analysis.

On the near end of the spectrum, an argument may be made for a conservative approach to grade I lesions. If properly collected and processed cytologic specimens obtained by selective catheterization—including catheter urine specimens, ureteral and/or pelvic washings, and brush biopsies of the lesion—show no cytologic evidence of significant atypicality, it is unlikely that the lesion is other than a low grade carcinoma. If this is in fact the case, the chances are less than 7 percent that the lesion is invasive and only slightly more than 2 percent that the lesion has extended to the level of the muscularis. Associated inapparent high grade abnormalities in adjacent urothelium are unlikely; if present, they will probably be manifest in the cytologic specimens, the situation will appear as one of "high grade" disease, and will be dealt with accordingly. With the advent of nephroureteroscopy, endoscopic biopsy specimens may obviously add to our ability to characterize these lesions at the outset.

On the opposite end of the spectrum, high grade transitional cell carcinomas, as well as the more unusual squamous and adenocarcinomas, are likely to be adequately characterized as such by preoperative cytologic or endoscopic biopsy examination, with appropriate surgery undertaken. An exciting development in this regard has been the study by Johansson and Wahlqvist,[28] who reported the results of a perifascial approach to removal of the upper tract, with adrenalectomy, versus the standard intrafascial nephroureterectomy for renal pelvic lesions. For *high grade* lesions, overall 5-year survival rates were 84 percent (perifascial) versus 51 percent (intrafascial), with particular note of a reduction in local recurrence in patients treated via the perifascial approach. Among patients with *high stage* malignancies, either confined to

or extending outside the kidney, the difference in 5-year survivals was even more striking: 74 percent (perifascial) versus 37 percent (intrafascial), with the latter figure comparable to those seen in other studies that used the standard intrafascial approach.

For intermediate grade lesions, the cytologic abnormalities preoperatively may not be nearly so striking as those of a high grade lesion, but specimens generally show more than the bland appearance associated with grade I lesions. In these cases, unless the lesion and remaining upper tract can be better characterized by endoscopic biopsy, the discretion of complete upper tract removal may be the better part of valor at the present time. A significant percentage of such lesions (approximately 30 percent) are more than superficially invasive at the time of surgery, with 20 percent or more showing significant associated urothelial abnormalities.

The benefits, if any, of lymphadenectomy at the time of surgery remain unsettled. McCarron et al.[39] noted the absence of metastatic disease in each of six patients with low stage renal pelvic tumors who had had lymph node dissections. Conversely, in six of seven patients who had high stage/high grade renal pelvic tumors, positive nodes were found on lymphadenectomy, and all six patients died with metastatic disease within 1 year. In the Memorial Hospital group of patients with ureteral primaries,[8] 10 of 16 with deeply invasive tumors had dissections of the pelvic and paraaortic nodes, and distant metastases were eventually noted in all cases. Despite these discouraging figures, however, as Batata and Grabstald[7] advised, the addition of routine node dissection to the surgery of deeply invasive upper tract tumors adds little if anything to the morbidity of the procedure, and until more systematic data are assembled the procedure should perhaps be continued. Long-term survivals in patients with positive nodes have been recorded,[28] and knowledge of nodal involvement may eventually prove of some help if effective adjunctive treatment is developed.

Preoperative irradiation, similar to that used for bladder carcinoma, has not been employed in any systematic fashion with upper tract disease, not only because of potential toxicity but also because of the basic difficulty in accurately establishing both the presence and the extent of upper tract malignancies to begin with.[39] The possible benefits of *postoperative* irradiation remain speculative, but this treatment should be given due consideration on a prospective basis, particularly as local recurrence following surgery of upper tract disease remains common (43 percent among those who died of their disease in Johansson's and Wahlqvist's report[28]), in contrast to present-day results with bladder cancer treated with a combined irradiation–surgery approach. Although the number of patients treated was small, a report by Brookland and Richter[15] suggested that at least local control may in fact be improved by postoperative irradiation.

The efficacy of topical chemotherapy has been examined only rarely in upper tract disease[58] with some anecdotal reports of success.[39] The difficulties encountered delivering such agents on a prolonged basis may be formidable, requiring either an indwelling catheter or repeated ureteral catheterization. Moreover, if the effects of the therapy are monitored indirectly, management becomes even more hazardous. With newer methods of direct endoscopic surveillance, this subject may be better explored; but for the present there are many unanswered questions regarding topical therapy in the upper tract.[26]

Finally, if upper tract tumors may be effectively characterized as low grade, endoscopic resection/fulguration may be attempted,[25] with direct laser therapy also having recently been employed with some success.[48]

Systemic chemotherapy of advanced upper tract disease per se has been the subject of only occasional reports, and generally the same agents used for bladder cancer have been employed. Unfortunately, results appear similar to those with advanced bladder cancer, i.e., median survivals of roughly 7 months, with a range of 4 to 14 months.[54,55] More recent reports of certain combined agent chemotherapy regimens[52] suggest that this picture may improve somewhat, however.

In summary, despite the many biologic similarities and identities between upper and lower tract urothelial malignancies, treatment regimens for the primary tumor remain different for various reasons. Foremost has been the relative inaccessibility of the upper tract compared to the bladder, with obvious problems in both initial diagnosis and follow-up. Second, removal of one upper tract simply does not have the same consequences for the patient as does a radical cystectomy, and the loss generally remains "transparent" to the patient if function of the opposite tract is normal. Third, unlike "conservative" surgery for bladder disease, total nephroureterectomy may in fact be technically simpler than at least some of the "conservative" surgical procedures for upper tract lesions, particularly for tumors above the distal ureter.[58]

Nonetheless, there is a movement toward more conservative treatment for upper tract disease; and as noted, it seems logical for low grade lesions. With the development of effective nephroureteroscopy, we may perhaps look forward to safer "conservative handling" of upper tract lesions with regard to better characterization initially as well as possible effective endoscopic therapy. The ability to monitor upper tract lesions directly may also afford a more rational setting for attempts at intensive topical therapy, which is proving to be of increasing success for bladder cancer. Even more novel "kidney-sparing" approaches have been evaluated, such as nephroureterectomy and autotransplantation of the kidney to open directly into the bladder[45] with cystoscopic accessibility for follow-up and topical therapy. In the final analysis, these recent developments are exciting, as the therapy of upper tract disease has been given little attention for the last 50 years. Multiinstitutional cooperative studies in particular, given the small number of patients with upper tract lesions, may indicate some new directions in what currently remain relatively uncharted waters.

REFERENCES

1. Althausen AF, Prout GR Jr, Daly JJ: Non-invasive papillary carcinoma of the bladder associated with carcinoma in situ. J Urol 116:575, 1976
2. Assor D: Inverted papilloma of the renal pelvis. J Urol 116:654, 1976
3. Aufderheide AC, Streitz JM: Mucinous adenocarcinoma of the renal pelvis: report of two cases. Cancer 33:167, 1974
4. Babaian RJ, Johnson DE: Primary carcinoma of the ureter. J Urol 123:357, 1980
5. Bagley DH, Huffman JL, Lyon ES: Combined rigid and flexible ureteropyeloscopy. J Urol 130:243, 1983
6. Bagley DH, Huffman JL, Lyon ES: Flexible ureteropyeloscopy: diagnosis and treatment in the upper urinary tract. J Urol 138:280, 1987
7. Batata M, Grabstald H: Upper urinary tract urothelial tumors. Urol Clin North Am 3:79, 1976
8. Batata MA, Whitmore WF Jr, Hilaris BS, et al: Primary carcinoma of the ureter: a prognostic study. Cancer 35:1626, 1975

9. Beahrs OH, Myers MH (eds): Manual for Staging of Cancer. 2nd Ed. American Joint Committee on Cancer. Lippincott, Philadelphia, 1983

10. Bennington JL, Beckwith JB: Tumors of the kidney, renal pelvis, and ureter. Atlas of Tumor Pathology. Fascicle 12, Second Series. Armed Forces Institute of Pathology, Washington, DC, 1975

11. Bloom NA, Vidone RA, Lytton B: Primary carcinoma of the ureter: a report of 102 new cases. J Urol 103:590, 1970

12. Blute RD Jr, Gittes RR, Gittes RF: Renal brush biopsy: survey of indications, techniques, and results. J Urol 126:146, 1981

13. Booth CM, Cameron KM, Pugh RCB: Urothelial carcinoma of the kidney and ureter. Br J Urol 52:430, 1980

14. Brawer MK, Waisman J: Papillary adenocarcinoma of ureter. Urology 19:205, 1982

15. Brookland RK, Richter MP: The postoperative irradiation of transitional cell carcinoma of the renal pelvis and ureter. J Urol 133:952, 1985

16. Chasko SB, Gray GF, McCarron JP Jr: Urothelial neoplasia of the upper urinary tract. p. 127. In Sommers SC, Rosen PP (eds): Pathology Annual, Part 2. Appleton-Century-Crofts, New York, 1981

17. Davis BW, Hough AJ, Gardner WA: Renal pelvic carcinoma: morphological correlates of metastatic behavior. J Urol 137:857, 1987

18. Di Cello V, Brischi G, Durval A, Mincione GP: Inverted papilloma of the ureteropelvic junction. J Urol 123:110, 1980

19. Droller MJ: Editorial comment. J Urol 127:25, 1982

20. Eriksson O, Johansson S: Urothelial neoplasms of the upper urinary tract: a correlation between cytologic and histologic findings in 43 patients with urothelial neoplasms of the renal pelvis or ureter. Acta Cytol (Baltimore) 20:20, 1976

21. Geisler CH, Mori K, Leiter E: Lobulated inverted papilloma of the ureter. J Urol 123:270, 1980

22. Grabstald H, Whitmore WF, Melamed MR: Renal pelvic tumors. JAMA 218:845, 1971

23. Hall L, Faddoul A, Saberi A, Edson M: The use of red cell surface antigen to predict the malignant potential of transitional cell carcinoma of the ureter and renal pelvis. J Urol 127:23, 1982

24. Heney NM, Nocks BN, Daly JJ, et al: Prognostic factors in carcinoma of the ureter. J Urol 125:632, 1981

25. Huffman JL, Bagley DH, Lyon ES, et al: Endoscopic diagnosis and treatment of upper-tract urothelial tumors: a preliminary report. Cancer 55:1422, 1985

26. Huffman JL, Morse MJ, Herr HW, Whitmore WF Jr: Consideration for treatment of upper urinary tract tumors with topical therapy. Urology, suppl. 4, 26:47, 1985

27. International Union Against Cancer: TNM Classification of Malignant Tumors. 4th Ed. Springer-Verlag, Berlin, 1987

28. Johansson S, Wahlqvist L: A prognostic study of urothelial renal pelvic tumors: comparison between the prognosis of patients treated with intrafascial nephrectomy and perifascial nephroureterectomy. Cancer 43:2525, 1979

29. Kakizoe T, Fujita J, Murase T, et al: Transitional cell carcinoma of the bladder in patients with renal pelvic and ureteral cancer. J Urol 124:17, 1980

30. Keating MA, Heney NM, Young HH II, et al: Ureteroscopy: the initial experience. J Urol 135:689, 1986

31. Kimball FN, Ferris HW: Papillomatous tumors of the renal pelvis associated with similar tumors of the ureter and bladder: review of literature and report of two cases. J Urol 31:257, 1934

32. Koyanagi T, Sasaki K, Arikado K et al: Transitional cell carcinoma of renal pelvis in an infant. J Urol 113:114, 1975

33. Leistenschneider W, Nagel R: Lavage cytology of the renal pelvis and ureter with special reference to tumors. J Urol 124:597, 1980

34. Li MK, Cheung WL: Squamous cell carcinoma of the renal pelvis. J Urol 138:269, 1987

35. Lundell C, Kadir S, Engel R, Nyberg LM: Concurrent renal cell and transitional cell carcinoma in a single kidney: a case report. J Urol 127:761, 1982

36. Lyon ES, Huffman JL, Bagley DH: Ureteroscopy and ureteropyeloscopy. Urology, suppl. 5, 23:29, 1984

37. Lyon ES, Kyker JS, Schoenberg HW: Transurethral ureteroscopy in women: a ready addition to the urological armamentarium. J Urol 119:35, 1978

38. Mahadevia PS, Karwa GL, Koss LG: Mapping of urothelium in carcinomas of the renal pelvis and ureter: a report of nine cases. Cancer 51:890, 1983

39. McCarron JP, Mills C, Vaughn ED Jr: Tumors of the renal pelvis and ureter: current concepts and management. Semin Urol 1:75, 1983

40. Mostofi FK, Sobin LH, Torloni H (eds): International Histological Classification of Tumours, No. 10: Histological Typing of Urinary Bladder Tumours. World Health Organization, Geneva, 1973

41. Murphy DM, Zincke H, Furlow WL: Primary grade I transitional cell carcinoma of the renal pelvis and ureter. J Urol 123:629, 1980

42. Murphy DM, Zincke H, Furlow WL: Management of high grade transitional cell cancer of the upper urinary tract. J Urol 125:25, 1981

43. Nocks BN, Heney NM, Daly JJ, et al: Transitional cell carcinoma of the renal pelvis. Urology 19:472, 1982

44. Parra G, Seery W, Khashu B, Cole AT: Retrograde brushing: improved technique using a catheter-tip deflector system. J Urol 117:693, 1977

45. Pettersson S, Brynger H, Henriksson C, et al: Treatment of urothelial tumors of the upper urinary tract by nephroureterectomy, renal autotransplantation, and pyelocystostomy. Cancer 54:379, 1984

46. Rubenstein MA, Walz BJ, Bucy JG: Transitional cell carcinoma of the kidney: 25-year experience. J Urol 119:594, 1978

47. Sadoughi N, Rubenstone A, Mlsna J, Davidsohn I: The cell surface antigens of bladder washing specimens in patients with bladder tumors, a new approach. J Urol 123:19, 1980

48. Schilling A, Bowering R, Keiditsch E: Use of the neodymium-YAG laser in the treatment of ureteral tumors and urethral condylomata acuminata. Eur Urol, suppl. 1, 12:30, 1986

49. Schulze S, Holm-Nielsen A, Ravn V: Inverted papilloma of the upper urinary tract. Urology 28:58, 1986

50. Seldenrijk CA, Verheggen WJHM, Veldhuizen RW, et al: Use of cytomorphometry and cytology in the diagnosis of transitional-cell carcinoma of the upper urinary tract. Acta Cytol (Baltimore), 31:137, 1987

51. Silverberg E, Lubera J: Cancer statistics, 1987. CA 37:2, 1987

52. Sternberg CN, Yagoda A, Scher HI, et al: Preliminary results of M-VAC (methotrexate, vinblastine, doxorubicin, and cisplatin) for metastatic transitional cell carcinoma of the urothelium. J Urol 133:403, 1985

53. Stragier M, Desmet R, Denys H, et al: Primary carcinoma in situ of renal pelvis and ureter. Br J Urol 52:401, 1980

54. Tannock IF, Gospodarowicz M, Evans WK: Chemotherapy for metastatic transitional carcinoma of the urinary tract: a prospective trial of methotrexate, adriamycin, and cyclophosphamide (MAC) with cis-platinum for failure. Cancer 51:216, 1983

55. Trindade A, Samuels ML, Logothetis CJ: Chemotherapy of carcinoma of renal pelvis: preliminary report. Urology 18:54, 1981

56. Wagle DG, Moore RH, Murphy GP: Primary carcinoma of the renal pelvis. Cancer 33:1642, 1974

57. Werth DD, Weigel JW, Mebust WK: Primary neoplasms of the ureter. J Urol 125:628, 1981

58. Whitmore WF Jr: Management of urothelial tumors of the upper collecting system. p. 181. In Skinner DG (ed): Urological Cancer. Grune & Stratton, New York, 1983

59. Wild RM Jr, Ladaga LE, Copeland JS, Schellhammer PF: Primary mucinous adenocarcinoma of the renal pelvis. Br J Urol 53:195, 1981

20

Nonepithelial Tumors of the Ureters and Urinary Bladder

David Brandes
Robert S. Katz

Nonepithelial tumors of the ureters and urinary bladder include a variety of benign and malignant histologic variants, all infrequent to rare. Benign tumors described in the bladder include leiomyoma, granular cell myoblastoma, hemangioma, giant cell tumor, paraganglioma (pheochromocytoma) and neurofibroma. Pheochromocytomas vary in their biologic behavior and can be either benign or malignant. Leiomyosarcoma and rhabdomyosarcoma are the most frequently encountered malignant tumors of the bladder. Lymphomas, including immunoblastic sarcoma, liposarcoma, and yolk sac tumor, are among the rarer malignant nonepithelial tumors described in this organ.

Benign or malignant nonepithelial tumors of the ureter are rare and account for less than 3 percent of all primary tumors of the ureter.[1] They essentially parallel those in the bladder and are discussed under the appropriate headings. Carcinosarcoma is described in Chapter 18.

BENIGN TUMORS

Leiomyoma

Benign nonepithelial bladder tumors are rare. Among them, leiomyoma is the most frequently observed, with approximately 155 having been de-

scribed in the literature.[55] According to their location in relation to the bladder wall, these tumors have been subclassified into intravesical, intramural, and extravesical varieties. In most cases the growth of the tumors is expansile, and they appear well encapsulated.

Symptoms may be absent in the case of intramural or extravesical tumors and they are often found incidentally at operation.[29a] Intravesical tumors may give rise to symptoms of urinary tract infection, hematuria, or urinary retention or occasionally pelvic pain.[29a,35a] The tumors can be diagnosed by radiologic imaging, intravenous pyelogram (IVP), cystoscopy, computed tomography (CT) scan, or ultrasound.[6a] It has been pointed out that the cytoscopic finding of an intact vesical mucosa overlying a mural mass should heighten suspicion of leiomyoma.[6a]

Histologically, the tumors present the typical arrangement of interlacing bundles of slender smooth muscle cells. The architectural arrangement of the cells may produce a nuclear palisading effect, as is seen in neurilemmomas. The nuclei are elongated and cigar-shaped, and can be seen contained within the central part of the elongated cells. Linear striations produced by intracytoplasmic fibrils can be observed. Masson trichrome stains smooth muscle cytoplasm bright red in contrast to the green staining of collagen. With the phosphotungstic acid hematoxylin stain the cytoplasm appears blue-purple.

Usually the histologic characteristics and staining properties described alone facilitate the distinction from such tumors as neurofibroma, neurilemomma, and dermatofibroma. The presence of pushing, well-circumscribed borders, the lack of nuclear pleomorphism, and the absence or rarity of mitotic figures suffice to distinguish these lesions from the malignant version of smooth muscle tumors. Rare tumors fall into the category of cellular leiomyoma, with the same diagnostic criteria applying to such lesions elsewhere in the body.[29a]

Because most tumors are well encapsulated, total enucleation seems to be the treatment of choice. Prognosis is excellent, particularly as no recurrences have been reported.[55]

Although extremely rare, leiomyomas have also been reported to occur in the ureter. Munir-Zaitoon[41] reported one case and reviewed the literature, which seems to contain about seven additional cases. The patients may present with flank and lower abdominal pain, hematuria, and filling defects with ureterectasis and caliectasis on IVP.

Granular Cell Myoblastomas

Fletcher et al.[14] reported one case of granular cell myoblastoma and reviewed four others cited in the literature. The tumor consisted of a 2-cm nodule that histologically revealed large polyhedral cells with eosinophilic granular cytoplasm, as seen in these tumors in other sites. Nuclei are small and dark with a pyknotic appearance. Unlike most normal smooth muscle cells and tumors of muscle cell origin, the cytoplasm of granular cell tumors does not stain with the periodic acid-Schiff (PAS) stain, thus revealing the absence of glycogen. There have been numerous electron microscopic studies of granular cell tumors in diverse organs. The tumor cells contain dense granules that presumably constitute autophagic types of secondary lysosomes, and the individual tumor cells are surrounded by distinct basal laminae.[16]

Although it was once generally agreed that these tumors were likely to be of muscle origin, many authors now favor a Schwann cell origin for the granular cell myoblastoma and suggest that these tumors should be called granular cell schwannomas.[12] This concept of neural origin of granular cell tumors is based on their more frequent occurrence in tissues other than muscle, their close association with peripheral nerves, and their histochemical and electron microscopic patterns, including positive staining with S-100 protein, a marker for Schwann cells. It has been suggested that granular cells are most likely Schwann cells with cytoplasmic alterations caused by a lysosomal defect of the nature of a storage disease, whereas others favor fibroblastic, histiocytic, or undifferentiated mesenchymal cells as the origin of granular neoplasia. Enzinger and Weiss[10] have discussed in detail the various views on the histogenesis of these tumors.

Christ and Ozzello[7] described a benign granular cell tumor in the urinary bladder of a 23-year-old woman in which they demonstrated myofilaments in the cytoplasm of the tumor cells. However, this particular tumor may represent granular cell changes in a leiomyoma.[10]

Most of the granular cell tumors in the urinary bladder are benign and can apparently be treated by local excision.[40] However, one case of malignant granular cell tumor of the urinary bladder was described by Ravich et al.[48]

Cavernous Hemangiomas

Cavernous hemangiomas are benign congenital tumors,[6c,20,55a] described predominantly in children and young adults,[26] that usually present with gross, painless hematuria.[6c,26] About 25 percent of cases are associated with cutaneous hemangiomas over the abdomen, perineum, genitalia, and thighs.[6c,55a] Histologically, the tumors are located in the mucosa of the bladder; they have dilated vascular spaces containing red blood cells and are lined by endothelium. Diagnosis by pelvic arteriography and scans, with removal of the lesion with a cuff of normal bladder, are the recommended procedures.[20,26]

Neurofibroma of the Bladder

Neurofibromatosis of the bladder is a rare condition, with only 75 cases reported in the literature.[58] The occurrence of neurofibromatosis in the genitourinary tract without other expressions of the disease in other parts of the body is rare.[31]

Clark et al.[8] reviewed 11 cases of bladder neurofibromatosis in children and reported a case in a 3-year-old male child. Two additional cases in children have subsequently been added to the literature by Kramer et al.[31]

It has been proposed that neurofibromas in genitourinary organs originate from the vesicoprostatic plexus in the male patient and from the ureterovaginal plexus in the female patient.[45] Grossly, the tumors tend to invade the entire thickness of the wall of the bladder, with extension to the adjacent organs in the pelvis.[8,58]

In most cases reported, the histopathology of bladder neurofibromatosis revealed a classic plexiform neurofibromatous configuration. Plexiform neurofibromas contain nerve fibers and intermixed fasicles of collagen and Schwann cells embedded in a mucinous matrix. Sometimes they have nodules resembling Verocay bodies.[31,58]

In cases where the urinary bladder is involved by neurofibromatosis, the patient may remain asymptomatic or may present with symptoms of urinary tract obstruction, e.g., urinary frequency, incontinence, and flank pain.[6b] Surgical treatment is performed according to the seriousness of the symptomatology and the extent of the tumor within the bladder. In cases of extensive involvement, radical excision of the bladder with permanent diversion has been recommended,[8] and 13- and 17-year survivals have been documented for two patients treated by such procedures.[8]

Plasma Cell Granuloma of the Bladder

Plasma cell granulomas occur almost exclusively in the lungs,[4] but one case has been reported in the bladder.[28] The tumor had produced dysuria and lower abdominal pain and was diagnosed by excretory urogram and ultrasonic transverse scan. Grossly, the tumor appeared as a moderately well defined multilobulated mass with a firm consistency. Although the lesion involved the entire wall of the bladder and part of the adjacent fibroadipose tissue, the bladder mucosa was intact.[28] Treatment was performed by an open abdominal resection. Histologically, the lesion consisted mainly of plasma cells. Kappa and lambda light chains and immunoglobulins A, G, and M (IgA, IgG, IgM) were demonstrated in the plasma cells, estab-

lishing the polyclonal, non-neoplastic nature of the lesion.[28]

The etiology of these lesions is not well established. In the lungs[4] it is believed they may represent chronic nonspecific inflammation, and the possibility of an immunologically determined pathogenesis has also been considered. Attempts to culture organisms and to stain mycobacteria and fungi have been negative.[4]

MALIGNANT TUMORS

Rhabdomyosarcomas

Rhabdomyosarcoma represents 4 to 8 percent of all malignancies in patients below the age of 15.[60] Its incidence in the general population is 1 per 4.5 per million per year for white children and 1 per 1.3 per million per year for black children. It is estimated that at least 350 new cases of rhabdomyosarcoma occur every year in the United States.[10] A study of the age distribution in 558 cases of rhabdomyosarcoma reviewed at the Armed Forces Institute of Pathology (AFIP) during 1970 to 1979[10] indicates that more than half of the cases are observed during the first 10 years of life, with a second peak between 15 and 20 years. In the younger group there is a preponderance of embryonal rhabdomyosarcomas, whereas in the older group alveolar rhabdomyosarcoma is the preponderant type.[10] In the cases observed at the AFIP, 190 of 558 (34 percent) were located in the genitourinary tract and retroperitoneum. The paratesticular region was the site of preference in 114 cases, followed by the retroperitoneum in 46 cases, the prostate in 15 cases, the urinary bladder in 10 cases, and the region of the common bile duct in 8 cases.

Thus around 20 percent of the rhabdomyosarcomas arise in the pelvic region, principally in the genitourinary tract.[11] In the urinary bladder rhabdomyosarcoma is the most frequent tumor in children under 10 years of age. Mostofi and Moss[39] reported 10 cases of rhabdomyosarcoma in children between 5 weeks and 9 years of age.

Ghavimi and co-workers[17] reported 27 cases of rhabdomyosarcoma of the bladder, prostate, uterus, and vagina in patients between 5 days and 30 years old. In this group there were 6 female patients with primary bladder rhabdomyosarcoma and 16 male patients with prostate, bladder, or retrovesical tumor involving the bladder neck. Fleishmann et al.[13] described 14 cases of embryonal rhabdomyosarcoma of the genitourinary organs, and in 3 of these patients the tumor was located in the prostate–bladder area.

CLINICAL PRESENTATION AND GROSS APPEARANCE

Ordinarily, these tumors originate in the submucosa on the posterior wall of the bladder. They preferentially involve the area of the trigone and bladder neck and cause lower urinary tract obstruction with secondary incontinence, infection, and possibly hematuria. They may be well circumscribed and multinodular, and on cut surface they appear glistening and gelatinous with a grayish color and areas of hemorrhage; sometimes they appear cystic. When these tumors are markedly gelatinous, are myxoid in composition, and form grapelike structures, they are known as botryoid-type embryonal rhabdomyosarcomas.

MICROSCOPIC APPEARANCE

According to the histologic and cytologic appearance of these tumors, they have been subclassified into four large categories: embryonal rhabdomyosarcoma, botryoid-type embryonal rhabdomyosarcoma, alveolar rhabdomyosarcoma, and pleomorphic rhabdomyosarcoma.[10] A correlation between histologic type and primary disease site was apparent from the results of the Intergroup Rhabdomyosarcoma Study.[35] Sixty-seven percent of the genitourinary lesions were classified as embryonal cell type. In 75 percent of those patients with botryoid-type tumors, the primary site was in the genitourinary tract.[35]

Special stains such as Masson-trichrome, PTAH, and iron–hematoxylin may serve to demonstrate intracellular myofibrils and cross striations. PAS stains with and without diastase are valuable, as glycogen is a constant feature in rhabdomyosarcoma cells. Immunocytochemical methods and immunoperoxidase techniques for the detection of myoglobin and myosin may be useful diagnostic tools. Staining for desmin may be particularly helpful.[22a] By electron microscopy it is possible to demonstrate thin (actin) and thick (myosin) filaments with cross-striations in later stages of differentiation of the tumor cells.[5]

Embryonal rhabdomyosarcoma occurs predominantly in children between birth and the age of 15 years. Embryonal rhabdomyosarcomas may be composed predominantly of undifferentiated round cells or may show various degrees of cellular differentiation toward the formation of rhabdomyoblasts (Figs. 20-1 and 20-2). In the well-differentiated areas distinct cross-striations can be seen in the tumor cells (Fig. 20-2). In some tumors the arrangement of the myofilaments at the periphery of the cytoplasm confers a tubular appearance resembling that of the tubular stage of fetal muscle development.

Botryoid-type rhabdomyosarcomas are simply a variant of the embryonal lesion. They are characterized by the gross presentation as grapelike polypoid masses

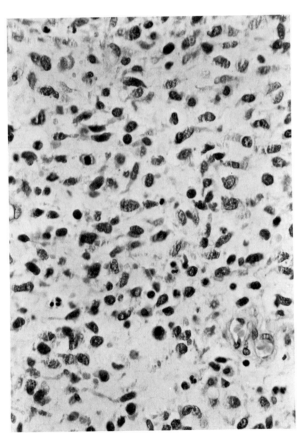

Fig. 20-1 Rhabdomyosarcoma of the bladder, embryonal type. Some cells are poorly differentiated with large pleomorphic nuclei and indistinct cytoplasm. The better differentiated cells are rounded or elongated rhabdomyoblasts with pink cytoplasm. ×390.

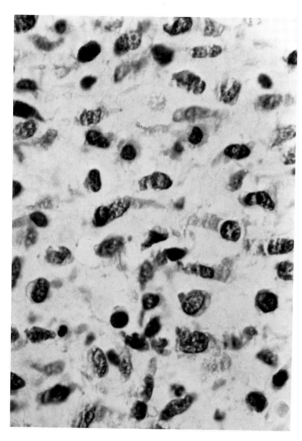

Fig. 20-2 Rhabdomyosarcoma. Higher magnification showing cross-striations in some of the cells (arrows). ×740.

with a shiny surface and a mucoid–myxoid appearance and consistency. This variant of the embryonal rhabdomyosarcoma is most frequently seen in hollow viscera such as the vagina and urinary bladder. A characteristic histologic feature is the presence of a dense zone of undifferentiated cells immediately below the surface epithelium, the Nicholson cambium layer. A superficial biopsy of the bladder mucosa may contain only this layer and convey an erroneous impression as to the nature and degree of differentiation of the tumor. In the more differentiated parts of the botryoid tumor, there are areas where elongated rhabdomyoblasts with cross-striations and strap-shaped and ribbon-shaped rhabdomyoblasts can be seen.

Alveolar and pleomorphic rhabdomyosarcomas are rare in the bladder and prostate. Their histologic appearance are described in Chapter 29.

STAGING

The staging system devised by the Intergroup Rhabdomyosarcoma Study[34,35] is summarized in Table 29-2.

TREATMENT

A marked improvement in survival rate and extension of the recurrence-free interval has been achieved with the development of combined protocols including surgery, radiation therapy, and chemotherapy. Bladder-prostate rhabdomyosarcomas, perhaps because they produce symptoms early, have much better survivals than rhabdomyosarcomas arising elsewhere in the pelvis.[45a] The Intergroup Rhabdomyosarcoma Study (IRS) carried out extensive multidisciplinary/multiinstitutional studies of the various modalities for the treatment of rhabdomyosarcoma.[23,25,34,47]

During the first period of the IRS trial (IRS-I), which included 54 patients with prostate–bladder rhabdomyosarcoma, the prevailing approach was to resect surgically primary tumor followed by radiation therapy and chemotherapy.[23,25] Chemotherapeutic agents included vincristine, actinomycin D, and cyclophosphamide, which were used for years in some cases. The overall survival rate for the bladder–prostate patients included in the IRS-I was 81 percent, which represented an improvement over patients previously treated by surgery alone.

In the IRS-II study[24,46] the primary surgical treatment consisted in tumor biopsy followed only by intense chemotherapy with vincristine, actinomycin D, and cyclophosphamide (VAC) in a repetitive monthly course schedule. Patients might then be subjected to surgical exploration to determine the extent of residual disease, which might be treated by adding radiotherapy to their regimen and continued VAC therapy. Approximately two-thirds of the patients were alive and relapse-free with a median follow-up of 2.7 years. A clear-cut advantage was that two-thirds of the patients were able to retain their bladders, the results being somewhat better than those attained in IRS-I, which included primary surgical treatment. The overall survival rate of the bladder–prostate for patients in IRS-II at the time of the report of Raney et al.[46] was 80 percent.

Ghavimi et al.[17] reported similar results in patients with rhabdomyosarcoma of the bladder treated by a combination of surgery, adjuvant chemotherapy, and two protocols of radiation therapy. They also stated that in their experience the patients who were treated by primary chemotherapy required subsequent use of radiation therapy, extensive surgical procedures or both in order to achieve a disease-free status.

Nodal metastases have an influence on prognosis. In a recent report from the Intergroup Rhabdomyosarcoma Study,[31a] 21 percent of bladder lesions had histologically proven nodal metastases. Three-year survival (for all sites) was 54 percent with nodal metastases versus 78 percent without. Interestingly, there was no difference between histologic types in the rate of nodal metastasis.

When all sites are considered, Hawkins and Camacho-Valasquez[22a] have found that tumors with cellular anaplasia, defined as nuclear enlargement, hyperchromasia, and abnormal mitoses, had a much higher mortality rate than those without (85 versus 30 percent).

Leiomyosarcoma of the Urinary Bladder

Sarcomas of the bladder in general are rare, accounting for approximately 0.5 percent of all bladder cancers. Among adults, leiomyosarcoma is the most frequent type, and yet only about 75 cases have been reported in the literature.[6,42,43,52,54] Leiomyosarcoma of the urinary bladder occurs predominantly in middle-aged or older adults,[6,52,57] without a clear-cut predominance in either sex. Leiomyosarcomas have also been found to occur in children. Weitzner[56] described a leiomyosarcoma of the bladder in a 14-year-old girl and reviewed seven other cases reported in the literature.

Grossly, the tumors involve the lamina propria and muscularis, and they tend to protrude into the lumen. Their consistency is firm and rubbery, but sometimes they have a mxyoid character. Histologically, the leiomyosarcomas are composed of fusiform, elongated cells arranged in interlacing spindlelike bundles. The well-differentiated leiomyosarcomas may show fasicles in which the cells tend to intersect each other at right angles. This fasicular arrangement becomes less conspicious as the degree of differentiation decreases (Fig. 20-3). Perinuclear vacuolation is a common feature in these tumors (Fig. 20-4). Nuclear palisading simulating neurilemmoma is also seen in

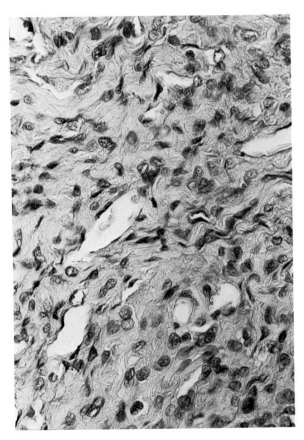

Fig. 20-3 Leiomyosarcoma of the bladder. The nuclei are pleomorphic, and the cytoplasm appears fibrilar in longitudinally sectioned areas. ×370.

some areas. A myxoid variant has been described in which spindle cells with myofilaments were distributed, often in stellate fashion through a myxoid matrix.[60a] Coexisting leiomyosarcoma and transitional cell carcinoma has also been described in the bladder.[6d]

Electron microscopy of leiomyosarcoma cells reveals the presence of cytoplasmic thin filaments, focal densities, dense plaques, and basal lamina material, which are also present in normal smooth muscle cells.[16] It has been suggested[38] that smooth muscle tumors, particularly the malignant varieties, may have a reduced number of such special structures as myofilaments, pinocytotic vesicles, dense plaques, and focal densities.

Immunoperoxidase studies reveal that these tumors stain positively for desmin, muscle-specific actin, as well as vimentin, but negatively for epithelial mem-

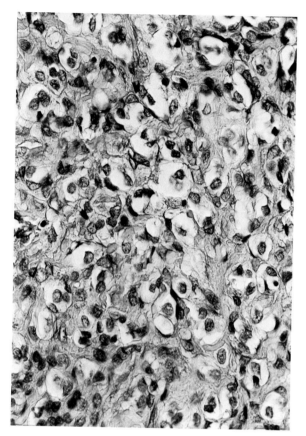

Fig. 20-4 Leiomyosarcoma. Detail of nuclear pleomorphism and perinuclear vacuolation. ×370.

brane antigen, this last serving to distinguish them from carcinosarcomas or poorly differentiated carcinomas.[56a]

Tumors with slight nuclear pleomorphism have been designated grade 1 lesions. The infiltrative nature of the margins distinguishes these tumors from leiomyomas. With increasing nuclear pleomorphism the grades assigned to these tumors range from grade 2 to grade 4.[30] The level of mitotic activity using the scale of 1 to 10 mitoses per 10 high power fields, the occurrence of necrosis, and nuclear atypia also constitute criteria for potential malignant behavior.

The treatment varies from partial to total cystectomy. Irradiation and chemotherapy have not been widely explored for treatment of leiomyosarcomas.[43,52]

Prognosis and assessment of survival varies in different series because of a lack of uniformity in the extension of tumor and treatment. Survival in the series of Swartz et al.,[52] which included patients treated by partial or radical cystectomy, with or without irradiation or chemotherapy, varies from weeks to 10 years.

The development of leiomyosarcoma of the bladder following cyclophosphamide therapy for Hodgkin's disease has been reported in two patients: one in a 17-year-old female and one in a 4.5-year-old boy.[50,51]

Leiomyosarcoma of the Ureter

Only 12 cases of primary leiomyosarcoma of the ureter have been reported in the literature.[31] There is a greater female/male ratio than for the bladder lesion, and the age at diagnosis is between 34 and 79 years.

Signs at presentation may include flank pain, hematuria, and hydronephrosis that may be documented by urography. The size of the tumors at the time of resection varies between 1.0 and 12.5 cm. Radical excision of the tumor seems to be the recommended procedure; radiotherapy is not recommended because of the tendency of these tumors to be radioresistant.[1,18] There are no series with sufficient numbers of cases to allow speculation about the general prognosis of these tumors.

Miscellaneous Rare Malignant Tumors

Primary lymphoma of the urinary bladder, though rare, is the third most frequent group of nonepithelial bladder tumors, after muscle tumors and pheochromocytoma. However, frequent is a relative term, for less than 50 cases have been published.[1a,3,21] to 42. Primary lymphomas in the bladder seem to occur predominantly during middle age and are more common in women.[28] Presentation usually includes hematuria, increased frequency of micturition, and dysuria. Grossly, lymphomas appear as round, nodular masses located in the submucosa with intact epithelium and are more frequently located at the base and the trigone.[3] The tumors likely originate from submucosal lymph follicles, which occur in follicular cystitis,[30] and histologically all lymphoma types may be observed in the bladder.[30] Because of their sensitivity to radiation, x-ray therapy appears to be the treatment of choice,[3,30] with approximately 50 percent of patients so treated surviving 5 years or more.[30]

On occasion, disseminated lymphomas directly involve the ureter[33] and produce urinary symptoms. More frequently, lymphoma in paraaortic and iliac nodes produces extrinsic compression and obstruction of the ureter.

A single case of immunoblastic sarcoma arising as a bladder primary tumor has been reported in a 62-year-old man who presented with nocturia and dysuria and showed pyuria and microscopic hematuria on urinalysis.[15]

A case of extramedullary plasmacytoma of the bladder was reported by Yang et al.,[59] who reviewed the literature and were able to find a single additional case of this rare localization of plasma cell tumors.

Taylor et al.[53] reported the first case of yolk sac tumor of the bladder, with a confirmed diagnosis by immunohistochemistry and electron microscopy. The first reported case of primary bladder liposarcoma was reported by Rosi et al.[49]

Other rare nonepithelial bladder malignancies recently reported have included angiosarcoma,[51a] malignant fibrous histiocytoma,[22a] malignant melanoma,[26a] lymphomatoid granulomatosis (angiocentric lymphoma),[10a] osteosarcoma,[60b] and malignant mesenchymoma,[53a] this last containing fibroleiomyomatous, myxomatous, osteoid, and cartilaginous elements. These lesions generally present, as do other bladder tumors, with hematuria and obstructive or irritative symptoms. Their histologic appearances can be characterized as being typical of such lesions when they occur elsewhere in the body.

Pheochromocytoma

CLINICAL PRESENTATION

Pheochromocytomas of the urinary bladder are infrequent tumors of unpredictable behavior, some behaving in benign fashion, others malignantly. Das et al.[9] described three of their own cases and discussed 97 additional cases reported in the literature. Among the 100 patients the female/male ratio was 3 : 2, and there was a relatively higher incidence during the second decade of life, with 15 patients less than 18 years of age.[9]

Clinically, most pheochromocytomas of the bladder are hormonally active. They may present with hypertension and characteristic attacks related to micturition, including headaches, palpitations, blurred vision, and sweating.[9] There is a known association between adrenal pheochromocytoma and neurofibromatosis, and this has also been reported with the bladder lesions.[6a]

Determination of urinary catecholamines and their metabolites, e.g., metanephrine and vanillylmandelic acid (VMA), is of diagnostic value because these levels are significantly elevated in most cases of urinary bladder pheochromocytoma.[9,22,29] This is particularly true of norepinephrine, which may show a 10- 20-fold increase.[9,29] A 70-fold increase of norepinephrine above baseline after micturition was noted in the case reported by Messerli et al.[36] Reports also indicate that some of the clinical symptoms, e.g., headaches, as well as the elevation of plasma norepinephrine and urinary VMA, are more significant in patients with the malignant variety of pheochromocytoma.[9,29]

PATHOLOGY

Pheochromocytomas of the urinary bladder apparently derive from chromaffin cells of intravesical or perivesical sympathetic plexuses.[9] Most of the tumors are poorly circumscribed. The histologic appearance (Figs. 20-5 and 20-6) is that of polyhedral cells, with acidophilic cytoplasm arranged in nests or as trabeculae surrounded by connective tissue strands containing blood vessels.[19] Pheochromocytomas usually produce a positive chromaffin reaction, a test performed by placing fresh tissue in either buffered dichromate, dichromate in Zenker fixative, or 10 percent potassium iodate in water or formalin solution. A positive reaction is a dark brown color in the tissues and the solution. Positive chromaffinity was established in four of the cases reviewed by Leestma and Price[32] and in the case reported by Jann-Brown et al.[27] The granular material in the adrenal medulla and pheochromocytomas that stains dark brown after dichromate or chromate acid fixation was originally thought to be epinephrine, but it was also shown later that some aromatic compounds containing two OH or NH_2 groups in an *ortho* or *para* position to one another may also produce a brown color after fixation with dichromate. It was also thought that the chromaffin reaction was due to reduction of dichromate to a yellow or brown compound owing to the incorporation of chromium into the chromaffin granules, but it was

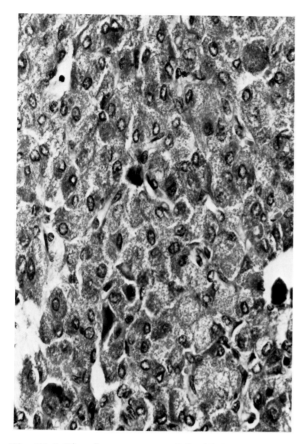

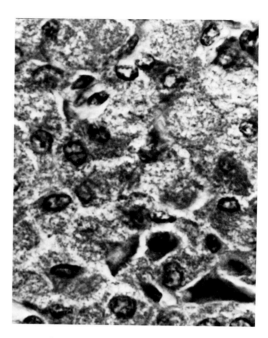

Fig. 20-6 Pheochromocytoma. Detail of characteristic cytoplasmic granularity. ×740.

Fig. 20-5 Pheochromocytoma of the bladder. Cells are polyhedral in shape, and the acidophilic cytoplasm has a granular appearance. ×370.

later shown that it was due to oxidation of the reactive material by dichromate.[44]

A modification of Schmorl's method has also been employed to demonstrate chromaffin granules in a case of pheochromocytoma[44] with tissues fixed in either dichromate-containing fixatives or formalin and stained with Giemsa. In nonchromated tissues the cytoplasm of chromaffin cells stains pink, but the color is green in postchromated tissues. Fontana's silver method for demonstrating chromaffin material was discussed by Leestma and Price.[32] Chromaffin granules appear dark brown by this method. In most of the cases in which either the chromaffin, Giemsa, or Fontana's stain (indicative of catecholamine activity in the cells) was positive, there was good correlation with the functional activity of the tumor, indicated by elevated urinary catecholamines or their metabolites.[32]

The chromaffin cells were seen by electron microscopy[27] to contain abundant dense granules and great numbers of mitochondria, including giant mitochrondria with remnants of laminar cristae.

Moyana and Kontozoglu[40a] have recently published an immunohistochemical study of three bladder paragangliomas. They found that all three stained positively for neuron-specific enolase, S-100 protein, serotonin, somatostatin, vasoactive intestinal polypeptide, and adrenocorticotropic hormone. They stained variably for calcitonin, gastrin, and glucagon. All of these are consistent with their neural crest derivation, and the hormonal activities of paragangliomas and carinoid tumors in other sites. They were negative for keratin, carcinoembryonic antigen, and epithelial membrane antigen, as befits their nonepithelial origin.

As with pheochromocytomas arising in other organs, the basis of establishing the benign or malignant nature of urinary bladder pheochromocytomas remains unresolved.[9] The ordinary histologic criteria of malignancy, e.g., pleomorphism, hyperchromasia, or mitoses, which would be applicable to other tumors, do not contribute to the differentiation between those pheochromocytomas that behave in a benign versus a malignant fashion. It has been claimed, however, that malignant pheochromocytomas may secrete larger amounts of dopamine and some of its metabolites, e.g., homovanillic acid or 3,4-dihydroxyphenylalanine.[2,37] The accumulation of dopamine may result from failure of N-methylation of norepinephrine.[9]

Leestma and Price analyzed the follow-up of 68 patients with pheochromocytoma of the urinary bladder. In a separate analysis of 24 cases presented for the first time by the authors, follow-up was possible in 15, ranging from 1 month to 17 years with an average of approximately 6 years. Recurrent or multifocal tumors at autopsy were seen in two cases. Except for these two cases, which may have represented the development of new tumors or metastases from the original tumor, none of the other cases showed metastases. For the other 34 cases reported in the literature, the follow-up ranged from none to as long as 7 years, with an average of 9 months. There was recurrence of the original tumor in eight cases. In three patients the tumors were considered malignant, with proved evidence of metastases. Treatments of choice include wedge resection or partial cystectomy.[32]

REFERENCES

1. Abeshouse BS: Primary benign and malignant tumors of the ureter. Am J Surg 91:237, 1956
1a. Aigen AB, Phillips M: Primary malignant lymphoma of urinary bladder. Urology 27:235, 1986
2. Anton AH, Greer M, Sayre DF, Williams CM: Dihydroxyphenylalanine secretion in a malignant pheochromocytoma. Am J Med 42:469, 1967
3. Aquilina JN, Bugeja TJ: Primary malignant lymphoma of the bladder: case report and review of the literature. J Urol 112:64, 1974
4. Bahadori M, Liebow AA: Plasma cell granulomas of the lung. Cancer 31:191, 1973
5. Bocher W, Stegner HE: Mixed müllerian tumors of the uterus: ultrastructural studies on the differentiation of rhabdomyoblasts. Virchows Arch [Pathol Anat] 365:337, 1975
6. Bohne AW, Urwiller RD, Pantos TG: Leiomyosarcoma of the urinary bladder with review of the literature. Henry Ford Hosp Med Bull 10:445, 1962
6a. Bornstein I, Charboneau JW, Hartman GW: Leiomyoma of the bladder: sonographic and urographic findings. J Ultrasound Med 5:407, 1986
6b. Brooks PT, Scally JK: Case report: bladder neurofibromas causing ureteric obstruction in von Recklinghausen's Disease. Clin Radiology 36:537, 1985
6c. Chandna S, Bhatnagar V, Mitra DK, Upadhyaya P: Hemangiolymphangioma of the urinary bladder in a child. J Ped Surg 22:1051, 1987
6d. Chen KTK: Coexisting leiomyosarcoma and transitional cell carcinoma of the urinary bladder. J Surg Oncol 33:36, 1986
7. Christ ML, Ozzello L: Myogenous origin of a granular cell tumor of the urinary bladder. J Clin Pathol 56:736, 1971
8. Clark SS, Marlett MM, Prudencio RF, Dasgupta TK: Neurofibromatosis of the bladder in children: case report and literature review. J Urol 118: 693, 1977
9. Das S, Bulusu NV, Lowe P: Primary vesical pheochromocytoma. Urology 21:20, 1983
10. Enzinger FM, Weiss SW: Rhabdomyosarcoma. p. 338. In: Soft Tissue Tumors. Mosby, St. Louis, 1983
10a. Feinberg SM, Leslie KO, Colby TV: Bladder outlet obstruction by so-called lymphomatoid granulomatosis (angiocentric lymphoma). J Urol 137:989, 1987
11. Fernandez CH, Sutow RW, Merino OR, George SL: Childhood rhabdomyosarcoma: analysis of coordinated therapy and results. AJR 123:588, 1975
12. Fisher ER, Wechsler H: Granular cell myoblastoma—a misnomer: EM and histochemical evidence concerning its Schwann cell derivation and nature (granular cell schwannoma). Cancer 15:936, 1962
13. Fleischmann J, Perinetti EP, Catalona WJ: Embryonal rhabdomyosarcoma of the genitourinary organs. J Urol 126:389, 1981
14. Fletcher MS, Aker M, Hill JT, et al: Granular cell myoblastoma of the bladder. Br J Urol 57:109, 1985
15. Forrest JB, Saypol DC, Mills SE, Gillenwater JY: Immunoblastic sarcoma of the bladder. J Urol 130:350, 1983
16. Ghadially FN: Diagnostic Electron Microscopy of Tumors. p. 128. Butterworth, London, 1980
17. Ghavimi F, Herr H, Jereb B, Exelby PR: Treatment of genitourinary rhabdomyosarcoma in children. J Urol 132:313, 1984
18. Gislason T, Arnarson OO: Primary ureteral leiomyosarcoma. Scand J Urol Nephrol 18:253, 1984
19. Glenner GG, Grimley PM: Tumors of the Extra-Adrenal Preganglion System (Including Chemoreceptors). Fascicle 9. Armed Forces Institute of Pathology, Bethesda, 1974
20. Gottesman JE, Seale RH: Cavernous haemangioma of the bladder. Br J Urol 55:450, 1983
21. Gupta DR, Gilmour AM, Ward JP: Primary malignant lymphoma of the bladder. Br J Urol 57:238, 1985
22. Hamberger B, Arner S, Backman KA, et al: Pheochro-

mocytoma of the bladder: a case report. Scand J Urol Nephrol 15:333, 1981

22a. Harrison GSM: Malignant fibrous histiocytoma of the bladder. Br J Urol 58:457, 1986

22b. Hawkins HK, Camacho-Velasquez JV: Rhabdomyosarcoma in children: correlation of form and prognosis in one institution's experience. Am J Surg Pathol 11:531, 1987

23. Hays DM, Raney RB, Lawrence W, et al: Bladder and prostatic tumors in the Intergroup Rhabdomyosarcoma Study (IRS-1): results of therapy. Cancer 50:1472, 1982

24. Hays DM, Raney RB, Lawrence W, et al: Primary chemotherapy in the treatment of children with bladder-prostate tumors in the Intergroup Rhabdomyosarcoma Study (IRS-II). J Pediatr Surg 17:812, 1982

25. Hays DM, Raney RB, Lawrence W, et al: Rhabdomyosarcoma of female urogenital tract. J Pediatr Surg 16:828, 1981

26. Hendry WF, Vinnicombe J: Haemangioma of bladder in children and young adults. Br J Urol 43:309, 1971

26a. Ironside JW, Timperley WR, Madden JW, et al: Primary malanoma of the urinary bladder presenting with intracerebral metastases. Br J Urol 57:593, 1985

27. Jann-Brown W, Barajas L, Waisman J, De Quattro V: Ultrastructural and biochemical correlates of adrenal and extra-adrenal pheochromocytoma. Cancer 29:746, 1972

28. Jufe R, Molinolo AA, Fefer SA, Meiss RP: Plasma cell granuloma of the bladder: a case report. J Urol 131:1175, 1984

29. Khan O, Williams G, Chisholm GD, Welbourn RB: Phaechromocytomas of the bladder. J R Soc Med 75:17, 1982

29a. Knoll LD, Segura JW, Scheithauer BW: Leiomyoma of the bladder. J Urol 136:906, 1986

30. Koss LG: Tumors of the Urinary Bladder. Fascicle 11, 2nd Series. Armed Forces Institute of Pathology, Washington, DC, 1975

31. Kramer SA, Barrett DM, Utz DC: Neurofibromatosis of the bladder in children. J Urol 126:693, 1981

31a. Lawrence W, Hays DM, Heyn R, et al: Lymphatic metastases with childhood rhabdomyosarcoma: a report from the Intergroup Rhabdomyosarcoma Study. Cancer 60:910, 1987

32. Leestma JE, Price EB: Paraganglioma of the urinary bladder. Cancer 28:1064, 1971

33. Lighthelm RJ, Lister TA: Malignant lymphoma of the ureter. Br J Urol 57:587, 1985

34. Maurer HM: The Intergroup Rhabdomyosarcoma Study (N.I.H.) — objectives and clinical staging of classification. J Pediatr Surg 10:977, 1975

35. Maurer HM, Moon T, Donaldson M, et al: The Intergroup Rhabdomyosarcoma Study: a preliminary report. Cancer 40:2015, 1977

35a. McLucas B, Stein JJ: Bladder leiomyoma: a rare cause of pelvic pain. Am J Obstet Gynecol 153:896, 1985

36. Messerli FH, Finn M, MacPhee AA: Pheochromocytoma of the urinary bladder: systemic hemodynamics and circulating catecholamine levels. JAMA 247:1863, 1982

37. Moloney GE, Cowdell RH, Lewis CL: Malignant phaeochromocytoma of the bladder. Br J Urol 38:461, 1966

38. Morales AR, Fineg, Horn RC Jr: Rhabdomyosarcoma: an ultrastructural appraisal. Pathol Annu 7:81, 1972

39. Mostofi FK, Moss WH: Polypoid rhabdomyosarcoma: sarcoma botryoides of bladder in children. J Urol 67:681, 1952

40. Mouradian JA, Coleman JW, McGovern JH, Gray GF: Granular cell tumor (myoblastoma) of the bladder. J Urol 112:343, 1974

40a. Moyana TN, Kontozoglu T: Urinary bladder paragangliomas: an immunohistochemical study. Arch Pathol Lab Med 112:70, 1988

41. Munir-Zaitoon M: Leiomyoma of ureter. Urology 27:50, 1986

42. Narayana AS, Loening S, Weimar GW, Culp DA: Sarcoma of the bladder and prostate. J Urol 119:72, 1978

43. Patterson DE, Barrett DM: Leiomyosarcoma of urinary bladder. Urology 21:367, 1983

44. Pearse AGE: Histochemistry: Theoretical and Applied. 3rd Ed. Vol. 2. p. 1059. Churchill Livingstone, Edinburgh, 1972

45. Pessin JI, Bodian M: Neurofibromatosis of the pelvic autonomic plexuses. Br J Urol 36:510, 1964

45a. Raney B, Carey A, Snyder H, et al: Primary site as a prognostic variable for children with pelvic soft tissue sarcomas. J Urol 136:874, 1986

46. Raney B, Hays D, Maurer, et al: Primary chemotherapy ± radiation therapy (RT) and/or surgery for children with sarcoma of the prostate, bladder or vagina: preliminary results of the Intergroup Rhabdomyosarcoma Study (IRS-II), 1978–1982 (abstract C-293). Proc Am Soc Clin Oncol 2:75, 1983

47. Raney RB Jr, Donaldson MH, Sutow WW, et al: Special considerations related to primary site in rhabdomyosarcoma: experience of the Intergroup Rhabdomyosarcoma Study, 1972–1976. Natl Cancer Inst Monogr 56:69, 1981

48. Ravich A, Stout AP, Ravich AR: Malignant granular cell myoblastoma involving the urinary bladder. Ann Surg 121:361, 1945

49. Rosi P, Selli C, Carini M Rosi MF: Myxoid liposarcoma of the bladder. J Urol 130:560, 1983

50. Rowland RG, Eble JN: Bladder leiomyosarcoma and

pelvic fibroblastic tumor following cyclophosphamide therapy. J Urol 130:344, 1983

51. Seo IS, Clark SA, McGovern FD, et al: Leiomyosarcoma of the urinary bladder: 13 years after cyclophosphamide therapy for Hodgkin's disease. Cancer 55:1597, 1985

51a. Stroup RM, Chang YC: Angiosarcoma of the bladder: a case report. J Urol 137:984, 1987

52. Swartz DA, Johnson DE, Ayala AG, Watkins DL: Bladder leiomyosarcoma: a review of 10 cases with 5-year followup. J Urol 133:200, 1985

53. Taylor G, Jordan M, Churchill B, Mancer K: Yolk sac tumor of the bladder. J Urol 129:591, 1983

53a. Terada Y, Saito I, Morohoshi T, Niijima T: Malignant mesenchyoma of the bladder. Cancer 60:858, 1987

54. Tripathi VNP, Dick VS: Primary sarcoma of the urogenital system in adults. J Urol 101:898, 1969

55. Vargas AD, Mendez R: Leiomyoma of bladder. Urology 21:308, 1183

55a. Vicente-Rodriguez J, Garat JM, Perea C, et al: Hémangiomes vésicaux. J Urol (Paris) 92:43, 1986

56. Weitzner S: Leiomyosarcoma of urinary bladder in children. Urology 12:450, 1978

56a. Wick MR, Brown BA, Young RH, Mills SE: Spindle-cell proliferations of the urinary tract: an immunohistochemical study. Am J Surg Pathol 12:379, 1988

57. Wilson TM, Fauver HE, Weigel JW: Leiomyosarcoma of urinary bladder. Urology 13:565, 1979

58. Winfield HN, Catalona WJ: An isolated plexiform neurofibroma of the bladder. J Urol 134:542, 1985

59. Yang C, Motteram R, Sandeman TF: Extramedullary plasmacytoma of the bladder: a case report and review of literature. Cancer 50:146, 1982

60. Young JL, Miller RW: Incidence of malignant tumors in U.S. children. J Pediatr 86:254, 1975

60a. Young RH, Proppe KH, Dickersin GR, Scully RE: Myxoid leiomyosarcoma of the urinary bladder. Arch Pathol Lab Med 111:359, 1987

60b. Young RH, Rosenberg AE: Osteosarcoma of the urinary bladder. Report of a case and review of the literature. Cancer 59:174, 1987

21
Urinary Tract Cytology

James W. Eagan, Jr.

For most practicing urologists and pathologists the term "urinary tract cytology" brings to mind almost immediately the diagnosis of urinary tract neoplasms. Obviously, many nonneoplastic disorders may also be reflected in the urinary cytology specimen, but the bulk of this chapter is devoted to the diagnosis of neoplastic diseases, urothelial neoplasms in particular.

In this regard, the advent of modern urinary tract cytology is most often dated to the 1945 paper by Papanicolaou and Marshall.[150] In fact, the appearance of malignant cells in urine had been noted in the literature quite some time before, and Grunze and Spriggs[71] credited Lambl[109] with having published the first reported observation of exfoliated cells from bladder cancer in 1856. Thus the technique of cytologic diagnosis of urinary tract malignancies has been around for well over 100 years and widely known for at least 40 years, certainly enough time to have been honed to a fine art. Well, not quite, according to the literature, and certainly not so according to some of our clinical colleagues.

Dr. George Prout, a urologist who has contributed much of value to the literature on urothelial malignancies, reflected on cytologic studies as aids in the management of early bladder lesions[159]:

Discussions among urologists are often earthy, and those about cytology often evoke the most pithy comments. The entire field of urinary cytology seems to be in a surprising state of disarray. When Dr. Papanicolaou's laboratory reported that a tumor was present, it was. Twenty years later, in teaching and community hospitals

alike, there is an immense difference in attitudes about urinary cytology. . . .

In a subsequent editorial on bladder cancer, Dr. Prout further observed[160]:

Cytology is an established technique used for the detection of transitional cell carcinoma. . . . Unhappily, this is irrelevant for many patients and their urologists because ad hoc inquiries suggest that only a third of the urologists in this country have access to good cytologic studies.

Indeed, there is much in the literature to support Prout's observations. In this chapter, we examine some of the reasons for this seeming "disarray," many of which are more of a philosophic than a scientific nature. First, however, we consider normal urinary cytology and certain nonneoplastic diseases that may be associated with characteristic cytologic findings.

NORMAL URINARY CYTOLOGIC FINDINGS

Under normal circumstances voided urine contains relatively few epithelial cells and few cells of other types, e.g., polymorphonuclear leukocytes, red blood cells, and macrophages. Under normal circumstances, however, urinary cytology preparations are usually not ordered by the clinician, and in the average hospital setting most patients for whom the test is performed have either a clinical suggestion of urinary tract disease, an abnormal urinalysis, or both. Thus the sparsely cellular "normal" urinary cytology preparation is unusual in day-to-day practice, and the numbers of both epithelial cells and nonepithelial cells in a given voided specimen may vary widely depending on the disease process. Specimens obtained by catheterization often yield a larger number of epithelial cells in particular, and irrigation specimens a greater number still.

Care must be taken to note the manner by which a specimen was collected for a number of reasons other than just an explanation of the "cellularity" of a given specimen. In particular, the pathologist must gain a "feel" for the natural degenerative changes that occur in cells from voided specimens, especially first morning specimens. These changes may result not only from the lengthy period a given exfoliated cell may have been separated from its nutrient supply but from the nature of the suspending medium as well. Although some of the solutes in urine may pass freely across cell membranes, complete equilibration of intra- and extracellular fluid would not be expected, and urine is often hypertonic, at times hypotonic, and rarely exactly isotonic to the intracellular fluid. Particularly in a hypertonic medium, urothelial cell nuclei may appear increasingly hyperchromatic as fluid is drawn into the surrounding medium, at times mimicking the hyperchromaticity of tumor cell nuclei. Also commonly present in irrigation and catheterization specimens, as well as for some time after any sort of instrumentation, are tissue fragments that may be misinterpreted as having been shed from a low grade papillary tumor.

The manner of specimen preparation may also have some effect on the cell yield and the individual cell characteristics. A number of methods of fixation, slide preparation, and staining may be employed. As with histologic preparations, each cytology method is equipped with its own set of artifactual distortions of which the pathologist must be aware and take into account in arriving at a diagnosis.

Normal Transitional ("Urothelial") Cells

Normal transitional cell epithelium, or *urothelium,* may be divided into three levels: superficial or "umbrella" cells, intermediate cells, and parabasal cells. In contrast to the situation with squamous epithelium, however, the latter two cell types are not readily distinguishable in urinary cytology preparations and urothelial cells are more practically separated into two categories: deep and superficial cells.

DEEP TRANSITIONAL CELLS

In voided specimens most of the normal deep transitional cells have an ovoid or rounded shape by the time of fixation (Fig. 21-1). There is considerable variation in size, with the smallest cells on the order of 10 to 15 μm in greatest diameter. In specimens obtained by catheterization or irrigation, some cells may have an elongated shape (Fig. 21-2). Harris et al.[74] noted that cells with a nonciliated columnar configuration were actually found in most bladder irrigation specimens. The authors cited other possible sources of these columnar cells, including the prostatic ducts and tubules, but suggested that at least some of the cells must be derived from the lining of the bladder itself. The frequency with which they are found in irrigation specimens certainly supports this idea, and many of these "columnar cells" are probably nothing more than elongated transitional cells that retain this shape during the short interval from irrigation to preparation.

Cytoplasm tends to stain uniformly, generally basophilic or intermediate in character, although on careful inspection a diffuse, fine vacuolation may be seen in most of the cells in voided specimens.[92] At times a lighter-staining outer rim is noted.

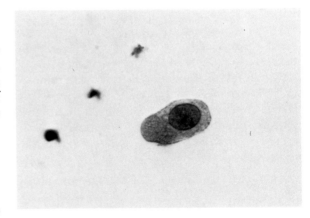

Fig. 21-1 Normal deep transitional cell from a voided specimen. Note the smooth nuclear contour and relatively uniform, finely granular chromatin. Papanicolaou. ×880.

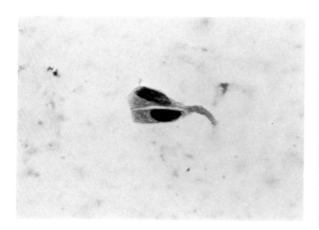

Fig. 21-2 Elongated transitional cells. These cells are a normal finding in irrigation and catheterization specimens. Papanicolaou. ×880.

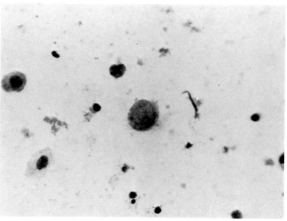

Fig. 21-4 Degenerated transitional cell (center). Markedly enlarged nucleus suggests possible neoplastic change, but virtual absence of cytoplasm indicates advanced cell degeneration. Such "naked nuclei" are not reliable for diagnosis. Papanicolaou. ×352.

The nucleus is ovoid in most cells, with lesser numbers showing rounded or slightly irregular contours. Chromatin is finely granular and uniformly dispersed throughout the nucleus. In degenerated states (Fig. 21-3) the chromatin may become densely hyperchromatic without an easily discernible pattern, or the nucleus may show varying degrees of central clearing with dense clumping of the chromatin around the periphery. Caution is urged in making any interpretation regarding the presence or absence of neoplasia

when such changes are prominent, as they signify a specimen too degenerated to be reliable for diagnosis. Similar caution is also in order when cell integrity cannot be clearly defined, and making judgments on nuclear characteristics when the cytoplasm is not clearly intact may also be hazardous (Fig. 21-4).

Nucleoli are infrequently seen, found in only 1 percent of normal deep cells.[92] If present, they are generally small, are basophilic, and often cannot be definitely distinguished from small chromocenters.

In catheterization and irrigation specimens, sheets of deep cells are common, presumably dislodged by the respective instrumentations (Fig. 21-5). Attached superficial cells may or may not be apparent. Although the presence of these tissue fragments may be startling, their benign nature may be recognized by such features as nuclear uniformity from one cell to the next, a relatively low nuclear/cytoplasmic (N/C) ratio, and the bland nuclear characteristics seen at higher power. Nuclear overlap, or "crowding," a feature that may be found with tumor fragments, is not usually present, but this phenomenon is seen on occasion in nonneoplastic settings.

All of the features described for transitional cells of deep origin are those noted in "normal" cells. It must be stressed that in reparative or reactive states, which are commonly encountered in the population of patients from a urologic service, many of the cytologic

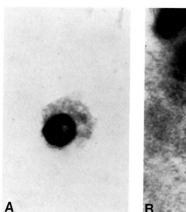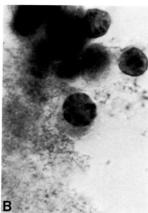

Fig. 21-3 Degenerated transitional cells. **(A)** Partially fragmented cell with karyopyknotic nucleus. Note the dense, hyperchromatic nuclear appearance, with little in the way of discernible nuclear detail. **(B)** Partially degenerated nucleus, with coarse clumping of chromatin along the nuclear membrane and central clearing. Papanicolaou. ×880.

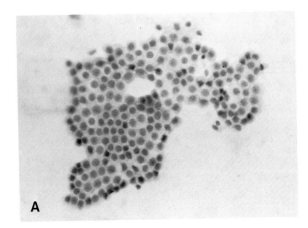

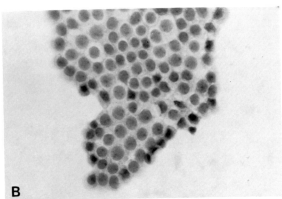

Fig. 21-5 Normal transitional cells. **(A)** Sheet of normal transitional cells, a common finding in specimens obtained with or following instrumentation. **(B)** Sheet of normal transitional cells. Note the bland nuclear features, relative nuclear uniformity, and low N/C ratio. **A,B,** Papanicolaou. **A,** ×220; **B,** ×352.

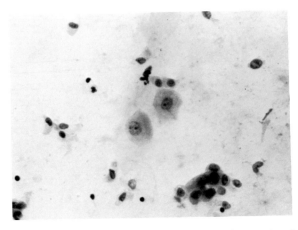

Fig. 21-6 Normal mononucleated superficial transitional cells (center). Note the relatively large size compared with surrounding deep transitional cells. Papanicolaou. ×352.

particularly in irrigation specimens, retaining convex/concave surface contours. The cytoplasm generally shows some degree of vacuolation, and individual vacuoles may coalesce, giving the cell a "clear" appearance.

There is nuclear enlargement that corresponds to the overall cell enlargement, a feature that may serve as a pitfall in cytologic diagnosis. The increase in nuclear size may be striking, particularly in "reactive"

features associated with urothelial malignancies may be seen to varying degrees. The subject of "reactive changes" is discussed in the section, Urothelial Neoplasms.

SUPERFICIAL TRANSITIONAL CELLS

Superficial transitional cells are present in voided specimens and are often prominent in catheterization urine specimens as well as those obtained by irrigation. The major difference between these and deeper cells is one of size, with superficial cells on the order of two to four times the diameter of deeper cells (Fig. 21-6) and at times considerably larger. Contours vary from ovoid to irregularly scalloped, with some cells,

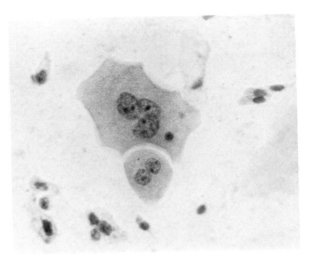

Fig. 21-7 Two multinucleated superficial transitional cells. Note the marked increase in cell and nuclear size of the upper cell in particular, compared not only to surrounding deep transitional cells but also to binucleated superficial cells below. Papanicolaou. ×387.

settings such as cystitis and lithiasis. It is here that one must take into account the N/C ratio, which most often remains low because of the usually generous amounts of cytoplasm in superficial cells. Binucleation is common; multinucleation is frequent (Fig. 21-7); and occasional cells of great proportions (more than 100 μm) that contain large numbers of nuclei may be seen. Koss[98] noted such cells to be particularly prominent in ureteral specimens. Renal pelvic specimens apparently show less striking populations of such cells, however.[74]

Despite the increase in nuclear size, nuclear contours are generally rounded or ovoid (Fig. 21-8). Chromatin dispersion in well preserved cells is uniform, with a finely granular appearance, but an increasingly coarse texture may be seen in reactive states. Nucleoli are often present and may be particularly prominent in reactive states. In multinucleated cells, nuclear size may vary from uniform to moderately disparate.

Perhaps the most important point concerning superficial cells is their lack of reliability in the diagnosis of urothelial neoplasia. According to Crabtree and Murphy,[26] such cells "differ chemically and ultrastructurally from other urothelial cells, are constantly exposed to urine, and are unimportant in the cytologic interpretation of urinary specimens"—observations with which I concur. In fact, "overinterpretation" of cytologic findings on the basis of changes *confined* to obvious superficial cells is one of the major causes of erroneous diagnosis of malignancy. One word of caution is in order here, however, and that is not to go to the opposite extreme and ignore all cells with concomitant nuclear and cytoplasmic enlargement and thereby a "normal" N/C ratio. Occasionally such cells are seen in the setting of high grade malignancy (Fig. 21-9); they are usually recognizable as other than just reactive superficial cells by numerous nuclear features of malignancy in addition to the nuclear enlargement.

Squamous Cells

One sees only occasional squamous epithelial cells in voided specimens from male patients, and they are generally derived from the distal urethra and meatus. They are often much more prominent in specimens from female patients, however. These cells may be from various sources: vaginal contamination; the distal urethra and meatus, which are also lined by squamous epithelium; and areas of squamous metaplasia in the trigonal area of the bladder.[98] Such metaplastic

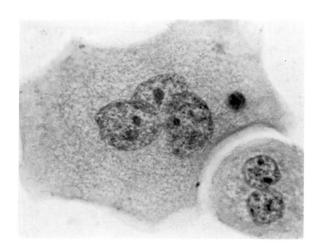

Fig. 21-8 High-power view of superficial cells depicted in Fig. 21-7. Note the marked nuclear enlargement but still relatively low N/C ratio. The larger cell shows a typical nuclear appearance for "reactive" superficial cells, with prominent nucleoli and slightly coarse but evenly distributed chromatin. Papanicolaou. ×880.

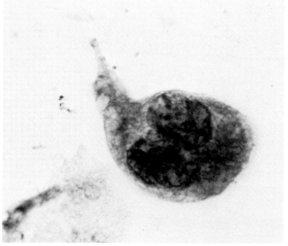

Fig. 21-9 Squamous carcinoma. Note the multinucleated malignant cell with relatively generous amount of cytoplasm. Nuclear features such as marked hyperchromaticity and a coarse, irregular chromatin pattern help to identify it as a malignant cell. Compare to the reactive superficial cell in Fig. 21-8. Papanicolaou. ×1012.

foci are quite common in the trigonal area of the bladder in normal women, and they have been found in excess of 80 percent of adult women with chronic recurrent cystitis.[147] Certain clinical conditions (e.g., paraplegia, with the commonly accompanying lithiasis and chronic urinary tract infections) and other infectious diseases (e.g., schistosomiasis) may be associated with prominent squamous metaplasia, with corresponding appearance of such cells in cytology specimens.

Squamous cells, whatever their origin, have an appearance distinct from that of normal urothelial cells (Fig. 21-10). They may be twice the diameter of the average mononuclear superficial cells but with a much more thinned cytoplasm. The cytoplasm usu-

ally stains basophilic or amphophilic but shows increasing degrees of acidophilia and finally "orangophilia"[62] if keratinization is present. Nuclei, generally smaller than those of superficial urothelial cells, are centrally placed, and the N/C ratio is comparatively low. The nuclei are again rounded to ovoid, with a finely or moderately granular to faintly fibrillar chromatin pattern, again with uniform dispersion. A decrease in nuclear size with an increase in chromaticity may be seen with increasing maturity and onset of keratinization. Nucleoli are generally inapparent and if prominent in cells with recognizable squamous differentiation should give rise to suspicion.[62]

Columnar Cells

Columnar cells (Fig. 21-11) are unusual in voided specimens but, as noted above, are actually found in most bladder irrigation specimens.[74] They are most often nonciliated, but a few ciliated cells are seen on occasion.[74] One possible source for columnar cells is the stratified or pseudostratified columnar epithelium lining the membranous and penile urethra in the male; similar epithelium is found at times in the female urethra. Areas of cystitis glandularis or cystica comprise another source. Various other sources of these cells are also cited, such as the lacunae of Morgagni, glands of Littré, and areas of surface mucous cell metaplasia.[74] Again, as they are seen with such

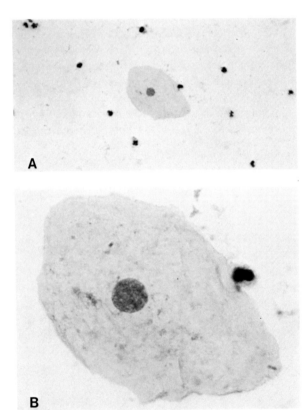

Fig. 21-10 Normal squamous cell. **(A)** Note the large size of the cell, with a relatively small nuclear size and the usual low N/C ratio. **(B)** Typically round to ovoid nucleus with a moderately granular chromatin pattern. The nucleus is usually smaller than that of superficial transitional cells, with nucleoli generally inapparent. Papanicolaou. **A,** ×352; **B,** ×880.

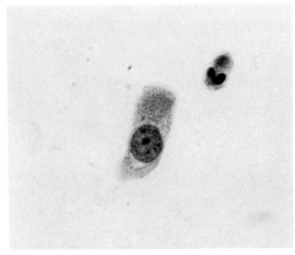

Fig. 21-11 Normal columnar cell in a bladder irrigation specimen. Papanicolaou. ×968.

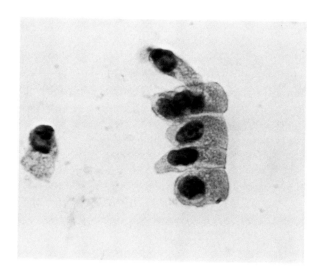

Fig. 21-12 Normal columnar cells. Tissue fragment found in a bladder irrigation specimen. Papanicolaou. ×968.

Another possible site of origin of cuboidal and columnar cells is the prostate, and such cells are often seen following prostatic massage.[98] In younger patients, spermatozoa in varying numbers may be present in the background (Fig. 21-13). Prostate cells tend to shed in clusters (Fig. 21-14) with round, small, evenly spaced nuclei.[98] These are often hyperchromatic compared to those of normal urothelial cells but still have uniform chromatin dispersion. Nucleoli are usually inapparent but are seen at times with prostatitis.[95] If present, they are generally smaller than those seen with carcinoma and are basophilic or amphophilic rather than eosinophilic. The columnar-cuboidal nature of prostatic cells may be recognized only around the periphery of the cell clusters and often is not discernible.

Cells and tissue fragments of seminal vesicle origin may also be present after prostatic massage[98] and, like their counterparts in tissue sections, may show disturbing nuclear features (Fig. 21-15). As with histologic preparations, one should carefully seek the characteristic granular yellowish pigment to correctly identify the origin of such cells.

Renal epithelial cells are rarely observed in cytology preparations in the absence of renal parenchymal disease, according to Schumann and Weiss.[169] These cells are said to vary from cuboidal in the proximal and

frequency in irrigation specimens, it might be presumed that many are in fact just elongated transitional cells. In irrigation specimens, columnar cells not only are seen individually but may also be shed in tissue fragments (Fig. 21-12). Cytoplasm stains basophilic to amphophilic. Nuclear chromatin is again most often finely granular and evenly dispersed, but disturbing hyperchromasia is noted at times.[74] Nucleoli are unusual, and if present, they are generally small.

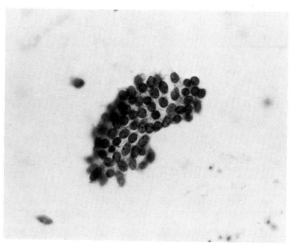

Fig. 21-14 Normal prostatic cells in a voided specimen after prostatic massage. These cells tend to shed in tight clusters; they have small, rounded nuclei that are relatively hyperchromatic compared to those of normal transitional cells. Papanicolaou. ×387.

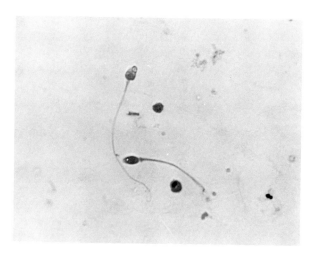

Fig. 21-13 Spermatozoa in a voided specimen after prostatic massage. Papanicolaou. ×968.

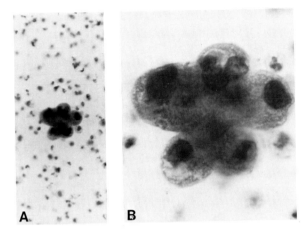

Fig. 21-15 Seminal vesicle cells in a voided specimen after prostatic massage. **(A)** Disturbing-appearing cell group, with inflammatory background. **(B)** Atypical, hyperchromatic nuclei, with irregular nuclear borders. Granular yellowish cytoplasmic pigment seen with routine Papanicolaou stain served to identify these cells as seminal vesicle in origin. Papanicolaou. **A,** ×220; **B,** ×880.

distal convoluted tubules and proximal collecting ducts to columnar in the terminal collecting ducts; but when they present in voided specimens in particular, they may assume much more rounded contours. Such cells may shed individually or in tissue fragments (Fig.

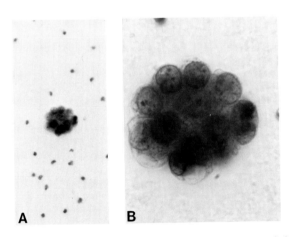

Fig. 21-16 Renal epithelial cells in a voided specimen. **(A)** Cell group, with inflammatory background. **(B)** Cluster of rounded renal epithelial cells with relatively large, but bland, round to ovoid nuclei. Such cells may retain their cuboidal-columnar shape in some instances, particularly in directly obtained specimens such as from fine needle aspirations. Papanicolaou. **A,** ×220; **B,** ×880.

21-16). The former may be difficult or impossible to identify as such and can appear similar to reactive urothelial cells. The latter may be seen with various renal parenchymal diseases and are much more easily identified as to origin when encasing castlike material.[169]

Inflammatory Cells

Inflammatory cells are present to a greater or lesser degree in many disease states and may be seen in very small numbers in the absence of any significant disease. The morphology is generally characteristic in well preserved specimens, with most of the usual cell types easily discerned (Fig. 21-17). Red blood cells are often seen in accompaniment, and they should always be noted in the report. The significance of increased numbers of the various cell types is not always certain, however.

Polymorphonuclear leukocytes are generally abundant with acute inflammatory conditions such as cystitis but may be equally numerous with malignant tumors. Whatever their relation (e.g., tumor necrosis, secondary infection) the inflammatory cells may, by sheer numbers, make difficult the identification of a smaller number of tumor cells scattered throughout.

Lymphocytes bespeak the same element of chronicity as elsewhere in the body. Their presence is nonspecific but, in conjunction with other parameters, may be of some help in specific clinical settings, e.g., monitoring renal transplant rejection (see below).

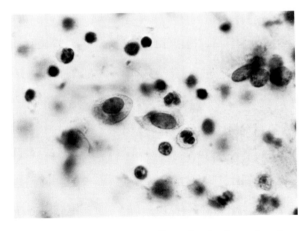

Fig. 21-17 Inflammatory cells. Polymorphonuclear leukocytes and lymphocytes are present, with some deep transitional cells also seen. Papanicolaou. ×880.

Eosinophils may be readily identified in well stained Papanicolaou preparations, by cell and granule size as well as color, with typical bilobed nuclei apparent. If there is doubt as to the nature of these cells, air-dried Romanowsky-stained preparations usually settle the issue, and other methods may be even more efficacious.[143] Their presence has been cited as an aid in the diagnosis of drug-induced acute interstitial nephritis,[113] although significant eosinophiluria may be seen with other disorders, such as rapidly progressive glomerulonephritis and acute prostatitis,[143] and in specimens from patients with recent bladder cauterization.[98] "Eosinophilic cystitis" is discussed below. Although unusual, eosinophiluria may be found with urothelial malignancies, with accompanying prominent infiltrates in histologic sections. The prognostic significance of this finding remains uncertain.

Histiocytic cells (Fig. 21-18) are also rarely present in normal urine but may be prominent in inflammatory states of various types. At times they can be confused with transitional cells, but generally they are even smaller, perhaps half the size of the average well preserved transitional cell. Larger cells, often multinucleated, are sometimes noted, however. The nuclei tend to be more vesicular or "open-faced" than in transitional cells, are usually located peripherally, and may be round or focally flattened; but when they have a reniform shape they are characteristic. Nucleoli are usually detectable in at least some cells. Vacuolated cytoplasm containing phagocytized material may be recognized, particularly in larger cells.

Another type of cell found commonly in urine specimens is the "red inclusion cell" (Fig. 21-19). These cells were described by Bolande[15] in children with viral diseases, and the inclusions therefore were initially thought to be of probable viral origin. In fact, such cells are rather common, with these eosinophilic bodies noted in 43 percent of 500 consecutive urinary specimens examined by Melamed and Wolinska.[124] The inclusion bodies are found most commonly in the cytoplasm and rarely in the nucleus; they vary from barely perceptible to as large as 15 μm in diameter. They are often rounded, simulating engulfed red blood cells in appearance, but they may assume elongated and other odd shapes. There appears to be no correlation with the type of disease, and the inclusions are thought to represent degenerated elements in epithelial cells, which commonly show other degenerated features, e.g., karyopyknosis. Of interest is the finding, on close inspection, of such epithelial inclusions in histologic material as well.[124]

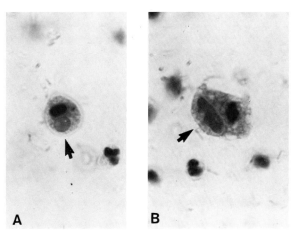

Fig. 21-19 "Red inclusion cells." **(A)** The rounded eosinophilic structure (arrow) appears similar to an engulfed red blood cell, and also may be mistaken for a viral cytoplasmic inclusion body. Note the typical degenerated appearing nucleus. **(B)** Red inclusions may assume odd shapes, such as the elongated structure in the left area of the cell (arrow). Again, degenerative nuclear changes are apparent. Papanicolaou. ×880.

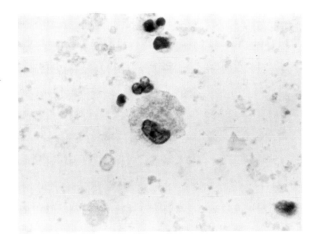

Fig. 21-18 Histiocyte. Note vacuolated cytoplasm and eccentric vesicular nucleus, with a single nucleolus. Papanicolaou. ×880.

Noncellular Constituents

As with routine urinalysis, a number of noncellular constituents may be found in urinary cytology specimens. Perhaps the most commonly seen artifactual element is lubricating jelly (Fig. 21-20), an excess of which can make microscopic examination arduous. Other elements, including crystals (Fig. 21-21), casts (Fig. 21-22), concentric lamellations presumably representing prostatic corpora amylacea[74] (Fig. 21-23), etc., may be present, and at least some may prove to be of diagnostic significance. These elements are often noted during routine urinalysis, but when present in cytology specimens they should be identified and recorded nonetheless. If casts are present, note should be made of any identifiable constituent cells.

Such elements may not be seen as frequently as in fresh urine specimens, presumably the result of disruption and dissolution in processing. Crystalline structures in particular may become more or less apparent than in fresh specimens during the pH modifications of processing.

NONNEOPLASTIC DISEASE

Numerous nonneoplastic diseases of the urinary tract may be reflected in the urinary cytology specimen, with findings varying in degree of specificity. Certain processes, e.g., bacterial cystitis, may be sug-

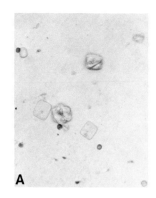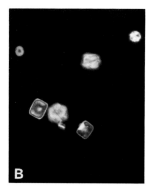

Fig. 21-21 Calcium oxalate crystals. Clear to translucent structures on routine microscopy **(A),** with their crystalline nature more apparent under polarized light **(B).** Papanicolaou. ×220.

gested by the cytologic changes, but definitive diagnosis obviously requires additional tests such as urinalysis and culture. Other processes, e.g., urinary tract cytomegalovirus infection, may result in virtually diagnostic findings.

In addition to searching for specific diagnostic features in nonneoplastic disease, the cytologist should take every opportunity to examine the accompanying changes in the urothelial cell population, which may range from those that are nondescript and nonalarming to changes that can mimic almost perfectly those seen with high grade urothelial malignancies. A firm knowledge of the type and degree of these "back-

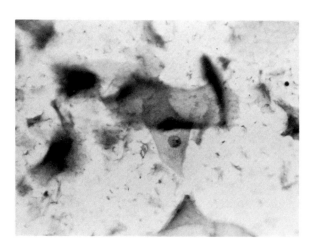

Fig. 21-20 Lubricating jelly in a catheterized urine specimen. Smudgy blue-purple aggregates tend to obscure the cellular constituents. Papanicolaou. ×220.

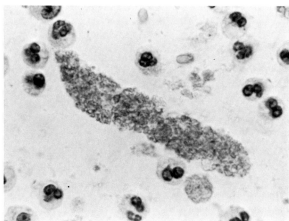

Fig. 21-22 Coarsely granular cast. Some areas show structures suggestive of red blood cell remnants. Papanicolaou. ×880.

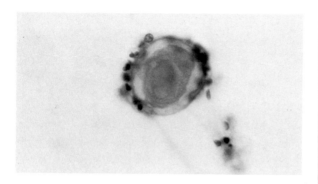

Fig. 21-23 Corpus amylaceum with a typical lamellated structure. Partial rim of degenerating inflammatory cells is present. Papanicolaou. ×387.

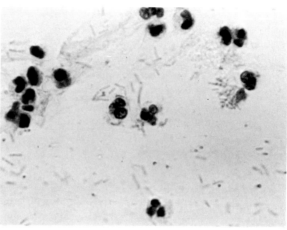

Fig. 21-24 Bacterial cystitis. Note the numerous rod-shaped bacteria, with predominantly acute inflammatory cells. Papanicolaou. ×880.

ground epithelial changes" in various nonneoplastic diseases is an invaluable asset to the pathologist. Indeed, without this asset, the diagnosis of malignancy may be a hazardous business.

Infections

The hallmark of infection is generally the appearance of inflammatory cells, varying in type and number depending on cause and chronicity. Certain infectious processes, however, e.g., upper tract viral infections, may be associated with little in the way of inflammatory exudate. Red blood cells commonly accompany, and at times overshadow, the inflammatory exudate.

BACTERIAL INFECTIONS

The most common entity in this category, acute bacterial cystitis, is usually reflected in the cytology specimen by a plethora of polymorphonuclear leukocytes and red blood cells, and occasional mononuclear cells as well (Fig. 21-24). Bacteria may be apparent, but as any medical intern entering a "floor lab" on a Monday morning knows, urine is a remarkably good culture medium, and the number of bacteria present may depend more on the length of time between collection and specimen processing than the severity of the infection.

As Koss[98] indicated, there may be considerable alteration in epithelial cells in the face of severe inflammation, whatever the cause, and some of the changes may suggest neoplastic alteration. Many epithelial

cells show degenerative changes (Fig. 21-25), including karyopyknosis with loss of fine nuclear detail, karyorrhexis, and cytoplasmic disruption. The pathologist should move cautiously when faced with such changes in the setting of severe inflammation. The safest course is to *never make a judgment* regarding neoplastic alteration strictly on the basis of cells with overt degenerative changes.

Obviously, this becomes problematic with the not infrequent neoplasms accompanied by significant in-

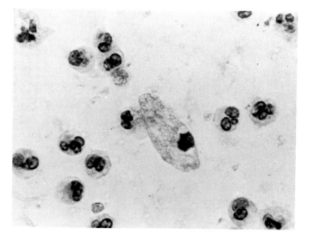

Fig. 21-25 Transitional cell with "reactive changes," related to inflammation. Note the irregular, hyperchromatic nucleus, atypical in appearance, but with poor nuclear detail indicative of degenerative change. Papanicolaou. ×880.

flammation, necrosis, or coexistent bacterial infections, and one should not totally discard the possibility of making a diagnosis of neoplasia just because there is a marked degree of inflammation and degeneration. However, judgments regarding possible neoplastic alteration should be based only on the appearance of cells that are obviously well preserved, and careful search most often delineates a number of such cells. Nonetheless, when a specimen shows severe inflammation and degeneration, one may not be able to arrive at an accurate diagnosis. This should be communicated to the clinician, for if it is possible to clear or reduce the inflammation by, for example, treating a concomitant infection, cytologic diagnosis may become much more reliable.

VIRAL INFECTIONS

Virtually any disseminated viral infection may affect the genitourinary system. The usefulness of cytology as a diagnostic tool in viral infections was suggested by Wyatt et al.[200] in cytomegalic inclusion disease in the pediatric population. The morphologic findings may be virtually diagnostic in some types of viral diseases, notably herpes and cytomegalovirus infections. Indeed, in unsuspected infections the cytopathologist may be the first to suggest a viral process, to be confirmed by serology, culture, or both. It is particularly important to be vigilant for evidence of such diseases in certain patient populations, notably infants, renal transplant patients, and other immunosuppressed groups, especially patients undergoing systemic chemotherapy and those with the acquired immunodeficiency syndrome (AIDS). Careful scrutiny of the cytology specimen for virus-associated changes is important, as not infrequently only a few cells in a given specimen show characteristic features.

Cytomegalovirus Infection

In the early stages of cytomegalovirus infection, viral inclusions may be small and distributed throughout both nucleus and cytoplasm,[98] and definitive diagnosis may be difficult or impossible. Later, with coalescence of the intranuclear inclusions, characteristic cells are seen (Fig. 21-26). They are commonly of renal tubular origin but may arise from other parts of the urinary tract during disseminated infection. They are usually enlarged, at times markedly so,

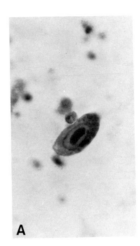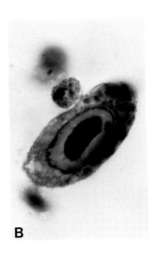

Fig. 21-26 Cytomegalic inclusion disease. **(A)** Note the marked cellular and nuclear enlargement. **(B)** Typical massive intranuclear inclusion body, with halo zone. Papanicolaou. **A,** ×352; **B,** ×880.

standing out even at low power, with a correspondingly enlarged nucleus distended by a single massive inclusion body. This inclusion usually stains uniformly basophilic to amphophilic, with a surrounding clear halo zone. Peripheral to the inclusion is densely packed chromatin material marginated along the nuclear membrane.

Other processes resulting in intranuclear inclusions also typically affect the renal tubular cell, including lead and cadmium poisoning, nephrotoxicity with drugs such as gentamicin, etc.[169] In such cases, however, prominent nuclear enlargement does not usually accompany the inclusions. Indeed, as the name cytomegalovirus implies, the finding of such *greatly enlarged cells* containing enlarged, inclusion-bearing nuclei is quite characteristic.

Herpes Virus Infection

Although the cytomegalovirus is a member of the herpes virus family, the morphologic appearance of infected cells is distinctly different from those seen with other viruses in this group. Among the remaining members of the family, herpes simplex is the most commonly encountered in practice, and here again the cytologic changes are distinctive. Although these alterations are uncommonly encountered in urinary specimens, occasional reports of such have appeared in the literature[119,152] in association with active genital herpes and in renal transplant patients.[17] In the former situation the finding of characteristic cells in urinary specimens may be ascribed to contamination from the genital lesions, although according to Person et al.,[152] the symptom of dysuria with active genital herpes may be indicative of a true associated herpes cystitis, particularly in cases of primary infection.

The cytologic alterations are similar to those seen in routine vaginal smears.[119] Most frequent are multinucleated giant cells, often containing three or more nuclei, with prominent nuclear molding and a characteristic "smokey" or "ground glass" appearance (Fig. 21-27A and B). Less commonly, medium-sized intranuclear inclusions are found, noticeably smaller than those seen in association with cytomegalovirus infections (Fig. 21-27C). A clear perinuclear halo is present. Such inclusions may be seen in either mon-

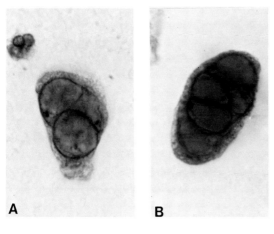

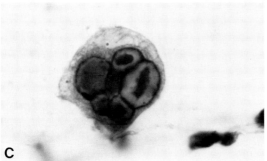

Fig. 21-27 Herpes virus infection. **(A,B)** Enlarged, multinucleated cells, with "ground glass" nuclei and prominent nuclear molding. **(C)** Multinucleated cell with features similar to those seen in **A** and **B,** but with medium-sized inclusions noted in some nuclei. Papanicolaou. ×880.

onucleated or multinucleated cells and are essentially pathognomonic when seen in association with the other nuclear features described above.

Human Polyoma Virus Infection

Human polyoma viruses (HPVs), similar to members of the herpes virus group, are DNA viruses. They belong to one of the major subgroups of the papova virus family, another subgroup of which includes the human papilloma virus. In 1971, human polyoma virus infection was noted in a renal transplant patient by Gardner and colleagues.[65] They isolated and characterized the virus from urine samples of a patient, "BK," after whom the virus was named. (Interestingly, in the same journal issue, Padgett et al.[149] described and characterized a similar papovalike virus cultured from the brain of a patient with progressive multifocal leukoencephalopathy, which they named the "JC" virus.) Subsequent to these reports, Coleman and co-workers[25] demonstrated serologic evidence of HPV infection in 38 percent of renal transplant patients and found prominent cytologic evidence of such infection in urinary specimens from 7 percent of these patients, with less striking evidence in a number more. Similar findings were recorded from Koss's laboratory[88,98,99] in both renal transplant and oncology patients, as well as in 2 to 3 percent of diabetic patients surveyed. HPV has also been described as a cause of intrinsic ureteral obstruction (see Ch. 13). It should be emphasized that these findings are not limited to such patients, and, in fact, episodic viruria may be seen in otherwise apparently healthy individuals for prolonged periods of time.[99]

Although the actual deleterious effects of the viral infection in the genitourinary tract may be uncertain in a given patient, awareness of this type of infection is important on another account: its ability to induce cytologic changes that may mimic those seen with urothelial malignancies.[98,103] These changes are best seen in membrane filter preparations.[24] The affected cells appear enlarged (25 to 35 μm), with ominous-appearing hyperchromatic nuclei, and they often stand out even at low power. In a few cells, a single large, homogeneous, basophilic inclusion may be seen to occupy most of the nucleus, at times with a clearly defined halo zone similar to that seen with cytomegalovirus infection. Much more frequently, however, the inclusion material seems to fill the entire nucleus, and, if a small halo zone is present, often it may be perceived only at the highest magnification under oil. This results in a cell with a disturbingly enlarged, hyperchromatic nucleus, and it is this form that is most commonly mistaken for a malignant cell (Fig. 21-28A and B). Infected cells are usually mononuclear, but multinucleated forms may also be seen (Fig. 21-28C).

Although the homogeneity of the hyperchromatic nucleus, compared to the more coarsely granular appearance of a true malignant nucleus, may give some clue that one is dealing with an HPV infection, distinction from malignant cells may not always be possible. Therefore when presented with such findings in an immunosuppressed patient, one must at least consider the possibility of polyoma virus infection, with confirmatory studies such as viral culture and electron

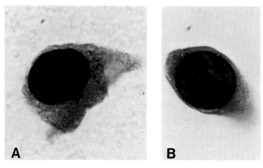

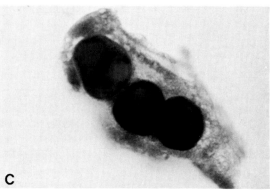

Fig. 21-28 Human polyoma virus (HPV) infection. **(A,B)** Enlarged mononucleated cells, with single huge inclusions occupying most of the nuclear area. Inclusions are homogeneous **(A)** to vaguely granular **(B)**. Chromatin is compressed around the nuclear membrane, and typical cells have an inapparent or only barely discernible halo zone. **(C)** Multinucleated HPV-infected cell. Compressed chromatin rims are better seen than in **A** and **B**. Papanicolaou. ×880.

microscopic evaluation considered.[24] Perhaps more disturbing, however, is the occurrence of such infections in patients with no evidence of immunosuppression. Koss[98] cited three such patients, in two of whom an erroneous diagnosis of carcinoma was made on the basis of the urinary cytology findings.

In fact, infection with human polyoma virus is probably much more common than is appreciated. Serologic studies have shown significant levels of antibody to both BK[64] and JC[148] virus in the general population, with infection acquired at a young age. Presumably, these subclinical infections during childhood may be the source of viruses that in later life lead to clinically apparent HPV infections following disturbances in the immune system. In addition to the usual vulnerable patient groups cited in this regard, the increasing population of AIDS patients must also be kept in mind, as these patients have already demonstrated susceptibility to active HPV infections in the form of progressive multifocal leukoencephalopathy. Therefore it will not be unexpected if we begin to see evidence of urinary tract HPV infection appearing in cytology specimens from this population as well.

TUBERCULOSIS

Although now rare in most Western countries, in many other parts of the world tuberculosis remains the most frequent cause of granulomatous inflammation of the urinary tract.[155] The urinary cytologic findings in 13 cases of bladder tuberculosis were reviewed by Piscioli and colleagues,[155] with all cases having been confirmed by culture and histologic evaluation.

The specimens typically showed an inflammatory background, with "epithelioid cells" seen in 5 of 13 cases. These cells were described as elongated in shape, with finely vacuolated cytoplasm and indistinct cell borders. Nuclei were variable in configuration, ranging from round or oval to "carrot-shaped," pale in color, with finely stippled chromatin. Large histiocytic cells were noted, usually with evidence of extensive phagocytosis. Multinucleated forms were found, in apparent transition to typical Langhans-type giant cells, with the latter seen in 11 of 13 cases. They most commonly showed characteristic peripheral localization of the nuclei, but occasional similar cells with central nuclei were noted as well. Although the authors discussed differential points between these and multinucleated surface urothelial cells, it appears that in some cases difficulty would be encountered in definitely distinguishing the two types of cell. As with histologic preparations, presumably one feature that helps in this respect is the peripheral localization of the nuclei in some of the Langhans-type cells.

Of interest in this study were atypical urothelial cells in the cytologic specimens, with changes ranging from rather mild to those closely mimicking malignancy. In the milder cases epithelial hyperplasia was found in biopsy specimens, with occasional cells having enlarged, hyperchromatic nuclei. In the more severe cases biopsies showed moderate to (in some cases) severe epithelial atypia, approaching the level of carcinoma in situ. Follow-up studies after treatment, however, revealed no evidence of tumor. Although this scenario may be less disturbing because of the relative rarity of urinary tract tuberculosis in many countries, increasing use of bacillus Calmette Guérin (BCG), with attendant granulomatous cystitis[107] and even prostatitis,[181] may prove to be a source of diagnostic difficulty for the cytologist. Urinary cytologic changes in this setting have not yet been well characterized, but the potential for seeing atypical features in these specimens presumably also exists.

FUNGAL INFECTIONS

Clinically significant fungal infections of the genitourinary tract are most commonly seen in immunocompromised patients and also occasionally in diabetics.[53,85,111,165] Most often such infections are part of a systemic process, with genitourinary tract involvement noted in approximately 6 percent of patients with disseminated fungal disease.[146] Isolated genitourinary tract infection is seen less commonly, however,[53,165] and may also be found in apparently previously healthy patients, particularly following the use of systemic antibiotics.[165] Various areas may be involved, either alone or in combination, with the prostate, kidney, and epididymis most commonly affected.[146] The bladder and ureters are involved less frequently, but are perhaps more likely to be recognized cytologically by dint of greater access of the organisms to the urinary pool.

Almost all of the common mycoses, including blastomycosis, cryptococcosis, candidiasis, aspergillosis, etc., have been reported,[53,146,170] with less common organisms, e.g., *Torulopsis glabrata,*[165] also implicated

on occasion. In most reports, the diagnosis has been made as the result of tissue examination, culture, or both. The frequency with which one sees genitourinary tract mycoses reflected in the urinary cytology specimens in such cases is essentially unknown.

In practice, identification of fungal organisms by cytologic means (Fig. 21-29) may be difficult. Frost[62] noted that even chronic fungal infections may cause a chiefly neutrophilic rather than a lymphocytic response, and that the presence of the former might suggest to the cytologist the use of special stains, e.g., periodic acid-Schiff (PAS) or methenamine silver, to more clearly delineate the organisms. If fungi are identified, their presence should always be mentioned in the cytology report. Obviously, the problem of contamination, either from other sources in the patient, notably the vagina, or less commonly during processing, must be considered, particularly for rather common organisms such as *Candida*. Certain findings, such as the presence of organisms in recognizable casts,[5] are of obvious diagnostic significance. The finding of organisms in great profusion should also arouse suspicion of true urinary tract infection, and at times even grossly recognizable "fungus balls" are passed via the urethra.[53] Considering the rarity of these infections in otherwise healthy individuals, the clinical setting must always be kept in mind.

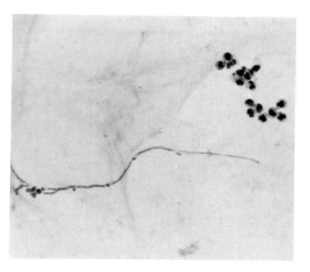

Fig. 21-29 Fungus in a voided specimen. The pseudohyphal form with budding is consistent with *Candida* species. Papanicolaou. ×387.

PARASITIC INFECTIONS

Various parasitic diseases may affect the urogenital tract,[75] either primarily or secondarily, with trichomoniasis the only one seen with any degree of frequency in the Western population. Among the parasitic diseases that may be diagnosed on the basis of urinary cytology, urinary schistosomiasis (bilharziasis) is of major importance in the Middle East in particular. Less commonly, other parasitic infestations, such as onchocerciasis and strongyloidiasis, may be marked by passage of organisms in the urine,[75] and one must be alert for the occasional unexpected parasite that crosses one's microscope stage (Fig. 21-30), preferably secured between two layers of glass. Only trichomoniasis and schistosomiasis are considered in detail here.

Trichomoniasis

Trichomoniasis most often involves the cervix and vagina in the female and is readily diagnosed on routine Papanicolaou smears. However, the organism may also be harbored in the male genitourinary system, with involvement of the urethra, seminal vesicles, prostate, or prepuce. Urethral and bladder involvement presumably also occur in the female, although vaginal contamination may be difficult to exclude in voided specimens. With urinary involvement, symptoms may vary from none at all to those of a "nonspecific urethritis," acute or chronic prostatitis, etc.[105a,183]

The organism responsible, *Trichomonas vaginalis,* is a flagellate protozoan. As with vaginal/cervical material, *T. vaginalis* may be seen in fresh urinary sediment or expressed prostatic fluid, wherein its characteristic frenzied motility may be observed. Relatively accurate diagnosis, however, may be made on the basis of cytologic examination of urine as well as prostatic secretions. The organism is generally ovoid, at times with a pointed protrusion at the flagellated end. It measures approximately 15 to 20 μm, although its size may be variable (Fig. 21-31). The flagellum itself is not seen in cytologic preparations. The cytoplasm has a light green tint with routine Papanicolaou staining and may contain minute but detectable eosinophilic granules. There is usually a single round to ovoid nucleus that is small, eccentrically placed, and generally pale in staining quality. It should be identified for accurate diagnosis, as degenerating cell forms of similar size, e.g., histiocytes, may be mistaken for trichomonads, particularly in the face of severe inflammation. If trichomonads are suspected but not proved cytologically, further evidence may be gained by examination of wet preparations. If necessary, various culture methods may be used to definitively identify the organism, and monoclonal antibody

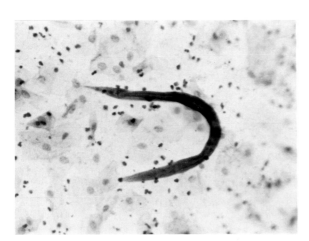

Fig. 21-30 Parasites. This larval form, not further characterized, is seen in a voided urine specimen. Papanicolaou. ×220.

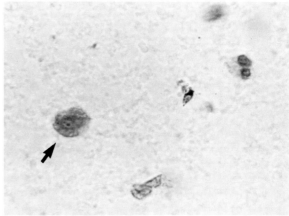

Fig. 21-31 Trichomoniasis. The organism (arrow) has a faintly staining ovoid nucleus. Compare its size with polymorphonuclear leukocyte in the upper right area. Papanicolaou. ×968.

identification techniques may perhaps supplant direct culture in the near future.[105b]

Urinary Schistosomiasis (Bilharziasis)

Of the various pathogenic species of schistosomes, *Schistosoma hematobium* is the major organism encountered in genitourinary tract disease in the populations of Africa and the Middle East, although *Schistosoma mansoni,* ordinarily implicated in gastrointestinal disease, may play a lesser role in these areas and the Western hemisphere as well.[75]

Infestation with *S. hematobium* most prominently involves the bladder and lower ends of the ureters, with deposition of ova resulting in an inflammatory reaction with secondary fibrosis and subsequent obstruction.[38] Associated mixed bacterial infection is frequent. In certain areas, notably Egypt, the subsequent development of bladder carcinoma is extremely common (see also Ch. 16).

Schistosoma hematobium ova are characteristic when seen in the urinary sediment, and quantitation of egg excretion in fresh sediments correlates with activity of disease.[175] The ova are also easily recognized in cytology preparations (Fig. 21-32A and B). They are ovoid in shape, measuring approximately $150 \times 80 \ \mu m$, and show a refractile rim surrounding a darker granular central area in those ova still bearing organisms. A distinctive terminal spine is apparent. An occasional

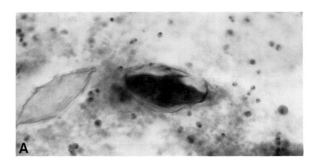
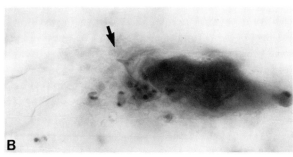
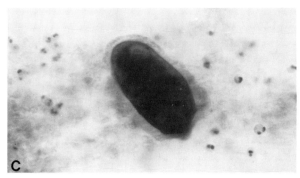

Fig. 21-32 Urinary schistosomiasis (bilharziasis). **(A)** The ovum in the center contains a darkly staining organism. An empty ovum is noted at left. **(B)** Terminal spine (arrow), typical of *S. hematobium.* **(C)** Hatched miracidium, with characteristic ciliary fringe. Papanicolaou. **A,C,** ×220; **B,** ×352.

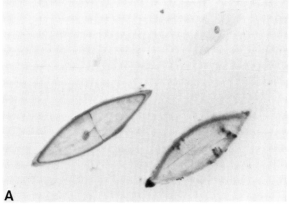
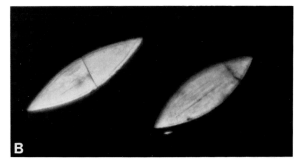

Fig. 21-33 Uric acid crystals — "lemon drop" form. Note the similarity to schistosomal ova **(A)**; Crystalline nature of the structures becomes readily apparent, however, when examined under polarized light **(B)**. Papanicolaou. ×220.

free miracidium, with its characteristic ciliary fringe, may also be noted (Fig. 21-32C).

Although schistosome ova are unlikely to be confused with other organisms or structures in the urine, one possible source of confusion — uric acid crystals — should be mentioned. Generally, they are pleomorphic, assuming various shapes and sizes. One distinct form is the "lemon drop" (Fig. 21-33A), which at first glance may be confused with a schistosome ovum. Examination under polarized light (Fig. 21-33B) readily resolves the issue, however.

Again, it is emphasized that such ova are best seen in fresh urinary sediment and, according to Koss,[98] they were not found in a series of 51 cytology specimens from patients with schistosomiasis in a study by Houston et al.[80] In that study numerous squamous cells were noted in many specimens, a reflection of the secondary squamous metaplasia common in patients with chronic involvement. The background is usually "inflammatory," as a result of the primary infestation as well as the accompanying bacterial infections. Urinary cytology may be a particularly effective diagnostic technique for the detection of bilharzia-associated malignancies,[36] however, most of which are squamous carcinomas.

Other Inflammatory Conditions of the Urinary Tract

EOSINOPHILIC CYSTITIS

Patients with eosinophilic cystitis generally present with frequency, urgency, dysuria, bladder pain not relieved by voiding, and in some instances urinary retention.[114] There is often a strong history of allergies or asthma, with food allergens most commonly implicated. The bladder may show an infiltrate of eosinophils in all layers, and Koss[98] noted that true "eosinophilic granuloma" formation, with simultaneous infiltration of eosinophils and macrophages, may occur. In such cases numerous eosinophils may be seen in urinary cytology specimens.[98] Cystoscopic findings may resemble those seen with carcinoma in situ, including erythema and raised plaques, with occasional proliferative-appearing lesions also noted. A report by Uyama et al.[188] of apparently similar changes confined to a ureteral segment indicates that such lesions are not limited to the bladder.

As noted earlier, eosinophiluria is not confined to patients with eosinophilic cystitis and may be found in a wide variety of clinical situations, including drug-induced interstitial nephritis, rapidly progressive glomerulonephritis, and acute prostatitis.

INTERSTITIAL CYSTITIS

According to Koss,[98] there are no specific cytologic findings in patients with interstitial cystitis (Hunner's ulcer), although recent reports have indicated that increased numbers of mast cells may be seen not only in biopsy material[50] but also in bladder washings from at least some patients with this disorder.[47] For definite recognition of these cells by their metachromatic granules, air-dried Romanowsky preparations or toluidine blue-stained smears are suggested. As with eosinophilic cystitis, clinical symptoms may be identical to those seen with carcinoma in situ of the bladder,[98] and cystoscopic findings may also be confused with those of intraepithelial malignancy.[47] However, patients with symptomatic carcinoma in situ most frequently shed sufficient abnormal cells to allow establishment of a cytologic diagnosis of malignancy.[47] In patients with interstitial cystitis, conversely, reactive-appearing epithelial changes, at most, would be expected.

MALAKOPLAKIA

Malakoplakia, which has been viewed as a manifestation of compromised inflammatory response, most commonly involves the urinary tract but may be seen in a surprising variety of other sites, notably the gastrointestinal tract and retroperitoneum.[178] Bladder involvement predominates, but the disease may occur virtually anywhere in the urinary tract. It is typically a disease of middle-aged women and may be associated with considerable morbidity and mortality.

On cystoscopic examination, variable-sized yellow-brown plaques are noted that are composed predominantly of aggregates of large epithelioid histiocytes[27,178] (von Hansemann cells) with an admixture of lymphocytes and plasma cells. Characteristic Michaelis-Gutmann bodies are seen intra- and extracellularly, although these structures may not be apparent in the early stages of the disease.[178] They are sharply demarcated, spheroid structures ranging from 5 to

10 μm in diameter, with a concentric lamellated ("owl eye") appearance; they stain positively with PAS as well as calcium and iron stains.[178] Various pathogenetic mechanisms of formation have been proposed for these structures, and it appears most likely that they result from mineralization of partially degraded bacteria,[108] most commonly *Escherichia coli.* (See also Ch. 8.)

Melamed,[121] in a cytology case report, noted that even in voided urine specimens prior to instrumentation, there were varying numbers of epithelioid cells with intracytoplasmic Michaelis-Gutmann bodies, identical in appearance to those seen in histologic section. The concentric ring appearance was best demonstrated in the largest structures, with others staining uniformly dark or with dark margins and a pale central area. Michaelis-Gutmann bodies were usually found in intact cells with normal nuclei, and therefore would not be confused with degenerated nuclei in cells undergoing karyorrhexis. Similar structures, according to Melamed,[121] are at times seen in patients with high urinary calcium but no evidence of malakoplakia. However, these structures are extracellular and therefore readily distinguished from the intracytoplasmic structures found in malakoplakia.

Urinary Tract Lithiasis

Urinary tract lithiasis may result in significant cytologic alterations, and the clinician should always inform the cytologist if calculi are present or suspected. An inflammatory background is common, with or without associated infection, and multinucleated epithelial cells are frequent.[10] Associated squamous metaplasia,[10] and at times glandular metaplasia,[167] may result in the shedding of corresponding cells in the cytology specimen. In fact, the presence of large numbers of squamous cells in a specimen from a male patient may suggest the possibility of clinically inapparent lithiasis.

Lithiasis as a cause of false-positive cytologic diagnoses is mentioned time and again in the literature with both conventional methods[10,56,164] and flow cytometry.[93] Calculus-associated abnormalities most commonly mimic those seen with intermediate grade transitional cell carcinoma.[10] Changes similar to those seen with high grade malignancies may also be encountered, and we have seen corresponding histologi-

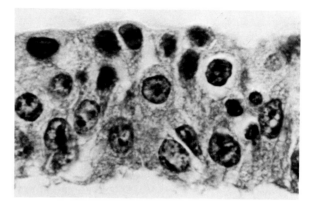

Fig. 21-34 Lithiasis-associated atypia. Renal pelvic mucosa from a kidney removed for a staghorn calculus. H&E. ×880.

cally alarming abnormalities in patients with long-standing calculi without supportive evidence for malignancy (Fig. 21-34). Cytologic abnormalities (Fig. 21-35) may include anisonucleosis, nuclear enlargement, irregularities of nuclear shape, nuclear hyperchromaticity, coarsely granular chromatin pattern, and appearance of nucleoli. Such changes are seen in mononucleated as well as multinucleated cells. Not infrequently, the number of epithelial cells is increased, and epithelial fragments similar to those

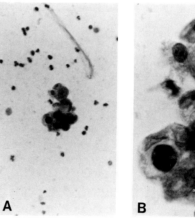
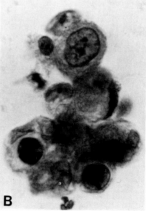

Fig. 21-35 Lithiasis-associated atypia. **(A)** Tissue fragment in a voided specimen, with inflammatory background. **(B)** The nuclei have atypical features, including anisonucleosis, hyperchromaticity, and focally prominent nucleoli. Papanicolaou. **A,** ×220; **B,** ×880.

seen following instrumentation may be present, presumably a result of shearing by the calculus. As with postinstrumentation specimens, such fragments may be mistaken for true papillary fragments, and their appearance in routine voided specimens may be worrisome.

Beyer-Boon et al.[10] discussed various points that may help differentiate calculus-associated changes from those of malignancy, such as the appearance of a large number of multinucleated cells, both abnormal and normal, in the former situation. These authors also discussed the possible etiologic relation between lithiasis and carcinoma (see also Ch. 16). They noted that despite some suggestive differentiating features, the combination of lithiasis and carcinoma in situ in particular may not be able to be excluded on cytologic grounds alone. The pathologist attempting to render a definitive diagnosis of malignancy in the setting of lithiasis should tread carefully. In some cases only careful clinical follow-up following stone removal can demonstrate that some rather alarming cytologic changes were in fact "reactive."[10]

Radiation

Radiation therapy is used for the treatment of bladder cancer, but until recently it was employed primarily as preoperative adjunctive treatment, with radical cystectomy performed shortly after. Of late, however, there has been a renewed interest in definitive radiotherapy for bladder cancer in certain patients, with "salvage cystectomy" for nonresponsive disease. In the situation of definitive radiotherapy and also when there is incidental urothelial involvement caused by radiation applied for nonurothelial malignancies, one must be aware of the cytologic changes that may occur.

Loveless[116] examined serial voided urine specimens from patients given definitive radiotherapy for bladder cancer as well as a group of patients who had had radiotherapy for other pelvic tumors. Radiation-associated changes appeared in urothelial cells at or near a predictable dose level. When the bladder was in the primary field, these changes occurred at about 2,800 rads; and when the bladder was secondarily involved by pelvic radiation concentrated elsewhere, changes appeared after approximately 3,500 rads, at about 3.5 weeks into therapy. As has been noted in biopsy stud-

ies, it is typically at this time that postradiation desquamation of urothelial cells begins to appear with accompanying hyperemia and edema.[46]

Radiation-associated changes in urinary cytology specimens are similar in many respects to those described in gynecologic material[129]. They include cellular and nuclear enlargement, nuclear hyperchromasia, multinucleation, and cytoplasmic vacuolation and polychromasia (Fig. 21-36). Loveless[116] noted that many of these changes are sometimes found in normal transitional cells, superficial cells in particular, and are therefore not completely reliable indicators of radiation effect. It was found with radiation, however, that such changes as hyperchromasia and cytoplasmic vacuolation became more exaggerated, and other findings, e.g., cytoplasmic polychromasia and nuclear

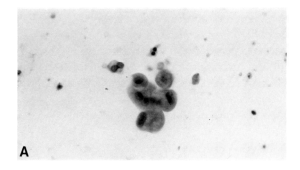

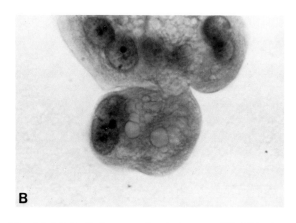

Fig. 21-36 Radiation-associated changes. **(A)** This tissue fragment stands out at low power because of cellular and nuclear enlargement. **(B)** Multinucleated and mononucleated cells show nuclear enlargement and corresponding cell enlargement, with retention of a low N/C ratio. Note the prominent cytoplasmic vacuolation. Papanicolaou. **A,** ×220; **B,** ×880.

pyknosis and karyorrhexis, also appeared. The single most reliable feature appears to be marked overall cell enlargement, with cell size averaging almost twice normal (and up to five times normal in some cells). Nuclear enlargement may be correspondingly striking, but the finding of such nuclei in greatly enlarged cells, with maintenance of a relatively low N/C ratio, is characteristic of radiation damage, as is also true of radiation-induced changes in gynecologic material.[46]

Obviously, similar changes indicative of cell damage may, and hopefully will, occur in irradiated tumor cells. In fact, the alterations may be even more pronounced, and some of the changes may lead to the impression of a higher histologic grade of tumor remaining in the cystectomy specimen than expected on the basis of prior biopsy results, a phenomenon not apparent in cystectomy cases without preoperative radiation.[140] These same alterations may prove to be a source of difficulty in the cytologic follow-up of patients who have undergone definitive radiotherapy. Nonetheless, in the subgroup of patients with persistent viable or recurrent tumor following radiation, a population of cells showing many of the *usual* features of malignancy will generally be noted.[116] A persistently high N/C ratio is of particular value for sorting out radiation-damaged versus malignant cells. If a well preserved subpopulation of such cells can be delineated that one would feel comfortable calling malignant in a nonirradiated patient, in all likelihood the patient indeed has residual or recurrent carcinoma.

In the experience of some authors,[11] radiation-induced changes are virtually always distinguishable from those of malignancy. For others[98] occasional borderline situations may be encountered, and in such situations Koss[98] advised withholding judgment until clear-cut evidence of cancer is obtained on subsequent samples of urine.

In the setting of incidental bladder irradiation, seen most commonly in women treated for cervical carcinoma, one should proceed with equal caution. Obviously, radiation exposure is potentially carcinogenic, and in this group of women the relative risk of developing bladder carcinoma is in fact increased compared to that of a similar population of nonirradiated women. Despite this fact, the actual number of women treated with radiation for cervical carcinoma who develop bladder carcinoma remains relatively small (see Chapter 16 for a more detailed discussion).

Chemotherapy

The morphologic effects of chemotherapeutic agents on urinary cytologic material may be divided into the two categories of how they are administered: topical and systemic. Although the former situation would be expected to be the most problematic for the cytopathologist because of the already proven urothelial malignancy, and also the direct application of the agents to the urothelium, it is systemic chemotherapy that actually poses the greater difficulties.

TOPICAL CHEMOTHERAPY

Various topical agents are used to treat superficial bladder cancer. They are generally employed as adjuncts to surgical resection but occasionally as primary agents, particularly for the treatment of diffuse carcinoma in situ. Thiotepa (triethylene thiophosphoramide)[96,176] remains the most commonly used drug in the United States at present, although more recent reports suggest that it may be supplanted by the increasing use of BCG therapy (see Chapter 18 for a more complete discussion of these agents). Mitomycin C[82,83,176] appears to be at least equally as effective as thiotepa but is considerably more expensive. Other drugs, e.g., doxorubicin,[13,176] are used much less commonly; and still others, e.g., epodyl,[163] have also proved efficacious but are not presently available for use in the United States.

Thiotepa and mitomycin C are alkylating agents, active in their native form. Therefore when used topically, each might be expected to interfere with DNA replication in a fashion similar to that of other drugs in their class such as cyclophosphamide and busulfan. If so, one would also expect the disturbing cytologic changes associated with the latter drugs; however, at least when administered topically, this has not proved to be the case. Murphy et al.[135] suggested that this may be the result of the agents acting in a relatively nonspecific toxic role when delivered topically rather than as specific inhibitors of DNA synthesis.

It has now been shown in a number of studies that neither thiotepa[34,135,141] nor mitomycin C[135] appears to produce cytologic changes that mimic those of malignancy. Instead, the changes following administration are generally similar to those seen in other "reactive" situations. Increased epithelial exfoliation is expected. Some of the individual cell alterations are similar to those seen following radiation exposure but are generally less exaggerated (Fig. 21-37). They include nuclear enlargement with corresponding overall cell enlargement, resulting in retention of a low N/C ratio, and degenerative cytoplasmic changes including vacuolation and fraying of the cell borders. Individual nuclei generally retain their round or ovoid shape but may become wrinkled, reflective of degeneration. A normal degree of nuclear chromaticity is usually seen, but occasional hyperchromatic nuclei may also be noted. According to Droller and Erozan,[34] such nuclei often show degenerative changes as well, with a smudgy appearance to the chromatin. As illustrated in Figure 21-37, most of these changes are seen in superficial cells, a point emphasized by Murphy et al.[135] When confined to such cells, the changes should not be confused with those of malignancy. It is only the appearance of cells with the more conventional features of malignancy that indicate persistent or recurrent disease in the patient with bladder cancer. Multiple studies[34,135,141] indicate that these cells are generally readily discernible from reactive cells. This fact is of particular note, as the effects of topical agents, epithelial denudation in particular, often render accurate cystoscopic and histologic eval-

uation difficult in these patients, with the burden of follow-up at times falling to the cytopathologist. In the study of Murphy et al.,[135] cytologic confirmation of recurrent tumor preceded histologic confirmation in 8 of 13 cases, with tumor cells appearing in the cytology specimen an average of 14 months before histologic confirmation.

SYSTEMIC CHEMOTHERAPY

Among systemic chemotherapeutic agents two are of particular note in urinary cytology: *cyclophosphamide* and *busulfan*. Both are alkylating agents, of the same family as thiotepa and mitomycin C, and both have been employed in the treatment of systemic malignancies. They have also been used to induce immunosuppression in the treatment of certain nonneoplastic disorders, e.g., lupus erythematosus and severe psoriasis, and as part of preprocedural regimens in patients undergoing bone marrow transplantation.

Of the two, cyclophosphamide has more clinically apparent effects on the urothelium, with hemorrhagic cystitis occurring in a small but significant number of patients treated.[9] Busulfan, conversely, has only rarely been implicated in the development of clinically apparent cystitis.[125] Both drugs, however, may be associated with widespread epithelial abnormalities, including striking alterations of the urothelium.[54,104,139]

Forni et al.[54] described the urothelial changes associated with cyclophosphamide therapy in detail. They noted some similarities to those seen following irradiation, most strikingly variable but sometimes marked cell enlargement, with corresponding nuclear enlargement (Fig. 21-38). In contrast to typical radiation effects, however, the nucleus appeared disproportionately enlarged in some cells, with an increase in the N/C ratio. The enlarged nuclei were often eccentric, slightly irregular in outline, and markedly hyperchromatic. Chromatin was sometimes coarsely granular but generally evenly distributed, resulting in a "salt and pepper" appearance. One or two nucleoli were often seen, sometimes large and frequently irregular in shape. Degenerative changes, including nuclear pyknosis and karyorrhexis, were noted in some cells. Again, similar to radiation effect, the cytoplasm showed marked vacuolation, at times containing particulate material or polymorphonuclear leuko-

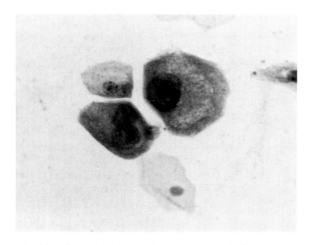

Fig. 21-37 Topical chemotherapy-associated changes in a patient treated with topical thiotepa. Note that changes typically are most prominent in superficial cells, with both nuclear and cell enlargement, retention of a low N/C ratio, some degree of nuclear hyperchromaticity, and loss of fine nuclear detail. Papanicolaou. ×352.

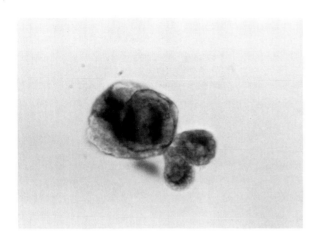

Fig. 21-38 Systemic chemotherapy-associated changes in a patient with a history of cyclophosphamide therapy for lymphoma. Occasional markedly atypical cells were noted in this urinary cytology specimen, with disproportionate nuclear enlargement, nuclear hyperchromaticity, and degenerative-type changes in both nucleus and cytoplasm. Papanicolaou. ×880.

cytes. According to other studies from Koss's laboratory,[98,104] the cytologic abnormalities encountered with busulfan are similar.

Such alterations may result in an extremely atypical urinary cytology picture which can be difficult or impossible to distinguish from that seen with carcinoma.[54] As noted in Chapter 16, at least for cyclophosphamide, the morphologic similarities have proved to be more than just "mimetic" at times, and a number of cases of urothelial carcinoma associated with a history of cyclophosphamide treatment have now been reported.[19,63,120] Most such patients have received more than 150 g of cyclophosphamide (total dose), with the average time lapse from treatment to discovery of urothelial malignancy approximately 7 years.[120]

It is of obvious importance for the cytopathologist to be aware of a history of such drug therapy, and one should move with caution diagnostically in this situation. It seems prudent to follow patients who have survived for lengthy periods after courses of cyclophosphamide with periodic cytologies. If abnormal cells are found, a combined diagnostic approach is suggested,[120] including cystoscopy, excretory urography, urinary cytology, and directed biopsy evaluation.

Renal Transplantation

Renal transplantation, once limited to a few major academic centers, is now relatively commonplace. It remains the most widely practiced and successful among major organ transplantations. Despite therapeutic improvements, graft rejection continues to be the most difficult problem for renal transplant recipients. Urinary cytology, in conjunction with other clinical and laboratory studies, has proved to be of some use for monitoring this complication, and in some centers it is supplemented by direct fine needle aspiration cytology.[76,77]

Allograft rejection has traditionally been divided into three phases[169]: (1) hyperacute rejection, occurring within minutes to hours posttransplantation; (2) acute rejection, occurring as early as 2 days posttransplantation, but potentially occurring episodically at any time during the life of the transplanted organ; and (3) chronic rejection, occurring progressively over the course of months to years posttransplantation. Hyperacute rejection generally results in rapid loss of the transplanted organ, and examination of the urinary sediment, if indeed urine is produced at all, is not a major consideration in clinical management. At the opposite end of the spectrum, chronic rejection results in gradual deterioration of graft function, with no specific therapy of value aside from control of acute episodes. It is in the intermediate form, acute rejection, where the cytopathologist may be of some value in clinical management of renal transplant patients.

Characteristic urinary cytologic findings have been proposed as indicative of acute graft rejection.[18,145,168,169] Such findings include the presence of increased numbers of lymphocytes (especially those demonstrating pyroninophilia[4,81]), tubular lining cells (particularly those with apparent degenerative changes), casts, and red blood cells set in a background of amorphous and cellular debris (Fig. 21-39). In a study by Bossen et al.,[18] such elements, usually in combination, were prominent in specimens taken during ten rejection episodes among nine patients but were found in none of 135 urinary specimens from 13 transplant patients with no evidence of rejection. Most reliable were the findings of increased numbers of lymphocytes and moderate numbers of tubular lining cells.

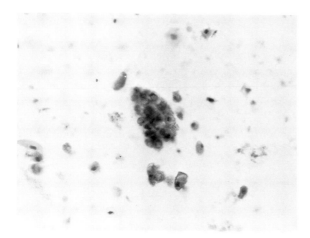

Fig. 21-39 Renal transplant rejection. Partially degenerated renal tubular cell cast and individual tubular lining cells are set in an inflamed, debris-laden background. Papanicolaou. ×220.

Some authors[86,168,169] have advocated the use of cytocentrifugation techniques, with quantitation of the various elements, reported as the number/per ten high power fields. The pattern of abnormalities seen in the urinary sediment may be of help in differentiating rejection episodes from other problems incurred by these patients, such as acute tubular necrosis and transplantation glomerulopathy.[86] Other investigators[81,184] have emphasized single facets, such as the degree of lymphocyturia, in the diagnosis of rejection episodes. However, reliance on single features for the diagnosis of rejection may be more likely to lead to false-positive diagnoses than is reliance on a profile of the various features in combination.[18] Methods to expand the information available, such as the subtyping of lymphocytes present,[185] are undergoing evaluation in an attempt to increase accuracy. This is of importance because one of the most valuable assets of cytology is that the suggestive findings may precede clinical and other laboratory evidence of rejection in many cases by days to weeks.[18,185] The obvious corollary, however, is that the diagnosis may thus not be substantiated by other means, and treatment of rejection episodes is not without hazard. For practical purposes, as advised by Schumann and Weiss,[169] sequential urinary evaluation of these patients may be of great help; and if performed at defined intervals, changes against the patients' own baseline findings may provide valuable information.

URINARY CYTOLOGY OF NEOPLASIA

Urothelial Neoplasms

There are numerous pros and cons regarding the value of urinary cytology in the diagnosis of urothelial malignancies. Among its many assets, the method would seem ideally suited to the diagnostic problem. That is, we are faced with the development of neoplastic change in a relatively inaccessible area, yet one that is bathed throughout its reaches by readily accessible fluid into which cells are shed that may indicate the presence of malignancy. As multifocal disease is so common with urothelial malignancy, this ability to "survey" virtually the entirety of the urothelium in a single specimen is obviously of great value.

Another asset of the method is that it can be performed with relatively simple, inexpensive equipment and supplies; and with a reasonably diligent approach on the part of the laboratory, excellent preparations can be obtained. This presumes of course that specimens are submitted expeditiously to the laboratory by the urologist.

Urinary cytology is also cost-effective if applied in the proper setting. It is considered ineffective as a screening procedure in the general population[126] because of the relatively low incidence of the disease and also the difficulty of diagnosing low grade malignancies. If limited to particular groups of patients, however, the yield is considerably increased. Examples include older patients with recent onset of signs and symptoms of urinary tract disease, patients with proved urothelial malignancies who are being followed posttherapy, and those in certain high risk groups such as workers exposed to urothelial carcinogens and those residing in areas of endemic bilharziasis.

Despite these many assets, as noted at the beginning of the chapter, cytology as a diagnostic tool in urologic oncology has been held in somewhat less than high esteem. Whatever the criticisms, virtually all are directed at one aspect of the technique: diagnostic accuracy. In simple terms, the foremost question the clinician asks of the pathologist when submitting a specimen is: "Is there or is there not evidence of malignancy?" Unfortunately, the reliability of "the answer" shows considerable variation in the literature.

El-Bolkainy[35] surveyed 17 reported series on the cytologic diagnosis of primary carcinoma of the bladder, with a combined total of close to 2,000 cases. The ability to identify by cytologic means those patients with malignant disease, as reflected by the "positivity" rates in the series considered, varied from a low of 44.7 percent to a high of 97.3 percent. Negative cytology results, in the presence of proved carcinoma, showed corresponding variation, ranging to as high as 48.7 percent. That is, on the poorest end of either scale, the diagnostic accuracy approached that which might be accomplished by a coin flip, without bothering with the trouble or expense of the urinary cytology examination. Moreover, if these figures were from academic laboratories with recognized expertise in the field, what must be going on in the community hospitals? Let us look at some of the reasons for these rather disturbing numbers.

First there are the *inherent limitations of the technique.* Numerous factors are operative here. One is that the success of the test is predicated on the fact that the lesion present is shedding sufficient cells into the medium to allow diagnosis. The cell yield may be improved by certain methods, irrigation for example, but even here sufficient *well preserved* cells may not be present in the cytology specimen for proper assessment. Also, it is unrealistic to believe that one is at no disadvantage when attempting to diagnose malignancies on the basis of cytologic versus histologic examination. Although the diagnostic accuracy of the two methods may approach equality in tumors demonstrating significant nuclear pleomorphism, it must be kept in mind that the majority of transitional cell carcinomas are of low and intermediate grade. Here nuclear pleomorphism is expected to be absent to (at most) moderate in degree, and the diagnosis often rests on architectural alterations that are simply not apparent in the cytologic preparation.

This brings us to perhaps the major problem area with the technique: the diagnosis of "low grade malignancies." In Chapter 18 the ongoing controversy concerning low grade papillary lesions was discussed at length. The controversy revolves around the fact that lesions designated grade I papillary transitional cell carcinomas rarely behave *per se* as malignancies. Nor by definition do they appear malignant at the individual cell level by conventional morphologic criteria. Some major centers, such as the Memorial Sloan-Kettering Cancer Center, still do not designate

such lesions as carcinomas. Most centers do, however, in accordance with major classifications of urothelial neoplasms.[97,128] Subtle cytologic features for the recognition of such lesions have been described by Murphy et al., but admittedly at the expense of a high false-positive rate, in the range of 10 to 14 percent.[136] Others[197] have not enjoyed even this degree of success.

Grade I papillary lesions account for one-fourth to one-third of all urothelial carcinomas encountered. Grade II papillary lesions, which have more recognizable but at times still subtle cytologic features, may account for an additional one-third or more of urothelial lesions. Therefore in 50 percent or more of urothelial carcinomas, the pathologist is faced with specimens that may show few if any of the conventional cytologic features of malignancy. This setting, then, is hardly one in which a high degree of diagnostic accuracy can be expected.

Another factor generating criticism from clinical colleagues is the *variability of expertise among cytopathologists* — a very real consideration. It is safe to say that few practicing pathologists would argue that their training in cytopathology was equal to that in histopathology, often because it has been given relatively short shrift in many anatomic pathology training programs. In urinary tract cytology in particular, both adequate training and experience are invaluable, as it remains one of the more difficult areas of diagnostic cytopathology. Nevertheless, it should not be thought of as some esoteric science that must be left in the hands of a few experts. This situation would be no more practical than suggesting that all patients with urothelial neoplasms should be cared for by the relative handful of urologists with real expertise in the field. In fact, with diligent attention to detail and the help of competent, well trained cytotechnologists, the practicing pathologist should be as adept at urinary tract cytodiagnosis as in other areas in cytopathology. Quality control is most important,[59] and continuous efforts to correlate cytologic and corresponding histologic material serve to improve diagnostic accuracy.

A final consideration concerns *"matters philosophical"* and their contribution to the "state of disarray" in cytopathology observed by Dr. Prout.[159] To return to El-Bolkainy's[35] review of the literature on the cytologic diagnosis of bladder carcinoma, it was of interest that most (9 of 17) reported series had only two diagnostic categories: negative and positive. The other eight series had an additional "inconclusive" category; and in all of these reports the percentages in the latter category were substantially less than those in the "positive" category. Presuming that low grade lesions were included in at least some of the series, these facts remain a mystery to me. If there is any area of diagnostic cytopathology in which an "inconclusive" category is a necessity, it is urinary cytology. Obviously, opinions on this issue vary enormously. In the literature, for example, one comes upon such phrases as "expansion of criteria for the diagnosis of urothelial malignancy" and "acceptable false-positive rates." We believe that such concepts, although perhaps of value in certain settings, have contributed greatly to the dissatisfaction with urinary cytology among our clinical colleagues. In our own laboratory, the category of "inconclusive for malignancy" is used more frequently than appears to be reflected in the literature. Although it is much more satisfying for both pathologist and clinician to establish a definitive diagnosis on the basis of each specimen, it is imperative to realize that one is not always dealing with a definitive situation. The pathologist must recognize when the cytology specimen is short of sufficient features to render a definite diagnosis of malignancy. The clinician in turn must be aware that an "inconclusive" diagnosis is indicative of a situation that must be closely followed and that may be further elucidated by repeat cytology examinations or histologic evaluation. Categoric designations in the diagnosis should be accompanied by a description of the findings whenever it may add to the diagnostic picture. The "inconclusive" category in particular should always be accompanied by a note indicating how closely (or how remotely) the features seen approach those of malignancy.

It is our belief that a *cytologic* diagnosis of "positive for malignancy" should be the equivalent of a *histologic* diagnosis of malignancy, with an "acceptable false-positive rate" of zero. This is not to say that occasional genuine and unavoidable false-positive diagnoses never occur, as they most certainly do, particularly in certain clinical settings such as lithiasis or prior systemic chemotherapy. For want of a better term, "false false-positives" are also encountered in cases where cytologic evidence of malignancy precedes the appearance of detectable lesions, with clinically apparent tumors following months to years later.

By maintaining this strict approach, we believe that the clinician may rely on the fact that a positive diagnosis for malignancy means just that, i.e., a definite area of malignant epithelial alteration is present somewhere in the urinary tract. In return for the increased degree of certainty, the clinician must recognize that the pathologist is making a positive diagnosis on the basis of features indicating at least an intermediate and most often a high grade malignancy, and that low grade lesions are likely to merit, at most, an inconclusive designation. We have no compunction about our diagnostic inabilities with low grade papillary lesions, as, with rare exceptions, they are not the ones that are killing our patients.

SPECIMENS

A great deal has been written about techniques for handling specimens (fresh or refrigerated versus fixed in various fashions), preparation of slides (smears versus membrane filters versus cytocentrifuge techniques), and staining (routine alcohol-fixed Papanicolaou versus air-dried Romanowsky). The only conclusion that can be drawn is that all authors seem to believe that their techniques are optimal and all others are comparatively second rate. We continue to use routine Papanicolaou-stained membrane filter preparations and sediment smears, but we recommend simply that one choose any given technique with which one is comfortable and then stick with it.

Among specimen types, the spontaneously voided specimen is obviously the most easily obtained and is useful for screening new patients and follow-up of patients with a history of urothelial neoplasms. Its major advantage is that it is obtained without the use of invasive procedures, with the usual attendant risks. Another advantage over irrigation and directed brushing specimens is its "survey" quality, presumably with the capacity to sample all areas bathed by the urinary pool. Disadvantages include cellular degenerative changes, contamination with material from other sites (notably the female genital tract), and the often sparse cell population, particularly in patients with low grade urothelial neoplasms.[164]

Although some authors[70] advise the use of the same specimen favored for routine urinalysis (the first voided morning specimen), others[164] believe that degenerative changes are most pronounced in these specimens and suggest that a specimen be collected later in the day, approximately 3 hours after the patient has last voided. The reason for the degenerative changes found in voided urine specimens is not clear. Traditionally it has been ascribed to the "hostile environment" urine presents to a cell. Urinary osmolarity and pH in particular may vary considerably from that to which deeper urothelial cells are usually exposed. Even immediate placement in fixative such as ethanol may do little to improve the situation, however, as many of the degenerative changes may well have taken place before the patient voids, and at least some of the changes presumably relate to the reason the cells exfoliated in the first place.[26] As a general rule, whatever the causes, cell details are usually least well preserved in voided specimens.

Despite the above, the diagnostic yield is relatively high with a single voided specimen, particularly when dealing with higher grade lesions. The yield may be maximized with the use of multiple serial specimens, generaly three taken on consecutive days.[103,151] Among 151 cases with positive cytologies, Koss et al.[103] were able to establish a diagnosis in 79 percent based on the first submitted specimen, but they detected an additional 14 and 7 percent on the second and third specimens, respectively.

Specimens obtained by catheterization or at cystoscopy largely circumvent the problem of specimen contamination. Obtaining specimens in this manner may also result in better cell preservation by decreasing the time cells are exposed to the degenerative effects of urine, particularly important in patients with partial obstruction who may have large residual urine volumes. These specimens offer no increase in cellular yield over the routine voided specimen, aside from cells directly dislodged by the catheter or cystoscope. This may be disadvantageous (see below), as such cells are often peeled off in intact strips, and may simulate papillary fragments of low grade transitional cell carcinoma. Moreover, lesions in the prostatic urethra may be bypassed in these specimens, and supplementing the work-up with voided specimens has been advocated for this reason.[33]

A third method of specimen collection is that of irrigation (washing, barbotage), generally applied for bladder evaluation but also useful in the upper tract. Excellent bladder specimens may be obtained by instillation of 50 ml of normal saline into the empty bladder via a catheter, followed by withdrawal and reinsertion, repeated five times.[52] The irrigant may

then be placed in a suitable fixative, e.g., an equal volume of 50 percent alcohol, or submitted fresh directly to the laboratory. We prefer the latter method, as do others.[136]

This method has the advantages of both augmented cell yield, presumably by forceful dislodgement of cells by the irrigation fluid, and better cell preservation,[61] as many of the cells present have been attached and viable up to the point of specimen collection, with no degenerative effects. In addition, background debris also appears reduced in comparison to catheterized urine specimens.[74]

As the result of these advantages, diagnostic accuracy appears to be improved compared to that with catheterization and voided urine specimens. Frable et al.[56] compared simultaneously submitted cystoscopic urine samples and irrigation specimens, and found that the cytologic diagnosis was the same for both types of material in 68 percent of their patients with bladder cancer. In the 32 percent of patients with a difference in diagnosis between the two sources, however, the irrigation specimens consistently indicated that a more severe lesion was present. When a voided urine specimen was available, such specimens appeared significantly less diagnostic in 65 percent of the cases when compared to the submitted bladder washings. Murphy et al.[133] also compared cystoscopic urine specimens with irrigation specimens but noted little consistent difference in either cell yield or preservation between the two techniques. These authors found diagnostic cells by both methods in most cases but did note that in 20 to 30 percent of the cases they could be identified only in the cystoscopically obtained urine specimens. Although acknowledging a greater diagnostic yield by the irrigation method alone when compared to catheterization methods alone, they advocated the use of the two techniques as complementary, a view with which I concur.

Among the disadvantages of irrigation specimens, the necessity for an invasive procedure is noted, although many such specimens are obtained at the time of cystoscopy, so this is not a major consideration. Confusion caused by "pseudopapillary fragments" as seen with catheter or cystoscopically obtained urine specimens is, if anything, even more exaggerated. Even experienced cytologists often have difficulty discerning true papillary fragments in these specimens. Finally, directed irrigation specimens lack the "survey" quality of urine specimens, although this trait may be an advantage in certain situations. For example, finding malignant transitional cells in a voided specimen in the face of a negative bladder irrigation would obviously direct further work-up to either the upper tract, urethra, or prostatic ducts.

TRANSITIONAL CELL CARCINOMA

Transitional Cell Carcinoma, Grade III

It is perhaps easiest to begin discussion of the cytologic diagnosis of urothelial malignancies with high grade transitional cell lesions, as these lesions display most prominently the abnormalities we traditionally associate with malignancies at other body sites. Moreover, cytologic diagnosis is often facilitated in cases of high grade neoplasia, as malignant cells are frequently present in abundance, particularly in comparison to specimens from patients with lower grade lesions. High grade papillary and nonpapillary tumors are considered together because, at the individual cell level, the features of malignancy are indistinguishable.

The emphasis, as with tumors at other sites, is on nuclear changes, with cytoplasmic features other than relative volume being of little help in deciding if a given cell is malignant. All of the "standard" cytologic abnormalities associated with malignant behavior may be seen to varying degrees in high grade transitional cell carcinomas, including nuclear enlargement, irregular nuclear borders, a high N/C ratio, nuclear hyperchromaticity, abnormal chromatin pattern, prominent nucleoli, etc.

Even with high grade neoplasms there is inevitably some degree of morphologic overlap with reactive cellular changes seen in nonneoplastic conditions, and certain nuclear features appear to be more characteristic of high grade transitional cell carcinoma than others. Here we refer to one of the best and easily one of the most painstaking studies of the cytology of transitional cell carcinoma — that of Kern,[92] who examined the cytologic features in urinary specimens from patients with carcinomas and compared them to control specimens from patients with no indication of urologic disease and specimens showing "benign atypia" in patients with cystitis. Overall, the individual characteristics of approximately 9,000 cells were observed and recorded, with planimetric measurements performed on close to 6,000 cells.

As illustrated in Table 21-1, adapted from Kern's data,[92] mean cell size in high grade transitional cell carcinoma was higher than in cases of reactive atypia but actually lower than in "normal" specimens. There was a wide range of sizes within each group, however, and superficial cells were not indicated as excluded, so presumably these cells account at least in part for the high mean size in normal specimens. Other cytoplasmic features recorded, e.g., cell shape and cytoplasmic vacuolation, were not helpful in identifying the cases of malignancy.

Among the nuclear features tabulated, cells showing multiple nucleoli, irregular nuclear shapes, and nuclear hyperchromasia appeared to be increased in number in the malignant cases, but they were also

Table 21-1 High Grade Transitional Cell Carcinoma: Comparative Cytologic Features

Parameter	High Grade Transitional Cell Carcinoma	Reactive Atypia	Normal Tissue
Cell size (mean μm^2)	235	181	341
Nuclear size (mean μm^2)	90	52	36
N/C ratio (mean)	0.383	0.287	0.106
Coarsely granular chromatin pattern (percent)	74	20	1
Macronucleoli (percent)	11	1	0
Multiple nucleoli (percent)	29	10	0
Irregular nuclear shape (percent)	75	51	43
Nuclear hyperchromasia (percent)	43	24	23

(Modified from Kern,[92] with permission.)

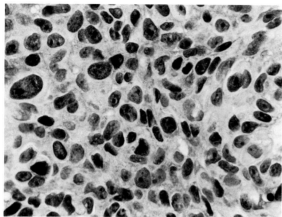

Fig. 21-40 Transitional cell carcinoma, grade III. H&E. ×300.

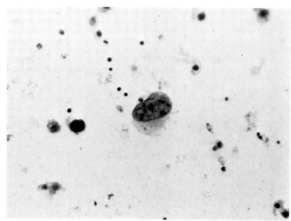

Fig. 21-41 Transitional cell carcinoma, grade III. Note the single markedly enlarged nucleus, with a high N/C ratio and multiple nucleoli. Papanicolaou. ×220.

seen in significant numbers in the normal and/or reactive categories. The best discriminating features of malignancy appeared to be *increased nuclear size, increased N/C ratio, a coarsely granular chromatin pattern, and the presence of macronucleoli.* One has only to look at the average histologic preparation from high grade transitional cell carcinoma (Fig. 21-40) to confirm such observations.

As noted in Table 21-1, the mean nuclear size in the cases of high grade malignancy was 2.5 times that seen in normals and almost twice the size seen in the reactive cases. The importance of this feature has been emphasized by others,[11] although in a computerized discriminant study between benign and malignant urothelial cells, Koss et al.[100] found no significant differences in nuclear size between benign and malignant cells. This study was performed on a small number of cells in each category, however. In fact, even in high grade malignancies, nuclear size from one cell to the next may be quite variable,[136] but the finding of even a few markedly enlarged nuclei *without* proportionate overall cell enlargement should immediately alert the pathologist to the possibility of high grade transitional cell carcinoma (Fig. 21-41).

This relation of nuclear size to cell size should always be taken into account in the diagnosis of urothelial malignancy. Superficial cell nuclei may become markedly enlarged in the face of various nonneoplastic stimuli, but there is generally a corresponding increase in overall cell size. Again it is emphasized that the sometimes disturbing nuclear features of such cells should be viewed in context. If compared only to nonsuperficial cells, malignant cells are at times even smaller than average-sized normal cells; therefore, in conjunction with the mean increase in nuclear size, a high N/C ratio may be of particular value for distinguishing benign from malignant cells[92,100] (Fig. 21-42).

The presence of multiple nucleoli, particularly if there is variation in size and shape from one nucleolus

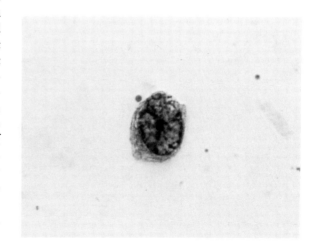

Fig. 21-42 Transitional cell carcinoma, grade III. This individual malignant cell has a markedly increased N/C ratio and irregular nuclear membrane folding in the superior aspect. Papanicolaou. ×960.

to the next in an individual nucleus, is a standard "worrisome" feature in cytology. As seen in Table 21-1, however, this feature is found in a significant number of reactive urothelial cells and may be particularly prominent in reactive superficial cells. Macronucleoli (Fig. 21-43), on the other hand, are only rarely seen in nonmalignant cells. In addition to size increase, irregular nucleolar contours are also characteristic of high grade malignancy. In contrast to the situation with other high grade tumors, however, we have found the presence of prominent nucleoli to be variable in high grade transitional cell carcinomas. Some cases may display all of the earmarks of a grade III tumor yet have unimpressive nucleolar abnormalities.

A final feature of malignancy that Kern[92] noted is a coarsely granular chromatin pattern (Fig. 21-44). Again, this may be seen in a minority of reactive cells, but this pattern is the rule rather than the exception in high grade malignancies. Although there is some disagreement among investigators as to the relative value of this feature, the coarsely granular chromatin pattern of high grade transitional cell carcinoma is nonetheless mentioned repeatedly in the literature[11,92,136,173] and by computerized analysis dense chromatin granularity appears to be the single most helpful feature for distinguishing malignant from benign urothelial cells.[100,102]

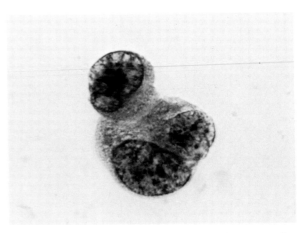

Fig. 21-44 Transitional cell carcinoma, grade III. Note the coarsely granular chromatin pattern and some degree of anisonucleosis in this tissue fragment. Papanicolaou. ×880.

Although high grade transitional cell carcinomas often shed single cells in predominance, tissue fragments of varying size are seen not infrequently (Fig. 21-44), particularly in cases of grade III papillary carcinoma. They may become much more prominent following instrumentation. In true fragments, marked variation in size or appearance from one nucleus to the next is another hallmark of high grade disease.

In the final analysis, however, it must be emphasized that in urinary cytology, as in all other areas of cytology, there is no single cellular feature that is 100 percent "diagnostic" of malignancy. All cytologic diagnoses, urothelial or otherwise, are necessarily the result of a composite impression of the many cell features encountered in a specimen, with studies such as that of Kern being of great help in deciding where in the composite to place emphasis.

Transitional Cell Carcinoma In Situ

Although some workers have extended their diagnostic criteria to include lower grade lesions[8] (a topic discussed more fully in Chapter 17), at least in cytopathology we prefer to limit this diagnosis to intraepithelial lesions that are the cytologic equivalents of invasive grade III transitional cell carcinoma, a view shared by others.[16,60,187] In this setting, cytology has proved to be an accurate diagnostic tool; and because

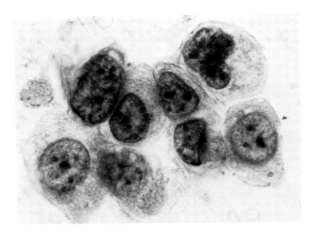

Fig. 21-43 Transitional cell carcinoma, grade III. Note the cluster of malignant cells with multiple nucleoli and occasional macronucleoli, some with irregular contours. Papanicolaou. ×880.

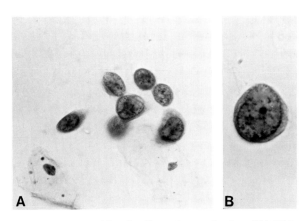

Fig. 21-45 Transitional cell carcinoma in situ. **(A)** This cluster of cells is from a patient with carcinoma in situ. Note the nuclear enlargement and high N/C ratio, relative uniformity of abnormal cells, and "clean" background. Such features suggest the possibility of carcinoma in situ, but *do not exclude* invasive disease (see text). **(B)** Individual cell with a high N/C ratio, moderately granular chromatin pattern, and single small nucleolus. Papanicolaou. **A,** ×352; **B,** ×880.

of difficulties in obtaining intact biopsy specimens, cytology often serves as the diagnostic cornerstone.[16,49] In fact, as noted above, a positive cytology may precede the appearance of any clinically detectable urothelial disease by months to at times years.

It would be of potential value if the cytopathologist could discriminate between carcinoma in situ (Fig. 21-45) and high grade invasive malignancy. Certain features, summarized by Shenoy et al.,[173] may be indicative of the presence of carcinoma in situ. They include a "clean" background, in contrast to the often inflamed, debris-ridden background of invasive disease, and also a paucity of nucleoli in the malignant-appearing nuclei, in contrast to the often prominent macronucleoli of other high grade lesions. Other authors have suggested that cells from carcinoma in situ tend to be more uniform than those from invasive tumors[166,198] and of relatively smaller size.[166] Some indicate clustering of cells as characteristic,[166] although others cite predominant shedding of single cells to be more frequent.[173]

All of the features cited have been seen in specimens from patients with no clinical or histologic evidence of anything more than carcinoma in situ, many of whom have been followed for years. However, even in those studies that have attempted a detailed analysis

to discriminate between carcinoma in situ and high grade invasive disease,[166,173] clear-cut discrimination has been lacking in at least some cases. Shenoy and colleagues,[173] for example, found that pure carcinoma in situ was mistaken for other high grade disease in approximately 50 percent of their cases. Rosa and co-workers[166] also cited cases in which invasive carcinoma either coexisted with, or developed in, patients who showed nothing more than findings thought typical for carcinoma in situ alone. These authors suggested that the cells shed from areas of carcinoma in situ may predominate in a given specimen, masking findings that may indicate the presence of coexistent invasive disease, a view with which I agree.

For practical purposes, the cytologist presented with a specimen that has large numbers of disturbing but relatively uniform cells with hyperchromatic nuclei, a coarsely granular chromatin pattern, and a high N/C ratio, set in a relatively "clean" background, can suggest that such findings are often indicative of the presence of carcinoma in situ. However, a disclaimer should be added that such findings in no way exclude the possibility of coexistent invasive disease.

Papillary Transitional Cell Carcinoma, Grade II

By definition, grade II transitional cell carcinomas have a papillary configuration (Fig. 21-46), as there is no corresponding nonpapillary carcinoma in most standard classifications of urothelial tumors. In histo-

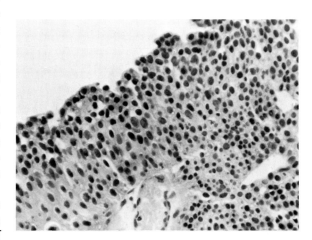

Fig. 21-46 Papillary transitional cell carcinoma, grade II. H&E. ×220.

Table 21-2 Intermediate Grade Transitional Cell Carcinoma:
Comparative Cytologic Features

Parameter	Intermediate Grade Transitional Cell Carcinoma	Reactive Atypia	Normal Tissue
Cell size (mean μm^2)	215	181	341
Nuclear size (mean μm^2)	78	52	36
N/C ratio (mean)	0.359	0.287	0.106
Coarsely granular chromatin pattern (percent)	60	20	1
Macronucleoli (percent)	7	1	0
Multiple nucleoli (percent)	16	10	0
Irregular nuclear shape (percent)	63	51	43
Nuclear hyperchromasia (percent)	39	24	23

(Modified from Kern,[92] with permission.)

logic material, similar alterations in flat mucosa would generally elicit a diagnosis of no more than "dysplasia" or "atypical hyperplasia." It is not surprising therefore that our ability to identify such lesions in cytologic preparations is much more limited than with high grade lesions.

Kern[92] found that cells from patients with intermediate grade papillary carcinomas showed trends similar to those with higher grade lesions but with less pronounced differences between them and cells shed from reactive atypias (Table 21-2). The major differentiating features again included increased nuclear size, increased N/C ratio, the presence of macronucleoli in a small number of cells, and a coarsely granular chromatin pattern. Evidence of nuclear enlargement and an increased N/C ratio is often most noticeable in tissue fragments, which may show apparent nuclear "crowding" (Fig. 21-47). Nuclear overlap, a feature thought to be characteristic of grade II lesions by Shenoy et al.,[173] may be present; but as seen in Figure 21-48, this feature may not be striking. Moreover, we have seen nuclear overlap in fragments found in obviouly nonmalignant circumstances (Fig. 21-49), so this finding must be viewed in context.

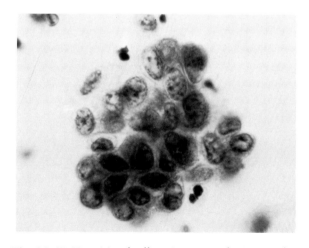

Fig. 21-47 Transitional cell carcinoma, grade II. Note the moderate increase in nuclear size, high N/C ratio, and areas of nuclear overlap in this tissue fragment. Papanicolaou. ×352.

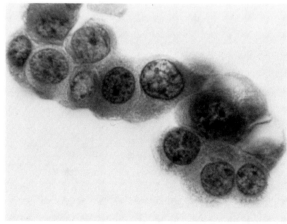

Fig. 21-48 Transitional cell carcinoma, grade II. In this tissue fragment the nuclear features are similar to those in Fig. 21-47 but nuclear crowding is less apparent. Papanicolaou. ×880.

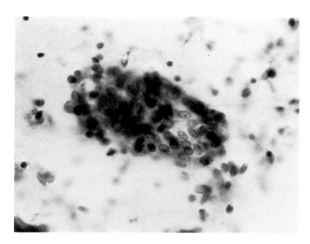

Fig. 21-49 Benign tissue fragment in a catheterization urine specimen. Note the prominent nuclear overlap but otherwise absence of any features to suggest malignancy. In particular, individual nuclei are quite bland in appearance. Papanicolaou. ×352.

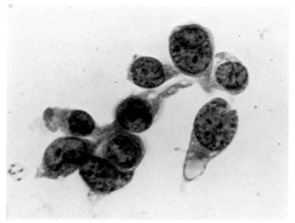

Fig. 21-50 Transitional cell carcinoma, grade II. Nuclear enlargement and a coarsely granular chromatin pattern are apparent but are of a lesser degree than seen in cells from the grade III lesion in Fig. 21-51. Note also the relatively more rounded nuclear contours in the intermediate grade cells, with irregularities generally limited to occasional notches and creases. Papanicolaou. ×880.

As an aside, one frequently sees reference in the literature to the value of finding "true papillary fragments" in the diagnosis of malignancy. It has been our impression, however, that in the absence of a well preserved inner fibrovascular core, which unfortunately is rarely shed with the surface epithelium intact, the designation of a curled bit of mucosa as "true papillary" versus "pseudopapillary" by the pathologist is much more a guess than a diagnosis. Nonetheless, whatever the tumor grade, the finding of such tissue fragments *in spontaneously voided urine specimens, in the absence of prior instrumentation,* is suspicious in and of itself. Even in this instance, however, it is important to remember that cell clusters may be seen in the presence of marked inflammation as well as lithiasis, with true tissue fragments particularly common in the latter situation.[98] Such fragments are the rule rather than the exception following instrumentation, and they are almost uniformly present in irrigation specimens.

Kern's analysis of individual cells in intermediate grade lesions noted "irregular nuclear shape" in a number of cells in all categories, malignant and otherwise, but the degree of nuclear membrane irregularity was not specified. The high percentages in this category, including 43 percent of cells from control specimens, suggest that relatively minor alterations were counted. If only more pronounced degrees of nuclear shape irregularities are taken into account, this feature may be of greater help in differentiating intermediate from high grade lesions. That is, in the former case, nuclei tend to be enlarged, with an increased N/C ratio and some degree of coarse granularity to the nuclear chromatin pattern, but they also tend to maintain a *relatively* rounded or ovoid nuclear contour (Fig. 21-50). Murphy et al.[136] cited the presence of one or two nuclear notches (on edge) or creases (en face) as characteristic of both low and intermediate grade transitional cell carcinomas. High grade lesions, conversely, often show more pronounced nuclear membrane irregularities, with sharp angulations and irregular contours in at least some cells (Fig. 21-51).

The chromatin pattern is also of value in differentiating intermediate from high grade transitional cell carcinoma. Whereas nuclei from both are coarsely granular, chromatin is somewhat less granular and relatively more evenly distributed in grade II lesions and more coarsely granular and unevenly distributed in high grade lesions, with nuclei from the latter at times showing prominent areas of parachromatin clearing.

Finally, relative nuclear size is of help in the differential between intermediate and high grade lesions. Although both have enlarged nuclei compared to those seen in reactive states, intermediate grade cells

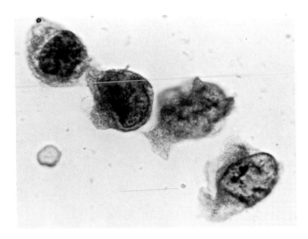

Fig. 21-51 Transitional cell carcinoma, grade III. Compare the features here to those seen in Fig. 21-50. Papanicolaou. ×880.

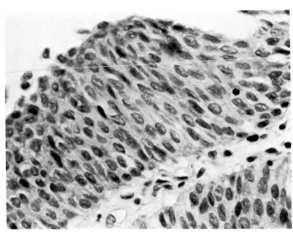

Fig. 21-52 Papillary transitional cell carcinoma, grade I. H&E. ×352.

show a more modest degree of nuclear enlargement. Moreover, there tends to be a greater degree of uniformity from one nucleus to the next, and the finding of even a few markedly and disproportionately enlarged nuclei is more often indicative of high grade rather than intermediate grade disease.

Because of the more subtle cytologic features of intermediate grade transitional cell carcinoma, it is not surprising that diagnostic accuracy for lesions in this category is noticeably less than for high grade lesions. In fact, many such cases do not have sufficient cytologic abnormalities for the pathologist to be comfortable in making a clear-cut diagnosis of malignancy. In such instances the case is best relegated to the "inconclusive" category, with a brief narrative as to how great (or small) is the suspicion of malignancy.

Papillary Transitional Cell Carcinoma, Grade I

Grade I lesions (Fig. 21-52) are essentially defined by their papillary configuration and increase in number of cell layers over the usual seven to ten found in normal urothelium. Individual cell abnormalities (Fig. 21-53), by definition, are minimal when compared to normal urothelial cells. As Kern's data[92] show (Table 21-3), the various characteristics of cells from patients with grade I transitional cell carcinoma closely approach those of cells in the "reactive atypia" category, and the problem is further compounded by

the fact that specimens from patients with low grade disease tend to be comparatively less cellular than those from patients with higher grade tumors.

Mean nuclear size is still somewhat greater compared to that of normal urothelial cells, as is the N/C ratio, but both values are essentially identical to those found in reactive cells. Irregularities of nuclear shape are more frequent than in either normal or reactive cells, but they tend to be of a more subtle nature,

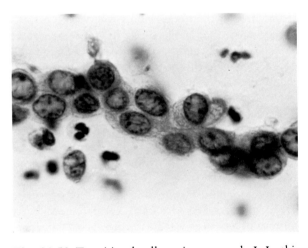

Fig. 21-53 Transitional cell carcinoma, grade I. In this tissue fragment there is a smaller increase in nuclear size, compared to that seen with intermediate and high grade malignant cells, and a more finely granular chromatin pattern. Papanicolaou. ×880.

Table 21-3 Low Grade Transitional Cell Carcinoma:
Comparative Cytologic Features

Parameter	Low Grade Transitional Cell Carcinoma	Reactive Atypia	Normal Tissue
Cell size (mean μm^2)	169	181	341
Nuclear size (mean μm^2)	54	52	36
N/C ratio (mean)	0.319	0.287	0.106
Coarsely granular chromatin pattern (percent)	48	20	1
Macronucleoli (percent)	4	1	0
Multiple nucleoli (percent)	14	10	0
Irregular nuclear shape (percent)	65	51	43
Nuclear hyperchromasia (percent)	37	24	23

(Modified from Kern,[92] with permission.)

generally consisting of the nuclear notching and creasing mentioned above.[136] A few nucleoli may be present, but they are generally of small size. With the vagaries of staining, many such structures may actually be nothing more than small chromocenters. Some increase in nuclear chromaticity may be apparent, but chromatin granules tend to be evenly distributed. (Again, Kern's criteria[92] in this category appear somewhat liberal, as chromatin granules in low grade transitional cell lesions usually approach the pattern of fine dispersion found in normal urothelial cells.[136,173])

Shenoy et al.[173] noted that although tissue fragments may be seen with low grade disease, the nuclear crowding and overlapping seen in intermediate grade lesions are not features seen in grade I lesions. Also, the same observations pertaining to differentiation of true versus pseudopapillary fragments with grade II tumors hold for grade I tumors, and this differential is most often a very subjective exercise.

As the reader will have gleaned by now, the deviations from normal and reactive cells exhibited in cytologic preparations from patients with low grade transitional cell carcinomas are extremely subtle and at times unrecognizable. Moreover, similar cytologic features have been seen in voided specimens from patients with quite dissimilar urologic lesions, such as nephrogenic adenoma.[186] Diagnostic accuracy figures (or perhaps better—inaccuracy figures) readily attest to these facts. Indeed many authorities in the field[11,45,61,92,98,173,197] essentially dismiss cytology as a method for definitive diagnosis of low grade lesions. Others, such as Murphy et al.,[136] have attempted to identify such lesions by cytologic means; but even

with their considerable diagnostic experience, low grade lesions resulted in positive or suspicious diagnoses in only three-fourths of their patients, at the expense of a false-positive rate of 10 to 14 percent. For the general pathologist, the cytologic diagnosis of low grade tumors is probably best limited to *suggesting* the possibility. Even then, realistic accuracy figures are probably attained only in certain settings, such as the appearance of some of the changes described above in serial cytologic preparations from patients being followed for recurrent low grade disease.

SQUAMOUS CARCINOMA

Pure squamous carcinomas account for a minority of urothelial malignancies in the Western world, with most studies indicating a frequency in the 5 to 10 percent range. Conversely, in other areas, particularly in certain regions with endemic bilharziasis, most cases are squamous carcinoma.[37] Some tendency to *focal* squamous or glandular differentiation in high grade transitional cell carcinoma in the Western population is not uncommon, however. In fact, if sufficient features to indicate such differentiation are noted in the cytologic preparation, one is very often dealing with a high grade carcinoma.[173]

The cytologic appearance of squamous carcinoma is similar to that of squamous carcinomas arising at other sites, and, particularly for lesions exhibiting prominent keratinization, it is quite distinct from the cytologic appearance of transitional cell carcinoma.

The specimen background is typically inflammatory, a reflection of the often advanced stage of these lesions at the time of initial diagnosis. Malignant cells tend to shed individually, but tissue fragments may be present, particularly after instrumentation. As with transitional cell carcinoma, the diagnosis of malignancy rests primarily on nuclear characteristics. With squamous lesions, one also sees an array of changes in the nuclei, with the emphasis on characteristic features somewhat different from transitional cell carcinoma. Nuclear variation, even within a single specimen, is often striking in comparison to that seen with transitional cell tumors (Fig. 21-54). The nuclei of

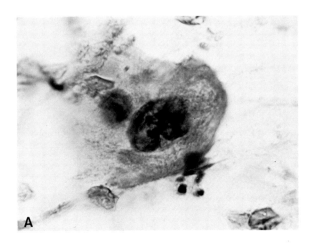

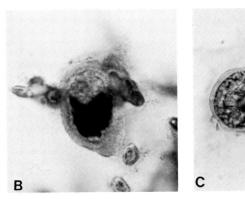

Fig. 21-54 Squamous carcinoma. Note the marked variability in the appearance of the malignant cells. **(A)** Markedly abnormal nucleus, with hyperchromaticity, dense chromatin clumping, and irregular parachromatin clearing. **(B)** Densely hyperchromatic nucleus, with markedly irregular nuclear contours. Note the demarcation of the outer and inner rims of cytoplasm, with formation of the so-called ectoendoplasmic border. **(C)** More rounded nucleus, with a high N/C ratio and abnormal chromatin pattern. Papanicolaou. ×880.

squamous carcinoma cells are often densely hyperchromatic, with a coarsely granular to (at times) almost karyopyknotic appearance. Irregular chromatin dispersion, with intervening areas of abnormal parachromatin clearing, may be noted. In contrast to transitional cell carcinomas, nuclear border irregularities may be much more pronounced, with irregular, jagged indentations in at least some cells. The appearance of prominent nucleoli in cells showing squamous differentiation is a worrisome feature, according to Frost.[62] In typical squamous carcinomas, we have found nucleolar formation to be variable, with some cells showing one or two macronucleoli, and others that are obviously malignant showing none at all.

The cytoplasmic features are most helpful in identifying the malignant cells as squamous rather than transitional cell in type. Malignant squamous cells often appear to have a more abundant cytoplasm than their transitional cell counterparts, with correspondingly lower N/C ratios. The latter may be more apparent than real, however. As with normal squamous cells, the cytoplasm of malignant squamous cells tends to be thinner than that of transitional or glandular epithelial cells; and if the third dimension of thickness could be accurately assessed, the comparative volumetric N/C ratios might be much closer than is apparent by routine light microscopy. Also of considerable help in optimally stained smears is the tinctorial quality of the cytoplasm. In contrast to the typical basophilic tint of transitional cells, malignant squamous cells tend to be more acidophilic or "orangeophilic," with increasing degrees of the reddish orange tint noted with increasing amounts of keratin formation. Another feature associated with squamous differentiation is the presence of a lighter staining, relatively demarcated outer rim of cytoplasm surrounding the darker staining central area, with the formation of the so-called "ectoendoplasmic border"[62] (Fig. 21-54B).

Cell shape in squamous carcinomas varies considerably, from cells of round or ovoid shape (Fig. 21-55), similar to malignant transitional cells, to rather bizarre forms with irregular cytoplasmic projections and elongations (Fig. 21-56). As with histologic diagnosis, the finding of an occasional "pearl" arrangement of cells (Fig. 21-57) is usually indicative of squamous differentiation.

In full bloom, squamous carcinomas of the urothelium are among those most readily diagnosed by cyto-

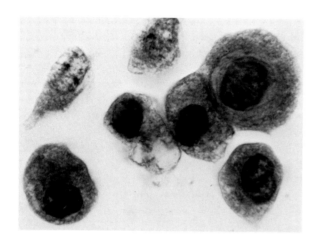

Fig. 21-55 Squamous carcinoma. These round to ovoid cells are similar to those seen with high grade transitional cell carcinoma. Papanicolaou. ×880.

logic means. Particularly in those situations wherein squamous carcinomas predominate, such as bilharzia-associated carcinoma, a high degree of diagnostic accuracy can be expected.[36]

ADENOCARCINOMA

Primary adenocarcinoma of urothelial origin is the least common of the standard epithelial malignancies, comprising usually only 1 to 2 percent of cases in most series. Two exceptions to this rule are the development of malignancy in the exstrophic bladder and in

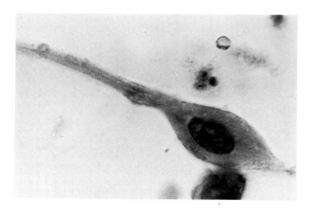

Fig. 21-56 Squamous carcinoma. Note the bizarre cell form. The appearance of such cells in an epithelial malignancy is very suggestive of squamous differentiation. Papanicolaou ×880.

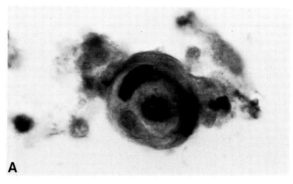

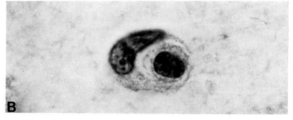

Fig. 21-57 Squamous carcinoma. Note the "pearl formations" with nuclear features of malignancy apparent. Papanicolaou. ×880.

urachal remnants, wherein adenocarcinomas are seen much more frequently. Again, it is stressed that *focal glandular differentiation* may be seen in otherwise typical transitional cell carcinomas, often high grade, and this may be reflected in the cytologic material examined in such cases.

As with squamous carcinomas, adenocarcinomas are most often deeply invasive at the time of diagnosis, with a corresponding inflammatory background noted in cytologic preparations. Cells shed from adenocarcinomas have a tendency to occur in tissue fragments or intact sheets (Fig. 21-58). This feature may also be seen with transitional cell carcinoma but is less common with squamous carcinomas. A columnar configuration is recognized at times,[98] but more poorly differentiated adenocarcinomas shed cells with an appearance that begins to merge with that seen in typical high grade transitional cell lesions.[6] Features helpful in distinguishing poorly differentiated adenocarcinomas from their transitional cell counterparts include the presence of prominent cytoplasmic vacuolation in at least some cells (Fig. 21-59), at times compressing the adjacent nucleus, and a tendency to show more "open-faced" nuclei that tend to retain a rounded contour. Nucleoli, whether single or multi-

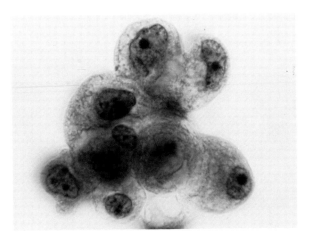

Fig. 21-58 Adenocarcinoma of the bladder. Features which may suggest adenocarcinomatous differentiation include the presence of tissue fragments, cytoplasmic vacuolation, and large, vesicular nuclei with one or more prominent nucleoli. Papanicolaou. ×880.

ple, are generally quite apparent, macronucleoli are frequently seen, and irregular nucleolar contours may be observed. As Frost[62] noted, however, prominent nucleolar abnormalities may be found with virtually any type of high grade malignancy and are not good discriminators of adenocarcinomatous differentiation.

In practice, some of our best examples of adenocarcinoma in urinary cytologic preparations have turned out to be nonurothelial primaries involving the urinary tract secondarily. Indeed, because of the relative paucity of primary urothelial adenocarcinomas, one should immediately question the possibility of metastatic disease from local or distant sites when confronted with a cytologic picture suggesting adenocarcinoma. Because of the small numbers of such cases, meaningful accuracy figures are difficult to come by. With the advanced stage of most such lesions, however, the cytologist will often be able at least to arrive at a "positive" diagnosis if not be able to definitely subclassify the lesion on purely cytologic grounds.

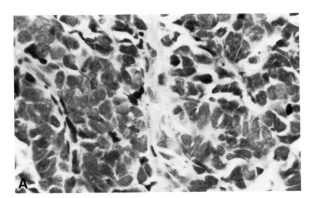

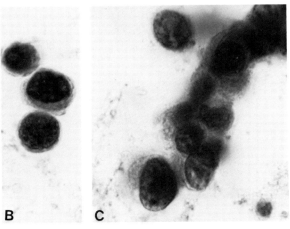

Fig. 21-60 Small cell undifferentiated carcinoma of the bladder. **(A)** Note the histologic similarity to small cell carcinoma of lung origin. **(B)** Individual cells with rounded, hyperchromatic nuclei and a very high N/C ratio. **(C)** The presence of true tissue fragments excludes certain other "round cell malignancies" such as lympho-hematopoietic neoplasms. **A,** H&E. ×352. **B,C,** Papanicolaou. ×880.

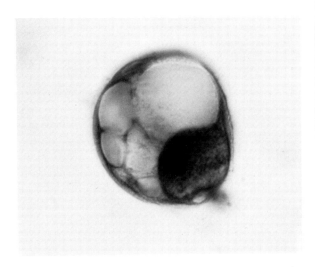

Fig. 21-59 Adenocarcinoma of the bladder. Note the prominent secretory vacuoles, with displacement of the nucleus to the side of the cell. Single large nucleolus is partially obscured. Papanicolaou. ×968.

UNDIFFERENTIATED CARCINOMA

Urothelial carcinomas that show essentially no evidence of differentiation along any of the traditional cell lines are uncommon, accounting for considerably less than 1 percent of all malignancies encountered. Such tumors are virtually always invasive at the time of diagnosis and may shed cells in great profusion. In cytology preparations, individual cells show varying amounts of cytoplasm, usually with a rather high N/C ratio. Nuclear pleomorphism ranges from little, with cells showing an appearance essentially identical to small cell undifferentiated lung primaries (Fig. 21-60), to prominent, with many or all of the usual features of malignancy (Fig. 21-61). It is only the former type, i.e., small cell undifferentiated carcinoma, that may have a characteristic cytologic appearance, and cells in many of the latter cases in fact turn out to have been shed from poorly differentiated carcinomas of the standard types that may be properly classified when histologic material becomes available.

Nonurothelial Neoplasms

Cells from tumors other than urothelial primaries are not often encountered in urinary cytology specimens. Among other genitourinary neoplasms, renal parenchymal and prostatic carcinomas are common in clinical practice, but neither sheds cells into the uri-

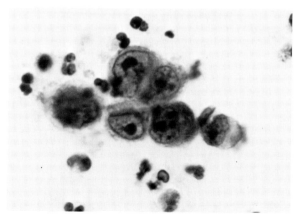

Fig. 21-61 Large cell undifferentiated carcinoma of the bladder. Such blatantly malignant cells may not allow categorization on the basis of cytology alone. At least some cases will be able to be classified subsequently on the basis of histologic material. Papanicolaou. ×880.

nary pool with any degree of frequency. Indeed, prior to the advent of fine needle aspiration techniques (see below), our experience with these lesions in the cytology laboratory had been relatively limited. Much less common primary tumors, e.g., nephroblastoma, lymphoma, and melanoma, are generally the subject of isolated case reports, with little in the way of systematic study available in the cytology literature. Metastatic tumors of all sorts may be encountered, but again they account for only a small percentage of malignancies found by urinary cytologic examination. Moreover, differentiating them as such strictly on the basis of urinary cytology is not possible. That is, virtually all types of malignancy, including all of the standard types of carcinoma, have been noted at one time or another as primary lesions in the genitourinary tract, and the total clinicopathologic picture must always be taken into account.

RENAL CELL CARCINOMA

Urinary cytopathologic examination is of limited value in the diagnosis of renal cell carcinoma because the tumors are not usually in direct contact with the urothelial surfaces until late in their courses, if at all, and therefore do not shed cells into the urinary pool. DeVoogt and Wielenga[32] found only one positive examination among urinary specimens from seven patients with renal cell carcinoma. Even with direct renal pelvic lavage, Leistenschneider and Nagel[110] found no positive results among their six cases of renal cell carcinoma, with only one case reaching the level of "atypia." These figures reflect the general experience, and urinary cytology rarely serves as an "early indicator" of renal cell carcinoma. Tumors break through into the pelvis most often at a late stage, often with accompanying inflammation, hemorrhage, and necrosis. These obscuring factors, plus a tendency of the tumor cells to degenerate once shed into the urine, make accurate diagnosis, and at times even mere suspicion of such tumors, quite difficult.[98] In fact, we have found that some of the best examples of well preserved renal cell carcinoma have proved to be metastases secondarily involving the bladder, a phenomenon occasionally reported in the literature.[162]

In renal cell carcinoma, well differentiated tumor cells may be difficult to recognize as such, with little in the way of nuclear abnormalities. Less well differentiated tumors may shed cells that have characteristics similar to those in histologic material (Fig. 21-62), with varying degrees of "clear cell" appearance sometimes serving as a diagnostic clue. On close inspection, this appearance is often found to result from a finely, rather than a coarsely, vacuolated cytoplasm. However, cells showing a more granular, basophilic appearance predominate in some cases. Well preserved cells usually retain a relatively rounded contour. Nuclei are generally large, are round or ovoid, and may be eccentrically placed, with a moderate increase in the N/C ratio. With higher grade tumors, irregular nuclear contours may be seen. Nuclei are commonly "open-faced," and many cells have a characteristic single, large, rounded nucleolus. With increasing degeneration, however, nuclei may become densely hyperchromatic, with nucleoli less and less apparent.

It is well to remember that none of the features noted in cells from renal cell carcinoma is particularly distinctive. Other malignancies, particularly adenocarcinomas of varied origin (Fig. 21-63), may mimic the appearance described above.[153] It is of greater concern that certain *nonmalignant lesions,* e.g., nephrogenic adenoma, may shed cells that may have not only prominent cytoplasmic vacuolation but significant nuclear atypia as well.[180] Thus caution is in order in rendering a diagnosis of renal cell carcinoma on the basis of urinary cytology, and most often the best one can do is to suggest the possibility.

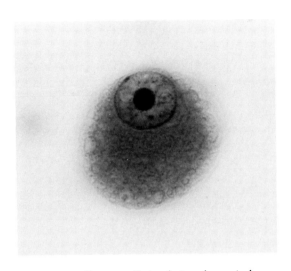

Fig. 21-63 Malignant cell simulating the typical appearance of renal cell carcinoma. This patient, however, proved to have a clear cell carcinoma of the prostatic utricle. Papanicolaou. ×968.

PROSTATIC CARCINOMA

Although involvement of the bladder neck and proximal urethra may be seen in a significant number of cases of prostatic carcinoma, it is unusual to find cytologic evidence of this tumor in spontaneously voided urine specimens. One possible explanation is the seeming resistance of the urothelium itself to tumor penetration despite direct spread to the underlying submucosa.[127] Improvement in diagnostic yield may be noted either with or after prostatic massage. Garret and Jassie[66] reported a series of cases in which secretions obtained by prostatic massage and postmassage voided urine specimens were examined. In patients with urinary tract symptoms, 33 of 149 were subsequently found to have prostatic carcinoma. In this group, diagnostic evidence of carcinoma was found in massage secretion specimens in 21.2 percent, with an additional 6 percent of specimens reported as suspicious. Surprisingly, postmassage voided urine specimens gave even better results, with positive and suspicious rates of 48.5 and 15.1 percent, respectively.

Prostatic adenocarcinoma cells, particularly those from low and intermediate grade tumors, tend to shed in groups (Fig. 21-64), and in some an acinar arrangement may be discerned (Fig. 21-65). Individual cells show varying amounts of basophilic cytoplasm. Nuclei often retain rounded contours and are enlarged,

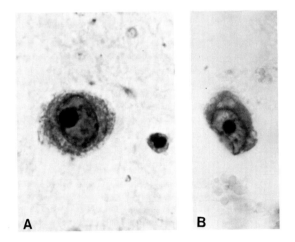

Fig. 21-62 Renal cell carcinoma. Note the varying degrees of cytoplasmic vacuolation and large, vesicular nuclei with solitary large nucleoli. Papanicolaou. ×880.

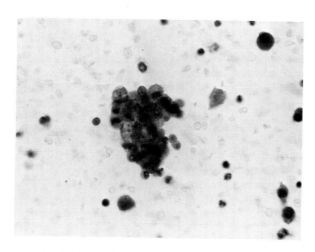

Fig. 21-64 Prostatic carcinoma. Note the nuclear crowding and overlap in this tissue fragment of malignant cells. Papanicolaou. ×352.

and the N/C ratio is increased. Chromatin texture varies, increasingly coarse in higher grade tumors, and nucleoli are generally prominent. With increasing tumor grade, the malignant cells become less cohesive, and the cytologic features begin to merge with those of other poorly differentiated malignancies. Again, as with other nonurothelial primaries, it is often the most aggressive, poorly differentiated prostatic tumors that are seen in spontaneously voided urine specimens, and the cytologic features of these lesions may not be sufficiently characteristic to reliably distinguish them from high grade urothelial lesions. Immunoperoxidase stains for prostate-specific antigen and prostatic acid phosphatase performed on cytocentrifuge preparations or cell block material may be of help in the differential diagnosis.

NEPHROBLASTOMA (WILMS' TUMOR)

Nephroblastoma, or Wilms' tumor, is the most common renal malignancy of childhood, with approximately two-thirds of cases occurring before the age of 5.[72] Hajdu[72] reviewed the cytologic findings in 32 cases, with diagnostic material obtained predominantly from pleural and peritoneal fluids in patients with metastatic disease. Three of the 32 cases yielded diagnostic cells by urinary cytology, however, and the morphologic findings were similar.

The material reflected the primitive appearance of nephroblastoma seen histologically. Cells tend to shed singly, but cell clusters may be found (Fig. 21-66), and truly cohesive groups help to differentiate the cells from those seen with lymphoreticular and hematopoietic neoplasms. Most cells varied from oval to short-spindled in shape, most often without discernible cytoplasm. Nuclear borders were distinct, with only slight irregularities, and chromatin appeared to be relatively uniformly distributed in a granular fashion, with occasional peripheral condensation. Nucleoli were prominent in some cells. Large mononuclear cells were also sometimes seen. In gen-

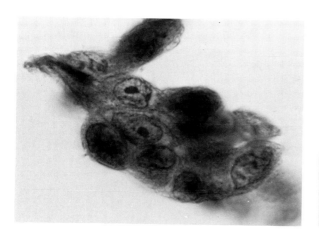

Fig. 21-65 Prostatic carcinoma. Note the enlarged nuclei with prominent nucleoli in this tissue fragment with acinar features. Papanicolaou. ×880.

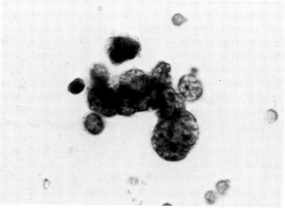

Fig. 21-66 Nephroblastoma. Note the primitive-appearing cells with very high N/C ratios, coarsely granular chromatin, and occasional nucleoli. Papanicolaou. ×880.

eral, the cytologic features bespeak a rather primitive tumor.

Although such cases are unusual in the cytology laboratory, the fact that hematuria is one of the most common presenting complaints among patients with Wilm's tumor is indicative that these lesions may be in communication with the urinary drainage system at the time of diagnosis. As the cells often seem to lack intact cytoplasm, they may be passed by as nothing more than degenerated epithelial cells. When the setting is proper, however, the cytopathologist must be alert to the possibility of this disorder. Differential diagnosis, according to Hajdu,[72] includes neuroblastoma, Ewing's sarcoma, and rhabdomyosarcoma. Differentiation from these other lesions may not be possible, and the cytopathologist is often limited to a diagnosis of "small cell malignant tumor," with a comment listing the various possibilities in the differential.

LYMPHOMA

Although most unusual, true primary lymphomas have been seen on occasion throughout the genitourinary tract,[90,174] and they may shed recognizable cells into the urinary pool. Much more frequently, however, such lesions are part of a systemic process. The urologist may be confronted with the problem of hematuria and renal failure in patients with known lymphoma; and among the various diagnostic possibilities, including drug effects and clotting disorders, direct involvement of the genitourinary tract by the lymphomatous process must also be considered.[193] The kidney is the organ most commonly involved by systemic lymphomas, although bladder spread has been noted in as many as 13 percent of patients in autopsy studies.[182] All of the standard types of lymphoma may be seen, with some reports showing a preponderance of non-Hodgkin's lymphomas[182] and others an approximately equal distribution between Hodgkin's and non-Hodgkin's lymphomas.[193]

The cytopathologist may be of help in the diagnosis of genitourinary lymphoma, whether primary or secondary. The cytologic appearance of these lesions in well preserved urine specimens is similar to that in other body fluids. Small cell or lymphocytic lymphomas shed cells that are usually somewhat larger than normal lymphocytes, with comparably high N/C ratios, but with moderately hyperchromatic nu-

clei that may have recognizable nuclear foldings and irregular nuclear protrusions (Fig. 21-67). Some cell aggregates may be found, but true tissue fragments are obviously lacking. Large cell or "histiocytic" lymphomas shed cells of noticeably greater size but still usually smaller than those seen with poorly differentiated epithelial malignancies. They have more vesicular nuclei, at times still rounded but at other times convoluted in shape, with basophilic to amphophilic nucleoli usually apparent. For patients with Hodgkin's disease, both classic Reed-Sternberg cells and variant types have been noted in urinary preparations.[14]

One must be wary of overinterpreting atypical nuclear changes in lymphoid cells seen in urinary cytology preparations, particularly in the presence of severe inflammation and degenerative changes. Even if the setting is suspicious, i.e., the patient has systemic lymphoma with genitourinary symptoms, the degree of nuclear abnormality may be such that a definitive diagnosis is not possible, and histologic studies may be necessary for confirmation.

PLASMACYTOMA

Rare extramedullary plasmacytomas of the genitourinary tract, such as the bladder lesion described by Yang et al.,[201] have been noted in the literature. In patients with systemic myeloma, evidence of genito-

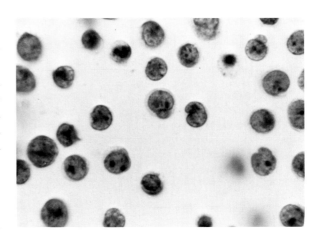

Fig. 21-67 Lymphoma. Individual cells show some degree of nuclear enlargement compared to normal lymphocytes and a high N/C ratio; prominent nuclear protrusions are apparent in some cells. Papanicolaou. ×880.

urinary "involvement" occurs principally in the form of renal insufficiency. Only a few cases are due to direct invasion by malignant plasma cells, however, with most cases of renal failure related to tubular damage and the development of "myeloma kidney."

As indicated by Geisinger et al.,[67] direct diagnosis of myeloma by exfoliative cytology is unusual, with only 6 of 126 such patients in their series showing diagnostic features in cytologic specimens, with all sources (pleural and peritoneal fluid, urine, etc.) considered. In fact, in their review of 20 years' experience, none of the urinary specimens from patients with myeloma showed positive findings. Nonetheless, in some cases of direct involvement of the genitourinary tract by primary or secondary plasma cell tumors, diagnostic cytologic changes may be found in the urinary sediment.[138,201] As with lymphoma, the cells shed singly; and particularly for the more poorly differentiated tumors, plasmacytic features may be so lacking that one thinks of other forms of lymphoma first.[67] "Working backward" may be of help, wherein one traces the morphologic lineage of the essentially undifferentiated malignant cells, through intermediate forms, to more recognizable plasmacytoid cells. At least some are seen to demonstrate nuclear eccentricity, with peripheral dispersion of the chromatin in clumps along the nuclear membrane. Recognizable hofs may be seen adjacent to the nuclei. Binucleate forms, with antipodal symmetric nuclei, may also be of diagnostic help.

The cytopathologist may be of service in diagnosing the myeloma kidney, as patients with this lesion may excrete "myeloma casts," which are seen as a castlike, laminated, waxy-to-granular matrix surrounded by reactive-appearing syncytial giant cells, with occasional renal tubular cells embedded in the cast matrix.[21] In one series[21] six of nine myeloma patients with renal failure demonstrated such casts, and none was observed in a larger group of myeloma patients without evidence of renal failure.

MELANOMA

Primary melanoma of the genitourinary tract is rare; and aside from external penile and vulvar lesions, most such cases involve the distal urethra.[142,144] Rare case reports of primary bladder melanomas have also appeared.[2,196] However, although not often clinically apparent, metastatic malignant melanoma involving the genitourinary tract is surprisingly common at autopsy.[28] Whatever the source, these lesions may shed distinctive cells into the urine (Fig. 21-68).[157,199] They are described as occurring singly, with large, sharply defined vesicular nuclei, often eccentric in position. Large acidophilic macronucleoli are commonly seen. Recognition of these features should prompt a search for the key diagnostic feature: fine to coarse brown-black cytoplasmic melanin granules.[157] The number of granules may vary from cell to cell, being generally sparse to moderate in many cells but almost obscuring the nucleus in some. Routine centrifuged sediments and cytospin preparations may afford cell block material for confirmatory histochemical or immunohistochemical staining. These additional diagnostic steps should be pursued when-

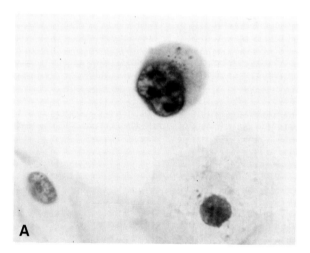

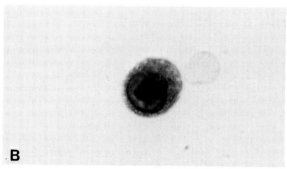

Fig. 21-68 Melanoma. **(A)** Cells are typically shed singly and have enlarged, eccentric, vesicular nuclei and prominent nucleoli. This cell shows sparse cytoplasmic pigment granules. **(B)** This more heavily pigmented cell has nuclear features that are partially obscured. Papanicolaou. ×968.

ever possible, as other pigmented cells, e.g., lipofuscin-containing renal tubular cells, occasionally cause confusion. These cells may show some degree of nuclear atypia as well, but they lack the distinctive nuclear features characteristic of melanoma described above.[157] At times, true *melanuria* is seen in the absence of actual melanoma cells in the urine,[157,189] but it typically occurs in patients with known systemic metastases with accompanying skin pigmentation, or "melanosis," a distinctive clinical picture.

METASTATIC TUMORS INVOLVING THE URINARY TRACT

The genitourinary system is not infrequently involved by local extension from adjacent primaries, e.g., those arising in the gastrointestinal tract and female genital tract, and it may obviously be involved by metastatic disease of varied origin. On rare occasions metastatic disease from an occult primary may first become apparent in the genitourinary tract and manifest in the urinary cytology preparation. The pathologist should be mindful of such a possibility when confronted with a tumor unusual in the urothelium, e.g., an adenocarcinoma (Fig. 21-69), and even more so when the possibility of a primary is rare, as in the case of lymphoma.

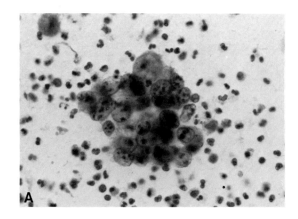

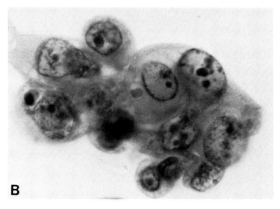

Fig. 21-70 Poorly differentiated malignant neoplasm found in a voided specimen. This tumor was difficult to categorize on the basis of cytologic features. It proved to be secondary involvement of the bladder by mesodermal mixed tumor of uterine origin. Papanicolaou. **A,** ×352; **B,** ×880.

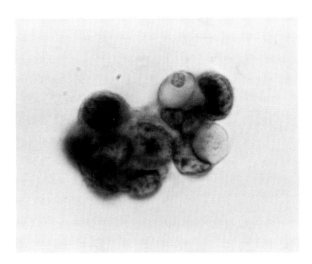

Fig. 21-69 Metastatic carcinoma. The patient had metastatic breast carcinoma secondarily involving the urinary tract. Cytologic features such as prominent cytoplasmic vacuolation suggest adenocarcinomatous differentiation. Papanicolaou. ×968.

Often, however, tumors aggressive enough to have insinuated themselves into the urinary tract are also high grade, poorly differentiated malignancies with little in the way of distinguishing features (Fig. 21-70). In such situations, cytologic diagnoses may be limited to generic terms, such as "poorly differentiated epithelial malignancy." It is then incumbent on the clinician to supply, whenever possible, adequate histologic material that may offer more definitive information to allow categorization of the tumor and a better opinion as to whether the tumor is likely to be primary or secondary. If the latter is more likely, it is obvious that all attempts must be made to exclude an occult primary elsewhere before proceeding with definitive urologic therapy.

EFFICACY OF CYTOLOGY IN THE DIAGNOSIS OF PRIMARY UROTHELIAL NEOPLASMS

Most reliable data on the efficacy of cytologic diagnosis are derived from studies of transitional cell carcinoma of the bladder, and the bulk of the discussion here is devoted to this topic. Difficulties associated with assessing the accuracy of cytology in the diagnosis of upper tract disease are outlined. Attention is also given to the occurrence and meaning of false-positive and false-negative diagnoses.

Bladder Carcinoma

In El-Bolkainy's[35] review of the cytology of bladder carcinoma, it was noted that the sensitivity of the technique showed wide variation from one published series to the next, ranging from a low of 44.7 percent to a high of 97.3 percent. This variation in figures is obviously disturbing; but as pointed out by the author and emphasized by other authorities,[103] studies from the literature are only roughly comparable for many reasons, which may be summarized as follows:

1. Many series encompass all patients with bladder carcinoma seen at a given institution and so include those with low grade papillary lesions, whereas other studies specifically exclude such patients. The resultant effects on accuracy figures are obvious.

2. Populations of patients in the various studies are often not clearly subdivided into those being seen for primary evaluation and those followed after a previously treated bladder carcinoma. The notable tendency for recurrent malignancy in the latter group of patients may obviously result in a positive bias in accuracy figures if they account for a significant percentage of the population studied.

3. The number of samples per patient is often not stated. For voided specimens and presumably for other specimen types, diagnostic accuracy is increased by the examination of multiple specimens versus only a single specimen.

4. In some instances the results of voided urinary specimens are not clearly separated from those based on other types of specimens, e.g., bladder washings, which may have a higher diagnostic yield.

5. Some series include nonurothelial tumors, e.g., renal carcinoma, prostatic carcinoma, and metastatic tumors, whereas others do not. The efficacy of urinary cytology in the diagnosis of such lesions, particularly the first two, is generally poor.

6. Inadequate documentation of the state of the remaining urothelium, as reflected in biopsy material from areas away from apparent primary lesions, is common. In cases of low grade papillary tumors, more serious abnormalities may be lurking in the cystoscopically "uninvolved" mucosa,[177] and overestimation of the efficacy of the method in the diagnosis of low grade tumors may result.

7. Some series only separate results into either positive or negative categories, whereas other series utilize an inconclusive category as well.

8. Cytologic criteria of malignancy presumably differ among the various series. More liberal criteria may increase sensitivity but generally at the expense of a decrease in specificity.

The last factor is the one that may contribute most to the variation in statistics from one study to the next. Examples of this phenomenon are seen in Tables 21-4 and 21-5, tabulations of cytology results for specimens from patients with low and intermediate grade carcinomas, respectively, in four representative series in the literature. All four studies were conducted by recognized authorities in the field of urinary cytology. Yet it appears that the first two laboratories, with high "false-negative" rates, are less adept at the diagnosis of low grade and intermediate grade malignancies than the last two laboratories. In fact, the disparities noted are probably most reflective of the variation of criteria for the cytologic diagnosis of low and intermediate grade malignancies, with the first two laboratories employing a conservative approach and the last two a relatively more liberal approach. This variation was, in turn, reflected in the rates of false positivity in the respective studies, i.e., the incidence of positive cytologic diagnosis in which no evidence of tumor could be found. The overall false-positive rate

Table 21-4 Results of Cytology: Grade I Carcinomas

Study	Negative (Percent)	Atypical (Percent)	Positive (Percent)
Farrow,[48] Rife et al.[164]	66.3	11.2	22.4
Esposti et al.[44]	85.7	14.3	0
Murphy et al.[136]	23.8	14.3	61.9
Shenoy et al.[173]	13.3	13.3	73.4

Table 21-5 Results of Cytology: Grade II Carcinomas

Study	Negative (Percent)	Atypical (Percent)	Positive (Percent)
Farrow,[48] Rife et al.[164]	25.4	12.7	61.9
Esposti et al.[44]	26.1	23.1	50.8
Murphy et al.[136]	0	22.7	77.3
Shenoy et al.[173]	0	11.5	88.5

Table 21-7 Results of Cytology: Carcinoma In Situ

Study	Negative (Percent)	Atypical (Percent)	Positive (Percent)
Farrow,[48] Rife et al.[164]	16.5	10.5	73.0
Koss et al.[103]	0	100.0	
Murphy et al.[136]	0	0	100.0
Shenoy et al.[173]	0	12.5	87.5

from the studies by Farrow, Rife, and co-workers[48,164] was 2.3 percent; and Esposti and colleagues[44] reported no false positives. Murphy's group,[136] conversely, had a false-positive rate of 10 to 14 percent and Shenoy et al.[173] a rate of 11 percent. Even this situation is not as clear-cut as it seems, however, a topic which we consider in more detail below.

As seen in Tables 21-6 and 21-7, the accuracy figures for grade III lesions and pure carcinoma in situ become much more respectable. A high percentage of such cases should yield sufficient evidence to diagnose malignancy; and with "atypical" and "positive" figures taken together, diagnostic rates should be at least in the neighborhood of 85 percent, with figures between 90 to 100 percent attainable.

With regard to invasive tumors, a somewhat peculiar but fortunate situation obtains with intermediate grade malignancies; that is, our ability to diagnose invasive intermediate grade lesions appears to be superior to that for noninvasive lesions. Esposti et al.[44] noted that none of 14 grade II tumors without suspected or proved invasion was cytologically reported as carcinoma. In contrast, 9 of 16 grade II lesions with suspected invasion and 24 of 35 lesions with frank invasion were cytologically classified as carcinoma. One possible explanation cited by the authors is that the number of cells shed from invasive tumors may be higher than the number shed from noninvasive

Table 21-6 Results of Cytology: Grade III Carcinomas

Study	Negative (Percent)	Atypical (Percent)	Positive (Percent)
Farrow,[48] Rife et al.[164]	6.1	9.8	84.1
Esposti et al.[44]	3.2	11.1	85.7
Murphy et al.[136]	0	6.3	93.7
Shenoy et al.[173]	9.3	5.5	85.2

tumors of the same grade. Another potential explanation is that the abnormal cells are shed from a more "disturbed" urothelium than is manifested in the obvious primary lesion, which also may at least in part account for the poorer prognosis in patients with grade II invasive disease versus those with noninvasive disease.

Whatever the explanation for our success in the cytologic diagnosis of invasive versus noninvasive lesions, it is apparent from the literature that our ability to detect the former cases, all grades included, by cytologic means is good, on the order of 92 to 93 percent.[44,103] In the transitional cell category, such invasive lesions are virtually all intermediate and high grade tumors. Moreover, these lesions, along with others readily detected by cytologic means (e.g., high grade carcinoma in situ and squamous and adenocarcinomas) presumably constitute the greatest threats to the health and life of the patient.

Renal Pelvic, Ureteral, and Urethral Carcinomas

The efficacy of cytology in the detection of urothelial carcinomas in the upper tract and urethra, particularly with voided or catheterization urine specimens, is difficult to assess. The major reason is the frequent occurrence of associated bladder carcinoma in patients with such lesions. For example, close to one-fourth of all upper tract carcinomas are discovered while the patient is being followed for a previously treated bladder carcinoma. Even in patients with no such history, approximately 7 to 10 percent of patients evaluated primarily for upper tract lesions are found to have concurrent bladder tumors, and subsequent bladder tumors occur in as many as 30 percent of patients following surgery for upper tract lesions. These facts suggest that many patients with upper tract malignancies already have abnormalities in the bladder uro-thelium to begin with, which may account for some or all of the abnormal cells seen in the cytology prepa-ration. Many studies on the cytology of upper tract lesions do not, and perhaps cannot, distinguish such interfering factors.

In one study, Eriksson and Johansson[39] reported the results of urinary cytology of voided specimens from 43 patients with upper tract carcinomas (30 renal pel-vic and 13 ureteral primaries). All but one patient had undergone preoperative cystoscopy to exclude asso-ciated bladder tumors. Their results, excluding three patients with unsatisfactory specimens, are shown in Table 21-8.

As with bladder carcinoma, approximately 86 per-cent of the specimens from patients with high grade upper tract lesions were reported as positive or atypi-cal. Again, there was variation of results, invasive versus noninvasive, from patients with intermediate grade tumors, with all of the five patients with inva-sive lesions reported as positive or atypical on cytol-ogy, versus only two of the ten patients with nonin-vasive lesions. All three patients with low grade tumors had negative cytology results.

Among the false negatives in the intermediate and high grade categories, a number of patients proved to have nonfunctioning kidneys on excretory urogra-phy. However, three patients with high grade carci-nomas did show positive urinary cytology despite ra-diologically nonfunctioning kidneys.

Attempts to localize lesions to the upper tract by directed catheterization, with either "drip collected urine specimens" or irrigation, have met with varied success; but basic diagnostic results appear to be supe-rior to those with simple voided specimens.[171] A good method is upper tract brushing, described by Gill et al.,[68,69] which may be even further improved with subsequent technical advances.[91] Presuming that a small catheter may be passed at all, it certainly appears to be the method of choice in patients with evidence of obstruction. It may yield not only material for cy-tology but also small tissue fragments for histologic evaluation, of particular value in the diagnosis of low grade papillary tumors. With the advent of nephrour-eteroscopy, however (see Ch. 19), direct histologic sampling of upper tract tumors may eventually re-place cytology for preoperative characterization of these lesions.

The cytologic diagnosis in voided urinary speci-mens of urothelial carcinomas occurring in the proxi-mal urethra presents a problem similar to that found with upper tract disease. That is, many such lesions are seen in association with bladder carcinomas, and it is not possible to localize the site of origin on the basis of the urinary cytologic findings. More distal lesions in the urethra show a greater propensity to squamous and glandular differentiation, although primaries yielding cytologically identical cells may also be found in the bladder and upper tract.

Localization of the cells to a urethral source may be attempted by the use of directed urethral swabbing, with either routine smears prepared and immediately fixed, or utilization of the soluble cellulose acetate swab technique described by Williams.[195] The latter technique, as with upper tract brushing, may yield not only excellent material for cytologic evaluation but also tissue fragments for histologic examination.

Such evaluation may be useful not only for primary urethral carcinomas but also in patients with bladder carcinoma, both before and after therapy. Urethral involvement in patients with high grade bladder le-sions may indicate a poorer prognosis, and such pa-

Table 21-8 Voided Urine Cytology versus Histology: Upper Tract Urothelial Carcinomas

Urinary Cytology Result	No. of Patients by Histologic Grade of Resected Tumor			
	0–I	II Noninvasive	II Invasive	III–IV
Negative	3	8	0	3
Atypical	0	2	3	2
Positive	0	0	2	17
Unsatisfactory	0	1	0	2

(From Eriksson and Johannson,[39] with permission.)

tients would be considered for total urethrectomy in conjunction with cystectomy. However, routine prophylactic urethrectomy in patients without evidence of involvement subjects many such patients to unnecessary additional surgery and precludes certain urinary diversion techniques.[79] Certainly in all cystectomy patients in whom the urethra is left intact, periodic urethral cytology examination should be considered.[79,198]

False-Negative and False-Positive Tests

The terms "false negative" and "false positive" are used frequently in the literature. "False negatives" are cases with proved carcinoma that have been reported as cytologically negative for tumor. "False positives," conversely, are cases reported as cytologically positive for malignancy that do not prove to have tumor by the usual corroborative means. Taken at face value, it seems that such measures would be clear indicators of the efficacy of the method. Unfortunately, however, their meaning is somewhat situational when applied to urinary cytology.

Here again, variability in the criteria for diagnosing malignancy of transitional cell lesions poses a basic problem. If one follows a liberal approach, false negatives are minimized but at the expense of an increased number of false positives. In the opposite direction, with a conservative approach, where one requires many of the "standard" cytologic features of malignancy before establishing a diagnosis, false positives are few, but false negatives necessarily increase.

With the liberal approach to diagnosis, the major cause of false-positive diagnosis is reactive changes encountered with various nonneoplastic processes. As we have seen from Kern's data,[92] the differences between cell characteristics in lower grade carcinomas and reactive atypias are small, and "overcalling" the cytologic findings in such instances account for many of the false-positive diagnoses.

Even with a conservative approach, however, there are still apparently "nonmalignant" situations that may be associated with cytologic alterations sufficient to elicit a diagnosis of carcinoma. As discussed above, the two most frequently mentioned in the literature are lithiasis[11,48] and prior treatment with systemic chemotherapeutic agents,[11] cyclophosphamide in particular.

Lithiasis is statistically the most likely to be encountered in daily practice; it accounted for most of the genuine false-positive diagnoses in the study of Beyer-Boon et al.[11] As these authors noted, in their cases removal of the stones was followed by disappearance of "malignant cells" from the patients' cytology specimens. Therefore it is important that a history of lithiasis be made known to the cytopathologist.

The situation with cyclophosphamide is less clear, for, as noted previously, numerous cases of urothelial carcinoma have been reported following administration of this drug (see Ch. 16). Four patients in the study of Beyer-Boon et al.[11] had been under treatment with cyclophosphamide for various nonurothelial malignancies, and all were found to have positive urinary cytologies. Two died from their original diseases, but the other two developed invasive bladder carcinomas during the course of treatment for their nonurologic malignancies. Thus the question of true versus false positivity in such patients may be answered only in the course of time.

A more general problem, discussed by Murphy,[130] is the confusion of false positives with "unconfirmed positives." The most common example is the situation wherein a positive cytology report is followed by cystoscopy, during which the clinician sees no apparent tumor. Momentarily the report then appears to be a "false positive" one, and indeed one of the possible explanations is a mistaken diagnosis on the part of the pathologist. However, it is often the least likely explanation, particularly in a laboratory where a conservative approach to diagnosis is followed. Much more commonly, the cytology reflects abnormalities in the "cystoscopically negative" urothelium. Even if representative biopsies prove to be negative, areas of significant urothelial abnormality may have been overlooked or be quite unrecognizable by cystoscopic means. Moreover, at least in voided specimens, the upper tract and the urethra may also be serving as sources for abnormal cells.

The importance of careful follow-up of such patients is demonstrated frequently in the literature.[3,48,78,164] In a series from the Mayo Clinic,[48,164] for example, 203 patients were found to have positive cytologies with initial negative cystoscopies. With careful reexamination and follow-up, including consideration of extraurinary tract sites, a striking majority of such patients (93.6 percent) proved subsequently to have malignant disease (Table 21-9). It is emphasized that confirmation of the cytologic find-

Table 21-9 Follow-up of Patients with Positive Cytology and Negative Cystoscopy

Diagnosis	Percent
Carcinoma	
Bladder	69.5
Kidney, ureter	4.4
Prostate	6.9
Cervix, vulva, endometrium	8.9
Other	3.9
Calculi	3.9
Undetermined	2.5

(Data from Farrow[48] and Rife et al.[164])

ings in these situations may take some time, and there are numerous references to prolonged periods of positive cytologies prior to the recognition of any apparent lesion. A good illustration of this point was the study by Heney et al.,[78] wherein nine such patients were followed at length. The presence of tumor was eventually confirmed in eight of the nine, with periods between cytologic diagnosis and clinical discovery of tumor ranging from 1 to 61 months (average 25 months). Seven of the eight had bladder carcinomas, all intermediate to high grade lesions, and five of these seven had progressed to muscle invasion by the time the lesions became clinically detectable.

False-negative diagnoses with a conservative approach will be high for grade I and at least a certain portion of grade II tumors, particularly those that are noninvasive. For grade III bladder lesions, false negatives are most often the result of "sampling problems," when the tumor fails to shed sufficient cells into the specimen obtained. For voided specimens it is again emphasized that the yield may be increased by evaluating multiple specimens.

For high grade upper tract lesions, obstruction of the tract may prevent adequate cellular material from reaching the voided specimen. Attempts at directed cytologic and/or histologic evaluation, following radiologic indication of obstruction, are then in order.

AUTOMATED CYTOLOGY ANALYSIS

Examination of cytologic material, as well as histologic material, is essentially an exercise in discriminant analysis wherein large numbers of morphologic features are observed and evaluated in comparison to similar features seen in cases of known outcome in the pathologist's experience. In this sense, the diagnostic workings of the pathologist's mind are similar to the workings of computers (although hopefully still of a degree of sophistication greater in at least some respects). Perhaps in part due to the recognition that some "human computers" do better than others, whether because of "programming," "data retrieval," or even day to day "power fluctuations," attempts at automated analysis of cytologic material were first reported during the mid-1960's.[89,194]

One technique is computerized analysis of cells based on the taxonomic intracellular analytic system (TICAS), introduced by Weid and colleagues.[194] The results of this analysis may be compared directly to those of routine cytology, as photometric scanning of routinely stained Papanicolaou preparations is performed, with the analysis based on light transmittance (or absorption) by individual cells and their constituents.[102] The system allows for quantitative evaluation of numerous cytologic features, many of which, e.g., cell and nuclear size and configuration, nuclear density, and chromatin dispersion, are the same features the cytopathologist evaluates by conventional light microscopy. Koss and co-workers[100-102] found that cells from a group of patients with known intermediate and high grade urothelial lesions could be reliably distinguished from benign urothelial cells by the technique, and that cells classified as "atypical" by visual estimation could be separated into two apparent groups, one clearly clustering with the benign cells evaluated, and the other clustering with the malignant cells. It would appear that this technique might prove useful not only in routine diagnostic work but also as an educational tool, wherein automatic recall of the various abnormal cells seen in a given smear would allow the light microscopist to compare his or her impressions with those of the computerized analysis of the specimen. Indeed, similar automated morphometric analysis has been used routinely in other areas of the laboratory, particularly for the evaluation of peripheral blood smears. At present, however, the technique as applied to routine cytologic diagnosis has not found widespread use as a diagnostic tool, although introduction of less expensive microcomputer-based versions may allow more practical application.[12] Another method of analysis, "interactive morphometry,"[118] wherein the examiner preselects populations of cells for similar morphometric measurements, has also been applied to urothelial neoplasms.[30,171] Again, however, similar to the fully automated method, the technique remains at the research stage.

A second approach, more commonly cited in the present literature, is automated flow cytometry (FCM). In conjunction with other emerging technologies, e.g., monoclonal antibody production, FCM has found increasing application in various areas of laboratory medicine (e.g., hematopathology and immunopathology), although utilization in cytopathology is still in the evolving stage.[117] With the technique, DNA content, either alone[58] or in conjunction with other parameters such as RNA content,[122,123] may be measured in as many as 10,000 cells per second.[117] This method allows rapid determination of various abnormalities in large cell populations, such as patterns of deviation from diploidy (e.g., triploidy and tetraploidy), the presence of aneuploid stem cell lines, and the presence of increased numbers of cells in the replicative phase.

The technique has been applied to tumor pathology from its inception,[89] and it has compared well with conventional cytologic analysis in a number of settings. Klein et al.,[93] for example, compared the results of FCM with those of routine cytology in a group of cystoscopically examined patients with known urothelial lesions and a group of 100 control patients requiring cystoscopy or surgery for nonneoplastic diseases of the bladder. Overall, FCM was found to at least equal conventional cytology in sensitivity and specificity. In the group of patients with known tumors at the time of the study, FCM was positive in 86 percent of those with noninvasive papillary carcinomas, 97 percent of those cases with flat carcinoma in situ, and 92 percent of those with invasive carcinoma, figures that compare favorably with those for routine cytology. Similar to conventional cytology, only about one-third of cases with low grade lesions were positive by FCM. Among the 36 cases of low grade lesions, six were found to have aneuploid cell lines, and two of these six patients developed flat carcinoma in situ during the relatively short follow-up of 12 months. Among the controls, there were only two false positive results among 100 cases, and both were for patients with severe cystitis and bladder calculi.

The technique appears to be particularly accurate in detecting patients with flat carcinoma in situ, with positive results for as many as 98 percent of cases,[94] presumably a reflection of the high incidence of an-

euploidy with such lesions. Conversely, results with low grade lesions, similar to the findings of Klein et al.,[93] have been relatively disappointing, with only a minority of cases detected. Obviously, as with any laboratory test, such diagnostic rates may be improved, depending on where the statistical cutoff point is set for a "malignant" diagnosis. Equally obvious is that an increased diagnostic rate of low grade lesions has its expense, with false positivity rates in excess of 30 percent reported in some studies.[31]

Various findings have been associated with potentially aggressive tumor behavior, in particular an increased fraction of cells with a hyperdiploid DNA complement and the appearance of an aneuploid stem cell line. Although the latter finding has been noted in a significant percentage of relatively nonaggressive tumors in other areas, e.g., low grade renal oncocytomas,[161] the recognition of an aneuploid cell population in a urothelial specimen is a worrisome situation. According to Melamed, (one of the founding fathers of FCM) and Klein[123]: "We have never seen a patient *without* a bladder tumor who had an aneuploid population in the bladder irrigation specimen."

Unfortunately, the converse does not hold true. That is, not all patients with aggressive or potentially aggressive urothelial tumors have obvious abnormalities of ploidy, and this problem remains one of the major pitfalls of the method.

Chin et al.[22] analyzed the results of FCM from a series of bladder tumors encompassing all stages and grades. In addition to bladder irrigation specimens, direct tumor samplings, either by biopsy or from cystectomies, were disaggregated to single cell suspensions, thereby ensuring that the cell populations studied were actually from the neoplasms in question.

As expected from other studies, the frequency of aneuploid cell populations increased with increasing tumor stage and grade. All noninvasive tumors, as well as all grade I tumors, were found to be diploid. Conversely, most of the high stage and the high grade tumors showed evidence of aneuploidy, and intermediate stage/grade lesions fell somewhere in between. However, of particular note was the fact that among all high stage lesions (T3 and T4), fully 25 percent appeared diploid; and among all grade III lesions, again almost one-fourth (23.1 percent) appeared diploid. Thus a significant number of aggressive lesions might not be detected by the method using this criterion; and the quantitative separation of peridiploid tumors, which may nonetheless have significant chromosome abnormalities, remains a problem. And if this is a problem in Western populations, it may be even more so in patients with bilharzia-associated carcinomas, most of which appear to be peridiploid.[1]

A further criticism is that FCM analysis has yet to be shown to offer definite *independent* predictive information when compared to conventional light microscopy. Murphy et al.,[132] for example, compared the results of conventional histologic grading to those of FCM analysis of disaggregated nuclei from the same tumor and found that the results of the FCM analysis appeared to offer no more prognostic information than histologic grading alone when evaluated in retrospect.

At the present time, at least with regard to urologic pathology, FCM must still be considered to be in a developmental stage and not yet ready for application to routine diagnostic work in the average hospital laboratory.[179] Although FCM has been rapidly developing over the past 10 years, techniques still vary considerably from one institution to the next, no definite protocol for FCM has been widely accepted or utilized, and numerous other practical issues have yet to be dealt with.[131,158] Even in its present state of development, however, many investigators[7,29,31,84,134] have found that it appears to be complementary to conventional cytology rather than just another method to accomplish the same end. That is, although each method may allow diagnosis of a similar number of cases, overlap is not necessarily complete, and the combination of the two techniques may yield accurate diagnostic results in more than 90 percent of cases. Technologic advances in FCM continue at a rapid pace,[117,172] and the method appears to hold great promise for the future, both as a primary tool and potentially in conjunction with other tools such as monoclonal antibodies, similar to the present flow cytometric methods used for evaluation of lymphoreticular neoplasms.

FINE NEEDLE ASPIRATION BIOPSY

The technique of fine-needle aspiration biopsy (FNA) has been applied in the practice of urology principally for the diagnosis of prostatic carcinoma and the evaluation of renal mass lesions, and it may also be of some use in the preoperative evaluation of lymph node status in patients with genitourinary malignancies. Broad coverage of the topic is beyond the scope of this chapter, and the above areas are dealt with only in brief. For a more complete discussion, the reader is referred to a number of fine monographs that deal with the technique in general, such as those of Frable,[55] Koss et al.,[105] and Linsk and Franzen,[112] as well as to the work of Kline[95] on FNA of the prostate.

Prostate Carcinoma

Tumor diagnosis by FNA dates back some 60 years in the United States,[73] and the first report specifically dealing with the diagnosis of prostate carcinoma is said to be that of Ferguson in 1930.[51] Despite this early beginning, enthusiasm for the technique has appeared only recently in the United States, and at present tissue core biopsy by either the transperineal or transrectal route remains the most commonly used diagnostic method.

In contrast, FNA has been widely practiced in Europe during the past few decades, having been refined and reintroduced by Franzen et al. in 1960.[57] Numerous reports attesting to the efficacy of the technique have been published, among the more notable those from Esposti and co-workers in Sweden.[40-43] Esposti's first major report appeared in 1966,[40] documenting the experience with 1,430 FNAs of the prostate in 1,110 patients. It was noted that the procedure, even upon repeat, was readily tolerated by the patients, with no major complications encountered in this large series. Tumor cells were found by FNA in approximately 30 percent of the group. A subset of 162 patients had both FNA and histologic material available for comparison, and 52 of 58 patients with histologically confirmed carcinoma had been diagnosed as positive on FNA, with an additional case reported suspicious. Although it was stated that no false-positive FNA diagnoses were made, three cases reported as positive by FNA had only benign prostatic hypertrophy on histologic examination. These disparities were ascribed to the tissue having been obtained by transurethral resection, presumably missing areas of peripheral malignancy, and the patients received hormonal treatment on the basis of the FNA findings alone.

As the technique has been embraced in the United States, it appears that the high expectations of the method set by our European colleagues are being met. Chodak et al.,[23] comparing FNAs with transperineal core biopsies from the same patients, found that the sensitivity of FNA in the diagnosis of prostatic carcinoma was 98 percent, compared to only 81 percent by the core biopsy method. Similar results were found by Carter and co-workers,[20] with a false-negative rate of 2.7 percent for FNA, compared to a 5.3 percent false-negative rate by core biopsy. Moreover, very good correlation was found between cytologic and histologic grading in the latter study.

The cytopathologist must be completely familiar with the appearance of normal and nonneoplastic prostatic tissue in FNA material prior to utilizing the method for the definitive diagnosis of prostatic malignancies. According to Kline,[95] the pattern of benign disease is usually apparent on low power examination, with relatively sparse cellularity and with those cells present most commonly arranged in cohesive sheets (Fig. 21-71A). The individual sheets show an orderly array of uniform cells in a "honeycomb"

pattern, with minimal nuclear overlap (Fig. 21-71B). Nuclei are round to ovoid, relatively evenly spaced, and uniform in size. Chromatin is evenly dispersed and finely granular, with occasional small chromocenters seen. Nulceoli are generally inapparent.

Differentiation of low grade carcinomas from benign prostatic disease may be difficult, and such cases account for many of the inconclusive and false-negative situations encountered.[95] Cellularity may be increased in low grade carcinomas compared to that seen with benign disease. Sheets of cells are still com-

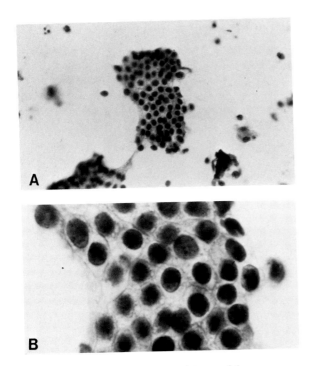

Fig. 21-71 Fine needle aspiration biopsy of the prostate — benign disease. **(A)** Relatively sparsely cellular specimen containing cohesive sheets of benign epithelium. **(B)** Uniform, bland-appearing nuclei arranged in a "honeycomb" pattern. Papanicolaou. **A,** ×242; **B,** ×968.

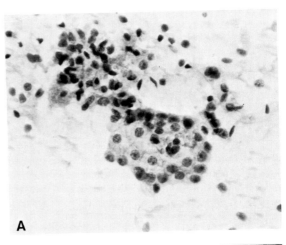

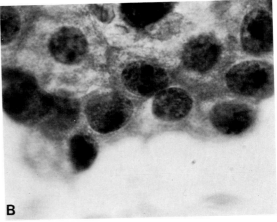

Fig. 21-72 Fine needle aspiration biopsy of the prostate — intermediate grade carcinoma. **(A)** Cellular specimen with malignant cells seen individually and in tissue fragments. **(B)** Tissue fragment, higher power view. Compare with Fig. 21-71B. Note the increased nuclear size, focal nuclear crowding, and prominent nucleoli. Papanicolaou. **A,** ×220; **B,** ×880.

monly present, but the degree of structural regularity begins to decrease, and some element of nuclear overlapping appears. Microacinar formation is a helpful diagnostic feature with these lesions.[95,115] At the individual cell level, overall cell and nuclear diameters are increased in at least some cells. Prominent nucleoli may now be noted in some cells, although this finding is not pathognomonic, as nucleoli are also seen on occasion in cells from patients with benign disease.[95]

Moderately and poorly differentiated carcinomas generally present a much easier task for the cytopathologist (Fig. 21-72). The cellularity of the specimen is often greatly increased compared to that seen with benign disease, with less cellular cohesion. Malignant cells, singly and in sheets, are now readily seen. In cell groups, nuclear overlap may be prominent. Anisocytosis and anisonucleosis are increased compared to well differentiated tumors, nuclear size is noticeably larger, and the N/C ratio is high in many cells. Other obvious features of malignancy, including nuclear membrane irregularity, abnormal chromatin distribution, etc. may be noted. Again, harking back to the typical histologic appearance of these tumors, prominent nucleoli are the rule.

There are a number of pitfalls in the diagnosis of prostatic aspirations, such as misinterpretation of the atypical-appearing seminal vesicle cells that are found in some specimens (Fig. 21-73) and overinterpreta-

tion of individual cell abnormalities in patients with, for example, inflammatory conditions or prior irradiation. For a discussion of these problems as well as a thorough pictorial representation, the reader is referred to Kline's monograph.[95]

Even with such problems taken into account, there is much to recommend FNA as a diagnostic method, and indeed one would have to concur with the sentiments expressed by Dr. Walsh in a recent editorial entitled: "Fine Needle Aspiration of the Prostate — Why has it taken so long to accept?"[191] The technique[95,115] is relatively simple, the equipment inexpensive, and the procedure well tolerated in most cases. Complications are few and generally of a minor nature, particularly compared to those associated with core biopsy.[23] Moreover, interference with subsequent surgery, which may be encountered with core biopsy, is minimized with FNA diagnosis.[23,191]

Despite the encouraging results now reported from many quarters, Walsh[191] pointed out that uncertainty about diagnostic accuracy is perhaps the major reason for reluctance to accept the technique by both clinician and pathologist. It has certainly been the prime hindrance to acceptance of diagnosis by FNA in other areas of the body, and one must appreciate the limitations of the technique in general, a topic discussed at length by Hajdu and Melamed.[73] One of the considerations with regard to FNA diagnosis noted by these authors — "aspiration samples should not be used in preference to larger biopsies when the latter can be easily and safely secured" — seems to speak for rather than against the use of FNA in the diagnosis of prostatic malignancies. In fact, all available data appear to indicate that the complications encountered with core biopsy of the prostate are considerably greater than those encountered with FNA, and the latter must be considered to be the safer of the two procedures. Moreover, the published figures indicate that the diagnostic accuracy rivals or surpasses that of core biopsy, and it seems that acceptance of the technique in the United States is indeed overdue. At the same time, a point of caution sounded by various authorities in the field is well taken[23,115]; that is, FNA of the prostate is a technique that takes some time to master, both in order to obtain adequate material and to arrive at an accurate diagnosis. At the outset, the clinician is urged to judiciously select those cases considered for the procedure, avoiding situations such as obvious prostatitis, where the cytologic findings may be diffi-

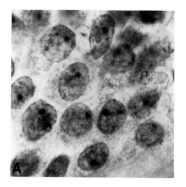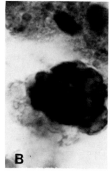

Fig. 21-73 Fine needle aspiration biopsy of the prostate — seminal vesicle cells. **(A)** Sheet of seminal vesicle epithelium with nuclei larger than those in typical benign prostatic epithelium and occasional nucleoli. Granular yellow pigment in the cytoplasm, which may be seen in Papanicolaou stained smears, allows identification of the origin of the cells. **(B)** Markedly atypical seminal vesicle cell. Failure to recognize the origin of such cells may lead to a mistaken diagnosis of malignancy. Papanicolaou. **A,** ×216; **B,** ×862.

cult to interpret and indeed the procedure is thought to be clinically contraindicated to begin with. Pathologists are urged not to overextend themselves at the microscope, particularly in attempts to diagnose well differentiated malignancies.[23] For those used to working with core biopsy material, a suitable in-house pilot study, wherein both core biopsy and FNA material are obtained at the same sitting, may be of great help in diagnostic correlation, and FNA probably adds little if any to the morbidity of the procedure.[20] It is only when both clinician and pathologist are completely comfortable with the technique that therapeutic decisions should be made on the basis of FNA material. In this regard the words of Dr. Fred Stewart, quoted by Hajdu and Melamed,[73] are well to remember: "Diagnosis by aspiration is as reliable as the combined intelligence of the clinician and pathologist makes it."

Renal Mass Lesions

Fine needle aspiration has proved of value in the diagnosis of renal mass lesions in many European centers.[87,106,190] In a report from Denmark, Juul et al.[87] documented their findings in a consecutive series of 301 FNAs of renal lesions performed over a 4-year period. The lesions were first characterized as solid masses by ultrasonography. Subsequent needle aspiration was guided by the same technique, although computerized tomography and fluoroscopy may serve equally well in this regard. A posterior approach was used, with an 18-gauge needle inserted through the skin and fascia serving as a guide sheath, through which a 23-gauge aspiration needle was inserted into the mass. Four or five passes were made in each case; and except for a few instances of transient hematuria, none requiring treatment, complications were not encountered.

Of the 301 patients, material sufficient for evaluation was obtained from 285 (95 percent). Of the malignant lesions encountered, 185 of 210 cases with adequate material were correctly diagnosed by FNA, with 25 reported as benign, giving a false-negative rate of 12 percent. Somewhat more disturbing, however, was the fact that 14 of 75 cases of benign disease were reported malignant by FNA, giving a false-positive rate of close to 20 percent. Six of these 14 cases proved to be inflammatory conditions, with benign cysts, adenomas, etc. accounting for the remaining eight. It is of particular note that all of the false-posi-

tive cases were diagnosed as relatively well differentiated adenocarcinomas on the basis of the FNA findings.

In another study, Murphy et al.[137] documented the results of 152 aspiration biopsies from a group of patients with various renal lesions, including suspected cysts and mass lesions in nonfunctioning kidneys. In all cases, attempts were made to obtain not only cytologic material but tissue fragments as well. Aspiration was initially performed with 20- to 22-gauge needles; if a solid mass was found and tissue was not obtained, aspiration was followed by introduction of an 18-gauge needle with a notched end, more suitable for extracting tissue fragments. Sufficient material for diagnosis was obtained in most of the cases. No significant complications were encountered despite use of the larger-bore needle. Confirmation of the clinical and radiologic findings in the two major categories of lesions (renal cysts and renal cell carcinomas) was accomplished in 90 of 92 and 29 of 35 cases, respectively. In those cases of solid tumor in which suitable material was obtained, 72 percent contained diagnostic material in both cytologic and histologic preparations, 20 percent in histologic preparations only, and 8 percent in cytologic preparations only. In the entire series, only one false-positive and one false-negative result were noted.

The cytologic findings in cases of benign renal cysts typically include cells with foamy cytoplasm, a low N/C ratio (less than 1:2), and round and regular nuclei with finely dispersed chromatin.[137] Nucleoli are either small or, more often, not seen at all. The cells usually occur singly, may contain brownish pigment, and are commonly set in a background of blood and cellular debris.

In contrast, cases of renal cell carcinoma (Fig. 21-74) more typically show cells in clusters, sheets, or papillary fragments, with homogeneous or foamy cytoplasm.[137] The N/C ratio is generally higher, with enlarged nuclei, round to oval in contour, and again relatively uniformly distributed granular chromatin. Prominent nucleoli were said to be present in all cells in the study of Murphy et al.[137] The background also usually consists of blood and necrotic debris.

Renal cell carcinoma is the most common tumor discovered by FNA of the kidney, although other tumors, e.g., transitional cell carcinomas of the pelvis, metastatic carcinomas, and lymphomas, may also be encountered.[137] It is perhaps in this area that FNA

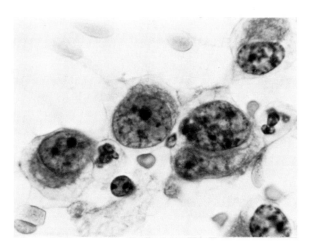

Fig. 21-74 Fine needle aspiration biopsy of the kidney — renal cell carcinoma. Note the large vesicular nuclei, with prominent nucleoli and some degree of cytoplasmic vacuolation and clearing. Papanicolaou. ×880.

may prove most useful. As pointed out by Juul et al.,[87] the mere finding of a solid renal mass lesion is considered an indication for open surgery in many centers; and because most of these lesions prove to be renal cell carcinomas, the FNA may be superfluous. It may prove helpful to confirm the diagnosis of renal cell carcinoma, however, particularly if maneuvers such as preoperative embolization are contemplated. As Murphy and colleagues[137] indicated, clinical situations are not always clear-cut, and FNA diagnosis may be pivotal to patient management in some cases. An example cited by these authors was a patient thought to have a primary renal neoplasm by computerized tomography (CT) scan, who turned out to have metastatic small cell undifferentiated carcinoma from the lung and thus was presumably spared unnecessary major surgery. A contrasting example was a woman with a history of breast carcinoma who had a renal mass initially thought likely to be a metastasis from her original tumor. It in fact proved, by FNA, to be a second primary, a transitional cell carcinoma of the renal pelvis. Thus the appropriate procedure, nephrectomy, was performed that might otherwise have been foregone.

It should be noted that enthusiasm for the technique is not universal. Wehle and Grabstald,[192] for example, documented one of the rare reported cases of needle tract seeding by renal adenocarcinoma and warned that FNA does not always contribute to

proper care of the patient. Prudent use of the technique is certainly in order. Both clinician and pathologist are urged to avoid the "Mount Everest approach" — sticking needles into things simply because they are there — but rather to contemplate what is to be gained by the procedure and how the patient's management might be altered by the findings. It must be kept in mind that false-positive and false-negative diagnoses do occur, and the hazards to the patients, although minimal, are not nonexistent. Despite the drawbacks, however, as illustrated by Murphy et al.,[137] FNA of renal mass lesions may afford a much more rational approach to therapy in selected clinical situations.

Lymph Node Staging

Bipedal lymphangiography has been used for many years in the preoperative assessment of nodal status in patients with genitourinary malignancies. As noted by Piscioli et al.,[154,156] the reported accuracy of the technique is variable, and these authors documented their experience with FNA of pelvic lymph nodes following lymphangiography. Their studies are of particular value in that all of the patients had subsequent lymphadenectomies, regardless of lymphographic or cytologic findings, in order to establish the reliability of the technique.

In a general study[156] of 71 patients thought initially to have localized prostatic, bladder, or penile cancers, these authors found the accuracy of FNA of the pelvic node groups to exceed that of lymphangiography alone, with positive cytologic findings in 21 of the 71 patients examined. Overall accuracy of FNA was reported as 93 percent, with a sensitivity of 81 percent and a specificity of 100 percent. An anterior approach was used for the needle aspirations, and despite obviously having to traverse a number of abdominal structures on the way to the lymph nodes to be aspirated, no complications were encountered in the entire series.

The technique is of particular value in that most of the major node groups likely to be involved by metastatic genitourinary malignancy may be sampled, with the high specificity rate particularly appealing. Certainly finding significant metastatic disease that involves the pelvic nodes should prove helpful, in that fruitless extirpative surgery may be avoided. Because of obvious sampling difficulties, false-negative results will be encountered, but the ability to more accurately stage at least a portion of patients with apparently localized disease would seem worth the effort.

REFERENCES

1. Abu Farha OM, Hamoud F, El-Garbawy M, et al: Cytogenetic study of carcinoma of bilharzial bladder. J Urol 133:300A, 1985
2. Ainsworth AM, Clark WH Jr., Mastrangelo M, Conger KB: Primary malignant melanoma of the urinary bladder. Cancer 37:1928, 1976
3. Allegra SR, Fanning JP, Streker JF, Corvese NM: Cytologic diagnosis of occult and "in situ" carcinoma of the urinary system. Acta Cytol (Baltimore) 10:340, 1966
4. Anderson JB, Nobbs GL, Hammonds JC: Urinary cytology and the early detection of renal allograft rejection. J Urol 136:10, 1986
5. Argyle C, Schumann GB, Genack L, Gregory M: Identification of fungal casts in a patient with renal candidiasis. Hum Pathol 15:480, 1984
6. Badalament RA, Cibas ES, Rueter VE, et al: Flow cytometric analysis of primary adenocarcinoma of the bladder. J Urol 137:1159, 1987
7. Badalament RA, Gay H, Whitmore WF Jr, et al: Monitoring intravesical bacillus Calmette-Guérin treatment of superficial bladder carcinoma by serial flow cytometry. Cancer 58:2751, 1986
8. Barlebo H, Sorensen BL, Soeborg Ohlsen, A: Carcinoma of the urinary bladder: flat intraepithelial neoplasia. Scand J Urol Nephrol 6:213, 1972
9. Bennett AH: Cyclophosphamide and hemorrhagic cystitis. J Urol 111:603, 1974
10. Beyer-Boon ME, Cuypers LHRI, deVoogt HJ, Brussee JAM: Cytological changes due to urinary calculi: a consideration of the relationship between calculi and the development of urothelial carcinoma. Br J Urol 50:81, 1978
11. Beyer-Boon ME, deVoogt HJ, van der Velde EA, et al: The efficacy of urinary cytology in the detection of urothelial tumours. Urol Res 6:3, 1978
12. Bibbo M, Dytch HE, Puls JH, et al: Clinical applications for an inexpensive, microcomputer-based DNA-cytometry system. Acta Cytol (Baltimore) 30:372, 1986
13. Blinst Italian Cooperative Group: Intravesical doxorubicin for the prophylaxis of superficial bladder tumors: a multicenter study. Cancer 54:756, 1984
14. Bocian JJ, Flam MS, Mendoza CA: Hodgkin's disease involving the urinary bladder diagnosed by urinary cytology: a case report. Cancer 50:2482, 1982
15. Bolande RP: Inclusion-bearing cells in the urine in certain viral infections. Pediatrics 24:7, 1959
16. Boon ME, Blomjous CEM, Zwartendijk J, et al: Carcinoma in situ of the urinary bladder: clinical presentation, cytologic pattern and stromal changes. Acta Cytol (Baltimore) 30:360, 1986
17. Bossen EH, Johnston WW: Exfoliative cytopathologic studies in organ transplantation. IV. The cytologic diagnosis of herpesvirus in the urine of renal allograft recipients. Acta Cytol (Baltimore) 19:415, 1975
18. Bossen EH, Johnston WW, Amatulli J, Rowlands DT, Jr: Exfoliative cytopathologic studies in organ transplantation. III. The cytologic profile of urine during acute renal allograft rejection. Acta Cytol (Baltimore) 14:176, 1970
19. Brenner DW, Schellhammer PF: Upper tract urothelial malignancy after cyclophosphamide therapy: a case report and literature review. J Urol 137:1226, 1987
20. Carter HB, Riehle RA, Jr., Koizumi JH, et al: Fine needle aspiration of the abnormal prostate: a cytohistological correlation. J Urol 135:294, 1986
21. Cheson BD, De Bellis CC, Schumann GB, Schumann JL: The urinary myeloma cast: frequency of detection and clinical correlations in 30 patients with multiple myeloma. Am J Clin Pathol 83:421, 1985
22. Chin JL, Huben RP, Nava E, et al: Flow cytometric analysis of DNA content in human bladder tumors and irrigation fluids. Cancer 56:1677, 1985
23. Chodak GW, Steinberg GD, Bibbo M, et al: The role of transrectal aspiration biopsy in the diagnosis of prostatic cancer. J Urol 135:299, 1986
24. Coleman DV: The cytodiagnosis of human polyomavirus infection. Acta Cytol (Baltimore) 19:93, 1975
25. Coleman DV, Gardner SD, Field AM: Human polyomavirus infection in renal allograft recipients. Br Med J 3:371, 1973
26. Crabtree WN, Murphy WM: The value of ethanol as a fixative in urinary cytology. Acta Cytol (Baltimore) 24:452, 1980
27. Curran FT: Malakoplakia of the bladder. Br J Urol 59:559, 1987
28. Das Gupta T, Grabstald H: Melanoma of the genitourinary tract. J Urol 93:607, 1965
29. Dean PJ, Murphy WM: Importance of urinary cytology and future role of flow cytometry. Urology 26:11, 1985
30. De Sanctis PN, Concepcion NB, Tannenbaum M, Olsson C: Quantitative morphometry measurements

of transitional cell bladder cancer nuclei as indicator of tumor aggression. Urology 29:322, 1987

31. DeVere White RW, Olsson CA, Deitch AD: Flow cytometry: role in monitoring transitional cell carcinoma of bladder. Urology 28:15, 1986

32. DeVoogt HJ, Wielenga G: Clinical aspects of urinary cytology. Acta Cytol (Baltimore) 16:349, 1972

33. Droller MJ: A rose is a rose is a rose, or is it? J Urol 136:1057, 1986

34. Droller MJ, Erozan YS: Thiotepa effects on urinary cytology in the interpretation of transitional cell cancer. J Urol 134:671, 1985

35. El-Bolkainy MN: Cytology of bladder carcinoma. J Urol 124:20, 1980

36. El-Bolkainy MN, Ghoneim MA, El-Morsey BA, Nasr SM: Carcinoma of bilharzial bladder: diagnostic value of urine cytology. Urology 3:319, 1974

37. El-Bolkainy MN, Mokhtar NM, Ghoneim MA, Hussein MH: The impact of schistosomiasis on the pathology of bladder carcinoma. Cancer 48:2643, 1981

38. Elsebai I: Parasites in the etiology of cancer— bilharziasis and bladder cancer. CA 27:100, 1977

39. Eriksson O, Johansson S: Urothelial neoplasms of the upper urinary tract: a correlation between cytologic and histologic findings in 43 patients with urothelial neoplasms of the renal pelvis or ureter. Acta Cytol (Baltimore) 20:20, 1976

40. Esposti PL: Cytologic diagnosis of prostatic tumors with the aid of transrectal aspiration biopsy: a critical review of 1,110 cases and a report of morphologic and cytochemical studies. Acta Cytol (Baltimore) 10:182, 1966

41. Esposti PL: Cytologic malignancy grading of prostatic carcinoma by transrectal aspiration biopsy: a five-year follow-up study of 469 hormone-treated patients. Scand J Urol Nephrol 5:199, 1971

42. Esposti PL, Elman A, Norlen H: Complications of transrectal aspiration biopsy of the prostate. Scand J Urol Nephrol 9:208, 1975

43. Esposti PL, Franzen S: Transrectal aspiration biopsy of the prostate: a re-evaluation of the method in the diagnosis of prostatic carcinoma. Scand J Urol Nephrol [Suppl] 55:49, 1980

44. Esposti PL, Moberger G, Zajicek J: The cytologic diagnosis of transitional cell tumors of the urinary bladder and its histologic basis: a study of 567 cases of urinary-tract disorder including 170 untreated and 182 irradiated bladder tumors. Acta Cytol (Baltimore) 14:145, 1970

45. Esposti PL, Zajicek J: Grading of transitional cell neoplasms of the urinary bladder from smears of bladder washings: a critical review of 326 tumors. Acta Cytol (Baltimore) 16:529, 1972

46. Fajardo LF, Berthrong M: Radiation injury in surgical pathology. Part I. Am J Surg Pathol 30:159, 1978

47. Fall M, Johansson SL, Aldenborg F: Chronic interstitial cystitis: a heterogeneous syndrome. J Urol 137:35, 1987

48. Farrow GM: Pathologist's role in bladder cancer. Semin Oncol 6:198, 1979

49. Farrow GM, Utz DC, Rife CC: Morphological and clinical observations of patients with early bladder cancer treated with total cystectomy. Cancer Res 36:2495, 1976

50. Feltis JT, Perez-Marrero R, Emerson LE: Increased mast cells of the bladder in suspected cases of interstitial cystitis: a possible disease marker. J Urol 138:42, 1987

51. Ferguson RS: Prostatic neoplasms: their diagnosis by needle puncture and aspiration. Am J Surg 9:507, 1930

52. Flanagan MJ, Miller A, III: Evaluation of bladder washing cytology for bladder cancer surveillance. J Urol 119:42, 1978

53. Flechner SM, McAninch JW: Aspergillosis of the urinary tract: ascending route of infection and evolving patterns of disease. J Urol 125:598, 1981

54. Forni AM, Koss LG, Geller W: Cytological study of the effect of cyclophosphamide on the epithelium of the urinary bladder in man. Cancer 17:1348, 1964

55. Frable WJ: Thin-needle aspiration biopsy. In Bennington JL (ed): Major Problems in Pathology. Vol. 14. Saunders, Philadelphia, 1983

56. Frable WJ, Paxson L, Barksdale JA, Koontz WW Jr: Current practice of urinary bladder cytology. Cancer Res 37:2800, 1977

57. Franzen S, Giertz G, Zajicek J: Cytological diagnosis of prostatic tumours by transrectal aspiration biopsy: a preliminary report. Br J Urol 32:193, 1960

58. Fried J, Perez AG, Clarkson BD: Rapid hypotonic method for flow cytofluorometry of monolayer cell cultures: some pitfalls in staining and data analysis. J Histochem Cytochem 26:921, 1978

59. Friedell GH: Urinary bladder cancer: selecting initial therapy. Cancer 60:496, 1987

60. Friedell GH, Hawkins IR, Nagy GK: Urinary bladder. p. 295. In Henson DE, Albores-Saavedra J (eds): The Pathology of Incipient Neoplasia. WB Saunders, Philadelphia, 1986

61. Friedell GH, Soto EA, Nagy GK: Cytologic and histopathologic study of bladder cancer patients. Urol Clin North Am 3:71, 1976

62. Frost JK: The Cell in Health and Disease: An Evalua-

tion of Cellular Morphologic Expression of Biologic Behavior. 2nd Revised Ed. Karger, Basel, 1986

63. Fuchs EF, Kay R, Poole R, et al: Uroepithelial carcinoma in association with cyclophosphamide ingestion. J Urol 126:544, 1981

64. Gardner SD: Prevalence in England of antibody to human polyomavirus (B.K.). Br Med J 1:77, 1973

65. Gardner SD, Field AM, Coleman DV, Hulme B: New human papovavirus (B.K.) isolated from urine after renal transplantation. Lancet 1:1253, 1971

66. Garrett M, Jassie M: Cytologic examination of post prostatic massage specimens as an aid in diagnosis of carcinoma of the prostate. Acta Cytol (Baltimore) 20:126, 1976

67. Geisinger KR, Buss DH, Kawamoto EH, Ahl ET, Jr.: Multiple myeloma: the diagnostic role and prognostic significance of exfoliative cytology. Acta Cytol (Baltimore) 30:334, 1986

68. Gill WB, Lu C, Bibbo M: Retrograde brush biopsy of the ureter and renal pelvis. Urol Clin North Am 6:573, 1979

69. Gill WB, Lu CT, Thomsen S: Retrograde brushing: a new technique for obtaining histologic and cytologic material from ureteral, renal pelvic and renal caliceal lesions. J Urol 109:573, 1973

70. Glashan RW, Wijesinghe DP, Riley A: The early changes in the development of bladder cancer in patients exposed to known industrial carcinogens. Br J Urol 53:571, 1981

71. Grunze H, Spriggs AI: Urine cytology I: What did Dr. Lambl say in 1856 about cancer cells in urine? Zeiss Inform Oberkochen 28:44, 1986

72. Hajdu SI: Exfoliative cytology of primary and metastatic Wilms' tumors. Acta Cytol (Baltimore) 15:339, 1971

73. Hajdu SI, Melamed MR: Limitations of aspiration cytology in the diagnosis of primary neoplasms. Acta Cytol (Baltimore) 28:337, 1984

74. Harris MJ, Schwinn CP, Morrow JW, et al: Exfoliative cytology of the urinary bladder irrigation specimen. Acta Cytol (Baltimore) 15:385, 1971

75. Hartman CR, Millar JW: Parasitic disease p. 515. In Devine CJ, Stecker JF, Jr. (ed): Urology in Practice. Little, Brown, Boston, 1978

76. Hayry P, von Willebrand E: Monitoring of human renal allograft rejection with fine-needle aspiration cytology. Scand J Immunol 13:87, 1981

77. Hayry P, von Willebrand E: Transplant aspiration cytology. Transplantation 38:7, 1984

78. Heney NM, Szyfelbein WM, Daly JJ, et al: Positive urinary cytology in patients without evident tumor. J Urol 117:223, 1977

79. Hickey DP, Soloway MS, Murphy WM: Selective urethrectomy following cystoprostatectomy for bladder cancer. J Urol 136:828, 1986

80. Houston W, Koss LG, Melamed MR: Bladder cancer and schistosomiasis: a preliminary cytological study. Trans R Soc Trop Med Hyg 60:89, 1966

81. Hrushesky W, Sampson D, Murphy GP: Lymphocyturia in human renal allograft rejection. Arch Surg 105:424, 1972

82. Huland H, Otto U, Droese M, Kloppel G: Long-term mitomycin C instillation after transurethral resection of superficial bladder carcinoma: influence on recurrence, progression, and survival. J Urol 132:27, 1984

83. Issell BF, Prout GR Jr, Soloway MS, et al: Mitomycin C intravesical therapy in noninvasive bladder cancer after failure on thiotepa. Cancer 53:1025, 1984

84. Jitsukawa S, Tachibana M, Nakazono M, et al: Flow cytometry based on heterogeneity index score compared with urine cytology to evaluate their diagnostic efficacy in bladder tumor. Urology 29:218, 1987

85. Johnson JR, Ireton RC, Lipsky BA: Emphysematous pyelonephritis caused by Candida albicans. J Urol 136:80, 1986

86. Jones DB, Rinas AC, Balachandran I, Steele C: Urinary cytology of renal transplantation. A.S.C.P. Check Sample Cont. Educ. Progr., Cytopathology No. C86-8 (C-158), 1986

87. Juul N, Torp-Pedersen S, Gronvall S, et al: Ultrasonically guided fine needle aspiration biopsy of renal masses. J Urol 133:579, 1985

88. Kahan AV, Coleman DV, Koss LG: Activation of human polyomavirus infection—detection by cytologic technics. Am J Clin Pathol 74:326, 1980

89. Kamentsky LA, Melamed MR, Derman H: Spectrophotometer: new instrument for ultrarapid cell analysis. Science 150:630, 1965

90. Kandel LB, McCullough DL, Harrison LH, et al: Primary renal lymphoma: does it exist? Cancer 60:386, 1987

91. Karlsen S: Improved technique for retrograde brushing in diagnosis of urothelial tumors of upper urinary tract. Urology 18:345, 1981

92. Kern WH: The cytology of transitional cell carcinoma of the urinary bladder. Acta Cytol (Baltimore) 19:420, 1975

93. Klein FA, Herr HW, Sogani PC et al: Detection and follow-up of carcinoma of the urinary bladder by flow cytometry. Cancer 50:389, 1982

94. Klein FA, Herr HW, Whitmore WF, et al: An evaluation of automated flow cytometry (FCM) in detection of carcinoma in situ of the urinary bladder. Cancer 50:1003, 1982

95. Kline TS: Guides to Clinical Aspiration Biopsy: Prostate. Igaku-Shoin, Tokyo, 1985

96. Koontz WW Jr, Prout GR Jr, Smith W, et al: The use of intravesical thio-tepa in the management of non-invasive carcinoma of the bladder. J Urol 125:307, 1981

97. Koss LG: Tumors of the urinary bladder. Atlas of Tumor Pathology. Fascicle 11, 2nd Series. Armed Forces Institute of Pathology. Washington, DC, 1975

98. Koss LG: Diagnostic Cytology and Its Histopathologic Bases. 3rd Ed. Lippincott, Philadelphia, 1979

99. Koss LG: BK viruria and hemorrhagic cystitis. N Engl J Med 316:108, 1987

100. Koss LG, Bartels PH, Bibbo M, et al: Computer discrimination between benign and malignant urothelial cells. Acta Cytol (Baltimore) 19:378, 1975

101. Koss LG, Bartels PH, Sychra JJ, Wied GL: Computer discriminant analysis of atypical urothelial cells. Acta Cytol (Baltimore) 22:382, 1978

102. Koss LG, Bartels PH, Wied GL: Computer-based diagnostic analysis of cells in the urinary sediment. J Urol 123:846, 1980

103. Koss LG, Deitch D, Ramanathan R, Sherman AB: Diagnostic value of cytology of voided urine. Acta Cytol (Baltimore) 29:810, 1985

104. Koss LG, Melamed MR, Mayer K: The effect of busulfan on human epithelia. Am J Clin Pathol 44:385, 1965

105. Koss LG, Woyke S, Olszewski W: Aspiration Biopsy. Cytologic Interpretation and Histologic Bases. Igaku-Shoin, Tokyo, 1984

105a. Krieger JN: Urologic aspects of trichomoniasis. Invest Urol 18:411, 1981

105b. Krieger, JN, Tam, MR, Stevens, CE, et al.: Diagnosis of trichomoniasis. Comparison of conventional wet-mount examination with cytologic studies, cultures, and monoclonal antibody staining of direct specimens. JAMA 259:1223, 1988

106. Kristensen JK, Holm HH, Rasmussen SN, Barlebo H: Ultrasonically guided percutaneous puncture of renal masses. Scand J Urol Nephrol [Suppl 15] 6:49, 1972

107. Lage JM, Bauer WC, Kelley DR, et al: Histological parameters and pitfalls in the interpretation of bladder biopsies in bacillus Calmette-Guérin treatment of superficial bladder cancer. J Urol 135:916, 1986

108. Lambird PA, Yardley JH: Urinary tract malakoplakia: report of a fatal case with ultrastructural observations of Michaelis-Gutmann bodies. Johns Hopkins Med J 126:1, 1970

109. Lambl W: Über harnblasenkrebs. Prager Vierteljahresschr f. Heilkunde 49:1, 1856

110. Leistenschneider W, Nagel R: Lavage cytology of the renal pelvis and ureter with special reference to tumors. J Urol 124:597, 1980

111. Lief M, Sarfarazi F: Prostatic cryptococcosis in acquired immune deficiency syndrome. Urology 28:318, 1986

112. Linsk JA, Franzen S (eds): Clinical Aspiration Cytology. Lippincott, Philadelphia, 1983

113. Linton AL, Clark WF, Driedger AA, et al: Acute interstitial nephritis due to drugs: review of the literature with a report of nine cases. Ann Intern Med 93:735, 1980

114. Littleton RH, Farah RN, Cerny JC: Eosinophilic cystitis: an uncommon form of cystitis. J Urol 127:132, 1982

115. Ljung B-M: Fine needle aspiration biopsy of the prostate gland: technique and review of the literature. Semin Urol 3:18, 1985

116. Loveless KJ: The effects of radiation upon the cytology of benign and malignant bladder epithelia. Acta Cytol (Baltimore) 17:355, 1973

117. Lovett EJ III, Schnitzer B, Keren DF, et al: Application of flow cytometry to diagnostic pathology. Lab Invest 50:115, 1984

118. Marchevsky AM, Gil J, Jeanty H: Computerized interactive morphometry in pathology: current instrumentation and methods. Hum Pathol 18:320, 1987

119. Masukawa T, Garancis JC, Rytel MW, Mattingly RF: Herpes genitalis virus isolation from human bladder urine. Acta Cytol (Baltimore) 16:416, 1972

120. McDougal WS, Cramer SF, Miller R: Invasive carcinoma of the renal pelvis following cyclophosphamide therapy for nonmalignant disease. Cancer 48:691, 1981

121. Melamed MR: The urinary sediment cytology in a case of malakoplakia. Acta Cytol (Baltimore) 6:471, 1962

122. Melamed MR, Darzynkiewicz Z, Traganos F, Sharpless T: Cytology automation by flow cytometry. Cancer Res 37:2806, 1977

123. Melamed MR, Klein FA: Flow cytometry of urinary bladder irrigation specimens. Hum Pathol 15:302, 1984

124. Melamed MR, Wolinska WH: On the significance of intracytoplasmic inclusions in the urinary sediment. Am J Pathol 38:711, 1961

125. Millard RJ: Busulfan-induced hemorrhagic cystitis. Urology 18:143, 1981

126. Morrison AS: Public health value of using epidemiologic information to identify high-risk groups for bladder cancer screening. Semin Oncol 6:184, 1979

127. Mostofi FK, Price EB Jr: Tumors of the male genital system. Fascicle 8, Second Series. Atlas of Tumor Pathology. Armed Forces Institute of Pathology, Washington, DC, 1973

128. Mostofi FK, Sobin LH, Torloni H (eds): International

Histological Classification of Tumours, No. 10: Histological Typing of Urinary Bladder Tumours. World Health Organization, Geneva, 1973

129. Murad TM, August C: Radiation-induced atypia: a review. Diagn Cytopathol 1:137, 1985

130. Murphy WM: Falsely positive urinary cytology: pathologists's error or preclinical cancer? J Urol 118:811, 1977

131. Murphy WM: DNA flow cytometry in diagnostic pathology of the urinary tract. Hum Pathol 18:317, 1987

132. Murphy WM, Chandler RW, Trafford RM: Flow cytometry of deparaffinized nuclei compared to histological grading for the pathological evaluation of transitional cell carcinomas. J Urol 135:694, 1986

133. Murphy WM, Crabtree WN, Jukkola AF, Soloway MS: The diagnostic value of urine versus bladder washing in patients with bladder cancer. J Urol 126:320, 1981

134. Murphy WM, Emerson LD, Chandler RW, et al: Flow cytometry versus urinary cytology in the evaluation of patients with bladder cancer. J Urol 136:815, 1986

135. Murphy WM, Soloway MS, Finebaum PJ: Pathological changes associated with topical chemotherapy for superficial bladder cancer. J Urol 126:461, 1981

136. Murphy WM, Soloway MS, Jukkola AF, et al: Urinary cytology and bladder cancer: the cellular features of transitional cell neoplasms. Cancer 53:1555, 1984

137. Murphy WM, Zambroni BR, Emerson LD, et al: Aspiration biopsy of the kidney: simultaneous collection of cytologic and histologic specimens. Cancer 56:200, 1985

138. Neal MH, Swearingen ML, Gawronski L, Cotelingam JD: Myeloma cells in the urine. Arch Pathol Lab Med 109:870, 1985

139. Nelson BM, Andrews GA: Breast cancer and cytologic dysplasia in many organs after busulfan (Myleran). Am J Clin Pathol 42:37, 1964

140. Neuman MP, Limas C: Transitional cell carcinomas of the urinary bladder: effects of preoperative irradiation on morphology. Cancer 58:2758, 1986

141. Nieh PT, Daly JJ, Heaney JA, et al: The effect of intravesical thio-tepa on normal and tumor urothelium. J Urol 119:59, 1978

142. Nissenkorn I, Servadio C, Avidor I, Marshak G: Malignant melanomas of female urethra. Urology 29:562, 1987

143. Nolan CR, III, Anger MS, Kelleher SP: Eosinophiluria—a new method of detection and definition of the clinical spectrum. N Engl J Med 315:1516, 1986

144. Oldbring J, Mikulowski P: Malignant melanoma of the penis and male urethra: report of nine cases and review of the literature. Cancer 59:581, 1987

145. O'Morchoe PJ, Riad W, Cowles LT, et al: Urinary cytologic changes after radiotherapy of renal transplants. Acta Cytol (Baltimore) 20:132, 1976

146. Orr WA, Mulholland SG, Walzak MP, Jr.: Genitourinary tract involvement with systemic mycosis. J Urol 107:1047, 1972

147. Packham DA: The epithelial lining of the female trigone and urethra. Br J Urol 43:201, 1971

148. Padgett BL, Walker DL: New human papovaviruses. Prog Med Virol 22:1, 1976

149. Padgett BL, Walker DL, ZuRhein GM, Eckroade RJ: Cultivation of papova-like virus from human brain with progressive multifocal leucoencephalopathy. Lancet 1:1257, 1971

150. Papanicolaou GN, Marshall VF: Urine sediment smears as a diagnostic procedure in cancers of the urinary tract. Science 101:519, 1945

151. Park C-H, Britsch C, Uson AC, Veenema RJ: Reliability of positive exfoliative cytologic study of the urine in urinary tract malignancy. J Urol 102:91, 1969

152. Person DA, Kaufman RH, Gardner HL, Rawls WE: Herpesvirus type 2 in genitourinary tract infections. Am J Obstet Gynecol 116:993, 1973

153. Peven DR, Hidvegi DF: Clear-cell adenocarcinoma of the female urethra. Acta Cytol (Baltimore) 29:142, 1985

154. Piscioli F, Pusiol T, Leonardi E, Luciani L: Role of percutaneous pelvic node aspiration cytology in the management of bladder carcinoma. Acta Cytol (Baltimore) 29:37, 1985

155. Piscioli F, Pusiol T, Polla E, et al: Urinary cytology of tuberculosis of the bladder. Acta Cytol (Baltimore) 29:125, 1985

156. Piscioli F, Scappini P, Luciani L: Aspiration cytology in the staging of urologic cancer. Cancer 56:1173, 1985

157. Piva AE, Koss LG: Cytologic diagnosis of metastatic malignant melanoma in urinary sediment. Acta Cytol (Baltimore) 8:398, 1964

158. Pritchett TR, Kanzler AW, Nichols PW, et al: A simple and practical technic for detecting cancer cells in urine and urinary bladder washings by flow cytometry. Am J Clin Pathol 84:191, 1985

159. Prout GR, Jr.: Introduction: management (control) of early bladder lesions. Cancer Res 37:2891, 1977

160. Prout GR, Jr.: Guest editorial: bladder cancer. J Urol 128:284, 1982

161. Rainwater LM, Farrow GM, Lieber MM: Flow cytometry of renal oncocytoma: common occurrence of

deoxyribonucleic acid polyploidy and aneuploidy. J Urol 135:1167, 1986

162. Remis RE, Halverstadt DB: Metastatic renal cell carcinoma to the bladder: case report and review of the literature. J Urol 136:1294, 1986

163. Riddle PR, Wallace DM: Intracavity chemotherapy for multiple non-invasive bladder tumours. Br J Urol 43:181, 1971

164. Rife CC, Farrow GM, Utz DC: Urine cytology of transitional cell neoplasms. Urol Clin North Am 6:599, 1979

165. Rohner TJ, Jr., Tuliszewski RM: Fungal cystitis: awareness, diagnosis and treatment. J Urol 124:142, 1980

166. Rosa B, Cazin M, Dalian G: Urinary cytology for carcinoma in situ of the urinary bladder. Acta Cytol (Baltimore) 29:117, 1985

167. Salm R: Combined intestinal and squamous metaplasia of the renal pelvis. J Clin Pathol 22:187, 1969

168. Schumann GB, Burleson RL, Henry JB, Jones DB: Urinary cytodiagnosis of acute renal allograft rejection using the cytocentrifuge. Am J Clin Pathol 67:134, 1977

169. Schumann GB, Weiss MA: Atlas of Renal and Urinary Tract Cytology and Its Histopathologic Bases. Lippincott, Philadelphia, 1981

170. Schwarz J: Mycotic prostatitis. Urology 19:1, 1982

171. Seldenrijk CA, Verheggen WJHM, Veldhuizen RW, et al: Use of cytomorphometry and cytology in the diagnosis of transitional-cell carcinoma of the upper urinary tract. Acta Cytol (Baltimore) 31:137, 1987

172. Shapiro HM: Technical developments in flow cytometry. Hum Pathol 17:649, 1986

173. Shenoy UA, Colby TV, Schumann GB: Reliability of urinary cytodiagnosis in urothelial neoplasms. Cancer 56:2041, 1985

174. Siegelbaum MH, Edmonds P, Seidmon EJ: Use of immunohistochemistry for identification of primary lymphoma of the bladder. J Urol 136:1074, 1986

175. Smith JH, Christie JD: The pathobiology of *Schistosoma haematobium* infection in humans. Hum Pathol 17:333, 1986

176. Soloway MS: Surgery and intravesical chemotherapy in the management of superficial bladder cancer. Semin Urol 1:23, 1983

177. Soloway MS, Murphy W, Rao MK, Cox C: Serial multiple-site biopsies in patients with bladder cancer. J Urol 120:57, 1978

178. Stanton MJ, Maxted W: Malacoplakia: a study of the literature and current concepts of pathogenesis, diagnosis and treatment. J Urol 125:139, 1981

179. Stephenson RA, Herr HW: Flow cytometry in urologic oncology. Urol Clin North Am 13:525, 1986

180. Stilmant M, Murphy JL, Merriam JC: Cytology of nephrogenic adenoma of the urinary bladder: a report of four cases. Acta Cytol (Baltimore) 30:35, 1986

181. Stilmant M, Siroky MB, Johnson KB: Fine needle aspiration cytology of granulomatous prostatitis induced by BCG immunotherapy of bladder cancer. Acta Cytol (Baltimore) 29:961, 1985

182. Sufrin G, Keogh B, Moore RH, Murphy GP: Secondary involvement of the bladder in malignant lymphoma. J Urol 118:251, 1977

183. Summers JL, Ford ML: The Papanicolaou smear as a diagnostic tool in male trichomoniasis. J Urol 107:840, 1972

184. Toma H: Experimental and clinical studies on prediction of acute renal allograft rejection. J Tokyo Womens Med Coll 51:704, 1981

185. Toma H, Ishida Y, Takahashi K, Ota K: The clinical value of active T-rosette-forming cells in urine after renal transplantation. J Urol 133:575, 1985

186. Troster M, Wyatt JK, Alen-Halagah J: Nephrogenic adenoma of the urinary bladder: histologic and cytologic observations in a case. Acta Cytol (Baltimore) 30:41, 1986

187. Utz DC, Farrow GM, Rife CC, et al: Carcinoma in situ of the bladder. Cancer 45:1842, 1980

188. Uyama T, Moriwaki S, Aga Y, Yamamoto A: Eosinophilic ureteritis? Regional ureteritis with marked infiltration of eosinophils. Urology 18:615, 1981

189. Valente PT, Atkinson BF, Guerry D: Melanuria. Acta Cytol (Baltimore) 29:1026, 1985

190. Von Schreeb T, Franzen S, Ljungqvist A: Renal adenocarcinoma: evaluation of malignancy on a cytologic basis: a comparative cytologic and histologic study. Scand J Urol Nephrol 1:265, 1967

191. Walsh PC: Fine needle aspiration of the prostate — why has it taken so long to accept? (editorial). J Urol 135:334, 1986

192. Wehle MJ, Grabstald H: Contraindications to needle aspiration of a solid renal mass: tumor dissemination by renal needle aspiration. J Urol 136:446, 1986

193. Weimer G, Culp DA, Loening S, Narayana A: Urogenital involvement by malignant lymphomas. J Urol 125:230, 1981

194. Wied GL, Bartels PH, Bahr GF, Oldfield DG: Taxonomic intra-cellular analytic system (TICAS) for cell identification. Acta Cytol (Baltimore) 12:180, 1968

195. Williams G: Cytological screening of the urethra. Br J Urol 40:703, 1968

196. Willis AJ, Huang AH, Carroll P: Primary melanoma of the bladder: a case report and review. J Urol 123:278, 1980

197. Wolinska WH, Melamed MR, Klein FA: Cytology of

bladder papilloma. Acta Cytol (Baltimore) 29:817, 1985

198. Wolinska WH, Melamed MR, Schellhammer PF, Whitmore WF, Jr.: Urethral cytology following cystectomy for bladder carcinoma. Am J Surg Pathol 1:225, 1977

199. Woodard BH, Ideker RE, Johnston WW: Cytologic detection of malignant melanoma in urine: a case report. Acta Cytol (Baltimore) 22:350, 1978

200. Wyatt JP, Saxton J, Lee RS, Pinkerton H: Generalized cytomegalic inclusion disease. J Pediatr 36:271, 1950

201. Yang C, Motteram R, Sandeman TF: Extramedullary plasmacytoma of the bladder: a case report and review of literature. Cancer 50:146, 1982

22

Anatomy, Embryology, and Physiology of the Testis and Its Ducts

James E. Wheeler

GROSS ANATOMY

The scrotum contains in separate compartments the paired male gonads, the testes, along with the excurrent duct system of each, the epididymis and vas deferens. The major blood vessels, nerves, lymphatics, and vas deferens run to or from the testis in a loosely connected bundle, the spermatic cord. As the testis descends into the scrotum (see Embryology, below), it brings with it a covering of mesothelial cells from the peritoneal cavity, which becomes the visceral layer of the tunica vaginalis. The parietal layer of the tunica vaginalis is the mesothelium-lined remnant of the processus vaginalis, an outpouching into the scrotum of the fetal peritoneal cavity (Fig. 22-1).

The testis is ovoid, 4 to 5 cm long, 3 cm in anteroposterior dimension, and 2.5 cm wide.[48] Measurements of the testis in vivo are complicated by the variable thickness of scrotal skin and the presence of the epididymis. Using caliper measurements over stretched scrotal skin Rundle and Sylvester[77] found that calculated testicular volume in more than 200 mentally deficient men was 31 ml (range 12 to 54 ml). Prior to 12 years of age, the volume averaged less than 5 ml, and the testicular growth spurt occurred between the 12th and 17th years. Takihara and his associates,[87] however, found the use of ellipsoidal rings more accurate when checked against orchiectomy specimens (correlation 0.81). In U.S. men, all with sperm counts of more than 40 million/ml, they determined testicular size at 24.8 ± 6 ml with a normal range of 17.4 to 31.9 ml. Accurate measurement may be important because of its correlation with function.[86]

Underneath the thin mesothelial layer of *tunica vaginalis* lies the tough white outer fibrous coat of the testis, the *tunica albuginea.* The gross anatomy of the testicular parenchyma as seen upon bisecting the testis is not impressive. It is soft and light tan with a finely granular surface. With fine forceps small groups of seminiferous tubules may be gently lifted up and extended to give some indication of their true length and the corresponding degree to which they are coiled. With fibrosis and atrophy, the parenchyma becomes paler, and tubules are less likely to be pulled out by the grasping forceps. The thin septa separating lobules of tubules may be seen with some difficulty. They radiate from the inner surface of the tunica albuginea to the upper part of the posterolateral margin of the testis. Here they meld with a poorly defined mass of fibrous connective tissue about 8 to 10 mm in diameter, the mediastinum testis *(organ of Highmore).*

935

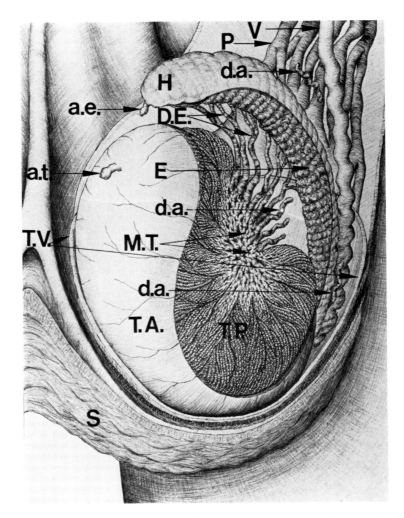

Fig. 22-1 Gross anatomy of testis and neighboring structures. A lateral portion has been cut away and the epididymis lifted slightly. The residual embryologic structures shown include the appendix epididymis (ae), appendix testis (at), and several possible locations for mesonephric remnants, the ductuli aberrantes (da). From the seminiferous tubules in the testicular parenchyma (TP), sperm pass to the epididymis (E) via the rete testis located in the mediastinum of the testis (MT) and the efferent ductules (DE). From the head (H) of the epididymis to the vas deferens (V), the 6 m duct is heavily coiled. Other structures shown include the fibrous white tunica albuginea (TA), the pampiniform plexus of veins (P), tunica vaginalis (TV), and scrotum (S). (From Silverberg SG (ed): Principles and Practice of Surgical Pathology. John Wiley, New York, 1982.)

In this structure the tubules drain through a network of channels, the *rete testis,* before anastomosing with efferent ductules. The epididymis is applied closely to the testis along its posterolateral margin, covered by its own layer of tunica vaginalis.

About 12 to 20 *efferent ductules* (each about 1 mm in diameter) may be dissected as they emerge from the mediastinum testis and coil to form the head of the epididymis. They drain into a single *epididymal duct (ductus epididymidis).* This duct, about 6 m in length, is tightly coiled to form the body and tail of the epididymis. By the time it exits the tail as the *vas deferens (ductus deferens)* its smooth muscle coat has become thicker, and it is now about 3 mm in diameter. The vas deferens runs up the medial side of the epididymis and becomes part of the spermatic cord, which passes through the superficial inguinal ring into the pelvis. It crosses the ureter to the posterior aspect of the bladder and then runs along the medial side of the seminal vesicle.

The *seminal vesicles* are paired, sacculated tubular structures that lie posterior to the prostate and bladder base. Each is about 5 cm long and 1.2 cm thick with a 3 cm³ capacity.[1,17] At the inferior end of each seminal vesicle there is a narrow outflow tract that is joined on its medial side by the entrance of the vas deferens, thereby forming the *ejaculatory duct.* The two ducts enter the prostate gland and then unite before debouching into the prostatic urethra at the verumontanum.

Embryologic remnants of the müllerian (paramesonephric) and wolffian (mesonephric) ducts are clinically important because of possible torsion. In about 90 percent of men, a 3- to 5-mm sessile or peduculated remnant of müllerian duct, the *appendix testis,* is found on the anterior superior surface of one or both testes about 1 cm inferior to the head of the epididymis. A wolffian remnant, the *appendix epididymis,* is of similar size and is found appended to the head of one or both epididymis in about 35 percent of men. Other remnants of aberrant ducts are rare.[74]

Arterial Blood Supply

The testis and spermatic cord are supplied by three arteries: the testicular *(internal spermatic)* artery, the artery of the vas deferens, and the artery of the cremasteric muscle (Fig. 22-2). Although occasional minute connections are present between these arteries, for practical purposes they should be looked on as end-arteries and guarded appropriately during surgery.

The *testicular artery* originates 2.5 to 5.0 cm below the renal artery ostium in about 85 percent of men. Origin may also take place from the aorta immediately above the renal arteries, from one of the renal arteries itself, or even from one of the arteries supplying the adrenal.[28] Although its path is relatively straight in the retroperitoneum, it divides below the inguinal orifice and then becomes somewhat coiled. This coiling, closely surrounded by the pampiniform plexus of veins, is a regular feature of the spermatic artery of many mammalian species and is only rela-

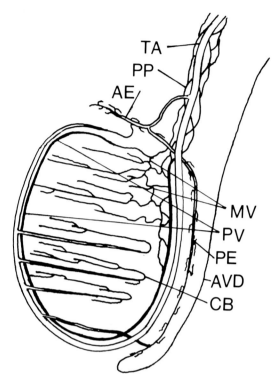

Fig. 22-2 Vascular supply of the testis. The epididymis and vas deferens are to the right; the free margin of the testis is to the left. Testicular (internal spermatic) artery (TA) and its branches are shown, including the anterior and posterior epididymal branches (AE; PE) and artery of the vas deferens (AVD). Note that the parenchyma is largely supplied by centripetal arterial branches (CB). The venous drainage collects in peripheral veins (PV) and in a plexus in the mediastinum (MV) before ascending about the TA in the pampiniform plexus (PP). Centripetal arteries are shown for the lower half of the parenchyma only; parenchymal veins are shown for the upper half only. Veins of the epididymis and vas deferens are not shown; see Ref. 36.

tively poorly developed in man.[83] A few minute branches may be given off to the covering of the spermatic cord.

Two epididymal branches arise from the testicular artery. A short anterior branch supplies the head of the epididymis, and the posterior branch runs along the epididymis supplying the body and the tail as far as the junction of the epididymis and vas deferens.[35,36,44]

After giving off the epididymal arteries, the testicular artery may remain single or divide into two or three branches that penetrate the tunica albuginea at the posterior border of the testis.[27,33] The vessels pass directly toward the lower pole of the testis and then, turning to run in a superior direction on the lateral and medial sides of the testis, give off parenchymal branches, many of which become recurrent as they approach the mediastinum. The microvasculature of the testis studied by corrosion casts[85] reveals a complicated network of intertubular and peritubular capillaries.[45]

Because of this typical arterial distribution pattern, the safest place to perform a testicular biopsy is anterosuperiorly, just below and anterior to the head of the epididymis. Although this area tends to be a safe zone, this pole is occasionally supplied in an aberrant fashion by small branches of the anterior epididymal artery.[40] Because of the possibility of a high division of the testicular artery, or even two testicular arteries, surgeons contemplating autotransplantation from the abdomen to the scrotum must take special care to identify the entire blood supply. The passage of the testicular arterial branches cannot be visualized underneath the tunica albuginea; hence a biopsy near the posterior-inferior pole or fixation to prevent torsion may permanently damage the critical end-artery system.

The *artery of the vas deferens* is a rather straight and minute artery originating as a branch of the superior vesical artery, which passes inferiorly along the vas deferens and may give off minute anastomotic branches to the testicular artery in its distal portion. At its end it often has a small anastomosis with the posterior epididymal artery and rarely vascularizes the posterior-inferior pole of the testis. Anastomoses between the artery of the vas deferens and the testicular artery[26] may be of crucial importance in the intrascrotal placement of an ectopic testis where the spermatic vessels appear to be too short. Transection of the testicular artery and vein with preservation of the artery of the vas permits sufficient flow to ensure testicular survival[12] and, at least experimentally, spermatogenesis.[67]

The *artery of the cremasteric muscle* supplies the covering of the spermatic cord and testis. It originates from the inferior epigastric artery. Its anastomoses are small and not of clinical significance. When mobilizing the testis and spermatic cord this small artery is usually ligated.

The external spermatic (*pudendal*) artery supplies the scrotal skin but may have small anastomoses with the arteries of the vas deferens.[35,83]

Venous Drainage

The *testicular (spermatic) veins* do not follow the arteries in the testicular parenchyma (Fig. 22-2). Some, running toward the mediastinum of the testis, interconnect and then pass out through the mediastinum, forming four to eight branches. Other venules extend in the parenchyma away from the mediastinum and then join beneath the tunica albuginea to pass around the inferior pole of the testis and join up with the other branches in the mediastinum testis. The branches exiting the mediastinum form a convoluted network about the testicular artery. This *pampiniform plexus* of thick-walled veins is joined by small venules from the head of the epididymis and another branch from the tail of the epididymis. The veins from the vas deferens may anastomose with the vein coming from the inferior portion of the epididymis as well as veins from the external spermatic system.[35]

Because of the high prevalence of varicocele, many data have been accumulated from testicular vein catheterization.[9,69] The left testicular vein usually enters the left renal vein about 4.6 cm from its junction with the inferior vena cava. The left testicular vein may be double (6 to 15 percent of the time) or may empty into the left renal vein branches rather than the main left renal vein itself (18 percent of cases). The right testicular vein is single and typically enters the inferior vena cava at about the level of L2, approximately 2.4 cm below the ostium of the right renal artery, but it may enter the right renal vein itself or the angle formed by the inferior vena cava and right renal vein (5 percent).

Venous valves are found in 70 percent (left) and 85 percent (right) of the testicular veins at or near their ostia with the renal veins or vena cava,[60] but many are not competent.[9]

Small anastomoses are frequent between the left testicular vein and the lumbar and perivertebral (40 percent) and colic (45 percent) veins as well as between the right testicular vein and the colic (37 percent) and perirenal (15 percent) veins. Occasional anastomoses to intercostal, periureteral, epigastric, and disk veins have been noted.[9]

Lymphatic Drainage

Lymphatic pathways, like venules, are a key consideration when considering spread of intratesticular tumors and infections. A rich system of minute lymphatic sinusoids and vessels are present in the testicular interstitium closely positioned between the tunica propria of the seminiferous tubules and the Leydig cells.[19] The lymphatic vessels collect at the dorsolateral margin of the testis in the hilum near the efferent ducts, and from there about a dozen lymphatic channels, up to 0.5 mm in diameter, run along in the spermatic cord.[58] As they proceed caudally in the cord they anastomose among themselves and decrease to four to six in number at the superficial inguinal ring. These larger lymph vessels have muscle fibers in their walls in the segments between valves.[58] The paths of lymphatic drainage from the testes, as reflected by tumor spread, are primarily to the retroperitoneal nodal areas.[71]

From the right testis the lymphatics drain into nodes lying between the bifurcation of the aorta and the renal vein. Occasional channels end in preaortic lymph nodes and precaval nodes. The nodes extend from L4 to T11 and occasionally communicate directly across the midline into lymph nodes lying on the left side.[6,93]

From the left testis lymphatics drain into nodes extending from the aortic bifurcation to near the level of the renal vein. They also run to preaortic nodes.

An occasional lymphatic vessel of the spermatic cord runs into an iliac lymph node.[11] Surgery in the region of the testis and cord, especially orchiopexy and herniorrhaphy, may initiate or augment lymphatic drainage to the inguinal nodes.[43]

Blue dye injected directly into the substance of the testis outlines superficial lymphatic pathways of both testis and epididymis as well as the branches of the lymphatics passing up into the spermatic cord.[93] Lipiodol injected into the cord rarely travels to iliac lymph nodes but does pass to lumbar, thoracic, and left supraclavicular lymph nodes.[93] The early filling of supraclavicular nodes explains why metastatic disease may present here when a testicular primary is still small.

Nerves

The nerve supply to the testis[56,57] and its appendages is autonomic and largely sympathetic. It is certainly responsible for the regulation of blood flow and thereby crucial for the integrity of the spermatogenic process.[83] Preganglionic fibers arising from lower thoracic and upper lumbar segments synapse in a number of posterior abdominal and pelvic ganglia before sending postganglionic fibers to the internal male genitalia. Renal and intermesenteric plexuses send branches to form the superior spermatic nerve, which accompanies the testicular artery along its course.[62,63] This nerve penetrates the testicular parenchyma and may have some influence over movement of seminiferous tubules, in addition to vasomotor functions.[83] Superior and inferior hypogastric plexuses give rise to the middle and inferior spermatic nerves, respectively. These autonomic fibers supply the epididymis and vas deferens. Parasympathetic fibers are apparently sparse. Afferent fibers pass in the reverse direction along the same paths as the efferent nerves.[63,64]

The phenomenon of referred pain to the testis from renal or ureteral calculi or other disease processes may be due to the close approximation of the genitofemoral nerve to the ureter or to the plexuses shared by the testis and upper urinary tract. The pain due to testicular trauma may actually originate from scrotal nerves.[97]

Damage to the spermatic plexus or some of the other lumbar sympathetics may cause vasodilation of testicular and epididymal blood vessels. This increased blood flow may raise testicular temperature and lead to degeneration of the parenchyma.[42] Spontaneous contractions of the testicular capsule and movements of the seminiferous tubules may also be under neural control. Whether the close anatomic relation between nerve endings and some of the Leydig cells influences testosterone release is not known.[83]

HISTOLOGY

Although van Leeuwenhoek first described spermatozoa in 1678, the histologic details of testicular parenchyma were not elucidated until the middle of the nineteenth century, and fine structure and architectural details are still being reported.[80] A section of normal adult testis (Fig. 22-3) is composed predominantly of cross sections of seminiferous tubules with vascular structures and Leydig cells in the intervening interstitium. Quantification of seminiferous tubules morphometrically has led to the determination that each testis in an infant boy contains approximately 90 m of seminiferous tubules (range 14 to 180 m). It increases in the 5- to 10-year-old[59] to 203 m (range

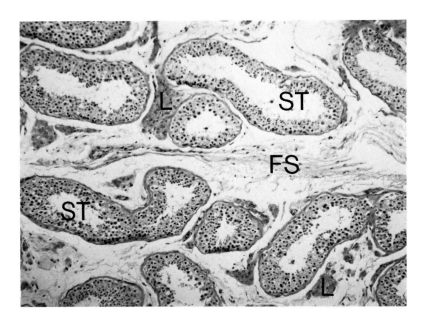

Fig. 22-3 Testicular parenchyma. Thin fibrous septa (FS) separate groups of seminiferous tubules (ST). Clusters of Leydig cells (L) are readily identified in the interstitium by their eosinophilic cytoplasm and central round nuclei.

138 to 330 m) and to 536 ± 148 m (range 299 to 981 m) in the adult.[46] Tubular diameter increases rather abruptly at puberty from about 50 to 60 μm to about 130 μm.[59] Germ cells increase from about 6 × 10^6 per testis in the newborn to 5-year-old to 43 × 10^6 in the 5- to 14-year-old and 750 × 10^6 in the 14- to 18-year-old.[59] Daily sperm production may be estimated[89,90] by histometric or testicular homogenization techniques at about 5.9 × 10^6 per gram of testicular parenchyma, or about 100 × 10^6 per testis.[38]

The *seminiferous tubules* are composed of an outer layer of myoid cells with a few collagen and elastic fibers, a middle layer composed of a thin basal lamina, and an inner layer of germinal epithelium composed of Sertoli cells, spermatogonia, and offspring of spermatogonia committed to differentiation toward mature spermatozoa (Fig. 22-4). The outer myoid layer consists of three to five layers of flattened myoid or contractile cells[75] that together with surrounding collagen and elastic fibers and the epithelial basement membrane make up the tunica propria.[32] These cells contain desmin-type intermediate filaments indicating their smooth muscle nature.[92] Laminin and type IV collagen form the basement membrane material around the myoid cells.[70] Laminin forms the base-

ment membrane of the germinal epithelium and may be synthesized by the Sertoli cells.[70]

The *Sertoli (supporting* or *nurse) cells*[82] have their base applied to the tubular basement membrane. The ovoid nucleus with a modest-sized red nucleolus is perpendicular to the basement membrane. A unique intracytoplasmic crystalloid, the Charcot-Böttcher body, may be noted in Sertoli cell cytoplasm in electron micrographs.[84] The spermatogonia with their round to slightly oval nuclei and nearly clear to light pink cytoplasm lie on the basement membrane between Sertoli cells. Electron microscopic examination demonstrates that Sertoli cells form multiple tight junctions that separate the spermatogonia below from the maturing spermatocytes above. Spermatogonia divide by mitosis to form primary spermatocytes, which migrate away from the basal lamina. Most of the cells seen in histologic sections are primary spermatocytes. Lengthy meiotic reduction divisions ensue in which two nuclear divisions take place with only one chromosomal division. The paired chromosomes of the pachytene stage are especially prominent (Fig. 22-4). The secondary spermatocytes rapidly mature to spermatids, which in turn acquire an acrosome and flagellum and shed cytoplasm before being released

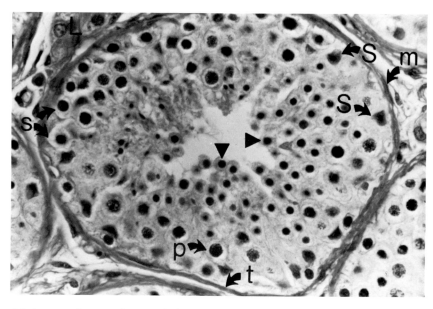

Fig. 22-4 Normal seminiferous tubule. Myoid cell nuclei (m) are visible in the thin tunica propria (t). Spermatogonia (s) lie next to the basement membrane and have a well defined cell membrane. Nuclei of Sertoli cells (S) are often convoluted and contain a small but distinct nucleolus. Primary spermatocytes are prominent (p). Maturing spermatids (arrowheads) are numerous at the edge of the tubular lumen. Leydig cells (L) lie in the interstitium. When fine detail of spermatogenesis is desired for light microscopy, 2-μm sections of plastic-embedded tissue are preferable to the parafin-embedded tissue shown here.

into the tubular lumen. The ultrastructural features of spermiogenesis have been worked out in detail and are discussed elsewhere.[17] During spermatogenesis the germ cells are largely surrounded and engulfed by intricate folds of Sertoli cell cytoplasm, and adjacent germ cells at the same maturation phase often are connected by intracellular bridges. The nature of the Sertoli–germ cell or germ cell–germ cell interactions are still largely unknown.

Rather than having a random organization, the seminiferous epithelium appears to be organized into spiral strips in a complex plan.[79,80] Through the critical process of spermatogenesis, some spermatogonia become committed to differentiation into spermatozoa. In this 64-day process[31] one spermatogonium, through mitosis and meiosis, may give rise to more than 250 sperm. The net biologic result of the process of spermiogenesis and contributions of the rest of the male duct system is an ejaculate of about 3 ml of semen containing 200 to 300 million spermatozoa.

Small zones of hypoplastic tubules may be found in one or both testes of more than 20 percent of normal

men.[30] They contain only Sertoli cells (Fig. 27-32), and because they decrease in frequency between age 15 and 39 they may represent a transient phenomenon.

The *interstitial (Leydig) cells*[47] are the most noticeable components of the interstitial tissue lying between the seminiferous tubules (Fig. 22-5). However, along with blood vessels and lymphatic channels, macrophages and mast cells are found in this area. The Leydig cells are of two morphologic forms: one large and round or polygonal, and the other small and spindly. The small spindly type may mature into the larger form. Both types have nearly round nuclei with prominent nuclear membranes and characteristic eosinophilic cytoplasm. From shortly after birth until puberty, Leydig cells are scanty, and only a few contain immunohistochemically demonstrable testosterone.[65] Some of the larger Leydig cells in adults contain one or more crystalloids described by Reinke[73] (Fig. 22-5). These elongated structures appear red on hematoxylin and eosin (H&E) staining. They are up to 20 μm long and 3 μm in maximum thickness,[17] and

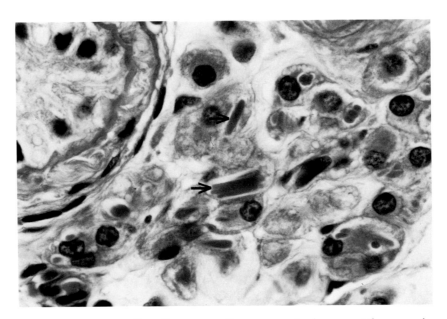

Fig. 22-5 Interstitium. Leydig cells are unusually numerous in the group. They are polygonal with prominent eosinophilic cytoplasm and nearly round nuclei. Reinke crystalloids of varying sizes and shapes are plentiful (arrows).

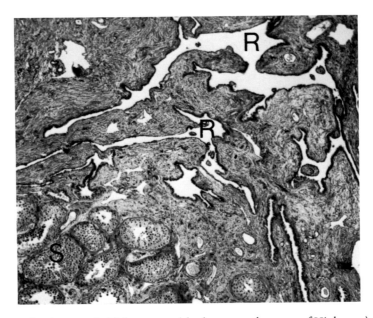

Fig. 22-6 Mediastinum testis. This structure (also known as the organ of Highmore) provides a fibrovascular support for the area in which the seminiferous tubules coalescence. These tubules (S) drain into the anastomosing ducts of the rete testis (R), which are lined by thin epithelium. These in turn empty into the efferent ductules, which lead to the epididymis.

contain proteinaceous and lipidic substances as yet poorly defined and of unknown significance. The major ultrastructural feature of Leydig cells is the presence of multiple smooth 80- to 200- mμ vesicles representing a form of smooth endoplasmic reticulum,[18] which is characteristic of steroid-producing cells. Gap junctions between adjacent Leydig cells may also be seen ultrastructurally.[61] Osmiophilic lipochrome pigment granules are also characteristic of Leydig cells.

The histology of the undescended testis is one of atrophic tubules, largely or totally absent germinal epithelium, and lipidic Leydig cells (see Ch. 23).[29]

As the loops of seminiferous tubules approach the mediastinum, they lose their germinal epithelium over a short segment. The spot where the Sertoli cell lining becomes replaced by low cuboidal epithelium marks the start of the *tubuli recti.*[17] These short tubules, which are less than 1 percent of the total seminiferous tubule length, soon blend into the anastomosing network of channels that forms the *rete testis* (Fig. 22-6). These channels are contained within the fibrovascular structure of the mediastinum testis and are lined by cuboidal cells.[17]

The dozen or so *ductuli efferentes* that pass from the rete to form the head of the epididymis are lined by alternating groups of ciliated and nonciliated cells and are surrounded by a thin muscular coat (Fig. 22-7A). Postpubertally elastic fibers appear in the coat of the ductuli efferentes as well as in the muscular coats of the remainder of the epididymis and vas. The efferent ductules empty into the epididymal duct, which is

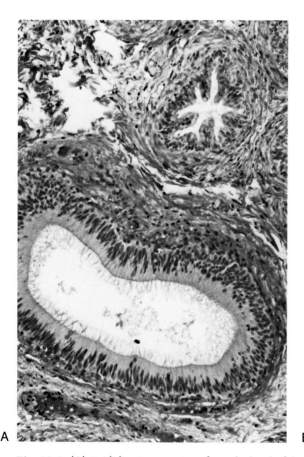
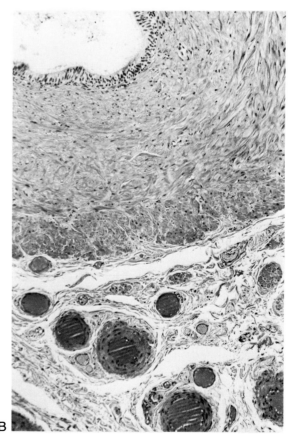

A

B

Fig. 22-7 (A) Epididymis. In sections from the head of the epididymis the coiled efferent ductules (top) have a thin muscular coat and undulating mucosa lined by ciliated and non-ciliated epithelial cells. The body and tail of the epididymis are composed of a single coiled duct (bottom) with a thick muscular coat and tall columnar epithelial cells. **(B)** The vas deferens (lumen at upper left) characteristically has three muscle layers and several folds of columnar epithelium. Note accompanying blood vessels (bottom).

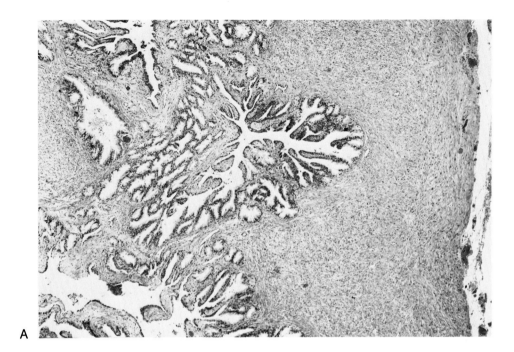

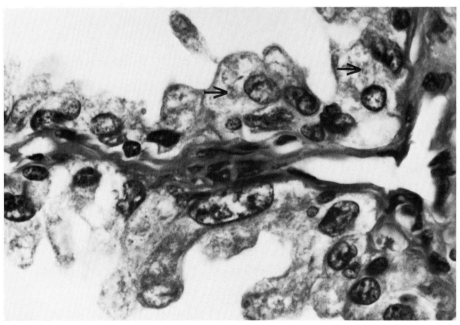

Fig. 22-8 Seminal vesicle. **(A)** This sacculated tube has a two-layered muscular coat lined by epithelium. **(B)** The columnar cells of the lining contain granules of lipochrome pigment (arrows). Occasional bizarre and enlarged nuclei, as shown here, are a normal histologic feature of seminal vesicular epithelium.

lined by tall columnar cells bearing nonmobile stereocilia and is surrounded by a thick muscular coat. This single duct, carrying the output of the testis, is tightly coiled throughout the body and tail of the epididymis. As the tail of the epididymis is approached, the epithelial cells become shorter and their nuclei more convoluted (Fig. 22-7B).

The *tail of the epididymis* blends into the *vas deferens,* characterized by loss of coiling and the presence of a stout muscular coat. This coat is formed of three layers of smooth muscle: outer and inner longitudinal layers and a central circular layer. The epithelial cells lining the lumen are somewhat shorter than those of the epididymis and is thrown up into low folds (Fig. 22-7C). The epithelial cells of adults often contain eosinophilic intranuclear inclusions.[8,51] Each *seminal vesicle* forms a sacculated tube with an inner circular and outer longitudinal smooth muscle coat. The epithelial lining, composed of nonciliated tall columnar cells containing lipochrome pigment (Fig. 22-8), rests on a lamina propria composed of numerous elastic fibers.[17]

EMBRYOLOGY

Y Chromosome

Differentiation of the testis appears to require genetic elements found on the Y chromosome as well as a gene on the X chromosome responsive to testosterone. Deletion of a portion of the short arm of the Y chromosome (p11.2 → pter) leading to a phenotypic female in an otherwise normal XY infant suggests that male-determining genes are located in this region.[52] Translocations of a minute but crucial portion of the Y chromosome to the X chromosome may be sufficient to cause maleness. This situation is seen characteristically in the XX "sex-reversed" mouse and may apply to XX human males and true hermaphrodites.[15,20] X to Y pairing with some crossover at meiosis may account for genetic exchange between the sex chromosomes.[55]

Undifferentiated Stage

At about 30 to 32 days after fertilization, when the embryo is 4.5 mm long (crown–rump), bilateral thickened regions of mesenchyme, the *gonadal ridges,* appear beneath the epithelium of the dorsal coelomic area between the mesonephros and root of the mesentery.[2] Some of these coelomic epithelial cells migrate into underlying mesenchyme to form the sex cords of the gonads, and they are joined there about 10 days later by germ cells migrating from the yolk sac via the dorsal mesentery.[96] The sex cords are then formed of cells that will differentiate into Sertoli cells, and germ cells with recognizably larger nuclei that will become spermatogonia.

A pair of longitudinal ducts form in the posterior coelomic cavity and stretch from the mesonephros and gonad caudally to the cloaca. The *mesonephric (wolffian) ducts* lie lateral to the *paramesonephric (müllerian) ducts.*

Testicular Differentiation

By day 42 the testicular sex cords form a branching mass that may be distinguished from fetal ovary (Fig. 22-9A), and by the seventh postfertilization week fibroblasts begin to form the tunica albuginea.[2] By the fourth month, the cords that merge at the mediastinum testis to form the rete testis extend to meet several mesonephric tubules. The testicular shape, originally an elongated ridge, becomes more ovoid by the fifth month. The sex cords have multiplied and are now termed seminiferous cords. They form loops that connect to the embryologic tubuli recti. The cords remain solid until gametogenesis begins at puberty. Mesenchymal cells between the cords differentiate into recognizable Leydig cells by 8 weeks[34] (Fig. 22-9B) and thereafter increase in size and number until week 17.[25] The enzyme that transforms androstenediol to testosterone, 3-hydroxysteroid dehydrogenase, is found in the gonadal ridge in the 14-mm embryo.[3]

Testicular Duct Differentiation

The developing testis appropriates many of the tubules as well as the duct of the fetal mesonephros to serve as the basis of its excurrent duct system. At around 8 weeks of fetal life, when mesonephric glomeruli are still readily identified (Fig. 22-9C), the mesonephric tubules lie near the mediastinum of the testis, and connections with the rete testis are formed during the fourth month.[2] The mesonephric tubules form the head of the epididymis and unite there into the common mesonephric duct (Fig. 22-10). This duct differentiates to form the body and tail of the

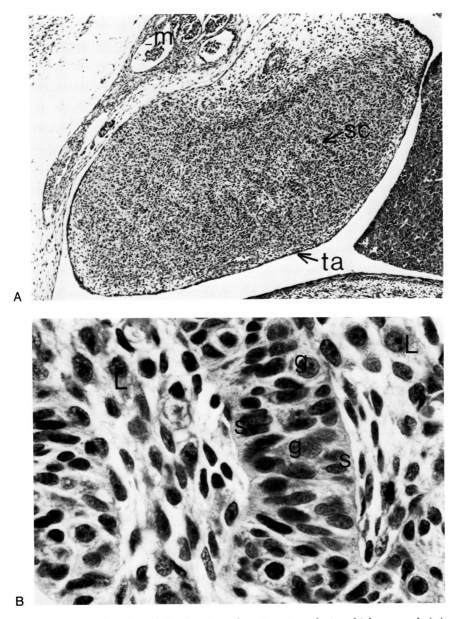

Fig. 22-9 Embryonal testis. **(A)** Fetal testis at about 7 to 8 weeks in which sex cords (sc) are visible beneath a distinct capsule that will become the tunica albuginea (ta). Mesonephric structures (m) are distinctly separate. The metanephros now forms the embryonal kidney. **(B)** Sex cords contain primitive gonocytes (g) with rounded nuclei and stromal cells (s) with elongated nuclei, which will become spermatogonia and Sertoli cells, respectively. Under the influence of maternal luteinizing hormone (LH) and human chorionic gonadotropin (hCG), the interstitial Leydig cells (L) become prominent *(Figure continues.)*

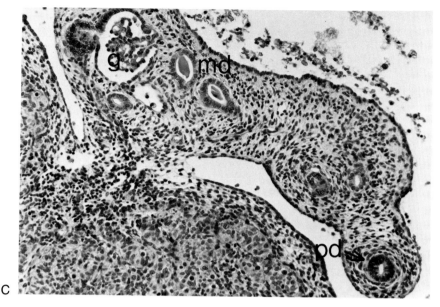

c

Fig. 22-9 *(Continued).* **(C)** Mesonephric structures include glomeruli (g), which later atrophy, and mesonephric (wolffian) ducts (md). Nearly all of the paramesonephric (müllerian) duct (pd) later regresses but is still present here.

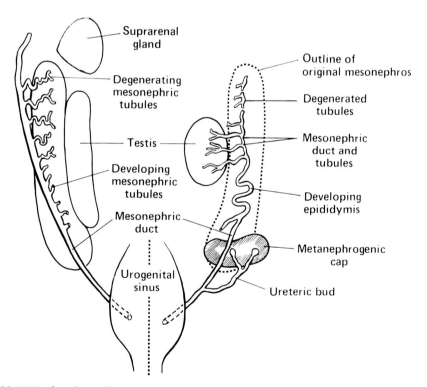

Fig. 22-10 Embryology of mesonephric duct. On the left side of the diagram the 5- to 6-week embryo contains an elongated embryonal testis next to the mesonephros. Developing mesonephric tubules drain into the mesonephric duct. On the right side of the diagram the testis at 8 weeks has an adult ovoid form. Mesonephric tubules extend into the hilum of the testis. The mesonephric duct begins to coil to form the epididymis.

epididymis as well as the vas deferens. The mesonephros may influence the differentiation of the gonad by donating cells that become Sertoli cells and possibly Leydig cells as well.[7,24]

Müllerian Duct Regression

Müllerian-inhibiting substance (MIS, also termed anti-müllerian hormone [AMH]) is a glycoprotein dimer[68] produced by fetal Sertoli cells that acts to cause regression of the müllerian duct system in male embryos only 51 days old.[39] Although the epithelial cells may not die, the basement membrane dissolves around the duct and a condensation of mesenchymal cells occupies the site of the former duct.[39] Testosterone is necessary for the action of MIS, which may work by dephosphorylating cell membranes.[37] Only the appendix testis and prostatic utricle survive in the adult as tiny remnants of the müllerian duct system.

Testicular Descent and Cryptorchidism

The developing testis lies at the cranial end of a columnar mass of mesenchymal cells that contains the mesonephric duct, and this cell mass becomes the abdominal gubernaculum. The gubernaculum is attached to the lower anterior abdominal wall where the inguinal canal later develops and is continuous with undifferentiated mesenchymal cells that pass through a gap in the developing abdominal musculature. Outside the abdominal muscles it connects with mesenchyme of the scrotal swelling. With body growth the testis remains attached by the vas deferens and gubernaculum to the anterior pelvic wall. The processus vaginalis, or outpouching of the peritoneal cavity, grows down into the scrotum around the sixth month. The cremasteric muscle differentiates around the processus, and the gubernaculum reduces in length. This structure, possibly with assistance from intraabdominal pressure,[21] tends to pull the testis from the abdominal cavity down into the scrotum by the seventh or eighth month of fetal life (Fig. 22-11). The epididymal portion of the former mesonephric duct lengthens and coils within the mesenchymal mass of the gubernaculum.

A testis that falters along the normal path of descent becomes a *cryptorchid testis;* it may be abdominal, in the inguinal canal, or at the external inguinal ring, de

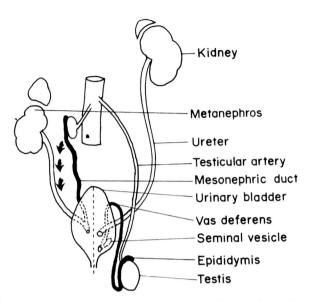

Fig. 22-11 Testicular descent. On the left side of the diagram, at 4 months of development the fetal testis with attached mesonephric duct lies adjacent to the developing kidney. Note the short testicular artery. On the right at 7 – 9 months the descending gonad has brought its duct and artery caudad down over the ureter. The vas deferens and ureter now open separately into the prostatic urethra and bladder.

pending on the degree of descent. Following descent through the external ring, a testis may become *ectopic* by coming to lie in an abnormal location, such as above the fascia of the external oblique muscle (*superficial inguinal* or *interstitial testis*), on the medial side of the upper femoral area *(femoral testis),* in the perineum, into the opposite hemiscrotum (*transverse testis),* or onto the penile shaft.[10] Low birth weight, maternal obesity, and intrauterine exposure to estrogens are risk factors for cryptorchidism.[16]

PHYSIOLOGY

The physiology of the male reproductive system is so interwoven with the functioning of the entire body that it is only outlined in this chapter. The interested reader may consult a number of detailed texts (especially that of Griffin and Wilson[23]) and reviews for a fuller treatment.[5,13,22,25,50,54,72,95] Normal functioning of the male system results in effective testosterone production and spermatogenesis. Although both pro cesses take place in the testis, they succeed only because of stimulation by pituitary hormones, which are subject to hypothalamic control.

Hypothalamic neurons secrete an active decapeptide, gonadotropin-releasing hormone (GnRH), also termed luteinizing hormone-releasing hormone (LHRH), which passes via the pituitary portal vein system to reach the anterior pituitary.[72] The neurons themselves may have receptors for testosterone and inhibin and therefore be subject to feedback control (Fig. 22-12). Gonadotropic cells, comprising 5 to 9 percent of the pituitary cell population[13] release both luteinizing hormone (LH) and follicle-stimulating hormone (FSH) in response to GnRH acting on cell receptors. The pulsatile nature of GnRH secretion is necessary for normal LH and FSH secretion. Although its ontogeny is not understood, some 8 to 14 pulses of varying amplitude occur every 24 hours stimulated by a pulse generator located in the hypothalamus and modified by hormonal feedback loops.[78] Pulsatile GnRH release results in pulsatile release of LH and FSH. These glycoproteins are each composed of two amino acid chains, identical 96-amino-acid α chains, and focally unique 115-amino-acid β chains. Although FSH has a larger carbohydrate moiety (32 percent versus 16 percent), both are believed to have some carbohydrate microheterogeneity, thereby possibly allowing for subtle receptor variations and hormonal actions.[13]

In the testis, FSH receptors are present on both Sertoli and Leydig cells. The FSH causes a rise in LH receptors in Leydig cells and acts on Sertoli cells to promote spermatogenesis, synthesis of androgen-binding protein (ABP), and the aromatase that converts testosterone to estradiol. The exact way in which FSH stimulates spermatogenesis is as yet unknown. ABP, by increasing the local androgen concentration in the tubule, may facilitate spermatogenesis.

Inhibin, the gonadal protein that provides inhibition of the pituitary secretion of FSH (Fig. 22-12), is produced by Sertoli cells.[14,53] In the pig, inhibin exists in two forms of heterodimer, A and B, which share identical α subunits (18,000 daltons) but different β subunits (13,800 to 14,700 daltons). A heterodimer formed of the different β subunits causes release of pituitary FSH and has been termed activin.[49]

Luteinizing hormone acts on the LH receptors of Leydig cells[98] to promote conversion of cholesterol to pregnenolone and then to testosterone. About 6 mg of testosterone is secreted per day resulting in peripheral blood levels of 250 to 1,000 ng/dl. Locally, testosterone acts with FSH on Sertoli cells to make possible spermatogenesis; it may also regulate production of inhibin by the Sertoli cell.[91]

Physiologically, testosterone acts peripherally on many tissues, in part through its derivative dihydrotestosterone (DHT). The cytosolic receptor protein for testosterone and DHT is coded for by an X chromosome locus.[25] The formation of DHT requires the enzyme 5α-reductase, and the enzyme's presence in fetal phallic and labioscrotal tissue makes DHT the hormone responsible for differentiation and growth of the penis and scrotum. 5α-Reductase is absent in the wolffian duct system, and testosterone is responsible for differentiation of the epididymis, vas deferens, and seminal vesicles. Plasma testosterone or its metabolites provide negative feedback to the Leydig cell through effects on the hypothalamus and pituitary gonadotrophs, and by down-regulating surface LH receptors on the Leydig cell.

The physiology of puberty is complex[94] but may be a process beginning with increased adrenal androgen production at 6 to 7 years of age (adrenarche). Prepubertal LH levels (about 2 to 4 mIU/ml) become modified by sleep-related surges of LH to adult levels (5 to 12 mIU/ml) at midpuberty. By the end of puberty, LH levels are elevated throughout the day and night, and the inconspicuous spindly stromal Leydig cells return to their perinatal state of prominence. FSH becomes elevated to a lesser degree (from about 6 mU/ml prepubertally to 10 mU/ml in the adult).[23] Seminiferous tubular length and diameter increase at puberty, as noted previously. The number of Sertoli cells per testis is uniform from birth to puberty; but as puberty approaches, Sertoli cell nuclei increase about 50 percent in size, and the number of nuclei per tubular cross section decreases.[64] The associated morphologic changes of puberty, including hair and muscle growth, and growth and development of the external genitalia and male accessory organs (prostate, seminal vesicles, epididymis), are dependent on the increased pubertal testosterone levels (from 100 ng/dl prepubertally to 500 ng/dl in the adult).

With advancing age (over 70 years) the Leydig cell population decreases in both number of cells and total cell volume. Thus a 20-year-old may have 2.5 cm³ of Leydig cells but a 60-year-old only 1.0 cm³.[41] Mul-

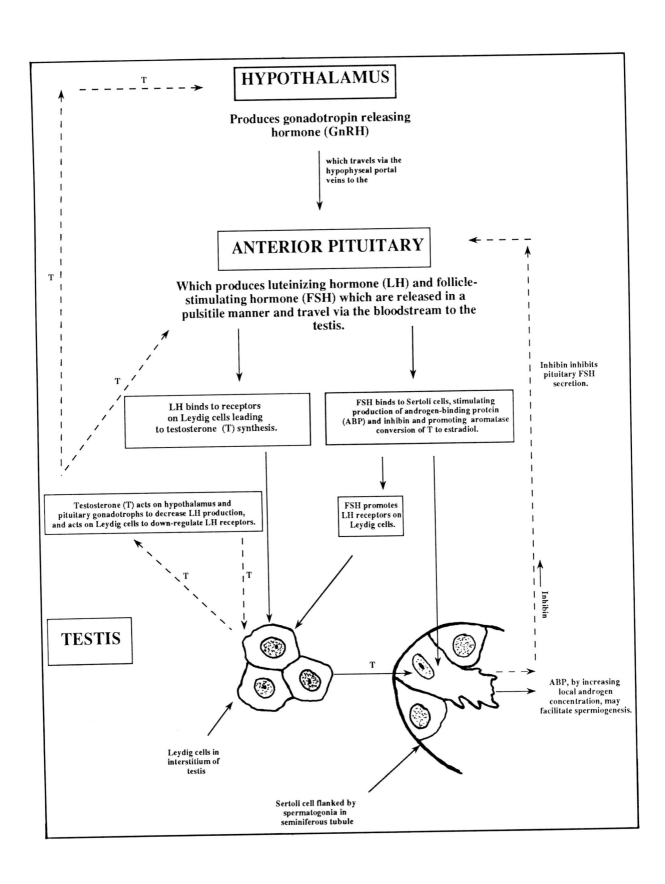

HYPOTHALAMUS

Produces gonadotropin releasing
hormone (GnRH)

which travels via the
hypophyseal portal
veins to the

ANTERIOR PITUITARY

Which produces luteinizing hormone (LH) and follicle-
stimulating hormone (FSH) which are released in a
pulsitile manner and travel via the bloodstream to the
testis.

Inhibin inhibits
pituitary FSH
secretion.

LH binds to receptors
on Leydig cells leading
to testosterone (T) synthesis.

FSH binds to Sertoli cells, stimulating
production of androgen-binding protein
(ABP) and inhibin and promoting aromatase
conversion of T to estradiol.

Testosterone (T) acts on hypothalamus and
pituitary gonadotrophs to decrease LH production,
and acts on Leydig cells to down-regulate LH receptors.

FSH promotes
LH receptors on
Leydig cells.

Inhibin

TESTIS

ABP, by increasing
local androgen
concentration, may
facilitate spermiogenesis.

Leydig cells in
interstitium of
testis

Sertoli cell flanked by
spermatogonia in
seminiferous tubule

tinucleated Leydig cells increase with age such that 5 percent of Leydig cells in men over age 50 have three or more nuclei.[66] Testosterone levels and sperm production undergo a mild decrease, but libido and procreative power may remain intact until death. With age, multinucleated Sertoli cells become a fairly common finding, possibly due to mitosis without cytokinesis,[81] and are most frequently seen in testes of patients with the Sertoli-cell-only syndrome.

The physiology of the male genital tract does not end with the testis. The epididymis has as its functions the concentration and storage of spermatozoa as well as sperm maturation and transport.[88] During the 12-day[76] 6-foot migration, the spermatozoa are exposed to epididymal fluid containing high concentrations of glycerylphosphorylcholine and carnitine. The microenvironment of high osmolality of these substances inhibits sperm motility while subtle changes in tail structure and acrosomal morphology are also occurring. Sperm removed from the head of the epididymis are generally infertile, whereas those in the tail or vas deferens are fully functional.[4,88] Secretory and absorptive activity is present from the rete testis through the epididymis to the vas deferens[8]; and much of the final volume of the ejaculate, including the fructose, represents the secretion product of the seminal vesicles.

REFERENCES

1. Aboul-Azm TE: Anatomy of the human seminal vesicles and ejaculatory ducts. Arch Androl 3:287, 1979
2. Backhouse KM: Development and descent of the testis. Eur J Pediatr 139:249, 1982
3. Baillie AH, Ferguson MM, Hart DM: Developments in Steroid Histochemistry. Academic Press, New York, 1966, p. 35
4. Brooks DE: Epididymal functions and their hormonal regulation. Aust J Biol Sci 36:205, 1983
5. Brown TR, Migeon CJ: Androgen receptors in normal and abnormal male sexual differentiation. Adv Exp Med 196:227, 1986
6. Busch FM, Sayegh ES, Chenault OW Jr: Some uses of lymphangiography in the management of testicular tumors. J Urol 93:490, 1965
7. Byskov AG, Grinsted J: Feminizing effect of mesonephros on cultured differentiating mouse gonads and ducts. Science 212:817, 1981
8. Chakraborty J, Nelson L, Jhunjhunwala J, et al: Intranuclear inclusion bodies in epithelial cells of human vas deferens. Arch Androl 2:1, 1979
9. Chatel A, Bigot JM, Dectot H, Helenon Ch: Anatomie radiologique des veines spermatiques: a propos de 152 phlebographies spermatique retrogrades. J Chir (Paris) 115:443, 1978
10. Concodora JH, Evans RA, Smith MJV: Ectopic penile testis. Urology 8:263, 1976
11. Cuneo B: Note sur les lymphatiques du testicule. Bull Soc Anat (Paris) 76:107, 1901
12. Datta NS, Tanaka T, Zinner NR, Mishkin FS: Division of spermatic vessels in orchiopexy: radionuclide evidence of preservation of testicular circulation. J Urol 118:447, 1977
13. Daughaday WH: The anterior pituitary. p. 568. In Wilson JD, Foster DW (eds): Williams Textbook of Endocrinology. Saunders, Philadelphia, 1985
14. De Jong F, Robertson DM: Inhibin: 1985 update on action and purification. Mol Cell Endocrinol 42:95, 1985
15. De la Chapelle A, Tippert P, Wetterstrand G, Page D: Genetic evidence of X-Y interchange in a human XX male. Cytogenet Cell Genet 37:436, 1984
16. Depue RH: Maternal and gestational factors affecting the risk of cryptorchidism and inguinal hernia. Int J Epidemiol 13:311, 1984
17. Dym M: The male reproductive system. p. 1000. In Weiss L (ed): Cell and Tissue Biology. Elsevier, New York, 1983
18. Fawcett DW, Burgos MH: Studies on the fine structure of mammalian testis. II. The human interstitial tissue. Am J Anat 107:245, 1960
19. Fawcett DW, Heidger PM, Leak LV: Lymph vascular system of the interstitial tissue of the testis as revealed by electron microscopy. J Reprod Fertil 19:109, 1969
20. Fellous M, Guellaen G, Bishop C, et al: Detection of male specific sequences in XX males and XX true hermaphrodites using probes derived from the human Y chromosome. Cytogenet Cell Genet 37:468, 1984
21. Frey HL, Rajfer J: Role of the gubernaculum and intra-abdominal pressure in the process of testicular descent. J Urol 131:574, 1984
22. Gorski RA: Sexual differentiation of the brain: possible

Fig. 22-12 Diagram of male reproductive physiology. Testosterone produced by the Leydig cells acts locally on the Sertoli cells to facilitate spermiogenesis and systematically as an anabolic steroid.

mechanisms and implications. Can J Physiol 63:577, 1985

23. Griffin JE, Wilson JD: Disorders of the testes and male reproductive tract. p. 259. In Wilson JD, Foster DW (eds): Williams Textbook of Endocrinology. Saunders, Philadelphia, 1985

24. Grinsted J, Aagesen L: Mesonephric excretory function related to its influence on differentiation of fetal gonads. Anat Rec 210:551, 1984

25. Grumbach MM, Conte FA: Disorders of sexual differentiation. p. 312. In Wilson JD, Foster DW (eds): Williams Textbook of Endocrinology. Saunders, Philadelphia, 1985

26. Harrison RG: The distribution of the vasal and cremasteric arteries to the testis and their functional importance. J Anat 83:267, 1949

27. Harrison RG, Barclay AE: The distribution of the testicular artery (internal spermatic artery) to the human testis. Br J Urol 20:5, 1948

28. Harrison RG, McGregor GA: Anomalous origin and branching of the testicular arteries. Anat Rec 129:401, 1957

29. Hedinger CE: Histopathology of undescended testes. Eur J Pediatr 139:266, 1982

30. Hedinger CE, Huber R, Weber E: Frequency of so-called hypoplastic or dysgenetic zones in scrotal and otherwise normal human testes. Virchows Arch [Pathol Anat] 342:165, 1967

31. Heller CG, Clermont Y: Kinetics of the germinal epithelium in man. Recent Prog Horm Res 20:545, 1964

32. Hermo L, Lalli M, Clermont Y: Arrangements of connective tissue components in the walls of seminiferous tubules of man and monkey. Am J Anat 148:433, 1977

33. Hodson N: The nerves of the testis, epididymis, and scrotum. p. 47. In Johnson AD, Gomes WR, Vandermark NL (eds): The Testis. Vol. I. Academic Press, New York, 1970

34. Holstein AF, Wartenberg H, Vossmeyer J: Zur Cytologie der pränatalen Gonadenentwicklung beim Menschen. Anat Embryol (Berl) 135:43, 1971

35. Hundeiker M: Untersuchungen über die vaskularisation des hoden. Forschr Med 89:403, 1971

36. Hundeiker M, Keller L: Die Gefässarchitekttur des menschlichen Hodens. Gegenbaur Morph Jahrb 105:26, 1963

37. Hutson JM, Fallat ME, Kamagata S, et al: Phosphorylation events during müllerian duct regression. Science 223:586, 1984

38. Johnson L, Petty CS, Neaves WB: A new approach to quantification of spermatogenesis and its application to germinal cell attrition during human spermiogenesis. Biol Reprod 25:217, 1981

39. Josso N, Picard J-Y: Anti-müllerian hormone. Physiol Rev 66:1038, 1986

40. Juskiewenski S, Vaysse P: Vascularisation artérielle du testicule et chirugie de l'ectopie testiculaire. Anat Clin 1:127, 1978

41. Kaler LW, Neaves WB: Attrition of the human Leydig cell population with advancing age. Anat Rec 192:513, 1978

42. King AB, Langworthy OR: Testicular degeneration following interruption of the sympathetic pathways. J Urol 44:74, 1940

43. Klein FA, Whitmore WF Jr, Sogani PC, et al: Inguinal lymph node metastases from germ cell testicular tumors. J Urol 131:497, 1984

44. Kormano M, Reijonen K: Microvascular structure of the human epididymis. Am J Anat 145:23, 1975

45. Kormano M, Suoranta H: Microvascular organization of the adult human testis. Anat Rec 170:31, 1971

46. Lennox B, Ahmad KN, Mack WS: A method for determining the relative total length of the tubules in the testis. J Pathol 102:229, 1970

47. Leydig F: Zur Anatomie der männlichen Geschlechtsorgane und Analdrüsen der Säugethiere. Z Wiss Zool 2:1, 1850

48. Lich R, Howerton LW, Amin M: Anatomy and surgical approach to the urogenital tract in the male. p. 3. In Harrison JH, Gittes RF, Perlmutter AD, et al (eds): Campbell's Urology. 4th Ed. Saunders, Philadelphia, 1978

49. Ling N, Ying S-Y, Ueno N, et al: Pituitary FSH is released by a heterodimer of the β-subunits from the two forms of inhibin. Nature 321:779, 1986

50. MacLusky NJ, Naftolin F: Sexual differentiation of the central nervous system. Science 211:1294, 1981

51. Madara JL, Haggitt RC, Federman M: Intranuclear inclusions of the human vas deferens. Arch Pathol Lab Med 102:648, 1978

52. Magenis RE, Tomar D, Brown MG, et al: Localization of male determining factors to the Y short arm, bands p11.2 → pter. Cytogenet Cell Genet 37:529, 1984 (abstract)

53. Mason AJ, Hayflick JS, Ling N, et al: Complementary DNA sequences of ovarian follicular fluid inhibin show precursor structure and homology with transforming growth factor-β. Nature 318:659, 1985

54. McEwen BS: Neural gonadal steroid actions. Science 211:1303, 1981

55. Miller OJ, Drayna D, Goodfellow P: Report of the committee on the genetic constitution of the X and Y chromosomes. Cytogenet Cell Genet 37:176, 1984

56. Mitchell GAG: The innervation of the kidney, ureter, testicle and epididymis. J Anat 70:10, 1935

57. Mitchell GAG: The innervation of the ovary, uterine tube, testis and epididymis. J Anat 72:508, 1938

58. Möller R: Arrangement and fine structure of lymphatic vessels in the human spermatic cord. Andrology 12:564, 1980

59. Müller J, Skakkebaek NE: Quantification of germ cells and seminiferous tubules by stereological examination of testicles from 50 boys who suffered from sudden death. Int J Androl 6:143, 1983

60. Nadel SN, Hutchins GM, Albertsen PC, White RI Jr: Valves of the internal spermatic vein: potential for misdiagnosis of varicocele by venography. Fertil Steril 41:479, 1984

61. Nagano T, Suzuki F: Freeze-fracture observations on the intercellular junctions of Sertoli cells and of Leydig cells in the human testis. Cell Tissue Res 166:37, 1976

62. Netter FH: The Ciba Collection of Medical Illustrations. Vol. 2. Reproductive System. Ciba, New York, 1965, p. 18

63. Netter FH: The Ciba Collection of Medical Illustrations. Vol 1. Nervous System, Part I. Anatomy and Physiology. Ciba, West Caldwell, NJ, 1983, p. 88

64. Nistal M, Abaurrea MA, Paniagua R: Morphological and histometric study on the human Sertoli cell from birth to the onset of puberty. J Anat 14:351, 1982

65. Nistal M, Paniagua R, Regadera J, et al: A quantitative morphological study of human Leydig cells from birth to adulthood. Cell Tissue Res 246:229, 1986

66. Nistal M, Santamaria L, Paniagua R, et al: Multinucleate Leydig cells in normal human testis. Andrologia 18:268, 1986

67. Noordhuisen-Stassen EN, Dijkstra G, Schamhardt HC, Wensing CJG: Compensatory development of a patent vascular supply to the testis after intraabdominal transection of its main blood vessels. Int J Androl 6:509, 1983

68. Picard J-Y, Tran D, Josso N: Biosynthesis of iodinated anti-müllerian hormone by fetal testes: evidence for the glycoprotein nature of the hormone and for its disulfide-bonded structure. Mol Cell Endocrinol 12:17, 1978

69. Pinsolle J, Drouillard J, Bruneton J-N, Grenier FN: Anatomical bases of testicular vein catheterization and phlebography. Anat Clin 2:191, 1980

70. Pöllänen PP, Kallajoki M, Risteli L, et al: Laminin and type IV collagen in the human testis. Int J Androl 8:337, 1985

71. Ray B, Hajdu SI, Whitmore WF Jr: Distribution of retroperitoneal lymph node metastases in testicular germinal tumors. Cancer 33:340, 1974

72. Reichlin S: Neuroendocrinology. p. 492. In Wilson JD, Foster DW (eds): Williams Textbook of Endocrinology. Saunders, Philadelphia, 1985

73. Reinke F: Beiträge zur Histologie des Menschen. Arch Micr Anat 47:34, 1896

74. Rolnick D, Kawanoue S, Szanto P, Bush IM: Anatomical incidence of testicular appendages. J Urol 100:755, 1968

75. Ross MH, Long IR: Contractile cells in human seminiferous tubules. Science 153:1271, 1966

76. Rowley MJ, Teshima F, Heller CG: Duration of transit of spermatozoa through the human male ductular system. Fertil Steril 21:390, 1970

77. Rundle AT, Sylvester PE: Measurement of testicular volume: its application to assessment of maturation, and its use in the diagnosis of hypogonadism. Arch Dis Child 37:514, 1962

78. Santen RJ, Bardin CW: Episodic luteinizing hormone secretion in man: pulse analysis, clinical interpretation, physiologic mechanisms. J Clin Invest 52:2617, 1973

79. Schulze W, Rehder U: Organization and morphogenesis of the human seminiferous epithelium. Cell Tissue Res 237:395, 1984

80. Schulze W, Riemer M, Rehder U, Hohne K-H: Computer-aided three-dimensional reconstructions of the arrangement of primary spermatocytes in human seminiferous tubules. Cell Tissue Res 244:1, 1986

81. Schulze W, Schulze C: Multinucleate Sertoli cells in aged human testis. Cell Tissue Res 217:259, 1981

82. Sertoli E: Dell'esistenza di particolari cellule ramificate nel canalicoli seminiferi del testicolo umano. Morgagni 7:31, 1865

83. Setchell BP: The Mammalian Testis. Cornell University Press, Ithaca, NY, 1978

84. Shovah AR, Suzuki Y, Gabrilove JL, Churg J: Ultrastructure of crystalloids in spermatogonia and Sertoli cells of normal human testis. J Ultrastruct Res 34:83, 1971

85. Takayama H, Tomoyoshi T: Microvascular architecture of rat and human testes. Invest Urol 18:341, 1981

86. Takihara H, Cosentino MJ, Sakatoku J, Cockett ATK: Significance of testicular size measurement in andrology. II. Correlation of testicular size with testicular function. J Urol 137:416, 1987

87. Takihara H, Sakatoku J, Fujii M, et al: Significance of testicular size measurement in andrology. I. A new orchiometer and its clinical application. Fertil Steril 39:836, 1983

88. Turner TT: On the epididymis and its function. Invest Urol 16:311, 1979

89. Van Dop PA, Kurver PHJ, Scholtmeijer RJ, et al: Cor-

relations between the quantitative morphology of the human testis and sperm production. Int J Androl 3:170, 1980

90. Van Dop PA, Scholtmeijer RJ, Kurver PHJ, et al: A quantitative structural model of the testis of fertile men with normal sperm counts. Int J Androl 3:153, 1980

91. Verhoeven G, Franchimont P: Regulation of inhibin secretion by Sertoli cell-enriched cultures. Acta Endocrinol (Copenh) 102:136, 1983

92. Virtanen I, Kallajoki M, Närvänen O, et al: Peritubular myoid cells of human and rat testis are smooth muscle cells that contain desmin-type intermediate filaments. Anat Rec 215:10, 1986

93. Wahlqvist L, Hultén L, Rosencrantz M: Normal lymphatic drainage of the testis studied by funicular lymphography. Acta Chir Scand 132:454, 1966

94. Waldhauser F, Weiszenbacher G, Frisch H, et al: Fall in nocturnal serum melatonin during prepuberty and pubescence. Lancet 1:362, 1984

95. Wilson JD: The endocrine control of sexual differentation. Harvey Lect 79:145, 1985

96. Witschi EW: Migration of the germ cells of human embryos from the yolk sac to the primitive gonadal folds. Contrib Embryol 32:67, 1948

97. Wollard HH, Carmichael EP: The testis and referred pain. Brain 56:293, 1933

98. Zipf WB, Payne AH, Kelch RP: Prolactin, growth hormone, and luteinizing hormone in the maintenance of testicular luteinizing hormone receptors. Endocrinology 103:595, 1978

23

Anomalies of the Testis

Frank Rudy

With the exception of cryptorchidism, congenital anomalies of the testes are rare occurrences. Other anomalies that may be encountered include the absence of one (monorchia) or both (anorchia) testes, the presence of more than two testes (polyorchidism), finding a testis in a position outside its normal course of descent (ectopia), and intrascrotal rests of adrenal or splenic tissue.

MONORCHIA AND ANORCHIA

The absence of one or both testes is encountered in approximately 3 percent of patients undergoing surgical exploration for presumed testicular maldescent.[14] Monorchia is estimated to occur with a frequency of 1 per 5,000 males and anorchia with a frequency of 1 per 20,000 males.[8] Although usually sporadic, heritable tendencies toward anorchia do exist; and monozygotic twins, both concordant and discordant for anorchia, have been reported.[12,72] In two families that have been described, one sibling had anorchia whereas the other sibling had monorchia.[81] Accompanying anomalies do not usually occur with anorchia, but monorchia may be associated with the syndrome of seminal vesicle cyst with ipsilateral renal dysgenesis[17] and abnormal fixation of the contralateral testis.[7] Compensatory hypertrophy of the remaining testis may occur in cases of monorchia.[47]

In those patients in whom one or both gonads are absent, an abnormal nodular structure, suspected of being testicular in origin, is often noted attached to a hypoplastic or normal vas deferens.[37] The epididymis may be normal or absent. On microscopic examination, these nodules consist of well circumscribed but nonencapsulated foci of loose or dense, highly vascularized fibrous connective tissue containing occasional nerves, smooth muscle bundles, and elastic fibrils.[37] Both seminiferous tubules and a covering tunica albuginea are lacking. Minute areas of calcification may be present (Fig. 23-1). In addition, small clusters of Leydig cells may be seen. The overall histologic appearance suggests that a testis previously existed here. Factors theoretically incriminated in the production of the testicular regression include infection, vascular accidents, torsion, teratogenic or toxic phenomena, and a mutant gene.

Anorchia is one form of the testicular regression syndrome, a group of disorders characterized by the absence of gonadal structures and varying degrees of external genital masculinization or müllerian duct regression in an XY individual (see Ch. 24). The varying clinical features of the testicular regression syndrome are due to loss of testicular function at different developmental stages. In patients classified as anorchic, excurrent ducts of mesonephric origin are always present, müllerian derivatives are typically absent, and the external genitalia are unambiguously male. These features indicate that the fetal testes in cases of anorchia were present and functioning during the critical period of intrauterine sexual differentiation but subsequently regressed in utero or postna-

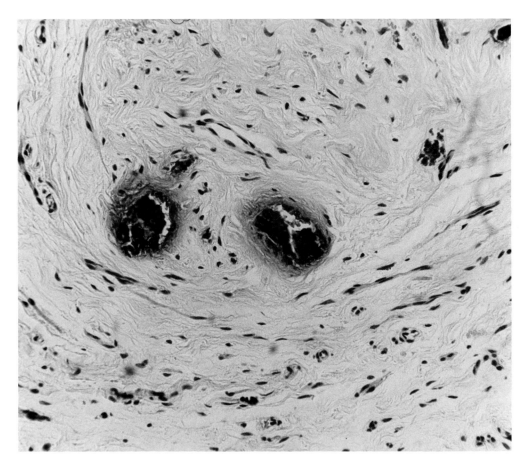

Fig. 23-1 Nodule encountered at a normal location of the testis. Calcification is evident in vascularized connective tissue. ×400.

tally.[52,69] Anorchia and "true agonadism," another variant of the testicular regression syndrome, have been observed to coexist in the same family.[40]

Anorchia results in failure of pubescent maturation. These individuals are typically tall, eunuchoid males with feminine body fat distribution and retarded bone age.[27] Failure to palpate testicular tissue in a phenotypic male suggests the need for additional preoperative studies prior to exploratory surgery. A buccal smear should be performed to avoid missing the totally masculinized female with congenital adrenal hyperplasia. Elevation of basal gonadotropin levels[38] and failure of significant (tenfold) testosterone response to gonadotropin stimulation indicate the absence of functioning testicular tissue and may obviate the need for exploration.[86]

In questionable cases thorough surgical exploration of the pelvis and abdomen may be required to exclude the presence of undescended testes. The standard treatment for agonadic boys is testosterone replacement at puberty, which leads to the appearance of male secondary sex characteristics and normal sexual function.[27] On one occasion a successful testicular transplant was performed, the donor being a normal identical twin.[79]

POLYORCHIDISM

Polyorchidism is a urologic curiosity, with only 53 cases reported in the world literature.[60] Although most are sporadic occurrences, familial polyorchidism has been observed.[82] Previously reported cases have included patients with three, four, and even five testes; however, only a maximum of four testes has been verified histologically.[80] The extra testis may be found below the normal testis within the scrotum, along the inguinal canal, or intraabdominally. In the most common type of anatomic relation, both ipsilateral testes have a separate epididymis, and a single vas deferens from the supernumerary testis joins the vas arising from the normal testis.[23a,60] Complete duplication, with a totally separate vas deferens, epididymis, and blood supply, has been observed in only two patients.[84,87] Polyorchidism may be associated with maldescent of the accessory or the ipsilateral normal testis, an indirect inguinal hernia, torsion,[20,23a] a hydrocele, epididymitis, or a varicocele. There are single case reports of testicular seminoma,[29] teratoma,[77] and

choriocarcinoma[77] in patients with polyorchidism, as well as one instance of a paratesticular rhabdomyosarcoma.[28]

Provided it is located within the scrotum, the mere presence of an extra testis does not require its removal. Although often palpable on physical examination, the clinical findings are inadequate to exclude an intrascrotal mass; therefore surgical exploration with biopsy, excision, or both may be required. Polyorchidism has been diagnosed before surgery with sonography and magnetic resonance.[5] In one unusual case, triorchidism was diagnosed after reexploration for unexpected fertility following a vasectomy.[33] The testicular histology appears to be related to the position of the supernumerary organ.[9] In most patients a scrotal location seems to ensure normal spermatogenesis. Abnormal findings in extrascrotal testes have

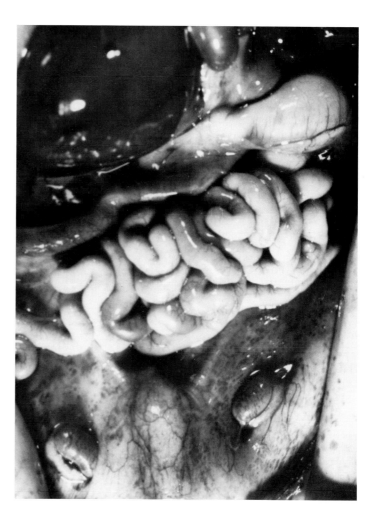

Fig. 23-2 Cryptorchidism. Bilateral intraabdominal testes are present in the pelvis in an infant with prune belly syndrome.

usually, but not always, included hypospermatogenesis, spermatogenic arrest, the Sertoli-cell–only syndrome,[20] and tubular atrophy.

CRYPTORCHIDISM

Descent of the testes takes place over a 7-month period, beginning at about the sixth week of gestation and finishing in some instances after birth. Testicular descent is a complex, incompletely understood process involving both hormonal and mechanical factors.[66] Hormonal factors include hypothalamic, pituitary, and gonadal hormones; and the mechanical forces involved in descent entail gubernacular and abdominal pressure as well as cremasteric factors.[45] Failure of complete testicular descent into the scrotum, with retention of the testis anywhere along its normal route of descent, is known as *cryptorchidism*. The incidence of cryptorchidism decreases from 10 percent at birth to about 3 percent by the end of the first month of life.[46,62] Descent occurs in most of the remaining cryptorchid boys during the first year, and only 0.3 to 0.4 percent of patients more than 1 year of age with maldescent have bilateral involvement; the remainder have unilateral cryptorchidism.[75] Inguinal testes are about four times more common than abdominal testes (Fig. 23-2). Arteriography has been successful in localizing nonpalpable undescended testes but has not been reported in young children. Because arteriography is associated with a low but definite risk, some prefer gonadal venography.[86] Laparoscopy has also been reported to be helpful in the search for impalpable testes.[76,86a] Computed tomography scans are also successful in localizing impalpable testes.[65] For bilateral undescended testes that are nonpalpable, one can administer human chorionic gonadotropin (hCG) followed by measurement of serum testosterone to ascertain the presence of testicular tissue.[70] This test, however, is not infallible, as some testes in young infants do not elaborate testosterone in response to hCG on initial testing but do so later in infancy.[42]

Cryptorchidism is commonly associated with other abnormalities such as hernias, duplication of the ureters,[22] hypospadias,[78] epididymal agenesis or atresia,[49,63] posterior urethral valves,[46] and meningomye-

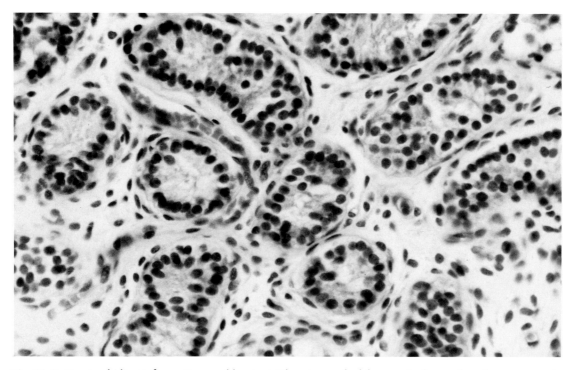

Fig. 23-3 Cryptorchid testis from a 9-year-old patient. There is a marked decrease in the number of spermatogonia. ×400.

locele.[45] With unilateral maldescent, the opposite testis may undergo compensatory hypertrophy.[47] Numerous genetic and congenital disorders are associated with a high incidence of cryptorchidism.[67,85] Cryptorchidism is seen particularly in association with mental retardation, especially in patients with cerebral palsy, 41 percent of whom are cryptorchid.[13] Prenatal exposure to diethylstilbestrol increases the risk of maldescent.[74] The exact cause of cryptorchidism is poorly understood. In a small percentage of cases it is believed to be a congenital, hereditary disorder, and in another small group a deficiency of gonadotropic hormonal stimulation appears to be re-

sponsible for gonadal maldescent. In most cases, however, it appears to represent an isolated, random, congenital anomaly or a mechanical obstruction to testicular descent.

There is no question about the adverse effects of maldescent on the testis, but the possible congenital nature of the changes and the age at which they become apparent are controversial. Ultrastructural alterations in the seminiferous tubules are evident as early as 1 year of age.[32] After age 2, cryptorchid testes reveal a progressive loss of spermatogonia, with almost 90 percent of cases showing complete loss or a significant decrease in the number of spermatogonia[51]

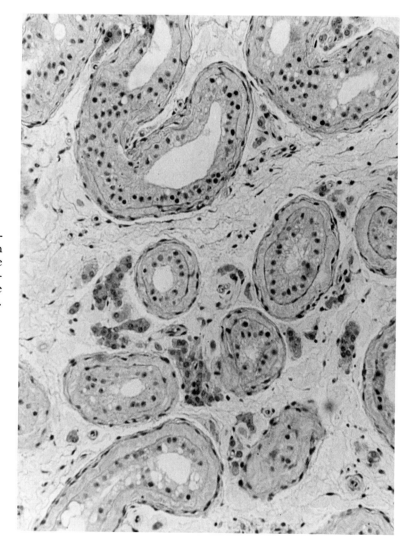

Fig. 23-4 Cryptorchid testis, postpubertal boy. There is partial hyalinization of the seminiferous tubules, which are mainly populated by Sertoli cells. Uninvolved clusters of Leydig cells are present in the fibrotic interstitium. ×225.

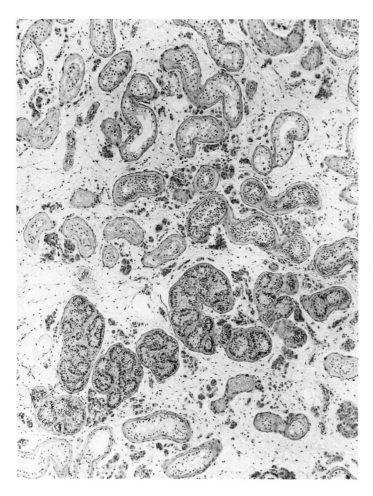

Fig. 23-5 Cryptorchid testis. Aggregates of seminiferous tubules lined by immature Sertoli cells are common in undescended testes from postpubertal males. ×60.

(Fig. 23-3). Tubular microliths may be evident.[58] There is a concomitant lack of maturation of Leydig and Sertoli cells.[56,68]

Furthermore, tubular diameters in undescended testes do not increase but, instead, sink below the normal range at the end of the second year of life, remaining at 40 to 50 μm until adulthood. In contrast, tubular diameters in normally descended testes grow steadily during puberty, reaching an average of 115 μm at 15 years of age. The prepubertal loss of germinal cells in cryptorchid testes is accompanied by hyaline thickening of the tubular basement membrane and tunica propria. Postpubertally, more profound changes occur, resulting in progressive atrophy of the germinal elements, eventual hyaline replacement of the seminiferous tubules, and increased interstitial connective tissue (Fig. 23-4). The number of Leydig cells may be decreased, increased, or normal. Rarely, they contain abundant lipid and resemble lipid-filled macrophages. A single case of intratesticular fatty metaplasia has been reported in a postpubertal cryptorchid testis.[36] Microscopic aggregates of immature tubules, sometimes called Pick's adenomas (Fig. 23-5), and collections of tubules lined by Sertoli cells are observed in almost one-half of the undescended testes in postpubertal males. These lesions are probably not truly neoplastic. In patients with unilateral cryptorchidism, testicular biopsies from the opposite, descended gonad are normal in 75 percent.[57] However, some patients have decreased spermatogonia and delayed maturation in the opposite testis as well.[26] Gonadotropin and testosterone levels are usually normal in patients with unilateral maldescent, but low testosterone and elevated gonadotropin levels may be encountered in those with bilateral cryptorchidism.[57,59] Interestingly, although most patients show diminution or disappearance of the germ cells, those that remain have nuclear diameters above normal as well as an increase in the DNA content.[54] Furthermore, histograms of the DNA distribution of these cells indicate that a substantial percentage have more than the normal diploid complement of DNA. One can only speculate on the possible contribution of these abnormal cells to the well recognized increase in germ cell malignancies in cryptorchid testes (see Ch. 27).

Data regarding the fertility of males with undescended testes following orchiopexy are unsatisfactory. It is believed that preservation of fertility can best be achieved by early orchiopexy, preferably at less than 2 years of age.[2,32] Although early orchiopexy appears to prevent subsequent deterioration in cryptorchid testes that initially show minimal histologic lesions, similar benefit may not occur in those with more significant changes.[57] Treatment before puberty has been reported to ensure fertility in 90 percent of cases of unilateral and 20 to 30 percent of bilateral cryptorchidism.[1] If surgery is performed after age 11, there is a 13 percent chance of fertility, a 56 percent incidence of sterility, and a high percentage of subfertility.[11] Increased gonadotropin levels in postpubertal boys who had a previous orchiopexy portend a poor prognosis for fertility.[3] Treatment with hCG has been attempted since the late 1930s in an effort to coax the testes down into the scrotum. It has been moderately successful, with statements in the literature to the effect that 50 percent of boys respond to this therapy.[42] However, one large series[24] puts a somewhat different slant on these overall data. Garagorri et al.[24] found that the chances of response to hCG improve with increasing age. Only 9 percent of those under 3 years responded with complete descent of the testes into the scrotum versus 32 percent descent in those aged 5 to 14 years. Attempts to bring the testis down with luteinizing hormone-releasing hormone (LHRH) were initially enthusiastically greeted, but double-blind studies have subsequently shown responses little greater than those with placebo.[41] Other studies, however, suggest that even when the testis does not descend the number of germ cells increases markedly, to near-normal levels.[32a] King[42] and more recently Chilvers et al.[10a] have reviewed the pros and cons of various therapeutic modalities.

Kogan et al.[44a,44b] have developed an experimental model of mechanical cryptorchidism in rats which should help define the chronology of loss of germinal epithelium and the optimal timing of orchiopexy.

(See Ch. 27 for a discussion of the relation between cryptorchidism and testicular tumors.)

ECTOPIC TESTES

Testicular ectopia refers to the presence of the testis in a position outside its normal course of descent. Backhouse,[4] who has extensively reviewed the embryology of testicular descent and maldescent, indicated that ectopia is often the result of gubernacular failure.[14] About 5 percent of maldescended testes are ectopic.[83] The principal sites of ectopia, in descending order of incidence, are the following: (1) the surface of the external oblique muscle (interstitial testis); (2) the femoral canal (femoral testis); (3) the ipsilateral ischial spine (perineal testis); (4) both gonads in one hemiscrotum (transverse testis);[25] and (5) the dorsal aspect of the base of the penis (pubic-penile testis). Rarely, the testis is in a preperitoneal position, deep to the abdominal muscles but superficial to the peritoneum,[55] or even between the internal and external oblique muscles.[70] Ectopic testes usually cannot be milked into the scrotum. Associated abnormalities include an indirect inguinal hernia, hypospadias, and hydrocele and may be the presenting problem. One case of transverse ectopia with an associated uterine structure representing a persistent müllerian duct has been described.[53a]

Testicular ectopia is frequently misdiagnosed as cryptorchidism, monorchia, or even a mass lesion. Histologically, ectopic testes are generally normal at birth but with time may undergo microscopic changes identical to those of the cryptorchid testis. A biopsy of the ectopic testis should be performed during surgical exploration; and if the testis is atrophic or cannot be placed in the scrotum, it should be excised. Germ cell tumors and carcinoma in situ have been reported in ectopic testes.[23,88]

PARATESTICULAR ADRENAL CORTICAL RESTS

Rests of adrenal cortical tissue in the region of the testis have been reported repeatedly since the original description by Dagonet in 1885.[15] In the 4-week-old embryo the adrenal and gonadal primordia and the mesonephros are located in close proximity. Adrenal cortical tissue, which may adhere to the gonad, appears to become separated from the main adrenal gland as the gonad descends.[16] An alternate theory is that the heterotopic adrenal tissue develops in situ from multipotential cells capable of forming cortical tissue.[30] Aberrant adrenal cortical tissue can be found anywhere along the course of the gonadal vessels, wolffian ducts, or their adult derivatives, or it may be adherent to the gonads.

The incidence of ectopic adrenal tissue in infants less than 1 year old is between 7.5 and 15.0 percent.[16,43] Adrenal rests are rare in adults and older children, suggesting that they frequently involute during infancy. Intrascrotal adrenal rests are most commonly found adjacent to the epididymis, in the connective tissue within the distal spermatic cord, in a hydrocele sac, or within or near the mediastinum testis.[16,73] There is a tendency for the ectopic adrenal to occur on the right side. There are no unequivocal reports of adrenal rests occurring within the testicular parenchyma. The rests range from 1 to 7 mm in diameter and are occasionally bilateral. Grossly, they appear as yellow, soft, semitranslucent nodules sur-

rounded by a delicate capsule. Microscopically, they contain zones of vacuolated cells mimicking the histologic appearance of the adrenal cortex, but no medullary component is present (Fig. 23-6). The zona fasciculata predominates, but zonae glomerulosa and reticularis may also be found.[48] The fetal provisional zone may be noted in adrenal rests in newborn infants.

In general, adrenal cortical rests do not require surgical excision. Most are found incidentally and rarely have any clinical significance. On rare occasions, the heterotopic adrenal tissue enlarges without known cause to form a clinically apparent tumor mass.[31] The accessory cortical tissue can undergo compensatory hypertrophy and modify the symptoms of adrenal insufficiency following destruction or extirpation of the adrenal glands.[73] The success of ablative adrenal surgery and therapy in some neoplastic diseases may depend on removal of all ectopic adrenal tissue that may be present.[48] Marked enlargement of paratesticular adrenal cortical nodules may occur in Nelson's syndrome [the development of an adrenocorticotropic hormone (ACTH)-producing pituitary tumor following bilateral adrenalectomy for Cushing's syn-

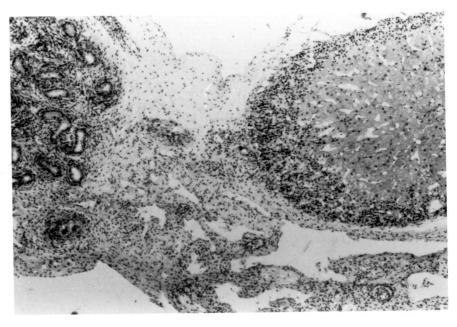

Fig. 23-6 Adrenal cortical rest. A paratesticular nodule composed of adrenal cortical cells (right) is present adjacent to the infantile epididymis (left). (From Silverberg SG (ed): Principles and Practice of Surgical Pathology. Wiley, New York, 1983.)

drome], the ACTH calling forth hyperplasia of these previously inapparent rests.[39] Such hyperplasia may also be seen with poorly controlled congenital adrenal hyperplasia.[44] Neoplasms arising in scrotal adrenal rests are usually adenomas, but a few reports of adrenal cortical carcinomas, sometimes endocrinologically active, have appeared in the literature.[53]

Difficulty may arise in distinguishing adrenal rests from Leydig cell tumors, but the latter tend to have a more eosinophilic, granular cytoplasm than adrenal cells whose cytoplasm is clear to finely vacuolar and often faintly basophilic. Should doubt persist, testicular venous hormone levels can settle the issue.

SPLENIC-GONADAL FUSION

Splenic-gonadal fusion consists in an abnormal connection between splenic tissue and the gonad or mesonephric structures. Fewer than 75 cases have been reported.[6,10,64] The condition shows a striking (12:1) male predominance, with only four cases having been reported in females.[34] In males the left testis is almost exclusively involved, and only a single case of a right scrotal spleen has been observed.[61]

The aberrant splenic tissue has generally been discovered incidentally at surgery or autopsy but may present clinically as an asymptomatic or symptomatic scrotal mass in patients of any age. When present, symptoms consist mainly of pain and tenderness, and they may develop following vigorous exercise due to splenic engorgement. The ectopic splenic tissue is subject to the same pathologic processes as the spleen, and enlargement of the scrotal-splenic tissue has been observed in patients with leukemia, malaria, mononucleosis, and other systemic infections.[61] In most cases both preoperative and intraoperative diagnoses have been incorrect. Technetium sulfur colloid scanning may be useful for locating the ectopic tissue.[50]

Two types of splenic-gonadal fusion have been identified. In the first type, termed *continuous fusion*,

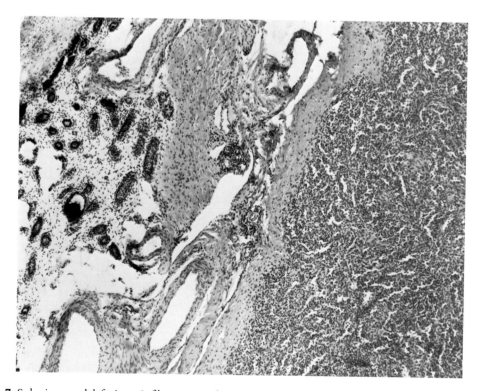

Fig. 23-7 Splenic-gonadal fusion. A fibrous capsule separates splenic tissue (right) from the testis (left). Focal seminiferous tubule calcification is evident. ×60.

the main spleen remains connected to the gonad by a continuous cord of tissue. The cord may be completely splenic, fibrous, or beaded with multiple nodular masses of splenic tissue. The cord generally arises from the upper pole of the spleen, extends all the way down the peritoneal cavity and into the inguinal canal, ending in an expanded mass of splenic tissue attached to the gonad, almost always the upper pole or the head of the epididymis. Bowel obstruction from extrinsic compression by the cord has been described.[35] In the second type, termed *discontinuous fusion,* aberrant splenic tissue is present as a discrete, encapsulated mass attached to the gonadal-mesonephric structures without any connection to the main spleen.

On gross examination, the scrotal-splenic tissue is usually located within the tunica vaginalis and is separated from the testis by a discrete fibrous capsule. Thus there is usually no intermingling with gonadal tissue (Fig. 23-7). The ectopic splenic tissue may be histologically normal or exhibit regressive changes including fibrosis, vascular thrombosis, and calcification.[21] The adjacent testicular tissue may be normal or reveal a spectrum of changes from mild atrophy, Leydig cell hyperplasia, and fibrosis to a complete absence of spermatogenesis. The most likely origin of splenic-gonadal fusion is the formation of an abnormal adhesion between the two primordia. It is assumed to occur between the fifth and eighth weeks of gestation because of the not infrequent association with limb bud anomalies, which are known to occur during this time span.[6] During caudal migration of the gonad the adhesion could lengthen and produce an intraperitoneal fibrous or splenic cord. Spontaneous rupture of the cord would result in transformation into the discontinuous type. Twenty percent of patients with continuous splenic-gonadal fusion have other congenital malformations such as limb deformities, micrognathia, and anal atresia.[61] Such malformations have not been reported in the discontinuous type. Splenic-gonadal fusion is often associated with cryptorchidism.[10,21]

In theory, splenic-gonadal fusion does not require treatment. Excision might be required if the ectopic spleen is symptomatic or involved in a disease process. In addition, scrotal splenic tissue may result in the failure of therapeutic splenectomy in cases of hypersplenism, necessitating removal of the spleen.[61] One case has been reported in which a testicular semi-oma occurred in a patient with splenic-gonadal fusion.[19]

REFERENCES

1. Albescu JZ, Bergada C, Cullem M: Male fertility in patients treated for cryptorchidism before puberty. Fertil Steril 18:829, 1971
2. Alpert PF, Klein RS: Spermatogenesis in the unilateral cryptorchid testis after orchiopexy. J Urol 129:301, 1983
3. Atkinson PM, Epstein MT, Rippon AE: Plasma gonadotropins and androgens in surgically treated cryptorchid patients. J Pediatr Surg 10:27, 1975
4. Backhouse KM: Embryology of testicular descent and maldescent. Urol Clin North Am 9:315, 1982
5. Baker LL, Hajek PC, Burkhard TK, Mattrey RF: Polyorchidism: evaluation by MR. AJR 148:305, 1987
6. Bearss RW: Splenic-gonadal fusion. Urology 16:277, 1980
7. Bellinger MF: The blind-ending vas: the fate of the contralateral testis. J Urol 133:644, 1985
8. Bobrow M, Gough MH: Bilateral absence of testes. Lancet 1:366, 1970
9. Butz RE, Croushore JH: Polyorchidism. J Urol 119:289, 1978
10. Ceccacci L, Tosi S: Splenic-gonadal fusion: case report and review of the literature. J Urol 126:558, 1981
10a. Chilvers C, Dudley NE, Gough MH, et al: Undescended testis: the effect of treatment on subsequent risk of subfertility and malignancy. J Pediatr Surg 21:691, 1986
11. Cittadina E, Gattuccio F, Gullo D: Fertility in treated cryptorchidism: evaluation during puberty and after puberty in surgically treated subjects. Acta Eur Fertil 10:15, 1979
12. Connors MH, Styne DM: Familial functional anorchidism: a review of etiology and management. J Urol 133:1049, 1985
13. Cortada X, Kousseff BG: Cryptorchidism in mental retardation. J Urol 131:674, 1984
14. Cromie WJ: Congenital anomalies of the testis, vas, epididymis, and inguinal canal. Urol Clin North Am 5:237, 1978
15. Dagonet J: Beritrage zur pathologischen Anatomie der Nebennieren des Menschen. Z Heilk 6:1, 1885
16. Dahl EV, Bahn RC: Aberrant adrenal cortical tissue near the testis in human infants. Am J Pathol 40:587, 1962
17. Das S, Amar AD: Ureteral ectopia into cystic seminal

vesicle with ipsilateral renal dysgenesis and monorchia. J Urol 124:574, 1980

18. D'Oplando C: Cited by Parks TG: Chromosome studies in polyorchidism. Br J Surg 54:113, 1967

19. Falkowski WS, Carter MF: Splenogonadal fusion associated with an anaplastic seminoma. J Urol 124:562, 1980

20. Feldman S, Drach GW: Polyorchidism discovered as testicular torsion. J Urol 130:976, 1983

21. Finkbeiner AE, DeRidder PA, Ryden SE: Splenic-gonadal fusion and adrenal cortical rest associated with bilateral cryptorchidism. Urology 10:337, 1977

22. Fram RJ, Garnick MB, Retik A: The spectrum of genitourinary abnormalities in patients with cryptorchidism, with emphasis on testicular carcinoma. Cancer 50:2243, 1982

23. Fujita J: Transverse testicular ectopia. Urology 16:400, 1980

23a. Gandia VM, Arrizabalaga M, Leiva O, Gonzalez RD: Polyorchidism discovered as testicular torsion associated with an undescended atrophic contralateral testis: a surgical solution. J Urol 137:743, 1987

24. Garagorri J-M, Job J-C, Canlorbe P, Chaussain J-L: Results of early treatment of cryptorchidism with human chorionic gonadotropin. J Pediatr 101:923, 1982

25. Gauderer WL, Grisoni ER, Stellato TA, et al: Transverse testicular ectopia (TTE). J Pediatr Surg 17:43, 1982

26. Gaudio E, Paggiarino D, Carpino F: Structural and ultrastructural modifications of cryptorchid human testes. J Urol 131:292, 1984

27. Glenn JF, McPherson HT: Anorchism: definition of a clinical entity. J Urol 105:265, 1971

28. Goldstein HH, Casilli AR: Rhabdomyosarcoma of the cremasteric muscle and concomitant polyorchidism. J Urol 41:453, 1939

29. Grechi G, Zampi GC, Selli C, et al: Polyorchidism and seminoma in a child. J Urol 123:291, 1980

30. Gruenwald P: Embryonic and postnatal development of the adrenal cortex, particularly the zona glomerulosa and accessory nodules. Anat Rec 95:391, 1946

31. Gualtieri T, Segal AD: Report of a case of adrenal-type tumor of the spermatic cord; a review of aberrant adrenal tissues. J Urol 61:949, 1949

32. Hadziselimovic F, Herzog B, Seguchi H: Surgical correction of cryptorchidism at two years: electron microscopic and morphologic investigation. J Pediatr Surg 10:19, 1975

32a. Hadziselimovic F, Huff D, Duckett J, et al: Long-term effect of luteinizing hormone-releasing hormone analogue (Buserelin) on cryptorchid testes. J Urol 138:1043, 1987

33. Hakami M, Mosavy SH: Triorchidism with normal spermatogenesis: an unusual cause for failure of vasectomy. Br J Surg 62:633, 1975

34. Halvorsen JF, Stray O: Splenogonadal fusion. Acta Paediatr Scand 67:379, 1978

35. Hines JR, Eggum PR: Splenic-gonadal fusion causing bowel obstruction. Arch Surg 83:887, 1961

36. Honore LH: Fatty metaplasia in a postpubertal undescended testis: a case report. J Urol 122:841, 1979

37. Honore LH: Unilateral anorchism; report of 11 cases with discussion of etiology and pathogenesis. Urology 11:251, 1978

38. Jarrow JP, Berkovitz GD, Migeon CT, et al: Elevation of serum gonadotrophins establishes the diagnosis of anorchism in prepubertal boys with bilateral cryptorchidism. J Urol 136:277, 1986

39. Johnson RE, Scheithauer B: Massive hyperplasia of testicular adrenal rests in a patient with Nelson's syndrome. Am J Clin Pathol 77:501, 1982

40. Josso N, Briard ML: Embryonic testicular regression syndrome: variable phenotypic expression in siblings. J Pediatr 97:200, 1980

41. Karpe B, Eneroth P, Ritzen EM: LHRH treatment in unilateral cryptorchidism: effect on testicular descent and hormonal response. J Pediatr 103:892, 1983

42. King LR: Optimal treatment of children with undescended testes (editorial). J Urol 131:734, 1984

43. Kirkbride MB: Embryonic disturbances of the testis. Arch Entwicklungsmeschn Organ 32:717, 1911

44. Kirkland RT, Kirkland JL, Keenan BS, et al: Bilateral testicular tumors in congenital adrenal hyperplasia. J Clin Endocrinol Metab 44:369, 1977

44a. Kogan BA, Gupta R, Juenemann KP: Fertility in cryptorchidism: further development of an experimental model. J Urol 137:128, 1987

44b. Kogan BA, Gupta R, Juenemann KP: Fertility in cryptorchidism: improved timing of fixation and treatment in an experimental model. J Urol 138:1046, 1987

45. Kropp KA, Voeller KKS: Cryptorchidism in meningomyelocele. J Pediatr 99:110, 1981

46. Krueger RP, Hardy BE, Churchill BM: Cryptorchidism in boys with posterior urethral valves. J Urol 124:101, 1980

47. Laron Z, Dickerman Z, Ritterman I, Kaufman H: Follow-up of boys with unilateral compensatory testicular hypertrophy. Fertil Steril 33:297, 1980

48. Mares AJ, Shkolnik A, Sacks M, Feuchtwanger MM: Aberrant (ectopic) adrenocortical tissue along the spermatic cord. J Pediatr Surg 15:289, 1980

49. Marshall FF, Shermeta DW: Epididymal abnormalities associated with undescended testis. J Urol 121:341, 1979

50. McLean GK, Alavi A, Ziegler MM, et al: Splenic-go-

nadal fusion: identification by radionuclide scanning. J Pediatr Surg, suppl., 16:649, 1981

51. Mengel W, Hienz HA, Sippe WG, et al: Studies on cryptoorchidism: a comparison of histological findings in the germinative epithelium before and after the second year of life. J Pediatr Surg 9:445, 1974

52. Mercer S: Agenesis or atrophy of the testis and vas deferens. Can J Surg 22:245, 1979

53. Morimoto Y, Hiwada K, Nanahoshi M, et al: Cushing's syndrome caused by a malignant tumor in the scrotum: clinical, pathologic and biochemical studies. J Clin Endocrinol 32:201, 1971

53a. Mouli K, McCarthy P, Ray P, et al: Persistent mullerian duct syndrome in a man with transverse testicular ectopia. J Urol 139:373, 1988

54. Muller J, Skakkebaek NE: Abnormal germ cells in maldescended testes: a study of cell density, nuclear size and deoxyribonucleic acid content in testicular biopsies from 50 boys. J Urol 131:730, 1984

55. Murphy DM, Butler MR: Preperitoneal ectopic testis: a case report. J Pediatr Surg 20:93, 1985

56. Nistal M, Paniagua R, Albaurrea MA, Santamaria L: Hyperplasia and the immature appearance of Sertoli cells in primary testicular disorders. Hum Pathol 13:3, 1982

57. Nistal M, Paniagua R, Diez-Pardo JA: Histologic classification of undescended testes. Hum Pathol 11:666, 1980

58. Nistal M, Paniagua R, Diez-Pardo JA: Testicular microliths in 2 children with bilateral cryptorchidism. J Urol 121:535, 1979

59. Nkuyama A, Statani H, Mizutani S, et al: Pituitary and gonadal function in prepubertal and pubertal cryptorchidism. Acta Endocrinol (Copenh) 95:553, 1980

60. Pelander WM, Luna G, Lilly JR: Polyorchidism: case report and literature review. J Urol 119:705, 1978

61. Pendse AK, Mathur PM, Sharma MM, et al: Splenicgonadal fusion. Br J Surg 62:624, 1975

62. Penny R: The testis. Pediatr Clin North Am 26:107, 1979

63. Priebe CJ, Holahan JA, Ziring PR: Abnormalities of the vas deferens and epididymis in cryptorchid boys with congenital rubella. J Pediatr Surg 14:834, 1979

64. Putschar WG, Manion WC: Splenic-gonadal fusion. Am J Pathol 32:15, 1956

65. Rajfer J, Tauber A, Zinner N, et al: Use of computerized tomography scanning to localize the impalpable testis. J Urol 129:972, 1983

66. Rajfer J, Walsh PC: Testicular descent. Urol Clin North Am 5:223, 1978

67. Randolph J, Cavett C, Eng G: Surgical correction and rehabilitation for children with "prune-belly" syndrome. Ann Surg 193:757, 1981

68. Re M, Micali F, Racheli T, Lannitelli M: Cryptorchid human testis after hCG treatment: histological study on Sertoli cells. Eur Urol 5:195, 1979

69. Reckler JM, Rose LI, Harrison JH: Bilateral anorchism. J Urol 113:869, 1975

70. Redman JF: Impalpable testes: observations based on 208 consecutive operations for undescended testes. J Urol 124:379, 1980

71. Redman JF, Brizzolara JP: An unusual case of testicular ectopia. J Urol 133:104, 1985

72. Ruvalcaba RHA, Gogue HP, Kelly VC: Discordance of congenital bilateral anorchia in uniovular twins: 17 years of observations on growth and development. Pediatrics 67:276, 1981

73. Schechter DC: Aberrant adrenal tissue. Ann Surg 167:421, 1968

74. Schottenfeld C: The epidemiology of cancer: an overview. Cancer 47:1095, 1981

75. Scorer CG: The descent of the testis. Arch Dis Child 39:605, 1964

76. Scott JES: Laparoscopy as an aid in the diagnosis and management of the impalpable testis. J Pediatr Surg 17:14, 1982

77. Scott KWM: A case of polyorchidism with testicular teratoma. J Urol 124:930, 1980

78. Shima H, Ikoma F, Terakawa T, et al: Developmental anomalies with hypospadias. J Urol 122:619, 1979

79. Silber SJ: Transplantation of a human testis for anorchia. Fertil Steril 30:181, 1978

80. Snow BW, Tarry WF, Duckett JW: Polyorchidism: an unusual case. J Urol 133:483, 1985

81. Summitt RL: Genetic forms of hypogonadism in the male. J Med Genet 3:1, 1979

82. Theodor R, Hertz M, Goodman RM: Symphalangism, short stature, skeletal anomalies, and accessory testis: a new malformation syndrome. J Med Genet 16:159, 1979

83. Thevathasau CG: Transverse ectopia of the testis. Aust NZ J Surg 37:93, 1967

84. Thiessen NW: Polyorchidism: report of a case. J Urol 49:710, 1943

85. Von Petrykowski W: Embryology of genital malformations: guidelines in diagnosis and treatment of intersex. Monogr Paediatr 12:1, 1981

86. Weiss RM, Glickman MG: Localization and management of nonpalpable undescended testes. Surg Clin North Am 60:1253, 1980

86a. Weiss RM, Seashore JH: Laparoscopy in the management of the nonpalpable testis. J Urol 138:382, 1987

87. Wescott JW, Dykhuizen RF: Polyorchidism. J Urol 98:497, 1967

88. Williams TR, Brendler H: Carcinoma in situ of the ectopic testis. J Urol 117:610, 1977

24

Disorders of Sexual Differentiation

Frank Rudy

Human anatomic sexuality and sexual differentiation may be conveniently classified into five categories: genetic sex, gonadal sex, ductal sex, hormonal sex, and genital sex. These factors normally combine to determine an individual's sex assignment. Aberrations of any of these normal determinants of sexual differentiation of the fetus may lead to intersex. Intersexuality refers to the presence of one or more contradictions of the morphologic criteria of sex and occurs in the broadest sense in about 1 percent of all newborn children.[141] The disorders of sexual differentiation can be classified according to the gonadal histology. Five major categories of intersex are recognized (Table 24-1): (1) testis plus ovary (true hermaphrodite); (2) testis only (male pseudohermaphrodite); (3) ovary only (female pseudohermaphrodite); (4) testis plus streak gonad (mixed gonadal dysgenesis); and (5) streak gonads only (gonadal dysgenesis).

During embryogenesis any disturbance of the various steps in normal sexual differentiation may be reflected clinically as a disorder of intersexuality; therefore the subject of abnormalities of sexual differentiation is justifiably regarded as complex and confusing. The clinical approach to these patients involves determining the individual's status with regard to each of the five categories of sexual differentiation and elucidating the basis of any discrepancies utilizing the principles of sexual development. Therefore a brief review of the mechanisms of normal sexual differentiation is appropriate (also see Ch. 22).

MECHANISMS OF NORMAL SEXUAL DIFFERENTIATION

Human male and female embryos develop in an identical fashion for approximately 40 days of gestation,[51] after which there is divergence of development resulting in the formation of the male and female phenotypes. The first step in the sequential process of sexual differentiation is establishment of the genetic sex at the time of fertilization, with the heterogametic complement (XY) being male and the homogametic state (XX) female. The genetic sex is then translated into the gonadal sex.

The embryonic gonad is bipotent, and under normal circumstances ovarian organogenesis inherently occurs in the absence of a functional Y chromosome.[88] Oocyte viability and ovarian structure seem to be maintained only in the presence of two intact X chromosomes.[119] Extragonadal female development occurs in the presence of an ovary or a streak gonad, or if no gonads are present. Therefore the female phenotype is viewed as being primarily inherent and as de-

967

Table 24-1 Characteristics of Intersex States

Diagnosis	External Genitalia	Karyotype	Gonads	Internal Ducts	Pubertal Change
True hermaphrodite	Ambiguous[a]	XX, XX/XY, XY, etc.	Ovary and testis	Müllerian and wolffian	Tendency to virilization
Male peudohermaphrodite					
Persistent müllerian duct syndrome	Cryptorchid male	XY	Testes	Müllerian and wolffian	Virilization
Defective testosterone synthesis	Ambiguous[b]	XY	Testes	Wolffian	Variable
Androgen insensitivity syndrome	Variable	XY	Testes	Wolffian (or none)	Variable
5α-Reductase deficiency	Female	XY	Testes	Wolffian	Virilization
Testicular dysgenesis	Ambiguous	XY, etc.	Testes (or none)	Wolffian with or without müllerian	Usually virilization
Female pseudohermaphrodite					
Congenital adrenal hyperplasia	Ambiguous	XX	Ovaries	Müllerian	Feminization (if treated)
Exposure to maternal estrogens, progestins, or androgens	Ambiguous	XX	Ovaries	Müllerian	Feminization
Mixed gonadal dysgenesis	Ambiguous	XO/XY, etc.	Testis and streak	Müllerian and wolffian	Usually virilization
Gonadal dysgenesis					
Turner's syndrome	Female	XO, etc.	Streaks	Immature müllerian	Eunuchoid
XX gonadal dysgenesis	Female	XX	Streaks	Immature müllerian	Eunuchoid
XY gonadal dysgenesis	Female	XY	Streaks	Immature müllerian	Eunuchoid or virilization

[a] Tendency toward maleness.
[b] Tendency toward femaleness.
(Modified from Allen,[5] with permission.)

veloping in a passive manner. In the presence of an XY sex chromosome constitution, the indifferent embryonic gonads develop as testes.

Evidence has begun to accumulate about the mechanism by which the Y chromosome induces testicular organogenesis. It appears that one or more loci on the Y chromosome determine a specific protein or set of proteins on the surface of the germ cell that, in turn, induces the gonadal ridges to differentiate into testes. It is postulated that this inducer is either a Y-determined histocompatibility antigen (H-Y antigen) or the product of a locus closely linked to the H-Y gene (Fig. 24-1). The H-Y antigen is a cell surface protein, originally identified in male rodents, that causes rejection of grafts by females of inbred strains.[37] H-Y antigen is thought to be disseminated in the embryo in a hormonelike fashion and to bind to two receptors: (1) the specific receptor of the gonad; and (2) nonspecific β_2-microglobulin stable membrane anchorage

sites that are present in all cells, gonadal and somatic.[143,144] Assuming a certain minimal threshold of H-Y antigen production, engagement of the disseminated H-Y molecules with the receptors and saturation of these receptors causes a change in membrane receptor configuration, thereby inducing the indifferent gonadal anlage to undergo testicular organogenesis.[142]

Genetic control of H-Y antigen expression is unclear, and the location of the H-Y structural gene is not known. Regulation of H-Y antigen expression is closely linked with the presence of an intact Y chromosome; however, there is increasing evidence that H-Y antigen is coded for by one or several autosomal gene loci that are under the regulatory control of genes in the pericentric region of the Y chromosome and in the short arm of the human X chromosome.[106,111,151] With this hypothesis, a locus on the Y gene may act as an inducer of the autosomal structural

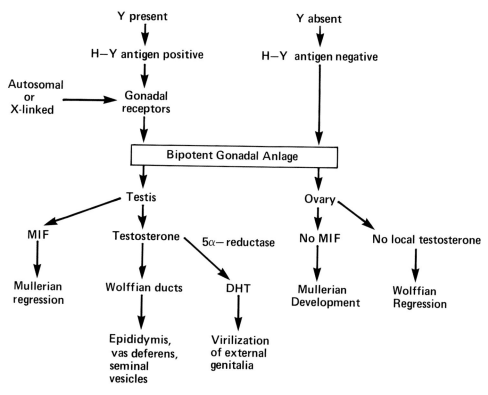

Fig. 24-1 Scheme of human sexual differentiation. MIF, müllerian inhibiting factor; DHT, dihydrotestosterone.

gene by suppressing an X chromosome repressor.[22,141] Therefore the H-Y phenotype per se may not be a valid marker for the Y chromosome.[145]

For testicular organogenesis to occur in the presence of the H-Y antigen, an additional gene, either autosomal or X-linked, must be present that determines the structure of the plasma membrane receptor for the H-Y antigen. It follows that failure of testicular organogenesis would result from reduced or absent synthesis of the H-Y antigen, synthesis of a faulty H-Y antigen, or anomalous binding characteristics of either the nonspecific anchorage sites or specific receptors. According to this scheme, the presence of testicular structures should always be associated with H-Y antigen expression, regardless of the karyotype or secondary sex phenotype.[89] Generally, serologically detectable H-Y antigen has been present whenever any degree of testicular differentiation has been found, even in the absence of a demonstrable Y chromosome.[55,115]

Data have shown that testicular tissue in patients with disorders of sexual development is not always associated with an X-Y+ phenotype.[118] This observation could indicate that: (1) H-Y antigen may not be responsible for testicular organogenesis; (2) H-Y antigen may not be the only inducer of testicular development; (3) H-Y antigen was present at a level too low to measure; or (4) X-Y antigen was present but was not serologically detectable owing to some alteration of the H-Y molecule or the cell surface.[55,118]

It has also been hypothesized that the H-Y molecules might compete with a blocking molecule for available H-Y receptors.[23,142] Occupation of the H-Y receptors by this second molecule would result in ovarian differentiation. A predominance of the H-Y antigen or the blocking molecule would lead to unambiguous testicular or ovarian differentiation, respectively.

The final process of sexual differentiation is the translation of gonadal sex into phenotypic sex, which is a direct consequence of the type of gonad formed. The testes actively induce masculine development (Fig. 24-1). Normal male differentiation requires that fetal testicular hormone secretion begin at about 8 weeks' gestation.[28,66,119] Timing is crucial, as the target cells are responsive to these developmental influences for only limited periods of time. Two sets of hormones are required: müllerian-inhibiting factor (MIF) and androgens. The first event in male phenotypic development is müllerian duct regression, which is brought about by MIF. MIF is an incompletely characterized protein elaborated by the Sertoli cells of the fetal testis. Müllerian duct regression appears to be a localized phenomenon, as the secretion of one testis has no effect on the contralateral müllerian duct.[36] Fetal testicular Leydig cells differentiate and produce testosterone. Testosterone secretion depends on the normal function of the steroidogenic enzymes. Data indicate that testosterone reaches all of the urogenital primordia by diffusion during early sexual differentiation (8 to 10 weeks).[119]

Testosterone exerts its effects on target cells in two major ways. First, high local concentrations of testosterone produced by the adjacent testis act directly to promote conversion of the wolffian duct into the epididymis, vas deferens, and seminal vesicle. Second, once inside the target cell, testosterone can be converted to dihydrotestosterone (DHT) by the enzyme 5α-reductase. DHT induces formation of the prostate from the urogenital sinus and virilization of the embryonic external genitalia. Furthermore, DHT is responsible for the development of most of the secondary sex characteristics at puberty.[51] Testosterone can also be aromatized to the potent estrogen 17β-estradiol, which may mediate some of its effects. Androgen action on target cells requires the presence of cellular receptors. In order to effect its biologic response, testosterone and DHT must bind to the same high-affinity androgen–receptor protein in the cytosol (Fig. 24-2). These hormone–receptor complexes then move into the nucleus where they interact with acceptor sites on the chromosomes. This interaction results in increased transcription of specific structural genes with subsequent appearance of new messanger RNA and proteins in the cell cytoplasm.[149] Intersexuality may result from deficient synthesis of MIF, testosterone, or DHT, or from defective androgen action on target cells. In the absence of testes, anatomic development is female in character. The müllerian ducts give rise to the fallopian tubes, uterus, cervix, and upper vagina. The wolffian system degenerates, and the external genitalia feminize. Female phenotypic differentiation does not require the presence of a gonad.

EVALUATION AND MANAGEMENT

Regardless of pathogenesis, intersex syndromes present in a limited number of ways. The individual may be found unexpectedly to have gonads or internal genitalia inappropriate for the putative sex. Other patients come to medical attention because of absent or heterosexual pubertal development. Most of the remaining patients present with ambiguous genitalia. Ambiguous genitalia may be defined as the presence of abnormal development of two or more external genital structures, i.e., phallus, urethral meatus, labioscrotal folds, urogenital folds, or vagina.[33] For the

TARGET CELL

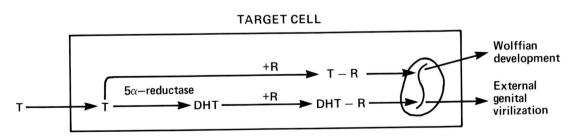

Fig. 24-2 Molecular mechanism of androgen action of target cell. T, testosterone; DHT, dihydrotestosterone; R, high-affinity androgen receptor protein; T-R and DHT-R, hormone receptor complexes. (Modified from Wilson et al,[149] with permission.)

evaluation of these defects, any infant with more than a single genital anomaly is considered to have a disorder of sexual differentiation until proved otherwise.[21] The presence of a single major anomaly and the association of common defects such as cryptorchidism, hypospadias, and inguinal hernias may also indicate the need for evaluation. The ambiguous genitalia of these cases tend to be similar, with an appearance intermediate on the spectrum between normal male and normal female phenotypes. Intersex must be distinguished from pseudointersex, the term applied to genital anomalies that arise from local dysgenetic influences rather than from aberrations in sexual developmental mechanisms.[119] Pseudointersex cases do not fall along the continuum between normal female and male development and often have other caudal or urologic abnormalities, e.g., bladder exstrophy.

To determine the one biologic error that underlies a single patient's problem may seem an overwhelming task and requires a multidisciplinary team approach. Obtaining a detailed history is the initial step in the evaluation of patients with intersexuality. Because many of the disorders are inherited, the family history must be probed.[95] A history of shock or vascular collapse during infancy suggests congenital adrenal hyperplasia. Hematuria, bleeding from a perineal orifice, or cyclic abdominal pain may indicate the presence of müllerian duct derivatives. Primary amenorrhea in a patient with a female phenotype raises the possibility of an androgen insensitivity syndrome. Proper investigation also requires a careful physical examination. External genital sex is the most amenable to clinical evaluation, but direct examination of the external genitalia is not infallible. The presence, shape, size, and position of all genital and gonadal structures should be determined. The size of the phallus and location of the urethral meatus must be documented, and the contents of any hernia should be carefully examined. Masses may represent gonads, gonadal tumors, or müllerian duct derivatives and are searched for by palpation of the scrotum, inguinal regions, and labioscrotal folds, as well as by deep abdominal and rectal examination. The presence of a gonad in the labioscrotal area is usually indicative of testicular tissue, as ovaries rarely descend.[147] Additional useful findings on physical examination include hyperpigmentation (often present in congenital adrenal hyperplasia), the distribution of pubic and genital hair, a palpable cervix, evidence of dehydra-

tion and failure to thrive, and the occurrence of other anomalies that may provide clues to associated syndromes.

Radiographic and endoscopic procedures are often required to adequately evaluate the urogenital sinus and internal ductal structures of intersex patients. Miniature fiberoptic endoscopes permit the evaluation of even young children.[38] The urethra, bladder, position of the vaginal opening, and the presence or absence of a cervix can be readily determined. Although the lower vagina may be present in many forms of intersexuality, the presence of a cervix excludes defects in testosterone and DHT synthesis and defective androgen action.[49] Laparoscopy may be employed to identify internal structures, e.g., the ovaries and uterus. A flush genitogram, voiding cystourethrogram, computed tomography (CT), and ultrasound studies may visualize the vagina, cervix, and uterus (Fig. 24-3). An exploratory laparotomy may be required to examine the internal genital ductal structures, biopsy the gonads for histologic identification, or assess abnormal masses. To obtain an adequate gonadal biopsy in an intersex case, it is mandatory that a generous, deep, longitudinal wedge of tissue be removed from all suspected gonadal structures. One-tenth to one-sixth of the gonad should be removed.

Laboratory studies should begin with chromosome and hormone determinations. A rapid approximation of the patient's sex chromosome complement can be obtained by examining buccal mucosal cells for Barr bodies and Y chromosome fluorescence. A Barr body is found in 20 percent or more of nuclei from cells from normal females and in less than 2 percent of cells from normal males.[147] It is important to recognize that lower Barr body counts may be found in normal female newborns during the first week of life and possibly in some infants with congenital adrenal hyperplasia.[119] Buccal smear study is a screening procedure, and a karyotype is obtained as early as possible to ascertain the exact chromosome complement and the presence of mosaicism and structural chromosome alterations. Genetic analysis of multiple tissues may be necessary to accurately determine mosaicism. Genetic sex is often critical for deciding the category of disorder to which the patient belongs and may affect decisions regarding the fate of gonadal tissue.

Plasma and urinary steroid determinations and serum electrolytes are invaluable laboratory tests. On the basis of these studies, the diagnosis of congenital

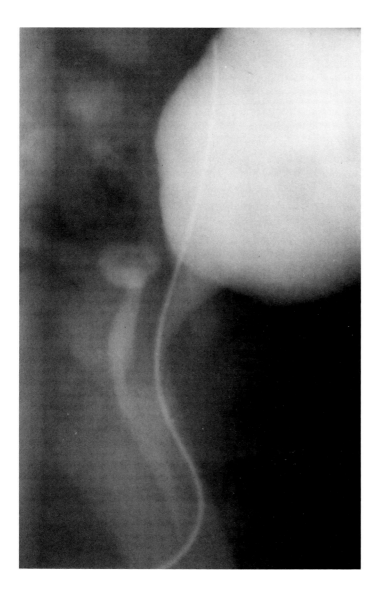

Fig. 24-3 True hermaphrodite. A vagina and uterus are visualized in this retrograde genitogram. The catheter is in the urethra. (Courtesy of Dr. Howard Snyder, Children's Hospital of Philadelphia.)

adrenal hyperplasia, the only life-threatening circumstances, may be confirmed or excluded. Assay of 17α-hydroxyprogesterone is supplanting urinary 17-ketosteroids and pregnanetriol levels as the hormonal measurement of choice to diagnose adrenocortical hyperplasia.[119] Additional steroid studies may be required to document high levels of plasma precursor hormones and reduced steroid levels beyond the specific enzymatic defect. In selected cases fibroblast cultures are necessary to assess androgen action.[13] Evaluation of the external genitalia for specific effects following exogenous hormonal stimulation may also

be rewarding. Determination of serum gonadotropins may indicate the absence of functional gonadal tissue if they are evaluated, but they do not provide information on the type of gonads present. Measurements of plasma sex steroids (testosterone, estrone, 17β-estradiol, and DHT) give little information in the basal state.[21] Stimulation of the patient with exogenous human chorionic gonadotropin (hCG) and subsequent sex steroid measurements may assist in elucidating the presence of specific gonadal components. The presence of functional testicular tissue can be detected by the testosterone response to hCG stimulation.[107] On a theoretical basis, the presence of ovarian tissue could be assessed by the hormonal response to appropriate gonadotropic stimuli. H-Y antigen determinations may be supportive evidence for the presence or absence of testes. The primary H-Y antigen assay currently employed is a cytotoxicity test using mouse sperm.[143]

Advances in techniques for prenatal diagnosis of a variety of conditions have increased the possibility of diagnosing some types of intersex in utero. By combining chromosome analysis in amniocytes with examination of the fetal genitalia using fetoscopy or sonography, it can be determined if the genitalia are appropriate to the genetic sex of the fetus.[39] Cultured amniocytes might be used to determine androgen receptor activity; and, at least theoretically, amniotic fluid steroid measurements might permit the diagnosis of specific inborn errors of testosterone synthesis.

When evaluating an intersex patient, the goal is not simply to determine "what it is" but to assign an appropriate sex of rearing.[74] Disorders of sexual differentiation in infants are considered medical and "social" emergencies, as there may be potentially lethal underlying metabolic abnormalities; and irreversible commitment to an inappropriate sex of rearing may occur, thereby precluding successful medical or surgical correction of the genital defects. Gender assignment is best made during the neonatal period because the psychosexual identity is generally considered fixed by 18 months to 2 years of age.[33,147] Final gender assignment is almost always based on the ability to define the anatomy and predict future development. When establishing the sex of rearing, the most important consideration is to achieve functional genitalia. The ultimate gender assignment may be appropriately contradictory to the genetic, gonadal, or internal ductal sex. Fertility is of secondary importance. Phallus adequacy is the major criterion for gender assignment. A phallic nomogram facilitates the determination of which phallus is likely to be adequate. A functional organ cannot be created from a clitoriform phallus. In general, the sex assignment is male in patients having a normal-sized penis (more than 2.5 cm in stretched length in a normal birth weight newborn) and no significant vagina.[33] When both a vagina and a well developed phallus are present, the findings on exploratory laparotomy and gonadal biopsy may be a major factor for fixing the gender. Individuals with an inadequate phallus should be reared as females regardless of the gonadal status. Surgical reconstruction of the external genitalia toward either a male or female appearance is best accomplished during infancy.[6] Although internal ductal structures that are contradictory to the assigned gender may be left in place, removal of these organs may be warranted for psychological reasons, particularly if other indications for a laparotomy are present.[33]

The final set of surgical considerations involves management of the gonadal elements in intersex patients. Gonadectomy is warranted if the gonad is a potential source of virilization at puberty in individuals reared as females, as may occur in those with dysgenetic testes, incomplete androgen insensitivity syndrome, mixed gonadal dysgenesis, or true hermaphroditism. Gonadectomy is also indicated if the gonad has an increased risk of malignant transformation, e.g., streak gonads and dysgenetic testes in intersex patients with a Y chromosome, testes in the androgen insensitivity syndrome, and undescended testes in older individuals.

TRUE HERMAPHRODITISM

True hermaphroditism, in which the individual possesses both testicular and ovarian tissue, is the rarest category of sexual ambiguity, accounting for less than 10 percent of the intersex population. Approximately 400 cases have been reported in the world literature,[139] with more than 50 of the documented cases occurring in African Bantus. True hermaphroditism is the most common form of intersexuality in this racial group.[52] Although most cases are sporadic, a number of families with more than one affected sibling have been described.[16,43] The pedigrees have suggested either an autosomal recessive genetic pattern or autosomal dominant inheritance with varying expression. Cytogenetic studies have demonstrated a 46,XX chromosome complement in 60 percent of true hermaphrodites, a 46,XX/46,XY mosaic or chimeric karyotype in 13 percent, a 46,XY pattern in 12 percent, and a variety of other mosaics in the remaining 15 percent.[27,30,40,139] Because on rare occasions the gonadal karyotype may be discordant with the peripheral blood karyotype, some instances of mosaicism or chimerism may go undetected.[63] True hermaphrodites often present with ambiguous genitalia during the newborn period. Gynecomastia in an individual reared as a male is the most common symptom in adolescents. Well developed breasts occurred in 70 percent of those who had reached puberty,[139] and three cases of breast carcinoma have been reported.[30] Other presenting complaints may include hematuria, perineal bleeding, cryptorchidism, amenorrhea, lower abdominal pain from endometriosis, inguinal hernia, abdominal tumor, asymmetrical gonadal enlargement, and torsion of müllerian duct derivatives and gonads.[27,53,104] Twenty percent of the reported cases were diagnosed before 5 years of age, 40 percent before age 15, and 75 percent before puberty.[104]

The appearance of the external genitalia of true hermaphrodites spans the full spectrum from a completely male to a completely female phenotype. A tendency toward maleness is evident, as 75 percent of reported cases were reared as males.[139] Indeed, absence of an enlarged phallus or clitoris is unusual, and only three cases have been described with normal female external genitalia.[104] The presence of a Y chromosome is more commonly associated with a male phenotype, whereas those with a female appearance have a greater tendency to lack a Y in their karyotype. The typical external genitalia consist of an enlarged phallus present in chordee, labioscrotal folds, and a perineal urogenital sinus (Fig. 24-4). A cryptorchid or normally descended gonad is palpable in many cases. A uterus, which can often be detected on rectal examination, is present in 87 percent of true hermaphrodites, and one-half of these individuals spontaneously menstruate.[139] Therefore in most patients sufficient DHT was produced during fetal life to partially virilize the external genitalia, but MIF secretion is deficient. Either virilization or feminization may occur at puberty depending on the dominant hormonal influence. Major somatic defects are found in about 4 percent of cases.[104]

Although on some occasions radiographic studies assist in the diagnosis, the definitive diagnosis of true hermaphroditism is established only by exploratory laparotomy and gonadal biopsy. The histologic examination of testicular tissue should demonstrate distinct seminiferous tubules, and the ovarian tissue must contain developing follicles. The presence of functional testicular elements may be determined by finding increased testosterone production following hCG stimulation.[47] The distribution of gonadal tissue, in decreasing order of frequency, is as follows: unilateral

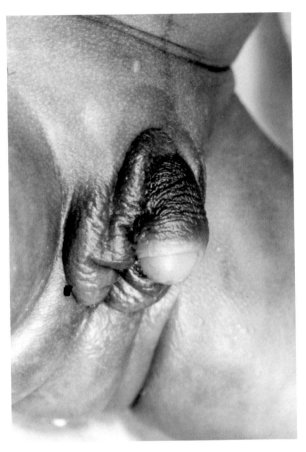

Fig. 24-4 True hermaphrodite. An enlarged phallus and labioscrotal folds give a masculine appearance to the external genitalia. (Courtesy of Dr. Howard Snyder, Children's Hospital of Philadelphia.)

ovary with contralateral testis, unilateral ovotestis with contralateral ovary, bilateral ovotestes, and unilateral ovotestis with contralateral testis.[139] When an ovary is present, it is most commonly found on the left side, whereas testicular tissue, either as a testis or an ovotestis, has a tendency to occur on the right side of the body.

The ovotestis is the most common gonad in true hermaphrodites. One-half are located intraabdominally, with the remaining 50 percent occurring in the inguinal canal or labioscrotal fold.[139] The ratio of ovarian to testicular elements in the ovotestis appears to determine its final anatomic location. The more testicular tissue that is present, the greater is the likelihood of descent. In 80 percent of cases the ovarian and testicular tissues are arranged in an end-to-end fashion, giving a diagnostic gross appearance (Fig. 24-5). In the remaining 20 percent the testicular component is in the hilar region of the gonad, making macroscopic diagnosis of an ovotestis more difficult. The ovarian portion of an ovotestis has a convoluted surface and is firm, whereas the testicular tissue is soft and shows a smoother, glistening surface. Generally, there is a distinct line of demarcation between the two types of gonadal tissue. Facilities for a frozen section should be available at laparotomy so that gonadal biopsies can be examined in doubtful cases. On histologic examination the ovarian tissue must contain developing follicles as well as ovarian stroma (Fig. 24-6). The ovarian portion of an ovotestis is usually histologically normal but may have a reduced number of primordial follicles. Evidence of ovulation is seen

in 50 percent of ovotestes.[118] The testicular portion of an ovotestis, which histologically resembles an infantile testis, should contain recognizable seminiferous tubules. Although occasionally relatively normal during the prepubertal period, progressive alterations develop subsequently. The main histologic changes include an absence of spermatogenesis, gradual disappearance of germ cells, the presence of abundant Sertoli cells in the lumens of the seminiferous tubules, and Leydig cell hyperplasia.[1,64,122,139] In adults hyalinization and tubular sclerosis ensue, and spermatogenesis is not observed.

The ovary, the second most common gonad in true hermaphrodites, is usually located in its normal anatomic position. When a gonad with the appearance of an ovary is encountered along the normal pathway of testicular descent, the possibility that it is an ovotestis

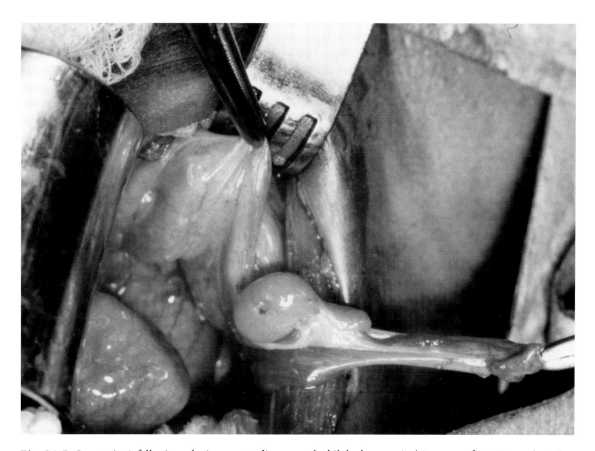

Fig. 24-5 Ovotestis. A fallopian tube is present adjacent to the bilobed ovotestis. (Courtesy of Dr. Howard Snyder, Children's Hospital of Philadelphia.)

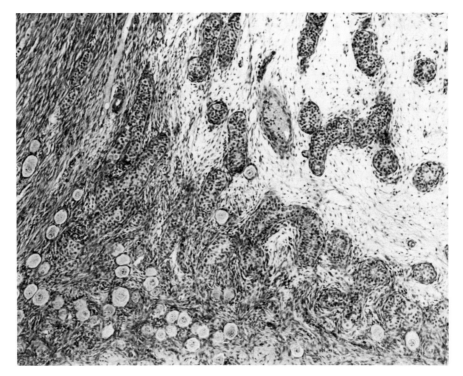

Fig. 24-6 Ovotestis. The ovarian portion (left) contains oocytes and a developing follicle. Immature seminiferous tubules populate the testicular tissue (upper right). ×60.

should be seriously considered. Most of the ovaries reveal either corpora lutea or corpora albicantia, indicating prior ovulation.

A testis is the least common gonad in true hermaphroditism and is histologically similar to the testicular portion of an ovotestis. There is a tendency for the testis to descend into the scrotum, although it may be found in the normal ovarian position. Spermatogenesis is present in 12 percent of cases.[139] Grossly, about two-thirds of the testes are smaller than normal. It appears that a testis is more likely to occur in a true hermaphrodite when the patient's karyotype includes a Y chromosome. Gonadal tumors have been noted in slightly more than 2 percent of true hermaphrodites.[139] Most have been dysgerminoma seminoma in type, but embryonal carcinoma, yolk sac tumor, mixed germ cell tumors, gonadoblastoma, Brenner tumor, mucinous cystadenoma, cystadenocarcinoma, and gynandroblastoma and other gonadal stromal tumors have also been reported.[30,33,101,139] The increased risk for the development of germ cell neoplasms may relate to the frequently cryptorchid loca-

tion of the testicular tissue. Nonneoplastic follicular and "chocolate" cysts of the ovary may also occur.[105]

The duct adjacent to a gonad corresponds to the histology of that gonad; hence an ovary is always associated with a fallopian tube and a testis with a vas deferens and epididymis. The duct accompanying an ovotestis may be either a fallopian tube or a vas deferens and appears to correlate with the ratio of testicular to ovarian tissue. The gross appearance of the duct may be misleading, as some ducts resemble a hypoplastic fallopian tube but are found on microscopic study to be wolffian in origin. Careful examination of the fallopian tube often reveals a congenitally closed osteal end, possibly the result of MIF production by the testicular portion of the ovotestis. A uterus is present in most true hermaphrodites, but it is generally incompletely developed.

Management of true hermaphrodites is a complex problem. Many escape detection at birth and are firmly entrenched in their gender role by the time the diagnosis is established. In these cases treatment is aimed at maintaining and enhancing their sex of rearing. Because most of them have a male assignment, reconstruction is toward masculinization if the phallus is of adequate size, with repair of the hypospadias and removal of all contradictory internal organs. If true hermaphroditism is diagnosed during the newborn period, more choices are available and the sex of rearing may be assigned on the basis of functional considerations and the findings at exploratory laparotomy.[116]

If there is a well developed phallus and a testis that can be placed in the scrotum, the child may be raised as a male with staged reconstructive procedures planned to be completed by 4 years of age.[16,147] The general absence of spermatogenesis in the testicular tissue may be attributed to its frequent ectopic location or the lack of XY germ cells. A second X chromosome is incompatible with the successful differentiation of definitive spermatogonia from primordial germ cells.[76] It is important to recognize that there are no documented cases of male fertility in a true hermaphrodite.[104]

Raising a newborn true hermaphrodite as a female usually gives the best functional results. Removal of all inconsistent internal organs, including all testicular tissue should be done at the time of the exploratory laparotomy in children who will be reared as females. Clitoridectomy may also be indicated. In individuals with bilateral ovotestes, partial gonadectomy has been employed to remove the testicular tissue with the subsequent occurrence of spontaneous menarche.[138] It is not always possible to distinguish testicular from ovarian tissue grossly; therefore if a partial gonadectomy is performed, the patient is followed by periodic hCG stimulation testing to check for residual testicular elements. Ovulation has been induced in true hermaphrodites using gonadotropin stimulation.[107] Pregnancies have been reported in true hermaphrodites raised as females; however, reproductive problems occurred in four of these cases.[102,148] It is of interest that all of the infants thus far reported have been male, and that all of the hermaphroditic mothers were 46,XX. It is hoped that with earlier recognition and treatment the prospects of fertility for both those reared as females and those raised as males will be improved.

The simultaneous occurrence of testicular and ovarian tissue in the same patient continues to intrigue investigators and is generally attributed to errors of synthesis, dissemination, or binding of H-Y antigen.[144] The striking laterality of gonadal elements in some and the polarization of testicular and ovarian tissue so characteristic of the ovotestis indicate a mosaicism of those factors that promote development of a testis versus an ovary from the gonadal anlage. Indeed, one report demonstrated that the cells cultured from the testicular portion of an ovotestis were H-Y antigen-positive, whereas those from the ovarian component were H-Y antigen-negative.[150] This finding implies that true hermaphroditism may be the result of H-Y⁺/H-Y⁻ mosaicism regardless of the karyotype. One would expect this situation to be the natural consequence of XX/XY chimerism or mosaicism, but most true hermaphrodites have an XX chromosome complement. Among several hypotheses to account for this finding is the possibility of reciprocal translocation of testicular determining genes from the Y to an X chromosome during paternal meiosis leading to an XX^Y offspring. Random lyonization could then account for the variable H-Y phenotype. Some propose that multiple H-Y genes are located on the Y chromosome,[127] and that when these genes are split by translocation of part of the Y to another chromosome the number of H-Y gene copies translocated may vary, with the result that a gene–dosage relation could determine the type of gonadal differentiation. It is still undetermined how a cell surface component, e.g., the H-Y antigen, which is thought to be released in a hormonal fashion, could be selectively excluded from a portion of the developing gonad.

MALE PSEUDOHERMAPHRODITISM

Male pseudohermaphroditism refers to the ambiguity of sexual differentiation in a patient who has testes as the only gonadal element. It is a heterogeneous group of disorders (Table 24-1) that includes the following: (1) persistent müllerian duct syndrome (hernia uteri inguinale), (2) defective testosterone synthesis (male andrenogenital syndrome); (3) androgen insensitivity syndrome (testicular feminization syndrome and its variants); (4) 5α-reductase deficiency (pseudovaginal perineoscrotal hypospadias); and (5) testicular dysgenesis. Male pseudohermaphroditism is frequently genetic in origin and may be associated with a variety of heritable defects. These conditions result from a greater variety of mechanisms and are less common disorders than female pseudohermaphroditism. The phenotypic aberrations that occur with this form of intersexuality result from decreasd production of MIF or androgenic hormones by the fetus, or from an inability to respond to these substances. The clinical phenotype is often not characteristic and may depend on the degree of the abnormality and the timing of its occurrence during fetal life. Proper gender assignment is sometimes difficult, for it may be impossible to predict what will occur during puberty. In the absence of a definitive diagnosis on genetic, endocrine, or biologic grounds, the major criterion for sex assignment rests on the degree of masculinization of the external genitalia that occurs in utero.

Persistent Müllerian Duct Syndrome (Hernia Uteri Inguinale)

Fewer than 100 cases have been reported in which persistent müllerian structures were found in an otherwise normal 46,XY phenotypic male.[11] The persistence of these structures is thought to result from an absence of MIF, production of a defective factor, or a lack of sensitivity to MIF by target organs.[83] MIF is probably not present in the postnatal or mature testis, and clinical testing for this factor is not available.[74] Although usually sporadic, several families have been reported with a pedigree consistent with either an autosomal recessive or an X-linked pattern of inheritance.[12] The typical presentation is that of a young man with an inguinal or scrotal hernia containing a uterus, fallopian tubes, and a cryptorchid testis (Fig. 24-7). Failure of descent of the contralateral testis may also occur. The testicular histology is appropriate for the patient's age and is initially normal[10]; however, subsequent changes may occur in these cryptorchid testes (see Ch. 21). The striking feature of cryptorchidism in the persistent müllerian duct syndrome suggests that MIF may play a role in the movement of the testes into the scrotum. In addition to müllerian derivatives, vasa deferentia are present bilaterally. The external genitalia are unambiguously male in appearance.

Sex assignment in patients with the persistent müllerian duct syndrome does not present a problem, as all of these patients are phenotypically male and are potentially fertile.[6] Removal of the cryptorchid testes

may be required, for replacement into the scrotum may be technically difficult, and gonadal germ cell tumors have been reported in a number of cases.[17,68,83,131] It is not yet clear whether the increased risk of gonadal neoplasia is the result of the factors that produce the defect in MIF synthesis or action or is secondary to the abnormal or absent testicular descent.

Defective Testosterone Synthesis (Male Adrenogenital Syndrome)

Adequate production of testosterone by the fetal testis is a prerequisite for normal masculinization of the internal and external genitalia. Five enzymes are essential for the synthesis of testosterone by the testicular Leydig cells (Fig. 24-8). Three of these enzymes (20,22-desmolase, 3β-hydroxysteroid dehydrogenase, and 17-hydroxylase) are also necessary for cortisol production; therefore deficiency of these enzymes would result in congenital adrenal hyperplasia as well as male pseudohermaphroditism. Defective synthesis of the other two enzymes (17,20-desmolase and 17-ketosteroid reductase) produce only inadequate virilization. Clinical examples of deficiencies of each of these enzymes have been observed in karyotypic males, as well as a case of multiple defects in steroid-biosynthetic enzymes occurring in a single patient.[108] These metabolic errors in testosterone biosynthesis are caused by autosomal or X-linked recessive mutations.[51]

Because male differentiation of the wolffian ducts requires high local concentrations of testosterone, there may be abnormal development of the wolffian derivatives. Low levels of DHT, a metabolite of testosterone, result in incomplete virilization of the external genitalia. Müllerian derivatives are absent, as there is normal production of MIF. The presence of a uterus and fallopian tubes in one patient with 17,20-desmolase deficiency remains unexplained.[49] The degree of masculinization of the external genitalia at birth and the degree of virilization that may occur at puberty depend on the severity of the enzyme deficiency and on the testosterone precursors that are produced. At birth, most patients are so phenotypically female that no consideration is given to a possible disorder of sexual differentiation. In these cases the diagnosis is not entertained until puberty when the

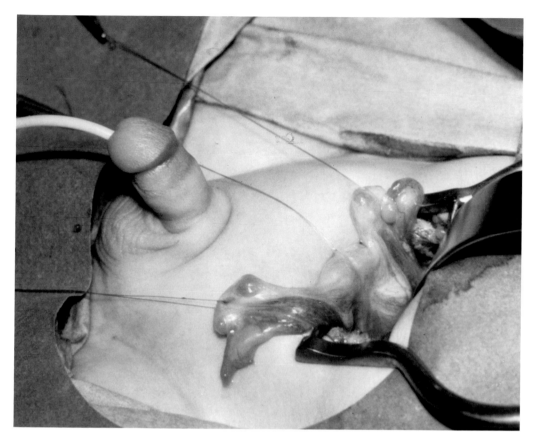

Fig. 24-7 Persistent müllerian duct syndrome. A uterus, fallopian tubes, and testes are evident. (Courtesy of Dr. Howard Snyder, Children's Hospital of Philadelphia.)

patient presents with amenorrhea or unexpected virilization. Individuals with enzyme defects that result in decreased mineralocorticoid or glucocorticoid secretion may present with adrenal insufficiency.

These disorders are diagnosed by demonstrating a low plasma testosterone level and an elevation of the steroid precursors on the proximal side of the enzyme block, a result of increased trophic hormone stimulation (Table 24-2). Plasma testosterone levels are normal in some patients with partial enzyme defects. Because testosterone levels are normally low in newborns, testosterone measurements during infancy may not be diagnostic. The hCG stimulation test may be used to assess testosterone synthesis before puberty. Depending on the degree of enzymatic deficiency, hCG stimulation would result in either no change or only a minimal increase in testosterone levels and penile size.[49] Theoretically, it might be possible to diagnose these metabolic errors prenatally based on concentrations of cortisol, testosterone, and appropriate precursors or abnormal metabolites in amniotic fluid.[99] Enzyme defects involving testosterone biosynthesis are characterized by the presence of Leydig cell hyperplasia secondary to increased gonadotropin production. Gonadal tumors observed in these patients have been variously interpreted as interstitial cell tumors, adrenal cortical rests, or hyperplastic cells from the testicular hilus.[41,71,100,112] There is evidence that these tumors may arise from pluripotential cells derived from the urogenital ridge from which both the adrenal cortex and testes develop.[44] Although there is no mention of carcinoma in the cases reported so far, the number of affected XY individuals is too small to ascertain the risk of malignancy in these patients.[78] Such individuals usually respond well to testosterone treatment and are raised as males when pos-

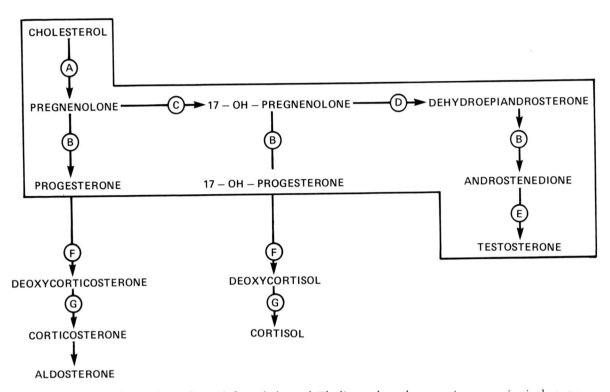

Fig. 24-8 Steps in biosynthesis of steroids from cholesterol. The line encloses those reactions occurring in the testes. The adrenal glands are capable of carrying out all these steps except the synthesis of testosterone from androstenedione. The adrenals also possess additional enzymes (F, G) that are required for the synthesis of glucocorticoids and mineralocorticoids. A, 20, 22-desmolase; B, 3β-hydroxysteroid dehydrogenase; C, 17-hydroxylase; D, 17, 20-desmolase; E, 17-ketosteroid reductase; F, 21-hydroxylase; G, 11β-hydroxylase. (Modified from Migeon,[86] with permission.)

Table 24-2 Abnormalities of Testosterone Biosynthesis

Deficient Enzyme	Progesterone	Cortisol	Aldosterone	Testosterone	Salient Features
20,22-Desmolase	↓	↓	↓	↓	Usually lethal in infancy Salt loss
3β-Hydroxysteroid dehydrogenase	↓	↓	↓	(DHEA ↑) ↓	Usually lethal in infancy Salt loss
17-Hydroxylase	↑	↓	(DOC ↑) ↓	↓	Hypertension Hyperkalemic alkalosis
17,20-Desmolase	N	N	N	↓	Remain infantile at puberty
17-Ketosteroid reductase	N	N	N	↓ (Δ⁴-dione ↑)	Virilization at puberty

DHEA, dehydroepiandrosterone; DOC, deoxycorticosterone; Δ^4-dione, androstenedione; ↓, decreased secretion; ↑, increased secretion; N, normal secretion. (Modified from Migeon,[86] with permission.)

sible.[49] When a patient is firmly established in a female gender role or when the genitalia are poorly virilized, it may be best to rear the child as a female.

20,22-DESMOLASE DEFICIENCY

A deficiency of 20,22-desmolase blocks the first step in steroidogenesis by which cholesterol is converted to pregnenolone, resulting in an inability to synthesize any of the biologically active steroids (Fig. 24-8). This disorder is termed congenital lipoid hyperplasia because of the accumulation of lipoid material within cells of the adrenal cortex and gonads. A similar disorder can be produced by administration of aminoglutethimide to the mother.[119] Affected XY individuals usually have completely female-appearing external genitalia, undescended testes, and normal regression of the müllerian ducts. The presence of wolffian-derived internal ducts in male survivors indicates some degree of testosterone synthesis. Shortly after birth the patients develop a severe electrolyte imbalance often resulting in death. This defect is probably incompatible with life unless appropriate glucocorticoid and mineralocorticoid replacement therapy is given. Urinary 17-ketosteroid and 17-hydroxycorticoid levels are low or undetectable (Table 24-2). The absence of 20-hydroxycholesterol and 20,22-dihydroxycholesterol after ACTH administration may be diagnostic.[119]

3β-HYDROXYSTEROID DEHYDROGENASE DEFICIENCY

Only a few patients with 3β-hydroxysteroid dehydrogenase (3β-HSD) deficiency have been described. Deficiency of 3β-HSD affects the production of all three classes of steroids. Catastrophic adrenal crisis may occur shortly after birth. A number of patients with partial deficiency of this enzyme have survived. Even when the defect is severe, some degree of masculinization of the external genitalia occurs, probably because of production of the weak androgen dehydroepiandrosterone. The typical external genitalia include a small phallus, second or third degree hypospadias, and partial fusion of the labioscrotal folds.[133] Gynecomastia is characteristic in those who survive until puberty. Exposure of the XY fetus to certain estrogens and synthetic progestins that share the ability to inhibit 3β-HSD may produce a similar syn-

drome.[119] 3β-HSD deficiency is diagnosed by finding increased urinary levels of Δ^5-steroids, e.g., pregnenolone and dehydroepiandrosterone, which occur in combination with pregnenetriol, a metabolite of 17-hydroxypregnenolone, and pregnenediol, a metabolite of pregnenolone.[87] 17-Ketosteroid excretion is increased.[69] Treatment with cortisol, glucose and saline, and mineralocorticoids may be required if these subjects are to survive the neonatal period.[97]

17-HYDROXYLASE DEFICIENCY

17-Hydroxylase (17-HD) deficiency is a rare congenital condition affecting both the adrenal glands and the gonads. First reported in XY individuals in 1970,[98] only 11 such cases are now described in the literature.[2] A defect in this enzyme blocks the synthesis of both sex hormones and cortisol (Fig. 24-8). Diminished cortisol levels lead to increased secretion of ACTH, which stimulates an overproduction of corticosterone and deoxycorticosterone, resulting in sodium and water retention, hypokalemic alkalosis, and hypertension.[136] Affected individuals typically present with primary amenorrhea and failure to develop secondary sex characteristics. The 46,XY patients with a complete deficiency of 17-HD are tall, often with eunuchoid body proportions, and have infantile feminized external genitalia with a blind-ending vagina.[78] If the deficiency is partial, the external genitalia are ambiguous.[86] The testes are usually situated in the inguinal canal and may be associated with inguinal hernias. Histologic examination reveals infantile testicular tissue with Leydig cell hyperplasia.[146] The seminiferous tubules contain only Sertoli cells and spermatogonia and may show thickened basement membranes.[91] Wolffian derivatives may be rudimentary, but müllerian structures are absent.

Laboratory studies demonstrate low to absent levels of plasma and urinary cortisol with resulting low levels of urinary 17-hydroxysteroids of 17-ketogenic steroids. Urinary 17-ketosteroids are also reduced. All patients have low values of both serum androgens and estrogens, whereas serum gonadotropins are elevated. The levels of steroid hormones not dependent on 17-hydroxy precursors such as progesterone, deoxycorticosterone, and corticosterone are increased. It is important to establish the diagnosis of 17-HD because impaired cortisol synthesis can be exacerbated by stress. Treatment with cortisol reduces the excess production of mineralocorticoid, thereby correcting the electrolyte disturbance and hypertension.[97]

17,20-DESMOLASE DEFICIENCY

In humans 17,20-desmolase deficiency is a rare cause of male pseudohermaphroditism. There are only a few reported cases of affected 46,XY individuals.[42,67] The patients thus far reported have a partial enzyme defect and ambiguous genitalia. A complete deficiency of this enzyme could be expected to give rise to a phenotypic female with features similar to those of XY subjects with 17-hydroxylase deficiency but without hypertension or electrolyte abnormalities.[78] Defective 17,20-desmolase activity is diagnosed based on the coexistence of increased levels of pregnenolone, 17-hydroxypregnenolone, progesterone and 17-hydroxyprogesterone, and low levels of dehydroepiandrosterone and androstenedione[24] (Fig. 24-8). 17,20-Desmolase is normally present in both testes and adrenals, and results of dynamic studies indicate that the enzyme defect affects both glands.[42]

17-KETOSTEROID REDUCTASE DEFICIENCY

The last enzyme in testosterone synthesis is 17-ketosteroid reductase (17-KR), which converts the relatively inactive androgen androstenedione to testosterone. Apparently, 17-KR exists in two forms, one of which is predominantly gonadal and the other widely distributed in peripheral tissues.[69] Data suggest that the two forms of the enzyme are under separate genetic control. There are reports of 10 cases of gonadal 17-KR deficiency, all of whom have been XY individuals.[78]

At birth, affected subjects may have only slightly masculinized external genitalia with the physical characteristics of pseudovaginal perineoscrotal hypospadias, and they are often raised as female.[85] Until puberty the phenotype resembles that of XY patients with 17-hydroxylase deficiency, and the patient may present with primary amenorrhea. Occasional patients show masculinization of the external genitalia at birth. Virilization, with clitoral enlargement and extensive hair growth on the face and body, occurs at puberty in patients with 17-KR deficiency.[25] They may also develop gynecomastia. The most characteristic biochemical finding is a marked increase in the

plasma androstenedione concentration[39] (Table 24-2). Plasma and urinary estrogen levels may be increased because of peripheral conversion from androgens. Pubertal masculinization is predominantly attributed to the conversion of high levels of androstenedione to testosterone by the peripheral form of 17-KR.[69] Testosterone levels in postpubertal patients range from low to low normal in male adults. Affected individuals thus far reported have been azoospermic and infertile. The testes have Leydig cell hyperplasia and hyalinized seminiferous tubules with few or absent spermatogonia.

Androgen Insensitivity Syndromes

The androgen insensitivity syndromes are a heterogeneous group of disorders having in common the essential feature of failure of androgen-dependent target cells to respond to circulating testosterone (Table 24-3). Studies of fibroblasts cultured from the genital skin of these patients have revealed that the underlying defects involve quantitative or qualitative changes in the intracellular high-affinity androgen receptors or possibly a postreceptor abnormality. For androgens to effect a cellular response, testosterone and its metabolite dihydrotestosterone must interact with cellular receptors, thereby initiating a series of postreceptor phases of androgen action (Fig. 24-2). Defects in the molecular mechanism of action of these androgens would result in abnormalities of external genital and wolffian duct differentiation, with the severity of the developmental aberrations dependent on the degree of the defect. Exogenous testosterone and hCG have little or no masculinizing effect on these patients.[49,54] Because MIF production by the fetal testis is unaffected, normal müllerian regression occurs except in rare cases.[137] Most of the disorders of androgen insensitivity result from single gene mutations.[51] The pedigrees of affected families indicate that inheritance is due to either an X-linked recessive or a male-limited autosomal dominant gene.[32]

The classic type of androgen insensitivity is the testicular feminization syndrome, a term first used by Morris in 1953.[92] This syndrome is a common cause of male pseudohermaphroditism. Patients with the *complete form of testicular feminization (CTF)* are characterized by a 46,XY karyotype and unequivocal female external genitalia at birth. A rare case of CTF

Table 24-3 Androgen Insensitivity Syndromes

Defect	Disorder	Phenotype	External Genitalia	Wolffian Ducts
Receptor disorders				
Receptor negative	CTF	Female	Female	Absent
Unstable receptor	CTF	Female	Female	Absent
Unstable receptor	ITF	Female	Ambiguous	Male
Receptor deficiency	RS	Male	IMD	Variable
Receptor-positive				
Uncertain	MP	Variable	Female to IMD	Variable

CTF, complete testicular feminization; ITF, incomplete testicular feminization; RS, Reifenstein syndrome; MP, male pseudohermaphroditism; IMD, incomplete male development. (Modified from Griffin,[51] with permission.)

with a 47,XXY chromosome complement has been described.[45] At puberty there is normal female breast development, and the general habitus and distribution of body fat are feminine. Virilization does not occur at puberty, and the clitoris is normal. Pubic and axillary hair is sparse or absent (Fig. 24-9). The internal genitalia are poorly formed, consisting of a shallow, blind-ending vagina and either absent wolffian derivatives or rudimentary cordlike structures that lead to testes located intraabdominally or in the inguinolabial area. The clinical presentation may occur prepubertally when a girl is found to have a hernia containing a cryptorchid testis. The remaining cases usually present later in life because of primary amenorrhea. Use of in vitro assays in fibroblasts cultured from genital skin have demonstrated that at least two receptor abnormalities can lead to the CTF syndrome: (1) an absence of androgen binding; and (2) unstable, thermolabile receptors with apparently one-half normal levels of binding[51] (Table 24-3). In those cases totally lacking androgen binding, it is unclear whether the receptor is truly absent or is structurally abnormal with respect to its ability to bind androgens.[86] Unstable, thermolabile receptors in other patients with CTF might be attributed to alterations in the tertiary structure of the mutant receptor proteins. CTF therefore appears to be the result of a mutation involving either the structural gene for the receptor or a regulatory gene that controls its activity.

Ten to fifteen percent of patients have a partial or *incomplete form of testicular feminization (ITF)*. Genital fibroblast studies in cases of ITF reveal the presence of unstable, heat-labile androgen receptors

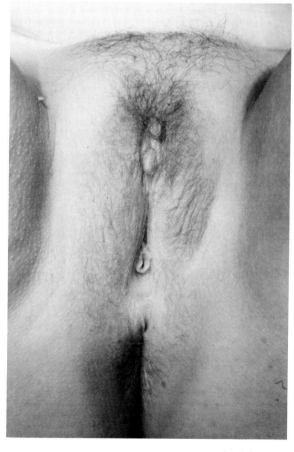

Fig. 24-9 Testicular feminization syndrome. The external genitalia are unequivocally female, but the pubic hair is sparse. (Courtesy of Dr. Howard Snyder, Children's Hospital of Philadelphia.)

with reduced binding capacity.[51] In most of the patients the family history is uninformative. In contrast to CTF, these individuals have ambiguity of the external genitalia, and some degree of masculinization as well as feminization occurs at puberty. Although the habitus and general appearance are feminine, there there is partial fusion of the labioscrotal folds and variable cliteromegaly. Gynecomastia is common at puberty but tends to be less marked than in those with CTF.[11] Wolffian duct derivatives are present in patients with ITF, but müllerian ductal structures are absent; the most common presentation is with primary amenorrhea. The vagina is short and blind-ending.

The incomplete and complete forms of testicular feminization syndrome do not occur in the same family and thus are distinct entities.[133] Partial virilization of the external genitalia and the presence of wolffian derivatives distinguish the incomplete from the complete form of the disorder.

The hormone profile in subjects with both forms of testicular feminization is in keeping with a defect occurring at the level of the androgen receptor. At puberty, plasma testosterone levels and rates of production by the testes are higher than normal,[51] the result of increased luteinizing hormone (LH) stimulation due to defective negative feedback regulation caused by resistance to the action of androgens at the hypothalamic-pituitary level. Coexisting high levels of testosterone and LH at puberty suggest the diagnosis of testicular feminization. In normal newborns and infants with testicular feminization, the serum concentrations of testosterone and LH are low; therefore the diagnosis of androgen insensitivity can be made only rarely during this period based on the serum levels of these hormones.[49,73] The existence of testicular feminization in a newborn can be surmised when stimulation with LH or hCG results in a significant rise in serum testosterone levels but no external genital masculinization. The diagnosis is confirmed by assaying genital skin fibroblasts for androgen receptors. These syndromes might be amenable to prenatal diagnosis based on receptor abnormalities in cultured amniocytes.[39]

The pubertal feminization seen in these individuals is explained by elevated estrogens, of both testicular and peripheral origin, which are unopposed by androgens.[69] In cases in which castration has been carried out before puberty, breast development has not occurred.[54] If testicular feminization is diagnosed

during infancy or childhood, the parents mustbe informed that although the patient is phenotypically female she will inevitably be amenorrheic and sterile. These individuals have normal female libidos, marry, and have normal sex lives.

It is important to differentiate CTF from ITF, for the management of the two disorders is different. In patients with CTF it is advisable to remove the testes because there is a 3.5 percent chance of testicular tumor development, usually seminoma, by 25 years of age and a 33 percent risk by the age of 50 years.[79,80] It is generally agreed that the gonads should not be removed until after puberty so that secondary female sex characteristics can develop. There appears to be little risk of malignancy in the testes prior to puberty. Because subjects with ITF virilize at puberty, gonadectomy should be performed in these patients prior to this age. The risk of gonadal tumor formation in ITF has not yet been established, but carcinoma in situ has been reported.[94,130] After orchidectomy in those with either form of testicular feminization, estrogen-replacement therapy should be instituted at the time of puberty. If the vaginal depth is inadequate, techniques may be used to increase its depth.

During the prepubertal period the testes are of normal size and histologically resemble testes from normal prepubertal males. In adults with CTF the seminiferous tubules are small and contain mostly Sertoli cells with few spermatogonia.[12] Spermatogenesis is lacking, and the Leydig cells are typically hyperplastic. In those with ITF, partial maturation of the germinal elements may occur.[85,94] In elderly patients, hyalinization and cystic areas may be noted.[70] Tumorlike masses of Sertoli and Leydig cells, perhaps best regarded as hamartomas,[93] and aggregates of tubules lined by Sertoli cells ("tubular adenomas") may impart a nodularity to the testes of patients with testicular feminization (Fig. 24-10). Except for their nodular appearance, postpubertally the gonads are similar to other cryptorchid testes. In addition, a testicular tumor resembling the sex cord tumor with annular tubules has been reported in a patient with androgen insensitivity.[114]

A variety of forms of intersexuality, originally termed incomplete male pseudohermaphroditism, type I, have been reclassified as disorders of androgen insensitivity. These disorders include the syndromes described by Lubs et al.,[75] Gilbert-Dreyfus et al.,[48] Reifenstein,[117] and Rosewater et al.[121] Lubs syndrome

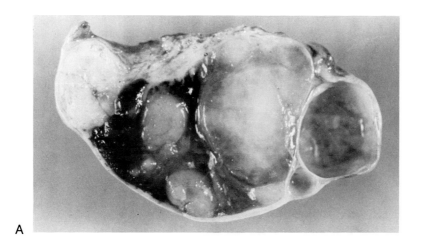

A

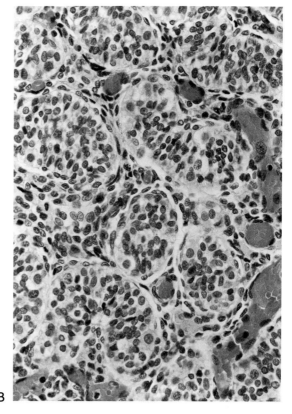

B

Fig. 24-10 Testicular feminization. **(A)** Large tan nodules extensively replace the testis. Focally intraoperative hemorrhage is apparent. **(B)** A tumorlike mass (right) is formed by tubules lined by Sertoli cells. Leydig cells can be seen between the tubules. **B**, ×250. (From Silverberg SG (ed): Principles and Practice of Surgical Pathology. J Wiley & Sons, New York, 1983.)

is characterized by a small phallus, bifid labioscrotal folds, and a single urogenital orifice. At puberty these children are eunuchoid. Patients with a small phallus, hypospadias, incomplete wolffian duct structures, and gynecomastia were described by Gilbert-Dreyfus et al. Phenotypic males with Reifenstein syndrome exhibit hypospadias, bifid scrotum, cryptorchidism, and gynecomastia. Gynecomastia and infertility are seen in those with Rosewater's syndrome. Perhaps the mildest disorder seen in this group are individuals who are phenotypically normal males and present with infertility[3,123] (see Ch. 23). Each of these disorders was originally held to be a distinct entity, but a number of pedigrees have been reported in which members of the same family exhibited variable appearances that incorporated the syndromes described above. As a group, these individuals have high plasma testosterone, estrogen, and LH levels and a partial androgen receptor deficiency without thermolability[51] (Table 24-3). The apparent X linkage and the common underlying receptor defect suggests that all of the syndromes of male pseudohermaphroditism, type I, represent variable manifestations of a single mutation and can be termed "Reifenstein syndrome."[51] Because different patients in the same family with "Reifenstein's syndrome" can manifest a spectrum of abnormalities, there must be other, as yet unidentified factors that modify hormone action in vivo. Psychological development in most cases is male, and treatment is directed at correcting the hypospadias and cryptorchidism. Disfiguring gynecomastia may require surgical intervention. Regardless of the phenotypic appearance, none of the patients described so far has been fertile.[119] Although azoospermia is the most common finding, sperms have been detected in the ejaculate of four patients.[140] In addition to defective spermatogenesis secondary to the receptor deficiency, some subjects also have an absence or hypoplasia of the wolffian derivatives, which may contribute to the infertility. The testes are small and on biopsy reveal normal Leydig cells and either germinal epithelial maturation arrest or scanty but normal spermatogenesis.[51,140]

A new category of androgen insensitivity has been identified that does not appear to involve androgen receptor deficiency. Although the first reported patients had a CTF phenotype, subsequent patients have had a range of abnormalities including ITF and an appearance similar to those with the Reifenstein syndrome.[51] These individuals are 46,XY and are clinically resistant to the actions of endogenous or exogenous androgens; yet standard fibroblast studies reveal normal amounts of androgen receptor and normal translocation of the hormone–receptor complex to the nucleus. Plasma testosterone and LH levels are increased or fall in the high normal range. The nature of the underlying defect in these "receptor-positive" cases is uncertain. It may involve a subtle qualitative receptor abnormality[110] or a defect in one of the postreceptor steps of androgen action. The management of these patients depends on the phenotype. Although most are reared as females and are castrated at puberty to prevent virilization, those with a "Reifenstein syndrome" appearance may be raised as males.

5α-Reductase Deficiency

The enzyme 5α-reductase is necessary for conversion of testosterone to DHT, which is required for virilization of the external genitalia in utero. Intersexuality due to a deficiency of this enzyme has in the past been referred to as *familial incomplete male pseudohermaphroditism, type II,* and *pseudovaginal perineoscrotal hypospadias.* The phenotype of pseudovaginal perineoscrotal hypospadias has also been associated with other disorders of sexual development.[69,85] 5α-Reductase deficiency was first reported in a number of families from the Dominican Republic,[59] and pedigree studies have revealed an autosomal recessive pattern of inheritance. At birth these 46,XY male pseudohermaphrodites have a female phenotype with a clitoruslike phallus, bifid scrotum, and a urogenital sinus, generally resulting in a female gender assignment[60] (Fig. 24-11). Bilateral testes, which are usually present in the inguinal canals or labioscrotal folds, may be palpable. The wolffian duct derivatives are

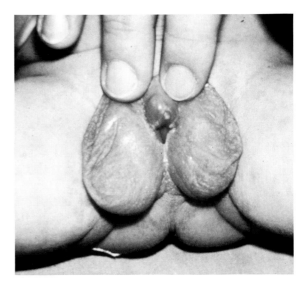

Fig. 24-11 Deficiency of 5α-reductase. A urogenital sinus is present beneath the clitoris-like phallus. The scrotum is bifid. (Courtesy of Dr. William Cromie, Albany Medical Center Hospital, Albany, NY.)

normal, as their differentiation depends on testosterone rather than DHT, but they empty into a blind-ending vagina. Müllerian inhibition is complete.

At puberty these individuals virilize and demonstrate marked phallic enlargement, deepening of the voice, increased muscle mass, and testicular descent. These patients, when raised as females, not only masculinize at puberty but frequently change their self-identification to male. Gynecomastia does not occur. It is of interest that certain male secondary sex characteristics, e.g., facial and body hair growth, acne, prostatic enlargement, and hairline recession, are not manifested. It therefore appears that some of the events of normal male masculinization at puberty are mediated by testosterone, whereas others are dependent on DHT. Affected individuals have erections and ejaculations, which also appear to be mediated by testosterone. Why the external genitalia of patients with 5α-reductase deficiency virilize at puberty but not during organogenesis remains unresolved. It may be the direct result of the high levels of testosterone that are normally present at puberty, or it may be due to conversion of a portion of the abundant testosterone to DHT by the action of the residual 5α-reductase demonstrable in all patients.[51]

The laboratory diagnosis of 5α-reductase deficiency can be made in adults on the basis of an increased plasma testosterone/DHT ratio, but in prepubertal patients these measurements must be preceded by hCG stimulation.[58,61] The ratio of 5α- and 5β-steroids, mainly androsterone and etiocholanolone, respectively, may provide a more sensitive test.[39] In normal individuals testosterone metabolism by the liver yields approximately equal amounts of 5α and 5β derivatives, whereas persons with a 5α-reductase deficiency have a markedly decreased 5α/5β ratio. Intermediate values have been observed in persons heterozygous for this enzyme deficiency, but they are clinically normal.[51,86] Abnormally low levels of 5α-reduced steroids are also seen in the urine of patients with acute intermediate porphyria.[9] The diagnosis can also be established by demonstrating decreased in vivo conversion of radiolabeled testosterone to DHT, diminished 5α-reductase activity in tissue biopsies, or deficient or abnormal enzyme activity in fibroblasts cultured from the genital skin.[61] Fibroblast studies have shown that the 5α-reductase enzyme is profoundly deficient in some families, is formed at a normal rate but with abnormal kinetic properties in

others, and is both deficient and kinetically abnormal in still others. No patient has a total absence of the enzyme. LH levels may be increased, suggesting a role for DHT in the negative feedback control of this gonadotropin.[81]

In persons raised as males and who have assumed a male gender, appropriate reconstructive genital surgery is performed along with repair of any coexisting cryptorchidism. In individuals reared as females and diagnosed before puberty, gonadectomy is performed to prevent disfiguring masculinization. The testes of these patients reveal arrest of spermatogenesis at the spermatid stage, with or without Leydig cell hyperplasia or thickening of the tunicas propria or basement membrane.[72,103] Large Reinke crystals may be seen in the Leydig cells. The serum follicle-stimulating hormone (FSH) concentration may be elevated, reflecting the depressed spermatogenesis seen in the testes. Complete spermatogenesis has been observed in some cases, but successful male fertility has not been reported.[86] Although an increased risk of malignancy might be expected in the frequently cryptorchid testes of these patients, gonadal neoplasms have not yet been reported for this entity.[12]

Testicular Dysgenesis

Broadly speaking, testicular dysgenesis refers to a wide spectrum of abnormal testicular development ranging from markedly hypoplastic gonads barely recognizable as testes to relatively minor abnormalities in well differentiated testes in patients with intersexuality. The internal and external genital abnormalities depend on the severity of the derangement of testicular development and the time of its occurrence during fetal life. Although the genitalia are ambiguous, there is a tendency toward a male phenotype. In addition to external genital ambiguity due to a deficiency of androgen production, patients may also have defective müllerian inhibition. These individuals have bilateral, frequently cryptorchid testes, and most have a 46,XY karyotype. A small number of cases with X0/XY mosaicism have been reported.[82] According to Jirasek,[62] who restricts this term to patients who also show failure of müllerian regression, typical dysgenetic testes are hypoplastic with an underdeveloped tunica albuginea, seminiferous tubule degeneration, peritubular hyalinization, and varying numbers of spermatogonia (Fig. 24-12). Regardless of

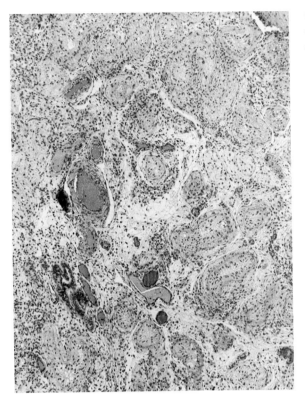

Fig. 24-12 Testicular dysgenesis. A 4-mm testis was removed from a patient with ambiguous genitalia. Scattered hyalinized tubules are present in the hypoplastic gonad. ×225.

the initial histologic appearance, dysgenetic testes tend to undergo further degeneration after puberty.[5] Dysgenetic testes, which may be closely related to streak gonads, are removed because of reports of gonadal neoplasms, including germ cell tumors and gonadoblastomas, in 15 percent of cases.[33,57,62,126]

Testicular dysgenesis comprises a heterogeneous group of disorders, the etiology of which has yet to be elucidated in most cases. One might include in this category those patients who have a selective absence or marked diminution of Leydig cells.[14,20,125] These individuals have cryptorchid testes and ambiguous, predominantly female-appearing external genitalia. Typically raised as females, they may present with primary amenorrhea and lack of breast development. A testicular biopsy is diagnostic, as it reveals a complete absence of Leydig cells even after intensive hCG stimulation. The seminiferous tubules, which may

undergo hyalinization after puberty, contain normal-appearing Sertoli cells and occasional immature germ cells. A loose myxoid interstitium may separate the tubules. This disorder is characterized by low testosterone levels that are unaffected by hCG stimulation or castration. LH concentrations are increased. It is essential in these cases to eliminate a primary deficiency of the enzymes responsible for testosterone biosynthesis. Leydig cell agenesis or hypoplasia may theoretically be due to an absence or decreased number of Leydig precursor cells or, alternatively, to an abnormality of hCG–LH receptors on these cells. It is of note that these patients have wolffian duct derivatives indicating some degree of androgen stimulation in utero.

The familial male pseudohermaphroditism syndrome described by Meyer et al.[85] and Keenan[69] may be a variant of testicular dysgenesis. These authors reported two families in which XY individuals were incompletely masculinized at birth but virilized markedly at puberty. Fibroblast studies indicated normal 5α-reductase and androgen receptor activity. Testicular biopsies showed a peculiar mosaic pattern with large areas of tubules containing only Sertoli cells adjacent to areas with active spermatogenesis. The gonadal histology suggests a primary testicular defect, although other etiologies cannot be excluded.

Finally, the group of disorders now classified under the term testicular regression syndrome[28,36] might be viewed as extreme examples of testicular dysgenesis. This syndrome includes patients previously categorized as having true agonadism,[26] gonadal agenesis,[8] embryonic testicular dysgenesis,[65] early fetal testicular dysgenesis,[84] rudimentary testes, and bilateral anorchia.[133] Although these disorders are usually sporadic, familial cases have been reported,[26] and more than one phenotypic expression has been described in members of the same family.[65] At laparotomy, no gonadal structures are identified in these patients, yet they exhibit varying degrees of external genital masculinization and/or müllerian duct regression, indicating that testes must have been present and functioning in part during intrauterine development. The serum concentration of testosterone is low and does not respond to hCG.[8] The clinical manifestations are the consequence of loss of testicular function at different times during embryonic or fetal sexual differentiation. Patients with bilateral anorchia, which is the result of an insult to testicular development occurring after 20 weeks' gestation, do not present with intersexuality, for the male phenotype is completed prior to the failure of testicular function (see Ch. 21). The reason for the absence of the gonads in these disorders is unclear. Proposed mechanisms include torsion or other trauma, genetic defects, teratogens, and defective anlage or connective tissue. In two cases studied thus far, the H-Y antigen was positive.[31,124]

FEMALE PSEUDOHERMAPHRODITISM

Female pseudohermaphroditism is characterized by an XX karyotype, bilateral ovaries, normal müllerian structures, absence of wolffian derivatives, and a wide range of ambiguity of the external genitalia. It results from exposure of the female fetus to excessive androgens in utero during critical periods of sexual differentiation. The degree of ambiguity depends on the amount and timing of the androgen exposure. Affected individuals typically have an enlarged clitoris, labial fusion, and a single common perineal orifice (Fig. 24-13). These patients should be raised as fe-

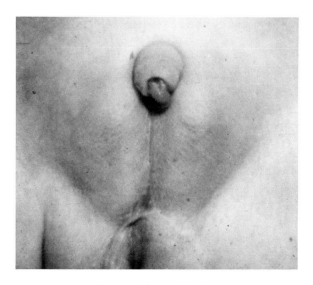

Fig. 24-13 Female pseudohermaphroditism. An enlarged clitoris, labial fusion, and a single perineal orifice are commonly seen in female subjects with congenital adrenal hyperplasia. (Courtesy of Dr. William Cromie, Albany Medical Center Hospital, Albany, NY.)

males but may require revision of the external genitalia, best accomplished before 2 years of age.[38] The excessive androgens may be of fetal origin or transferred to the fetus from the mother by way of the placenta. Endogenous fetal hyperandrogenemia is caused by congenital adrenal hyperplasia, the most common form of intersexuality.

Deficiencies of three enzymes, 21-hydroxylase, 11β-hydroxylase, and 3β-hydroxysteroid dehydrogenase may result in female pseudohermaphroditism. These disorders are inherited in an autosomal recessive fashion. The clinical picture arises from a deficiency of the enzyme products and from accumulation of precursor metabolites, i.e., androgens (Fig. 24-8). In addition to virilization, a deficiency of either 21-hydroxylase or 3β-hydroxysteroid dehydrogenase is commonly associated with salt wasting and addisonian crisis, whereas hypertension accompanies a deficiency of 11β-hydroxylase.

Exogenous etiologies of female pseudohermaphroditism include exposure of the fetus to maternal estrogens or progestins, which may block 3β-hydroxysteroid dehydrogenase activity, or exposure to maternal androgens arising from a hormone-producing tumor, luteoma of pregnancy, or therapeutic administration. For a more detailed discussion of female pseudohermaphroditism, the reader is referred to a number of excellent reviews.[5,87,97,119]

MIXED GONADAL DYSGENESIS

Mixed gonadal dysgenesis (MGD) has been reported to be the second most common cause of ambiguous genitalia in the neonate, ranking only after congenital adrenal hyperplasia.[38] The classic syndrome is characterized by the presence of a dysgenetic testis on one side and a contralateral streak gonad. Also included in this entity are individuals with: (1) a streak on one side and a gonadal tumor on the other; (2) absence of one gonad with a contralateral streak, testis, or gonadal tumor; (3) bilateral streaks with recognizable rudimentary testicular elements in at least one; and (4) bilateral testes capped with streak material.[4,115]

Mixed gonadal dysgenesis may be recognized in the neonate because of ambiguous, often asymmetric, external genitalia. Although there is extreme variability in the external genital phenotype, affected individuals tend to present with one of two types of external genital ambiguity.[118] In the first group the external genitalia are more masculine in appearance with a bifid scrotum or rugated, often asymmetric labioscrotal folds. The asymmetry is the result of varying degrees of descent of the unilateral testis. In this group a hypospadiac phallus is also present. The second form of external genitalia in these patients consists of normal, female-appearing labia with an enlarged clitoris (Fig. 24-14). This group of patients may go unrecognized at birth unless the clitoral enlargement is of sufficient magnitude to arouse suspicion. Sixty percent of such patients have been reared as females.[5] The development of heterosexual virilization at puberty, due to testicular androgenic function, may raise the question of intersex in these subjects. Approximately one-third of those with MGD who are less than 147 cm tall exhibit stigmata of Turner's syndrome.[18]

In the classic form of MGD, a unilateral testis is present and rarely exceeds 2 cm in maximal diameter. In most patients there is partial or complete descent, sometimes associated with an indirect inguinal hernia. The testis may vary from a rudimentary structure with primitive tubules to a normal-appearing prepubertal gonad containing spermatogonia.[5] Typically, there is disorganization of the superficial cortex and hilar zone.[118] Advanced spermatogenic maturation is lacking. Postpubertally, the seminiferous tubules may contain only Sertoli cells, and basement membrane thickening and hyalinization may occur.[18] The con-

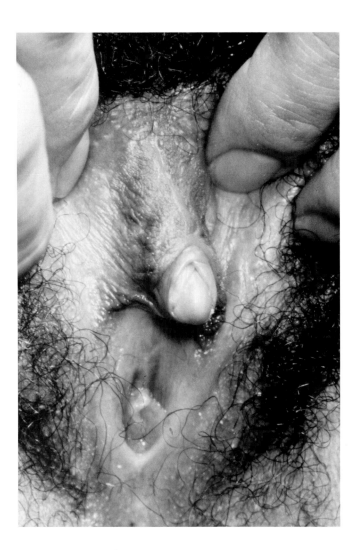

Fig. 24-14 Mixed gonadal dysgenesis. Clitoral hypertrophy is present, but the external genitalia are otherwise typically female. (Courtesy of Dr. Howard Snyder, Children's Hospital of Philadelphia.)

tralateral streak gonad in these subjects consists grossly of an elongated, firm, white or yellow fibrous band usually situated at the site normally occupied by an ovary. On occasion it is present in an indirect inguinal hernia as part of a hernia uteri inguinale. It is composed predominantly of fibrous connective tissue showing spindle-shaped cells often arranged in whorls (Fig. 24-15). The overall pattern resembles ovarian cortical stroma. In contrast to the gonadal streaks seen in Turner's syndrome, the streaks in patients with MGD may contain structures suggestive of primitive seminiferous tubules or clumps of granulosa cells. Mesonephric remnants may also be present. In addition, the streak may contain clusters of interstitial cells with abundant eosinophilic cytoplasm, representing either hilus or Leydig cells.[132]

The bilateral gonadal abnormalities are reflected in incomplete inhibition of müllerian development and incomplete support of wolffian duct differentiation. Although almost always abnormally formed, persistence of müllerian derivatives is a striking feature of MGD. The uterus is typically attenuated, fibrous, or without an apparent lumen.[118] Most of the patients have bilateral fallopian tubes despite the presence of one testis, indicating an abnormality in the production of MIF (Fig. 24-16). Differentiated wolffian duct structures are also commonly present and are more frequently found accompanying the testis. The presence or absence of a vas deferens or a fallopian tube does not correlate well with the histology of the testis. It is not clear whether the deficiencies in the development of the wolffian ducts and external genitalia are the result of deficient production of testosterone or of a delay in its secretion.

No specific laboratory tests are available to diagnose MGD. Testosterone and 17-ketosteroid levels tend to be in the normal range, whereas gonadotropins may be normal or slightly increased.[18] The diagnosis of this disorder is based on surgical exploration and gonadal histology. Once the diagnosis of MGD is established, it is advisable to rear these patients as females, as almost all have a uterus and vagina, and most are inadequately masculinized.[147] If the person is raised as a male, it must be recognized that he will be infertile, frequently of short stature, and often require multiple procedures for reconstruction of the external genitalia. Gonadoblastomas occur in about one-third of patients with MGD, and in 30 percent of cases the tumor becomes overgrown by a malignant germ cell

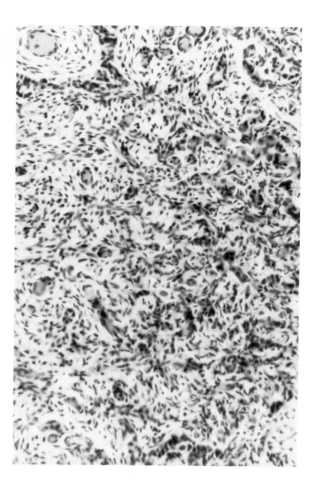

Fig. 24-15 Streak gonad. Irregular strands of gonadal stromal cells with hyperchromatic round nuclei are separated by a background stroma of paler spindle-shaped cells. ×284.

tumor, usually a dysgerminoma.[118] There is some evidence that patients with MGD who exhibit stigmata of Turner's syndrome may be at lower risk.[18,29] The small size of many of these tumors makes the clinical diagnosis difficult. It is of interest that the tumor generally involves the testis rather than the streak gonad, although bilateral neoplasms may also develop. Virilization or breast development in a patient with MGD, when occurring outside the normal period of puberty, usually indicates the presence of a gonadal tumor.[35] It has been postulated that persistent gonadotropin stimulation, dystrophic gonadal somatic cells, and the presence of germ cells in an unphysiologic environment may all be factors contributing to the high risk

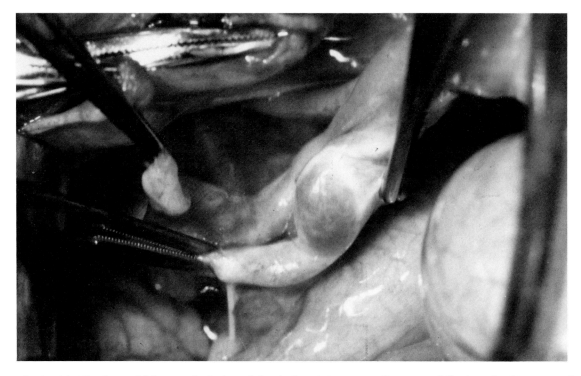

Fig. 24-16 Mixed gonadal dysgenesis. An intraabdominal testis is present adjacent to a fallopian tube. (Courtesy of Dr. Howard Snyder, Children's Hospital of Philadelphia.)

of gonadal neoplasia in these patients. Early prophylactic gonadectomy is recommended in persons with MGD. It also prevents pubertal masculinization. Exogenous female hormones can be administered at the age of puberty in those patients who are reared as females; but if the uterus is left in place, they must be carefully followed for the development of endometrial carcinoma to which they may be prone.[118] Five patients with MGD have been reported who also developed a Wilms' tumor, suggesting a defect in the urogenital ridge.[113]

Karyotypic analysis of MGD subjects typically reveals 45,X0/46,XY mosaicism, but it may be nondiagnostic (i.e., 46,XY; 45,X0) or demonstrate a multiple mosaic pattern.[35,74] Unless multiple tissues are examined, mosaicism may be overlooked. This disorder probably represents a cytogenetic sex chromosome anomaly that occurs early in embryogenesis. It is tempting to speculate that the asymmetric gonadal development in these individuals is the result of segregation of two distinct cell lines on separate sides of the body. This situation has been reported in one case of

MGD, with the testis typing as H-Y antigen-positive and the streak X-Y antigen-negative,[89] but it has not been observed in other patients.[35,118] The gonadal laterality in MGD therefore remains an enigma.

GONADAL DYSGENESIS

The term gonadal dysgenesis refers to intersex cases with bilateral streak gonads. Although this group of patients is heterogeneous, they share certain clinical features, including female but infantile external and internal genitalia, absence of differentiated mesonephric structures, primary amenorrhea, sparse pubic and axillary hair, usually undeveloped breasts, lack of secondary sexual characteristics, an atrophic vaginal smear, and castrate levels of gonadotropins.[15,56] The diagnosis is usually not suspected until puberty and can be established with certainty only by finding bilateral gonadal streaks at laparotomy (Fig. 24-17).

A variety of somatic anomalies occur in some patients with gonadal dysgenesis. The occurrence of so-

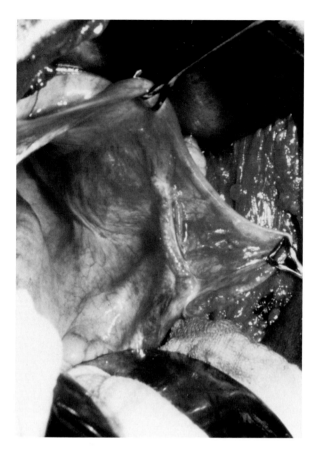

Fig. 24-17 Gonadal dysgenesis. A streak gonad can be seen along the broad ligament. The clamp is on the uterine fundus. (Courtesy of Dr. William Cromie, Albany Medical Center Hospital, Albany, NY.)

matic stigmata tend to depend on the karyotype; therefore these patients can be classified according to the chromosome complement (Table 24-1). Gonadal dysgenesis cases may be categorized into those with sex chromosome abnormalities (accounting for about two-thirds of the patients) and subjects who are chromosomally competent, including patients with 46,XX and those with 46,XY genotypes.[135] In general, these individuals should be reared as females, as they are phenotypically female and lack functioning testes.

Turner's syndrome is the classic form of gonadal dysgenesis. The clinical incidence of this sporadic disorder is estimated to be 1 per 2,700 women; however, most of the affected embryos are spontaneously aborted, and the incidence of this abnormality at con-

ception may approach 1 per 100.[11,12] Cytogenetic evaluation of these patients reveals a spectrum of chromosome abnormalities including 45,X0, mosaics with a 45,X0 cell line, and a variety of deletions and structural rearrangements of the X chromosome.[15,135] When identifying these patients as having Turner's syndrome, the exact chromosome complement should be specified for clarity.

Turner's syndrome is associated with a characteristic phenotype. These individuals are typically short in stature and have nuchal webbing, a low set hairline, a shield-shaped chest, and a variety of facial abnormalities. Cardiovascular and renal malformations constitute more serious somatic anomalies. Not every developmental abnormality is present in every Turner's patient.

After birth the gonads are merely fibrous streaks, devoid of germ cells, follicles, or their remnants. The streak gonads lack reproductive or hormonal function. Sections of 45,X0 gonads have revealed a normal population of germ cells before 3 months of gestation.[129] During subsequent intrauterine development, follicular formation is deficient and the oocytes degenerate, resulting in the formation of streak gonads. It appears, therefore, that two genetically intact X chromosomes are required for final development of the adult ovary.

The absence of germ cells in these gonads after birth may explain the rarity of gonadal neoplasms associated with this condition.[77] Although rare, gonadal tumors, including gonadoblastoma, hilus cell tumor, and dysgerminoma, have been reported in patients with this syndrome.[34,134] Gonadectomy is advisable in those whose karyotype includes a Y chromosome, as this group appears to be at increased risk for the development of a gonadal malignancy. Endometrial carcinoma has occurred in women with Turner's syndrome who underwent long-term estrogen treatment.[120]

There are two disorders associated with bilateral gonadal streaks and a normal karyotype. The first is *46,XX gonadal dysgenesis.* These patients usually present with primary amenorrhea, a eunuchoid habitus, and lack of secondary sexual development, but they do not have the short stature or other somatic anomalies of Turner's syndrome. Their streak gonads are identical to those seen in Turner's syndrome.[135] More than 130 such patients have been described.[4] At least 13 families with this disorder are known, with pedigrees suggesting an autosomal recessive mode of inheritance.[12] In several instances the parents were consanguineous. In certain families XX gonadal dysgenesis occurs with nerve deafness, and rare families are reported with microcephaly and arachnodactyly or other somatic abnormalities.[12,50] Some of these cases may be due to undetected mosaicism. This disorder appears to be etiologically heterogeneous. Familial aggregates suggest a gene mutation that prevents activation of the second X chromosome, leading to germ cell atresia, as occurs in Turner's syndrome. Sporadic cases may represent new mutations or, alternatively, environmental factors such as infections or autoimmunity.[4] The disorder does not appear to carry an increased risk for the development of gonadal tumors.[134]

The second form of chromosomally competent gonadal dysgenesis consists in patients with bilateral streak gonads and a 46,XY karyotype, or *46,XY gonadal dysgenesis*. Affected individuals are eunuchoid in appearance with an infantile female phenotype comparable to that seen in other varieties of gonadal dysgenesis. Failure of testicular development before the secretion of MIF and testosterone accounts for the genital findings. Signs of virilization may be present, e.g., deepening of the voice, hirsutism, temporal balding, and cliteromegaly.[88] There are varying degrees of breast development in these persons. Turner's syndrome stigmata are typically lacking but when present suggest an undetected mosaicism. Approximately 150 cases of XY gonadal dysgenesis, also known as Swyer's syndrome, have been reported.[19] Slightly less than one-third of these patients belong to families with more than one affected member. Although an X-linked recessive or male-limited autosomal dominant inheritance pattern has been found in several families, segregation analysis suggests the existence of a separate autosomal recessive form.[128] Further heterogeneity is indicated by the coexistence of campomelic dwarfism or renal parenchymal disease in a few patients. The streak gonads of subjects with XY gonadal dysgenesis may contain various abortive testicular or ovarian elements capable of steroid production.[88]

It is therefore possible that the reasons for the formation of streak gonads in these patients vary. Testicular constituents appear to form only if a Y-containing cell line is present or the H-Y antigen is produced.[109] Therefore the presence of testicular ele-

ments in the streak gonads of Turner's syndrome patients with an X0 karyotype indicates undetected mosaicism or expression of the H-Y antigen despite a pure X0 constitution. Studies have shown that some individuals with XY gonadal dysgenesis are H-Y antigen-negative, whereas others are positive.[106] Occasionally, this is due to variable degrees of deletion of the short arm of the Y chromosome. There is probably further heterogeneity within each of these subgroups, and patients with intermediate H-Y antigen titers have been found. H-Y antigen negativity could result from a mutation affecting either a structural or a regulatory gene involved in the production of this testicular organizer. In this situation the gonads would develop as ovaries but would degenerate into gonadal streaks due to the absence of a second X chromosome. It is of interest that the streaks in patients H-Y antigen-negative and who have XY gonadal dysgenesis do not exhibit testicular structures,[90] and that they do not show signs of virilization.[88] The formation of streak gonads in H-Y antigen-positive subjects suggests a disturbance in binding of the antigen to gonad-specific receptors, possibly resulting from a mutation that affects the receptor or the H-Y molecule. Alternative explanations include production of a functionally inert H-Y antigen, secretion of subthreshold amounts of this antigen, the presence of an inhibitor of the H-Y antigen, failure of germ cell migration, and a defective gonadal anlage. A teratogen or other environmental factor may be the etiology of nonfamilial cases and, by acting locally on the urogenital ridge, might also affect renal development.[46] The time of occurrence, duration, and severity of the defect might determine the presence or absence of virilization and partial testicular differentiation in H-Y antigen-positive individuals.

Patients with XY gonadal dysgenesis are predisposed to develop gonadal neoplasms, including germ cell tumors, gonadoblastoma, and Brenner tumor.[96,126,134] Virilization, breast development, and hypertension may result from endocrinologically active cells in a gonadoblastoma.[77,133] The reported incidence of gonadal tumors varies between 25 and 80 percent with this form of gonadal dysgenesis, with most of the tumors occurring after puberty.[88] The risk of gonadal neoplasia is not confined to patients with an XY karyotype but extends to any patient with gonadal dysgenesis and a cell line containing a Y chromosome. There is some evidence that H-Y antigen-positive subjects may be more prone to develop gonadal tumors than are those who are antigen-negative.[7,88,90,106]

Because H-Y negativity does not ensure freedom from gonadal neoplasia, prophylactic gonadectomy is recommended in all patients with gonadal dysgenesis and a Y chromosome.[77] The presence of testicular elements in the streak gonads of some of these individuals might increase their tumor risk. Prolonged gonadotropin stimulation could lead to unregulated proliferation of residual germ cells. It is also possible that the gene or genes determining XY gonadal dysgenesis also determine susceptibility to neoplastic transformation.

REFERENCES

1. Aaronson IA: True hermaphroditism: a review of 41 cases with observations on testicular histology and function. Br J Urol 57:775, 1985
2. Abad L, Parrilla JJ, Marcos J, et al: Male pseudohermaphroditism with 17α-hydroxylase deficiency. Br J Obstet Gynaecol 87:1162, 1980
3. Aiman J, Griffin JE, Gazak JM, et al: Androgen sensitivity as a cause of infertility in otherwise normal men. N Engl J Med 300:223, 1979
4. Aleem FA: Familial 46,XX gonadal dysgenesis. Fertil Steril 35:317, 1981
5. Allen TD: Disorders of sexual differentiation. Urology 7:1, 1976
6. Altwein JE: Surgical treatment of intersex. Monogr Paediatr 12:62, 1981
7. Amice V, Amice J, Bercovici JP, et al: Gonadal tumor and H-Y antigen in 46,XY pure gonadal dysgenesis. Cancer 57:1313, 1986
8. Aono T, Kurachi H, Kinugasa T, et al: Endocrine and androgen-receptor studies in a patient with XY gonadal agenesis. Obstet Gynecol 54:762, 1979
9. Bardin CW, Wright W: Androgen receptor deficiency: testicular feminization, its variants, and differential diagnosis. Ann Clin Res 12:236, 1980
10. Beheshti M, Churchill BM, Hardy BE, et al: Familial persistent müllerian duct syndrome. J Urol 131:968, 1984
11. Belman AB, Kaplan GW: Genitourinary problems in pediatrics. Major Probl Clin Pediatr 23:1, 1981
12. Bercu BB, Schulman JD: Genetics of abnormalities of sexual differentiation and of female reproductive failure. Obstet Gynecol Surv 35:1, 1980
13. Berkovitz GD, Lee PA, Brown TR, Migeon CJ: Etiologic evaluation of male pseudohermaphroditism in infancy and childhood. Am J Dis Child 138:755, 1984
14. Berthezene F, Forest MG, Grimaud JL, et al: Leydig-cell agenesis: a cause of male pseudohermaphroditism. N Engl J Med 295:969, 1976
15. Bosze P, Laszlo J: The streak gonad syndrome. Obstet Gynecol 54:544, 1979
16. Braren V, Warner JJ, Burr IM, et al: True hermaphroditism: a rational approach to diagnosis and treatment. Urology 15:569, 1980
17. Brooks CGD: Familial occurrence of persistent müllerian structures in otherwise normal males. Br Med J 1:771, 1973
18. Brosman SA: Mixed gonadal dysgenesis. J Urol 121:344, 1979
19. Brosnan PG, Lewandowski RC, Toguri AG, et al: A new familial syndrome of 46,XY gonadal dysgenesis with anomalies of ectodermal and mesodermal structures. J Pediatr 97:586, 1980
20. Brown DM, Markland C, Dehner LP: Leydig cell hypoplasia: a cause of male pseudohermaphroditism. J Clin Endocrinol Metab 46:1, 1978
21. Brown DR: Disorders of sexual differentiation. Minn Med 63:485, 1980
22. Buhler EM: A synopsis of the human Y-chromosome. Hum Genet 55:145, 1980
23. Byskov AG, Grinsted J: Feminizing effect of mesonephros on cultured differentiating mouse gonads and ducts. Science 212:817, 1981
24. Campo S, Moteagudo C, Nicolau G, et al: Testicular function in prepubertal male pseudohermaphroditism. Clin Endocrinol (Oxf) 14:11, 1981
25. Caufriez A: Male pseudohermaphroditism due to 17-ketoreductase deficiency: report of a case without gynecomastia and without vaginal pouch. Am J Obstet Gynecol 154:148, 1986
26. Cleary RE, Caras J, Rosenfield RL, Young PCM: Endocrine and metabolic studies in a patient with male pseudohermaphroditism and true agonadism. Am J Obstet Gynecol 128:862, 1977
27. Cook WA, Gashti E: Asymmetrical gonadal enlargement in adolescent true hermaphrodite with bilateral ovotestes. Urology 13:63, 1979
28. Coulam CB: Testicular regression syndrome. Obstet Gynecol 53:44, 1979
29. Davidoff F, Federman DD: Mixed gonadal dysgenesis. Pediatrics 52:725, 1973
30. Decker JP, Lerner HJ, Schwartz I: Breast carcinoma in a 46,XX true hermaphrodite. Cancer 49:1481, 1982
31. DeMarchi M, Campagnoli C, Chiringhello B, et al:

Gonadal agenesis in a phenotypically normal female with positive H-Y antigen. Hum Genet 56:417, 1981

32. De Sai M, Colberg C, Ranney B, Johnson C: Testicular feminization: patient report and brief review of the literature. SD J Med 33:29, 1980

33. Dinner M, Danish RK: Intersex problems: their clinical recognition, evaluation, and management. Surg Annu 11:403, 1979

34. Dominguez CJ, Greenblatt RB: Dysgerminoma of the ovary in a patient with Turner's syndrome. Am J Obstet Gynecol 83:674, 1962

35. Donahue PK, Crawford JD, Hendren WH: Mixed gonadal dysgenesis, pathogenesis, and management. J Pediatr Surg 14:287, 1979

36. Edman CD, Winters AJ, Porter JC: Embryonic testicular regression: a clinical spectrum of XY agonadal individuals. Obstet Gynecol 49:208, 1977

37. Eichwald EJ, Silmser CR: Untitled communication. Transplant Bull 2:148, 1955

38. Eickenberg HU, Mellin P, Walz KA, Ringert RH: Evaluation and management of the child with ambiguous genitalia. Monogr Paediatr 12:55, 1981

39. Fichman KR, Migeon BR, Migeon CJ: Genetic disorders of male sexual differentiation. Adv Hum Genet 10:333, 1980

40. Fitzgerald PH, Donald RA, Kirk RL: A true hermaphrodite dispermic chimera with 46,XX and 46,XY karyotypes. Clin Genet 15:89, 1979

41. Fore WW, Bledsoe T, Weber DM, et al: Cortisol production by testicular tumors in adrenogenital syndrome. Arch Intern Med 130:59, 1972

42. Forest MG, Lecornu M, De Peretti E: Familial male pseudohermaphroditism due to 17-20-desmolase deficiency. J Clin Endocrinol Metab 50:826, 1980

43. Fraccaro M, Tiepolo L, Zuffardi O, et al: Familial XX true hermaphroditism and the H-Y antigen. Hum Genet 48:45, 1979

44. Franco-Saenz R, Antonipillai I, Tan SY, et al: Cortisol production by testicular tumors in a patient with congenital adrenal hyperplasia (21-hydroxylase deficiency). J Clin Endocrinol Metab 53:85, 1981

45. Gerli M, Migliorini G, Bocchini V, et al: A case of complete testicular feminization and 47,XXY karyotype. J Med Genet 16:480, 1979

46. Gertner JM, Kauschansky A, Gresker DW, et al: XY gonadal dysgenesis associated with the congenital nephrotic syndrome. Obstet Gynecol, suppl., 55:66, 1980

47. Ghandchi A, Mozaffarin G, Abramzadeh R: Evaluation of hypothalamo-pituitary-gonadal axis in true hermaphroditism. Int J Fertil 24:120, 1979

48. Gilbert-Dreyfus S, Sebaoun CA, Belaisch J: Étude d'un cas familial d'androgyrodisme avec hypospadias grave, gynécomastie et hyperestrogénie. Ann Endocrinol (Paris) 18:93, 1957

49. Glassberg KI: Gender assignment in newborn male pseudohermaphrodites. Urol Clin North Am 7:409, 1980

50. Granat M, Reiter A, Dar H, Sharf M: 46,XX gonadal dysgenesis associated with congenital nerve deafness. Int J Gynaecol Obstet 17:231, 1979

51. Griffin JE, Wilson JD: The syndrome of androgen resistance. N Engl J Med 302:198, 1980

52. Grouse LD: The Y chromosome and primary sexual differentiation. JAMA 245:1953, 1981

53. Gupta AS, Dhruva AK, Kothari LK, Patni MK: A rare case of true hermaphroditism with an unusual presentation. Int Surg 64:83, 1979

54. Hammar B, Michowitz M, Solowiezczyk M: Testicular feminization syndrome. Am Surg 46:457, 1980

55. Haseltine FP, Genel M, Crawford JD, Breg WR: H-Y antigen negative patients with testicular tissue and 46,XY karyotype. Hum Genet 57:265, 1981

56. Hersh JH, Kable WT, Yen FF, et al: A case of familial XY gonadal dysgenesis. Fertil Steril 34:599, 1980

57. Hung W, Randolp JG, Chandra R, Belman AB: Gonadoblastoma in dysgenetic testis causing male pseudohermaphroditism in newborn. Urology 17:584, 1981

58. Imperato-McGinley J, Gautier T, Pichardo M, Shackleton C: The diagnosis of 5α-reductase deficiency in infancy. J Clin Endocrinol Metab 63:1313, 1986

59. Imperato-McGinley J, Guerrero L, Gautier T, et al: Steroid 5α-reductase deficiency in man: an inherited form of male pseudohermaphroditism. Science 186:1213, 1974

60. Imperato-McGinley J, Peterson RE, Gautier T, Sturla E: Male pseudohermaphroditism secondary to 5α-reductase deficiency. J Steroid Biochem 11:637, 1979

61. Imperato-McGinley J, Peterson RE, Leshin M, et al: Steroid 5α-reductase deficiency in a 65-year-old male pseudohermaphrodite: the natural history, ultrastructure of the testis, and evidence of inherited enzyme heterogeneity. J Clin Endocrinol Metab 50:15, 1980

62. Jirasek JE: Testicular dysgenesis syndromes. Birth Defects 7:159, 1971

63. Johnson JE, Byrd JR, McDonough PG: True hermaphroditism with peripheral blood and gonadal karyotyping. Obstet Gynecol 54:549, 1979

64. Jones HW, Ferguson-Smith MA, Heller RH: Pathologic and cytogenetic findings in true hermaphrodites, report of 6 cases and review of 23 cases from the literature. Obstet Gynecol 25:435, 1965

65. Josso N, Briard ML: Embryonic testicular regression syndrome: variable phenotypic expression in siblings. J Pediatr 97:200, 1980

66. Jost A: A new look at the mechanisms controlling sex differentiation in mammals. Johns Hopkins Med J 130:38, 1972

67. Kaufman FR, Costin G, Goebelsmann U, et al: Male pseudohermaphroditism due to 17,20-desmolase deficiency. J Clin Endocrinol Metab 57:32, 1983

68. Kazin E: Intra-abdominal seminomas in persistent müllerian duct syndrome. Urology 26:290, 1985

69. Keenan BS: Pseudovaginal perineoscrotal hypospadias: genetic heterogeneity. Urol Clin North Am 7:393, 1980

70. Khodr GS: An elderly patient with testicular feminization. Fertil Steril 32:708, 1979

71. Kirkland RT, Kirkland JL, Keenan BS, et al: Bilateral testicular tumors in congenital adrenal hyperplasia. J Clin Endocrinol Metab 44:369, 1977

72. Kuttenn F, Mowszowicz I, Wright F, et al: Male pseudohermaphroditism: a comparative study with the complete form of testicular feminization. J Clin Endocrinol Metab 49:861, 1979

73. Lee PA, Brown TR, La Torre HA: Diagnosis of the partial androgen insensitivity syndrome during infancy. JAMA 255:2207, 1986

74. Lippe BM: Ambiguous genitalia and pseudohermaphroditism. Pediatr Clin North Am 26:91, 1979

75. Lubs HA, Vilar O, Bergenstal DM: Familial male pseudohermaphroditism with labial testes, partial feminization, endocrine studies and genetic aspects. J Clin Endocrinol Metab 19:1110, 1959

76. Lyon MF: Mechanisms and evolutionary origins of variable X-chromosome activity in mammals. Proc R Soc Lond (Biol) 187:243, 1974

77. MacMahon RA, Cussen LJ, Walters WAW: Importance of early diagnosis and gonadectomy in 46,XY females. J Pediatr Surg 15:642, 1980

78. Madan K, Schoemaker J: XY females with enzyme deficiencies of steroid metabolism. Hum Genet 53:291, 1980

79. Manuel M, Katayama KP, Jones HW: The age of occurrence of gonadal tumors in intersex patients with a Y chromosome. Am J Obstet Gynecol 124:293, 1976

80. Marshall DG, Valentine GH: Testicular feminization syndrome (androgen insensitivity). J Pediatr Surg 16:465, 1981

81. Martini L, Celotti F, Serio M: 5α-Reductase deficiency in humans: support to the theory that 5α-reduction of testosterone is an essential step in the control of LH secretion. J Endocrinol Invest 2:463, 1979

82. McDonald M, Vinson RK, Diokno AC: Testicular tumor in male pseudohermaphrodite with X/XY chromosomal mosaicism. Urology 13:295, 1979

83. Melman A, Leiter E, Perez JM, et al: The influence of neonatal orchiopexy upon the testis in persistent müllerian duct syndrome. J Urol 125:856, 1981

84. Messinis IE, Nillius SJ: 46,XY male pseudohermaphroditism due to early foetal testicular dysgenesis. Acta Endocrinol (Copenh) 98:308, 1981

85. Meyer WJ, Keenan BS, De Lacerda L, et al: Familial male pseudohermaphroditism with normal Leydig cell function at puberty. J Clin Endocrinol Metab 46:593, 1978

86. Migeon CJ: Male pseudohermaphroditism. Ann Endocrinol (Paris) 41:311, 1980

87. Mininberg DT, Levine LS, New MI: Current concepts in congenital adrenal hyperplasia. Invest Urol 17:169, 1979

88. Moltz L, Schwartz U, Pickartz H, et al: XY gonadal dysgenesis: aberrant testicular differentiation in the presence of H-Y antigen. Obstet Gynecol 58:17, 1981

89. Moreira-Filho CA, Amaral AT, Otto PG, et al: H-Y antigen expression in a case of mixed gonadal dysgenesis. Hum Genet 57:366, 1981

90. Moreira-Filho CA, Toledo SPA, Bragnolli VR, et al: H-Y antigen in Swyer-syndrome and the genetics of XY gonadal dysgenesis. Hum Genet 53:51, 1979

91. Morimoto I, Maeda R, Izumi M, et al: An autopsy case of 17-α hydroxylase deficiency with malignant hypertension. J Clin Endocrinol Metab 56:915, 1983

92. Morris JM: The syndrome of testicular feminization in male pseudohermaphroditism. Am J Obstet Gynecol 65:1192, 1953

93. Mostofi FK: Histologic Typing of Testis Tumours. International Histologic Classification of Tumours, No. 16. World Health Organization, Geneva, 1976

94. Muller J: Morphometry and histology of gonads from twelve children and adolescents with the androgen insensitivity (testicular feminization) syndrome. J Clin Endocrinol Metab 59:785, 1984

95. Muram D, Dewhurst J: Inheritance of intersex disorders. Can Med Assoc J 130:121, 1984

96. Muzsnai D, Feinberg M: Mixed endodermal sinus tumor of the ovary in a Swyer's syndrome patient. Gynecol Oncol 10:230, 1980

97. Nelson DH: The adrenal cortex: physiological function and disease. Major Probl Intern Med 18:1, 1980

98. New MI: Male pseudohermaphroditism due to 17-alpha-hydroxylase deficiency. J Clin Invest 49:1930, 1970

99. New MI: Prenatal diagnosis of congenital adrenal hy-

perplasia. p. 187. In Vallet L, Porter I (eds): Genetic Mechanisms of Sexual Development. Academic Press, New York, 1979

100. Newell ME, Lippe BM, Ehrlich RM: Testis tumors associated with congenital adrenal hyperplasia: a continuing diagnostic and therapeutic dilemma. J Urol 117:256, 1977

101. Nichter LS: Seminoma in a 46,XX true hermaphrodite with positive H-Y antigen. Cancer 53:1181, 1984

102. Nihoul-Fekete C, Lortat-Jacob S, Josso N: Preservation of gonadal function in true hermaphroditism. J Pediatr Surg 19:50, 1984

103. Okon E, Livni N, Rosler A, et al: Male pseudohermaphroditism due to 5α-reductase deficiency: ultrastructure of the gonads. Arch Pathol Lab Med 104:363, 1980

104. O'Neil G: Case report—a true hermaphrodite presenting with hypospadias and an undescended testicle. Aust NZ J Obstet Gynaecol 21:47, 1981

105. Overzier C: Hermaphroditismus p. 227. In Overzier C (ed): Die Intersexualitat. Thieme, Stuttgart, 1961

106. Passarge E, Wolf U: Genetic heterogeneity of XY gonadal dysgenesis (Swyer syndrome): H-Y antigen-negative XY gonadal dysgenesis associated with inflammatory bowel disease. Am J Med Genet 8:437, 1981

107. Perez-Palacios G, Carnevale A, Escobar N, et al: Induction of ovulation in a true hermaphrodite with male phenotype. J Clin Endocrinol Metab 52:1257, 1981

108. Peterson RE, Imperato-McGinley J, Gautier T, Shackleton C: Male pseudohermaphroditism due to multiple defects in steroid-biosynthetic microsomal mixed-function oxidases. N Engl J Med 313:1182, 1985

109. Pickartz H, Moltz L, Altenahr E: XY (H-Y⁺) gonadal dysgenesis. Virchows Arch [Pathol Anat] 389:103, 1980

110. Pinsky L, Kaufman M, Summitt RL: Congenital androgen insensitivity due to a qualitatively abnormal androgen receptor. Am J Med Genet 10:91, 1981

111. Puck SM, Haseltine FP, Francke U: Absence of H-Y antigen in an XY female with campomelic dysplasia. Hum Genet 57:23, 1981

112. Radfar N, Bartter FC, Easley R, et al: Evidence for endogenous LH suppression in a man with bilateral testicular tumors and congenital adrenal hyperplasia. J Clin Endocrinol Metab 45:1194, 1977

113. Rajfer J: Association between Wilms tumor and gonadal dysgenesis. J Urol 125:388, 1981

114. Ramaswamy G, Jagadha V, Tchertkoff V: A testicular tumor resembling the sex cord with annular tubules in a case of the androgen insensitivity syndrome. Cancer 55:1611, 1985

115. Rao CS, Vaidza RA, Patel ZM, Ambani LM: Role of H-Y antigen in gonadal differentiation. Indian J Med Res 73:342, 1981

116. Raspa RW, Subramaniam AP, Romas NA: True hermaphroditism presenting as intermittent hematuria and groin pain. Urology 28:133, 1986

117. Reifenstein EC: Hereditary familial hypogonadism. Proc Am Fed Clin Res 3:86, 1947

118. Robboy SJ, Miller T, Donahoe PK, et al: Dysgenesis of testicular and streak gonads in the syndrome of mixed gonadal dysgenesis. Hum Pathol 13:700, 1982

119. Rosenfield RL, Lucky AW, Allen TD: The diagnosis and management of intersex. Curr Probl Pediatr 7:1, 1980

120. Rosenwaks Z, Wentz AC, Jones GS, et al: Endometrial pathology and estrogens. Obstet Gynecol 53:403, 1979

121. Rosewater S, Gwinup G, Hamwi GJ: Familial gynecomastia. Ann Intern Med 63:377, 1965

122. Roth LM, Cleary RE, Hokum WL: Ultrastructure of an ovotestis in a case of true hermaphroditism. Obstet Gynecol 48:619, 1976

123. Schulster A, Ross L, Scommegna A: Frequency of androgen insensitivity in infertile phenotypically normal men. J Urol 130:699, 1983

124. Schulte MJ: Positive H-Y antigen testing in a case of XY gonadal absence syndrome. Clin Genet 16:438, 1979

125. Schwartz M, Imperato-McGinley J, Peterson RE, et al: Male pseudohermaphroditism secondary to an abnormality in Leydig cell differentiation. J Clin Endocrinol Metab 53:123, 1981

126. Scully RE: Gonadoblastoma, a review of 74 cases. Cancer 25:1340, 1970

127. Selden JR, Wachtel SS, Koo GC, et al: Genetic basis of XX male syndrome and XX true hermaphroditism: evidence in the dog. Science 201:644, 1978

128. Simpson JL, Blagowidow N, Martin AO: XY gonadal dysgenesis: genetic heterogeneity based upon clinical observations: H-Y antigen status and segregation analysis. Hum Genet 58:91, 1981

129. Singh RP, Earr DH: The anatomy and histology of X0 human embryos and fetuses. Anat Rec 155:369, 1966

130. Skakkebaek NE: Carcinoma in situ of testis in testicular feminization syndrome. Acta Pathol Microbiol Scand 87:87, 1979

131. Snow BW, Rowland RG, Seal GM, Williams SD: Testicular tumor in patient with persistent müllerian duct syndrome. Urology 26:495, 1985

132. Sohval AR: Hermaphroditism with "atypical" or "mixed" gonadal dysgenesis. Am J Med 36:281, 1964

133. Summitt RL: Genetic forms of hypogonadism in the male. Prog Med Genet 3:1, 1979

134. Teter J, Boczkowski K: Occurrence of tumors in dysgenetic gonads. Cancer 20:1301, 1967

135. Tho PT, McDonough PG: Gonadal dysgenesis and its variants. Pediatr Clin North Am 28:309, 1981

136. Tvedegaard E, Frederiksen V, Olgaard K, et al: Two cases of 17α-hydroxylase deficiency—one combined with complete gonadal agenesis. Acta Endocrinol (Copenh) 98:267, 1981

137. Ulloa-Aguirre A, Mendez JP, Angeles A, et al: The presence of müllerian remnants in the complete androgen insensitivity syndrome: a steroid hormone mediated defect? Fertil Steril 45:301, 1986

138. Valdes E, del Castillo CF, Gutierrez R, et al: Endocrine studies and successful treatment in a patient with true hermaphroditism. Acta Endocrinol (Copenh) 91:184, 1979

139. Van Niekerk WA, Retief AE: The gonads of human true hermaphrodites. Hum Genet 58:117, 1981

140. Viinikka J, Hammond GL, Hortling H, et al: The clinical and endocrine evaluation of a pubertal boy with incomplete male pseudohermaphroditism type 1. Ann Clin Res 13:34, 1981

141. Von Petrykowski W: Embryology of genital malformations: guidelines in diagnosis and treatment of intersex. Monogr Paediatr 12:1, 1981

142. Wachtel SS: Immunologic aspects of abnormal sexual differentiation. Cell 16:691, 1979

143. Wachtel SS: Primary sex determination H-Y antigen and the development of the mammalian testis. Arthritis Rheum 22:1200, 1979

144. Wachtel SS: The dysgenetic gonad: aberrant testicular differentiation. Biol Reprod 22:1, 1980

145. Wachtel SS, Koo GC, Breg WR, Genel M: H-Y antigen in X,i (Xq) gonadal dysgenesis: evidence of X-linked genes in testicular differentiation. Hum Genet 56:183, 1980

146. Waldhausl W, Herkner K, Nowotny P, Bratusch-Marrain P: Combined 17α-18-hydroxylase deficiency associated with complete male pseudohermaphroditism and hypoaldosteronism. J Clin Endocrinol Metab 46:236, 1978

147. Walsh PC, Hensle T, Wigger HJ: Ambiguous genitalia in a child. Urology 14:405, 1979

148. Williamson HO, Phansey SA, Mathur RS: True hermaphroditism with term vaginal delivery and a review. Am J Obstet Gynecol 141:262, 1981

149. Wilson JD, George FW, Griffin JE: The hormonal control of sexual development. Science 211:1278, 1981

150. Winters SJ, Wachtel SS, White BJ, et al: H-Y antigen mosaicism in the gonad of a 46,XX true hermaphrodite. N Engl J Med 300:745, 1979

151. Wolman SR, McMorrow LE, Roy S, et al: Aberrant testicular differentiation in 46,XY gonadal dysgenesis: morphology, endocrinology, serology. Hum Genet 55:321, 1980

25
Male Infertility

Frank Rudy

In the United States approximately 15 percent of marriages do not produce progeny.[146] Evaluation of a couple for infertility is warranted if conception has not occurred after 1 year of unprotected coitus. Eighty-five percent of fertile couples achieve pregnancy within this period, and one-half of the remaining 15 percent do so within the next year without treatment.[158] The alternative of adoption is much less readily available today, so it is critical that physicians gain expertise in managing infertile couples. Both partners should undergo initial evaluation simultaneously. Despite thorough evaluation of the barren couple, the cause of the infertility cannot be determined in 10 percent of cases.[130] Among infertile couples in whom a causative factor can be assigned, the male partner is wholly or partially responsible for about one-half of the cases.[117]

ANALYTIC TECHNIQUES

Semen Analysis

Semen analysis has yielded important information in the study of infertile men. Three semen specimens, obtained at 2- to 6-week intervals, are evaluated.[128] Semen samples are collected after a period of abstinence, preferably 48 to 72 hours, and are examined within 45 to 90 minutes. If the seminal vesicles are present, the sample clots on emission, and it then liquefies within 20 to 60 minutes provided prostatic

proteolytic enzymes are effective. Seminal fructose, which is produced solely by the seminal vesicles, provides the substrate for the coagulation of semen and may be measured directly or by using Selivanoff's reagent.[52,87] Failure of the semen to coagulate with ejaculation is evidence of absent seminal vesicles. The results of semen analysis are compared with the normal values proposed by MacLeod,[91] which include a volume of 2 to 5 ml, sperm concentration of more than 20 million per milliliter, a motility of more than 40 percent, and more than 60 percent normal sperm forms. The number of immature cells must not exceed 4 percent, and the number of tapering forms must not exceed 10 percent.

Sperm motility is the most significant parameter of semen quality. The use of plastic specimen containers may adversely affect sperm motility.[152] Studies suggest that the point at which the sperm count is considered oligospermic may have to be lowered to less than 10 million milliliter.[151] Indeed, Ross[128] has stated that in his experience pregnancies occur more frequently in the partners of men with low semen densities (fewer than 20 million sperms per milliliter) and good sperm motility and morphology than in men with high sperm counts and low sperm motility. Morphology, paradoxically, seems not to be as important as motility. A Danish 20-year follow-up study[25] found that in patients with up to 60 percent morphologically abnormal spermatozoa there was no reduction in clinical fertility. Those with 60 to 80 percent abnormal forms had reduced fertility, and beyond 80 percent fertility was markedly reduced. The standard semen analysis may not reliably indicate male fertility in all cases, for some men with normal semen and normal partners are unable to induce pregnancy.

Cross-species in vitro fertilization techniques may prove to be a more accurate measure of male fertility.[128] These techniques involve separating the sperm from the seminal plasma to "capacitate" the sperm. The sperm are then mixed with zona-free hamster ova and observed for penetration of the ova, comparing the results with those of a normal subject of known fertility.[22,129] There is a high degree of correlation of ova penetration with the semen analysis of patients of known fertility.[36,82] These techniques also permit the demonstration that the viscous seminal plasma of some infertile patients has the capacity to markedly reduce the penetration of fertile donors, compared to their own seminal plasma.[36]

Hormone Levels

In addition to semen analysis, measurements of serum testosterone, follicle-stimulating hormone (FSH), and luteinizing hormone (LH) are useful tests for evaluating infertile men (Fig. 25-1). Serum testosterone is low in men with hypogonadotropism and those with failure of Leydig cell function. A decrease in libido and potency are the earliest symptoms of a low serum testosterone concentration. By the time diminished sexual hair or musculature or less than normal virilization are seen, a severe deficiency of testosterone exists. If testosterone deficiency occurs before puberty, the patient manifests eunuchoid proportions. Serum FSH and LH levels are reduced in

hypogonadotropic patients, with secondary hypogonadism resulting from the hypothalamic or pituitary dysfunction. The association of increased serum LH and low serum testosterone is indicative of some degree of Leydig cell failure and is encountered in approximately 30 percent of men with more severe testicular damage.[43] An increased LH concentration with a normal testosterone level denotes a state of compensated Leydig cell failure with the normal testosterone level being maintained at the expense of increased LH production.[60] Although typically an indicator of primary gonadal failure, the combination of increased LH and low testosterone can exceptionally be the consequence of secretion of an abnormal LH level, in which case the testicular response to human chorionic gonadotropin or exogenous LH is normal.[15] Increased serum LH levels with increased testosterone suggest androgen insensitivity in otherwise normal men.[6]

Serum FSH concentration is of considerable importance, for it provides a useful index of the state of the seminiferous epithelium. Provided the hypothalamic–pituitary–testicular axis is intact, increased FSH levels usually indicate severe impairment of spermatogenesis, presumably because of failure of the epithelium to produce adequate feedback signals to control FSH production. Elevated FSH levels are found in 30 percent of patients consulting for infertility.[158] Although generally associated with a poor prognosis, elevation of serum FSH is occasionally found in patients with mild oligospermia or even normal sperm counts. Prolactin measurements are warranted in infertile men. Hyperprolactinemia is encountered in 2 to 4 percent of infertile men, and appropriate treat-

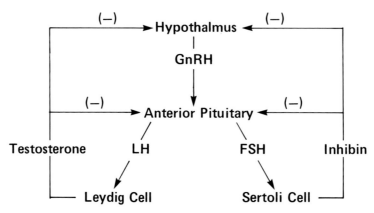

Fig. 25-1 Hypothalamic–pituitary–testicular axis. GnRH, gonadotropin-releasing hormone; LH, luteinizing hormone; FSH, follicle-stimulating hormone.

ment may lead to improvement in the sperm count and fertility.[139,164]

Dehydroepiandrosterone and 17-α-hydroxyprogesterone levels should be determined, for elevation of these substances helps to identify a group of patients with partial or subclinical adrenal dysfunction, with 11- or 21-hydroxylase deficiency and mild to moderate decreases in serum testosterone.[128,129] Additional laboratory studies that may be required in selected infertile men include a complete blood count, urinalysis, blood urea nitrogen, creatinine, buccal smear, immunologic studies, and karyotype. The incidence of cytogenetic abnormalities in men with infertility has been reported to vary from 2 to 21 percent.[151] Chromosome abnormalities are encountered more frequently in azoospermic or severely oligospermic men.[58,151] Supernumerary chromosomes and chromosome mosaics, translocations, and deletions have been reported.[151]

Anti-sperm Antibodies

Spermatozoa are antigenically different from the man producing them, possibly because they do not develop until puberty and are normally shielded from the immune system by the blood–testis barrier. Anti-sperm antibodies, including agglutinating, cytotoxic, and sperm-immobilizing antibodies, can be found in the serum of about 2 percent of fertile and 8 to 13 percent of subfertile men[58]; however, the relation of these antibodies may be more common in the presence of sperm-immobilizing rather than sperm-agglutinating antibodies.[151] Return of fertility can occur following long-term administration of immunosuppressants such as corticosteriods to patients with anti-sperm antibodies.[69,153] Pregnancy may also occur when the sperm from a man with anti-sperm antibodies are first washed in a physiologic buffer and then inseminated into the female partner.[79,157] Commonly used immunologic studies for the detection of anti-sperm antibodies are the Kibrik sperm agglutination test,[84] the Franklin-Dukes sperm agglutination test,[55] and the Isojima sperm-immobilizing test.[75]

Testicular Biopsy

Charney first advocated testicular biopsy in 1940,[32] but the use of testicular biopsy as a diagnostic procedure for infertility has not been universally accepted. Some reserve testicular biopsy for azoospermic men in

order to differentiate primary testicular failure from obstruction, whereas others believe that biopsy offers a guide to diagnosis, prognosis, and choice of treatment in oligospermic as well as azoospermic men.[31,59,106] In the presence of pyospermia or marked elevation of serum FSH levels, testicular biopsy may be unwarranted.[87,136] Although the two testes of most men show essentially similar histologic features, differences are encountered with sufficient frequency to make biopsy of both the preferred method.[109] An open testicular biopsy is best performed in connection with a formal scrotal exploration in order to properly evaluate the testes as well as the epididymis, vas, and other accessory genital structures. Needle aspiration of the testes has been employed in infertile men,[169] as have incisional and needle biopsies.[37] Testicular biopsies should be placed in Bouin's fixative with a minimum of handling. In addition to histologic evaluation, cytogenetic and biochemical studies may be performed,[111] as may flow cytometry.[29]

To properly interpret a testicular biopsy, one must carefully evaluate the number and size of the seminiferous tubules, the thickness of the tubular basement membrane, the state of the germinal epithelium, the presence or absence of peritubular and interstitial fibrosis, and the condition of the Leydig cells and blood vessels. The seminiferous tubular basement membrane and tunica propria can be differentiated using a combination of the periodic acid methenamine silver technique with Masson's trichrome. A quantitative assessment of spermatogenesis can also be employed.[78]

A given biopsy may show one of several well delineated defects but may also reveal a combination of defects or a histologic pattern that does not fall into an easily defined category. Furthermore, the same morphologic lesion may be produced by a variety of agents, and the same agent may lead to the develop-

Table 25-1 Morphologic Classification of Testicular Biopsies from Infertile Men

Normal histology
Immature testes in adults
Sloughing of immature cells
Hypospermatogenesis
Maturation arrest
Sertoli-cell–only syndrome
Peritubular fibrosis and tubular hyalinization

ment of different histologic lesions under different sets of circumstances. Nevertheless, the morphologic classification shown in Table 25-1 is practical and applicable to most testicular lesions.

MORPHOLOGIC CLASSIFICATION

Normal Histology

Normal histology refers to a morphologic appearance of the testis in which spermatogenic activity resembles that seen in normal postpubertal men (Fig. 25-2). Basement membrane thickening and interstitial fibrosis are absent. Normal or essentially normal testicular histology is most commonly encountered in azoospermic men with obstruction of the excurrent ducts of the testes (Table 25-2).

DUCTAL OBSTRUCTION

Obstructive azoospermia comprises 7 to 14 percent of cases of male infertility.[127,167] In most series obstruction is not associated with significant changes in

Table 25-2 Conditions Association with Normal Histology on Testicular Biopsy

Ductal obstruction
  Congenital
  Acquired
Idiopathic azoospermia
Varicocele
Absence of dynein arms (Kartagener's syndrome)
Anti-sperm antibodies
Seminiferous tubule hypercurvature
Branching of seminiferous tubules
Isolated impaired sperm motility
Sampling error
Toxic, metabolic, or infectious agents

serum testosterone or gonadotropin levels or with alterations in testosterone concentration in the seminal plasma; however, elevations of LH and total serum androgens and decreases in total serum estrogens and progesterone have been reported.[1,125] Obstruction of the excurrent testicular ducts may be congenital or acquired.

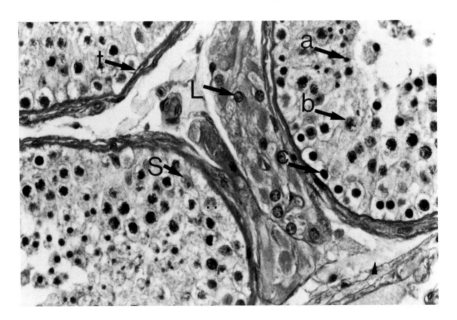

Fig. 25-2 Normal testis. Portions of three seminiferous tubules are seen. These tubules show a normal population of spermatogenic cells. A thin tunica propria surrounds each tubule, and Leydig cells are evident in the interstitium. (Silverberg SG (ed): Principles and Practice of Surgical Pathology. Wiley, New York, 1983.)

Congenital Obstruction

Congenital obstruction is usually caused by atresia of the distal portion of the epididymis or the adjoining part of the vas deferens.[59] Failure of anatomic union between the testis and epididymis, which may result from fibrolipomatous tissue compressing the ductuli efferentes, and total absence of the epididymides or vasa have been described.[58,87,113,114] If the patient's masculinization and testicular development are otherwise normal, nonpalpable vasa combined with an ejaculate of small volume that lacks fructose and fails to coagulate indicates bilateral absence of the vasa and seminal vesicles. Ductal obstruction may also be caused by solitary or multiple cystic dilatations in the epididymis (Fig. 25-3). These cysts may be secondary to in utero exposure to such substances as diethylstilbestrol and can produce extrinsic compression.[58,87] In addition to epididymal cysts, a variety of other genital abnormalities have been reported to occur with increased frequency in men exposed to diethylstilbestrol in utero, including testicular hypoplasia, cryptor-chidism, capsular induration of the testis, decreased penile length, hypospadias, urethral stenosis, varicocele, and monorchism.[21,163]

There is a strong link between obstructive azoospermia and chronic sinopulmonary infections, the association being known as *Young's syndrome.*[67,68,73a,168] This syndrome is much more frequent than previously realized and may constitute as many as 3.3 percent of all cases of infertility.[67] Typically these patients have a long history of upper respiratory tract infections, with varying mixtures of chronic bronchitis and chronic sinusitis, from early childhood that often ameliorate somewhat after adolescence. The infections are sufficiently severe to produce abnormalities on x-ray films of the paranasal sinuses in most of the patients, frequently with abnormal chest films as well. Patients are typically azoospermic but with normal or near-normal testicular biopsies and normal testosterone levels. There is dilatation of the head of the epididymis, which is filled with sperm, whereas the remaining epididymis is obstructed by inspissated secretions. Neville et al.[110] looked at the opposite side of

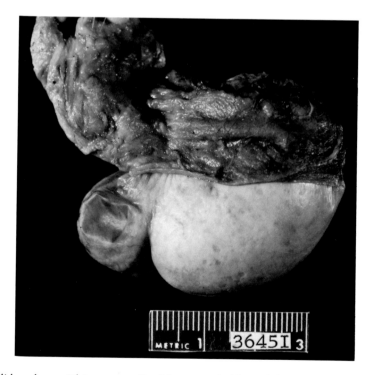

Fig. 25-3 Epididymal cyst. This cyst was lined by recognizable epididymal epithelium and filled with degenerating sperm.

the coin and confirmed that among patients with obstructive azoospermia there was a marked excess of respiratory problems compared with a control population.

Young's syndrome must be distinguished from two other conditions having a prominent respiratory component. First is the immotile cilia syndrome seen in patients with *Kartagener's syndrome,* where normal numbers of sperm, all immotile, are produced (see below). Second is *cystic fibrosis,* where there are obvious abnormalities in sweat and pancreatic secretions (see Ch. 28). Genitourinary tract anomalies abound in patients with cystic fibrosis. Holsclaw[72] summarized the lesions in men as an absence of the body of the epididymis, blind-ending efferent ducts, and absent or hypoplastic vas deferens. Although the testicular histology may be normal in involved children,[23] testicular biopsy usually reveals maturation arrest, with or without interstitial fibrosis.[47,81] Excurrent duct obstruction, usually high in the caput epididymis, with normal testicular biopsies has been observed in infertile men with a history of childhood bronchiectasis.[44]

Acquired Blockage

Acquired blockage may be due to infection or surgical interruption of the ductal system. Among infectious causes, gonorrheal epididymitis is the most common, with obstruction typically occurring in the distal epididymis and the adjacent proximal vas deferens[167] (Fig. 25-4). Tuberculous epididymitis also leads to ductal obstruction, and scarring often involves the vasa, seminal vesicles, and ejaculatory ducts in addition to the epididymides. Nonspecific pyogenic infections, often originating in the prostate, can lead to occlusion of the vas deferens, epididymis, or both. In endemic areas chronic filarial infection may be instrumental in obstructing the vasa.[130] However, nonpyogenic infections with agents such as mycoplasma, cytomegalovirus, or gram-positive commensals, probably seldom if ever are responsible for infertility,[155] and gram-negative organisms only infrequently. The clinical utility of routine screening of semen for *Ureaplasma urealyticum* has yet to be established.[105] To tie infection to infertility there must be symptomatic, culture-proved infection with verified pyospermia (the latter of which may be difficult to demonstrate conclusively).

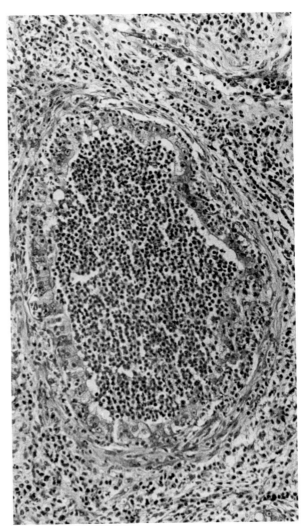

Fig. 25-4 Gonorrheal epididymitis. The epididymal lumen and interstitium are heavily infiltrated by acute and chronic inflammatory cells. ×230.

Surgical occlusion of the vas may be voluntary, or it may result from accidental ligation. Injuries to the vasa may be sustained during bilateral hernia repair, orchiopexy, or pelvic surgery for ureteral calculi in the region of the terminal ureter. Ejaculatory duct obstruction may occur secondary to transurethral procedures on the prostate or around the verumontanum.

Patients with obstructive lesions are potentially surgical candidates. The results of vasovasotomy and vasoepididymostomy are steadily improving with new microsurgical techniques. Spermatozoa arriving from the ductuli efferentes into the head of the epididymis acquire motility only gradually during their course through the epididymis. For this reason it has been thought that vasoepididymostomy should be performed as distally as possible to allow for maximal spermatozoal motility. After microscopic vasoepididymostomy to the mid or distal corpus of the epididymis, more than 80 percent of patients may recover a normal sperm count, with sperm motility returning to normal within 5 months.[144] Vasoepididymostomy to the head of the epididymis may also be successful, but sperm motility does not recover until 1 to 2 years after surgery.[145] It appears that a compensatory mechanism eventually allows sperm from the caput to exhibit normal motility. Lesions from genitourinary tract tuberculosis are usually not treatable because of extensive seminal pathway involvement.[58] Regardless of the etiology, obstruction of the vas or epididymis generally has no significant long-term adverse effect on the germinal epithelium or Leydig cells. Preservation of the germinal epithelium appears to be due to the ability of the epididymis to enlarge in order to accommodate the accumulating sperm, and to phagocytize and resorb disintegrated spermatozoa. Distension of the occluded vas with increased intraluminal pressure is known to occur following vasectomy, and animal studies have shown atrophy of the testicular germinal tissue, presumably resulting from backpressure on the seminiferous tubules.

Alterations Postvasectomy

Testicular biopsies in men performed shortly after vasectomy have revealed widespread degeneration of the germinal epithelium, thickening of the tubular basement membranes, arrest of spermatogenesis at the primary spermatocyte stage, and increased intertubular connective tissue.[48,64] More marked and widespread histologic changes may be observed in men vasectomized after 50 years of age. Occasionally, slight dilation of the seminiferous tubules, hypospermatogenesis, and sloughing of immature germinal epithelial cells are found in cases of ductal obstruction.[3,167] Ultrastructural analysis of testicular tissue from vasectomized monkeys has demonstrated focal seminiferous epithelial alterations consisting of extensive infoldings and duplication within the basal

lamina, as well as the presence of Sertoli cell cytoplasm.[30] The latter finding suggests a possible increase in the phagocytic activity of the Sertoli cells. In man, regeneration of the seminiferous epithelium appears to occur spontaneously, as biopsies obtained at longer intervals after vasectomy reveal essentially normal architecture with active spermatogenesis.[48,64] Available data strongly suggest that vasectomy has no significant immediate or long-term effects on the complex interrelations between the pituitary and the endocrine tests.

Vasectomy-reversal operations leads to return of sperm to the ejaculate in 30 to 98 percent of patients, with subsequent pregnancy rates varying widely, from 10 percent to as high as 68 percent.[8] Sperm may not appear in the ejaculate for as long as 6 months after a vasovasostomy. Vasectomy results in division of the inferior spermatic nerve that innervates the vas. An intact sympathetic nerve supply is probably essential for the transport of sperm from the epididymis at the time of ejaculation. Attempts at vasovasostomy may fail to restore fertility because iatrogenic factors during the original vasectomy may prevent regeneration of the sympathetic nerve supply. These factors include removal of a large segment of the vas, placement of a suture or clip close to the sheath around the stump of the vas, and a marked inflammatory reaction with scarring in response to the operative trauma.

Despite a technically successful vasovasostomy, patients may still exhibit poor fertility manifested by oligospermia, decreased motility, and a high proportion of abnormal forms. The etiology of the poor semen quality and the marked discrepancy between the presence of sperm after vasovasostomy and pregnancy rates remain obscure. It has been suggested that these effects might be caused by the development of an immune response to sperm following vasectomy. Vasectomy clearly results in sperm antibody production in 50 to 75 percent of subjects.[8,153] Sperm-agglutinating antibodies are most frequently found.[27] High antibody titers, although not a contraindication to vasectomy reversal, may be a poor prognostic sign. Postvasectomy studies have failed to demonstrate evidence of cell-mediated immunity to spermatozoa.[77]

The presence of circulating anti-sperm antibodies following vasectomy raises the possibility of systemic effects. More severe atherosclerosis has been shown to develop in vasectomized monkeys than in controls, but to date there is no conclusive evidence of systemic disease or an autoimmune phenomenon as a result of vasectomy in humans.[27]

IDIOPATHIC AZOOSPERMIA

Normal testicular histology has been observed in azoospermic men without evidence of hormonal disturbances or seminal tract obstruction. The proposed explanation for this paradoxical finding is that the absorption rate of sperm, mainly by the epididymis, exceeds the rate of sperm production in these patients.[94]

KARTAGENER'S SYNDROME

Kartagener's syndrome is characterized by situs inversus, recurrent sinopulmonary infections, and infertility. The latter two problems are related in most cases to an absence of dynein arms in the cilia of the respiratory epithelium and the sperm flagella,[44,88] although the sperm are normal in number. Young's syndrome, with obstructive azoospermia, is also marked by recurrent respiratory infections, but does not have situs inversus and cilia and flagellar structures are normal, although the cilia function poorly. Recently an intermediate form, with situs inversus, normal sperm flagella, but aplasia of nasal cilia, has been described,[96a] suggesting a possible link between Young's and Kartagener's syndromes. Decreased sperm motility with normal counts has also been attributed to faulty maturation or storage of spermatozoa during their journey through the epididymis, as well as to biochemical abnormalities of the seminal plasma.[28,49,94]

SEMINIFEROUS TUBULE HYPERCURVATURE

A common finding in otherwise normal-appearing biopsy specimens from oligospermic men is hypercurvature of the seminiferous tubules.[13,14]

Recognition of hypercurvature depends on identification of certain characteristic shapes of seminiferous tubules, i.e., "figure 8" profiles and grazing profiles, which are commonly present with hypercurvature and are comparatively rare in normal controls. "Figure 8" profiles, which are symmetrical, double circular tubule profiles formed by a common

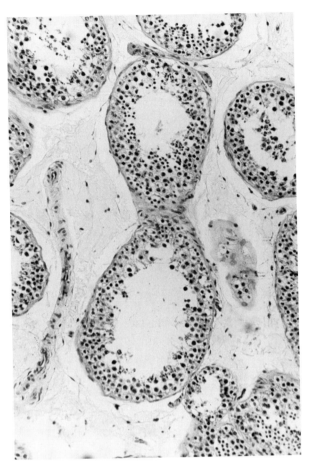

Fig. 25-5 "Figure 8" profile. A double-barrel lumen is produced by a transverse section through a bend in a seminiferous tubule. ×178.

element of wall, are produced by a transverse section through a band (Fig. 25-5). The finding of at least four "figure 8" profiles per ten high power fields establishes the diagnosis of hypercurvature. Grazing profiles are sections consisting of seminiferous wall without lumen (Fig. 25-6). Roughly one-half the area of the profile must be lamina propria, and progression toward the lumen cannot extend beyond the Sertoli cells and the first germinal layer. Four grazing profiles per ten ×100 fields indicates hypercurvature.

Abnormal contractile activity of myoid cells within the tubular lamina propria or the testicular tunica, structural compression, traction, and obstruction are potential causes of tubular hypercurvature. Averback suggested that the excessive curvature might impede sperm transport.[13,14]

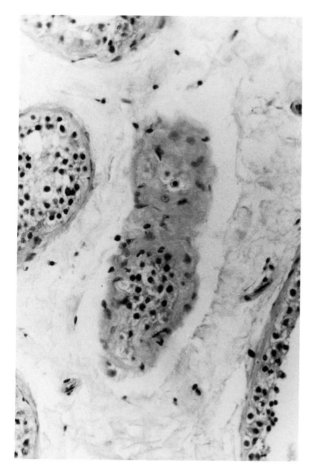

Fig. 25-6 Grazing profile. A lumen is not seen, and most of the tubule is composed of tunica propria. ×284.

Branching of the Seminiferous Tubules

Branched seminiferous tubules have been described in an otherwise normal biopsy from an oligospermic patient with chronic respiratory infection[12] (Fig. 25-7).

Other Causes

Occasionally, biopsies from men with oligospermia reveal a surprisingly normal appearance that is inexplicable. Some of these patients are found to have a varicocele. Additional explanations for oligospermia with a normal biopsy include anti-sperm antibodies, sampling error, and toxic, metabolic, or infectious effects on the testes that do not manifest histologically.

Immature Testes in Adults

In a small percentage of cases testicular biopsy specimens from infertile adult men are histologically identical to those from prepubertal testis.[167] Such testes are composed of small, lumenless, immature seminiferous tubules lined by numerous immature Sertoli cells and lesser numbers of undifferentiated germinal elements (Fig. 25-7). There is little evidence of maturation of germ cells beyond the stage of spermatogonia or primary spermatocytes. Ultrastructural study reveals absence of the specialized Sertoli cell junctional complexes that form the blood–testis barrier.[57] The tunica propria is thin and delicate. As in the prepubertal testis, there are no peritubular elastic fibers, indicating absent or inadequate stimulation of the testes by pituitary gonadotropins at puberty. Characteristically, mature Leydig cells are absent in the intertubular areas, but numerous immature and poorly developed Leydig cell precursors resembling undifferentiated mesenchymal cells may be present.

This histologic picture is seen in cases of prepubertal hypothalamic or pituitary dysfunction and in prepubertal androgen excess (Table 25-3). The common denominator in these conditions is diminished or absent gonadotropin secretion. Although representing only a small fraction of patients with infertility, these disorders may be amenable to specific therapy.

PREPUBERTAL HYPOTHALAMIC–PITUITARY DYSFUNCTION

Gonadal failure secondary to prepubertal hypothalamic–pituitary dysfunction may be caused by organic lesions in the region of the hypothalamus or pituitary, inadequate or absent hypothalamic gonadotropin-releasing hormone (GnRH), or pituitary failure to produce gonadotropins.[122,151,169] The clomiphene citrate stimulation test is abnormally low in patients with either hypothalamic or pituitary diseases, whereas administration of GnRH increases FSH and LH levels in most patients with hypothalamic disease but fails to do so when a pituitary disorder is responsible for the hypogonadism.[156] Organic lesions include tumors, cysts, or trauma to the sella turcica or suprasellar area. Patients with organic lesions eventually develop panhypopituitarism and exhibit sexual infantilism, lack of somatic growth, and varying degrees of thyroid and adrenal hypofunction.

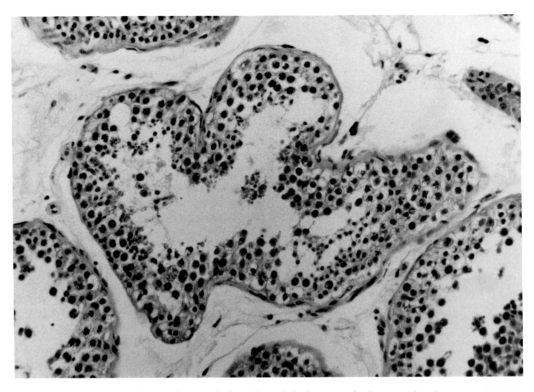

Fig. 25-7 Branching of seminiferous tubules. The tubule has a markedly convoluted contour. ×336.

Idiopathic hypogonadotropic hypogonadism, a collection of congenital conditions of unknown etiology, is associated with LH or FSH deficiency sometimes accompanied by deficient secretion of other pituitary hormones.[149]

HYPOGONADOTROPIC EUNUCHOIDISM

Combined deficiency of both FSH and LH, a type of hypogonadotropic hypogonadism referred to as hypogonadotropic eunuchoidism, is a sporadic or familial congenital disorder in which serum testosterone and gonadotropin levels are low. These patients give a history of never having undergone normal puberty. They are typically tall and eunuchoidal in build with small prepuberty-sized testes of normal consistency, absent ejaculations, and generalized diminished body hair growth. Although two additional variants are recognized, one with isolated LH deficiency, only the classic form of hypogonadotropic eunuchoidism

with combined deficiency of both gonadotropins reveals typical immature testicular histology.[96,122,165]

Kallmann's Syndrome

Kallmann's syndrome, a genetic disorder defined as hypogonadotropic eunuchoidism with anosmia, may have an X-linked or autosomal dominant mode of transmission.[120] There is a variable association with a cleft lip and palate, cryptorchidism, craniofacial asymmetry, deafness, and color blindness. This syndrome appears to be the least severe form of the holoprosencephaly–hypopituitarism complex, a spectrum of developmental anomalies associated with impaired midline cleavage of the embryonic forebrain, aplasia of the olfactory bulbs and tracts, and midline dysplasia of the face. Microscopically, the testes are prepubertal in appearance and may reveal foci of interstitial fibrosis[17,120] (Fig. 25-9). A testicular seminoma has been reported in a patient with Kallman's syndrome.[7]

The etiology of hypogonadotropic eunuchoidism

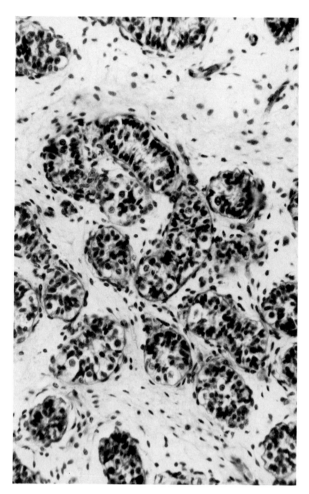

Fig. 25-8 Immature testis in an adult. The lumenless, immature tubules contain spermatogonia with round nuclei surrounded by a halo of clear cytoplasm. The remaining intratubular cells are immature Sertoli cells. Spermatogenic maturation and mature Leydig cells are not evident. ×300.

Table 25-3 Conditions Associated with Immature Testes in Adults
Abnormalities of hypothalamic–pituitary function
Prepubertal panhypopituitarism
Congenital
Acquired
Hypogonadotropic eunuchoidism
Kallmann's syndrome
Laurence–Moon–Biedl syndrome
Prader–Willi syndrome
Prepubertal androgen excess
Androgen-producing tumor
Adrenogenital syndrome
Exogenous androgen administration

response to hCG stimulation in Kallmann's syndrome have raised the possibility of concomitant pituitary and Leydig cell defects.[17,18]

OTHER CONGENITAL SYNDROMES WITH HYPOGONADOTROPIC HYPOGONADISM

Laurence–Moon–Biedl Syndrome

The Laurence–Moon–Biedl syndrome appears in a familial pattern and is characterized by growth retardation, mental deficiency, polydactyly, obesity, retinitis pigmentosa, and hypogonadotropic hypogonadism.[17,151]

Prader–Willi Syndrome

The cardinal features of the Prader–Willi syndrome are mental retardation, neonatal muscle hypotonia, uncontrollable hyperphagia with massive obesity, infantile external genitalia, impaired temperature regulation, small usually crytorchid testes, and hypogonadotropism. Testicular biopsies from postpubertal men have revealed prepuberty-appearing testes; however, normal adult testicular histology, interstitial cell defects, tubular atrophy, hyalinization, and absence of germinal epithelium have also been reported.[66,76] Although most studies of the hypogonadism of the Prader–Willi syndrome have concluded that the basic defect is hypothalamic, there is also evidence for a primary gonadal abnormality. Treatment with clomiphene citrate in one patient

with or without anosmia is unclear. In most patients the endocrinologic abnormalities are presumed to be secondary to a lack of GnRH, as the pituitary–gonadal axis can be stimulated by exogenous GnRH.[151] Long-term administration of GnRH may induce potency, virilization, and spermatogenesis. In addition, testosterone therapy has been used to obtain secondary sexual development, and human chorionic gonadotropin (hCG) and human menopausal gonadotropin administration have been employed to induce fertility.[39] Variable pituitary response to GnRH administration and diminished plasma testosterone

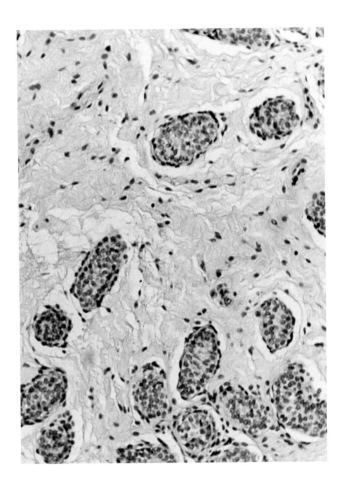

Fig. 25-9 Kallmann's syndrome. Immature seminiferous tubules are separated by an expanded, fibrotic interstitium. ×250.

with this syndrome resulted in the development of physical signs of puberty and normal spermatogenesis on repeat testicular biopsy.[66]

PREPUBERTAL ANDROGEN EXCESS

Androgen excess acts by suppressing pituitary gonadotropin secretion, leading to secondary testicular failure. Most cases of prepubertal androgen excess are endogenous in nature and either are due to an androgen-producing tumor of the adrenal cortex or testis or, alternatively, are associated with one of the biochemical variants of the adrenogenital syndrome.[165] Prepubertal administration of exogenous androgen produces the same picture of testicular maturation failure. Endogenous or exogenous estrogen excess can also cause secondary testicular failure by suppressing pituitary gonadotropin secretion, but the offending

disorders occur predominantly during the postpubertal period (see below).

Sloughing of Immature Cells

Sloughing of immature cells into the lumens of the seminiferous tubules is a common finding in the testes of oligospermic men.[3,138] The tubules are either normal or slightly reduced in diameter, and the central lumens are lost. The obliterated lumens contain sloughed spermatogenic cells consisting primarily in spermatocytes admixed with mature elements (Fig. 25-10). In these cases the orderly pattern of spermatogenesis is often disrupted, and the seminiferous epithelium has a jumbled, disorganized appearance. Progressive sloughing may produce hypocellularity of the germinal epithelium so that the center of the tubule, which contains numerous desquamated cells,

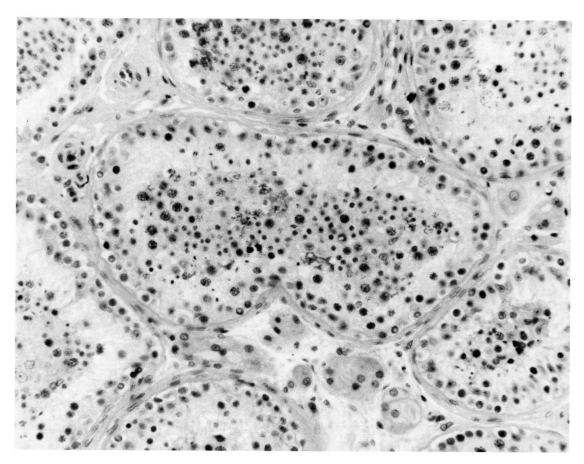

Fig. 25-10 Sloughing of immature cells. Immature seminiferous tubules are separated by an expanded, fibrotic intersitium. ×250.

appears more cellular than the periphery. Scattered tubules revealing complete spermatogenesis are often present. Mild degrees of peritubular fibrosis may be seen, and collagenous deposits may occur in intertubular areas. Leydig cells are usually present in normal numbers. Cases should be assigned to this group only if 50 percent or more of the tubules are affected, as focal tubular sloughing is seen in some cases of hypo-

Table 25-4 Conditions Associated with Sloughing of Immature Cells in Testicular Biopsy

Varicocele
Idiopathic sloughing
Prior vasectomy
Mumps orchitis

spermatogenesis.[99] This histologic picture is characteristically seen in patients with a varicocele[9,50,138] but can also be seen in the absence of varicocele or other identifiable cause (Table 25-4). A similar pattern has been reported in previously vasectomized men[3] and occasional patients with a history of mumps orchitis.[138] Patients with sloughing of immature cells may respond to therapy with clomiphene citrate.

VARICOCELE

A varicocele consists of abnormal tortuosity and dilation of the veins of the pampiniform plexus within the spermatic cord that results from free reflux of venous blood secondary to incompetence of the valves in the internal spermatic vein (Fig. 25-11). The incidence of varicocele in the general population is

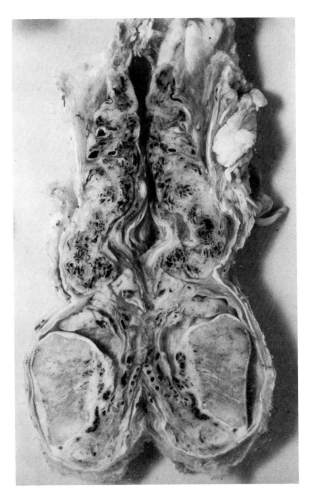

Fig. 25-11 Varicocele. Impressive gross specimen, showing marked engorgement of vessels along the spermatic cord. Note that the dilatation extends actually into the testis (left).

about 15 to 20 percent.[8] From 21 to 39 percent of men seeking evaluation for infertility have a clinical varicocele[63] and an even greater number may have a subclinical varicocele.[108] Smokers and men exposed to diethylstilbestrol in utero appear to be at increased risk for the development of a varicocele.[85,149] Among patients with varicocele, oligospermia is nine times more common among smokers than among nonsmokers.[84a]

Etiology of Infertility

A variety of mechanisms have been proposed to explain the infertility seen in these patients, and they have been well reviewed by Turner.[154] Any hypoth-

esis must explain the bilateral effects of a varicocele on spermatogenesis. The most widely accepted cause for the impaired spermatogenesis in patients with varicocele is increased intrascrotal temperature. In man the testis maintains euthermia by convection heat loss through the scrotal skin, a mechanism probably regulated by dartos and cremasteric activity.[132] In addition, there is evidence that a countercurrent heat exchange mechanism exists between the internal spermatic artery blood and venous blood returning via the internal spermatic vein and the pampiniform plexus.[170] Retrograde venous blood flow would nullify this heat exchange as would a marked increase in blood flow, which would tend to "wash out" the countercurrent mechanism. Elevated temperature in the contralateral testis might occur as a consequence of a gradient effect through the scrotal septum. There is also evidence for some degree of cross-collateral circulation between the two sides,[26,53] which may be of importance in explaining the contralateral temperature elevation. Induced intrascrotal hyperthermia has been shown to impair spermatogenesis in man, and thermography has demonstrated increased testicular temperature in varicocele patients.[19] Furthermore, a drop in intrascrotal temperature may follow varicocelectomy.[170]

Confirming and amplifying these observations are animal models of varicocele, in which the left renal vein is partially constricted, shunting blood into the left testicular vein.[35,62,83] Testicular blood flow measurements indicate a 34 percent increase in blood flow, not only in the primarily affected left testis but also in the right testis. There is also a rise in temperature from 34.4° to 35.3°C, bilaterally. If these data are applicable to man, they suggest that (1) the increase in temperature is probably due to washout of the countercurrent gradient, such as happens in the kidney, and (2) there are more substantial alterations in blood flow to the opposite testis than had previously been thought. The animal models resemble the human model also in that development of a seminal stress pattern and bilateral defects in spermatogenesis are seen on testicular biopsy.[35,83]

Another theory is that the varicocele's effect is due to a substance of renal or adrenal gland origin that is noxious to spermatogenesis and is carried to the testis by retrograde internal spermatic vein blood flow, reaching the contralateral testis by collateral vessels. Steroids and catecholamines have been incriminated, but no consistent data have substantiated this theory.[124] Other theories for the etiology of the varicocele effect continue to be argued in the literature and include Leydig cell dysfunction, hypoxia of the germinal epithelium,[20] epididymal dysfunction,[19] and an immunologic factor.[61]

Clinical and Radiographic Picture

A varicocele is a common finding in adolescent boys, reaching a peak incidence at 15 years of age. Usually the disorder is asymptomatic, but it may be associated with diminished testicular size. Many varicoceles are palpable with the patient in an upright position. Having the patient perform a sudden Valsalva maneuver while standing may permit detection of a varicocele that is otherwise not palpable. Using this diagnostic maneuver, bilateral varicoceles are found in 15 percent of affected patients, and a unilateral left-sided lesion is found in most of the remaining 85 percent.[8] Unilateral right varicoceles are rare. Incompetence of internal spermatic vein valves with resulting varicocele formation is presumed to be more common on the left side because of the right-angle drainage of the left internal spermatic vein into the left renal vein. In contrast, the right internal spermatic vein usually drains obliquely into the vena cava.

The size of the varicocele bears no relation to its effects on spermatogenesis or to the likelihood of improvement in semen quality or subsequent pregnancy rates after varicocelectomy. Therefore the "subclinical" varicocele that is not palpable becomes an important entity in infertile patients. The doppler examination[63] and thermography[121] are useful noninvasive techniques for detecting nonpalpable varicoceles. Retrograde internal spermatic vein venography is the most precise method for diagnosing small varicoceles. Venographically demonstrable varicoceles have been reported in a significant number of infertile men who did not have a clinical varicocele[108] (Fig.25-12). Venography has revealed varicoceles of the cremasteric vein and mixed varicoceles involving both internal spermatic and cremasteric veins.[27] Multiple internal spermatic veins have also been noted. Furthermore, venographic studies have shown that right-sided subclinical varicoceles may be almost as common as left-sided clinical varicoceles, suggesting that the bilateral effects of a left-sided varicocele may be caused by unrecognized bilateral reflux. In some of these patients the right internal spermatic vein enters directly into the right renal vein. Bilateral varicoceles can also be the result of cross-circulation from the left to the

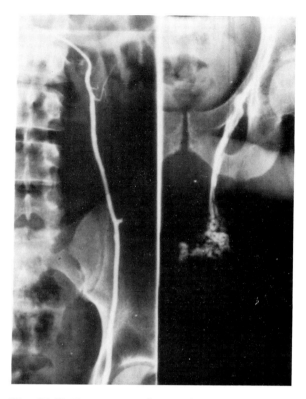

Fig. 25-12 Venogram. Reflux in the left internal spermatic vein is demonstrated by a venogram in a patient with a subclinical varicocele. (From Narayan et al.,[108] with permission.)

right side when valvular incompetence on the left side is the primary abnormality.[19] Radioisotope scanning has also been utilized to detect subclinical varicoceles.[161]

Hormone Levels

Serum FSH, LH, and testosterone levels are usually normal in varicocele patients.[124] FSH elevation may be seen in azoospermic or severely oligospermic patients. Leydig cell dysfunction has been demonstrated in severely oligospermic tissue.[160] Furthermore, serum LH is increased in some patients with varicoceles despite normal testosterone levels, indicating a degree of compensated Leydig cell failure.[116] These studies suggest that serum testosterone levels may not be a sufficiently sensitive index of Leydig cell function and indicate that Leydig cell dysfunction may be a factor in varicocele-induced infertility.

Semen Analysis

The presence of a varicocele may be suspected based on the results of semen analysis. The initial change in the spermiogram consists in a reduction of sperm motility, but it is soon followed by the appearance of the classic "stress pattern" consisting in oligospermia, poor semen motility, increased numbers of abnormal spermatozoa including tapering forms, and the presence of immature cells of the germinal line.[92] In one study, sperm concentration ranged from 64 million/ml for normal men, to 45 million/ml in fertile men with varicoceles, to a low of 19 million/ml for infertile men with varicoceles.[105a] Correlation between the spermiogram and testicular histology is not always possible. Spermatologic changes can be found in 65 to 93 percent of men with varicoceles.[71] The "stress pattern" is not diagnostic of a varicocele,[16] as it can also be induced by antispermatogenic agents, certain viral diseases, allergic reactions, and endocrinopathies.[19,27] Infertile men with varicocele have a higher incidence of poor penetration on sperm penetration assay than fertile men with or without varicocele.[121a]

Biopsy Findings

Testicular biopsies of affected children have demonstrated a progression of histologic changes.[71] Desquamation of immature spermatozoa and their preceding stages coupled with disorganization of the maturational sequence of the germ cell layers are seen in the seminiferous tubules. If the varicocele continues to exert its effect, peritubular fibrosis and a reduction in the number of secondary spermatocytes develop. Severe tubular damage may proceed to total depletion of the germ cells with concomitant reduction in the tubular diameter. Degenerative cytoplasmic and nuclear changes occur in the Sertoli cells, and tubular sclerosis progresses. The same changes are seen in adults with varicoceles, though in more severe form. Ultrastructural changes include abnormalities in spermatid orientation, nuclear morphology, and Sertoli–germ cell junctional complexes.[28] Leydig cells are usually present in normal numbers but on occasion are hyperplastic.[116] Vascular changes have been described and may be confined to the venular side of the vasculature or may involve pre- and post-capillary vessels.[10,71] These vascular alterations consist in luminal narrowing due to proliferation of enlarged endothelial cells, vessel wall and periadventitial fibrosis, and occasionally myoepithelial proliferation. It has been suggested that the resulting vascular occlusion may contribute to Leydig cell or germinal epithelial dysfunction.

Testicular changes in varicocele patients are not restricted to the typical appearance of premature sloughing of germinal epithelium but, instead, may show maturation arrest at the primary spermatocyte or spermatid stage, normal histology, a Sertoli-cell–only pattern, or tubular and peritubular fibrosis.[19] Even in patients with a unilateral varicocele both testes are adversely affected, though the changes may be less pronounced on the contralateral side.

Therapy

The conventional treatment for a varicocele is high ligation of the internal spermatic vein.[49] Percutaneous treatment by instillation of a sclerosing agent and spermatic vein embolization has also been employed.[27,121] The role of spermatic vein ligation in children remains controversial. Early surgical intervention might avert progressive and irreversible testicular damage; however, the mere presence of a varicocele is not an indication for surgery. Other possible causes for the infertility must first be excluded. If no abnormality is found and the varicocele is associated with a semen "stress pattern," varicocelectomy may be warranted. It must be remembered that varicoceles are occasionally caused by venous obstruction due to tumor or other abnormalities that produce extrinsic venous compression.[20]

Varicocelectomy results in improvement in the semen quality in 60 to 80 percent of patients with a subsequent pregnancy rate of 30 to 55 percent.[19,108,114a] Varicocelectomy in teenage patients can reverse the testicular growth failure associated with varicoceles.[82a] Improvement in sperm motility is generally more profound than improvement in sperm count or morphology. The best results are seen in cases of oligospermia rather than azoospermia, although azoospermia does not rule out the possibility of improvement in semen quality.[40] In patients with preoperative counts less than 10 million per milliliter, Amelar and Dubin recommended empiric postoperative treatment with hCG.[8] Attempts to improve spermatogenic potential are usually unsuccessful in patients with markedly diminished testicular volume, in those with FSH levels more than twice normal, and in the presence of bilateral Sertoli-cell–only syndrome. Preoperative biopsies showing marked sloughing, tubular fibrosis, or Leydig cell hyperplasia have all been associated with reduced pregnancy rates.[97] The finding of elevated preoperative gonadotropin and prolactin responses to GnRH and thyrotropin-releasing hormone, respectively, may be associated with an increased likelihood of improvement in the semen following varicocele repair.[73] In most patients failure of a varicocelectomy to achieve its goal results from irreversible testicular damage caused by the varicocele or by factors unrelated to the varicocele. Cremasteric incompetence, high cross-collaterals, and multiple internal spermatic veins are recognized causes of surgical failure of varicocele ligation.[27,88a] Intraoperative venography may be particularly helpful in assuring that all veins and collaterals are ligated.[88a,169a]

Mulcahy[104] has reported a simple and interesting approach to the treatment of patients with varicocele, oligospermia and reduced motility, or both. The patient applies a small pack of ice to the scrotum nightly, held in place by jockey-type underwear, to provide local testicular hypothermia. The effects on the patients' love life were not reported, but there was at least a twofold increase in sperm count (from 22 million to 65 million per milliliter) and corresponding increases in sperm motility (from 32 to 51 percent) in 65 percent of patients subjected to such therapy. This approach serves to underline the deleterious effects of hyperthermia on sperm production.

Hypospermatogenesis

Hypospermatogenesis, also called *germinal cell hypoplasia,* is a common histologic finding in testicular specimens from biopsies performed for infertility.[28,45,99,166] Seminiferous tubule diameter is usually within normal limits but may be slightly diminished. All of the normal spermatogenic cells are present in approximately normal proportions, but the number of each variety is reduced (Fig. 25-13). The consequence is overall thinning of the germinal epithelium, often accompanied by luminal enlargement. The least affected cases show only a slight quantitative change from normal, but in more severe cases only scanty precursors and spermatozoa are seen. In these more severe cases the paucity of germinal cells causes the Sertoli cells to be more conspicuous, creating a picture resembling the Sertoli-cell–only syndrome (see

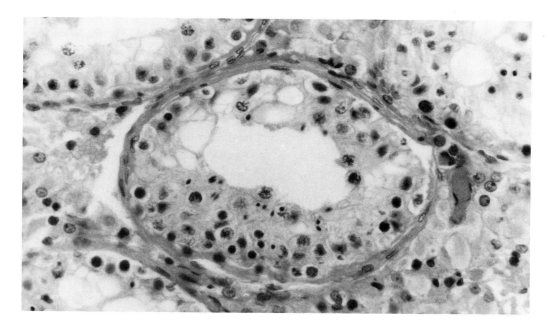

Fig. 25-13 Hypospermatogenesis. Although all of the normal germinal epithelial cells are present, they are reduced in number. The tunica propria and Leydig cells are unaffected. ×504.

Table 25-5 Conditions Associated with Hypospermatogenesis on Testicular Biopsy

Malnutrition
Chronic wasting illness
Advancing age
Exposure to excessive heat
Idiopathic hypospermatogenesis
Down's syndrome
XXY/XY
Antecedent febrile illness
Exposure to insecticides
Ductal obstruction
Glucocorticoid excess
Hypothyroidism
Fertile eunuch syndrome
Chemotherapy
Hyperprolactinemia

below); and in fact, some cases of the Sertoli-cell–only syndrome may represent the end-stage of germinal cell hypoplasia. Occasional tubules may contain sloughed immature spermatogenic cells. The tunica propria is generally not thickened, and the Leydig cells are usually normal in appearance. Affected patients are oligospermic, and in most cases serum gonadotropins and testosterone levels are normal.[165] Patients with a hypocellular specimen may respond to treatment with hCG[87] or clomiphene citrate.[159]

This histologic picture may result from a variety of causes, as shown in Table 25-5. Testicular histology is not generally helpful in identifying the causative agent, which instead must be ascertained by a careful history and physical examination combined with appropriate laboratory studies. Patients with hypothyroidism may have reduced fertility, and the only abnormality on biopsy is hypoplasia of the germinal epithelium. Thyroxine replacement often restores fertility.[165] Hypospermatogenesis is a common finding in patients treated with alkylating agents or combination chemotherapy (see below).[150]

FERTILE EUNUCH SYNDROME

Fertile eunuch syndrome, also known as the *Pasqualini syndrome,* is a form of hypogonadotropic eunuchoidism. It is one of the few causes of hypospermatogenesis that may be suspected histologically. The patients usually present with failure to progress through puberty and exhibit the clinical signs of eunuchoidism and variable secondary sexual development. On physical examination, however, the testes are normal or near normal in size. With this syndrome, FSH secretion is normal, LH production is deficient to varying degrees, and serum testosterone levels are low.[142,158] It is presumed that the amount of LH secreted by such patients is sufficient to assist FSH in promoting spermatogenesis to varying extents although insufficient to sustain normal levels of androgen in the peripheral tissues or to bring about full development of the secondary sex characteristics. The etiology of the isolated partial deficiency of LH is unclear. Testicular biopsy reveals either near-normal spermatogenesis or hypospermatogenesis. Leydig cells are absent or inapparent. The ejaculate contains small numbers of sperm.

Treatment with hCG frequently improves spermatogenic activity and increases testosterone production, thereby stimulating completion of male development.[151] Some have advised therapy with a mixture of LH and FSH.

Spermatogenic Maturation Arrest

Maturation arrest is present in 12 to 32 percent of testicular biopsies in infertile men.[150] With this condition the spermatogenic process fails abruptly to progress beyond one of the early stages of maturation. The point of arrest varies among patients but is constant in all the tubules of a given patient. The most common finding is failure of spermatogenesis to proceed beyond the primary spermatocyte level; less commonly, arrest can occur at the spermatogonial, secondary spermatocyte, or spermatid stages (Fig. 25-14). The preceding cell types are present in normal

Fig. 25-14 Maturation arrest. **(A)** Failure of spermatogenesis to proceed beyond the primary spermatocyte stage, shown here, is the most common finding in patients with a maturation block. **(B)** Germ cell maturation abruptly ceases at the spermatid level. **A,** ×679 **B,** ×372.

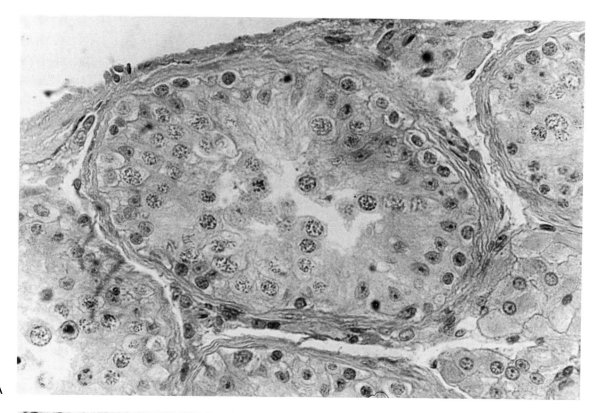

A

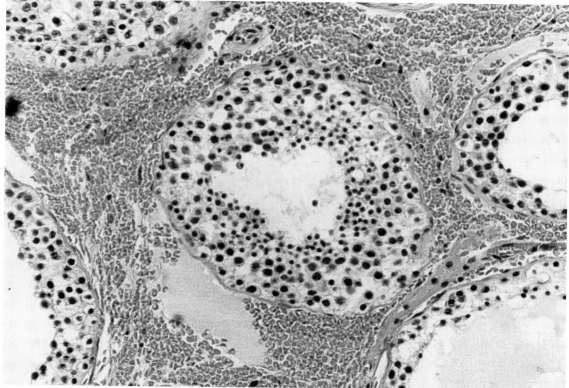

B

amounts, whereas cell types beyond the arrested stage are absent or are present in small numbers. The arrested cells, whatever the stage of their development, may be increased in number and can be found sloughed into the tubular lumens. Electron microscopy reveals degenerative nuclear and cytoplasmic changes in late pachytene spermatocytes.[150] Tubular diameter is usually within normal limits, and no light microscopic abnormalities are generally detectable in the Sertoli cells, basement membranes, tunica propria, or Leydig cells. An accumulation of cytoplasmic glycogen and abnormally dilated cisternae have been described in the Sertoli cells.[123] Areas of spermatogenic arrest have been described in association with testicular atrophy with tubular hyalinization, suggesting that some cases of tubular hyalinization may be the end-stage of maturation arrest.[150]

Clinically, patients with maturation arrest are either azoospermic or markedly oligospermic. Plasma gonadotropins and testosterone are generally normal. FSH may be elevated with severe arrest.[165] In most patients the cause is indeterminable, but a defect in chromosome synapse or meiotic division has been proposed.[9] Other possible causes include cogenital or acquired defects in Sertoli cell function[112] and defective action of gonadotropic hormones.[9]

The histologic picture of maturation arrest has been associated with a large variety of conditions (Table 25-6). Thorough clinical evaluation is mandatory for elucidation of possible causes. Although the testicular histology does not permit ascertainment of a specific etiology, maturation arrest at the secondary spermatocyte stage is most commonly seen in cases of *heat damage* to the testes.[9] Some of these patients have a documented chronic occupational exposure to a high-temperature environment. A few have a history of a severe and prolonged antecedent febrile illness.[95,165]

Decreased testicular function occurs in more than one-half of men with *traumatic paraplegia*.[102] Spermatogenic arrest is commonly found with paraplegia, but testicular atrophy with tubular hyalinization has also been described. The abnormal spermatogenesis is thought to be secondary to increased gonadal temperature due to interruption of the lumbar sympathetic nerve supply. Absence of the cremasteric reflex may further impair temperature regulation.

Gonadal and sexual disturbances are commonly encountered in patients with *glucocorticoid excess* of either endogenous or exogenous origin. Affected patients are oligospermic, and testicular biopsy reveals either maturation arrest or hypospermatogenesis.[165] When the glucocorticoid excess is corrected, improvement in sperm counts and fertility may occur.

Although the *XYY syndrome* affects approximately 0.21 percent of the male population, the relation of this chromosome abnormality to testicular insufficiency remains poorly defined.[151] Sperm counts vary from normal to azoospermic. Hormone levels may be normal, or elevated gonadotropins and low testosterone may be encountered.[74,151] Histologic examination of the testes may reveal maturation arrest, Sertoli-cell–only syndrome (see below), or tubular hyalinization and sclerosis.[74,131,147] Affected individuals are tall and may exhibit antisocial behavior.

Rosewater's syndrome is a rare, inherited abnormality in which the affected individual is hypogonadal with congenital gynecomastia. The phallus and prostate are small, but the testes are of normal size and show maturation arrest and a decrease in the number of

Table 25-6 Conditions Associated with Spermatogenic Maturation Arrest on Testicular Biopsy

Idiopathic arrest	Exposure to excessive heat
XYY	Exposure to noxious chemicals
Varicocele	Postpubertal gonadotropin deficiency
Abnormal meiosis	Prior vasectomy
Down's syndrome	Mumps orchitis
Uremia	Glucocorticoid excess
Rosewater's syndrome	Isolated FSH deficiency
Cystis fibrosis	Sickle cell anemia
Androgenital syndrome	Chemotherapy
Antecedent febrile illness	Spinal cord injury

Leydig cells. This syndrome results from an abnormality in the action of androgen on target cells and is a mild form of familial, incomplete male pseudohermaphroditism, type I[151] (see Ch. 24). Gonadotropin therapy has had limited success in the treatment of maturation arrest.[58] In patients with arrest at the spermatid level, testosterone rebound therapy may be effective[87]; however, testosterone administration may cause prolonged suppression of spermatogenesis and should be avoided.[128]

Sertoli-Cell—Only Syndrome

The Sertoli-cell—only syndrome, also known as *germinal aplasia* or *Del Castillo's syndrome,* is encountered in about 3 percent of biopsy specimens from infertile men.[151] It is characterized by the absence of germinal epithelium without impairment of Sertoli or Leydig cells. The seminiferous tubules are decreased in diameter and are devoid of germ cells, being lined exclusively by a single layer of elongated Sertoli cells (Fig. 25-15). Although aligned vertically to the basement membrane of the tubules, their apices may be inclined to one side, producing an appearance resembling "windswept treetops."[148] The cytoplasm of the Sertoli cells often contains large numbers of fat vacuoles. In some cases of Sertoli-cell—only syndrome,[164a] as well as postpubertal cryptorchid testes,[28a] the Sertoli cell cytoplasm contains coarse eosinophilic granules that are PAS-positive and diastase resistant and may be so numerous as to push the nucleus aside. These granules are thought to represent secondary lysosomes, though the origin within them is speculative.[164a] A high proportion of the tubules may be lined by immature Sertoli cells.[112] Ultrastructural abnormalities of Sertoli cell junctions have been described.[134] In rare biopsies a few tubules may contain residual germ cells, consisting predominantly of spermatogonia or spermatocytes. The tubular basement membrane is normal or minimally thickened, and characteristically the tunica propria is unremarkable. Leydig cells are usually present in normal numbers but are occasionally increased or decreased. The Leydig cell cytoplasm may be multivacuolated.[115] Although an infrequent patient may have a few sperm in the ejaculate, azoospermia is the rule. The Sertoli-cell—only syndrome comprises about 17 percent of all cases of azoospermia.[1] These patients are potent but infertile and usually have well developed secondary

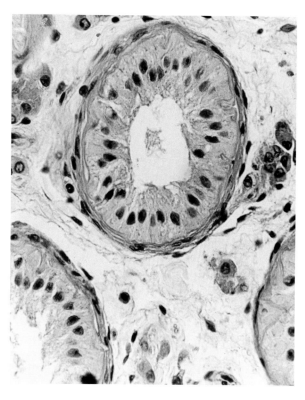

Fig. 25-15 Sertoli-cell—only syndrome. The seminiferous tubule is lined solely by elongated Sertoli cells. The Leydig cell population and tunica propria appear normal. ×300.

sex characteristics. The size of the testes may be slightly decreased. Most have normal serum LH and testosterone levels, but FSH is almost invariably increased as a response to the absence or near absence of spermatogenesis. There is a statistically significant correlation between the BW 35 HLA-B locus and germ cell aplasia.[80] The Sertoli-cell—only syndrome is currently untreatable.

This syndrome has been regarded as a congenital defect — hence the name germinal cell aplasia — and has been related to failure of the primitive germ cells to migrate from the yolk sac wall to the developing gonadal primordia.[46] The presence of immature Sertoli cells in many of the tubules supports the theory of a congenital defect. Although some cases may be congenital in origin, it seems probable that the Sertoli-cell—only syndrome is the end result of more than one pathologic process.

This histologic picture has been associated with a variety of conditions, as shown in Table 25-7. Testic-

Table 25-7 Conditions Associated with Sertoli-Cell–Only Syndrome on Testicular Biopsy

Idiopathic (? congenital) syndrome	Uremia
Chemotherapy	Irradiation damage
Klinefelter's syndrome with mosaicism	Adrenogenital syndrome
XYY	Mumps orchitis
Down's syndrome	Isolated FSH deficiency
Varicocele	Hyperprolactinemia

ular histology is not generally helpful for elucidating a specific etiology, although hyperplasia of the Leydig cells and basement membrane thickening in conjunction with the Sertoli-cell–only pattern are suggestive of 17-ketosteroid dehydrogenase or reductase deficiency.[38]

CHEMOTHERAPEUTIC AGENTS

The improved survival rate of patients with cancer, including those treated during their reproductive years, has stimulated interest in the effects of cancer chemotherapy on fertility. Among the commonly used cytotoxic drugs, alkylating agents, particularly cyclophosphamide and chlorambucil, have been most frequently associated with the development of infertility.[133] (Cyclophosphamide has also been used extensively in the treatment of glomerulonephritis and nephrotic syndrome.) Some drugs, e.g., doxorubicin,[42] seem to have less impact on sperm production than others. The occurrence of infertility in men receiving single alkylating agents is dose-related. Total doses of less than 6 mg of cyclophosphamide may produce oligospermia, but azoospermia is infrequently seen until 6 to 10 mg of the drug has been administered.[133] Although azoospermia commonly occurs in patients treated with a total dose of chlorambucil of more than 400 mg, lesser doses may produce progressive but reversible oligospermia. Combination chemotherapy has profound effects on spermatogenesis. More than 80 percent of men treated with the MOPP regimen (mechlorethamine, vincristine, procarbazine, and prednisone) for Hodgkin's disease become azoospermic or severely oligospermic. Information on the testicular effects of the new agents is incomplete.

The literature on the effects of chemotherapy on gonadal function in children is contradictory and complex owing to the variable introduced by the continuum of sexual development present in these patients. The data suggest that the prepubertal testis may be more resistant to the effects of alkylating agents than is the adult gonad.[119] Other authors[70] have found that there is no good relation between the abnormal morphology and the age at therapy, prepubertal testes suffering as extensively as postpubertal ones. However, a threshold drug dose appears to exist above which germinal epithelial injury will occur in the prepubertal testis. In contrast, antineoplastic drugs administered during puberty may have profound effects on the germinal epithelium and Leydig cell function.[24]

There are common histologic features in the testis that appear to be largely independent of the type of drug or drugs used but related to the total dose of therapy administered. Cytotoxic drugs predominantly affect the germinal epithelium resulting in germ cell depletion and the Sertoli-cell–only syndrome.[70,133,140,141,143] Occasional tubules contain residual germ cells. Hypospermatogenesis is present in some biopsy specimens,[150] and others have a pattern of peritubular fibrosis associated with germ cell depletion.[70,100,150] Maturation arrest has also been reported in patients treated with chemotherapeutic agents.[126] Regardless of the severity of the germinal epithelial changes, the Sertoli and Leydig cells remain morphologically normal in appearance, although Leydig cell hyperplasia may be present.

Clinically, there may be diminished testicular volume, severe oligospermia or azoospermia, decreased sperm motility, increased numbers of abnormal sperm forms, and infertility.[41] FSH levels are often markedly increased, particularly in azoospermic men. Normal or low serum testosterone levels in conjunction with increased LH levels in many of these men indicates a degree of Leydig cell dysfunction.[56,162] This dysfunction may manifest as gynecomastia, decreased libido, or changes in the secondary sexual characteristics in adults.[133,140,141]

Data on the frequency of recovery of spermatogenesis and fertility after cessation of the chemotherapy are incomplete. Recovery is likely related to the total dose, type of drug, and perhaps most importantly the duration of time off therapy. The reports of recovery of spermatogenesis in patients treated with single cytotoxic agents are encouraging. Treatment with combination regimens may produce more long-lasting azoospermia than does single-agent therapy, but recovery is possible. Recovery of spermatogenesis is unpredictable; but even in patients showing the Sertoli-cell–only pattern on biopsy occasional spermatogonia may remain, suggesting a potential for recovery. The age at which the chemotherapy is administered may be a factor.[141] Combined cytotoxic and radiation injury to the testes may preclude recovery. Long-term follow-up studies are needed to assess the ultimate impact of chemotherapy on testicular function. To date, the risk of chromosome abnormalities in the sperm of men who do recover is unknown. Flow cytometry studies of sperm nuclei from patients who recovered from multiagent chemotherapy did not detect sperm chromatin abnormalities; however, one of the men did father a child with multiple congenital malformations.[54]

Peritubular Fibrosis and Tubular Hyalinization

Although nearly every testicular biopsy contains a few tubules that show peritubular fibrosis, generalized thickening of the peritubular tissue is rarely seen in the testes of fertile men. This process may involve the tunica propria only, in which case there are increased numbers of peritubular fibroblasts, or it may be confined to a band of hyalinized material between the basement membrane and tunica propria. In other biopsy specimens the basement membrane may be involved in the hyalinized band, or both tunica propria and basement membrane may show sclerotic changes. The germinal epithelium is damaged by the interposition of fibrous tissue between it and its vascular supply. When these changes are present in more than 10 percent of the seminiferous tubules, fertility is almost invariably reduced.[109]

The fibrotic process may be essentially regional, or it may be widespread, with many tubules showing variable degrees of fibrosis or hyalinization. The fibrosis is often progressive, eventually involving larger numbers of tubules. It appears that the sperm-producing capacity of the testis is impaired to a degree proportional to the extent and severity of the fibrotic process.

The spermatogenic epithelium is more sensitive than the Sertoli cells to testicular fibrosis. With increasing fibrosis and hyalinization, there is a progressive loss of germinal epithelium (Fig. 25-16), followed by atrophy of the Sertoli cells. Finally, both germ cells and Sertoli cells disappear, and the lumens

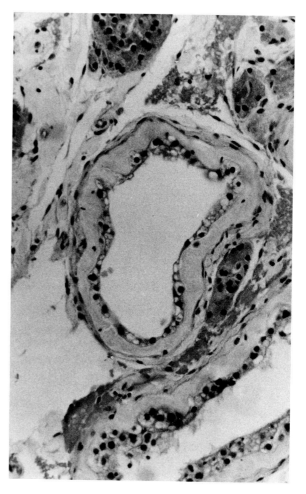

Fig. 25-16 Tubular hyalinization. A thick hyalinized band is interposed between the atropic germinal epithelium and small spindle-shaped cells of the tunica propria. ×300.

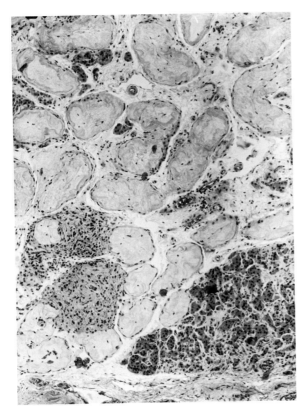

Fig. 25-17 Klinefelter's syndrome. The seminiferous epithelium is entirely replaced by hyalinized material. Prominent aggregates of Leydig cells are present. × 49.

of the tubules may be obliterated by abundant hyalinized material (Fig. 25-17). As this process progresses, the tubules are gradually reduced in diameter. Elastic fibers deposited at puberty in response to pituitary gonadotropin stimulation are generally present around the seminiferous tubules. Leydig cells occur in variable but usually reduced numbers. The intertubular areas contain unusual amounts of collagenous tissue and fibroblasts. Even in advanced cases some tubules show only partial fibrosis or are relatively undamaged.

Peritubular fibrosis and tubular hyalinization is a nonspecific picture that can be seen in a large variety of pathologic conditions (Table 25-8), the more important of which are discussed in the following sections. It is probable that other morphologic patterns of testicular damage may eventuate in this end-stage testis. Unfortunately, there is no treatment for patients with peritubular fibrosis and tubular hyalinization.[87]

KLINEFELTER'S SYNDROME

The syndrome of hypogonadal men with small, firm testes, gynecomastia, a tendency toward eunuchoid build, and increased gonadotropins was originally described by Klinefelter et al. in 1942.[86] It is a relatively common cause of frank hypogonadism, with an estimated incidence of 1 per 500 male newborns.[151] Patients with classic Klinefelter's syndrome have small testes and poorly developed secondary sexual characteristics. About two-thirds of these patients have an XXY karyotype, with the remaining patients having various combinations of poly-X and poly-Y or chromosome deletions and mosaicisms.[142,151] Klinefelter's syndrome may be caused by nondisjunction and may be attributable to advanced paternal or maternal age.

Table 25-8 Conditions Associated with Peritubular Fibrosis and Tubular Hyalinization on Testicular Biopsy

Idiopathic disturbance	Decreased testicular vascular supply
Klinefelter's syndrome	Myotonic muscular dystrophy
Adrenogenital syndrome	Varicocele
XYY	Alcoholism
Mumps orchitis	Diabetes mellitus
Reifenstein's syndrome	Cystic fibrosis
Postpubertal androgen or estrogen excess	Spinal cord injury
Irradiation damage	Chemotherapy
Postpubertal hypopituitarism	Androgen insensitivity in otherwise normal men
Testicular trauma	Hyperprolactinemia

Patients usually seek medical advice because of delayed completion of puberty, gynecomastia, eunuchoidism, or infertility. These signs typically appear sometime after puberty when the intrinsically abnormal testes, unable to respond to gonadotropin stimulation, begin to undergo regressive changes. The testes fail to increase in size and, instead, become firm and smaller because of progressive seminiferous tubule fibrosis and hyalinization. Plasma LH and FSH levels are markedly elevated, and the testosterone level is either within the normal range or low. Patients with an XXY chromosome complement are typically azoospermic, but spermatozoa and even fertility have been observed.[11] Fertile patients are most likely mosaics.

The presence of abnormal numbers of X chromosomes in testicular tissue is the basis for the pathologic changes observed in the seminiferous tubules and Leydig cells.[165] In prepubertal testes a decrease in the number of spermatogonia in the tubules is the only abnormality. The arrival of puberty brings about the alterations that lead to the typical histologic pattern of this syndrome. The earliest derangement noted in postpubertal testes is a reduction in spermatogenic activity. The loss of germ cells is associated with thickening of the tunica propria and is followed by atrophy of the Sertoli cells. Eventually, both germ cells and Sertoli cells are lost, and the lumens of the tubules become obliterated by the thickened, hyalinized, and contracted tunica propria (Fig. 25-17). Finally, the tubules are converted to shrunken collagenous cords. At first these changes do not affect all of the seminiferous tubules equally, and in the early stages the involvement is uneven and patchy. Ultimately, virtually all the tubules are sclerosed. The number of Leydig cells is characteristically increased, but whether it represents true hyperplasia or is a consequence of condensation due to decreased testicular volume is still debated.[4,51,166] Despite their hyperplastic appearance, Leydig cell function is impaired, as the serum testosterone level is low despite an elevated LH level. Histologically, the Leydig cells are immature and show progressive cytoplasmic degeneration as well as failure of appearance of the normal secretory changes. On ultrastructural study, a large proportion of the Leydig cells reveal abnormal differentiation.[115] The peritubular elastic fibers that normally appear during pubertal maturation are absent or markedly diminished, reflecting the congenital nature of the syndrome. In mosaics, biopsies reveal less severe fibrosis, and the tubules contain more mature germ cells than in the classic form.[118]

There is treatment for the infertile state associated with Klinefelter's syndrome. Data suggest that patients with this condition are predisposed to the development of germ cell tumors of extragonadal origin.[98]

Reifenstein's syndrome, a type of incomplete androgen insensitivity, is clinically similar to Klinefelter's syndrome, but these patients have a normal karyotype. They usually exhibit a male phenotype, perineal hypospadias, bifid scrotum, gynecomastia, high gonadotropin levels, and azoospermia. The testes show a marked histologic resemblance to Klinefelter's syndrome.[151]

MUMPS ORCHITIS

Orchitis is a rare complication of mumps parotitis in children, but when it does occur most patients recover without gonadal sequelae. When testicular infection occurs at puberty or during adult life, permanent damage to the germinal epithelium often results.[127] About one-third of patients with mumps orchitis are bilaterally affected, and 50 percent of the involved testes will become atrophic. There is no convincing evidence that any form of therapy is effective for preventing the testicular atrophy and subsequent sterility.

In the subacute and chronic phases the interstitial tissue is infiltrated by lymphocytes (Fig. 25-18). There are progressive chronic tubular changes consisting in loss of germ cells and tubular hyalinization and sclerosis. Tubular involvement is not uniform throughout the testes, some tubules being more affected than others. Elastic fibers are present around the seminiferous tubules. The Leydig cells appear to be less susceptible to the mumps viris and are nearly intact.

Because of the progressive nature of the chronic changes, the full extent of the damage may not become evident until 10 to 20 years after the acute infection. A history of mumps orchitis is necessary to confirm the histologic diagnosis. Affected patients are oligospermic or azoospermic, and FSH levels are increased. LH and testosterone levels are generally normal.

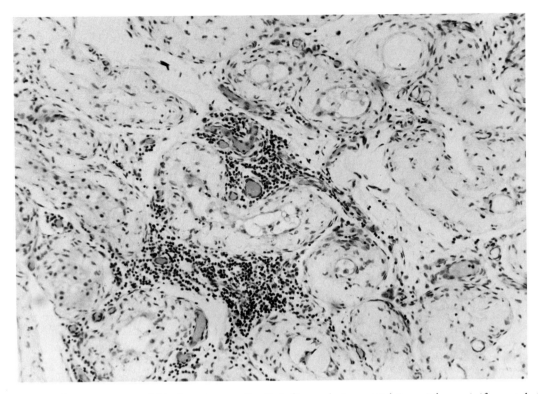

Fig. 25-18 Chronic mumps orchitis. Lymphocytes focally infiltrate the interstitial tissue. The seminiferous tubules are converted to collagenous cords. ×210.

POSTPUBERTAL HYPOGONADOTROPIC HYPOGONADISM

If hypogonadotropism occurs during the postpubertal period, the seminiferous tubules, having already attained the full development associated with normal puberty, do not revert to their prepubertal appearance. Instead, the tubules show regression of spermatogenesis, a progressive loss of germ cells, reduction in diameter, and gradual thickening and hyalinization of the tunica propria.[88,156] The Leydig cells are characteristically shriveled and inconspicuous, and serum testosterone levels are decreased. The Leydig cells often contain lipochrome pigment but scarcely any crystalloids of Reinke.

Gonadal failure secondary to hypogonadotropism may be due to a hypothalamic or pituitary disorder. Causes include a space-occupying lesion in or near the pituitary or hypothalamus, trauma to the pituitary fossa, or hypophysectomy.

Therapeutic intervention may restore spermatogenesis if begun early enough. Treatment typically includes hCG, alone or in combination with human menopausal gonadotropin or FSH.[43,127]

ANDROGEN AND ESTROGEN EXCESS

Androgen and estrogen excesses act primarily by suppressing pituitary gonadotropin secretion. Most cases of estrogen excess, e.g., estrogen-producing tumors of the adrenal cortex or testis, occur during the postpubertal period. In particular, weightlifters and other atheletes may take androgens because of their anabolic effects on skeletal muscle, without realizing their deleterious effect on the testis. Endogenous or exogenous excess of androgens may also occur postpubertally. When excess androgen or estrogen levels develop during the postpubertal period, histologic changes occur in the testes that are identical to those seen with postpubertal hypogonadotropic hypogonadism. Unless the sex hormone elevation is corrected before all spermatogonia are lost, no recovery is possible.

RADIATION-INDUCED CHANGES

Improvements in survival of cancer patients who undergo radiation therapy during their reproductive years has required an evaluation of the possible undesirable consequences of the unavoidable gonadal irradiation that occurs in some of these cases. The different germ cell stages have varying sensitivities to radiation.[65] Spermatids are extremely resistant, spermatocytes are relatively resistant, and spermatogonia are sensitive to the effects of radiation.[34] Spermatogonia are damaged at doses of 10 rads or more. In most instances human gonadal exposures are insufficient to cause permanent sterility.[89] After undergoing testicular irradiation, the patient remains fertile until the postspermatogonial germ cells are depleted. This stage is followed by a phase of sterility, the length of which varies. Complete recovery may occur within 9 to 18 months after doses of 100 rads or less, but recovery may not occur until 5 years or more after doses of 400 to 600 rads.[89] The dosage at which permanent sterility results is probably in excess of 600 rads. Following doses of this magnitude, the germ cells degenerate and are eventually lost, leaving tubules that are lined only by Sertoli cells. The tubular diameter decreases, and the tunica propria progressively thickens. Eventually, there is total sclerosis of the lumens. The Leydig cells are usually preserved, and testosterone and LH levels are normal. Pituitary FSH secretion is increased as a consequence of the loss of the germinal epithelium.

ALCOHOLISM

Chronic alcoholism has been associated with profound gonadal failure, apparently resulting from combined hypothalamic–pituitary and testicular dysfunction.[2] The hypogonadism is characterized by testicular atrophy due to germ cell depletion accompanied by peritubular fibrosis and hyalinization. These patients have increased conversion of testosterone to estradiol as well as some evidence of primary Leydig cell failure.[44]

UREMIA

Chronic renal failure is frequently associated with decreased libido, impotence, and impaired spermatogenesis.[107] Azoospermia or severe oligospermia occurs in most patients with end-stage renal failure. Histologic changes include loss of germinal epithelium, thickening of the tubular basement membranes, and tubular hyalinization.[135] Spermatogenic maturation arrest has been observed in other cases. Plasma testosterone is decreased, and LH levels are increased. There is evidence of altered hypothalamic–pituitary feedback sensitivity and primary gonadal damage in uremic men.[103]

MYOTONIC MUSCULAR DYSTROPHY

Myotonic muscular dystrophy is characterized by progressive muscle weakness and atrophy, myotonia, cataracts, mental retardation, and frontal baldness. Hypogonadism occurs in about 80 percent of patients.[103] The testicular failure appears to be primarily gonadal. The Leydig cells are generally spared, but seminiferous tubular damage occurs, ranging from abnormal spermatogenesis to complete tubular fibrosis.

ANDROGEN INSENSITIVITY IN OTHERWISE NORMAL MEN

Androgen insensitivity has been identified in some patients with severe oligospermia or azoospermia.[5,6,137] These phenotypic males have abnormal wolffian duct structures, elevated plasma LH and testosterone levels, and less than half-normal amounts of androgen receptors in genital skin fibroblasts. A testicular biopsy in one affected individual revealed peritubular hyalinization and seminiferous tubules lined only by Sertoli cells.[6] An androgen insensitivity index, the product of the serum testosterone (nanograms per milliliter) and LH (milli-international units per milliliter) concentrations has been proposed to identify these patients. An index of more than 200 suggests androgen insensitivity. Studies indicate that this index identifies only 30 percent of phenotypically normal, infertile men who have androgen insensitivity.[5] The remaining 70 percent can be diagnosed only by performing androgen-binding capacity studies on scrotal skin fibroblasts. These patients are not amenable to therapy.

HYPERPROLACTINEMIA

Hyperprolactinemia may be idiopathic or may be associated with a variety of pathologic states, including a pituitary or hypothalamic tumor, drug use (tranquilizers, neuroleptics, and antihypertensives), hypothyroidism, excessive exogenous estrogens, chest trauma, choriocarcinoma of the testis, adrenocortical tumors, metastatic renal carcinoma, and renal insufficiency.[139,164] Men with markedly elevated serum prolactin may present with loss of libido, impotence, hypogonadotropic hypogonadism, glactorrhea, or infertility. Clinical manifestations other than infertility are usually lacking in those with mild increases in serum prolactin. The pathophysiology of hyperprolactinemia-induced infertility in men is not well understood. Nonetheless, hyperprolactinemia is encountered in 2 or 4 percent of men with idiopathic oligospermia, and treatment with bromocriptine may improve the semen quality.[164] Testicular biopsy in these men may show thickening of the tunica propria accompanied by a reduction in the number of germ cells, hypospermatogenesis, or the Sertoli-cell–only syndrome.

REFERENCES

1. Abdalla MI, Ibrahim II, Rizk AM, et al: Endocrine studies of azoospermia. II. Serum steroid levels in obstructive azoospermia. Arch Androl 3:63, 1979
2. Abel EL: A review of alcohol's effects on sex and reproduction. Drug Alcohol Depend 5:321, 1980
3. Agarwal VP, Singh H, Chaudhury SK: Testicular biopsy in azoospermia; a morphologic appraisal. Indian J Med Sci 28:285, 1974
4. Ahmad KN, Lennox B, Mack WS: Estimation of the volume of Leydig cells in man. Lancet 2:461, 1969
5. Aiman J, Griffin JE: The frequency of androgen resistance as a cause of infertility in men. Endocrinology, suppl., 108:263, 1981
6. Aiman J, Griffin JE, Gazak JM, et al: Androgen insensitivity as a cause of infertility in otherwise normal men. N Engl J Med 300:223, 1979
7. Albers DD, Males JL: Seminoma in hypogonadotropic hypogonadism associated with anosmia (Kallmann's syndrome). J Urol 126:57, 1981
8. Amelar RD, Dubin L: Surgical management of male infertility. Clin Obstet Gynecol 22:221, 1979
9. Amelar RD, Dubin L, Walsh PC: Male Infertility. Saunders, Philadelphia, 1977
10. Andres TL, Triner TD, Lapenas DJ: Small vessel alterations in the testis of infertile men with varicocele. Am J Clin Pathol 76:378, 1981
11. Arce B, Padron S: Spermatogenesis in Klinefelter's syndrome. Reproduction 4:177, 1980
12. Averback P: Branching of seminiferous tubules associated with hypofertility and chronic respiratory infection. Arch Pathol Lab Med 104:361, 1980
13. Averback P: Histopathological diagnosis of hypercurved seminiferous tubules. Histopathology 4:75, 1980
14. Averback P, Wright DGD: Seminiferous tubule hypercurvature: a newly recognized common syndrome of human male infertility. Lancet 1:181, 1979
15. Axelrod L, Neer RM, Kliman B: Hypogonadism in a male with immunologically active biologically inactive luteinizing hormone an exception to a venerable rule. J Clin Endocrinol Metab 48:279, 1979
16. Azodeji O, Baker HWG: Is there a specific abnormality of sperm morphology in men with varicoceles? Fertil Steril 45:839, 1986
17. Bardin CW, Ross GT, Rifkind AB, et al: Studies of the pituitary-Leydig cell axis in young men with hypogonadotropic hypogonadism and hyposmia: comparison with normal men, prepuberal boys, and hypopituitary patients. J Clin Invest 48:2046, 1969
18. Batrinos ML, Panitsa-Faflia C, Pitoulis S, Petraki N: Pituitary-gonadal function in three relatives presenting with Kallman's syndrome. Horm Res 12:79, 1980
19. Belker AM: The varicocele and male infertility. Urol Clin North Am 8:41, 1981
20. Berger OG: Varicocele in adolescence. Clin Pediatr 19:810, 1980
21. Bibbo M, Gill WB: Screening of adolescents exposed to diethylstilbestrol in utero. Pediatr Clin North Am 28:379, 1981
22. Binor Z, Sokoloski JE, Wolf DP: Penetration of the zona-free hamster egg by human sperm. Fertil Steril 33:321, 1980
23. Blanc WA, Franciosi R, Wigger HJ: Pathology of the organs of reproduction in cystic fibrosis. I. Testes and prostate in prepubertal and early pubertal cases. p. 13. In: Cystic Fibrosis Club Abstracts. Cystic Fibrosis Foundation, Atlanta, 1965
24. Blatt J, Poplack DG, Sherins RJ: Testicular function in boys after chemotherapy for acute lymphoblastic leukemia. N Engl J Med 304:1121, 1981
25. Bostofte E, Serup J, Rebbe H: Relation between morphologically abnormal spermatozoa and pregnancies

obtained during a twenty-year follow-up period. Int J Androl 5:379, 1982

26. Brown JS, Dubin L, Becker M, Hotchkiss RS: Venography in the subfertile man with varicocele. J Urol 98:388, 1967

27. Caldamone AA, Cockett ATK: Recent advances in male infertility research. Urol Clin North Am 8:63, 1981

28. Cameron DF, Snyde FE, Ross MH, et al: Ultrastructural alterations in the adluminal testicular compartment in men with varicocele. Fertil Steril 33:526, 1980

28a. Chan KW, Ma LT: Eosinophilic granular cells in a cryptorchid testis. Arch Pathol Lab Med 111:877, 1987

29. Chan SL, Lipshultz LI, Schwartzendruber D: Deoxyribonucleic acid (DNA) flow cytometry: a new modality for quantitative analysis of testicular biopsies. Fertil Steril 41:485, 1984

30. Chapman ES, Heidger PM, Harrison RM, et al: Vasectomy in rhesus monkeys. Anat Rec 192:41, 1978

31. Charny CW: Reflections on testicular biopsy. Fertil Steril 14:610, 1963

32. Charny CW: Testicular biopsy: its value in male sterility. JAMA 115:1429, 1940

33. Charny CW: Treatment of male infertility. p. 649. In Behrman JJ, Kestner RW (eds): Progress in Infertility. Little, Brown, Boston, 1968

34. Clarke SJ, Resnick MI: Infertility following radiation and chemotherapy. Urol Clin North Am 5:531, 1978

35. Cockett ATK, Al-Juburi A, Altebarmakian V, et al: The varicocele: new experimental and clinical data. Urology 15:492, 1980

36. Cohen J, Mooyaart M, Vreeburg JTM, Zeilmaker GH: Fertilization of hamster ova by human spermatozoa in relation to other semen parameters. Int J Androl 5:210, 1982

37. Cohen MS, Warner RS: Needle biopsy of testes: a safe outpatient procedure. Urology 29:279, 1987

38. Craig JM: The pathology of infertility. Pathol Annu 10:299, 1975

39. Cunningham GR: Medical treatment of the subfertile male. Urol Clin North Am 5:537, 1978

40. Czaplicki M, Bablock L, Janczewski Z: Varicocelectomy in patients with azoospermia. Arch Androl 3:51, 1979

41. Da Cunha MF, Meistrich ML, Hage MM, et al: Temporary effects of AMSA (4'-(9-acridinylamino) methanesulfon-m-anisidide) chemotherapy on spermatogenesis. Cancer 49:2459, 1982

42. Da Cunha MF, Meistrich ML, Hubert LR, et al: Active sperm production after cancer chemotherapy with doxorubicin. J Urol 130:927, 1983

43. De Kretser DM: Endocrinology of male infertility. Br Med Bull 35:187, 1979

44. De Kretser DM: The effects of systemic disease on the function of the testes. Clin Endocrinol Metab 8:487, 1979

45. De Kretser DM, Burger HG, Fortune D, et al: Hormonal, histological and chromosomal studies in adult males with testicular disorders. J Clin Endocrinol Metab 35:392, 1972

46. Del Castillo EB, Trabucco A, de la Balze FA: Syndrome produced by absence of germinal epithelium without impairment of Sertoli or Leydig cells. J Clin Endocrinol 7:493, 1947

47. Denning CR, Sommers SC, Quigley HJ: Infertility in male patients with cystic fibrosis. Pediatrics 41:7, 1968

48. Derrick FC, Glover WL, Kanjuparamban Z, et al: Histologic changes in the seminiferous tubules after vasectomy. Fertil Steril 25:649, 1974

49. Dubin L, Amelar RD: Varicocele. Urol Clin North Am 5:563, 1978

50. Dubin L, Hotchkiss RS: Testes biopsy in subfertile men with varicocele. Fertil Steril 20:50, 1969

51. Dykes JRW: Histometric assessment of human testicular biopsies. J Pathol 97:429, 1969

52. Eliasson R: Biochemical analyses of human semen in the study of the physiology and pathophysiology of the male accessory genital glands. Fertil Steril 19:344, 1968

53. Etriby AA, Ibrahim AA, Mahmoud KZ, Elhaggar S: Subfertility and varicocele. I. Venogram demonstration of anastomosis sites in subfertile men. Fertil Steril 26:1013, 1975

54. Evenson DP, Zalmen A, Welt S, et al: Male reproductive capacity may recover following drug treatment with the L-10 protocol for acute lymphocytic leukemia. Cancer 53:30, 1984

55. Franklin RR, Dukes CD: Antispermatozoal antibody and unexplained infertility. Am J Obstet Gynecol 89:6, 1964

56. Friedman NM, Plymate SR: Leydig cell dysfunction and gynaecomastia in adult males treated with alkylating agents. Clin Endocrinol (Oxf) 12:553, 1980

57. Furuya S, Kumamoto Y, Ikegaki S: Blood-testis barrier in men with idiopathic hypogonadotropic eunuchoidism and postpuberal pituitary failure. Arch Androl 5:361, 1980

58. Fuselier HA, Beckman EN: Azoospermia: diagnosis and management. South Med J 74:731, 1981

59. Girgis SM, Etriby A, Ibrahim AA, et al: Testicular biopsy in azoospermia. Fertil Steril 20:467, 1969

60. Glass AR, Vigersky RA: Leydig cell function in idiopathic oligospermia. Fertil Steril 34:144, 1980

61. Golumb J, Vardinon N, Homonnai ZT, et al: Demonstration of antispermatozoal antibodies in varicocele-related infertility with an enzyme-linked immunosorbent assay (ELISA). Fertil Steril 45:397, 1986

62. Green KF, Turner TT, Howards SS: Varicocele: reversal of the testicular blood flow and temperature effects by varicocele repair. J Urol 131:1208, 1984

63. Greenberg SH: Varicocele and male infertility. Fertil Steril 28:699, 1977

64. Gupta AS, Kothari LH, Dhruva A, Bapna R: Surgical sterilization by vasectomy and its effect on the structure and function of the testes in man. Br J Surg 62:59, 1975

65. Hahn EW, Feingold BS, Simpson L, Batata M: Recovery from aspermia induced by low-dose radiation in seminoma patients. Cancer 50:337, 1982

66. Hamilton CR, Scully RE, Kliman B: Hypogonadotropinism in Prader-Willi syndrome: induction of puberty and spermatogenesis by clomiphene citrate. Am J Med 52:322, 1972

67. Handelsman DJ, Conway AJ, Boylan LM, Turtle JR: Young's syndrome: obstructive azoospermia and chronic sinopulmonary infections. N Engl J Med 310:3, 1984

68. Hendry WF, Knight RK, Whitfield HN, et al: Obstructive azoospermia: respiratory function tests, electron microscopy, and results of surgery. Br J Urol 50:598, 1978

69. Hendry WF, Stedronska J, Hughes L: Steroid treatment of male subfertility caused by antisperm antibodies. Lancet 2:498, 1979

70. Hensle TW, Burbige KA, Shepard BR, et al: Chemotherapy and its effect on testicular morphology in children. J Urol 131:1142, 1984

71. Hienz HA, Voggenthaler J, Weissbach L: Histological findings in testes with varicocele during childhood and their therapeutic consequences. Eur J Pediatr 133:139, 1980

72. Holsclaw D: Reproductive abnormalities of males with cystic fibrosis. p. 1. In: Problems in Reproductive Physiology and Anatomy in Young Adults with Cystic Fibrosis. Atlanta, Cystic Fibrosis Foundation, 1975

73. Hudson RW, Perez-Marrero RA, Crawford VA, McKay DE: Hormonal parameters in incidental varicoceles and those causing infertility. Fertil Steril 45:692, 1986

73a. Hughes TM, Skolnick JL, Belker AM: Young's syndrome: an often unrecognized correctable cause of obstructive azoospermia. J Urol 137:1238, 1987

74. Ishida H, Isurugi K, Fukutani, et al: Studies on pituitary-gonadal endocrine function in XYY men. J Urol 121:190, 1979

75. Isojima S, Li TS, Ashitaka Y: Immunologic analyses of sperm-immobilizing factor found in sera of men with unexplained sterility. Am J Obstet Gynecol 101:677, 1968

76. Jeffcoate WJ, Laurance BM, Edwards CRW, Besser GM: Endocrine function in the Prader-Willi syndrome. Clin Endocrinol (Oxf) 12:81, 1980

77. Jenkins IL, Muir VY, Blacklock NJ, et al: Consequences of vasectomy: an immunological and histological study related to subsequent fertility. Br J Urol 51:406, 1979

78. Johnsen SG: Testicular biopsy scorecount: a method for registration of spermatogenesis in human testes: normal values and results in 335 hypogonadal males. Hormones 1:2, 1970

79. Jones WR: Immunologic infertility — fact or fiction. Fertil Steril 33:577, 1980

80. Kamidono J, Matsumoto O, Ishigani J, et al: Infertility and HLA antigen — male infertility and infertile couples. Andrologia 12:317, 1980

81. Kaplan E, Schwachman H, Perlmutter AD, et al: Reproductive failure in males with cystic fibrosis. N Engl J Med 279:65, 1968

82. Karp LE, Williamson RA, Moore DE, et al: Sperm penetration assay: useful test in evaluation of male fertility. Obstet Gynecol 57:620, 1981

82a. Kass EJ, Belman AB: Reversal of testicular growth failure by varicocele ligation. J Urol 137:475, 1987

83. Kay R, Alexander NJ, Baugham WL: Induced varicoceles in rhesus monkeys. Fertil Steril 31:195, 1979

84. Kibrick S, Belding DL, Merrill B: Methods for the detection of antibodies against mammalian spermatozoa. II. A gelatin agglutination test. Fertil Steril 3:430, 1952

85. Klaiber EL, Broverman DM, Vogel W: Increased incidence of testicular varicoceles in cigarette smokers. Fertil Steril 34:64, 1980

86. Klinefelter HF, Reifenstein EG, Albright F: Syndrome characterized by gynecomastia, aspermatogenesis without aleydigism and increased excretion of follicle-stimulating hormone. J Clin Endocrinol 2:615, 1942

87. La Nasa JA: Office evaluation of the infertile couple. Urol Clin North Am 7:121, 1980

88. Levin HS: Testicular biopsy in the study of male infertility. Hum Pathol 10:569, 1979

88a. Levitt S, Gill B, Katlowitz N, et al.: Routine intraoperative post-ligation venography in the treatment of the pediatric varicocele. J Urol 137:716, 1987

89. Lushbaugh CC, Casarett GW: The effects of gonadal irradiation in clinical radiation therapy: a review. Cancer 37:1111, 1976

90. MacLeod J: Further observations on the role of vari-

cocele in human infertility. Fertil Steril 20:545, 1969

91. MacLeod J: Human male infertility. Obstet Gynecol 26:335, 1971

92. MacLeod J: Seminal cytology in the presence of varicocele. Fertil Steril 16:735, 1965

93. Maguire LC, Dick FR, Sherman BM: The effects of anti-leukemic therapy on gonadal histology in adult males. Cancer 48:1967, 1981

94. Makler A, Geresh I: An attempt to explain occurrence of patent reproductive tract in azoospermic males with tubular spermatogenesis. Int J Fertil 24:246, 1979

95. Marmor D, Elefant E, Dauchez C, Roux C: Semen analysis in Hodgkin's disease before the onset of puberty. Cancer 57:1986, 1986

96. Maroulis GB, Parlow AF, Marshall JR: Isolated follicle-stimulating hormone deficiency in man. Fertil Steril 28:818, 1977

96a. Matwijiw I, Thliveris JA, Faiman C: Aplasia of nasal cilia with situs inversus, azoospermia and normal sperm flagella: a unique variant of the immotile cilia syndrome: J Urol 137:522, 1987

97. McFadden, MR, Mehan DJ: Testicular biopsies in 101 cases of varicocele. J Urol 119:372, 1978

98. McNeil MM, Leong A, Sage RE: Primary mediastinal embryonal carcinoma in association with Klinefelter's syndrome. Cancer 47:343, 1981

99. Meinhard E, McRae CU, Chisholm GD: Testicular biopsy in evaluation of male infertility. Br Med J 3:577, 1973

100. Miller DG: Alkylating agents and human spermatogenesis. JAMA 217:1662, 1971

101. Moon KH, Bunge RG: Observations on the biochemistry of human semen. I. Fructose. Fertility 19:186, 1968

102. Morley JE, Distilber LA, Lissos I, et al: Testicular function in patients with spinal cord damage. Horm Metab Res 11:679, 1979

103. Morley JE, Melmed S: Gonadal dysfunction in systemic disorders. Metabolism 28:1051, 1979

104. Mulcahy JJ: Scrotal hypothermia and the infertile man. J Urol 132:469, 1984

105. Naessens A, Foulon W, Debrucker P, et al: Recovery of microorganisms is semen and relationship to semen evaluation. Fertil Steril 45:101, 1986

105a. Nagao RR, Plymate SR, Berger EB, et al.: Comparison of gonadal function between fertile and infertile men with varicoceles. Fertil Steril 46:930 1986

106. Nagler HM, Thomas AJ: Testicular biopsy and vasography in the evaluation of male infertility. Urol Clin North Am 14:167, 1987

107. Nakamura H, Matsushita K, Baba S: Gonadal function after renal allotransplantation. Transplant Proc 11:63, 1979

108. Narayan P, Amplatz K, Gonzalez R: Varicocele and male subfertility. Fertil Steril 36:92, 1981

109. Nelson WO: Interpretation of testicular biopsy. JAMA 151:449, 1953

110. Neville E, Brewis R, Yeates WK, Burridge A: Respiratory tract disease and obstructive azoospermia. Thorax 38:929, 1983

111. Nieschlag E, Wickings EJ, Mauss J: Endocrine testicular function in vivo and in vitro in infertile men. Acta Endocrinol (Copenh) 90:544, 1979

112. Nistal M, Paniagua R, Abaurrea MA, Santamaria L: Hyperplasia and the immature appearance of Sertoli cells in primary testicular disorders. Hum Pathol 13:3, 1982

113. O'Connor JJ: Surgical correction of male sterility. Surg Gynecol Obstet 110:649, 1960

114. O'Connor VJ: Mechanical aspects and surgical management of sterility in men. JAMA 153:532, 1953

114a. Okuyama A, Nakamura M, Namiki M, et al.: Surgical repair of varicocele at puberty: preventive treatment for fertility improvement. J Urol 139:562, 1988

115. Paniagua R, Nistal M, Bravo MP: Leydig cell types in primary testicular disorders. Hum Pathol 15:181, 1984

116. Pasqualini T, Chemes H, Coco R, et al: Testicular function in varicocele. Int J Androl 3:679, 1980

117. Paulsen CA: The testes. p. 323. In Williams RH (ed): Textbook of Endocrinology. Saunders, Philadelphia, 1968

118. Paulsen CA, Gordon DL, Carpenter RW, et al: Klinefelter's syndrome and its variants: a hormonal and chromosomal study. Recent Prog Horm Res 24:321, 1968

119. Pennisi AJ, Grushkin CM, Lieberman E: Gonadal function in children with nephrosis treated with cyclophosphamide. Am J Dis Child 129:315, 1975

120. Pervaiz N, Hagedoorn J, Mininberg DT: Electron microscopic studies of testes in Kallman syndrome. Urology 14:267, 1979

121. Pochaczevsky R, Lee WJ, Mallett E: Management of male infertility: roles of contact thermography, spermatic venography, and embolization. AJR 147:97, 1986

121a. Plymate SR, Nagao RR, Muller CH, Paulsen CA: The use of sperm penetration assay in evaluation of men with varicocele. Fertil Steril 47:680, 1987

122. Rabinowitz D, Cohen M, Rosenman E: Germinal aplasia of the testis associated with FSH deficiency of hypothalamic origin. Clin Res 22:346A, 1974

123. Re M, Carpino F, Familiari G, et al: Ultrastructural

characteristics of idiopathic spermatidic arrest. Arch Androl 4:283, 1979

124. Rege N, Phadki A, Bhatt J, et al: Serum gonadotropins and testosterone in infertile patients with varicocele. Fertil Steril 31:413, 1979

125. Richards IS, Davis JE, Lubell I: Current status of endocrinologic effects of vasectomy. Urology 18:1, 1981

126. Richter P, Calamer JC, Morgenfeld MC, et al: Effect of chlorambucil on spermatogenesis in the human with malignant lymphoma. Cancer 25:1026, 1970

127. Rife CC: Medical treatment of the infertile male. Urol Clin North Am 8:195, 1981

128. Ross LS: Diagnosis and treatment of infertile men: a clinical perspective. J Urol 130:847, 1983

129. Ross LS: Routine hormonal screening of infertile men: it is worthwhile. J Urol 126:756, 1981

130. Sahoo SK, Samal KC: Male infertility — an overview. Q Med Rev 31:15, 1980

131. Santen RJ, de Kretser DM, Paulsen CA, Vorhees J: Gonadotrophins and testosterone in the XYY syndrome. Lancet 2:371, 1970

132. Sayfan J, Adam YG, Soffer Y: A new entity in varicocele subfertility: the "cremasteric reflux." Fertil Steril 33:88, 1980

133. Schilsky RL, Lewis BJ, Sherins RJ, Young RC: Gonadal dysfunction in patients receiving chemotherapy for cancer. Ann Intern Med 93:109, 1980

134. Schleiermacher E: Ultrastructural changes of the intercellular relationship in impaired human spermatogenesis. Hum Genet 54:391, 1980

135. Schmitt GW, Shehadeh I, Sawin CT: Transient gynecomastia in chronic renal failure during chronic intermittent hemodialysis. Ann Intern Med 69:72, 1968

136. Schoysman R: The interest of testicular biopsy in the study of male infertility. Acta Eur Fertil 11:1, 1980

137. Schulster A, Ross L, Scommegna A: Frequency of androgen insensitivity in infertile phenotypically normal men. J Urol 130:699, 1983

138. Scott R, Rourke A, Yates A, et al: The results of 100 small tissue biopsies of testes in male infertile patients. Postgrad Med J 52:693, 1976

139. Segal S, Yaffe H, Laufer N, Ben-David M: Male hyperprolactinemia: effects on fertility. Fertil Steril 32:556, 1979

140. Shalet SM: Effects of cancer chemotherapy on gonadal function of patients. Cancer Treat Rev 7:141, 1980

141. Shamberger RC, Serins RJ, Rosenberg SA: The effects of postoperative adjuvant chemotherapy and radiotherapy on testicular function in men undergoing treatment for soft tissue sarcoma. Cancer 47:2368, 1981

142. Sherins RJ: Male infertility. p. 715. In Harrison JH (ed): Campbell's Urology. Saunders, Philadelphia, 1978

143. Sherins RJ, Olweny CLM, Ziegler JL: Gynecomastia and gonadal dysfunction in adolescent boys treated with combination chemotherapy for Hodgkin's disease. N Engl J Med 299:12, 1978

144. Silber JJ: Microscopic vasoepididymostomy: specific microanastomosis to the epididymal tubule. Fertil Steril 30:565, 1978

145. Silber SJ: Vasoepididymostomy to the head of the epididymis: recovery of normal spermatozoal motility. Fertil Steril 34:149, 1980

146. Simons FA: Human infertility. N Engl J Med 255:1140, 1956

147. Skakkebaek NE, Philip J, Mikkelsen M, et al: Studies on spermatogenesis, meiotic chromosomes, and sperm morphology in 2 males with a 47,XYY chromosome complement. Fertil Steril 24:645, 1970

148. Sniffen RC, Howard RP, Simmons FA: The testis. III. Absence of sperm cells: sclerosing tubular degeneration: "male climacteric." Arch Pathol 51:293, 1951

149. Snyder PJ: Endocrine evaluation of the infertile couple. Urol Clin North Am 5:451, 1978

150. Soderstrom KO, Suominen J: Histopathology and ultrastructure of meiotic arrest in human spermatogenesis. Arch Pathol Lab Med 104:476, 1980

151. Steinberger E: Management of male reproductive dysfunction. Clin Obstet Gynecol 22:187, 1979

152. Strickland DM, Ziaya PR: Reduced sperm motility in plastic containers. Lab Med 18:310, 1987

153. Talwar GP, Nas RK: Immunological control of male fertility. Arch Androl 7:177, 1981

154. Turner TT: Varicocele: still an enigma. J Urol 129:695, 1983

155. Ulstein M, Capell P, Holmes KK, Paulsen CA: Nonsymptomatic genital tract infection and male fertility. p. 355. In Hafez ESE (ed): Human Semen and Fertility Regulation in Men. Mosby, St. Louis, 1976

156. Urry RL: Pathophysiologic principles of male infertility. Urol Clin North Am 8:3, 1981

157. Urry RL, Middleton RG: Modern concepts in the diagnosis and treatment of male infertility. Urol Clin North Am 13:455, 1986

158. Vermeulen A, Comhaire F, Vandeweghe M: Hormonal exploration of male infertility. Acta Eur Fertil 10:105, 1979

159. Wang C, Chan CW, Wong KK, Yeung KK: Comparison of the effectiveness of placebo, clomiphene citrate, mesterolone, pentoxifylline, and testosterone rebound therapy for the treatment of idiopathic oligospermia. Fertil Steril 40:358, 1983

160. Weiss DB, Rodrigues-Rigau L, Smith KD, et al: Ley-

dig cell density and function and their relation to gonadotropins in infertile oligospermic men with varicocele. Isr J Med Sci 15:556, 1979

161. Wheatly JK, Fajman WA, Witten FR: Clinical experience with the radiosotope varicocele scan as a
screening method for the detection of subclinical varicoceles. J Urol 128:57, 1982

162. Whitehead E, Shalet SM, Blackledge G, et al: The
effects of Hodgkin's disease and combination chemotherapy on gonadal function in the adult male. Cancer
49:418, 1982

163. Whitehead ED, Leither E: Genital abnormalities and
abnormal semen analysis in male patients exposed to
diethylstilbestrol in utero. J Urol 125:47, 1981

164. Wong TW, Jones TM: Hyperprolactinemia and male
infertility. Arch Pathol Lab Med 108:35, 1984

164a. Wong TW, Strauss FH, Foster LV: Cytoplasmic
granular change of sertoli cells in two cases of sertoli-
cell-only syndrome. Arch Pathol Lab Med 112:200,
1988

165. Wong TW, Straus FH, Jones TM, Warner NE: Pathological aspects of the infertile testes. Urol Clin
North Am 5:503, 1978

166. Wong TW, Straus FH, Warner NE: Testicular
biopsy in the study of male infertility. I. Testicular
causes of infertility. Arch Pathol 95:151, 1973

167. Wong TW, Straus FH, Warner NE: Testicular
biopsy in the study of male infertility. III. Pretesticu-
lar causes of infertility. Arch Pathol 98:1, 1974

168. Young D: Surgical treatment of male infertility. J
Reprod Fertil 23:541, 1970

169. Zajicek J: Testes and epididymis. Monogr Clin Cytol
7:104, 1979

169a. Zaontz MR, Firlit CF: Use of venography as an aid in
varicocelectomy. J Urol 138:1041, 1987

170. Zorgniotti AW: Testes temperature, infertility, and
the varicocele paradox. Urology 16:7, 1980

26

Non-neoplastic Disorders of the Testis

Frank Rudy

ACUTE ORCHITIS

Acute orchitis occurs most commonly as a result of urethritis, cystitis, or seminal vesiculitis, with testicular involvement being due to spread of the infection along the vas deferens and epididymis. In these cases there is usually an associated epididymitis, and the testis is rarely solely involved. Other pathways whereby acute orchitis may develop include metastatic hematogenous and lymphatic spread of an infection remote from the testis. Patients with acute orchitis present with fever and a painful, enlarged, firm testis. Radionuclide testicular angiography appears to be a rapid and accurate means of distinguishing epididymo-orchitis from testicular torsion.[5] Aspiration biopsy reveals fibrin, granulocytes, phagocytes, and cell detritus.[66]

When a diagnosis of orchitis is made, one must search for the specific offending organism. The list of possible etiologic agents is long, as almost every known infectious process has been reported to involve the testis. Sexually transmitted organisms, including *Chlamydia trachomatis, Neisseria gonorrhoeae,* and possibly *Ureaplasma urealyticum,* appear to account for most cases of epididymo-orchitis in men less than 35 years of age, whereas common gram-negative bacilli secondary to urinary tract infections are the most likely agents in older men.[4] The common bacterial agents are *Escherichia coli, Klebsiella* sp., *Pseudomonas* sp., *Hemophilus influenzae,*[23] *Proteus mirabilis,* streptococci, staphylococci, *Neisseria meningitidis,*[63] *Salmonella,* and *Shigella.* Viral pathogens have also been implicated by laboratory, clinical, and epidemiologic studies. Mumps and Coxsackie viruses appear to be the most common causes of viral orchitis.[50,51] Testicular involvement has also been associated with many other viral illnesses such as smallpox, varicella, rubella, infectious mononucleosis, dengue, phlebotomus fever, lymphocytic choriomeningitis, and influenza.[27,47,51] Bat salivary gland virus has been reported as a cause of orchitis in two laboratory workers.[57] ECHO virus 9 has been considered a possible cause of orchitis,[53] and ECHO virus 6 has clearly been shown to produce orchitis.[64] Adenoviruses have also been implicated.[44] With most viral orchitis, subsequent atrophy of the affected testis is common. There is questionable association between vaccinia and lymphogranuloma venereum, a chlamydial infection, and orchitis.[51] On rare occasions other bacteria,[65] viruses, fungi, rickettsiae, chlamydiae, or parasites[45] may cause acute orchitis.

The pathology of the involved testis depends on the nature of the offending organism. With acute orchitis the testis is swollen and firm. The inflammatory reaction is characterized by intense interstitial infiltration

1035

by neutrophils, lymphocytes, and plasma cells with intratubular exudation and seminiferous epithelial damage (Fig. 26-1). Neutrophils are usually, but not invariably, more prominent in cases of bacterial orchitis than in orchitis with a viral etiology. Although rarely present, a careful search for viral inclusions should be undertaken. Treatment only rarely produces a surgical specimen, unless, as can happen, a testis is removed because of formation of a large, destructive abscess. In that case, anaerobic culture is considered. Sufficient sections must be taken to rule out a largely necrotic malignant tumor.

CHRONIC ORCHITIS

Untreated or inadequately treated acute orchitis may persist in a chronic form. One or both testes may be involved in a focal or diffuse fashion. Histologically, the testis displays a chronic interstitial inflammatory infiltrate, fibrosis, tubular degeneration, and peritubular hyalinization (Fig. 26-2). The etiology of the chronic orchitis is often difficult or impossible to ascertain from the testicular changes, and one is faced with a testis in the end-stage of inflammation without a clue as to the cause.

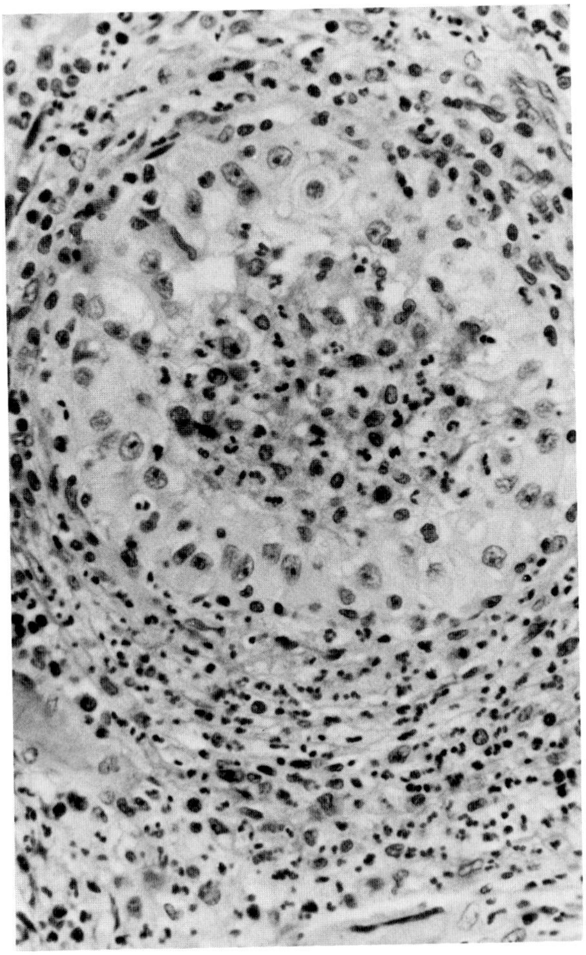

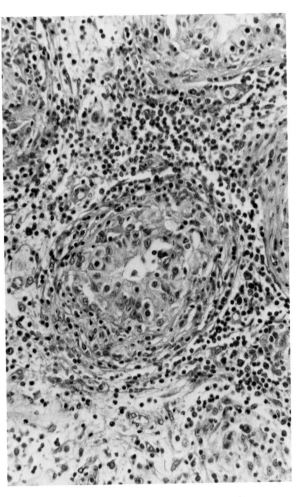

Fig. 26-1 Acute bacterial orchitis. An interstitial infiltrate of neutrophils is accompanied by an intratubular exudate. The germinal epithelium is damaged. ×600.

Fig. 26-2 Chronic orchitis. Mononuclear inflammatory cells infiltrate the interstitium. A few lymphocytes and plasma cells have extended into the tubular epithelium. Spermatogenesis is absent. ×400.

GRANULOMATOUS ORCHITIS

Granulomatous orchitis results from a heterogeneous group of chronic inflammatory diseases. Based on the microscopic picture, granulomatous orchitis may be subclassified into three types: (1) idiopathic, showing primary involvement of the seminiferous tubules with secondary involvement of the interstitium; (2) interstitial granulomatous orchitis with secondary tubular involvement, most often due to an infectious agent; and (3) granulomatous lesions characterized by the presence of Michaelis-Gutmann bodies (malakoplakia). In advanced cases it may be impossible to distinguish between the first two types.

Idiopathic Granulomatous Orchitis (Intratubular Orchitis)

Idiopathic granulomatous orchitis is a relatively uncommon condition that is most prevalent during the fifth and sixth decades of life.[37] The patients may present with either acute, painful testicular swelling that fails to respond to antibiotics[31] or the insidious development of testicular induration. A history of urinary tract infection, prostatectomy, inguinal surgery, or trauma is common. Clinically, the lesions are often confused with tuberculosis or neoplasm.[18]

The involved testis is usually grossly enlarged, firm, and covered by a thickened tunica albuginea. The cut surface is nodular or homogeneous in appearance, varying in color from gray to yellow. On microscopic examination, the outlines of the seminiferous tubules are still discernible in most cases. There is destruction of the germinal epithelium and replacement by an admixture of large epithelioid cells, lymphocytes, plasma cells, and occasional multinucleated giant cells (Fig. 26-3). A network of hyperplastic reticulin surrounds the tubular basement membranes, and in advanced cases marked peritubular fibrosis is evident. The interstitium contains a polymorphous cell infiltrate composed of lymphocytes, epithelioid cells, and rarely giant cells. Distinct granuloma formation does not generally occur in the interstitium. The origin of the large intratubular epithelioid cells is disputed. Some regard them as histiocytic in origin,[19] whereas others believe they represent transformed Sertoli cells.[41]

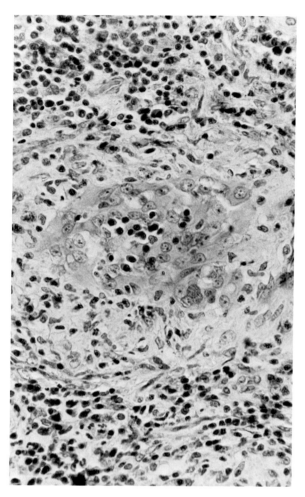

Fig. 26-3 Idiopathic granulomatous orchitis. The seminiferous tubular epithelium is completely replaced by large epithelioid cells. Plasma cells and lymphocytes are present in the interstitial tissue and affected tubule. ×600.

The etiology of this form of granulomatous orchitis remains obscure. A granulomatous reaction to lipid substances released by the disintegration of sperm is favored.[3,32] Previous injury and urinary tract infection are regarded as predisposing factors and may initiate a granulomatous reaction by causing extravasation of sperm. Other proposed etiologies include thrombosis of the pampiniform plexus[19] or an autoimmune phenomenon.[9] Two patients have been successfully treated with steroids.[13]

Granulomatous Orchitis of Known Etiology (Interstitial Orchitis)

A definite etiology is often identifiable in cases of granulomatous orchitis showing primary interstitial involvement. The differential diagnosis of this type of granulomatous orchitis includes tuberculosis,[20,37] atypical *Mycobacterium* infection,[31] syphilis,[16] fungal infection, brucellosis,[37] sarcoidosis,[46] lepromatous leprosy,[1] and foreign body reaction.[48] A similar interstitial pattern has been described in a patient in whom bilateral granulomatous orchitis was the presenting manifestation of an idiopathic systemic granulomatosis (possibly lymphomatoid granulomatosis).[33] The testicular histology depends on and is often suggestive of the underlying etiologic agent. The characteristic feature is the presence of granulomas, with or without necrosis, in the testicular interstitium (Fig. 26-4). Except in advanced or severe cases, tubular involvement is not prominent. Pertinent special stains and a careful history frequently permit a definite diagnosis, although cultural evidence is best.

Malakoplakia

Testicular malakoplakia is an uncommon granulomatous inflammatory condition, generally regarded as an unusual response to a gram-negative bacillary infection.[15,17] Since its initial description in the testis in 1958,[26] 30 cases have been reported, 7 of which had concomitant involvement of the epididymis.[38] The mean age at the time of diagnosis is 49 years, and patients typically present with painful testicular swelling.[38] The testis is enlarged, and the cut surface is either homogeneously yellow to brown, or nodular with white streaks of fibrous tissue.[7] Abscesses and areas of infarction may be observed.

Microscopic findings are characteristic and consist of intratubular and interstitial sheets of large epithelioid cells with abundant eosinophilic cytoplasm (von Hansemann cells).[61] Typical inclusions, called Michaelis-Gutmann bodies, are found within and outside the von Hansemann cells.[39] Michaelis-Gutmann bodies may be periodic acid-Schiff (PAS)-, von Kossa-, or iron stain-positive. These bodies appear to

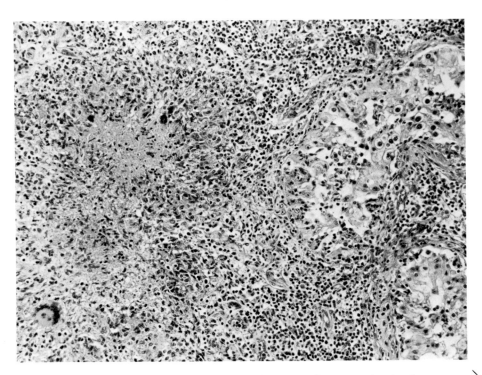

Fig. 26-4 Tuberculous orchitis. A caseating granuloma is evident. Special stains demonstrated numerous acid-fast bacilli. ×60. (Courtesy of Dr. Kenneth Zinsser.)

be giant phagosomes exhibiting intraphagosomal calcification[52] (see also Ch. 8).

Lesions Confused with Granulomatous Orchitis

Granulomatous orchitis is most commonly confused with lymphoma. With granulomatous orchitis the infiltrate is polymorphous and lacks atypical cells. The tubular involvement consists in replacement of the germinal epithelium by a mixed cellular infiltrate containing bland epithelioid cells. With lymphoma,

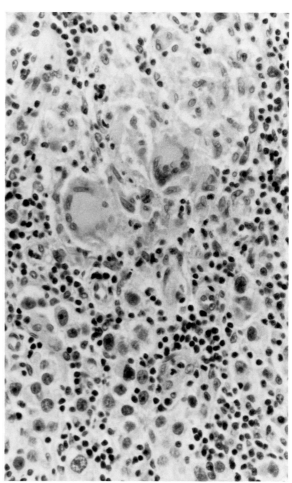

Fig. 26-6 Seminoma with a granulomatous reaction. A poorly formed granuloma with Langhans giant cells occupies the left side of the field. Large seminoma cells with hyperchromatic nuclei and prominent nucleoli are admixed with lymphocytes (right). Stains for glycogen may facilitate identification of the seminoma cells. ×600.

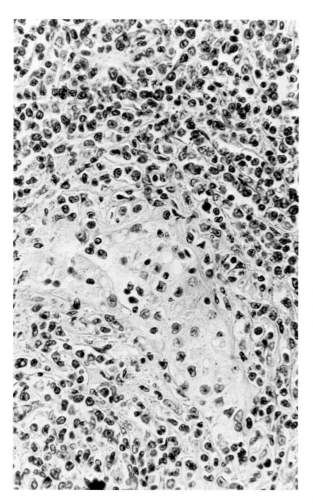

Fig. 26-5 Lymphoma. A damaged seminiferous tubule is surrounded by a cytologically malignant lymphoid infiltrate. Immunocytochemical techniques should be employed in difficult cases. ×400.

the cellular infiltrate is mainly of a single cell type, shows cellular atypia, and is predominantly interstitial (Fig. 26-5). The tubules reveal compressive atrophy and are invaded only late in the course of the lymphomatous process.[58]

Occasionally, granulomatous orchitis, in its early stages, mimics a Sertoli cell tumor. The main differential feature is the mixed inflammatory infiltrate of granulomatous orchitis, a change not seen in Sertoli cell tumors. Granulomatous orchitis may also have a superficial resemblance to seminoma with a granulomatous reaction; however, the classic "seminoma cell" is absent in the former condition (Fig. 26-6).

INFARCTION, HEMORRHAGE, AND TORSION

Testicular hemorrhage and infarction may occur during torsion, trauma, hypercoagulable states, polycythemia, leukemia, polyarteritis nodosa (Fig. 26-7), vena caval thrombosis, compression of the spermatic cord by an incarcerated hernia, or systemic embolization from bacterial endocarditis, or in association with

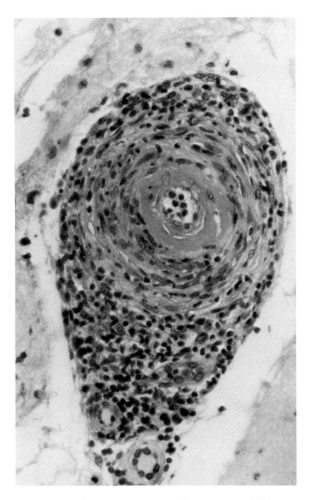

Fig. 26-7 Polyarteritis nodosa. Inflammation of all layers of the wall of this small artery is seen. Fibrinoid necrosis is present in the intima. ×600. (Courtesy of Dr. James Wheeler.)

a gonadal tumor.[22,40,49,62] The patients generally have painful, diffuse, testicular swelling, but focal testicular infarction may clinically simulate a tumor. Idiopathic testicular infarction, which may affect one or both gonads, is seen mainly in newborns.[30] At exploration torsion is not encountered, but it is likely that the lesion results from preexisting torsion with spontaneous correction; birth trauma is an alternative explanation. Idiopathic testicular infarction in older boys is typically focal and may result from trauma or vascular rupture during straining (Fig. 26-8).

The most common cause of testicular infarction is torsion with resultant compromise in testicular blood flow. Although torsion has been described in patients of all ages,[6] including men in their sixties, the two peak periods of occurrence are during the perinatal period and around the age of puberty.[24,56] There are two types of testicular torsion. The less common form is extravaginal torsion secondary to twisting of the spermatic cord and the entire tunica vaginalis. Extravaginal torsion occurs mainly during the prenatal or perinatal period and is presumed to be due to inadequate fixation of the tunica vaginalis to the scrotal wall, allowing the entire intrascrotal contents to rotate. There is bluish discoloration of the scrotum, and the testis is enlarged and firm but nontender. Rarely, both testes are affected.[34a] Although the problem may not be recognized until after birth, it appears that in most cases the torsion has occurred in utero. Chances of early recognition in this group are poor. Therefore there is usually little hope of preserving the testis.[30] Subsequent contralateral torsion does occasionally occur, so some authors recommend an orchiopexy on the other side.[34a,42]

Torsion of the spermatic cord within the tunica vaginalis (intravaginal torsion) is the more common form. This second type is traditionally thought to be found principally in pubertal and prepubertal boys, with adults only rarely affected. However, studies are changing our views on this point. In Nigeria 57 percent of cases of torsion in a large series occurred in men over age 20, and 9 percent were over age 30.[60] In a series from Vancouver, British Columbia, 26 percent were over age 21 and 10 percent over 30 years old.[35] Torsion has been reported recently in a 62 year old man.[1a] The type of torsion seen is the result of a congenital abnormality in which the tunica vaginalis covers the entire epididymis and extends high on the spermatic cord, so that the testis and epididymis are

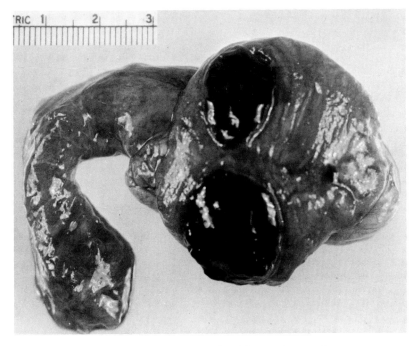

Fig. 26-8 Idiopathic testicular infarction. A localized hemorrhagic infarct was encountered in the testis of this 10-year-old boy.

suspended from an elongated or redundant mesorchium (bell and clapper deformity) (Fig. 26-9). In a rare variant, elongation occurs between the testis and epididymis, producing total or partial separation of these two structures, thereby permitting torsion of the testis.[10] The anatomic defect encountered with intravaginal torsion is frequently bilateral.

In these patients there is also a spiral insertion of cremasteric muscle fibers extending to the lowest point of the spermatic cord.[42] Strong contraction of the muscle may provide the force that actually causes rotation of the freely movable testis. A study from Ireland is of interest in this regard. There, at least, torsion is much more frequent in cold weather, 87 percent of the cases occurring on days when the temperature was less than 2°C, representing only 23.6 percent of days.[55] The authors suggested that the cold was responsible for contraction of the dartos or cremasteric muscles, producing the torsion.

The most common presentation is that of an adolescent or preadolescent boy with acute, painful scrotal swelling associated with nausea or emesis. The pain may also be experienced in the abdomen, flank, or groin. Inflammation of the scrotal skin increases with

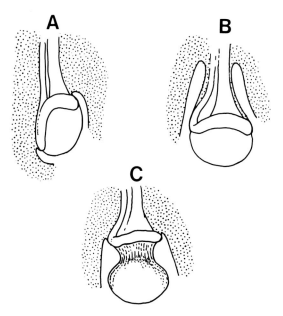

Fig. 26-9 Suspension of the testis. **(A)** Normal suspension of the testis. **(B)** High extension of the tunica vaginalis producing a bell and clapper deformity. **(C)** An elongation exists between the testis and epididymis, allowing torsion of the testis.

the duration of torsion, and so severe inflammation is an ominous sign. There is often a history of previous similar but milder attacks that resolved spontaneously. A testis riding high in the scrotal sac plus a thickened cord and an anterior or lateral position of the epididymis are highly suggestive of torsion.[21] No aspects of the history, physical examination, or laboratory tests are consistently discriminatory to distinguish testicular torsion from other, more benign intrascrotal conditions. Therefore surgical exploration has classically been recommended in males presenting with acute scrotal swelling. The use of doppler ultrasonic studies[29] and isotope scanning[28] may aid in making this difficult differential diagnosis.

At exploration the testis is usually characterized by congestion and edema with some evidence of hemorrhage. The normally glistening surface of the tunica albuginea may be dull owing to the presence of a fibrinous exudate. Microscopic findings depend on the degree of rotation and the duration of vascular compromise. With incomplete venous occlusion, there is interstitial congestion and edema accompanied by desquamation of the germinal epithelium.[2] Total obstruction of venous return results in greater congestion and eventual venous infarction with massive hemorrhage and necrosis. Rapid infarction develops if arterial blood flow is obliterated, producing a picture of coagulation necrosis often with only acellular, ghostlike tubules remaining (Fig. 26-10). Animal experiments have revealed slight damage to germinal epithelium after 2 hours of ischemia, severe damage after 4 hours, and a total loss of germinal elements after 6 hours.[8] The Leydig cells are somewhat more resistent to ischemia, with severe damage occurring after 8 hours and total loss only after 10 hours.

Testicular torsion is a surgical emergency, requiring prompt exploration and detorsion to preserve viability. An increased index of suspicion and an aggressive surgical approach have resulted in improved testicular salvage rates, ranging from 55 to 78 percent in some series.[56] In general, a conservative approach has been taken to orchidectomy if there was any hope of residual germ cell or endocrine function; however, to prevent significant atrophy, a corrective procedure should be performed within 8 hours or less of the onset of the symptoms.[2] The intraoperative use of fluorescein dye given intravenously may assist the surgeon in assessing testicular viability.[54]

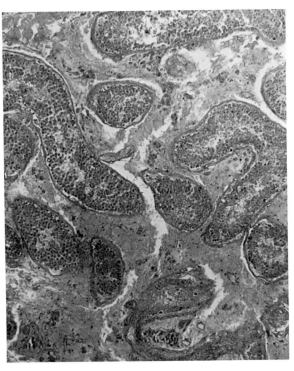

Fig. 26-10 Torsion. Necrotic ghostlike tubules in a testis removed 12 hours following the onset of testicular pain. ×250.

With torsion of the testis as many as 68 percent of the testes "saved" by surgery develop secondary atrophy.[34] There is a correlation between the duration of torsion and the degree and likelihood of subsequent atrophy. Although one would expect fertility to be normal in patients treated for unilateral torsion, it is not generally the case.[34] Even when detorsion has been done 4 hours or less after the onset of symptoms, the semen analysis is abnormal in one-half of the patients.[2] Elevated follicle-stimulating hormone and luteinizing hormone levels are present in individuals with a pathologic semen analysis.

Patients with a history of unilateral torsion seem to have bilateral testicular abnormalities. Follow-up biopsies of the opposite testis in cases of unilateral torsion have revealed hypospermatogenesis.[2] Experimentally, the degree of damage of the contralateral testis may be directly related to the severity of damage of the twisted gonad, which in turn parallels the duration of the torsion.[12,14,43] There is also experimental evidence to suggest that orchiectomy, rather than detorsion, results in less ultimate damage to the contralateral testis, hour for hour of torsion, and better preserves fertility.[14]

These clinical and experimental observations suggest that the torsion-induced damage leads to breakdown of some blood–testis barrier, with release into the circulation of some antigen that provokes an immune response directed against the opposite testis. Experimentally, there is support for this notion in that torsion is invariably followed by contralateral damage, particularly to the germ cell elements, whereas simple ligation of the cord carrying the testicular blood supply is not followed by any damage.[11] Equally, it has been shown that anti-sperm antibodies alone are not responsible for the contralateral damage.[11] However, cytotoxic anti-testis antibodies have been recognized in rats after ischemic damage.[36] Therefore the response seems to be more against the testis than the sperm. The possibility of a contribution of cellular immunity is suggested by the observation in another setting that experimental allergic orchitis can be transferred to other animals by lymphoid cells.[59] Thus it is conceivable that both arms of the immune system play a role in the damage to the contralateral testis. Alternatively, the infertility in patients with unilateral torsion might be the result of a pathologic process involving the testes that antedated the torsion.[25]

Because clinical experience tends to parallel these experimental observations, it has been suggested that serious consideration be given to the inadvisability of leaving a markedly damaged testis in the body, as doing so may have adverse effects on the contralateral testis.[12]

(Recently, however, two experimental studies of testicular torsion in the rat have challenged the accepted concept of contralateral testicular damage.[29a,59a] None of the various durations of torsion or other experimental therapeutic maneuvers had any deleterious effect on spermatogenesis in the contralateral testis. These studies will surely prompt reexamination of the situation in man.)

REFERENCES

1. Aktar M, Ashraf M, Mackey DM: Lepromatous leprosy presenting as orchitis. Am J Clin Pathol 73:712, 1980
1a. Alfert HJ, Canning DA: Testicular torsion in a 62-year old man. J Urol 138:149, 1987
2. Bartsch G, Frank S, Marberger H, Mikuz G: Testicular torsion: late results with special regard to fertility and endocrine function. J Urol 124:375, 1980
3. Berg JW: An acid-fast lipid from spermatozoa. Arch Pathol 57:115, 1954
4. Berger RE, Alexander EF, Harnisch JP, et al: Etiology, manifestations and therapy of acute epididymitis: prospective study of 50 cases. J Urol 121:750, 1979
5. Boedecker RA, Sty JR, Jona JZ: Testicular scanning as a diagnostic aid in evaluating scrotal pain. J Pediatr 94:760, 1979
6. Brewer ME, Glasgow BJ: Adult testicular torsion. Urology 27:356, 1986
7. Brown RC, Smith BH: Malakoplakia of the testes. Am J Clin Pathol 47:135, 1967
8. Burton JA: Atrophy following testicular torsion. Br J Surg 59:422, 1972
9. Capers TH: Granulomatous orchitis. Am J Clin Pathol 34:139, 1960
10. Cass AS, Cass BP, Veeraraghavan K: Immediate exploration of the unilateral acute scrotum in young male subjects. J Urol 124:829, 1980
11. Cerasaro TS, Nachtsheim DA, Otero F, Parsons CL: The effect of testicular torsion on contralateral testis and the production of antisperm antibodies in rabbits. J Urol 132:577, 1984
12. Chakraborty J, Jhunjhunwala J, Nelson L, Young M: Effects of unilateral torsion of the spermatic cord on the contralateral testis in human and guinea pig. Arch Androl 4:95, 1980
13. Chilton CP, Smith PJB: Steroid therapy in the treatment of granulomatous orchitis. Br J Urol 51:404, 1979
14. Cosentino MJ, Nishida M, Rabinowitz R, Cockett ATK: Histological changes occurring in the contralateral testes of prepubertal rats subjected to various durations of unilateral spermatic cord torsion. J Urol 133:906, 1985
15. Csapo Z, Kuthy E, Lantos J, et al: Experimentally induced malakoplakia. Am J Pathol 79:453, 1975
16. Dao AH, Adkins RB: Bilateral gummatous orchitis. South Med J 73:954, 1980
17. Dionne GP, Bovill EG, Seemayer TA: New fine structural observations in testicular malakoplakia. Urology 5:828, 1975
18. Elicker ER, Evans AT: Granulomatous orchitis. J Urol 113:199, 1975
19. Fajardo LF, Dueker GE, Kosek JC: Light and electron microscopic observations on granulomatous orchitis. Invest Urol 6:158, 1968
20. Ferrie BG, Rundle JSH: Tuberculous epididymo-orchitis: a review of 20 cases. Br J Urol 55:437, 1983
21. Flanigan RC, DeKernion JB, Persky L: Acute scrotal

pain and swelling in children: a surgical emergency. Urology 17:51, 1981

22. Fossum BD, Woods JC, Blight EM: Cavernous hemangioma of testis causing acute testicular infarction. Urology 18:277, 1981

23. Greenfield SP: Type B Hemophilus influenza epididymo-orchitis in the prepubertal boy. J Urol 136:1311, 1986

24. Guiney EJ, McGlinchey J: Torsion of the testis and the spermatic cord in the newborn. Surg Gynecol Obstet 152:273, 1981

25. Hadziselimovic F, Snyder H, Duckett J, Howards S: Testicular histology in children with unilateral testicular torsion. J Urol 136:208, 1986

26. Haukohl RS, Chinchinian H: Malakoplakia of the testicle: report of a case. Am J Clin Pathol 29:473, 1958

27. Hermansen MC, Chusid MJ, Sty JR: Bacterial epididymo-orchitis in children and adolescents. Clin Pediatr 19:812, 1980

28. Holder LE, Martire JR, Schirmer HKA: Clinical applications of testicular radionuclide angiography and scrotal scanning. JAMA 245:2526, 1981

29. Iuchtman M, Zoireff L, Assa J: Doppler flowmeter in the differential diagnosis of the acute scrotum in children. J Urol 121:221, 1979

29a. Janetschek G, Heilbronner R, Schactner W, et al: Unilateral testicular disease: effect on the contralateral testis (morphometric study). J Urol 138:878, 1987

30. Johnston JH: The acute scrotum in childhood. Practitioner 223:306, 1979

31. Kahn RI, Mcaninch J: Granulomatous disease of the testis. J Urol 123:868, 1980

32. Kisbenedek L, Nemeth A: Granulomatous orchitis and spermatic granuloma. Int Urol Nephrol 7:141, 1975

33. Klein FA, Vick CW, Schneider V: Bilateral granulomatous orchitis: manifestation of idiopathic systemic granulomatosis. J Urol 134:762, 1985

34. Krarup T: The testes after torsion. Br J Urol 50:43, 1978

34a. LaQuaglia MP, Bauer SB, Eraklis A, et al: Bilateral neonatal torsion. J Urol 138:1051, 1987

35. Lee LM, Wright JE, McLoughlin MG: Testicular torsion in the adult. J Urol 130:93, 1983

36. Lewis-Jones DI, Moreno de Marval MJ, Harrison RG: Impairment of rat spermatogenesis following unilateral experimental ischemia. Fertil Steril 38:482, 1982

37. Lynch VP, Eakins D, Morrison E: Granulomatous orchitis. Br J Urol 40:451, 1968

38. McClure J: Malakoplakia of the testis and its relationship to granulomatous orchitis. J Clin Pathol 33:670, 1980

39. Michaelis L, Gutmann C: Über Einschlusse in Blasentumoren. Z Klin Med 47:208, 1902

40. Mostofi FK: Testis, scrotum, and penis. p. 1013. In Anderson WAD, Kissane JM (eds): Pathology. 7th Ed. Mosby, St. Louis, 1977

41. Mostofi FH, Price EB: Tumors of the male genital system. Atlas of Tumor Pathology. Fascicle 8, 2nd Series. Armed Forces Institute of Pathology, Washington DC, 1973

42. Muschat M: The pathological anatomy of testicular torsion: explanation of its mechanism. Surg Gynecol Obstet 54:758, 1932

43. Nagler HM, Deitch AD, White RV: Testicular torsion: temporal considerations. Fertil Steril 42:257, 1984

44. Naveh Y, Friedman A: Orchitis associated with adenoviral infections. Am J Dis Child 129:257, 1975

45. Nistal M, Santana A, Paniaqua R, Palacios J: Testicular toxoplasmosis in two men with the acquired immunodeficiency syndrome (AIDS). Arch Pathol Lab Med 10:744, 1986

46. Opal SM, Pittman DL, Hofeldt FD: Testicular sarcoidosis. Am J Med 67:147, 1979

47. Preblud SR, Dobbs HI, Sedmak GV, et al: Testalgia associated with rubella infection. South Med J 73:594, 1980

48. Pugh JI, Stringer P: Glove-powder granuloma of the testis after surgery. Br J Surg 60:240, 1973

49. Purpon I, Albores-Saavedra J: Testicular infarction. Int Surg 58:740, 1973

50. Quast U, Hennessen W, Widmark RM: Vaccine induced mumps-like diseases. Dev Biol Stand 43:269, 1979

51. Riggs S, Sanford JP: Viral orchitis. N Engl J Med 266:990, 1962

52. Rinaudo P, Damjanov I, Stoesser B: Malacoplakia of testis. Int Urol Nephrol 9:249, 1977

53. Sanford JP, Sulkin SE: Clinical spectrum of echovirus infection. N Engl J Med 261:1113, 1959

54. Schneider HC, Kendal AR, Karafin L: Fluorescence of testicle: an indication of viability of spermatic cord after torsion. Urology 5:133, 1975

55. Shukla RB, Kelly DG, Daly L, Guiney EJ: Association of cold weather with testicular torsion. Br Med J 285:1459, 1982

56. Smith SP, King LR: Torsion of the testis: techniques of assessment. Urol Clin North Am 6:429, 1979

57. Sulkin SE, Burns KF, Shelton DF, Wallis C: Bat salivary gland virus: infections of man and monkey. Tex Rep Biol Med 20:113, 1962

58. Suseelan AV, Mbonu OO: Idiopathic granulomatous orchitis. Jpn J Surg 9:76, 1979

59. Tung KSK, Unanue ER, Dixon FJ: Pathogenesis of experimental allergic orchitis. I. Transfer with immune lymph node cells. J Immunol 106:1453, 1967

59a. Turner TT: On unilateral testicular and epididymal torsion: no effect on the contralateral testis. J Urol 138:1285, 1987

60. Udeh FN: Testicular torsion: Nigerian experience. J Urol 134:482, 1985

61. Von Hansemann: Uber Malakoplakie der Harnblase. Virchows Arch [Pathol Anat] 173:302, 1903

62. Waldbaum RS, Borden D, Cohen D, et al: Venous infarction of the testis owing to vena caval thrombosis. J Urol 116:259, 1976

63. Weinstein LW, Carcillo J, Scott SJ, Simon GL: Paratyphoid orchitis. Diagn Microbiol Infect Dis 1:163, 1983

64. Welliver RC, Cherry JD: Aseptic meningitis and orchitis associated with echovirus 6 infection. J Pediatr 92:239, 1978

65. Wheeler JS, Gulkin DJ, O'Connell J, Winters G: Nocardia epididymo-orchitis in an immunosuppressed patient. J Urol 136:1314, 1986

66. Zajicek J: Testis and epididymis. Monogr Clin Cytol 7:104, 1979

27

Testicular Tumors

James E. Wheeler

Most testicular masses are malignant tumors. In nearly 20 percent of intrascrotal masses surgically explored,[321] however, the patient is found to have a benign paratesticular or testicular process. Recognition of this possibility by the examining physician may allow for gonadal preservation in selected cases and may offer at least a modicum of hope to the preoperative patient.

Hydrocele and acute testicular torsion have characteristic signs and symptoms that make their diagnosis readily apparent in most cases. Other lesions, however, clinically simulate the swelling and occasional discomfort of a malignant tumor. These include (1) benign intratesticular and paratesticular tumors, especially epidermoid cyst and adenomatoid tumor (see Ch. 29)[321]; (2) benign intraparenchymal inclusion cyst[26]; (3) chronic orchitis and granulomatous processes (see Ch. 26); (4) infarction attributable to necrotizing vasculitis (see Ch. 26)[26]; (5) malignant paratesticular tumors (see Ch. 29); (6) fibrous pseudotumor of the tunica (see Ch. 29); and (7) as detailed in Chapter 26, a wide variety of infections by bacterial, fungal, parasitic, mycobacterial, or spirochetal organisms. Because some of these processes are part of a generalized process, careful patient evaluation may give some indication of a nonneoplastic process. Diagnostic maneuvers, besides physical examination and transillumination, include high-resolution ultrasound and radionucleide scan.

Ultrasound offers the possibility of detecting a testicular lesion too small to palpate. Sonographic exam-ination of testicular masses currently is prone to a high false-positive rate for malignancy owing to a multiplicity of benign conditions that can give rise to a hypoechoic study.[12,13,290] but false-negatives are uncommon.[87] Scan using Tc^{99m} sodium pertechnetate is highly useful in the rapid diagnosis of testicular torsion but offers little help in the diagnosis of testis tumors.[127]

On scrotal exploration, an inguinal approach with control of the spermatic vessels, careful intraoperative examination (Fig. 27-1), and biopsy in selected cases may spare the testis in as many as 75 percent of patients with benign lesions.[321]

Processing of Testicular Specimens

Proper photography of freshly bisected testis is difficult owing to the marked bulging of tumor. If a hemitestis is fixed in formalin, it may be later resected to provide a smooth surface of tumor with surrounding testis.

Although formalin is used for fixation in most laboratories, we prefer Bouin's fixative. The shrinkage artifact of fixation caused by formalin alone is countered by the acetic acid present in Bouin's solution and the picric acid results in brighter and more vivid staining of the histologic sections. Immunohistochemical staining may also be enhanced by Bouin's fixative. For flow cytometric examination of fixed or embedded tumor cell nuclei, however, formalin fixation is highly preferable.

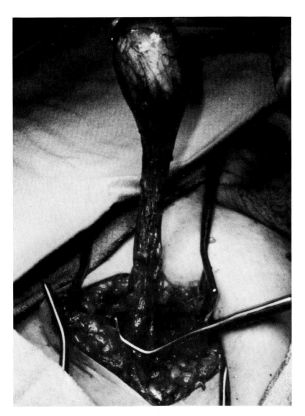

Fig. 27-1 Intraoperative examination of the testis. An inguinal approach and atraumatic control of the vascular supply permits careful intraoperative examination of a suspected testicular neoplasm. (Courtesy of Dr. H. Snyder.)

BENIGN TUMORS AND EPIDERMOID CYSTS

Epidermoid Cyst

This benign cystic lesion may account for between 1 and 3 percent of all testicular tumors.[261,265] Although patients range in age from 3 to 77, 86 percent of them are between 10 and 39 years old.[265] Reported cases have been in whites and orientals; cases in blacks were not found in a comprehensive review.[265] Patients present with a painless mass or have an incidentally found mass in 85 percent of cases, and the average duration of symptoms is over two years. Bilateral epidermoid cysts are rare, but reported.[284] There is one report of cyst in association with Gardner's syndrome.[141] The mean age, racial distribution, slight right-sided predominance, and occasional association with cryptorchidism are similar in patients having

epidermoid cysts and germ cell tumors; however, no definite relationship between the two has been demonstrated.[265]

On gross examination of the bisected testis, the cyst is well delineated and round with a thin wall and contains a cheesy, often laminated, material (Fig. 27-2). Microscopically, the cyst wall consists of stratified keratinizing squamous epithelium resting on a thin layer of fibrous tissue that may be focally calcified (Fig. 27-3).

Focally, rupture of the cyst wall will release keratin into the surrounding parenchyma and cause a vigorous inflammatory and foreign-body giant cell reaction. Since teratomas can have a substantial epidermoid component, generous sampling and careful microscopic examination of the cyst wall is necessary to rule out the presence of adnexal structures or tera-

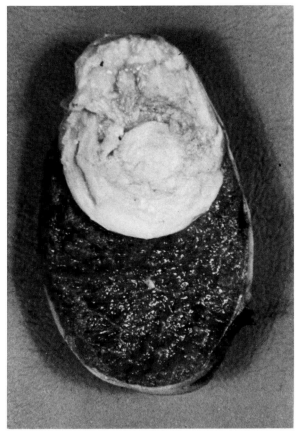

Fig. 27-2 Epidermoid cyst. This well-delineated benign tumor is filled with white debris exfoliated from the squamous lining. (Courtesy of Dr. A.J. Steinberg.) (From Wheeler et al.,[339a] with permission.)

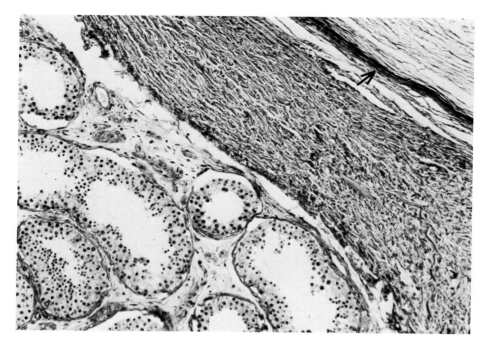

Fig. 27-3 Epidermoid cyst. Mature keratinizing squamous epithelium at upper right (arrow) lines the cyst and exfoliates anucleate squames into the cyst cavity. Note the fibrous cyst wall and the lack of skin adnexal structures or other non-squamous elements, the presence of which would indicate a teratoma with metastatic potential.

tomatous elements that may not be sampled on a single piece sampled for frozen section.[48] Any histologically mature element other than squamous epithelium categorizes the lesion as a mature teratoma (see below). A discovery of a nearby testicular scar also implies that the cyst may represent the remains of a burned-out germ cell tumor. The difficulty in sampling intraoperatively makes orchiectomy the operation of choice and makes frozen section unnecessary, although occasionally there may be a role for conservative surgery.[29,261]

Other Benign Testis Tumors

Rare cases have been reported of benign intratesticular mesenchymal tumors, including fibroma,[26] neurofibroma,[187] benign hemangioendothelioma,[109] hemangioma,[165,228] leiomyoma,[128] and lipoma.[217]

Careful gross examination should rule out origin in the testicular adnexal structures, where these mesenchymal lesions are more common. Thorough histologic examination is necessary ascertain that the apparently benign lesion does not merely represent part of a focally well-differentiated teratoma.

BRENNER TUMOR

This benign epithelial tumor most likely arises from metaplasia of mesothelium near the epididymal–testicular groove and is found as a paratesticular mass in that area.[103] (See Ch. 28.)

ADENOMATOID TUMOR (BENIGN MESOTHELIOMA)

This benign paratesticular tumor may invade the testis, necessitating treatment by orchiectomy. It is fully discussed in Chapter 29.

MELANOTIC HAMARTOMA (RETINAL ANLAGE TUMOR, NEUROECTODERMAL TUMOR)

This rare benign pigmented tumor involves the epididymis in male infants (see Ch. 29) and has been reported to have been primary in testis in two instances.[217]

GERM CELL TUMORS

Over 90 percent of testis tumors are malignant germ cell tumors, and any consideration of their pathology must take into account their incidence, geographic and age differences, histogenesis, proposed schemes of classification and staging, and etiologic factors. The patterns of tumor spread, prognosis, and response to modern therapy are clearly of major importance to anyone who wishes to understand their clinical behavior and to treat patients with testicular tumors.

Incidence

Incidence figures from the United States indicate a gradual rise in testicular tumors from less than 2.0/100,000 males prior to World War II to approximately 2.6/100,000 males in the early 1960s.[57] Comparing incidence data from England and Wales from 1911 through 1915 with incidence from 1971 through 1975 show an even more dramatic rise[71]; the death rate more than tripled in spite of presumably better therapy. Testicular cancer more than doubled its incidence in Denmark between 1943 and 1982, and especially increased in young men.[233] Although the figure of approximately 5,400 new testis cancer cases estimated to occur each year in the United States[271] gives some overall indication of the importance of the general disease category, it tells one nothing about the population at special risk for development of a testis tumor.

Geographically, there is a marked difference in incidence from country to country and even from state to state. Denmark (4.9/100,000 males), Norway, New Zealand, and California have incidence rates nearly twice that of New York State (2.3/100,000 males), Sweden, and Canada, and even this is far greater than such locations as Japan (0.7–1.2/100,000 males), Puerto Rico, and Nigeria.[264]

Racial differences are striking, with the incidence in Detroit and San Francisco Bay area 3.5 and 4.0/100,000 white males, respectively, versus only 0.8 and 1.0/100,000 black males in the same region.[17,288] In children below the age of 15, the incidence in whites and blacks is nearly identical at one case per million.[347] Hawaiian whites (5.0/100,000 males), Hawaiian Japanese (1.1/100,000 males), and Hawaiian Filipinos (0.2/100,000 males) are also af-

fected significantly differently.[49] Data from numerous locations[333] indicate that testicular cancer incidence is generally, but not always, appreciably higher in rural than in urban areas of a given community. The possible confounding variables that might account for this, such as social or economic class, diet, and exposure to carcinogens, have not been considered in these particular data, however.

Men in professional and semiprofessional occupations and skilled nonmanual jobs have a significantly higher age-adjusted incidence of testicular carcinomas than those in unskilled, partially skilled, or skilled manual occupations,[54] by a ratio of nearly two to one.

Although testicular tumors may occur in the infant, the incidence becomes appreciable in the 20 to 25 year old group, peaks at age 30 to 45, and thereafter decreases until about age 80 when there is a late rise, possibly due to lymphoma.

Etiology

CRYPTORCHIDISM

The one currently well-recognized antecedent of testicular carcinoma is cryptorchidism.[89,116] Whereas only 0.4 percent of men in the general population have cryptorchidism, 12.5 percent of testicular cancers originate in men with corrected or uncorrected cryptorchidism.[23] Abdominal testes are at higher risk than inguinal ones.[155] Almost all germ cell tumors developing in abdominal testes are seminomas, whereas tumors developing intrascrotally after orchiopexy are predominantly (72 percent) nonseminomatous. Inguinal testes have an intermediate level (37 percent) of nonseminomatous lesions.[22] Whereas early orchiopexy has been the longstanding practice, both to preserve testicular fertility and prevent later development of carcinoma, recent evidence fails to indicate that it does either.[22,243]

BILATERALITY

Patients with a germ cell tumor in one testis run a thousand-fold increased risk of a contralateral malignancy,[14,210] which may vary from 1.5[14] to 5 percent.[76]

Synchronously discovered tumors comprise about 22 percent of bilateral lesions. Metachronous tumor may occur many years later, only 57 percent of them being found within the first five years of followup.[76] From an etiologic point of view, the incidence of cryptorchidism in these patients is over 20 percent.[76]

Besides an increased incidence of subsequent contralateral testis cancer, the incidence of subsequent bladder cancers, leukemia, and lymphoma is also increased.[234]

CARCINOGENS

A linkage between environmental carcinogens and testicular carcinoma has not been well established. Many compounds tested in laboratory animals have been associated with testicular tumors, most of them apparently benign.[287] Testicular fibrosarcoma has been induced in rats with nickel sulfide, and the incidence of interstitial cell tumors (in Fischer rats which are frequently spontaneous), has been somewhat increased with a variety of compounds.[287] One testicular seminoma was found among 50 male B6C3F1 mice treated with anilazine 1000 ppm in diet for two years and another in a similar group of mice given 75 mg/kg of pivalolactone by stomach tube three times a week for two years.[287]

The inability to provoke germ cell tumors with the overwhelming majority of carcinogens tested raises the question of whether the blood–testis barrier prevents the compounds from reaching the germ cells, or whether the germ cells are, in fact, relatively resistant to carcinogenic compounds.

Although seminoma has been reported in men exposed to DES in utero,[62,192] insufficient data are available to confirm other than a chance association. Experimentally, DES does not appear to provoke any increase in testicular cancer in laboratory animals.[287]

TRAUMA

Nineteenth century accounts of patients with a testicular tumor frequently record a history of a blow to the area and suggest trauma as a etiologic factor. Even now, a history of trauma may be elicited in 8 to 25 percent of patients.[43] Certainly a testis enlarged by an unsuspected tumor would be in a better than usual position to be traumatized, and trauma might well cause bleeding into an unsuspected tumor with rapid enlargement. However, trauma as an etiologic factor is unproven experimentally.

GENETICS

Testicular tumors have been reported in identical twins,[202,352] brothers,[10] and in fathers and sons.[176] There is a reported association of stromal tumors, especially of the Sertoli cells, with the Peutz–Jeghers syndrome[344] that may have a genetic basis. There is some association as well between testicular cancer and urogenital development anomalies,[89,309] and polythelia.[99] Chromosomal analysis of testicular tumors[331] discloses that most tumors have a high modal number of chromosomes (51 to 61), and that all cell lines studied have numerical and structural changes in the q (long) arm of chromosome 1. There are commonly three to five copies of the q arm or one to four breaks that localize preferentially at p12, p22, p36, and q12. A recent study has confirmed 1q abnormalities and also found changes in chromosomes 12 and 7.[16] Chromosomal studies on germ cell tumors in situ (see below) have not been reported, hence the earliest chromosomal changes are still unknown.

MUMPS

Although testicular tumor has been reported following mumps orchitis,[338] careful case control studies[119,213] find no significant association.

RADIATION

Radiation received by the testes of most individuals today is almost invariably attributable to exposure to diagnostic x-rays. Barium enemas, lumbar and lumbosacral spine examinations, intravenous pyelograms, and hip examinations account for most incidental gonadal exposure.[323] The "genetically significant dose" is defined as "the gonadal dose which, if received by every member of the population, would result in the same genetic effect to the population as the doses which are actually received by individuals within the population."[323] In 1964 in the United States this was approximately 55 mrads per person per year, nearly all (96 percent) from radiologic studies. It was estimated that reduction of the x-ray beam to the size of the film would lower this to 19 mrads,[323] and since this study major efforts to lower radiation exposure have been made.

Severe radiation injury to the gonads, such as that received by atomic bomb victims, may result in profound germ cell loss and testicular atrophy, but because no increase in subsequent testicular tumors has been reported,[126] we lack data to link tumor incidence to dosage. No major study of the effect of prenatal radiation on the incidence of testicular cancer has been done, but a pilot study suggests that there is no significant increase.[192]

HORMONAL FACTORS

Case control studies suggest the possibility of a somewhat increased risk to patients who have been exposed to "hormones" before birth or whose mothers had increased nausea and vomiting during pregnancy[119] possibly owing to elevated maternal human chorionic gonadotropin (hCG) levels.

OTHER

Increased testicular heat, associated with brief (jockey) undershorts is associated with an increased incidence of testicular cancer.[192]

Histogenesis and Classification

Our understanding of the histogenesis and development of germ cell tumors has been put on a firmer basis by individuals such as Stevens[281,282] and Pierce.[241] Teilum's comparative analysis of ovarian and testicular lesions[301,302] and strong efforts by the World Health Organization and experts in several countries have led to classification schemes that better reflect our current knowledge. It is clear that testicular germ cell tumors originate from abnormal germ cells within the seminiferous tubules (see the section on germ cell tumors in situ) and, usually after invasion of the stroma, remain in an undifferentiated state or proceed, at least focally, to differentiate toward recognizable embryonal or extraembryonal tissues (Fig. 27-4).

Germ cell tumors have been classified many ways over the past few decades. Although we use the scheme proposed by the World Health Organization in 1977 (Table 27-1), one should note that it does not

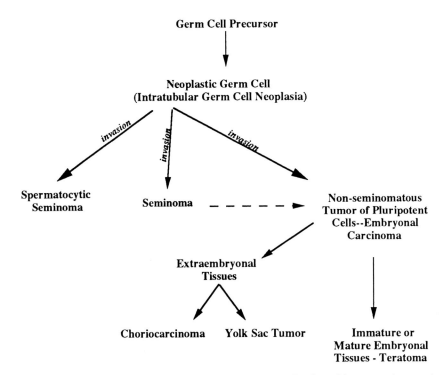

Fig. 27-4 Proposed inter-relationship of germ cell tumors. The dotted line provides a pathway for the development of nonseminomatous elements within a seminoma. There is no evidence for transformation of spermatocytic seminoma into seminoma, or vice versa.

Table 27-1 World Health Organization Classification of Testicular Germ Cell Tumors

Tumors of one histological type
  Seminoma
  Spermatocytic seminoma
  Embryonal carcinoma
  Yolk sac tumor (endodermal sinus tumor)
  Polyembryoma
  Choriocarcinoma
  Teratomas
    Mature
    Immature
    With malignant transformation
Tumors of more than one histological type
  Embryonal carcinoma and teratoma (teratocarcinoma)
  Choriocarcinoma and any other type (specify type)
  Other combinations (specify)

From Mostofi et al.,[218] with permission.

include a category of in-situ tumor and only the spermatocytic variant of seminoma is included.

For easier comprehension of the British literature, Table 27-2 lists the comparative British terminology. Thoughtful criticisms of both schemes have appeared in the last few years.[136,328] One hopes that an integration of the histologic appearance of the tumor with its immunohistochemical characteristics and serum tumor markers can be devised that would relate optimally to biological behavior and expected response to therapy.

Markers

Identification of specific proteins made by certain testicular tumors and released into the blood stream may be exceedingly useful, both in tumor diagnosis and in tumor therapy. These so-called "biological marker proteins" should be looked for and quantitated prior to operation in each patient with a suspected testicular tumor; they may be used postoperatively to follow the efficacy of therapy.[174]

The chief markers in current use are human chorionic gonadotropin (hCG), and α fetoprotein (AFP). An elevated serum level of hCG may be found in a wide variety of tumors (e.g., carcinoma of the stomach, pancreas, lung, liver, and melanoma[42,112] as well as in normal pregnancy, hydatidiform mole, and choriocarcinoma), but in a patient with a testicular mass an elevated hCG level strongly suggests the presence of a germ cell tumor containing either isolated syncytiotrophoblastic giant cells or foci of choriocarcinoma.

AFP is normally produced only by fetal liver and yolk sac but may be found in a number of tumors, especially hepatic, pancreatic, and biliary carcinoma, and with benign liver regeneration. Elevated levels may be seen in patients with liver metastases from these tumors. In a patient with presumed testicular tumor, elevated AFP levels suggest strongly that yolk sac elements are present, but levels may also be elevated when only more primitive embryonal elements are present.

The histologic cellular composition of the germ cell tumor profoundly influences the likelihood of serum marker production. Seminoma typically is not associated with AFP production but 7 to 15 percent[53,145] of these patients do have an elevated serum hCG level, nearly all of which contain demonstrable syncytiotrophoblasts. Most embryonal carcinomas and teratocarcinomas are associated with AFP or hCG production, or both, while only a minority of teratomas produce either marker.[145] Yolk sac tumors typically produce AFP, but rarely, if ever, hCG, while choriocarcinomas all produce hCG but no AFP.

Because only 80 to 90 percent of testicular tumors produce these marker proteins the clinician must not exclude tumor in their absence. In addition, metastatic disease may not contain marker-producing cells,

Table 27-2 Testicular Germ Cell Tumor Classification: Comparison of American and British Terms

American	British
Teratoma mature	Teratoma differentiated (TD)
Teratoma immature	Malignant teratoma intermediate (MTI)
Embryonal carcinoma	Malignant teratoma undifferentiated (MTU)
Choriocarcinoma	Malignant teratoma trophoblastic (MTT)

or the marker-producing cells may be selectively killed by chemotherapy, leaving behind viable tumor, which may progress without positive serum markers. This does not represent "false-negative" markers[340] but is a reflection of the well-known heterogeneity of tumor cell populations.

Human chorionic gonadotropin (hCG) is a 45,000 D glycoprotein. Analysis is typically performed on serum, but concentrated 24 hour urine specimens[92] and pleural and ascitic fluid[64] may contain hCG. Accuracy depends on the ability to separate clearly the β subunit of hCG from that of luteinizing hormone (LH), since the α subunits of each are identical. Using a double antibody radioimmunoassay, males normally have a serum level of hCG below 1 ng/ml (5 milli-international units/ml).[146] Impurity of the antibody used or lack of antibody specificity may give rise to false-positive and false-negative results, especially in patients with elevated LH levels.[149] Hence, a reliable laboratory is essential, and laboratory results must be correlated with the clinical picture and repeated if necessary.

A more sophisticated approach to hCG reveals that in addition to intact hCG molecules, some tumors secrete free α- and β-chains of hCG, and that there is probably heterogeneity among hCG molecules secreted from different sites, depending on the degree of glycosylation.[198]

Radioactively labelled antibodies to hCG have been used experimentally to localize but not, as yet, successfully treat foci of tumor not detected by other methods.[146] Intravenously injected antibody labelled with ^{131}I appears to bind selectively to tumor sites in patients with elevated hCG levels. Antibodies to AFP may also be used successfully for immunodetection of metastatic sites of tumors producing AFP, although some of the positivity may be due to nonspecific tumor localization.[101]

Following removal of the testicular tumor any elevation in serum hCG level should return to normal in the absence of metastases. Although the serum half life of hCG is roughly 24 hours, catabolism may be variable in sick or postoperative patients, and it may be more realistic to state that the hCG half life may vary in various patients between 18 and 30 hours.[175] AFP half life is about 4 to 6 days with a mean of about 5 days. Abrupt lowering of marker levels immediately postoperatively and abrupt increase during induction chemotherapy are likely artifacts of therapy,[175] there-fore *serial* marker values over weeks and months are required to accurately assess tumor status. A simple plot of marker values against time on semi-log paper allows the clinician to detect deviations from expected decay[188] and may allow for a prompt change in therapy if there is appreciable change from straight line marker decay (Fig. 27-5).

Moderate elevation of hCG (10 to 20 ng/ml) after apparently curative therapy has been claimed to be due to marihuana smoking[94] and one patient had persistence of AFP elevation without known cause long after what appeared to be curative chemotherapy.[246] Nevertheless, failure of an elevated level of hCG or AFP to drop with surgery and chemotherapy is very strong evidence that residual viable tumor is present, and is considered by most clinicians as sufficient evidence to warrant further vigorous therapy.

The limitation of these markers is most evident with seminomas, which are all negative for AFP and hCG except for those few with syncytiotrophoblastic giant cells.

A potentially useful serum marker for seminoma has been found in placenta-like alkaline phosphatase (PLAP).[173] Nearly two thirds[137] to 90 percent[312] of seminoma patients have significant elevation of serum PLAP levels, with a fall to normal levels after therapy. However, as many smokers, nontestis tumor patients, and 21 to 33 percent of nonseminomatous testis tumor patients also have elevated serum PLAP levels, the test may be more useful for following a known seminoma patient than for primary diagnosis. Immunohistochemically, PLAP is localized mainly to cell membranes of seminoma and syncytiotrophoblastic cells, with slight staining of embryonal carcinoma and negative staining of yolk sac, teratoma, and cytotrophoblast.[315] Intratubular carcinoma stains positive in 80 percent to over 90 percent of cases.[132,137]

An elevated serum ferritin level has been found in many patients with pure seminoma,[308] but the finding is limited in usefulness because levels are also elevated in other testicular germ cell tumors, as well as in leukemias, lymphomas, and carcinomas of the breast, bowel, and lung.[117,308] Further, serial determinations of serum ferritin levels in patients with testicular carcinoma have not yet been proven of value. Histologically, positive staining for ferritin in pure seminomas may be obtained with immunoperoxidase techniques using rabbit antisera to isoferritins of both human liver and heart.[61]

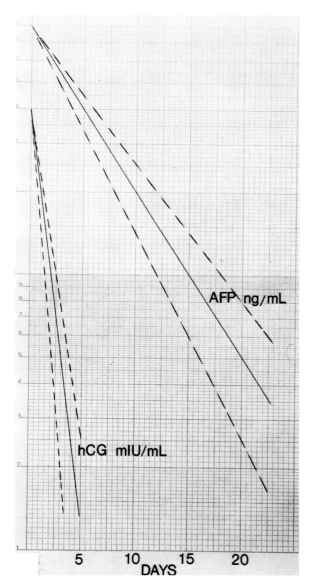

Fig. 27-5 Semi-log representation of decay of serum markers α-fetoprotein (AFP) and human chorionic gonadotropin (hCG). Straight line decay within the limits of biologic variability implies total or near total ablation of tumor cells producing the marker. Note the differing rates of disappearance: 5 ± 1 day half-life for AFP and 24 ± 6 hour half-life for hCG.

Elevated serum lactic dehydrogenase (LDH) levels may be found in over 60 percent of patients with metastatic germ cell tumors.[38] LDH appears to operate as an independent variable of prognostic significance.[37,325] Since elevation may occur both in semi-

nomatous and nonseminomatous germ cell tumors, as well as in numerous malignant and nonmalignant conditions,[353] specific LDH isoenzymes have been examined in the search for greater specificity.[40] Testicular tumors of all histologic types typically have elevated serum levels of isoenzyme LDH 1, which is composed of four heart-type (H) subunits,[186] in contrast to other malignancies in which one, two, or three muscle-type (M) subunits are present.[102] LDH 1 has been demonstrated immunohistochemically in 85 percent of testicular germ cell tumors tested, including all seminomas.[224]

Although serum LDH levels may be useful in monitoring treatment of advanced nonseminomatous disease,[39] their use may lie especially in their ability to follow patients with seminoma,[185] where serum AFP is normal and serum hCG uncommonly elevated.[147] However, their usefulness as a prognostic indicator or as an aid in monitoring therapy has not yet been proven.

Carcinoembryonic antigen has been also examined as a serum marker of possible usefulness. Because its level is usually not raised and because CEA, when raised, may be due to so many malignant and nonmalignant causes, its use cannot be routinely recommended.[39]

Other proposed markers in patients include hemoglobin F,[68,159] α_1-antitrypsin,[25,124] specific β_1-glycoprotein (SP$_1$),[144] and placental lactogen.[245] Although histochemically one may stain certain areas of some testicular tumors for each of these substances, it remains to be demonstrated that, as one group claims,[139] "addition of further tumor markers to the already established ones, AFP and hCG, may result in greater certainty in diagnosis, monitoring, and prognostic evaluation of patients with testis tumors."

Substances secreted by testicular germ cell tumors may cause various signs and symptoms. One individual with embryonal carcinoma had clinical signs of hyperthyroidism with elevated plasma TSH-like activity that responded to tumor chemotherapy.[278] Synthesis of the factor by the tumor was postulated, but recurrent tumor did not result in recurrent hyperthyroidism.

Gynecomastia or breast tenderness is found in about 10 percent of patients with stage IIc and III disease at presentation, and is present in one fourth of those whose hCG level is over 100 mIU/ml.[311] It is likely due both to elevated hCG and circulating estrogens,

Table 27-3 Staging of Testicular Tumors Among Various Institutions

Stage	Memorial Sloan–Kettering[a]	UCLA[b]	Royal Marsden[c]	Massachusetts General[d]
Stage I (or A)		Tumor Limited to Testis		
Stage II (or B)				
Regional node metastasis				
II A (B1)	Microscopic metastases	Microscopic metastases	Metastases < 2 cm	Metastases < 2 cm
II B (B2)	Microscopic metastases, completely resected	Metastases < 3 cm	Metastases 2–5 cm	Metastases > 2 cm
II C (B3)	Microscopic metastases, incompletely resected	Bulky retroperitoneal disease	Metastases > 5 cm	—
Stage III (or C)				
Distal node metastases				
III A (C1)	Distant lymph nodes involved	—	Supraclavicular or mediastinal nodes	Supraclavicular or mediastinal nodes
III B (C2)	Lung metastases	—		
III C (C3)	Multiple organ metastases	—		
Stage IV	—	—	Extralymphatic metastases	Disseminated tumor

Data from [a]Barzell et al.,[21] [b]de Kernion,[74] [c]Hendry et al.,[120] and [d]Donohue et al.[80]

especially estrone.[280] The estrogens arise from aromatization of dehydroepiandrosterone and androstenedione of possible tumor origin.[164] There is a significantly poorer prognosis of the patients with breast symptoms, independent of the serum hCG.[311]

Staging

Treatment and prognosis are heavily dependent on proper staging, which may be clinical or surgical. The staging systems in Table 27-3 are among those in common use. The first two (Memorial Sloan–Kettering and UCLA) are for surgical, and the latter two for clinical staging. Additional schemes besides these are in use.[151] Computerized tomography and lymphangiography of the retroperitoneum have negative rates of about 40 percent.[84,183] Careful mapping of involved nodes demonstrates that right testis tumors spread preferentially (93 percent) to the inter-aortocaval zone just below the left renal vein. Left testis primaries spread to the pre-aortic and left para-aortic areas most commonly (87 percent).[80] The lymphatics of the spermatic vein are involved in about 15 percent of patients, but iliac areas are uncommonly tumor positive.[80] Supraclavicular node biopsy is probably not useful in the absence of clinical suspicion.[206]

Germ Cell Tumors In Situ

Reasonably clear identification of an in-situ precursor lesion for germ cell tumors as confirmed by followup has been made only in the past 15 years. In 1972 Skakkebaek[273] reported that two men with histologically abnormal intratubular cells on testicular biopsy had developed an ipsilateral infiltrating germ cell tumor 16 months and 4.5 years later. Earlier observations[19,77,200,343] had noted these atypical cells and had postulated a precursor role on morphologic grounds. Histologically, nuclei of these intratubular cells were reported to be enlarged, the chromatin was coarsely and irregularly clumped, and mitoses were common. DNA content measured spectrophotometrically was abnormally high. A subsequent larger study involved biopsies from 50 men aged 18 to 30 with a history of cryptorchid testis and orchiopexy.[166] Four patients had abnormal intratubular cells with or without an infiltrating germ cell tumor indicating a clinically significant (8 percent) incidence of in-situ carcinoma.

A further study[222] of boys aged 8 to 18 with maldescended testes revealed many with abnormal and enlarged intratubular cells. Long-term followup is needed to identify the risk of this finding, especially since not all investigators have confirmed it.[221] If confirmed, the optimal age of biopsy, probably after puberty, and the risks and benefits will need careful analysis. If intratubular tumor involves as much as 10 percent of the testis, because of its multifocal nature a 3 mm biopsy should detect it in most cases.[31]

There is a known increased risk to the contralateral testis in patients with a testicular germ cell tumor. Biopsies of 250 such patients revealed in-situ carcinoma in 13 (5 percent), two of whom developed invasive tumor 21 and 46 months later.[30] The average latent period between the development of phenotypically abnormal intratubular germ cells and invasive tumor is not known. It may be as long as 10 years, but typically is from 2 to 5 years after an abnormal biopsy.[31,133]

The finding of in-situ carcinoma adjacent to infiltrating tumor in 93 of 99 patients with germ cell tumors (89 percent of seminomas and 99 percent of nonseminomas) strongly supports the concept that abnormal intratubular cells are the precursors of invasive disease.[140] Although intratubular syncytiotrophoblastic cells may be noted on rare occasions in in-situ carcinomas,[217] the intratubular cells associated both with seminomas and nonseminomas usually appear similar on hematoxylin and eosin staining. The periodic acid-Schiff stain reveals that virtually all cases contain glycogen in the atypical intratubular germ cells as defined by diastase-sensitivity. Only rarely (2 percent of cases) do intratubular tumor cells stain immunocytochemically for hCG, CEA, or ferritin, and none has stained for AFP.[60] This leads to speculation that many germ cell tumors may differentiate only upon penetration of the tubular basement membrane and interaction with the stromal components.

Whereas no grossly visible lesion is to be expected, microscopically one may find a spectrum ranging from normal-sized seminiferous tubules with only rare scattered abnormal cells to distended tubules with massive replacement by tumor cells (Fig. 27-6).

The cells of in-situ carcinoma are larger than normal, with abundant clear cytoplasm, and tend to be adjacent to the basement membrane; their nuclei are also enlarged, round or irregular, and hyperchromatic. The abnormal cells may be admixed with normal

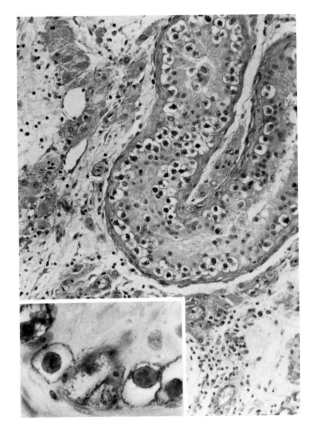

Fig. 27-6 Carcinoma in situ. Large cells with nuclear atypia, enlargement and hyperchromatism and clear cytoplasm lie adjacent to the basement membrane in the initial stages of the process. The cell membrane stains positively for the presence of placental-like alkaline phosphatase (inset). (Inset, courtesy of Dr. J.E. Tomaszewski.)

germ cells, with Sertoli cells only,[262] or may replace all normal cells. In contrast to normal germ cells, intratubular neoplastic germ cells express placenta-like alkaline phosphastase activity when stained immunohistochemically in over 90 percent of cases.[132] This has been proposed as a useful diagnostic marker.[2,137] Ultrastructural studies[6] show the cells to contain dense-cored vesicles and accumulations of granular electron-dense material "nuages" in the cytoplasm, consistent with germ cell origin. In addition, and in distinction to normal spermatogenesis, intercellular bridges linking the neoplastic germ cells to Sertoli cells are absent.[104] The early stages of tumor cell emigration from the tubules have been examined ultrastructurally.[262] Carcinoma in situ may be found

accompanied by early stromal invasion without a frank tumor mass, so-called microinvasive carcinoma (Fig. 27-7).[326] Histologically abnormal germ cells are noted in the stroma. An accompanying lymphocytic infiltrate is frequently present, and its presence should raise the suspicion of early invasion when abnormal intratubular cells are seen. The prognosis of microinvasive disease appears excellent; appropriate treatment is unknown, but regional lymph node irradiation has been given in two cases.[326] There is an anecdotal report of apparently successful treatment of carcinoma in situ by chemotherapy,[324] but elsewhere one notes that sequential bilateral germ cell tumors occurred despite chemotherapy.[88]

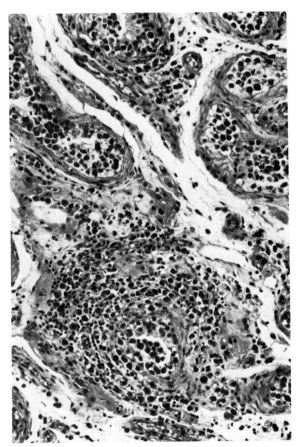

Fig. 27-7 Carcinoma in situ with early invasion. Seminiferous tubules are largely filled with atypical germ cells, some of which have invaded the stroma. The infiltrate of lymphocytes is characteristic.

Seminoma

Seminoma comprises approximately 40 percent of all germ cell tumors. It is virtually nonexistent before the age of 10,[238] and occurs most commonly between the ages of 25 and 55, with a peak incidence at about 35.

CLINICAL PRESENTATION

Whereas the presenting complaint of a man with seminoma is most often that of testicular mass, nearly half have some local discomfort or pain as well. In a few cases, the symptoms are related to metastases to retroperitoneal or supraclavicular nodes, or to the lungs, or to weight loss or anemia. Exophthalmos is a rare manifestation of seminoma.[300]

GROSS PRESENTATION

The typical seminoma seen has already resulted in gross testicular enlargement, but the tunica albuginea is normally intact and the epididymis usually grossly uninvolved. On section the tumor typically bulges above the surrounding tan testicular parenchyma and appears lobulated and rather well delineated without any capsule (Fig. 27-8). It is typically white or pinkish-white, but if a heavy mononuclear cell infiltrate is present it may appear tan. It may be focally soft or necrotic, but does not usually appear hemorrhagic or cystic. The presence of either of these features or of focal firmness or calcification is strongly suggestive of a nonseminomatous germ cell component. The alert clinician, when reviewing the case with the pathologist, will check to make certain that a minimum of eight to ten areas of tumor are sampled to rule out a nonseminomatous component. Certainly, if the tumor is 7 to 8 cm in diameter or larger, additional sampling may be required. Preoperative elevation of serum hCG or AFP is another indication for more extensive sampling.

MICROSCOPIC PRESENTATION

The classic microscopic pattern of seminoma is one composed of a sheet of large regular polygonal cells separated by thin fibrous septa into lobules (Fig. 27-9). These lobules typically contain a few dozen up to a hundred or so cells. At least 80 percent of semi-

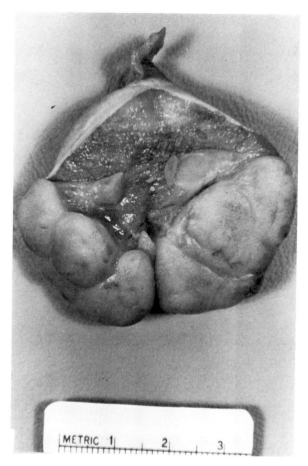

Fig. 27-8 Seminoma. The pure seminoma has a clearly defined but non-encapsulated border. It is off-white, and if heavily infiltrated by lymphocytes, tan. Note lack of cysts or hemorrhage which might indicate a nonseminomatous component. (Courtesy of Dr. A.J. Steinberg.) (From Wheeler et al.,[339a] with permission.)

nomas contain a readily apparent lymphocytic infiltrate, especially prominent about the septa, composed largely of T cells.[5] Total absence of lymphocytes should raise the suspicion of possible embryonal carcinoma. The commonest variation on this pattern is one caused by infiltrating histiocytes that may nearly totally obscure the underlying pleomorphic tumor cells. Histiocytes may have a somewhat pale vacuolated cytoplasm, but often appear more eosinophilic and epithelioid, forming a frank granulomatous reaction in half of the cases (Fig. 27-10).[152] Although a similar granulomatous response may be seen in testicular ter-

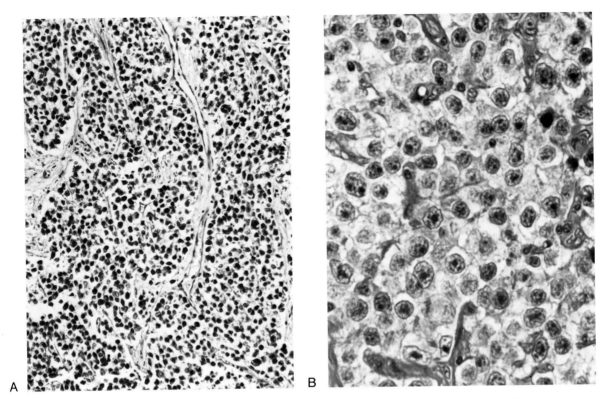

A   B

Fig. 27-9 Seminoma. **(A)** The rather uniform neoplastic cell population is formed into lobules by delicate fibrous septa. A lymphocytic infiltrate is typical but may be absent, as here. **(B)** High magnification reveals rather uniform polygonal tumor cells with clear cytoplasm, crisp and prominent nuclear membranes, and coarsely clumped nuclear chromatin. PLAP, PAS, and Vimentin stains will be positive, Keratin almost always negative.

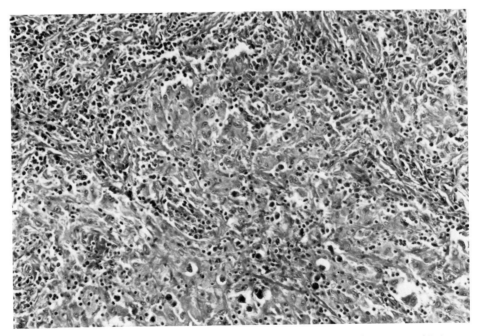

Fig. 27-10 Seminoma. A marked granulomatous reaction is present with numerous histiocytes and lymphocytes and occasional giant cells. Residual tumor cells may be difficult to find or even absent on a given section.

atomas,[307] it is far more characteristic of seminoma and may be a diagnostic clue in metastatic foci.[254]

At least some necrosis is present focally in most tumors, but fibrosis is seen in only 15 percent.[152] Leydig cells in nontumor areas may appear prominent, but whether this is true hyperplasia or merely a reflection of relative tubular atrophy and fibrosis has not been determined by a careful morphometric study.

One or more germ cell tumors of differing histologic type may be found focally in an otherwise typical seminoma[293] or in metastases from what is believed to have been a pure seminoma.[44,217] The question of what constitutes a pure seminoma, and whether other germ cell tumors may occasionally originate directly from a histologically classic seminoma, has not been settled definitively. The likelihood of a continuum between seminoma and yolk sac carcinoma,[251] or between anaplastic seminoma and embryonal carcinoma, the random distribution of syncytiotrophoblastic giant cells in some seminomas, and the heterogeneity of staining for intermediate filaments,[75] tend to support the idea that a seminoma cell may retain pluripotent capabilities.

BEHAVIOR

Seminoma is an actively growing tumor. Perfusion studies of removed tumorous testes yield a potential doubling time for the proliferating portion of tumor of about five days.[250] Seminoma metastasizes primarily via the lymphatics and later hematogenously. Retroperitoneal lymph node involvement usually precedes mediastinal and supraclavicular nodal disease. The lungs, liver, kidney, bone, and brain, as well as other sites, are involved in descending order of frequency.[44,201] Death from respiratory insufficiency and sepsis from secondary infections constitute the major cause of death.[44] Late recurrences after therapy are uncommon since the great majority of patients are cured, but 20 percent of those that do recur appear after two years (in contrast to only 4 percent late recurrence in nonseminomatous tumors).[354] Recurrences after many years are rarely reported,[194,332] and because of the bilaterality of some testis tumors, a secondary primary must be excluded.[59] Likewise, in primary seminoma both of the retroperitoneum[52] and of the mediastinum,[51] tumors nearly exclusively of men, an occult testicular primary must be excluded.[18,35] Histologic factors influencing prognosis

have been sought for diligently,[152,168] but the overriding factor is the stage of disease.[152]

TREATMENT AND PROGNOSIS

The exquisite radiosensitivity of seminoma makes radiation the treatment of choice. This results in 5-year survival rates of 97 percent in stage I and 86 percent in stage II.[269] The 25 percent of patients presenting with higher-stage disease have a sufficiently high relapse rate with radiation alone that systemic chemotherapy is currently advocated.[339] This may result in sustained complete remission in 90 percent of patients. Treatment for a second primary germ cell tumor after a seminoma is complicated by previous therapy[59] and must be individualized. The content of alkaline phosphatase isozymes is greatly elevated in seminoma tissue[125] and the serum level of one of them, placenta-like alkaline phosphatase (PLAP) (as noted earlier), may be used to follow the course of therapy.

SEMINOMA WITH SYNCYTIOTROPHOBLASTIC GIANT CELLS OR POSITIVE hCG TITER

When Dixon and Moore illustrated the rather frequent presence of syncytiotrophoblastic giant cells in otherwise typical seminomas in 1952,[77] the histogenesis was not understood and the prognostic implications were unknown. The former is still true; the latter is becoming clearer.

The clinical presentation and gross appearance of the tumor are the same as for typical seminoma, except for gynecomastia in some patients. Histologically, one may find syncytiotrophoblastic giant cells in some 5 to 14 percent of all seminomas.[53,77,145,289,304] The cells stain positively with antibodies to hCG[170] and are presumed to account for the elevated hCG level found in most of these patients. Although the assumption has been in the past that an elevated hCG without syncytiotrophoblastic giant cells merely reflected sampling problems with the tumor, exhaustive sampling occasionally fails to identify giant cells,[93] and some recent evidence[258,351] exists that mononuclear hCG-producing cells could be responsible. On the other hand, an elevated AFP strongly implies an undiscovered focus of yolk sac tumor, and indicates the need for extensive further tumor sampling[147] and treatment appropriate for a nonseminomatous tumor.

Any gross areas of a seminoma resembling petechial hemorrhages should be carefully searched microscopically for syncytiotrophoblastic giant cells. These cells are quite characteristic, with irregular cell outlines, eosinophilic or amphophilic cytoplasm, and multiple, often clumped nuclei (Fig. 27-11). They are frequently vacuolated and often appear to line blood-filled spaces. They should not be confused with the giant cells of a granulomatous reaction. Staining for hCG should solve any diagnostic ambiguity.

Although the initial prognostic data indicated a worse prognosis for seminomas with syncytiotrophoblastic giant cells,[216] more recent information,[204,211,289,329] fails to support a worse outcome. It should be emphasized that the presence of syncytiotrophoblastic giant cells is quite different from a focus of choriocarcinoma with demonstrable areas of both syncytiotrophoblastic and cytotrophoblastic cells. With syncytiotrophoblastic giant cells the serum hCG β subunit is typically on the order of 20 to 70 MIu/ml,[204] while with focal choriocarcinoma it is usually far higher. The metastatic potential and incidence of lethal outcome is far higher with a focus of true choriocarcinoma.

SPERMATOCYTIC SEMINOMA

This germ cell tumor is of importance because it may be confused with lymphoma or other tumors of poor prognosis, and because spermatic seminoma itself carries an excellent prognosis.

Clinical

In the large series reported by Talerman[295] the incidence of spermatocytic seminoma was 13 in 292 seminomas (4.4 percent) or 2.6 percent of all germ cell tumors. The mean age of men affected is reported at 55 to 60 with a range of 30 to 87,[295] although in Masson's original series[203] two of the patients were 25 and 26 years old. Bilaterality has been reported in at least four patients,[255,295] either synchronously[255] or up to 20 years later.

The patients typically present with painless testicular swelling of a few weeks' to several years' duration, or the enlarged testis may be found only incidentally on routine physical examination. All serum markers thus far examined (AFP, hCG, LDH) have been negative.[295]

Gross Examination

Radical orchiectomy is the typical specimen obtained for suspected tumor. On section the spermatocytic seminoma has a well-delineated outline and may even appear encapsulated. Although the usual size is 4 to 5 cm in diameter, some have been reported up to 15 cm. The tumor is soft and grayish-white to yellow. Edema is characteristic and causes the surface to appear gelatinous or mucoid. In the larger tumors one may see small mucoid-appearing cysts, and rarely there may be focal hemorrhage and necrosis.[295] Only the largest tumors involve the epididymis. Occasionally the tumor appears to consist of two or three separate nodules.

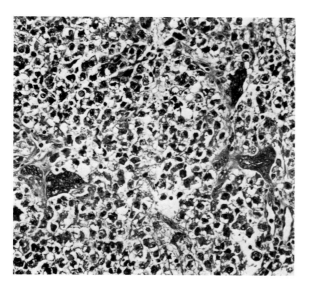

Fig. 27-11 Seminoma with syncytiotrophoblastic giant cells. The multinucleated giant cells have a more irregular cell outline and more hyperchromatic nuclei than those seen with a granulomatous reaction. Blood-filled spaces may lie adjacent to the syncytiotrophoblast. The presence of any accompanying cytotrophoblast indicates focal choriocarcinoma.

Microscopic

The initial low-power impression is one of a sheet of small cells suggestive of lymphoma or a leukemic infiltrate (Fig. 27-12). Any stromal support present

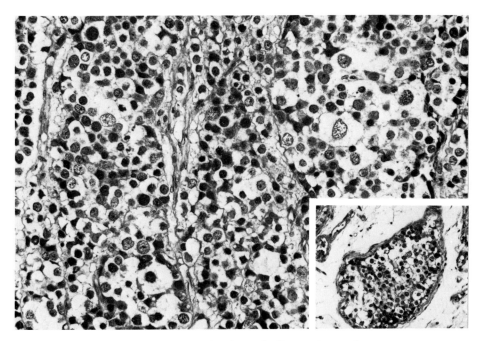

Fig. 27-12 Spermatocytic seminoma. The sheet of cells seen here at low power may suggest lymphoma, but the presence of intratubular disease (as shown in the inset), cell cohesion, and the mixture of cell types noted at higher magnification are helpful in arriving at the correct diagnosis.

tends to be quite delicate and inconspicuous, and a lymphocytic infiltrate is not present.

The growth pattern of spermatocytic seminoma is distinctive owing to prominent involvement of the seminiferous tubules. These are enormously expanded and are filled with neoplastic cells. Tubular rupture in more than one area may explain the occurrence of two or more gross nodules of tumor in a single testis.

On higher power three rather distinctly different cell types may be noted (Fig. 27-13). Most of the cells are 6 to 8 μm in diameter with condensed dark chromatin. The larger cells have a vesicular nucleus with granular filamentous clumped chromatin and an inconspicuous nucleolus. The filamentous chromatin is strongly reminiscent of the spireme configuration of meiosis. The nuclear outline of the small, dark and larger, vesicular cells is classically quite round. Larger, frequently multinucleated giant cells are present, ranging up to 50 to 100 μm in diameter, but these form only a very small proportion of the total tumor population. Their nuclei tend to be oval with irregular clumped chromatin and the cytoplasm of the giant cells is eosinophilic.

Intracellular glycogen is absent or barely detectable, in contrast to typical seminomas. Mitoses are rare, and this finding coupled with the spireme nuclear pattern and diversity of nuclear forms led Masson[203] to suggest that the tumor was a neoplastic mimic of the normal process of spermatogenesis. The smallest cells are compared with spermatogonia; the larger cells were likened to primary spermatocytes in leptotene. Some cells suggested degenerating secondary spermatocytes. When tested with lectins histochemically, however, spermatocytic seminomas do not react with the lectins, which recognize spermatids,[179] weakening the spermatogenesis analogy. Immunohistochemical staining reveals lack of placenta-like alkaline phosphatase activity, unlike classical seminomas and embryonal carcinomas,[11,132] and this finding has led to uncertainty concerning its histogenesis.[223]

Electron microscopic study[256,298] confirms some features of spermatogenesis but offers distinctions from it. The nuclei of most intermediate-sized cells lack indentations. A large nucleolus is present, with a central amorphous area and a larger nucleolonema (convoluted thread-like structure) similar to sperma-

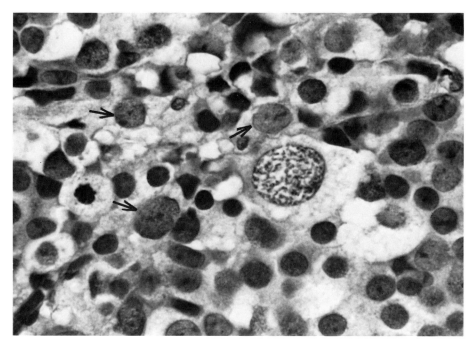

Fig. 27-13 Spermatocytic seminoma. Three cell types are present in this tumor: small dark lymphocyte-like cells, medium-sized cells with granular or filamentous chromatin (arrows), and one of the rare large or giant cells with "spireme-like" chromatin. (From Wheeler et al.,[339a] with permission.)

togonia.[256] Most cells have homogeneously granular chromatin, but a few have thread-like chromatin resembling the leptotene stage of meiosis.[256] Golgi has been described both as prominent[256] and as not well demonstrated,[298] but all observers agree that rough endoplasmic reticulum is scarce. Of special interest is the finding of the zona adherens type of cell junction and intercellular bridges similar to those seen between spermatocytes and spermatids in normal spermatogenesis.

Prognosis

The natural history of spermatocytic seminoma is almost certainly totally benign. The only patients with tumors reported to have had fatal metastatic disease have been shown on review either to most likely have had a tumor of hematopoietic origin,[255] or to have had insufficient documentation of metastases and no reported autopsy findings.[203]

Many patients have been subjected to postorchiectomy lymph node radiation[295] in spite of the absence of proven metastases, and it is not truly known

whether the tumor is even radiosensitive. Eleven patients treated with surgery only[330] have had 10 years of mean followup without sign of metastatic disease.

Rosai notes that this tumor shares many features with canine testicular seminomas: it occurs in older individuals, with a relatively high incidence of bilaterality, and is rarely if ever malignant; nor is it associated with other germ cell tumors (unlike typical seminoma). Two recent reports do note association of spermatocytic seminoma with a sarcomatous component,[85,310] a fact previously only incidentally illustrated.[217]

ANAPLASTIC SEMINOMA

Variation in the degree of histologic anaplasia in seminomas has been known to exist for many years and was, in fact, illustrated in the first AFIP Fascicle.[77] The practice of trying to separate typical from anaplastic seminomas was apparently started at Walter Reed about that time, based upon anaplasia, pleomorphism, and an increased mitotic rate, which has now become codified as an average of three or more mitoses per high-power field.

Clinical Presentation

Clinically an anaplastic seminoma presents as a typical seminoma with swelling, occasional pain, or, in about 10 percent, with symptoms secondary to distant metastases.[217] The age range is similar to that of typical seminomas.

Pathological Examination

The gross appearance of anaplastic and typical seminomas is similar. Microscopically, nuclear anaplasia and increased mitoses are the most important findings (Fig. 27-14). The frequency of pyknotic nuclei in seminomas simulating mitoses, and the wide interobserver variation in mitotic counts in other tumors,[272]

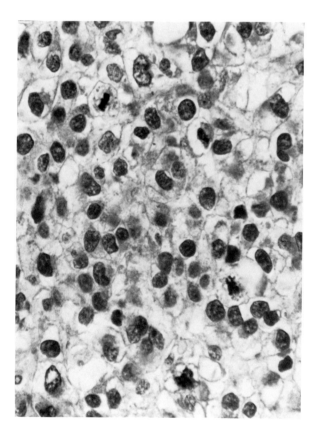

Fig. 27-14 Anaplastic seminoma. Cellular and nuclear pleomorphism is more prominent than that seen in a typical seminoma, and mitoses are abundant.

suggest that the diagnosis of anaplastic seminomas should be eyed with some skepticism. Although as recently as 1984[58] the mitotic count delineating an anaplastic seminoma was considered three or more per high-power field, von Hochstetter[327] found that 87 percent of the seminomas he analyzed contained three or more, and 10 percent of the tumors contained six or more mitoses per high-power field, with a high-power field defined as 0.152 mm^2. The boundary between anaplastic seminoma and embryonal carcinoma may present diagnostic difficulties owing to anaplasia and what Nochomovitz wryly terms "provocative pseudoglandular patterns"[229] in some seminomas. Immunohistochemical staining of intermediate filaments[209,252] in germ cell tumors indicates that seminomas are vimentin positive in most cells, whereas embryonal carcinomas are cytokeratin positive.[24] A few cells in each tumor, however, may stain for the other component.

Ultrastructural analysis of an anaplastic seminoma proved to be similar to typical seminomas.[143]

Prognosis

Whereas initially it appeared that the biologic behavior of the anaplastic group was perhaps not very different from typical seminoma,[196] additional studies[153,156,217] have provided evidence for a worse prognosis. When corrected for stage, however,[196,231] the treatment, radiosensitivity, and prognosis of typical and anaplastic seminoma appear similar. Attempts to examine the biological behavior of this lesion has been hampered by small numbers in one series,[153] inclusion of patients with elevated hCG in another,[236] and referral selection in still another.[58]

Current therapy for seminoma is sufficiently good that it may never become possible to prove that anaplastic seminomas are prognostically worse than typical seminomas of the same stage.

Embryonal Carcinoma

Embryonal carcinoma is a highly malignant tumor in which histologically primitive cells form the sole element or a prominent histologic component of many nonseminomatous germ cell tumors. At the outset it must be pointed out that the British literature often uses the term *undifferentiated malignant teratoma* for the World Health Organization's (WHO) classification term of embryonal carcinoma. (See Table 27.2) Although we use the WHO classification here, the frequent observation of transitions between and combinations of embryonal carcinoma and malignant teratoma (so-called teratocarcinoma) should make the rationale for the British system clearer. Another area of possible confusion is the fact that yolk sac tumors of childhood have, in previous years, been referred to as "infantile embryonal carcinoma." These are classified as yolk sac tumors and discussed in that section.

Both microscopic and experimental studies[241] demonstrate that the component cells of embryonal carcinoma retain the ability to differentiate toward somatic or extraembryonic structures. Because of these frequent admixtures of teratomatous elements, yolk sac or choriocarcinoma, careful pathologic examination is necessary.

Patients are usually in the 20 to 35 year age range and present with local or metastatic complaints common to all patients with testicular germ cell tumors. It is rarely, if ever, found in children below 12 years of age,[114] but may be found in old age.

Gross section of the testis reveals a grayish, soft, and often focally necrotic or hemorrhagic mass (Fig. 27-15). Multiple sections are necessary to rule out other differentiated components or an accompanying seminoma. Microscopically the tumor cells tend to form sheets with or without clefting or papillary formation (Fig. 27-16). The cell outlines are inconspicuous so as to simulate a syncytium, the cytoplasm is weakly eosinophilic, and the nuclei large and pleomorphic, with coarse chromatin clumping and frequent mitoses (Fig. 27-17). Nucleoli may be multiple. Embryonal carcinoma typically lacks the lymphocytic infiltrate seen with most seminomas. In 10 to 20 percent of cases the tumor at the time of removal has already invaded the epididymis.[217]

Ultrastructural examination confirms the undifferentiated nature of embryonal carcinoma. Only a few organelles are present, with occasional rudimentary microvilli and desmosomes.[242] Some cells show further differentiation, with well-developed desmosomes and microvilli.

Metastases to retroperitoneal nodes occur early, and over half of the tumors are at least stage II when first diagnosed.[79] Nonseminomatous tumors of the right testis, when metastatic, most commonly (93 percent) involve the interaortocaval zone immediately below

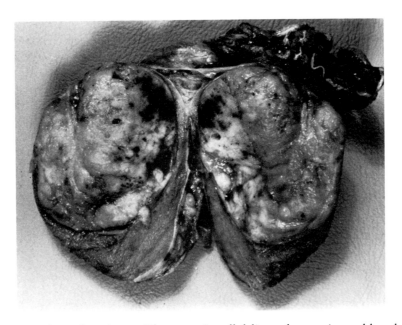

Fig. 27-15 Embryonal carcinoma. The tumor is well delineated on section and largely gray-white with focally variegated coloration due to areas of necrosis and hemorrhage. Multiple sections may be needed to rule out other histologic patterns. (Courtesy of Dr. A.J. Steinberg.) (From Wheeler et al.,[339a] with permission.)

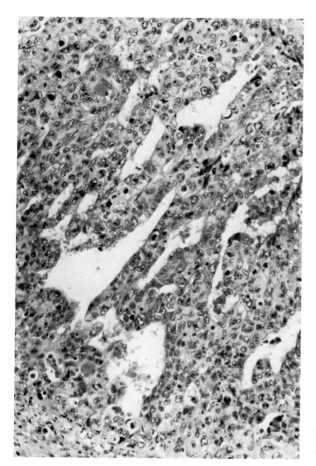

Fig. 27-16 Embryonal carcinoma. Tumor cells are fully anaplastic with nuclear pleomorphism and indistinct cell membranes. Trabecula of cells may be separated by clefts. Cytoplasm is usually amphophilic.

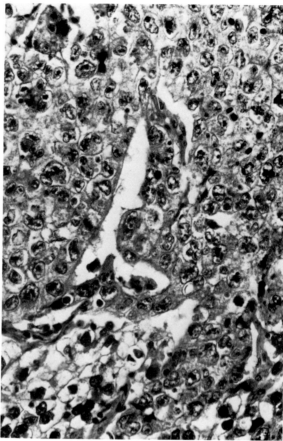

Fig. 27-17 Embryonal carcinoma. High magnification emphasizes the nuclear anaplasia and irregular chromatin distribution. A seminomatous component in the tumor is responsible for the cells at bottom with contrasting clear cytoplasm.

the left renal vein; left testis tumors spread to the pre-aortic (88 percent), and left para-aortic (86 percent) zones.[80] Blood-borne metastases to lungs, liver, pleura, bones, and gastrointestinal tract are commonly found at autopsy, most of which contain embryonal carcinoma (96 percent). However, areas of histologic teratoma (8 percent) and choriocarcinoma (5 percent) may be expressed in metastases.[217]

The previously poor prognosis of embryonal carcinoma has been immeasurably ameliorated by modern chemotherapy. Three year survival rates of 35 percent in the early 1970s, 50 percent for clinical stage I and II lesions, and nearly 0 percent for stage III tumors,[41]

have become 95 to 98 percent survival for stages I and II lesions and over 40 percent survival for stage III tumors.[150]

Patients with all histologic types of non-seminomatous germ cell tumors are commonly lumped together when amassing survival statistics. This may be helpful in acquiring sufficient numbers to compare treatments, but one should note that the presence of histologically verified embryonal carcinoma is a strong predictor of metastases.[150] Vascular invasion and extension to the epididymis or spermatic cord are two other indicators of probable metastasis in stage I disease.[150]

Teratoma

Nearly 30 percent of all testicular tumors contain a component of teratoma, in which neoplastic cells differentiate toward endodermal, mesodermal, or ectodermal structures. Teratomas may be divided into three types, those found in infants, those in adults with histologically mature elements, and those in adults with histologically immature elements.[70,248]

Studies on the origin of testicular teratomas[184] have noted the presence of a Y chromosome in addition to one or more X chromosomes in virtually all cases. This is taken as evidence of origin through mitotic activity without an antecedent meiotic division.

Histologically Mature Teratomas

Histologically mature teratomas comprise about 5 percent (2 to 9 percent[83]) of germ cell tumors and are found almost exclusively in children. Half of the infants with a testicular teratoma present with a mass lesion before the age of 2 years.[47] The bisected testis reveals a characteristic gross variegated appearance with cysts with or without hair, firm cartilage or bone, and foci of sebaceous material in a whitish stromal matrix. Dark pigment may be noted secondary to tissue simulating the retinal choroid. Microscopically, a variety of tissues of ecto-, meso-, and endodermal origins are found (Fig. 27-18). Skin and its adnexal structures may be jumbled with nodules of cartilage and bone. Respiratory epithelium may be underlain by mesodermal tissues so as to replicate bronchial structure, and colonic mucosa may overlie submucosa and muscle layers. Pancreatic tissue is absent,[285] but thyroid tissue may be prominent.[335] Histologic immaturity may be present, but this does not confer malignancy upon the tumor; behavior is invariably benign. In contrast to many adult teratomas, embryonal, yolk sac, and choriocarcinomatous components are absent.

Between the age of 5 years, when the last of the infant teratomas is seen,[47] and the onset of puberty, when the adult teratomas begin to appear, too few cases are reported to evaluate histology or behavior.

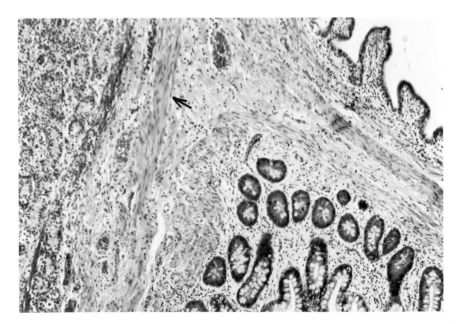

Fig. 27-18 Teratoma, infantile. Note the mature glands at lower right and smooth muscle (arrow) in this lesion from a 2-year-old boy. Immature testis is at left.

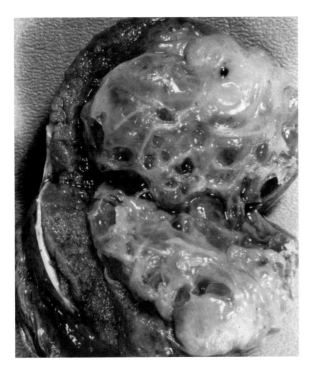

Fig. 27-19 Teratoma. On section the tumor is well delineated without gross evidence of necrosis. The presence of cysts, seen here, or palpable cartilage, is a good gross clue to the presence of teratoma. (Courtesy of Dr. A.J. Steinberg.) (From Wheeler et al.,[339a] with permission.)

Teratomas with Histologically Mature or Immature Elements

These forms of teratoma are reported from age 12 on,[214] with a mean of about 30 years.[8] Mature teratomas are rare in adults, but have a gross appearance when bisected similar to those of childhood (Fig. 27-19). Microscopically, the varied tissues seen are histologically mature. Gastrointestinal epithelium in these lesions may contain argentaffin-positive cells staining immunohistochemically for serotonin, somatostatin, glucagon, or pancreatic polypeptide.[46] The clinical course is distinctly different from childhood teratoma in that metastases to regional lymph nodes or lungs may occur. These may appear histologically mature[172,274] or may contain an embryonal,[83] yolk sac, or immature teratomatous component.[297]

The metastatic interval may range up to 18 years.[83] Talerman[297] suggests that those tumors in adults which metastasize have immature elements which are responsible for their behavior, and that those which are totally mature should be considered benign. This places a strong burden upon the responsible pathologist to study any apparently mature teratoma in great detail with multiple blocks.

Immature Teratomas

Frankly immature teratomas are much more common in adults. The gross appearance may be similar to mature teratoma, but owing to the frequent association with embryonal or extragonadal germ cell components (see the section on mixed germ cell tumors), they may be softer, necrotic, or hemorrhagic. Microscopically, the tissues are histologically immature; a cellular spindle cell stroma may contain nodules of cartilage with nuclear pleomorphism or glands of uncertain histologic nature with epithelial cells lacking normal polarity and having nuclear atypia (Fig. 27-20). Regional lymph nodes or distant metastases may contain the histologic pattern of any nonseminomatous germ cell tumor.

A few cases have been described in which, following chemotherapy of teratoma, a mesodermal component, usually embryonal rhabdomyosarcoma, has survived and progressed as a pure or mixed sarcoma, usually in pulmonary nodules or retroperitoneal lymph nodes.[3,318] In some instances[3] no sarcomatous component is identified in the primary tumor; in others,[318] atypical stromal cells are seen. Other sarcomatous histologic patterns noted include myxoid liposarcoma, epithelioid leiomyosarcoma, neuroblastoma, angiosarcoma,[316] chondrosarcoma, and alveolar rhabdomyosarcoma.[4] Carcinomas characterized by gland formation, distinct cell borders, and mucicarmine positivity may also differentiate from metastatic teratoma, and must be distinguished from the more chemotherapeutically treatable embryonal carcinoma.[317] A more common finding after chemotherapy is the presence of residual or growing masses, especially in retroperitoneum or lungs.[191,320] On resection, these may prove to consist solely of histologically mature tissue, in which case the prognosis is excellent.[189] Patients with residual immature teratoma in resected nodes also may have a good prognosis, but the presence of other elements such as em-

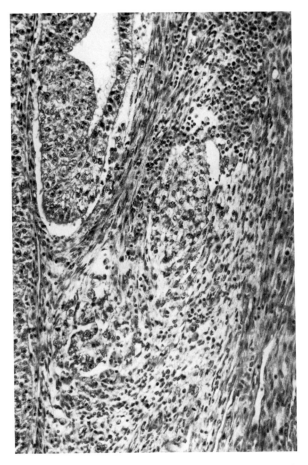

Fig. 27-20 Teratoma. Histologically immature glands with intervening spindle cell stroma is apparent. Careful tumor sampling and histologic study is often required to reveal an embryonal component with the attendant worse prognosis.

bryonal carcinoma, yolk sac or choriocarcinoma or seminoma is associated with over 90 percent recurrence rates.[320]

CARCINOID

Testicular carcinoids, like their more common ovarian counterparts, may be of metastatic origin, may originate as part of a testicular teratoma, or may originate as a "pure" primary testicular carcinoid. Seventy percent of reported cases[28,299] appear to be primary pure carcinoids, whereas the others are metastatic or are associated with a teratoma.

Primary pure carcinoids are found in men aged 22 to 71 and present as a unilateral testicular mass, often without tenderness or pain. No carcinoid syndrome is reported except for in the largest lesion reported (8 cm).[345] On section the circumscribed lesion is usually 3 or 5 cm in diameter and yellow-tan.

Microscopically, except for foci of central necrosis, the tumor has an insular pattern composed of islands or nests of compact uniform cells with round nuclei and coarsely clumped chromatin. Occasionally one may note small acinar formations. Argentaffin staining is positive, and ultrastructure reveals membrane-bound dense granules. Fluorescence characteristic of serotonin is present in ultraviolet light.[299] Metastases occurred in 2 of 25 reported cases, and there was one death.[28]

Carcinoid associated with teratoma has been found in men aged 22 to 58, where it may be a major or very minor component of an otherwise unremarkable tumor. Careful gross and histologic study of any testicular carcinoid is indicated, to search for underlying teratomatous elements. It may be that any primary testicular carcinoid should be regarded as presenting one-sided development of teratoma. The prognosis is good.

Carcinoids metastatic to the testis may appear grossly and microscopically identical to primary carcinoids, and reported cases are of gastrointestinal, typically ileal, origin.[28] Therefore, following orchiectomy and discovery of a carcinoid, radiographic examination of the small bowel may be indicated. Most of the patients with metastatic disease, however, succumb within a year or two of widespread disease.

RHABDOMYOSARCOMA

A rare testicular tumor composed of malignant striated muscle cells has been described.[9] Because of the greater frequency of rhabdomyosarcoma of the spermatic cord (Ch. 29), any such testicular lesion should be accepted as primary only after thorough cord examination. Most of the older reports in the literature are not very specific about findings in the spermatic cord. The reported ages have ranged from 4 to 60 years,[72] and the biological behavior has been benign[9] but is usually malignant. If such a tumor exists as a testicular primary, it appears logical to think of it as a monophasic development of a teratoma, for teratomas both with major and minor rhabdomyosarcomatous components are recognized.

Yolk Sac Carcinoma (Endodermal Sinus Tumor)

This germ cell tumor is seen either as a histologically pure lesion in early childhood, or as a more or less histologically prominent part of an adult testicular tumor. Microscopically the tumor patterns are similar to those seen in extraembryonic membranes and yolk sac endoderm in early embryonic development.[301]

In childhood, where in the past it was known also as *orchioblastoma, infantile embryonal carcinoma,* and *adenocarcinoma of infantile testis,* it is by far the commonest testicular tumor.[47,110,114] Children range in age from infancy to 5 years old.[294] The bisected tumor is grossly yellowish-white (Fig. 27-21) and nonencapsulated. Its texture may vary from soft to firm with cystic areas. A wide variety of histologic patterns may be present to confuse the pathologist; cysts, large or small, are a useful common denominator. Papillary, glandular alveolar, and micro- and macrocystic patterns (Fig. 27-22) are said to be more common among

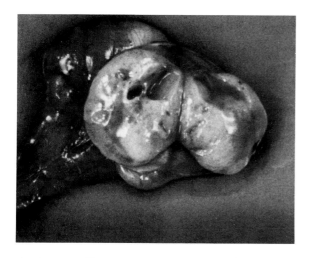

Fig. 27-21 Yolk sac carcinoma. On section, this 17 month old child's tumor is distinctly yellowish and well delineated but not encapsulated. (Courtesy of Dr. J. Chatten, Children's Hospital of Philadelphia.)

infants.[296] Metastases occur to regional and distal nodes, lungs, and liver.

Children less than 2 years old often, but not always,[259] do well, whereas those over 2 years old tended to die of the disease before the advent of modern chemotherapy.[240] Survival is now nearly always attainable.[110,114] Retroperitoneal node dissection is controversial owing to a low incidence of metastasis (4[47] to 14[81] percent) in most series, the presence of an excellent tumor marker (AFP) for recurrent or residual disease, and the ability to successfully treat metastatic tumor with chemotherapy.[167]

Yolk sac carcinoma of the adult testis is, in thoroughly studied cases, always found in association with other germ cell elements,[296] even in the 7 percent of nonseminomatous germ cell tumors in which it is the predominant element. Small foci of yolk sac tumor are readily overlooked, but a high index of suspicion and careful sampling will reveal foci in nearly 45 percent of all nonseminomatous germ cell tumors.[296] Serum AFP levels in patients without metastatic disease have ranged up to 6,100 mg/ml, whereas with metastases levels have surpassed 35,000 ng/ml and appear to be proportional both to the amount of tumor and the relative proportion of it consisting of yolk sac elements.[296]

The gross appearance of a yolk sac tumor is dependent to some extent on the admixed germ cell tumor components, but is typically grayish-white and soft, with a mucoid surface and focal areas of hemorrhage and necrosis.[297] Histologically, a wide variety of patterns may be seen, often within a single specimen (Figs. 27-22, 27-23). The microcystic (reticular) and solid patterns are most common, being found in over 80 to 90 percent of cases; whereas, the papillary (festoon) pattern is seen in about 50 percent, and the polyvesicular vitelline pattern in less than 10 percent.[319] This last pattern mimics cystic structures formed during the embryonic development from the primary to the secondary yolk sac,[301] and are ironically scarce in most specimens. Schiller–Duval bodies, neoplastic perivascular structures, resemble the endodermal sinuses of the rat placenta, and are diagnostic of yolk sac carcinoma (Fig. 27-23A). They are also uncommon. Microcystic and other patterns may focally blend into small enteric-type epithelial glands, and these glands are frequently associated with areas of hepatic-like differentiation.[136,319]

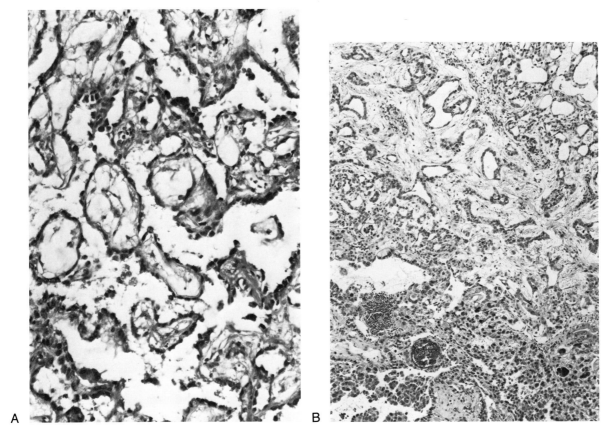

A   B

Fig. 27-22 Yolk sac carcinoma (endodermal sinus tumor). **(A)** Edematous and nearly acellular myxoid stroma and cystic spaces with thin linings of tumor cells are frequent in childhood tumors. **(B)** A pale myxomatous stroma is present at upper center in which cystic spaces are lined by tumor cells. More solid areas at bottom blend into tumor indistinguishable from embryonal carcinoma.

Histologically these hepatic-like areas are characterized by trabeculae and solid nests of polygonal cells with eosinophilic cytoplasm. The nuclei are round with a large nucleolus (Fig. 27-23B).[319] Hepatic-like areas may stain for ferritin, albumin, and transferrin in addition to AFP,[138] and cells positive for hemoglobin A and F have also been identified, reminiscent of the red blood cell formation typically first seen in the embryonic yolk sac.[7]

Yolk sac tumor elements metastasize in the same pattern as other nonseminomatous germ cell tumors. Their prognosis, however, is appreciably worse. In a recent follow-up of patients with bulky stage III nonseminomatous disease, two thirds of those without yolk sac elements were alive and well, whereas only one third of those with similar bulk disease with yolk sac foci were doing well.[190]

Choriocarcinoma

Pure choriocarcinoma is very rare as a pure germ cell tumor of the testis, occurring only in about one case in 300.[215] As a component of carefully studied nonseminomatous germ cell tumors, however, choriocarcinoma may be found in about 15 percent.[296] Any gross focus of hemorrhage seen on section of a germ cell tumor may represent an area of choriocarcinoma (Fig. 27-24), and such foci should be well represented in samples for histologic study. Microscopically, multinucleated syncytiotrophoblastic cells are found apparently randomly admixed with mononuclear cytotrophoblasts. Close inspection, however, reveals that syncytiotrophoblasts typically line most of the blood-filled spaces and are adjacent to hemorrhagic areas, presumably related to the same angioin-

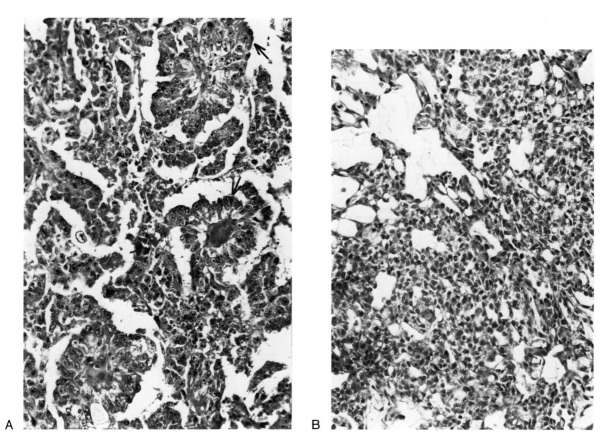

A   B

Fig. 27-23 Yolk sac carcinoma. **(A)** The Schiller-Duval body (arrows) characteristic of this tumor is a glomerular-like structure with a loose or myxoid fibrovascular core covered by a mantle of tumor cells which projects into a cystic space. **(B)** Even in solid areas of tumor, small cystic spaces are apparent. Some solid areas may have hepatoid differentiation.

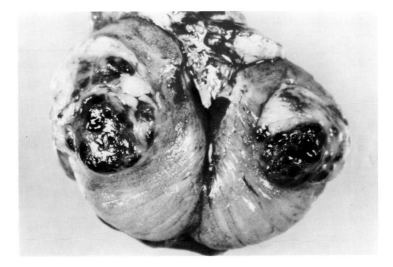

Fig. 27-24 Choriocarcinoma. Germ cell tumors containing pure choriocarcinoma are extremely rare. The grossly hemorrhagic portion of this lesion contained numerous areas of choriocarcinoma, but other areas sampled contained seminoma, embryonal carcinoma, and teratoma, emphasizing the need for generous sampling.

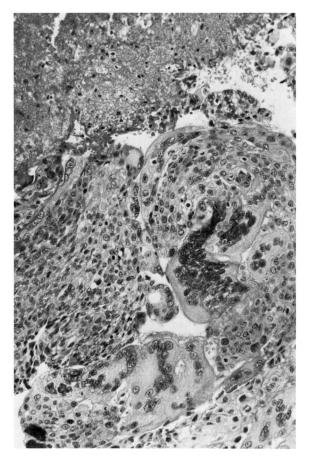

Fig. 27-25 Choriocarcinoma. Cytotrophoblast has distinct cell membranes with pale cytoplasm; syncytiotrophoblast has a much more amphophilic or eosinophilic slightly granular or vacuolated cytoplasm with atypical hyperchromatic nuclei lying in a syncytium.

vasive property shown in the normal blastocystic implantation of pregnancy. The cytotrophoblast cells have a crisp cell membrane around almost clear cytoplasm and a rather vesicular nucleus. The syncytiotrophoblastic nuclei are often irregular and hyperchromatic and the syncytiotrophoblastic cytoplasm eosinophilic or amphophilic with vacuoles (Fig. 27-25). These giant cells are distinctly different from the benign giant cells associated with a granulomatous reaction, which have uniform, bland nuclei. Immunohistochemical staining positivity for hCG will be positive only in the former.

Spread of tumors with a choriocarcinomatous component occurs as in the other germ cell tumors. The syncytiotrophoblastic cells continue to produce hCG when present in metastases, giving an excellent serum tumor marker (see above) for clinical followup. Patients with pure testicular choriocarcinoma formerly had an almost invariably rapidly lethal course, whereas those with a major choriocarcinomatous component had a survival of less than 20 percent at 2 years.[217] Modern chemotherapy may improve this grim record.[45] In patients dying of nonseminomatous germ cell tumors, the choriocarcinomatous component is most prone to be present in brain metastases.[44]

POLYEMBRYOMA

Rarely within a nonseminomatous germ cell tumor a histologic component will form structures reminiscent of presomite embryos.[282] This may be a form of differentiation by embryonal cells, but evidence of somite formation and further stages of normal embryonal differentiation has not been noted. Microscopically, the best-defined embryoid bodies are composed of two or three layers of primitive embryonal-like cells in a slightly curved disc delineated on the convex side by a crescentic space and on the concave side by a yolk sac-like vesicular space. The significance and prognosis of this histologic pattern is unknown.

MIXED GERM CELL TUMORS

About 40 percent of all germ cell tumors are found, when studied carefully, to be formed of two or more histologic components.[215] With careful gross sectioning of the primary tumor and liberal histologic sampling, and with knowledge of preoperative serum AFP and hCG levels, one may hope to identify all significant histologic patterns. Nonetheless, metastases from what had been thought to be a pure seminoma may be found to contain a variety of nonseminomatous patterns. Any confirmed elevation in serum AFP level should be taken to mean that there is a focus of yolk sac tumor that must be treated, even if not identified histologically. Likewise, any hCG elevation implies, at a minimum, isolated syncytiotrophic tumor cells and quite possibly a focus of choriocarcinoma.

Embryonal carcinoma frequently shows attempts at somatic differentiation, and the combination of embryonal carcinoma and teratoma is known as teratocarcinoma. Its behavior and prognosis are similar to the more malignant embryonal component.

GERM CELL TUMOR REGRESSION: THE TESTICULAR SCAR

Extragonadal germ cell tumors, especially those in the retroperitoneum[35,50] are often discovered to be associated with a testicular scar with calcification or hemosiderin-laden macrophages, with or without the presence of atypical cells. Other cases of disseminated germ cell tumor are associated with hematoxylinophilic bodies containing DNA and protein debris in seminiferous tubules.[19,217] The occasional presence of atypical cells or frankly malignant foci in some cases of testicular scar supports the idea that total regression of the primary lesion is possible in testicular germ cell tumors. The scar is typically only 3 or 4 mm in size[50] and nonpalpable. Ultrasound may help reveal the lesion. Testes of patients with fatal cases of extragonadal germ cell tumor should be minutely examined for a site of possible origin. These scars are often perihilar, but may be located anywhere in the testis.[217] Besides fibrous tissue and hemosiderin, a few chronic inflammatory cells may be present. The intratubular hematoxylinophilic bodies may be noted independent of a scar (Fig. 27-26) and are rounded with a granular or amorphous consistency.

Far commoner than the finding of a scar is the finding of areas within an otherwise unremarkable seminoma where only rare tumor cells, often pyknotic, are identifiable amid an overwhelming granulomatous reaction.

Spontaneous regression of metastatic testicular tumors is rare, with only a dozen or so cases reported.[220]

COMPLICATIONS AND PATHOLOGY OF TREATMENT

Current treatment of testicular nonseminomatous germ cell tumors by inguinal orchiectomy is commonly followed by retroperitoneal node dissection and chemotherapy. This has resulted in high survival rates,[342] but the morbidity of the treatment is substantial.

Retroperitoneal dissection, besides operative morbidity and cost, usually results in retrograde ejaculation and resulting infertility. Antegrade ejaculation

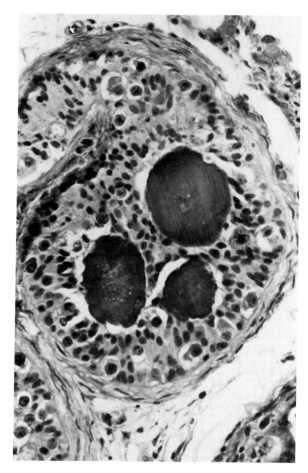

Fig. 27-26 Hematoxylinophilic bodies. These intratubular basophilic rounded bodies may be associated with testicular scars. (From Wheeler et al.,[339a] with permission.)

may be restored in some patients with oral α-sympathomimetics,[227] but much interest and controversy centers about the role of watchful waiting (without node dissection) in stage I nonseminomatous tumors,[96,122,154,182,253] a less-than-total node dissection,[148,244] or, in stage II tumors, chemotherapy followed by selective node dissection.[189]

The use of high-dose multiagent potent chemotherapy calls for superior clinical experience and meticulous patient care. The four drugs currently in greatest use are cis-platinum, vinblastine or etoposide, and bleomycin. Cis-platinum ($PtCl_2H_6N_2$) is a heavy metal complex that causes inter- and intrastrand crosslinks in DNA. It is excreted by the kidney with appreciable renal toxicity. As the compound is myelosuppressive and may cause irreversible neurotoxicity, including ototoxicity, frequent evaluation is necessary. Anaphylactic reactions may occur. Vinblastine is a plant alkaloid that blocks amino acid metabolism and interferes with nucleic acid synthesis. Its use results in leukopenia with immunosuppression and loss of hair. Neurologic and gastrointestinal adverse reactions may occur. Etoposide is a podophyllotoxin derivative which inhibits DNA synthesis. Its toxicity appears to be less than that of vinblastine,[342] but myelotoxicity is still a major limiting side effect. Bleomyin is a mixture of bacterial-derived glycopeptides that interfere with DNA synthesis. It is largely secreted in the urine. Pulmonary toxicity with hyaline membrane formation resulting in septal fibrosis and pulmonary insufficiency is a hazard of bleomycin not always dose related. Skin and mucus membrane toxic effects are common, and idiosyncratic reactions may occur.

Radiation for seminoma may cause moderate leukopenia or thrombocytopenia, but is generally very well tolerated.[269,270]

EXTRAGONADAL GERM CELL TUMORS

Both seminomatous and nonseminomatous germ cell tumors have been described as primary in a number of extragonadal sites, many of which are located in midline areas. The pineal gland, mediastinum, sacrococcygeal area, and retroperitoneum are the most frequent sites. Of special interest to the urologist is the finding on followup that most patients with retroperitoneally located tumors, nearly all of whom are male, eventually are shown to have a testicular scar, atypical intratubular testicular germ cells, or a frankly invasive but nonpalpable testicular tumor.[35,232] Because the testes of patients with extragonadal germ cell tumors may be palpably normal, ultrasonic examination of the testes is suggested as a more sensitive diagnostic procedure.

GONADAL STROMAL TUMORS

Gonadal stromal tumors (sex cord-stromal, Sertoli–Leydig cell tumors) comprise only some 2 to 6 percent of all testicular tumors.[215] Even though a recent detailed book on testicular tumors entirely omit-

Table 27-4 World Health Organization Classification of Testicular Sex Cord-Stromal Tumors

Well-differentiated forms
Leydig cell tumor
Sertoli cell tumor
Granulosa cell tumor
Mixed forms
Incompletely differentiated forms

From Mostofi et al.,[218] with permission.

ted them from discussion,[79] their frequent endocrinologic manifestations and high rate of curability make them of special interest to clinicians, whereas their homologies to ovarian stromal tumors, varied gross and microscopic appearances, and difficulties in differential diagnosis are of interest to pathologists.

The World Health Organization's classification of sex cord-stromal tumors (Table 27-4) is over 10 years old,[218] and may perhaps be improved by indicating additional stromal lesions whose pathology has been somewhat clarified in recent years (Table 27-5).

Virtually no data are available on geographic distribution or variation of incidence of these tumors, nor

Table 27-5 Sex Cord-Stromal Classification (Proposed)

Leydig cell tumor
Well differentiated
Moderately or poorly differentiated
Sertoli cell tumor
Well differentiated
Moderately or poorly differentiated
Large cell calcifying variant with or without CAPS[a] syndrome
Mixed forms
Well differentiated
Moderately or poorly differentiated
Nontumoral stromal-like lesions:
Hyperplastic adrenal cortical rest
Nodular hyperplasia of Sertoli cells in testicular feminization
Immature Sertoli cell rests
Granulosa cell tumor
Juvenile variant
Adult type

[a] Cardiac myxoma, adrenal hyperplasia, pituitary adenoma, Sertoli cell tumor.

have etiologic factors been identified. In the laboratory the Fischer 344 strain of rats has a very high frequency of spontaneous Leydig cell tumor, typically preceded by nodular Leydig cell hyperplasia.[313] Estradiol acts in a susceptible mouse strain to induce Leydig cell tumors, perhaps related to estrogen receptor protein present in the Leydig cells. This receptor is lacking in the Leydig cells of a resistant strain.[131] Dogs acquire Leydig cell tumors that rarely are malignant.[63] Sertoli cell tumors are one of the most frequent testicular lesions of dogs, and are frequently feminizing owing to estrogen production by the neoplastic Sertoli cells.[55,63] Only 2 of 138 canine tumors in one study metastasized, however.[63] Sertoli cell tumors may be induced in rat ovaries with the carcinogen N-ethyl-N-nitrosourea.[283] None of these potential animal models, however, has been clearly related to gonadal stromal tumors in humans.

Leydig Cell Tumors

Leydig cell (interstitial cell) tumors comprise the great majority of all stromal tumors of the testis. Since the first clear description of a Leydig cell tumor in 1895,[260] several hundred cases have been reported.[161] Only rarely are the tumors bilateral,[86] or familial.[157] The neoplastic Leydig cells usually produce testosterone, and, in some well-studied cases, estradiol and progesterone.[67] Either precocious development of secondary sexual characteristics in children or gynecomastia (present in 30 percent of adults) may be the presenting complaint.[161] Lesions may be so small as to

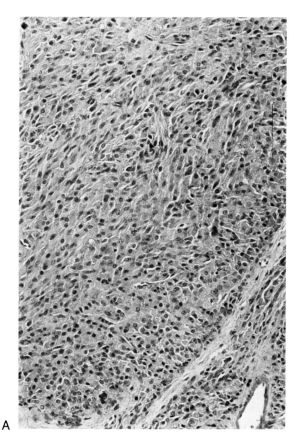
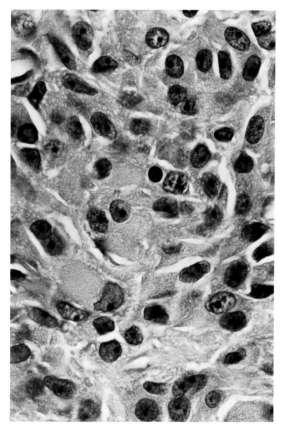

Fig. 27-27 Leydig cell tumor. **(A)** Sheets of eosinophilic polygonal cells have round to slightly oval nuclei similar to normal Leydig cells. **(B)** At higher magnification the similarity to Leydig cells is more apparent. Reinke crystalloids, not seen here, may be present. Occasionally these tumors may have highly lipidic cytoplasm which will appear clear or vacuolated on routine sections.

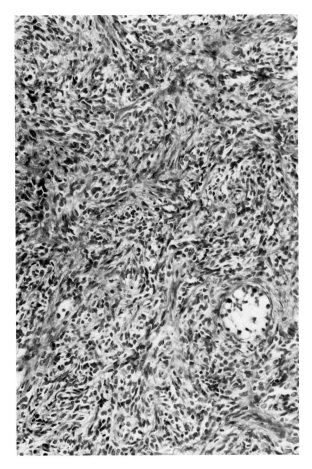

Fig. 27-28 Gonadal stromal tumor. Most of the tumor is composed of nonspecific spindle cells of stromal origin, with only occasional recognizable Leydig cells.

be nonpalpable, and ultrasound[67] or spermatic vein catheterization with hormone determinations[27] may be necessary to localize the tumor. The most common complaint, however, is testicular mass.

The mean patient age is in the mid 40s, but the tumor has been reported in children as young as 2 and men as old as 90.

On gross examination of the bisected testis the usual Leydig cell tumor is 2 or 3 cm in diameter (range 0.5 to 10 cm[161]) and characteristically brown, but may be yellowish-brown, red-brown, dark brown, or yellowish-gray. Microscopically, it is composed of nests, trabeculae, or sheets of polyhedral cells with eosinophilic cytoplasm and one or more round or oval vesicular nuclei (Fig. 27-27A). The cytoplasm may con-

tain a sufficient quantity of lipid to render it vacuolated and pale (Fig. 27-27B). Only in about a third of the cases are Reinke crystalloids identifiable.[161]

Besides Leydig cells, many tumors also contain variable numbers of spindle cells (Fig. 27-28). These cells contain myofilaments analogous to contractile peritubular cells of the testis.[105] If the great majority of cells are spindly, the term *gonadal stromal tumor* is preferable to Leydig cell tumor.

Ultrastructurally, smooth endoplasmic reticulin, lipochrome pigment, mitochondria, and membraneous whorls are prominent cytoplasmic features.[158] Ultrastructural diagnostic differences between androgenic and estrogenic tumors have not been identified.[275] Immunohistochemical staining for intermediate filaments reveals vimentin positivity.[208]

About 7 to 10 percent of Leydig cell tumors pursue a malignant course. Careful evaluation reveals these to be characterized by increased cellular atypia, an increased mitotic rate, and evidence of infiltrating margins with vascular permeation.[161] Other than metastases, however, there is no absolute delineator for malignant Leydig cell tumors. Patients with malignant-behaving tumors tend to be older, with a mean age near 60 years (range 20 to 82).[106] Regional lymph nodes are the primary site of metastatis in three fourths of the cases, with lung, liver, and bone lesions following in frequency.[106] A bare majority of patients have androgen or estrogen elevation.[73,106] Whereas 22 percent of patients with malignant tumors are found to have metastases at the time of presentation, nearly 60 percent do not have evidence of spread for over a year. Median survival is 2 years (mean 4 years), and radiation and chemotherapy are only anecdotally helpful.[106]

HYPERPLASIA OF ADENOCORTICAL REST

A testicular mass found in a patient with congenital adrenal hyperplasia may represent a Leydig cell tumor or a hyperplastic rest of adrenal cortical tissue.[90,226,322] Preoperative diagnosis of the latter condition should lead to appropriate glucocorticoid treatment and obviate the need for surgery. Whereas at least one such tumor carefully studied by light and electron microscopy appeared to be a typical Leydig cell tumor, biochemical studies showed it capable of 11β-hydroxylation and cortisol production, abilities unique to adrenal cortical tissue.[90] It may be, as proposed,[268] that Leydig cells and adrenal cortical cells arise from a common urogenital ridge precursor so that properties of each may be occasionally shared.

Sertoli Cell Tumors

Sertoli cell tumors are typically small, 1 to 2 cm in diameter, but if neglected over years may grow to 15 cm in size (800g). Patients with Sertoli cell tumors are usually in the 20 to 50 year age range, but tumors have been found from childhood to old age. There may be an association with the Peutz–Jegher's syndrome.[344] On section the gross tumor is usually yellowish-white, yellowish-gray, or yellowish-tan and tends to be well delineated and slightly raised from the surrounding testicular tissue (Fig. 27-29). Cystic degeneration may occur in the larger tumors, but the smaller ones are typically solid and firm. When solid they may be distinguished grossly from seminomas, which will usually be larger, softer, and grayer; when cystic, they will tend to be less variegated than teratomas. Those gritty on section will likely prove to be of the large cell calcifying variety (see below).

Microscopically, one should identify cells forming well to poorly defined tubular structures (Fig. 27-30). Bands of fibrous tissue may be prominent. Focally the tumor may be composed of undifferentiated spindle cells of gonadal stroma. The tubules may be highly differentiated and surrounded by a clearly defined basement membrane. They are composed of cells with oval vesicular nuclei and distinct reddish nucleoli similar to those seen in normal seminiferous tubules. Usually the tubules do not have a lumen. Immunohistochemical study reveals cytokeratin positivity, in contrast to the vimentin positivity of normal Sertoli cells.[209] Intratubular growth of neoplastic-ap-

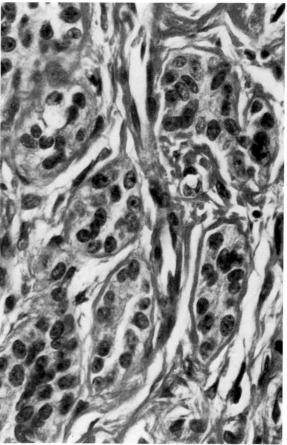

Fig. 27-30 Sertoli cell tumor. Small tubular arrangements of neoplastic Sertoli cells are apparent. The lack of mitoses and nuclear anaplasia suggest a probable benign behavior.

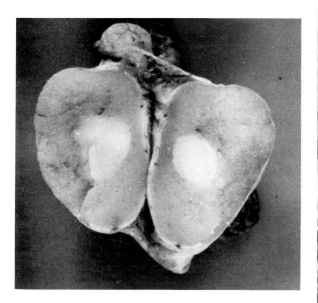

Fig. 27-29 Sertoli cell tumor. This white rather well delineated mass had no hormonal effects. It is too small grossly to be a typical germ cell tumor, and Leydig cell tumors are usually quite brown. (Courtesy Dr. J. Chatten.) (From Wheeler et al.,[339a] with permission.)

pearing Sertoli cells is seen in an occasional case, indicating that at least some, if not all, of these tumors originate by in-situ transformation.[247] If admixtures of Leydig cells are present, the lesion is termed a Sertoli–Leydig cell tumor.

If nearly the entire tumor is composed of undifferentiated spindle-shaped stromal cells with minimal evidence of focal differentiation toward recognizable Sertoli cells, it would appear best to use the less committal diagnostic term of undifferentiated gonadal stromal tumor.

Malignant Sertoli cell tumors are rare.[178,291] Although they constitute some 12 percent[247] of reported Sertoli cell tumors, one suspects that there is disproportionate reporting of the malignant variety and that the real incidence of malignancy is under 10 percent. The patients reported with malignant tumors have ranged in age from 8 to 79.[178] The tumors have generally been quite large (7 to 15 cm) when removed, with histologically demonstrated pleomorphism, some mitotic activity, and occasional evidence of lymphatic involvement. No single feature or combination of gross or microscopic findings has yet been shown to be absolutely predictive of biologic malignancy.

Metastatic spread appears to be primarily lymphatic, with tumor deposits in iliac, periaortic and inguinal lymph nodes. Bone metastases were prominent in at least one case.[129]

Estrogen may be produced by Sertoli cell tumors in sufficiently large amounts to cause gynecomastia and loss of libido.

Electron microscopic study of Sertoli cell tumors[100] reveals intertubular collagen and a basement membrane partially surrounding many cells. Numerous desmosomes connect the tumor cells, which contain both smooth and rough endoplasmic reticulum and frequent lipid droplets.

LARGE CELL CALCIFYING SERTOLI CELL TUMOR

A histologic variant of Sertoli cell tumors with important clinical features has been recognized recently. In the largest series reported of these large cell calcifying Sertoli cell tumors,[247] 11 of 12 patients were under 20 years old, 6 had bilateral and frequently multifocal tumors, and 3 had isosexual precocity. The association of this tumor with adrenal hyperplasia, pituitary adenoma, cardiac myxoma, and testicular Leydig cell nodules[247,257,334] may eventually be proven significant.

These large cell calcifying tumors are typically yellow on section, and are often gritty owing to the presence in about half of them of nodules or plaques of calcification, located either in intratubular or extratubular tumor sites (Fig. 27-31). The tumor cells are large (12 to 35 μm),[247] with abundant eosinophilic finely granular cytoplasm and slightly oval vesicular nuclei with one or two small to occasionally prominent nucleoli. Mitoses are generally lacking. The tumor cells grow in tubules, cords, and trabeculae in a loose myxoid or dense collagenous stroma with a variable lymphocytic infiltrate (Fig. 27-31). Due to the large size and eosinophilia of the cytoplasm, these tumors may be confused with Leydig cell tumors. Ultrastructural studies[237] confirm Sertoli cell features, with abundant cytoplasmic smooth endoplasmic reticulum, lipid, and demonstrable crystalline cytoplasmic Charcot–Böttcher bodies in at least one case.[334] These bodies appear to be unique to Sertoli cells.

Intratubular growth is prominent in many of these tumors and is accompanied by prominent thickening of the tubular basement membrane. The membrane material may protrude inward to form intratubular tufts and nodules.[247]

One of the large cell calcifying tumors that had increased pleomorphism and four mitoses per 10/hpf later metastasized to lymph nodes and bone.

OTHER SERTOLI CELL LESIONS

Two additional Sertoli cell abnormalities must be distinguished from Sertoli cell tumor. Testes removed from patients with a male genotype but female phenotype secondary to unresponsive end organ receptors to gonadal androgens (testicular feminization) will be nodular on section owing to hyperplasia of tubules composed almost entirely or entirely of immature Sertoli cells (Fig. 24-10). These nodules may enlarge to form tumors up to 14 cm (910g) in size, with focal hemorrhage and necrosis.[56] Such lesions are commonly referred to as *adenomas* (*tubular adenoma of Pick*[239]).

Undescended testes in otherwise normal males[277] may harbor small collections of tubules lined by immature Sertoli cells; a study of apparently normal descended testes reveals such lesions to be present in over 20 percent of specimens (Fig. 27-32).[118] If large

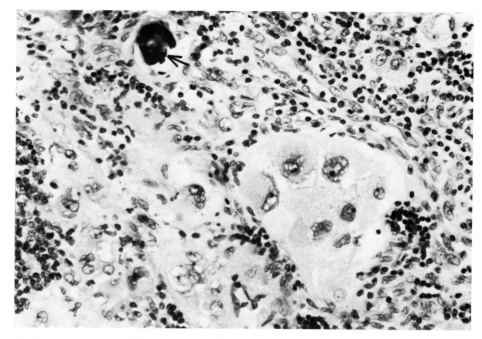

Fig. 27-31 Large cell calcifying Sertoli cell tumor. Tumor cells are very large, with correspondingly enlarged nuclei and prominent nucleoli. Focal calcification (arrow) is a feature of these tumors. A lymphocytic infiltrate may be seen. (Case courtesy of Dr. I. Damjanov.)

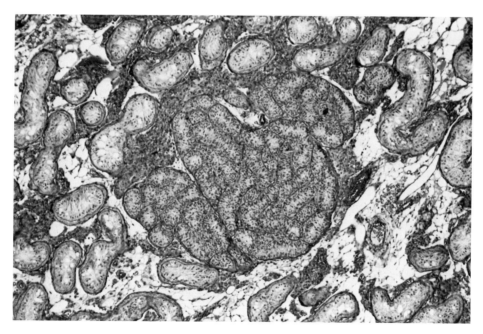

Fig. 27-32 Sertoli cell nodule. This collection of small tubules is not a tumor, but an anatomic variant. Note lack of compression of surrounding structures.

enough, these tubular aggregates may form a visible white nodule.

Other Sex Cord-Stromal Tumors

GRANULOSA CELL TUMORS

Granulosa cell tumors are exceedingly rare in the adult testis[177,178] and only slightly more common in infants. The juvenile variant has been found in a 30-week fetus[65] and in infants up to 4.5 months old. The tumors are grayish-yellow on section and up to 5 cm in diameter[177] with a nodular solid or cystic appearance. Microscopically, the cells contain rather uniform, ovoid to round, vesicular nuclei, usually lacking a nuclear groove, and a moderate amount of eosinophilic pale cytoplasm. Tumor cells in the cystic tumors form follicular structures (Fig. 27-33), some of which are surrounded by prominent thecal cell layers with abundant eosinophilic cytoplasm. This appearance is identical to that described in the juvenile granulosa cell tumor of young women.[348] Despite occasionally high mitotic rates (up to 24 per 10 hpf), none of these tumors has yet behaved in a malignant fashion.[177] This juvenile variant has also been described in testes of a few infants with gonadal dysgenesis and ambiguous genitalia.[349]

Unlike the juvenile variant, those rare granulosa cell tumors found in adults may be associated with gynecomastia.[219] The gross appearance of the tumor is similar to the juvenile variety, but microscopically the nuclei show the characteristic nuclear grooving, and Call–Exner bodies, characteristic of ovarian granulosa cell tumors, may be present (Fig. 27-34).[178]

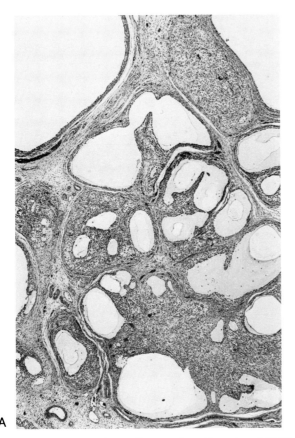
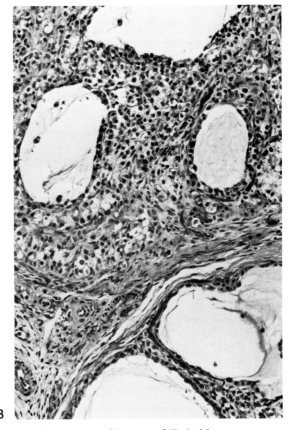

A   B

Fig. 27-33 Granulosa cell tumor, juvenile variant. **(A)** The well defined borders of the cystic follicle-like structures are apparent at low magnification. **(B)** Tumor cells have pale cytoplasm and small ovoid nuclei. The basophilic follicular fluid may stain positively for mucin.

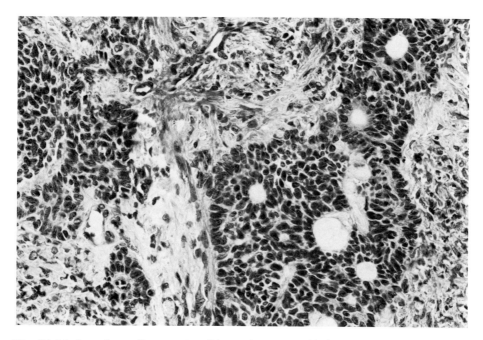

Fig. 27-34 Granulosa cell tumor. Small hyperchromatic cells form cords and follicle-like arrangements. There is a background of non-specific stromal cells.

EXTRATESTICULAR GONADAL STROMAL TUMOR

A single case of apparently extragonadal Sertoli–Leydig cell tumor has been found in the pelvis of a 40-year-old man with normally descended testes.[205] Because of the normal anatomic presence of nests of Leydig cells in the spermatic cord, it is not surprising that on occasion they may become neoplastic.[341]

Gonadoblastoma

This lesion, a mixed germ cell–sex cord-stromal tumor, is almost invariably found in patients with some form of gonadal dysgenesis. Although the patient's genotype usually is 45X/46XY or XY, only 20 percent of the patients are phenotypically male. Phenotypic females often present in adolescence owing to amenorrhea, and infants with ambiguous genitalia may have gonadoblastomas discovered at a few months of age.[69] Pheontypic males present in childhood or early adolescence with hypospadias, and more than a third will have a vagina.[263] Gynecomastia is frequent. At abdominal exploration a uterus is noted, and half the patients have bilateral fallopian

tubes. In the others, a tube is present unilaterally. Male structures, such as prostate, epididymis and vas deferens are present in about half the patients.[263] Gonadoblastoma will frequently obscure the nature of underlying gonad, but all phenotypic males have at least some recognizable testicular tissue. A streak gonad may be found opposite to the gonadoblastoma. The karyotype is most often 45X/46XY. The Y chromosome, which normally has a fluorescent long arm, may be nonfluorescent[66] or fluorescent.[193]

Aside from infertility and the anatomic abnormalities, the chief clinical problem faced is development of a frank germ cell tumor within the gonadoblastoma. Because the dysgenetic gonads in phenotypic males are almost invariably found in the pelvis, the tumor may grow 6 to 8 cm in diameter before being recognized clinically. The gonadal surface is lobulated and smooth and the tumor yellow-brown on section, with focal and occasionally very prominent calcifications (Fig. 27-35). Sectioning and sampling must be liberal owing to the high incidence of development of malignant tumors.

Microscopically, gonadoblastomas have a characteristic nesting pattern, with a peripheral palisade of

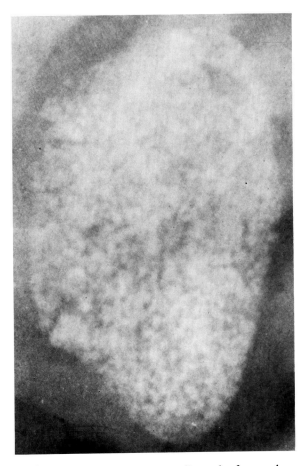

Fig. 27-35 Gonadoblastoma. A radiograph of a gonad replaced by gonadoblastoma reveals nearly confluent foci of calcification.

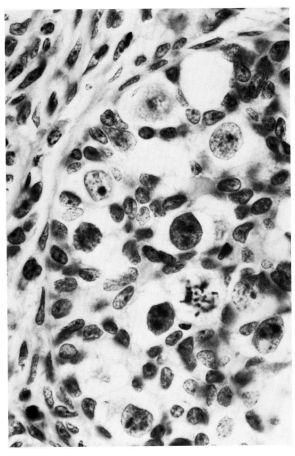

Fig. 27-36 Gonadoblastoma. A tumor nodule is composed of a mixture of large atypical germ cells with prominent nucleoli invested with smaller ovoid stromal nuclei. Background stroma is present at left.

stromal cells that encloses a mixture of germ cells and smaller stromal cells (Fig. 27-36). The nuclei of the germ cells are rather large, round, and vesicular; those of the stromal cells tend to be compressed, carrot-shaped, and more hyperchromatic. Stromal cells orient around eosinophilic masses of laminated basement membrane-like material.[33,134] Focal calcification with hydroxyapatite is a frequent feature in these masses.[95]

A gonadoblastoma may be looked upon as a premalignant lesion; half of them at the time of diagnosis harbor a germ cell tumor, and careful microscopic examination of others may detect proliferation of germ cells suggestive of an early seminoma.[111] Of the germ cell tumors reported with gonadoblastoma, seminoma (dysgerminoma) is by far the most common, but more highly malignant tumors such as embryonal carcinoma, yolk sac (endodermal sinus) tumors, choriocarcinoma, and teratocarcinomas have also been found.[263] We and others have seen the underlying gonadoblastoma overlooked owing to overgrowth of the secondary germ cell tumor. A radiograph of the specimen may help locate the characteristic calcifications, and a habit of generous sampling may fortuitously find a diagnostic area. Clinical recognition of abnormal genitalia also will raise the index of suspicion. The implications for the contralateral gonad are important, and prompt removal is indicated to avoid later germ cell tumor development.

Gonadal neoplasms of mixed germ cell and sex cord stromal derivatives, other than gonadoblastoma, are rarely reported.[36,292]

The prognosis of patients with gonadoblastoma is excellent, provided that germ cell tumor has not developed. The behavior of germ cell tumors developing in a gonadoblastoma is similar to those developing in a testis, except for the readier access to the abdominal cavity.

LYMPHOMA

Unilateral or bilateral testicular involvement with lymphoma is one of the commonest causes of an enlarged testis in men over 50. In some of the earliest large series reported[1] of men with testicular lymphomas, nearly all patients (91 percent) had histiocytic lymphoma, and all died, usually within a few months. Subsequent reports[78,235,314] on selected patient populations confirmed the high frequency of the histiocytic subtype (74 to 83 percent) and a poor prognosis, especially if generalized disease appeared within six months. However, several patients survived for over 5 years, indicating that the tumor may behave as if it were primary in the testis. It is very uncommon as a primary neoplasm in those under 35 years of age, but a few well-documented cases have been seen in children.[337] Childhood testicular disease, if carefully followed, may prove to be the presenting sign of underlying leukemia.[135]

The typical patient with testicular lymphoma is about 65 years old, with asymptomatic testicular swelling, possibly associated with pain.[135] There are commonly systemic signs of disease,[235] such as fever or weight loss, and no history of testicular maldescent, trauma, or inflammation. Radiologic examination often reveals abdominal, especially para-aortic, lymph node involvement.[82,303] Further workup should include bone marrow biopsies and careful inspection of the skin, central nervous system, and Waldeyer's ring.[78] Serum hCG and AFP will be negative. Patients presenting with bilateral testicular masses, with rare exception,[14,210] have diffuse lymphoma with a poor long-term prognosis.[20] Orchiectomy may be necessary, even though systemic disease is confirmed, if only to control an awkward or even painful mass.

On gross examination, the tunica is intact but the epididymis may be grossly involved.[1,160] On section

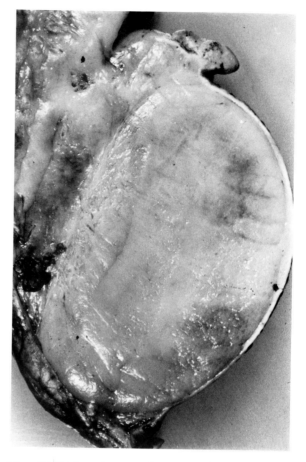

Fig. 27-37 Lymphoma. The cut surface is diffusely grayish-white with obliteration of parenchymal detail. Note involvement of epididymis and adjacent cord. (From Wheeler et al.,[339a] with permission.)

(Fig. 27-37) the testis is replaced by a fish-flesh, grayish-white to brown, diffuse cellular infiltrate, typically without necrosis or hemorrhage. Discrete nodules may occur, and pose a problem in a gross differential diagnosis.[160] Microscopically, like leukemia, lymphoma cells diffusely infiltrate the interstitium, compressing but only rarely involving the seminiferous tubules (Fig. 27-38). The less common types of lymphoma to involve the testis, such as poorly differentiated lymphocytic lymphoma, must be distinguished from leukemia histologically and by examination of peripheral blood and bone marrow. The rare testicular lymphomas of childhood are typically lymphocytic in children less than 5 years of age,[337] with leukemic or generalized dissemination within

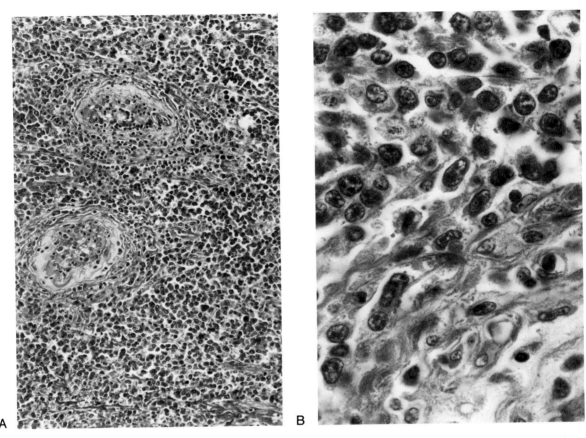

A

B

Fig. 27-38 Diffuse histiocytic (large cell) lymphoma. **(A)** Malignant cells heavily infiltrate the interstitium, with relative sparing of seminiferous tubules. **(B)** Irregular dark clumped chromatin with a high nuclear to cytoplasmic ratio characterize the lymphoma cells on the left. A remnant of seminiferous tubule in lower right is only minimally infiltrated by tumor.

months or years. Older children (8 to 12 years old) tend to have histiocytic rather than lymphocytic disease.

Survival relates best to stage of disease; with para-aortic lymph node involvement it is about 6 months, whereas without it median survival may exceed 5 years. Late recurrences are uncommon.[303] Bilaterality, either synchronous or metachronous, is much commoner than in germ cell tumors and is associated with a poor prognosis.[20]

Malignant plasmacytoma is rare. Patients may present months or years after plasmacytoma elsewhere with a testicular plasmacytoma,[276,279] or the testicular plasmacytoma may present as the initial symptom of multiple myeloma.[181] It is rare even at autopsy.[115] A testis with plasmacytoma is grossly en-

larged (Fig. 27-39) with firm fleshy tumor microscopically infiltrating and obliterating the normal parenchyma (Fig. 27-40). Occasionally tubules may be invaded. The nuclei of the tumor cells show moderate to marked pleomorphism with mitoses, which differentiates plasmacytomas from the mature plasmacytic infiltrate of interstitial orchitis. Anaplastic seminoma or embryonal carcinomas may enter the differential diagnosis.[181] However, the lack of cohesion of the malignant plasma cells and their eccentric nuclei should distinguish them from the germ cell tumors, which typically have a more centrally located nucleus with evidence of cellular cohesion. Touch preparations of the lesion at the time of frozen section may be helpful in elucidating cytologic detail. The patients usually are over 40 and often anemic. The

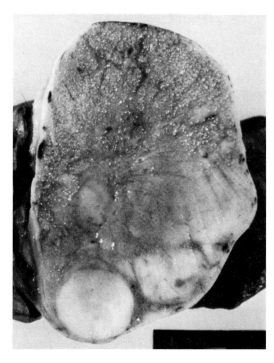

Fig. 27-39 Plasmacytoma. On section of the testis a nodule of tumor is noted at lower left. A more diffuse infiltrate of tumor is present in the lower half of the specimen.

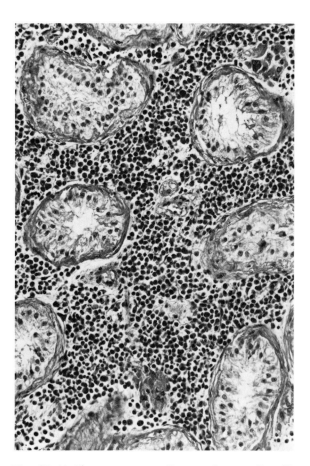

Fig. 27-40 Plasmacytoma. Malignant plasma cells infiltrate interstitium with sparing of seminiferous tubules.

marrow may or may not be involved at the initial presentation. The serum should be examined for a monoclonal immunoglobulin spike.

Hodgkin's disease of the testis is extremely rare.[107] Burkitt's lymphoma presenting in the testis is also rare.[235,314]

LEUKEMIA

Leukemia, especially acute lymphoblastic leukemia of childhood, commonly involves the testis: at the time of first diagnosis, as a site of clinical or subclinical relapse, and as a finding at autopsy.[207] Of the relatively few patients biopsied prior to treatment, approximately 20 percent will have involvement by clusters of diffuse infiltrates of neoplastic lymphoblasts.[162] Involvement may also be found during what appears to be complete clinical remission.[15,163] Testicular relapse is currently seen in about 5 to 8 percent of boys in clinical remission, either as a palpable infiltrate or, more commonly, as a microscopic finding on bilateral wedge biopsies.[15,199,225,305] There is some correlation of testicular relapse with pretreatment lymphoadenopathy, and relapse while still under treatment presages a poorer prognosis.[225] Although the testis is a frequent first site of relapse,[305] elective biopsy to detect relapse has little, if any, clinical value.[163,249]

At autopsy testicular involvement is seen in nearly two thirds of patients with acute leukemia and nearly one fourth of those with chronic leukemia.[98,169]

At the time of biopsy, extra care must be taken by the surgeon to avoid pressure on the tissue, as leukemic cells are exquisitely sensitive to crush artifact. The pathologist may wish to obtain improved morphologic detail through plastic embedding and 1 μm

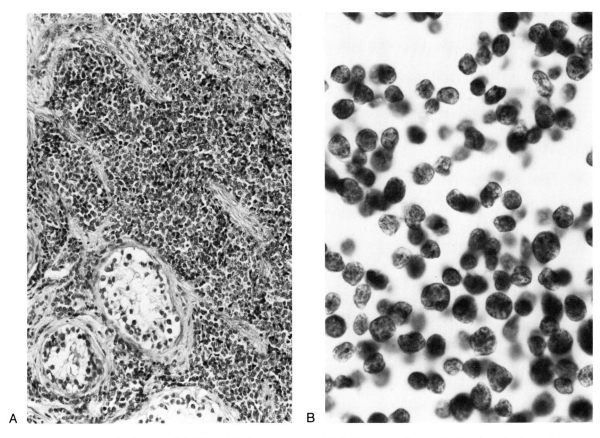

Fig. 27-41 Acute leukemia of childhood. **(A)** A monomorphic infiltrate preferentially involves the interstitium. **(B)** A touch preparation from the fresh specimen reveals malignant nuclear detail of the leukemic cells.

sections.[108] Infiltrating lymphoblasts may then more easily be distinguished from those merely transiting interstitial capillaries, and minimal infiltrates become diagnostic.

Histologically, leukemic cells infiltrate in the interstitium between the seminiferous tubules or form small interstitial clusters. The cytologic appearance will naturally reflect that of the underlying type of leukemia (Fig. 27-41). The differential diagnosis may include lymphoma, seminoma, and interstitial orchitis. Microscopic examination of the peripheral blood will almost always indicate the true diagnosis in the case of leukemia, but the blood count itself may be normal.[142] Bone marrow examination may be useful in selected cases. Poorly fixed, sectioned, and stained material may resemble a spermatocytic or ordinary seminoma.[142] Infiltrative interstitial orchitis will characteristically be granulomatous and polymorphic. Careful and gentle touch preparations at the

time of biopsy may provide helpful differential cytologic detail (Fig. 27-41B).

Following chemotherapy for leukemia there is typically severe depression of the germ cells, but eventual recovery follows in a majority of young patients,[34,195,266] despite frequent histologic evidence of some interstitial fibrosis and tubular basement membrane thickening.[121,180] In adults, germ cell survival is noted in about 65 percent of treated patients.[169] Testicular radiation for leukemia, however, causes irreversible infertility, although Leydig cell function may remain.[267,286]

RETE TESTIS

Benign and malignant tumors of the rete testis are rare, and like similar tumors in the mouse,[346] are papillary adenomas,[91,123] or carcinomas.[97,230,350] These lesions are discussed in detail in Chapter 29.

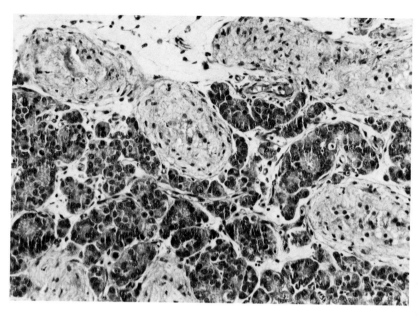

Fig. 27-42 Metastatic carcinoma. Early development of a focus of metastatic prostate carcinoma shows the typical interstitial location of the tumor and the characteristic pattern of small proliferating acini.

METASTATIC TUMORS

It is distinctly rare for tumor primary elsewhere in the body to present initially as a testicular mass, but over 100 patients with solid tumors have been reported with significant secondary testicular involvement.[113] Mechanisms of proposed metastatic spread include arterial embolism, retrograde lymphatic growth, retrograde venous extension, and spread via the vas deferens and epididymis.[130] Transperitoneal seeding via a communicating hydrocele may also occur.[212] A prospective autopsy study found that 2.5 percent of all males with solid neoplasms had one or more metastatic deposits in the testis when carefully examined at postmortem,[306] but it is not clear if any of them were noted clinically. Metastatic prostate carcinoma provides nearly one third of the reported cases, followed in frequency by carcinoma of the lung, melanoma, colon, and kidney.[113] Neuroblastoma may involve the testis more frequently than previously thought.[171] Metastatic prostate and kidney carcinomas are the two most likely to present as a primary testicular mass.[113]

To distinguish primary from secondary tumors, it is helpful to note that the mean age of patients with metastatic tumor is 57, 25 years older than the average patient with a primary germ cell or stromal tumor.[113]

Grossly, the testis may be involved by one or more nodules, or may be diffusely and subtly infiltrated. Metastatic tumors tend to infiltrate the interstitium with extensive vascular and lymphatic infiltrates (Fig. 27-42), but rarely there may be a pattern of seminiferous tubule involvement.[32] Mucicarmine positivity and the absence of suspected teratomas strongly supports metastatic disease, whereas positive immunohistochemical staining for AFP and hCG highly favors a testicular primary.[113] Survival after diagnosis is usually less than a year.[336] Secondary involvement with leukemia is quite common, as noted in the discussion of that disease.

REFERENCES

1. Abell MR, Holtz F: Testicular and paratesticular neoplasms in patients 60 years of age and older. Cancer 21: 852, 1968
2. Aguirre P, Scully RE, Dayal Y, DeLellis RA: Placenta-like alkaline phosphatase in germ cell tumors of the ovary and testis. Lab Invest 52: 2A, 1985

3. Ahlgren AD, Simrell CR, Triche TJ, et al: Sarcoma arising in a residual testicular teratoma after cytoreductive chemotherapy. Cancer 54: 2015, 1984

4. Ahmed T, Bosl GJ, Hajdu SI: Teratoma with malignant transformation in germ cell tumors in men. Cancer 56: 860, 1985

5. Akaza H, Kobayashi K, Umeda T, Niijima T: Surface markers of lymphocytes infiltrating seminoma tissue. J Urol 124: 827, 1980

6. Albrechtsen R, Nielsen MH, Skakkebaek NE, Wewer U: Carcinoma in situ of the testis. Some ultrastructural characteristics of germ cells. Acta Pathol Microbiol Immunol Scand Sect A 90: 301, 1982

7. Albrechtsen R, Wewer U, Wimberley PD: Immunohistochemical demonstration of a hitherto undescribed localization of hemoglobin A and F in endodermal cells of normal human yolk sac and endodermal sinus tumor. Acta Pathol Microbiol Scand 88: 175, 1980

8. Alderdice JM, Merrett JD: Factors influencing the survival of patients with testicular teratoma. J Clin Pathol 38: 791, 1985

9. Alexander F: Pure testicular rhabdomyosarcoma. Br J Cancer 22: 498, 1968

10. Anderson KC, Li FP, Marchetto DJ: Dizygotic twinning, cryptorchism, and seminoma in a sibship. Cancer 53: 374, 1984

11. Aquirre P, Scully RE, Dayal Y, DeLellis RA: Placenta-like alkaline phosphatase in germ cell tumors of the ovary and testis. (Abstract) Lab Invest 52: 2A, 1985

12. Arger PH: Scrotum. p. 406. In Coleman BG (ed): Genitourinary Ultrasound: a Text/Atlas. Igaku-Shoin Medical Publishers, New York, 1988

13. Arger PH, Mulhern CB Jr., Coleman BG, et al: Prospective analysis of the value of scrotal ultrasound. Radiology 141: 763, 1981

14. Aristizabel S, Davis JR, Miller RC, et al: Bilateral primary germ cell testicular tumors. Report of four cases and review of the literature. Cancer 42: 591, 1978

15. Askin FB, Land VJ, Sullivan MP, et al: Occult testicular leukemia: Testicular biopsy at three years continuous complete remission of childhood leukemia: A Southwest Oncology Group study. Cancer 47: 470, 1981

16. Atkin NB, Baker MC: Chromosome analysis of three seminomas. Cancer Genet Cytogenet 17: 315, 1985

17. Austin DF, Bragg K, Snyder M, et al: Cancer Incidence in San Francisco Bay Area 1973–1977. In Waterhouse J, Muir C, Shanmugaratnam K, Powell J (eds): Cancer Incidence in Five Continents. Vol. IV, International Agency for Research on Cancer, Lyon, 1982

18. Azzopardi JG, Hoffbrand AV: Retrogression in testicular seminoma with variable metastasis. J Clin Pathol 18: 135, 1965

19. Azzopardi JG, Mostofi FK, Theiss EA: Lesions of testes observed in certain patients with widespread choriocarcinoma and related tumors. The significance and genesis of hematoxylin-staining bodies in the human testis. Am J Pathol 38: 207, 1961

20. Bach DW, Weissbach L, Hartlapp JH: Bilateral testicular tumor. J Urol 129: 989, 1983

21. Barzell WEI, Whitmore WF, Jr.: Neoplasms of the testis. p. 1143. In Harrison JH, Gettes RF, Perlmutter AD, et al. (eds): Campbell's Urology. 2nd Ed., Vol. 2, Saunders, Philadelphia, 1979

22. Batata MA, Chu FCH, Hilaris BS, et al: Testicular cancer in cryptorchids. Cancer 49: 1023, 1982

23. Batata MA, Whitmore WF, Jr., Chu FCH, et al: Cryptorchidism and testicular cancer. J Urol 124: 382, 1980

24. Battifora H, Sheibani K, Tubbs RR, et al: Antikeratin antibodies in tumor diagnosis and distinction between seminoma and embryonal carcinoma. Cancer 54: 843, 1984

25. Beilby JOW, Horne CHW, Milne GD, Parkinson C: Alpha-fetoprotein, alpha-1-antitrypsin, and transferrin in gonadal yolk sac tumours. J Clin Pathol 32: 455, 1979

26. Belville WD, Insalaco SJ, Dresner ML, Buck AS: Benign testis tumors. J Urol 128: 1198, 1982

27. Bercovici J-P, Nahoul K, Tater D, et al: Hormonal profile of Leydig cell tumors with gynecomastia. J Clin Endocrinol Metab 59: 625, 1984

28. Berdjis CC, Mostofi FK: Carcinoid tumors of the testis. J Urol 118: 777, 1977

29. Berger Y, Srinivas V, Hajdu SI, Herr HW: Epidermoid cysts of the testis: Role of conservative surgery. J Urol 134: 962, 1985

30. Berthelsen JG, Skakkebaek NE, von der Maase H, et al: Screening for carcinoma in situ of the contralateral testis in patients with germinal testicular cancer. Br Med J 285: 1683, 1982

31. Berthelsen JG, Skakkebaek NE: Value of testicular biopsy in diagnosing carcinoma in situ of the testis. Scand J Urol Nephrol 15: 165, 1981

32. Binkley WF, Seo IS: Metastatic transitional cell carcinoma of the testis. A case report. Cancer 54: 575, 1984

33. Bjersing L, Cajander S: Ultrastructure of gonadoblastoma and disgerminoma (seminoma) in a patient with XY gonadal dysgenesis. Cancer 40: 1127, 1977

34. Blatt J, Poplack DG, Sherins RJ: Testicular function in boys after chemotherapy for acute lymphoblastic leukemia. N Engl J Med 304: 1121, 1981

35. Bohle A, Studer UE, Sonntag RW, Scheidegger JR:

Primary or secondary extragonadal germ cell tumors? J Urol 135: 939, 1986

36. Bolen JW: Mixed germ cell–sex cord stromal tumor. A gonadal tumor distinct from gonadoblastoma. Am J Clin Pathol 75: 565, 1981

37. Bosl GJ, Geller NL, Cirrincione C, et al: Multivariate analysis of prognostic variables in patients with metastatic testicular cancer. Cancer Res 43: 3403, 1983

38. Bosl GJ, Geller NL, Cirrincione C, et al: Serum markers in patients with metastatic germ cell tumors of the testis: A 10 year experience. Am J Med 75: 29, 1983

39. Bosl GL, Lange PH, Nochomovitz LE, et al: Tumor markers in advanced non-seminomatous testicular cancer. Cancer 47: 572, 1981

40. Boyle LE, Samuels ML: Serum LDH activity and isozyme patterns in nonseminomatous germinal (NSG) testis tumors. Proc Am Assoc Cancer Res 18: 278, 1977

41. Bradfield JS, Hagen RO, Ytredal DO: Carcinoma of the testis: An analysis of 104 patients with germinal tumors of the testis other than seminoma. Cancer 31: 633, 1973

42. Braunstein GD, Vaitukaitis JL, Carbone PP, Ross GT: Ectopic production of human chorionic gonadotrophin by neoplasms. Ann Intern Med 78: 39, 1973

43. Braunstein GD, Friedman NB, Sacks SA, et al: Germ cell tumors of the testis. West J Med 126: 362, 1977

44. Bredael JJ, Vugrin D, Whitmore WF, Jr: Autopsy findings in 154 patients with germ cell tumors of the testis. Cancer 50: 548, 1982

45. Brigden ML, Sullivan LD, Comisarow RH: Stage C Pure Choriocarcinoma of the Testis: A potentially curable lesion. Ca 32: 82, 1982

46. Brodner OG, Grube D, Helmstaedter V, et al: Endocrine GEP-cells in primary testicular teratoma. Virchows Arch Pathol Anat 388: 251, 1980

47. Brosman SA: Testicular tumors in prepubertal children. Urology 13: 581, 1979

48. Buckspan MB, Skeldon SC, Klotz PG, Pritzker KPH: Epidermoid cysts of the testicle. J Urol 134: 960, 1985

49. Burch TA, King WJ, Mimura LS, et al: Cancer incidence in Hawaii 1973–1977. In Waterhouse J, Muir C, Shanmugaratnam K, Powell J (eds): Cancer Incidence in Five Continents. Vol. IV. International Agency for Research on Cancer, Lyon, 1982

50. Burt ME, Javadpour N: Germ-cell tumors in patients with apparently normal testes. Cancer 47: 1911, 1981

51. Bush SE, Martinez A, Bagshaw MA: Primary mediastinal seminoma. Cancer 48: 1877, 1981

52. Buskirk SJ, Evans RG, Farrow GM, Earle JD: Primary retroperitoneal seminoma. Cancer 49: 1934, 1982

53. Butcher DN, Gregory WM, Gunter PA, et al: The biological and clinical significance of hCG containing cells in seminoma. Br J Cancer 51: 473, 1985

54. Cancer Statistics Registrations: Cases of diagnosed cancer registered in England and Wales, 1980. Her Majesty's Stationery Office, London, 1983

55. Capen CC, Martin SL: Ultrastructural evaluation and pathophysiology of testicular Sertoli cell neoplasms from dogs with a syndrome of hyperestrogenism. p. 384. In Arceneaux CJ (ed): Proceedings, Thirty-first Annual Meeting of the Electron Microscopy Society of America. Claitor's Publishing Division, Baton Rouge, 1973

56. Case Records of the Massachusetts General Hospital (Case 8-1977). N Engl J Med 296: 439, 1977

57. Clemmensen J: Testis cancer incidence-suggestion of a world pattern. Int J Androl 4(suppl): 111, 1981

58. Cockburn AG, Vugrin D, Batata M, et al: Poorly differentiated (anaplastic) seminoma of the testis. Cancer 53: 1991, 1984

59. Cockburn AG, Vugrin D, Batata M, et al: Second primary germ cell tumors in patients with seminoma of the testis. J Urol 130: 357, 1983

60. Coffin CM, Weing S, Dehner LP: Frequency of intratubular germ cell neoplasia with invasive testicular germ cell tumors. Histologic and immuno-cytochemical features. Arch Pathol Lab Med 109: 555, 1985

61. Cohen C, Shulman G, Budgeon LR: Immunohistochemical ferritin in testicular seminoma. Cancer 54: 2190, 1984

62. Conley GR, Sant GR, Ucci AA, Mitcheson HD: Seminoma and epididymal cysts in a young man with known diethylstilbestrol exposure in utero. JAMA 249: 1325, 1983

63. Cotchin E: Testicular neoplasms in dogs. J Comp Pathol Therap 70: 232, 1960

64. Couch WD: Combined effusion fluid tumor marker assay, carcinoembryonic antigen (CEA) and human chorionic gonadotropin (hCG) in the detection of malignant tumors. Cancer 48: 2475, 1981

65. Crump WD: Juvenile granulosa cell (sex cord-stromal) tumor of fetal testis. J Urol 129: 1057, 1983

66. Curtis WRS, White BJ, Lucky AW, et al: Gonadal dysgenesis with mosaicism and a nonfluorescent Y chromosome: Report of two cases with correlation of clinical, pathological, and cytogenetic findings. Am J Obstet Gynecol 136: 639, 1980

67. Czernobilsky H, Czernobilsky B, Schneider HG, et al: Characterization of a feminizing testicular Leydig cell tumor by hormonal profile, immunocytochemistry, and tissue culture. Cancer 56: 1667, 1985

68. Dainiak N, Hoffman R: Hemoglobin F production in testicular malignancy. Cancer 45: 2177, 1980

69. Damjanov I, Klanber G: Microscopic gonadoblas-

toma in dysgenetic gonad of an infant. An ultrastructural study. Urology 15: 605, 1980

70. Damjanov I: The pathology of human teratomas. p. 23. In Damjanov I, Knowles BB, Solter D (eds): The Human Teratomas. Experimental and Clinical Biology. Humana Press, Clifton, NJ, 1983
71. Davies JM: Testicular cancer in England and Wales: Some epidemiological aspects. Lancet 1: 928, 1981
72. Davis AE, Jr: Rhabdomyosarcoma of the testicle. J Urol 87: 148, 1962
73. Davis S, DiMartino NA, Schneider G: Malignant interstitial cell carcinoma of the testis: Report of two cases with steroid synthetic profiles, response to therapy, and review of the literature. Cancer 47: 425, 1981
74. de Kernion JB: Quoted by Johnson DE. p. 140. In Donohue JP (ed): Testis Tumors. Williams & Wilkins, Baltimore, 1983
75. Denk H, Moll R, Weybora W, et al: Intermediate filaments and desmosomal plaque proteins in testicular seminomas and non-seminomatous germ cell tumours as revealed by immunohistochemistry. Virchows Arch Pathol Anat 410: 295, 1987
76. Dieckmann K-P, Boeckmaun W, Brosig W, et al: Bilateral testicular germ cell tumors. Report of nine cases and review of the literature. Cancer 57: 1254, 1986
77. Dixon FJ, Moore RA: Tumors of the male sex organs. In: Atlas of Tumor Pathology. Armed Forces Institute of Pathology, Washington, DC, 1952
78. Doll DC, Weiss RB: Malignant lymphoma of the testis. Am J Med 81: 515, 1986
79. Donohue JP (ed): Testis Tumors. Williams & Wilkins, Baltimore, 1983
80. Donohue JP, Zachary JM, Maynard BR: Distribution of nodal metastases in non-seminomatous testis cancer. J Urol 128: 315, 1982
81. Drago JR, Nelson RP, Palmer JM: Childhood embryonal carcinoma of testes. Urology 12: 499, 1978
82. Duncan PR, Checa F, Gowing NFC, et al: Extranodal non-Hodgkin's lymphoma presenting in the testicle. A clinical and pathologic study of 24 cases. Cancer 45: 1578, 1980
83. Dunn D, Hertel B, Kennedy BJ: The management of mature teratoma of the testicle. J Urol 117: 259, 1977
84. Ehrlichman RJ, Kaufman SL, Siegelman SS, et al: Computerized tomography and lymphangiography in staging testis tumors. J Urol 126: 179. 1981
85. Floyd C, Ayala AG, Logothetis CJ, Silva EG: Spermatocytic seminoma with associated sarcoma of the testis 61:409, 1988
86. Flynn PT, Severance AO: Bilateral interstitial-cell tumors of the testis. Cancer 4: 817, 1951
87. Fournier GR, Jr, Laing FC, Jeffrey RB, McAninch JW: High resolution scrotal ultrasonography: A highly sensitive but nonspecific diagnostic technique. J Urol 134: 490, 1985
88. Fowler JE, Jr, Vugrin D, Cvitkovic E, Whitmore WF, Jr: Sequential bilateral germ cell tumors of the testis despite interval chemotherapy. J Urol 122: 421, 1979
89. Fram RJ, Garnick MB, Retik A: The spectrum of genitourinary abnormalities in patients with cryptorchism, with emphasis on testicular carcinoma. Cancer 50: 2243, 1982
90. Franco-Saenz R, Antonipillai I, Tan S-Y, et al: Cortisol production by testicular tumors in a patient with congenital adrenal hyperplasia (21-hydroxylase deficiency). J Clin Endocrinol Metab 53: 85, 1981
91. Fukunaga M, Aizawa S, Furusato M, et al: Papillary adenocarcinoma of the rete testis. A case report. Cancer 50: 134, 1982
92. Fukutani K, Libby JM, Panko WB, Scardino PT: Human chorionic gonadotropin detection in urinary concentrates from patients with malignant tumors of the testis, prostate, bladder, ureter, and kidney. J Urol 129: 74, 1983
93. Fukutani K, Yokoyama M, Mohri N: Increased human chorionic gonadotropin levels in spermatic vein blood of seminoma patients. Jpn J Clin Oncol 12: 181, 1982
94. Garnick MB: Spurious rise in human chorionic gonadotropin induced by marihuana in patients with testicular cancer. N Engl J Med 303: 1177, 1980
95. Garvin AJ, Pratt-Thomas HR, Spector M, et al: Gonadoblastoma: Histologic, ultrastructural and histochemical observations in five cases. Am J Obstet Gynecol 125: 459, 1976
96. Gelderman WAH, Koops HS, Sleijfer DTh, et al: Orchidectomy alone in stage I nonseminomatous testicular germ cell tumors. Cancer 59: 578, 1987
97. Gisser SD, Nayak S, Kaneko M, Tchertkoff V: Adenocarcinoma of the rete testes: A review of the literature and presentation of a case with associated asbestosis. Hum Pathol 8: 219, 1977
98. Givler RL: Testicular involvement in leukemia and lymphoma. Cancer 23: 1290, 1969
99. Goedert JJ, McKeen EA, Javadpour N, et al: Polythelia and testicular cancer. Ann Intern Med 101: 646, 1984
100. Goellner JR, Myers RP: Sertoli cell tumor. Case report with ultrastructural findings. Mayo Clin Proc 50: 459, 1975
101. Goldenberg DM, Kim EE, DeLand F, et al: Clinical studies on the radioimmunodetection of tumors containing alpha-fetoprotein. Cancer 45: 2500, 1980

102. Goldman RD, Kaplan NO, Hall TC: Lactic dehydrogenase in human neoplastic tissues. Cancer Res 24: 89, 1964

103. Goldman RL: A Brenner tumor of the testis. Cancer 26: 853, 1970

104. Gondos B: Intratubular germ cell neoplasia: Ultrastructure and pathogenesis. p. 21. In Talerman A, Roth LM (eds): Pathology of the Testis and Its Adnexa. Churchill Livingstone, New York, 1986

105. Greco MA, Feiner HD, Theil KS, Mufarrij AA: Testicular stromal tumor with myofilaments: Ultrastructural comparison with normal gonadal stroma. Human Patol 15: 238, 1984

106. Grem JL, Robins HI, Wilson KS, et al: Metastatic Leydig cell tumor of the testis: Report of three cases and review of the literature. Cancer 58: 2116, 1986

107. Hamlin JA, Kagan AR, Friedman NB: Lymphomas of the testicle. Cancer 29: 1352, 1972

108. Hargreaves H, Brynes R, Hawkins H: Detection of minimal infiltrates in testicular biopsies of boys with acute lymphoblastic leukemia. (Abstract) Lab Invest 46: 34A, 1982

109. Hargreaves HK, Scully RE, Richie JP: Benign hemangioendothelioma of the testis: Case report with electron microscopic documentation and review of the literature. Am J Clin Pathol 77: 637, 1982

110. Harms D, Janig U: Germ cell tumours of childhood. Report of 170 cases including 59 pure and partial yolk-sac tumours. Virchows Arch Pathol Anat 409: 223, 1986

111. Hart WR, Burkons DM: Germ cell neoplasms arising in gonadoblastomas. Cancer 43: 669, 1979

112. Hattori M, Fukase M, Yoshimi H, et al: Ectopic production of human chorionic gonadotropin in malignant tumors. Cancer 42: 2328, 1978

113. Haupt HM, Mann RB, Trump DL, Abeloff MD: Metastatic carcinoma involving the testis. Clinical and pathologic distinction from primary testicular neoplasms. Cancer 54: 709, 1984

114. Hawkins EP, Finegold MJ, Hawkins HK, et al: Nongerminomatous malignant germ cell tumors in children: A review of 89 cases from the pediatric oncology group, 1971–1984. Cancer 58: 2579, 1986

115. Hayes DW, Bennett WA, Heck FJ: Extramedullary lesions in multiple myeloma. Review of literature and pathologic studies. Arch Pathol 53: 262, 1952

116. Hayes HM Jr, Wilson GP, Pendergrass TW, Cox VS: Canine cryptorchism and subsequent testicular neoplasia: case-control study with epidemiologic update. Teratology 32: 51, 1985

117. Hazard JT, Drysdale JW: Ferritinaemia in cancer. Nature 265: 755, 1977

118. Hedinger CE, Huber R, Weber E: Frequency of so-called hypoplastic or dysgenetic zones in scrotal and otherwise normal human testes. Virchows Arch Pathol Anat 342: 165, 1967

119. Henderson BE, Benton B, Jing J, et al: Risk factors for cancer of the testis in young men. Int J Cancer 23: 598, 1979

120. Hendry WF, Barrett A, McElwain TJ, et al: The role of surgery in the combined management of metastases from malignant teratomas of the testis. Br J Urol 52: 38, 1980

121. Hensle TW, Burbige KA, Shepard BR, et al: Chemotherapy and its effect on testicular morphology in children. J Urol 131: 1142, 1984

122. Herr HW, Whitmore WF, Jr, Sogani PC, et al: Selection of testicular tumor patients for omission of retroperitoneal lymph node dissection. J Urol 135: 500, 1986

123. Herschman BR, Ross MM: Papillary cystadenoma within the testis. Am J Clin Pathol 61: 724, 1974

124. Heyderman E: Multiple tissue markers in human malignant testicular tumors. Scand J Immunol 8(Suppl.8): 119, 1978

125. Hirano K, Domar UM, Yamamoto H, et al: Levels of alkaline phosphotase isozymes in human seminoma tissue. Cancer Res 47: 2543, 1987

126. Hiroshima and Nagasaki: The physical, medical, and social effects of the atomic bombings. The Committee for the Compilation of Materials on Damage Caused by the Atomic Bombs in Hiroshima and Nagasaki. Basic Books, New York, 1981

127. Holder LE, Melloul M, Chen D: Current status of radionuclide scrotal imaging. Semin Nucl Med 11: 232, 1981

128. Honore LH, Sullivan LD: Intratesticular leiomyoma: A case report with discussion of differential diagnosis and histogenesis. J Urol 114: 631, 1975

129. Hopkins GB, Parry HD: Metastasizing Sertoli cell tumor (androblastoma). Cancer 23: 463, 1969

130. Howard DE, Hicks WK, Scheldreys EW: Carcinoma of the prostate with simultaneous bilateral testicular metastases: Case report with special study of routes of metastases. J Urol 78: 58, 1957

131. Huseby RA: Demonstration of a direct carcinogenic effect of estradiol on Leydig cells of the mouse. Cancer Res 40: 1006, 1980

132. Hustin J, Collette J, Franchimont P: Immunohistochemical demonstration of placental alkaline phosphatase in various states of testicular development and in germ cell tumours. Int J Androl 10: 29, 1987

133. Ishida H, Isurugi K, Nijima T, et al: Carcinoma in situ of germ cells and subsequent development of an invasive seminoma in a hyperprolactinaemic man. Int J Androl 6: 229, 1983

134. Ishida T, Tagatz GE, Okagaki T: Gonadoblastoma. Ultrastructural evidence for testicular origin. Cancer 37: 1770, 1976

135. Jackson SM, Montessori GA: Malignant lymphoma of the testis: Review of 17 cases in British Columbia with survival related to pathological subclassification. J Urol 123: 881, 1980

136. Jacobsen GK: Histogenetic considerations concerning germ cell tumours. Morphological and immunohistochemical comparative investigation of the human embryo and testicular germ cell tumours. Virchows Arch Pathol Anat 408: 509, 1986

137. Jacobsen GK, Norgaard-Pedersen B: Placental alkaline phosphatase in testicular germ cell tumours and in carcinoma-in-situ of the testis. An immunohistochemical study. Acta Pathol Microbiol Immunol Scand 92: 323, 1984

138. Jacobsen GK, Jacobsen M: Possible liver cell differentiation in testicular germ cell tumours. Histopathology 7: 537, 1983

139. Jacobsen GK, Jacobsen M, Clausen PP: Distribution of tumor-associated antigens in the various histologic components of germ cell tumors of the testis. Am J Surg Pathol 5: 257, 1981

140. Jacobsen GK, Henriksen OB, von der Maase H: Carcinoma in situ of testicular tissue adjacent to malignant germ-cell tumors: A study of 105 cases. Cancer 47: 2660, 1981

141. Jalota R, Middleton RG, McDivitt RW: Epidermoid cyst of the testis in Gardner's syndrome. Cancer 34: 464, 1974

142. Jampol ML, Ohnysty J: Acute leukemia seen as testicular tumor. NY State J Med 67: 1903, 1967

143. Janssen M, Johnson WH: Anaplastic seminoma of the testis. Ultrastructural analysis of three cases. Cancer 41: 538, 1978

144. Javadpour N: The value of biologic markers in diagnosis and treatment of testicular cancer. Semin Oncol 6: 37, 1979

145. Javadpour N: The role of biologic tumor markers in testicular cancer. Cancer 45: 1755, 1980

146. Javadpour N, Kim EE, DeLand FH, et al: The role of radioimmunodetection in the management of testicular cancer. JAMA 246: 45, 1981

147. Javadpour N, McIntire KR, Waldmann TA: Human chorionic gonadotropin (HCG) and alpha-fetoprotein (AFP) in sera and tumor cells of patients with testicular seminoma. A prospective study. Cancer 42: 2768, 1978

148. Javadpour N, Moley J: Alternative to retroperitoneal lymphadenectomy with preservation of ejaculation and fertility in stage I non-seminomatous testicular cancer. A prospective study. Cancer 55: 1604, 1985

149. Javadpour N, Soares T: False-positive and false-negative alpha-fetoprotein and human chorionic gonadotropin assays in testicular cancer: A double blind study. Cancer 48: 2279, 1981

150. Javadpour N, Young JD, Jr: Prognostic factors in non-seminomatous testicular cancer. J Urol 135: 497, 1986

151. Johnson DE: Clinical Staging. p. 131. In Donohue, JP (ed): Testis Tumors. Williams & Wilkins, Baltimore, 1983

152. Johnson DE, Gomez JJ, Ayala AG: Histologic factors affecting prognosis of pure seminoma of the testis. South Med J 69: 1173, 1974

153. Johnson DE, Gomez JJ, Ayala AG: Anaplastic seminoma. J Urol 114: 80–82, 1975

154. Johnson DE, Lo RK, von Eschenbach AC, Swanson DA: Surveillance alone for patients with clinical stage I non-seminomatous germ cell tumors of the testis: Preliminary results. J Urol 131: 491, 1984

155. Johnson DE, Woodhead DM, Pohl DR, Robinson JR: Cryptorchidism and testicular tumorigenesis. Surgery 63: 919, 1968

156. Kademian M, Bosch A, Caldwell WL, Jaeschke W: Anaplastic seminoma. Cancer 40: 3082, 1977

157. Kaufmann E: Ueber Zwischenzellengeswulste des hodens und reine tubulare Adenoma. Dtsh Med Wochenschr 34: 803, 1908

158. Kay S, Fu Y-S, Koontz WW, Chen ATL: Interstitial cell tumor of the testis. Tissue culture and ultrastructural studies. Am J Clin Pathol 63: 366, 1975

159. Kellen JA, Bush RS, Malkin A: Alkali-resistant hemoglobin (HbF) in cancer patients. Cancer 45: 1448, 1980

160. Kiely JM, Massey BD, Jr, Harrison EG, Jr, Utz DC: Lymphoma of the testis. Cancer 26: 847, 1970

161. Kim I, Young RH, Scully RE: Leydig cell tumors of the testis. A clinicopathological analysis of 40 cases and review of the literature. Am J Surg Pathol 9: 177, 1985

162. Kim TH, Hargraves HK, Brynes RK, Hawkins HK, et al: Pretreatment testicular biopsy in childhood acute lymphocytic leukemia. Lancet 2: 657, 1981

163. Kim TH, Hargreaves HK, Chan WC, et al: Sequential testicular biopsies in childhood acute lymphocytic leukemia. Cancer 57: 1038, 1986

164. Kirschner MA, Cohen FB, Jespersen D: Estrogen production and its origin in men with gonadotropin-producing neoplasm. J Clin Endocrinol Metab 39: 112, 1974

165. Kleiman AH: Hemangioma of the testis. J Urol 51: 548, 1944

166. Krabbe S, Skakkebaek NE, Bethelsen JG, et al: High incidence of undetected neoplasia in maldescended testis. Lancet 1: 999, 1979

167. Kramer SA, Wold LE, Gilchrist GS, et al: Yolk sac

carcinoma: An immunohistochemical and clinico-pathologic review. J Urol 131: 315, 1984

168. Kreider JW, Bartlett GL, Butkiewicz BL: Relationship of tumor leukocytic infiltration to host defense mechanisms and prognosis. Cancer Metastasis Rev 3: 53, 1984

169. Kuhajda FP, Haupt HM, Moore GW, Hutchins GM: Gonadal morphology in patients receiving chemotherapy for leukemia. Evidence for reproductive potential and against a testicular tumor sanctuary. Am J Med 72: 759, 1982

170. Kurman RJ, Scardino PT, McIntire KR, et al: Cellular localization of alpha-fetoprotein and human chorionic gonadotropin in germ cell tumors of the testes using an indirect immunoperoxidase technique. A new approach to classification utilizing tumor markers. Cancer 40: 2136, 1977

171. Kushner BH, Vogel R, Hajdu SI, Helson L: Metastatic neuroblastoma and testicular involvement. Cancer 56: 1730, 1985

172. Kusuda L, Leidich RB, Das S: Mature teratoma of the testis metastasizing as mature teratoma. J Urol 135: 1020, 1986

173. Lange PH, Millan JL, Stigbrand T, et al: Placental alkaline phosphatase as a tumor marker for seminoma. Cancer 42: 3244, 1982

174. Lange PH, Raghaven D: Clinical applications of tumor markers in testicular cancer. p. 111. In JP Donahue (ed): Testis Tumors. Williams & Wilkins, Baltimore, 1983

175. Lange PH, Vogelgang NJ, Goldman A, et al: Marker half-life analysis as a prognostic tool in testicular cancer. J Urol 128: 708, 1982

176. Lapes M, Iozzi L, Ziegenfus WD, et al: Familial testicular cancer in a father (bilateral seminoma - embryonal cell carcinoma) and son (teratocarcinoma). A case report and review of the literature. Cancer 39: 2317, 1977

177. Lawrence WD, Young RH, Scully RE: Juvenile granulosa cell tumor of the infantile testis. A report of 14 cases. Am J Surg Pathol 9: 87, 1985

178. Lawrence WD, Young RH, Scully RE: Sex cord-stromal tumors. p. 67. In Talerman A, Roth LM (eds): Pathology of the Testis and Its Adnexa. Churchill Livingstone, New York, 1986

179. Lee M-C, Talerman A, Oosterhuis JW, Damjanov I: Lectin histochemistry of classic and spermatocytic seminoma. Arch Pathol Lab Med 109: 938, 1985

180. Lendon M, Hann IM, Palmer MK, et al: Testicular histology after combination chemotherapy in childhood for acute lymphoblastic leukaemia. Lancet 2 439, 1978

181. Levin HS, Mostofi FK: Symptomatic plasmacytoma of the testis. Cancer 25: 1193, 1970

182. Liebundgut U, Biedermann C, Landmann C, Obrecht JP: Orchiektomie allein beim malignen Hodenteratom Stadium I? Schweiz Med Wochenschr 114: 820, 1984

183. Lien HH, Kolbenstvedt A, Telle K, et al: Comparison of computed tomography, lymphography, and phlebography in 200 consecutive patients with regard to retroperitoneal metastases from testicular tumor. Radiology 146: 129, 1983

184. Linder D: The origin of teratomas. p. 68. In Damjanov I, Knowles BB, Solter D (eds): The Human Teratomas. Experimental and Clinical Biology. Humana Press, Clifton, NY, 1983

185. Lippert MC, Javadpour N: Lactic dehydrogenase in the monitoring and prognosis of testicular cancer. Cancer 48: 2274, 1981

186. Liu F, Fritsche HA, Trujillo JM, Samuels ML: Serum lactate dehydrogenase isoenzyme 1 in patients with advanced testicular cancer. Am J Clin Pathol 78: 178, 1982

187. LiVolsi VA, Schiff M: Myxoid neurofibroma of the testis. J Urol 118: 341, 1977

188. Lo RK, Johnson DE: A graphic method to analyze serum tumor marker decay in nonseminomatous testis tumors. J Urol 131: 896, 1984

189. Logothetis CJ, Samuels ML, Selig DE, et al: Primary chemotherapy followed by selective retroperitoneal lymphoadenectomy in the management of clinical stage II testicular carcinoma: A preliminary report. J Urol 134: 1127, 1985

190. Logothetis CJ, Samuels ML, Trindade A, et al: The prognostic significance of endodermal sinus tumor histology among patients treated for stage III nonseminomatous germ cell tumors of the testis. Cancer 53: 122, 1984

191. Logothetis CJ, Samuels ML, Trindade A, Johnson DE: The growing teratoma syndrome. Cancer 50: 1629, 1982

192. Loughlin JE, Robboy SJ, Morrison AS: Risk factors for cancer of the testis (letter). N Engl J Med 303: 112, 1980

193. Lukusa T, Fryns JP, van den Berghe H: Gonadoblastoma and Y-chromosome fluorescence. Clin Genet 29: 311, 1986

194. Maatman T, Bukowski RM, Montie JE: Retroperitoneal malignancies several years after initial treatment of germ cell cancer of the testis. Cancer 54: 1962, 1984

195. Maguire LC, Dick FR, Sherman BM: The effects of anti-leukemic therapy on gonadal histology in adult males. Cancer 48: 1967, 1981

196. Maier JG, Sulak MH, Mittemeyer BT: Seminoma of the testes: Analysis of treatment success and future. Am J Roentgenol 102: 596, 1968

197. Maier JG, Mittemeyer BT, Sulak MH: Treatment and prognosis in seminoma of the testis. J Urol 99: 72, 1968

198. Mann K, Karl H-J: Molecular heterogeneity of human chorionic gonadotropin and its subunits in testicular cancer. Cancer 52: 654, 1983

199. Marboe CC, Hensle TW, Wigger HJ: Testicular biopsies following therapy for acute leukemia in childhood. (Abst.) Lab Invest 46: 10P, 1982

200. Mark GJ, Hedinger C: Changes in remaining tumor-free testicular tissue in cases of seminoma and teratoma. Virchows Arch Pathol Anat, 340: 84, 1965

201. Martin LSJ, Woodruff MW, Webster JH, Pickren JW: Testicular seminoma: A review of 179 patients treated over 50 years. Arch Surg 90: 306, 1965

202. Martin WMC, Dane TEB: Testicular germ cell tumors in monozygotic twins: Case report and review of the literature. J Urol 134: 765, 1985

203. Masson P: Etude sur le séminome. Rev Canad Biol 5: 361, 1946

204. Mauch P, Weichselbaum R, Botnick L: The significance of positive chorionic gonadotropins in apparently pure seminoma of the testis. Int J Radiat Oncol Biol Phys 5: 887, 1979

205. Maurer R, Taylor CR, Schmucki O, Hedinger CE: Extratesticular gonadal stromal tumor in the pelvis. A case report with immunoperoxidase findings. Cancer 45: 985, 1980

206. McCauley RL, Javadpour N: Supraclavicular node biopsy in staging of testicular carcinoma. Cancer 51: 359, 1983

207. Medical Research Council Working Party on Leukemia in Childhood: Testicular disease in acute lymphoblastic leukemia in childhood. Br Med J 1: 334, 1978

208. Miettinen M, Talerman A, Wahlstrom T, et al: Cellular differentiation in ovarian sex-cord-stromal and germ-cell tumors studied with antibodies to intermediate-filament proteins. Am J Surg Pathol 9: 640, 1985

209. Miettinen M, Virtanen I, Talerman A: Intermediate filament proteins in human testis and testicular germ-cell tumors. Am J Pathol 120: 402, 1985

210. Miles BJ, Kiesling VJ, Jr, Belville WD: Bilateral synchronous germ cell tumors. J Urol 133: 679, 1985

211. Mirimanoff RO, Shipley WU, Dosoretz DE, Meyer JE: Pure seminoma of the testis: The results of radiation therapy in patients with elevated human chorionic gonadotropin levels. J Urol 134: 1124, 1985

212. Moore JB, Law DK, Moore EE, Dean CM: Testicular mass: An initial sign of colon carcinoma. Cancer 49: 411, 1982

213. Morrison AS: Some social and medical characteristics of Army men with testicular cancer. Am J Epidemiol 104: 511, 1976

214. Mosli HA, Carpenter B, Schillinger JF: Teratoma of the testis in a pubertal child. J Urol 133: 105, 1985

215. Mostofi FK: Testicular tumors. Cancer 32: 1186, 1973

216. Mostofi FK: Pathology of germ cell tumors of the testis. Cancer 45: 1735, 1980

217. Mostofi FK, Price EB: Tumors of the male genital system. Second Series, Fascicle 8. Atlas of Tumor Pathology. Armed Forces Institute of Pathology, Washington, DC, 1973

218. Mostofi FK, Sobin LH: International histological classification of tumours. No. 16. In Histological Typing of Tumours of the Testis. World Health Organization, Geneva, 1977

219. Mostofi FK, Theiss EA, Ashley DJB: Tumors of specialized gonadal stroma in human male patients. Androblastoma, Sertoli cell tumor, granulosa-theca cell tumor of the testis, and gonadal stromal tumor. Cancer 12: 944, 1959

220. Mueh JR, Greco CM, Green MR: Spontaneous regression of metastatic testicular carcinoma in a patient with bilateral sequential testicular tumor. Cancer 45: 2908, 1980

221. Muffly KE, McWhorter CA, Bartone FF, Gardner PJ: The absence of premalignant changes in the cryptorchid testis before adulthood. J Urol 131: 523, 1984

222. Muller J, Skakkebaek NE: Abnormal germ cells in maldescended testis: A study of cell density, nuclear size, and deoxyribonucleic acid content in testicular biopsies from 50 boys. J Urol 131: 730, 1984

223. Mueller J, Skakkebaek NE, Parkinson MC: The spermatocytic seminoma: Views on pathogenesis. Int J Androl 10: 147, 1987

224. Murakami SS, Said JW: Immunohistochemical localization of lactate dehydrogenase isoenzyme 1 in germ cell tumors of the testis. Am J Clin Pathol 81: 293, 1984

225. Nesbit ME, Jr, Robinson LL, Ortega JA, Sather HN, et al: Testicular relapse in childhood acute lymphoblastic leukemia: Association with pretreatment patient characteristics and treatment. A report for Children's Cancer Study Group. Cancer 45: 2009, 1980

226. Newell ME, Lippe BM, Ehrlich RM: Testis tumors associated with congenital adrenal hyperplasia: A continuing diagnostic and therapeutic dilemma. J Urol 117: 256, 1977

227. Nijman JM, Jager S, Boer PW, et al: The treatment of ejaculation disorders after retroperitoneal lymph node dissection. Cancer 50: 2967, 1982

228. Nistal M, Paniaqua R: Testicular and Epididymal Pathology. Thieme-Stratton, New York, 1984, p 327

229. Nochomovitz LE: Final comments. p. 293. In Donohue JP (ed): Testis Tumors. Williams & Wilkins, Baltimore, 1983

230. Nochomovitz LE, Orenstein JM: Adenocarcinoma of the rete testis. Case report, ultrastructural observations, and clinicopathologic correlates. Am J Surg Pathol 8: 625, 1984

231. Nochomovitz LE, De La Torre RFE, Rosai J: Pathology of germ cell tumors of the testis. Urol Clin North Am 4: 359, 1977

232. Osler W: Abdominal tumours associated with disease of the testicle. Lancet 1: 1409, 1907

233. Osterlind A: Diverging trends in incidence and mortality of testicular cancer in Denmark, 1943–1982. Br J Cancer 53: 501, 1986

234. Osterlind A, Rorth M, Prener A: Second cancer following cancer of the male genital system in Denmark, 1943–1980. Natl Cancer Inst Monogr 68: 341, 1985

235. Paladugu RR, Bearman RM, Rappaport H: Malignant lymphoma with primary manifestation in the gonad. A clinicopathologic study of 38 patients. Cancer 45: 561, 1980

236. Percarpio B, Clements JC, McLeod DG, et al: Anaplastic seminoma. An analysis of 77 patients. Cancer 45: 2510, 1979

237. Perez-Atayde AR, Nunez AE, Carroll WL, et al: Large-cell calcifying Sertoli cell tumor of the testis. An ultrastructural, immunocytochemical, and biochemical study. Cancer 51: 2287, 1983

238. Perry C, Servadio C: Seminoma in childhood. J Urol 124: 932, 1980

239. Pick L: Ueber adenoma der mannlichen und weiblichen Keimdruse bei Hermaphroditismus verus und spurius. Berl Klin Wochenschr 42: 502, 1905

240. Pierce GB Jr, Bullock WK, Huntington RW, Jr: Yolk sac tumors of the testis. Cancer 25: 644, 1970

241. Pierce GB Jr: Teratocarcinoma: Model for a developmental concept of cancer. Curr Top Dev Biol 2: 223, 1967

242. Pierce GB Jr: Ultrastructure of human testicular tumors. Cancer 19: 1963, 1966

243. Pike MC, Chilvers C, Peckham MJ: Effect of age at orchidopexy on risk of testicular cancer. Lancet 1: 1246, 1986

244. Pizzocaro G, Salvioni R, Zanoni F: Unilateral lymphadenectomy in intraoperative stage I non-seminomatous germinal testis cancer. J Urol 134: 485, 1985

245. Porteus IB, Beck JS, Pugh RCB: Localization of human placental factor in malignant teratoma of testis. J Pathol Bacteriol 95: 527, 1968

246. Pritchett TR, Skinner DG: Embryonal carcinoma with falsely positive elevation of serum alpha-fetoprotein after curative therapy: A case report. J Urol 131: 970, 1984

247. Proppe KH, Scully RE: Large cell calcifying Sertoli

248. Pugh RCB, Cameron KM: Teratoma. p. 199. In Pugh RCB (ed): Pathology of the Testis. Blackwell, Oxford, 1976

249. Pui C-H, Dahl GV, Bowman WP, et al: Elective testicular biopsy during chemotherapy for childhood leukaemia is of no clinical value. Lancet 2: 410, 1985

250. Rabes HM, Schmeller N, Hartmann A, et al: Analysis of proliferative compartments in human tumors. II. Seminoma. Cancer 55: 1758, 1985

251. Raghavan D, Sullivan AL, Peckham MJ, Neville AM: Elevated serum alphafetoprotein and seminoma. Clinical evidence of a histologic continuum? Cancer 50: 982, 1982

252. Ramaekers F, Feitz W, Moesker O, et al: Antibodies to cytokeratin and vimentin in testicular tumour diagnosis. Virchows Arch Pathol Anat 408: 127, 1985

253. Read G, Johnson RJ, Wilkinson PM, Eddleston B: Prospective study of followup alone in stage I teratoma of the testis. Br Med J 287: 1503, 1983

254. Richter HJ, Leder L-D: Lymph node metastases with PAS-positive tumor cells and massive epithelioid granulomatous reaction as diagnostic clue to occult seminoma. Cancer 44: 245, 1979

255. Rosai J, Silber I, Khodadoust K: Spermatocytic seminoma. I. Clinicopathologic study of 6 cases and review of the literature. Cancer 24: 92, 1969

256. Rosai J, Khodadoust K, Silber I: Spermatocytic seminoma. II. Ultrastructural study. Cancer 24: 103, 1969

257. Rosenzweig JL, Lawrence DA, Vogel DL, et al: Adrenocorticotropin-independent hypercortisolemia and testicular tumors in a patient with a pituitary tumor and gigantism. J Clin Endocrinol Metabol 55: 421, 1982

258. Roth A, Le Pelletier O, Cukier J: Cryptocarcinome trophoblastique à cellules mononucléés sécrétrices d'hormones gonadotrophiques chorioniques bêta dans les séminomes. Valeur pronostique. Presse Med 12: 2801, 1983

259. Roth LM, Panganiban WG: Gonadal and extragonadal yolk sac carcinomas. A clinicopathologic study of 14 cases. Cancer 37: 812, 1976

260. Sacchi E: Di un caso di giantismo infantile (pedomacrosomia) con tumore del testicolo. Arch Ortop Milano 12: 305, 1895

261. Schlecker BA, Siegel A, Weiss J, Wein AJ: Epidermoid cyst of the testis: A surgical approach for testicular preservation. J Urol 133: 610, 1985

262. Schulze C, Holstein AF: On the histology of human seminoma. Development of the solid tumor from intratubular seminoma cells. Cancer 39: 1090, 1977

263. Scully RE: Gonadoblastoma. A review of 74 cases. Cancer 25: 1340, 1970

264. Segi M: Graphic Presentation of Cancer Incidence by State and by Area and Population. p. 27. In Segi M (ed): Segi Institute of Cancer Epidemiology, Nagoya, Japan, 1977

265. Shah KH, Maxted WC, Chun B: Epidermoid cysts of the testis: A report of three cases and an analysis of 141 cases from the world literature. Cancer 47: 577, 1981

266. Shalet SM, Hann IM, Lendon M, et al: Testicular function after combination chemotherapy in childhood acute lymphoblastic leukemia. Arch Dis Child 56: 275, 1981

267. Shamberger RC, Sherins RJ, Rosenberg SA: The effects of postoperative adjuvent chemotherapy and radiotherapy on testicular function in men undergoing treatment for soft tissue sarcoma. Cancer 47: 2368, 1981

268. Shanklin DR, Richardson AP, Rothstein G: Testicular hilar nodules in adrenogenital syndrome. Am J Dis Child 106: 243, 1963

269. Shipley WU: The role of radiation therapy in the management of adult germinal testis tumors. p. 48. In Einhorn LH (ed): Testicular Tumors. Masson, New York, 1980

270. Shipley WU: Radiation therapy for patients with testicular and extragonadal seminoma. p. 224. In JP Donohue (ed): Testis Tumors. Williams & Wilkins, Baltimore, 1983

271. Silverberg E, Lubera JA: Cancer Statistics 1983. Am Cancer Society, New York, 1983

272. Silverberg SG: Reproducibility of the mitosis count in the histologic diagnosis of smooth muscle tumors of the uterus. Hum Pathol 7: 451, 1976

273. Skakkebaek NE: Possible carcinoma-in-situ of the testis. Lancet 2: 516, 1972

274. Snyder RN: Completely mature pulmonary mestastasis from testicular teratocarcinoma. Cancer 24: 810, 1969

275. Sohval AR, Churg J, Gabrilove JL: Ultrastructure of feminizing testicular Leydig cell tumors. Ultrastruct Pathol 3: 335, 1982

276. Soumerai S, Gleason EA: Asynchronous plasmacytoma of the stomach and testis. Cancer 45: 396, 1980

277. Stalker AL, Hendry WT: Hyperplasia and neoplasia of the Sertoli cell. J Pathol Bacterol 64: 161, 1950

278. Steigbigel NH, Oppenheim JJ, Fishman LM, Carbone PP: Metastatic embryonal cancer of the testis associated with elevated plasma TSH-like activity and hyperthyroidism. N Engl J Med 271: 345, 1964

279. Steinberg D: Plasmacytoma of the testis. Report of a case. Cancer 36: 1470, 1975

280. Stepamas AV, Samaan NA, Schultz PN, Holoye PY: Endocrine studies in testicular tumor patients with and without gynecomastia. Cancer 41: 369, 1978

281. Stevens LC: The development of transplantable teratocarcinomas from intertesticular grafts of pre- and post implantation mouse embryos. Dev Biol 21: 364, 1970

282. Stevens LC: Embryonic potency of embryoid bodies derived from transplantable testicular teratoma of the mouse. Dev Biol 2: 285, 1960

283. Stoica G, Koestner A, Capen CC: Testicular (Sertoli's cell)-like tumors of the ovary induced by N-ethyl-N-nitrosourea (ENU) in rats. Vet Pathol 22: 483, 1985

284. Strahlberg M, Brown JS: Concommitant bilateral epidermoid cysts of the testis. J Urol 109: 343, 1973

285. Suda K, Mizuguchi K, Hebisawa A, et al: Pancreatic tissue in teratoma. Arch Pathol Lab Med 108: 835, 1984

286. Sullivan MP, Perez CA, Herson J, et al: Radiotherapy (2500 rad) for testicular leukemia: Local control and subsequent clinical events: A Southwest Oncology Group Study. Cancer 46: 508, 1980

287. Survey of Compounds Which Have Been Tested for Carcinogenic Activity. 1978 Volume. U.S. Government Printing Office, Washington, 1980

288. Swanson GM, Brennan MJ: Cancer Incidence in Detroit 1973–1977. p. 344. In Waterhouse J, Muir C, Shanmugaratnam K, Powell J (eds): Cancer Incidence in Five Continents. Vol. IV, International Agency for Research on Cancer, Lyon, 1982

289. Swartz DA, Johnson DE, Hussey DH: Should an elevated human chorionic gonadotropin titer alter therapy for seminoma. J Urol 131: 63, 1984

290. Tackett RE, Ling D, Catalona WJ, Melson GL: High resolution sonography in diagnosing testicular neoplasms: Clinical significance of false positive scans. J Urol 135: 494, 1986

291. Talerman A: Malignant Sertoli cell tumor of the testis. Cancer 28: 446, 1971

292. Talerman A: A distinctive gonadal neoplasm related to gonadoblastoma. Cancer 30: 1219, 1972

293. Talerman A: Yolk sac tumor associated with seminoma of the testis in adults. Cancer 33: 1468, 1974

294. Talerman A: Germ cell tumors of the testis. p. 175. In Fenoglio CM, Wolff M (eds): Progress in Surgical Pathology. Vol. I. Masson, New York, 1980

295. Talerman A: Spermatocytic seminoma. Clinicopathological study of 22 cases. Cancer 45: 2169, 1980

296. Talerman A: Endodermal sinus (yolk sac) tumor elements in testicular germ-cell tumors in adults: Comparison of prospective and retrospective studies. Cancer 46: 1213, 1980

297. Talerman A: Germ cell tumors. p. 29. In Talerman A, Roth LM (eds): Pathology of the Testis and Its Adnexa. Churchill Livingstone, New York, 1986

298. Talerman A, Fu YS, Okagaki T: Spermatocytic seminoma. Ultrastructural and microspectrophotometric observations. Lab Invest 51:343, 1984

299. Talerman A, Gratama S, Miranda S, Okagaki T: Primary carcinoid tumor of the testis. Case report, ultrastructure, and review of the literature. Cancer 42: 2696, 1978

300. Taylor JB, Solomon DH, Levine RE, Ehrlich RM: Exophthalmos in seminoma. Regression with steroids and orchiectomy. JAMA 240: 860, 1978

301. Teilum G: Special Tumors of Ovary and Testis and Related Extragonadal Lesions: Comparative Pathology and Histological Identification. Munksgaard, Copenhagen, 1971

302. Teilum G: Classification of testicular and ovarian androblastoma and Sertoli cell tumors. A survey of comparative studies with consideration of histogenesis, endocrinology, and embryological theories. Cancer 11: 769, 1958

303. Tepperman BS, Gospodarowicz MK, Bush RS, Brown TG: Non-Hodgkin's lymphoma of the testis. Radiology 142: 203, 1982

304. Thackray AC, Crane WAJ: Seminoma. p. 164. In RCB Pugh (ed): Pathology of the Testis. Oxford, Blackwell, 1976

305. Tiedemann K, Chessels JM, Sandland RM: Isolated testicular relapse in boys with acute lymphoblastic leukaemia: Treatment and outcome. Br Med J 285: 1614, 1982

306. Tiltman AJ: Metastatic tumours in the testis. Histopathology 3: 31, 1979

307. Tiltman AJ: Granulomatous reaction in testicular teratomas. S Afr Med J 67: 1231, 1974

308. Tisman G, Wu SG, Hittle T: Serum ferritin as a parameter of response to cancer chemotherapy. Clin Res 25: 580A, 1977

309. Tollerud DJ, Blattner WA, Fraser MC, et al: Familial testicular cancer and urogenital developmental anomalies. Cancer 55: 1849, 1985

310. True LD, Otis, CN, Del prado W, et al: Spermatocytic seminoma of testis with sarcomatous transformation. A report of five cases. Am J Surg Pathol 12: 75, 1988

311. Tseng A, Horning SJ, Freiha FS, et al: Gynecomastia in testicular cancer patients. Prognostic and therapeutic implications. Cancer 56: 2534, 1985

312. Tucker DF, Oliver RTD, Travers P, Brodmer WF: Serum marker potential of placental alkaline phosphastase-like activity in testicular germ cell tumours evaluated by H17E2 monoclonal antibody assay. Br J Cancer 51: 631, 1985

313. Turek FW, Desjardins C: Development of Leydig cell tumors and onset of changes in the reproduction and endocrine system of aging in F344 rats. J Nat Cancer Inst 63: 969, 1979

314. Turner RR, Colby TV, MacKintosh FR: Testicular lymphomas: A clinicopathologic study of 35 cases. Cancer 48: 2095, 1981

315. Uchida T, Shikata T, Iino S: Immunohistochemical localization of placental and intestinal alkaline phosphatase. p. 185. In DeLellis R (ed): Advances in Immunohistochemistry. Masson, New York, 1984

316. Ulbright TM, Clark SA, Einhorn LH: Angiosarcoma associated with germ cell tumors. Hum Pathol 16: 268, 1985

317. Ulbright TM, Goheen MP, Roth LM, Gillespie JJ: The differentiation of carcinomas of teratomatous origin from embryonal carcinoma. A light and electron microscopic study. Cancer 57: 257, 1986

318. Ulbright TM, Loehrer PJ, Roth LM, et al: The development of non-germ cell malignancies within germ cell tumors. A clinicopathologic study of 11 cases. Cancer 54: 1824, 1984

319. Ulbright TM, Roth LM, Brodhecker CA: Yolk sac differentiation in germ cell tumors. A morphologic study of 50 cases with emphasis on hepatic, enteric and parietal yolk sac features. Am J Surg Pathol 10: 151, 1986

320. Ulbright TM, Roth LM: Evaluation of germ cell tumors following chemotherapy. p. 231. In Talerman A, Roth L (eds): Pathology of The Testis And Its Adnexa. Churchill Livingstone, New York, 1986

321. Upton JD, Das S: Benign intrascrotal neoplasms. J Urol 135: 504, 1986

322. Urban MD, Lee PA, Plotnick LP, Migeon CJ: The diagnosis of Leydig cell tumors in childhood. Am J Dis Child 132: 494, 1978

323. U.S. Public Health Service: Population dose from X-rays. U.S. 1964. Estimates of gonad and genetically significant dose from the Public Health Service X-ray Exposure Study. Public Health Service Publication 2001, U.S. Government Printing Office, Washington, DC, 1969

324. Von der Masse H, Berthelsen JG, Jacobsen GK, et al: Carcinoma-in-situ of testis eradicated by chemotherapy. (Letter) Lancet 1: 98, 1985

325. Von Eyben FE: Lactate dehydrogenase and its isoenzymes in testicular germ cell tumors: An overview. Oncodevel Biol Med 4: 395, 1983

326. Von Eyben FE, Mikulowski P, Busch C: Microinvasive germ cell tumors of the testis. J Urol 126: 842, 1981

327. Von Hochstetter AR: Mitotic count in seminomas — an unreliable criterion for distinguishing between classical and anaplastic types. Virchows Arch Pathol Anat 390: 63, 1981

328. Von Hochstetter AR, Hedinger CE: The differential diagnosis of testicular germ cell tumors in theory and practice. A critical analysis of two major systems of classification and review of 389 cases. Virchows Arch Pathol Anat 396: 247, 1982

329. Von Hochstetter AR, Sigg C, Saremaslani P, Hedinger C: The significance of giant cells in human testicular seminomas. A clinicopathological study. Virchows Arch Pathol Anat 407: 309, 1985

330. Walter P: Seminome spermatocytaire. Etude de 8 observations et revue de la littérature. Virchows Arch Pathol Anat 386: 175, 1980

331. Wang N, Trend B, Bronson DL, Fraley EE: Nonrandom abnormalities in chromosome 1 in human testicular cancers. Cancer Res 40: 796, 1980

332. Warhol M, Nickoloff B, Weinberg D: Seminoma metastasis to the terminal ileum after a 17-year disease-free interval. Cancer 52: 1957, 1983

333. Waterhouse J, Muir C, Shanugaratnam K, Powell J (eds): Cancer Incidence in Five Continents. Vol. IV, International Agency for Research on Cancer, Lyon, 1982

334. Waxman M, Damjanov I, Khapra A, Landau SJ: Large cell calcifying Sertoli tumors of the testis. Cancer 54: 1574, 1984

335. Waxman M, Vuletin JC, Pertschuk LP, et al: Pleomorphic atypical thyroid adenoma arising in struma testis: Light microscopic, ultrastructural and immunofluorescent studies. Mt Sinai J Med 49: 13, 1982

336. Weitzner S: Survival of patients with secondary carcinoma of prostate in the testis. Cancer 32: 447, 1973

337. Weitzner S, Gropp A: Primary reticulum cell sarcoma of testis in a 12 year old. Cancer 37: 935, 1976

338. West AB, Butler MR, Fitzpatrick J, O'Brien A: Testicular tumors in subfertile men: Report of 4 cases with implications for management of patients presenting with infertility. J Urol 133: 107, 1985

339. Wettlaufer JN: The management of advanced seminoma. Semin Urol 11: 257, 1984

339a. Wheeler JE, Rudy FR: The testis, paratesticular structures, and external male genitalia. p. 1147. In Silverberg SG (ed): Principles and Practice of Surgical Pathology. Wiley, New York, 1983

340. White R de V, Karian S, Hong WK, Olsson CA: Testis tumor markers: How accurate are they? J Urol 125: 661, 1981

341. Wilkins L: Ectopic Leydig cell tumor in cord. p. 233. In Wilkins L (ed): The Diagnosis and Treatment of Endocrine Disorders in Childhood and Adolescence. 3rd Ed. Charles C Thomas, Springfield, IL, 1965

342. Williams SD, Birch R, Einhorn LH, et al: Treatment of disseminated germ-cell tumors with cisplatium, bleomycin, and either vinblastine or etoposide. N Engl J Med 316: 1435, 1987

343. Willis RA: Pathology of Tumours. 2nd Ed. CV Mosby, St Louis, 1953

344. Wilson DM, Pitts WC, Hintz RL, Rosenfeld RG: Testicular tumors with Peutz-Jeghers syndrome. Cancer 57: 2238, 1986

345. Wurster K, Brodner O, Rosner JA, Grude D: A carcinoid occurring in the testis. Virchows Arch Pathol Anat 370: 185, 1976

346. Yoshitomi K, Morii S: Benign and malignant epithelial tumors of the rete testis in mice. Vet Pathol 21: 300, 1984

347. Young JL Jr, Ries LG, Silverberg E, et al: Cancer incidence, survival, and mortality for children younger than age 15 years. Cancer 58: 598, 1986

348. Young RH, Dickersin GR, Scully RE: Juvenile granulosa cell tumor of the ovary. A clinicopathologic analysis of 125 cases. Am J Pathol 8: 575, 1984

349. Young RH, Lawrence WD, Scully RE: Juvenile granulosa cell tumor—another neoplasm associated with abnormal chromosomes and ambiguous genitalia. A report of three cases. Am J Surg Pathol 9: 737, 1985

350. Young RH, Scully RD: Miscellaneous neoplasms and non-neoplastic lesions. p. 93. In Talerman A, Roth L (eds): Pathology of the Testis and Its Adnexa. Churchill Livingstone, New York, 1986

351. Zarabi MC, Rupani M: Human chorionic gonadotropin-secreting pure dysgerminoma. Hum Pathol 15: 589, 1984

352. Zevallos M, Snyder RN, Sadoff L, Cooper JF: Testicular neoplasm in identical twins. A case report. JAMA 250: 645, 1983

353. Zondag HA, Klein F: Clinical applications of lactate dehydrogenase isoenzymes: Alterations in malignancy. Ann NY Acad Sci 151: 578, 1968

354. Zwaveling A, Soebhag R: Testicular tumors in the Netherlands. Cancer 55: 1612, 1985

28

Paratesticular Structures: Nontumorous Conditions

Gary S. Hill
Claire Billey-Kijner

The testicular adnexa, or paratesticular structures, include the epididymis, ductus deferens and spermatic cord, seminal vesicles, and ejaculatory ducts, plus sundry other vestigial remnants, such as the appendix testis. These structures tend not to attract much interest from pathologists. On the one hand, the specimens they see most frequently, segments of vas deferens at vasectomy, are almost always normal, and on the other hand, the most common ailments of the testicular adnexa, hydroceles and varicoceles, very seldom produce pathologic specimens. Nonetheless, these paratesticular structures occasionally yield fascinating and challenging diagnostic problems, particularly in the realm of tumors.

DEVELOPMENTAL ANOMALIES

Embryology

The embryology of the testis and testicular adnexa is described in some detain in Chapter 22. The following is a brief resumé of the more important events as they relate to the development of the paratesticular structures. The testis and head of the epididymis arise from the genital ridge, whereas the epididymal body and tail, vas deferens, and ejaculatory duct develop from the mesonephros.[2,39,51,79] The seminal vesicles develop from a lateral diverticulum of the caudal end of the mesonephric duct. During early life, the testes are located in the dorsal part of the abdominal cavity, and the left testicle is near the spleen. A large part of the cranial portion of the mesonephric duct disappears, but a blunt end may persist as the appendix of the epididymis, while other structures from the caudal end may remain as the vasa aberrans and paradidymis. The paramesonephros, or müllerian duct, disappears in the male, but may also leave remnants, such as the appendix testis (Fig. 28-1).

During the eighth month of gestation, the testis migrates down to the scrotum, preceded by an evagination of the peritoneum, the processus vaginalis. Just before birth, the saccus vaginalis becomes obliterated. This obliteration begins at the inguinal end and proceeds downwards, so that the peritoneum surrounding the testis is separated entirely from the general peritoneal cavity and becomes the tunica vaginalis.

A failure in any of the embryologic processes, be it problems in growth, migration, or regression, may result in abnormalities, notably absence, atresia, or ectopia of the vas, epididymis, or spermatic cord, or more commonly, vestigial ducts or cysts attached to these structures.

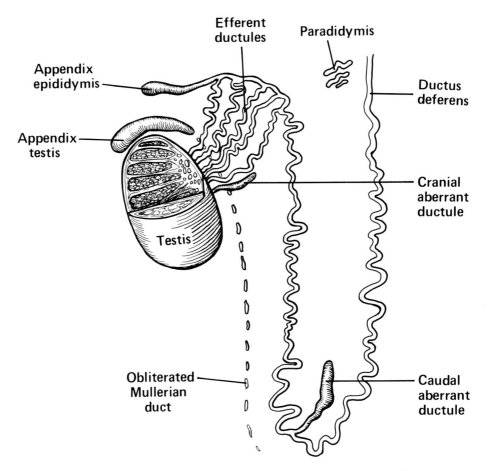

Fig. 28-1 Testicular adenexa. Diagram showing the relationships of testis and paratesticular structures, including the variably present vestigial remnants (appendix testis, appendix epididymis, paradidymis, cranial and caudal aberrant ductules, and the obliterated müllerian duct).

Atresias and Duplications

The various types of paratesticular anomalies may be unilateral or bilateral and may result from abnormal development of the genital ridge or the adjacent wolffian structures, or from failure of fusion of the various parts of the testicular adenexa. Abnormal development of the genital ridge results in atresia or hypoplasia of the testis and head of the epididymis. This is often associated with abnormal development of wolffian structures as well, leading to absence or adjacent hypoplasia of the body and tail of the epididymis and/or vas deferens (Fig. 28-2). Some cases of congenital aplasia of the vas deferens, with or without renal agenesis, appear to be autosomal recessive.[128] Lack of connection between the testis and head of the epididymis or between the head and body of the epididymis has also been described.[78] These anomalies may be associated with ectopia of the testis, epididymis or vas deferens. They are also often associated with renal malformations such as hypoplasia or dysplasia and appear to be more frequent in cryptorchid boys with congenital rubella.[111]

Maldevelopment of seminal vesicles[101] results in hypoplasia, agenesis, or cyst formation. Unilateral agenesis of the seminal vesicles may be associated with renal agenesis,[29] but this is more frequent in defects of the vas deferens or epididymis.

Abnormal development of the ureteral bud may result in ectopic termination of the ureter in the epididymis, vas deferens, seminal vesicle, or ejaculatory duct.[26,43,104] Congenital cysts of the seminal vesicles

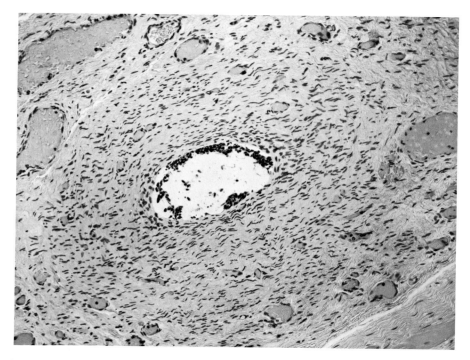

Fig. 28-2 Atresia, vas deferens. In this infant, the vas deferens was normal in its proximal reaches, but tapered and ended abruptly. The wall is thinned, consisting mainly of fibrous tissue, and the epithelium is pyknotic. ×128.

are almost always associated with ipsilateral renal agenesis as well.[6,25,99] They are solitary and occur mostly in the third decade of life.[99] They contain variable amounts of pale brown or yellow viscid fluid, are usually monolocular,[25] and are lined by flat-to-cuboidal epithelium lying on a thin or thick and fibrous wall. Lipofuscin may be present in the epithelial cells.

Duplication of the epididymis, vas deferens, or seminal vesicles is rare, but may occur[62,115] and does not generally seem to be associated with significant clinical problems.

Agenesis, atresia, or failure of fusion of the various components of the genital tract, when bilateral, would obviously result in sterility. The only other significant problems arise from associated lesions, such as renal dysplasia, cystic fibrosis (see below), or testicular ectopia.

CYSTIC FIBROSIS

Cystic fibrosis[65,138] is accompanied in the majority of cases by sterility. This is generally due to a partial or total atresia of the derivatives of the mesonephric duct and/or to abnormalities in testicular function. The vas deferens is absent, atretic, or otherwise abnormal; the epididymis may be normal, absent, or rudimentary. In the latter case there is atrophy of the tail or the body of the epididymis (Fig. 28-3), while the seminal vesicles are dilated or absent. The testes may also present abnormalities of development, notably absence, atrophy, or abnormalities of spermatogenesis.

Ectopias

ECTOPIC EPIDIDYMIS AND SCROTUM

Ectopic epididymal tissue has been described in retroperitoneal or intrarenal positions[4] and is anterior to the testes in 10 to 15 percent of men.[5] This may be associated with sterility in the case of failure of fusion between epididymis and testis. A *lateral or suprainguinal scrotum* is generally associated with ipsilateral upper urinary tract anomalies and probably results from a gubernacular defect.[36]

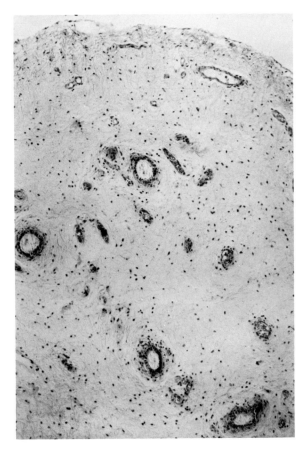

Fig. 28-3 Epididymal agenesis in cystic fibrosis. Epididymis from a youth dying of cystic fibrosis. There is near-total atresia, with only a few vestigial tubules and scattered inflammation in a sea of connective tissue. ×81.

SCROTAL ADRENAL AND SPLENIC RESTS

Intrascrotal ectopic adrenal rests are primarily of interest to the surgeon.[24,83,100,134] The adrenal glands arise from ectodermal and mesodermal tissue near the mesonephric bodies, and migration of adrenal rests with the testis and cord seems to be a fairly common event.[39] As many as 1 percent of the children operated on for inguinal hernia or undescended testis have accessory adrenal cortical tissue along the spermatic cord.[77] These rests usually involute in early life, but may persist and be functional, so that their removal can result in adrenal insufficiency.[39,83] They are small, sometimes umbilicated nodules, yellow-orange and firm, resembling fat lobules. Adrenal rests are usually located near the inguinal ring, but may be found near the epididymis (Fig. 28-4).[5] They generally consist of cortical tissue (fasciculata and glomerulosa) and only rarely of medullary tissue.[5] On rare occasions tumors may develop in adrenal rests.[38,134] More frequently, adrenal rests develop into tumorlike masses in adrenogenital syndrome and Nelson's syndrome.

Paratesticular accessory spleen[149] is also frequently associated with an indirect inguinal hernia and occasionally with an incomplete descensus of the testis. They occur on the left side, the ectopic splenic tissue having adhered to the left testis early in embryologic development and migrated with it. As such, splenic

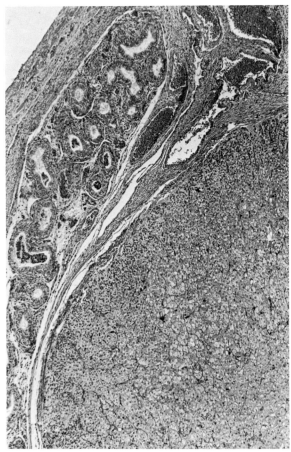

Fig. 28-4 Adrenal rest, scrotum. This rather large adrenal rest, composed entirely of cortex, is nestled next to the epididymis (above) in this newborn infant. ×138.

remmants may be encountered at any point along the path of descent of the testis, for example perivesically,[152b] but those that have strayed that far usually go on to the scrotum with the testis.

The splenic rest is a small, beefy red, encapsulated mass, easily dissected from neighboring structures, and is located along the cord or next to the testicle (splenogonadal fusion). Usually it is attached to the upper pole of the testis, but it may be attached to the lower pole or even lie within the testis. In some cases, the splenic rest is linked to the normal spleen by a cordlike structure composed of fibrous tissue, sometimes containing some amount of splenic tissue. This is called *continuous type* splenic ectopia. In the discontinuous type, the ectopic spleen lacks any connection with the normal spleen.[84] Because of its origin early in embryologic development, there is a high incidence of associated anomalies, particularly limb defects.

ECTOPIC RENAL PARENCHYMA

Ectopic renal parenchyma, with tubules and glomeruli, may on rare occasion be found in the scrotum. Two spermatic cord Wilms' tumors have been reported in children. One way lying adjacent to an ectopic focus of renal parenchyma with renal tubules and immature glomeruli.[103] The other occurred in a child exposed in utero to phenytoin.[140]

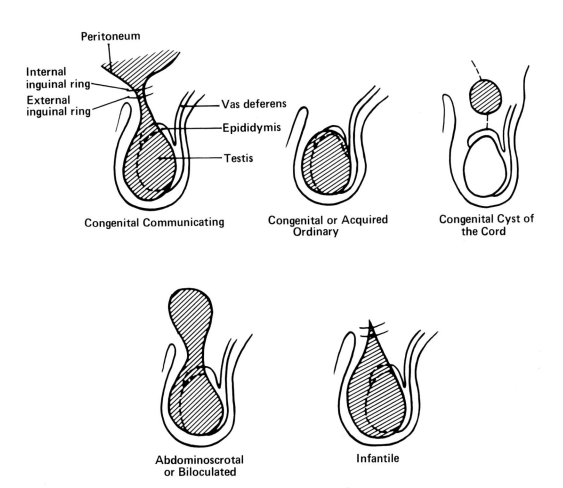

Fig. 28-5 The principal types of hydroceles.

Congenital Hydroceles

Persistence of the processus vaginalis is responsible for the congenital type of inguinal hernia and is frequently associated with cryptorchidism. Congenital inguinal hernias most commonly contain portions of bowel. Rarely, they may contain urinary bladder (cystocele) or kidney.[148]

When the processus vaginalis does not completely seal off, peritoneal fluid accumulates in the tunica vaginalis, creating a congenital communicating hydrocele (Fig. 28-5).[49,101] The congenital cyst of the cord (hydrocele of the cord) results from a localized remnant of the processus vaginalis, while the abdominoscrotal hydrocele or hydrocele en bissac is a pouch communicating between the scrotum and peritoneal cavity. The upper end of an infantile hydrocele lies in the internal inguinal ring but does not communicate with the peritoneal cavity. All congenital forms of hydrocele are filled with serous clear fluid and lined by mesothelium.[16] Infection may occur as a result of a tap; by local spread of organisms from an adjacent orchitis, epidymitis, or peritonitis; or by the lymphohematogenous route.[118] (See hydrocele infections below.)

Remnants of the Müllerian and Wolffian Ducts

REMNANTS OF THE PARAMESONEPHRIC OR MÜLLERIAN DUCT

Appendix Testis

The appendix testis is by far the most common embryonal remnant. It represents the vestigial cranial portion of the müllerian duct. It has been found in 80 percent to 92 percent of patients in careful autopsy studies.[120,136]

The appendix testis is located at the upper pole of the testis, beneath the end of the head of the epididy-

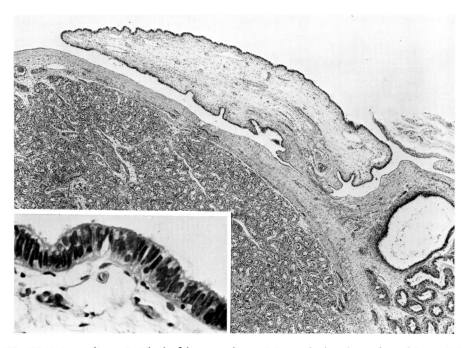

Fig. 28-6 Appendix testis. The leaflike appendix testis is attached to the surface of the testis in this infant. On its underside are numerous indentations; when more developed later they may give the impression of glands within the appendix testis. **Inset** High-power view of the columnar epithelium lining the racemose infoldings of the appendix testis. In some specimens cilia may be seen. ×28 and ×320.

mis, but it may be attached to the groove between the epididymis and testis or to both the testis and epididymis. The appendix testis is usually pedunculated. Although it is usually a small smooth sphere measuring a few millimeters in diameter, it may be a leaflike structure 2 or 3 cm long.[98] Occasionally, it overlies a cyst of the tunica vaginalis.

The surface of the appendix testis is lined by a cuboidal-to-columnar epithelium (Fig. 28-6) in continuity with the mesothelium of the tunica vaginalis. Its irregular surface often sends invaginations into the superficial stroma, appearing as tubules in cross-section. The epithelium usually consists of a single layer of columnar or tall cuboidal cells. Their nuclear/cytoplasmic ratio is high, and their nuclei are usually dense and hyperchromatic, but without atypia. Their slightly basophilic cytoplasm contains granules of glycogen. Although Sundarasivarao in his major study of müllerian remnants[136] considers that those columnar cells are not ciliated, occasional but definite cilia may be seen. Most often, the apical surfaces of these cells are irregular as a result of artifact or secretions. Here, as in other vestigial structures, lipofuscins are absent.

The core of the appendix testis is made of loose and richly vascularized connective tissue containing a few mononuclear cells, with scattered smooth muscle bundles. Sometimes the number of fibroblasts is increased, either diffusely or around tubules. Rarely, the connective tissue is hyalinized or focally calcified.

In approximately 40 percent of patients, the appendix testis contains tubular remnants of the müllerian duct, free of any connection with the surface epithelium. These müllerian remnants are sometimes cystic and filled by mucoid material, their folded and branched epithelium resembling the mucosa of the fallopian tube;[61] hence the name *hydatid of Morgagni* is sometimes applied to these structures.

Other Müllerian Remnants

Other müllerian remnants are occasionally seen in or near the epididymis and rarely in inguinal hernia sacs and spermatic cords.[144] They consist of small nests or small cysts of columnar or polyhedral cells with large, hyperchromatic nuclei. They may be surrounded by smooth muscle. One case of müllerian vestigial papilloma has been described in the literature.[23]

WOLFFIAN REMNANTS

Appendix Epididymis

The appendix epididymis, derived from cranial mesonephric collecting tubules, is found in approximately one-fourth to one-third of autopsy cases.[120,136] It is a pedunculated cyst, usually arising from the anterosuperior end of the epididymis and filled with clear fluid (Fig. 28-7).[98] Histologically, the inner wall of the cyst is lined by a layer of cells similar to those of the epithelium of the appendix testis, although more frequently ciliated. This epithelium lies on a thin wall of loose or hyalinized connective tissue, lined on the serosal surface by mesothelium. The cyst contains a mucoid material which is periodic acid-Schiff (PAS) and alcian blue positive.

Other Wolffian Remnants

Rarer than the appendix epididymis, the *vasa aberrans,* also called the cranial and *caudal aberrant ductules,* are a small group of tubules located between the testis and the body of the epididymis. The *ductus aberrans inferior* (or duct of Haller) is usually connected to the epididymis and ranges in length from 3.5 to 35 cm.[51] Its diameter is usually the same throughout, averaging a few millimeters. Rarely, it has no connection to the epididymis. The *ductus aberrans superior* arises near the rete testis and is similar to the inferior aberrant ductules. The *paradidymis* (organ of Giraldés) is a group of coiled tubules, sometimes pedunculated, arising in the spermatic cord near the head of the epididymis.[98] The vasa aberrans and paradidymis are derived from the vestigial caudal mesonephric collecting tubules. These remnants are lined by columnar cells similar to those of the previously described appendix epididymis and appendix testis.

LESIONS OF MÜLLERIAN AND WOLFFIAN REMNANTS

All of these pedunculated structures are subject to spontaneous torsion, but the appendix testis is by far the most frequently involved.[40,133] Clinically, the vast

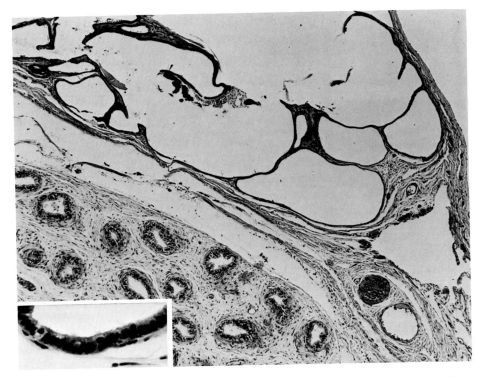

Fig. 28-7 Appendix epididymis. The structure is cystic, with an interior lining (inset) similar to but simpler than that of the appendix testis. ×14 and ×320.

majority of patients are young boys, 6 to 14 years old, with the peak incidence at age 10 to 12 years. The symptoms vary from none at all to severe pain, typically setting in after vigorous activity. Torsion of the appendix testis is often misdiagnosed as a testicular torsion, acute epididymitis, or even acute appendicitis.[101]

Macroscopically, the appendix testis is at first red, swollen, and hemorrhagic and later becomes black and necrotic. The inflammatory process sometimes elicits a hydrocele. Infarction is followed by sclerosis, resulting in a small dense hyaline structure. The appendix may detach from its base at any stage to float free in the hydrocele fluid. Histologically, the pattern is one of hemorrhagic infarction, followed by inflammation and fibrosis.

Cystic enlargement of the ductus aberrans inferior and of the paradidymis (or possibly ductus aberrans) has been reported in young men by Wollin et al.[152a] They speculated that the hormonal changes at puberty and resulting secretion caused these blind remnants to become cystically enlarged.

DEGENERATIVE CHANGES

Pseudomalignant Epithelial Cells; Nuclear Inclusions

Scattered epithelial cells of bizarre appearance are sometimes encountered in the epithelium of the epididymis, seminal vesicles, and ductuli efferentes, mainly in older persons, and are not necessarily associated with cancer.[75] These cells are enlarged, with marked variation in the size of the nuclei and of the cell overall (Fig. 28-8). The nuclei become hyperchromatic with irregular contours, and later pyknotic as the cell is shed into the lumen. In addition to these pleomorphic cells, multinucleated epithelial cells are also found in the ejaculatory ducts, epididymis, and seminal vesicles (Fig. 28-9).[32,75] They are probably polyploid and prepyknotic.[89,94]

These atypical cells may be encountered in aspiration biopsy smears of the prostate,[32,72] and rarely even in vaginal smears.[89] The presence of lipofuscins helps distinguish them from truly malignant cells. Lipofu-

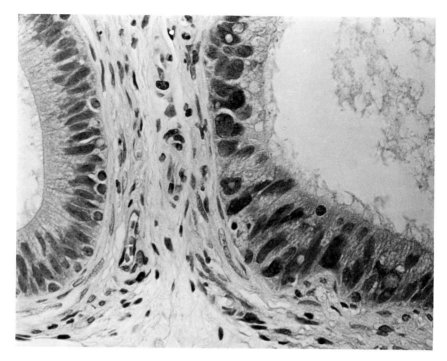

Fig. 28-8 Bizarre nuclei with nuclear inclusions, epididymis. Compare the irregular and pleomorphic nuclei in the right-hand tubule with the more normal ones on the tubule on the left. Such nuclei are a normal finding in the epididymis and have no connotation of malignancy. Numerous nuclear inclusions are also seen; some are clear, while others contain an eosinophilic, PAS-positive material. ×380.

scins are yellow-brown pigments present in the epididymis and seminal vesicles from puberty on, accumulating with increasing age.[89,137] They stain brown with hematoxylin and eosin and with Papanicolaou stain and blue-green with the May-Grünwald-Giemsa stain. They are also characterized by orange-red autofluorescence.

The origin and significance of these epithelial changes are unknown, and different explanations — physiological, degenerative, or viral changes — have been proposed. Because of the blurred cytoplasm and cell membranes and the suggestion of degenerative nuclear changes, the degeneration hypothesis is particularly attractive, but there is little direct evidence to support it.

Nuclei with vacuoles or apparent inclusions are commonly found in the epithelium of the epididymis and may also occur in the vas deferens.[82] The somewhat granular, slightly eosinophilic inclusion stains red with PAS, is negative or only slightly positive after diastase digestion, and is negative for alcian blue.

It seems likely that it represents a real intranuclear glycogenic inclusion, as is sometimes seen in the liver, but it may represent a cytoplasmic pseudoinclusion, similar to the Dutcher bodies seen in the cells of Waldenström's macroglobulinemia.

Calcifications and Calculi

Most often discovered at autopsy, and sometimes recognizable as nodules on radiographs, calcification of the muscularis of the vas deferens (Fig. 28-10) is generally associated with diabetes mellitus. It is found in approximately 15 percent of aged diabetics.[96,126] It is sometimes bilateral and may involve the seminal vesicles as well. As with Mönckeberg's medial sclerosis, it occurs focally, is not associated with inflammation or fibrosis, and may extend circumferentially around the lumen. The calcific deposits are of variable size and shape. The calcium may appear to precipitate directly on or in the smooth muscle cells, whose ghosts may be recognizable. Also, as with Möncke-

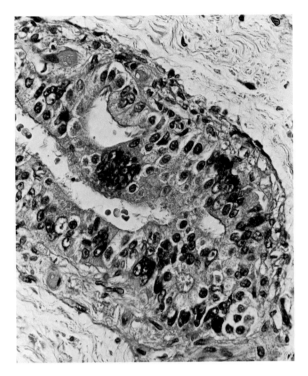

Fig. 28-9 Giant cells, epididymis. In addition to some nuclear pleomorphism, the epididymal epithelium in this older patient has several giant cells (more properly, nuclear syncytia). ×330.

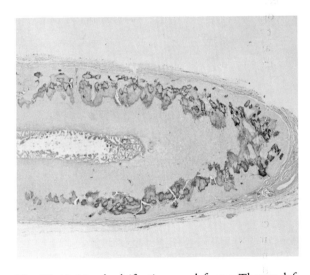

Fig. 28-10 Mural calcification, vas deferens. The vas deferens in this elderly diabetic shows extensive calcification of the muscularis, probably originating either in or directly on the individual smooth muscle cells. ×7.0.

berg's medical sclerosis, there may be foci of metaplastic ossification.[126]

Calcifications related to chronic inflammation are different. They consist of small deposits, which may also ossify, but which are scattered randomly through the wall and associated with fibrosis and/or an inflammatory exudate. This pattern of calcification has no association with diabetes.

Calculi occur in the vas deferens and, more frequently, in the seminal vesicles.[126] They are brown, single or multiple, and range from 1 mm to 1 cm. They are composed of phosphates and carbonates around an organic nidus.[31] Formation of calculi is favored by obstruction and chronic inflammation, and their presence tends to perpetuate the inflammation, in a vicious circle.

Amyloidosis of Seminal Vesicles

Amyloidosis of the seminal vesicles[17,74,108] is more common than generally realized among older men. McDonald and Heckel[87] found 2 cases in a study of 167 consecutive autopsies of male patients, while Bursell[14] described 33 cases in a study of 178 autopsies. He concluded that its incidence increases with age, as none of his patients under 46 years of age showed seminal vesicle amyloidosis, as opposed to 34 percent in the group of patients over 76 years old. These results were confirmed by Pitkänen et al.[108] who found that 21 percent of males over 75 years old had seminal vesicle amyloidosis, mostly of the senile type.

Seminal vesicle amyloidosis is almost always bilateral and symmetric and is generally a part of senile amyloidosis, in which deposits are found variably in the brain, the islands of Langerhans, the aorta, and the heart (in this latter case with concomitant vascular and pulmonary involvement).

Symptoms are generally absent, but when present may consist of local pain or, rarely, microscopic hematuria resulting from focal hemorrhage.[87]

Macroscopically, the seminal vesicles are normal and may be stained black by iodine if the deposits are substantial. Microscopically, the amorphous, eosinophilic, homogeneous deposits thicken the basement membranes and usually form distinct subepithelial lumps (Fig. 28-11). They are sometimes seen seemingly free in the lumen. By contrast, deposits in the

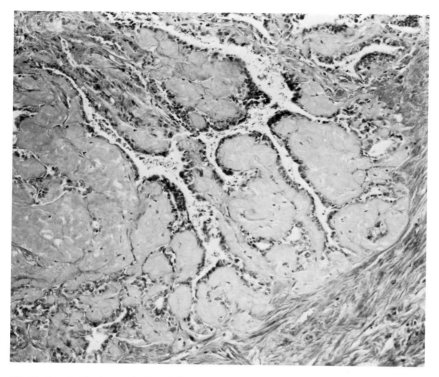

Fig. 28-11 Amyloidosis, seminal vesicles. Massive deposits in the subepithelial zone and basement membranes, probably a part of senile amyloidosis. ×156.

vascular walls or smooth muscle suggest possible systemic amyloidosis, rather than senile amyloidosis.

The deposits are stained red by Congo red with characteristic apple green birefringence on polarization. They also stain specifically with thioflavine and are metachromatic with crystal violet and toluidine blue, although these latter stains are often difficult to interpret if the deposits are less than massive.

Senile amyloidosis of the seminal vesicles has unique histochemical properties and does not belong to any clear-cut group, such as light chain-derived or serum amyloid protein-derived amyloid.[108] Its composition is not yet entirely established.

Eosinophilic Hyaline Bodies

These interstitial bodies are round, oval, or sometimes irregular and are located in the muscle layer of the seminal vesicle. These structures, which may reach 15 nm to 20 nm in diameter, have a hyaline quality, and they stain red with hematoxylin and eosin (H&E) and Masson's trichrome, pink with PAS,

and blue with luxol fast blue. They do not stain with phosphotungstic acid–hematoxylin, methyl green pyronin, Feulgen, Alcian blue at pH 2.5, or Congo red. They may arise from hyaline degeneration of smooth muscle fibers, since transitional forms with pyknotic nuclei may be observed. Their significance is not known.[75]

CYSTIC, INFLAMMATORY, AND OTHER NONTUMOROUS CONDITIONS

Hydrocele

By far the most frequent cause of increased scrotal volume is hydrocele, an accumulation of serous liquid in the cavity of the tunica vaginalis, which normally contains only a few drops.[12,49,102,125] Hydroceles may be congenital, idiopathic, or secondary to trauma, tumors, or inflammation. They may also be due to any cause of generalized edema[118] or to certain viral lesions such as infectious mononucleosis,[55] and exceptionally may be due to myxoedema.[63]

The fluid varies in quantity from a few milliliters to more than 300 ml and may compress the testis, with resulting interstitial edema and tubular alterations (Fig. 28-12). When long-standing, a voluminous hydrocele may lead to testicular atrophy.[12,118] The fluid is generally clear, pale yellow to amber, and without odor. It may take on a hemorrhagic character in cases of tumor or inflammation, and in the latter situation it may become cloudy or frankly purulent. Occasionally, a detached necrotic appendix testis is found floating in the fluid. Other unusual bodies include scrotal pearls or scrotal mice, which are loose fibrous bodies resulting from fibrinous deposits or from a sclerosed detached appendix testis; multifaceted cholesterol stones;[20,61,80] or even microfilaria.[143]

The tunica vaginalis, which is smooth and supple in congenital hydroceles, may take on various appearances in hydroceles of other causes. The tunica becomes red, roughened, and covered with fibrin in cases of acute inflammation resulting from gonorrheal epididymitis or infection secondary to a tap.[12] Tuberculosis of the tunica vaginalis is usually associated with an epididymal or peritoneal infection in a patient in whom the processus vaginalis has incompletely involuted.

Chronic inflammation renders the tunica whitish and fibrous. It may be uniformly thickened or perhaps multinodular with a pseudotumoral appearance (Fig. 28-13) (see Ch. 29). It often shows fibrous adhesions to neighboring structures or a polycystic structure as a result of loculation of fluid between adhesions. It may also contain calcifications.

Hydrocele fluid is comparable to the liquid of pleural or peritoneal effusions, and examination of this fluid sometimes yields a cytologic diagnosis.[64] Microscopic study of the walls often permits identifi-

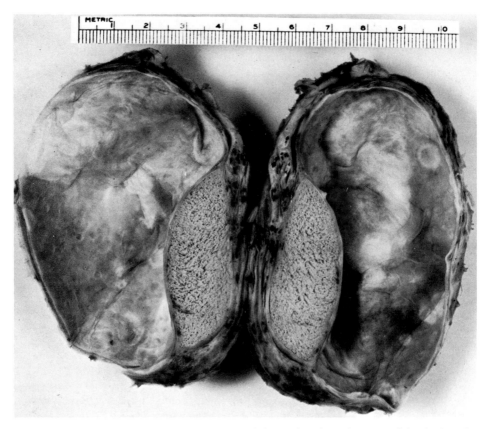

Fig. 28-12 Hydrocele. Despite the large size and the evident long duration of this hydrocele, there is only modest testicular atrophy. The individual testicular tubules are readily recognizable.

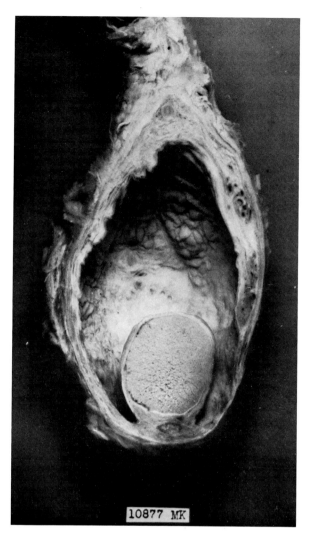

Fig. 28-13 Chronic hydrocele. The greatly thickened wall of this hydrocele sac is lined by nodular excrescences representing an admixture of reactive proliferative mesothelium, inflammation, and fibrous tissue.

cation of the reason for their thickening. The tunica vaginalis shows congestion and fibrinopurulent exudate in cases of acute inflammation. Fibrosis and sclerosis, a mononuclear infiltrate of variable extent, and possible calcific deposits are seen in cases of chronic inflammation. Sometimes foreign body granulomas directed against cholesterol crystals[80] are present.

In rare infants, the hydrocele is accompanied by marked thickening of the tissues or by a frank scrotal mass (*meconium periorchitis*,[27] *meconium granuloma*,[58] or

meconium vaginalitis[91]) secondary to meconium-induced chronic inflammation. In this situation there appears to have been an antenatal perforation of the colon, with spillage of meconium that eventually percolates through the still-open processus vaginalis into the scrotum. There it elicits a brisk foreign body response and scarring. Grossly, there are multiple orange-brown to green nodules on the tunica vaginalis. Microscopically, the nodules are composed of loose myxoid fibrous tissue with scattered lymphocytes and macrophages. There macrophages and associated foreign body cells may contain bile,[58] cholesterol, squames, and even lanugo hairs,[27] all derived from the meconium.[11] In almost all cases the bowel perforations seem to have closed spontaneously before birth, leaving only focal calcifications on abdominal films as evidence of their occurrence. Interestingly, only one of the 24 cases thus far reported has had cystic fibrosis.[27]

In other cases, foreign body granulomas surround particles of talc, appearing as Maltese crosses by polarized light. These are mute testimony to prior surgical interventions, in some instances as much as 45 years earlier.[56,92] Talc granulomas may also rarely be seen in the epididymis or the vas deferens.

The microscopic appearance of specific inflammations, tumors, etc., are described in the corresponding sections below.

Although the mechanism of hydroceles associated with acute inflammation, that is, exudation, is well understood, that of other categories of hydrocele is less so. Some investigators[119] suggest that the fluid is formed primarily by the visceral layer of the tunica vaginalis and is reabsorbed by the parietal layer and that hydroceles occur when the resorptive ability of the parietal layer is less than the amount of fluid produced. According to this hypothesis, congenital hydroceles, usually resorbed during the first year of life, would be due to an immaturity of the reabsorbing lymphatics in the parietal layer. In tumors and chronic inflammation, the lymphatics might be partially blocked, compromised by fibrosis, or invaded by the proliferation.[102] Irritation of the tunica by an underlying tumor also represents a possibility in the genesis of these lesions.

Treatment is etiologic.[119] For congenital hydrocele, it consists of puncture, dissection of the tunica, or eversion of the sac. Aspiration and reinjection have also been proposed.[15]

Cysts of Rete Testis, Epididymis, and Vas Deferens

Cysts are not infrequently found in the epididymis or along the course of the vas deferens as an incidental finding at autopsy in older men. Only rarely are they palpable, much less symptomatic, during life. By contrast, only one definite example of a rete testis cyst has been described, presenting as an asymptomatic testicular mass in a 66-year-old man.[140a]

In the epididymis, the acquired cysts generally are the result of tubular obstruction with dilatation of tubules adjacent to the obstruction (Fig. 28-14). The dilated tubules are filled variably with viable and degenerating sperm. Such cysts can be distinguished from those in Young's syndrome[54] by the absence of a history of recurrent sinopulmonary infections. Also, in Young's syndrome the tubules in the head of the epididymis are consistently dilated and filled with sperm, whereas those of the middle and tail are of normal caliber and filled with yellowish, amorphous debris. In age-related cysts, the dilatation is much more irregularly distributed. (Young's syndrome is discussed in Ch. 25.)

In the vas deferens, the cysts take the form in many instances of an "aneurysmal" dilatation of the lumen, and in others they appear to represent small diverticula (Fig. 28-15). The reason for their occurrence is not clear.

Spermatoceles are most frequent in the epididymis, but may occur in other structures, particularly the tunica vaginalis. They are discussed in detail below.

Cysts of the Seminal Vesicles

Most cysts of the seminal vesicles are congenital and are associated with ipsilateral renal agenesis[26,66] (see above). More rarely, they are acquired as a result of an inflammatory stenosis.[6] Seminal vesicle cysts are

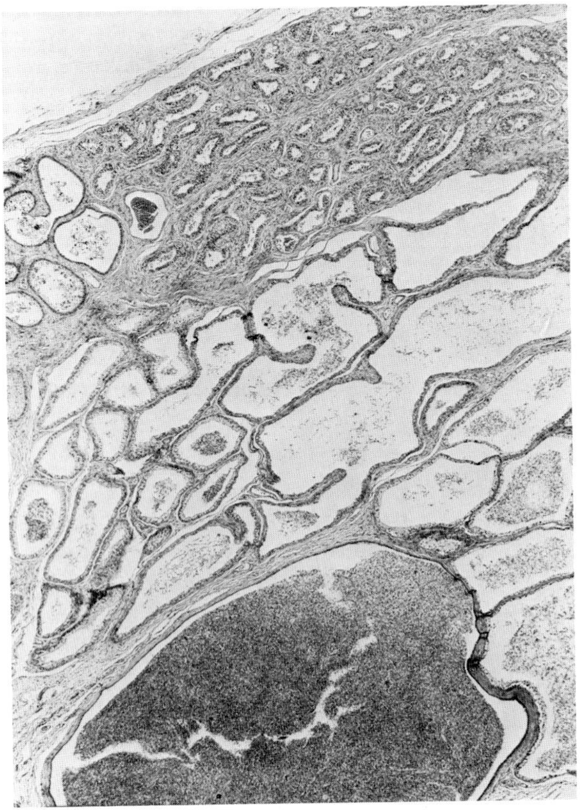

Fig. 28-14 Epididymal cyst. The cyst below is basically a grossly dilated epididymal tubule, probably the result of obstruction. Lesser degrees of dilatation are seen adjacent. ×24.

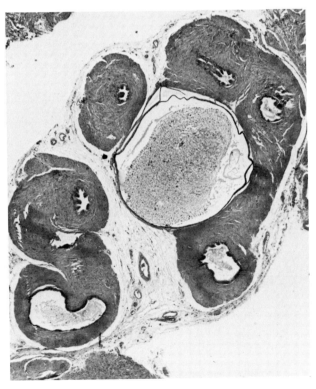

Fig. 28-15 Cyst of vas deferens. Such small cysts, many actually cystic diverticula, are common at autopsy in older individuals. Other tubules show lesser degrees of dilatation. ×14.

soft fluctuant masses located between the rectum and the base of the bladder. Their symptomatology is scant, consisting of perineal discomfort, pain on ejaculation,[66] dysuria, and rarely, urinary retention.[30] The treatment consists of aspiration or excision.

Histologically, these cysts often have a relatively thick fibrous wall, with scattered foci of chronic inflammation. Depending on the size of the cyst and the degree of inflammation, the epithelial lining varies from essentially normal seminal vesicle epithelium, with clear columnar cells containing lipofuscin granules, to flattened epithelium, to total disruption of the epithelium by the inflammation.

Epididymitis

Epididymal inflammation, or epididymitis, is rarely an isolated occurrence.[91,97] Usually, it occurs in the setting of genitourinary inflammation or a systemic disorder, but it may also be of traumatic origin. The clinical presentation differs according to the etiology. Epididymal infection takes place most often by retrograde or lymphatic routes and more rarely by hematogenous spread. Retrograde spread was long debated, but is now generally accepted. It occurs by vesicoepididymal reflux of urine, which may be substantial, and if so, is frequently accompanied by recurrent infections. Direct extension from a scrotal, testicular, or retroperitoneal infection is also possible. Epididymitis in infants is uncommon and usually is associated with significant anomalies of the urinary tract, such as ectopic ureteral orifices, with resulting reflux.[130a,142,150] Urine cultures are typically negative unless such anomalous communications exist.[130a]

The testicular involvement in cases of epididymo-orchitis is generally secondary to that of the epididymis, and isolated orchitis is less frequent than an isolated acute epididymitis.

ACUTE EPIDIDYMIS

Generally unilateral, acute epididymitis[71,118,121,125] seems to occur slightly more frequently on the right side. Painful swelling of the epididymis is observed, accompanied by reddening and edema of the overlying scrotum. The process initially begins toward the tail of the epididymis and extends to involve the entire organ and even the testicle (epididymo-orchitis) or the tunica, provoking a hydrocele. The whole may be converted to an abscess with fistula formation, but this is fortunately rare. If untreated, acute epididymitis may resolve, but its course is frequently marked by recurrences and it may progress to chronicity.

ACUTE PURULENT (BACTERIAL) EPIDIDYMITIS

Numerous organisms may cause acute purulent epididymitis. In infants and children coliform organisms are most frequent.[130a] *Neisseria gonorrheae* and *Chlamydia trachomatis* (see below) predominate among young men, whereas *Escherichia coli* and *Pseudomonas* are more frequent among patients over age 35 and are usually associated with urinary tract infections.[8,89a,93] Other pyogenic organisms include *Aerobacter aerogenes, Klebsiella, Streptococcus, Staphylococcus, Pneumococcus, Neisseria meningitidis, Haemophilus influenzae,* and other gram-positive cocci. Hematogenous disease, which is rare, is predominantly meningococcal or pneumococcal.

In patients with gonococcal infections, the process may be relatively asymptomatic and the epididymis may serve as a silent reservoir of infection.[41]

Grossly, the epididymis is swollen and red, with a dull, granular surface sometimes showing petechiae or a fibrous exudate. The vas deferens is often involved, and if so it will be thickened and edematous. Extension to the tunica leads to hydrocele formation.[91]

On cut section, the wall is thickened and the lumens contain thick whitish exudate, or there may be multiple small abscesses. Fistulas to other peritesticular tissues or rupture of the epididymis do occur, but are rare.

In acute epididymitis, the epididymis itself is seldom seen by the pathologist. More frequently, smears of the accompanying urethal exudate are seen; these are often diagnostic when examined by Gram stain, which may reveal the characteristic intracellular, gram-negative diplococci diagnostic of gonorrhea or, less frequently, other bacteria.

Histologically, acute epididymitis is most often characterized by vascular congestion and interstitial edema, associated with a mixed leukocyte infiltrate, and tubular alterations (Fig. 28-16). The inflammatory elements, including polymorphs, lymphocytes, plasma cells, and macrophages, infiltrate the connective tissue, surround the epididymal tubules, and insinuate themselves between the epithelial cells to reach the lumens. Elongated macrophages with large

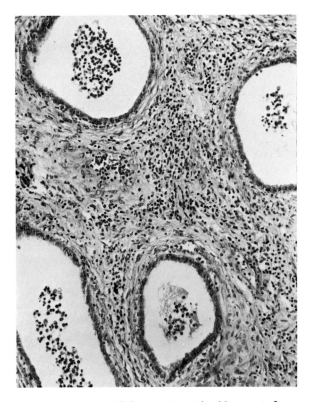

Fig. 28-16 Acute epididymitis. Considerable acute inflammation is present in the tissue around the epididymal tubules, as well as in the lumen. There is early fibrosis of the peritubular tissue. ×130.

hyperchromatic nuclei may be scattered through the interstitium, and may take on a pseudoepithelial appearance.

The epididymal tubules are sometimes completely destroyed by abscess formation, but more frequently there is simple compression or dilatation of the tubules. The lining epithelium shows alternating normal and focally desquamated zones. Squamous metaplasia or regeneration, as indicated by a layer of cuboidal cells with basophilic cytoplasm beneath the desquamated necrotic epithelium, may be present.

In some cases, coalescence of microabscesses and pooling of purulent material is so extensive as to destroy the whole organ. Such extensive suppuration is generally not a feature of gonorrhea, however. More typically, gonorrhea is marked by formation of multiple minute abscesses or of widespread inflammatory edema.[12] Vascular lesions may also be observed, with microhemorrhages or thromboses, particularly venous, leading in some cases to epididymotesticular

infarction, which must be distinguished from torsion of the spermatic cord.[70]

The inflammation extends in 50 percent of cases to the tunica vaginalis, causing a fibrinous or fibrinopurulent exudate between the layers, sometimes with a serous, serosanguinous, or even purulent effusion. Testicular involvement may lead to fibrosis with tubular atrophy, and hence, if bilateral, to sterility.

CHLAMYDIA TRACHOMATIS EPIDIDYMITIS

Chlamydia trachomatis (serotypes D–K) is responsible for a large number of cases of epididymitis occurring in young men.[9] However, chlamydial epididymitis is seldom, if ever, diagnosed by pathologists. In a study performed on 90 endometrial biopsies, in which the pathologic lesions might be expected to parallel those in the epididymis, Winkler et al.[152] found four cases of certain chlamydial infection, confirmed by immunoperoxidase stains. They were characterized by extensive inflammatory infiltrate, admixing neutrophils, lymphocytes, and many plasma cells, with associated stromal necrosis and reparative cellular atypias of the epithelium. Chlamydial inclusions were only occasional and were not identified as such on H&E since they were often obscured by inflammation and stromal necrosis and resembled degenerated nuclei or other cytoplasmic vacuoles. The inclusions, identified by immunoperoxidase, consisted of rounded cytoplasmic vacuoles with fine, irregular, granular basophilic stippling. Positive immunoperoxidase stain was a prerequisite for the diagnosis.

VIRAL EPIDIDYMITIS—MUMPS

The only common, clinically significant viral infection of the epididymis is mumps orchiepididymitis. However, overwhelming systemic infection by cytomegalovirus may leave its traces in the form of occasional viral nuclear inclusions in the epithelial cells. In addition, one may occasionally see large, granular or hyaline nuclear inclusions closely resembling viral inclusions, perhaps accompanied by mild acute or chronic inflammation, in a grossly normal, asymptomatic epididymis. At present, however, there is no evidence either for or against a viral origin for these inclusions.

Mumps orchitis[19,44,81,91] is accompanied in 85 percent of cases by acute epididymitis. Clinically, there is severe scrotal pain with swelling, generally unilateral, that begins several days after the parotid gland infection. It appears that the epididymis is clinically affected before the testicle.

Macroscopically, the testicle is bluish and the epididymis and tunical albuginea are congested. An accompanying hydrocele is often present.

Microscopically, the epididymal architecture is preserved, particularly the tubules, whose epithelium is basically intact. There is interstitial vascular congestion with occasional hemorrhagic areas, edema, and most strikingly, a predominantly lymphocytic inflammatory infiltrate. Leukocytes are not seen between the epithelial cells, but sometimes the lumens contain desquamated epithelial cells, cellular debris, and even rare aggregates of polymorphonuclear leukocytes, presumably resulting from the testicular inflammation. The testicular involvement consists of an initial interstitial edema, followed by acute inflammation, with interstitial and tubular neutrophilic, lymphocytic, and histiocytic infiltrate.[97]

TRAUMATIC EPIDIDYMITIS

This is usually due to contusion or scrotal injury and is nearly always accompanied by involvement of the testis and tunica vaginalis. Congestion and hemorrhages are common. These range from petechiae to extensive hemorrhage, sometimes associated with a hematocele. There may be associated edema and swelling, occasionally with rupture of the testicle or epididymis.[154] The lesions tend to resolve if small, but suppuration may supervene, as well as thrombosis and testicular infarction.

Chronic Epididymitis

Chronic epididymitis[97,118,125] develops in the wake of recurrent acute attacks. Clinically, it may present as epididymal induration, sometimes causing a sensation of discomfort, or may only be recognized during clinical evaluation for sterility.

Macroscopically, the epididymis is indurated, fibrous and in some cases dilated tubules may be visible as small cysts. Small whitish nodules several millimeters in diameter correspond to the spermatic granulomas which may be associated with lesion. A chronic periorchitis often accompanies chronic epididymitis.

Microscopically, diffuse and/or destructive interstitial fibrosis may be infiltrated by lymphocytes, plasmacytes and macrophages in variable proportions, numbers and distribution (Fig. 28-17). The tubular epithelium may have a low cuboidal, basophilic appearance suggestive of repair in some areas, marked vacuolization in others, and may even show squamous metaplasia. The lumens may be empty or filled with normal or altered sperm, with cholesterol clefts admixed (Fig. 28-18), and/or oval concentric or hyaline concretions, similar to prostatic corpora amylacea, also called sympexions of Robins. Somtimes foreign body granulomas are seen in the lumens and interstitium, directed against the cellular debris or against the granular material. The fibrotic interstitial tissue may also contain small calcifications and macrophages,

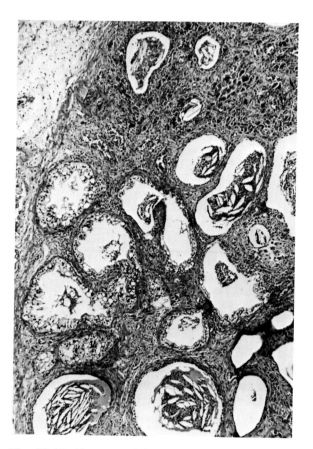

Fig. 28-17 Chronic epididymitis. Prominent peritubular infiltrate with large macrophages in the interstitium. Epididymal epithelium is markedly vacuolated in some locations (left) Tubular stasis with degeneration of sperm and leukocytes, marked by cholesterol clefts and amorphous debris. ×51.

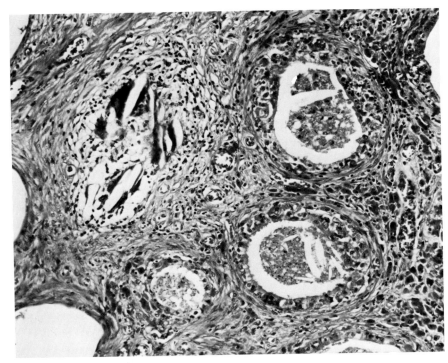

Fig. 28-18 Chronic epididymitis. Higher power showing interstitial infiltrate, degeneration of luminal contents with cholesterol clefts, and epithelial inflammation with dissolution of tubules on right. ×140.

which may be foamy or filled with debris, particularly hemosiderin or lipofuscin. There may also be hemorrhages, cysts, spermatoceles, and spermatic granulomas resulting from obstruction (see below). Lastly, yet other foreign body granulomas directed toward exogenous substances such as silicone may be associated with this lesion.

Xanthogranulomatous inflammation has been reported in one case of *E. coli*-induced epididymitis in a 60-year old diabetic.[149a] The destructive inflammatory infiltrate was composed predominantly of large foamy histiocytes typical of those seen in xanthogranulomatous pyelonephritis (see Ch. 8), admixed with lymphocytes and plasma cells. No structures suggestive of Michaelis-Gutmann bodies were identified.

SPERMATIC GRANULOMA

Found in about 2.5 percent of autopsies,[76] the spermatic granuloma[18,46,48] involves primarily the epididymis, particularly its upper pole, and the spermatic cord and is unusual in the testes. Nowadays, the great majority of cases are seen postvasectomy, since it is a common complication (15 percent to 42 percent of cases) of vasectomy.[131] The etiologic factors in other cases include a history of trauma, chronic epididymitis, or granulomatous orchitis. Vasitis nodosa is accompanied by spermatic granulomas in about one-third of cases.[129] The common thread in all these situations appears to be breakdown of the tubular basement membranes, with extravasation of sperm.

Clinically, the spermatic granuloma may pass totally unnoticed, but the majority of patients complain of pain and swelling, often of some months' duration.[46] Alternately, it may present as a mass lesion, simulating a testicular neoplasm.[34]

Macroscopically, it is usually recognized as a small, yellowish, firm nodule ranging from a few millimeters to 2 cm to 3 cm in diameter.

Histologically, its appearance is very variable. At the onset, the extravasation of sperm induces a neutrophilic exudate followed by a granulomatous response in which interstitial masses of sperm are mixed with epithelial cells, macrophages, polymorphs; and lymphocytes.[1] The sperm is actively phagocytosed by spermiophages, a generic term for the macrophages, epithelioid cells, polymorphs, and to a lesser degree, multinucleated giant cells that engulf sperm (Fig. 28-19). These lesions age much as other granulomata do, with progressive fibrosis and loss of inflammatory cells. The sperm, however, are fairly indigestible, for they may appear in relatively advanced lesions.

Pathogenesis

Extravasation of sperm into the interstitial tissue does not always lead to inflammation, since it is observed as an isolated phenomenon in 10 percent of autopsies. The factors leading to inflammation in some instances and not in others are not clear. Spermatic granulomas are rare in cauterization of the vas deferens [18] and occur primarily in cases of cord ligation, most particularly when this is done with nonresorbable sutures. It has been suggested that a foreign body reaction initiates the inflammation and that an autoimmune component is associated. However, experiments on vasectomized rats demonstrating that the appearance of spermatic granulomas does not change after immunosuppression[13] are against the autoimmune hypothesis.

According to Phillips,[107] the granulomatous inflammation results from release of yellow-brown pigments (identified since as ceroids) from the sperm. This acid-fast, autofluorescent lipid produces a granulomatous reaction when injected into hamsters.[7] Its acid-fast character permits the recognition of sperm and their degradation products in lesions in which they would not otherwise be evident.

TUBERCULOSIS

Relatively frequent until the 1950s, genital involvement by tuberculosis is now rare.[33,116,132,135,151] The epididymis is the principle site of involvement, and the testis is affected only secondarily.[118] Tuberculous epididymitis is associated in 80 percent of cases with tuberculosis elsewhere in the urinary tract (i.e., kidney, prostate, and seminal vesicles) and is found in

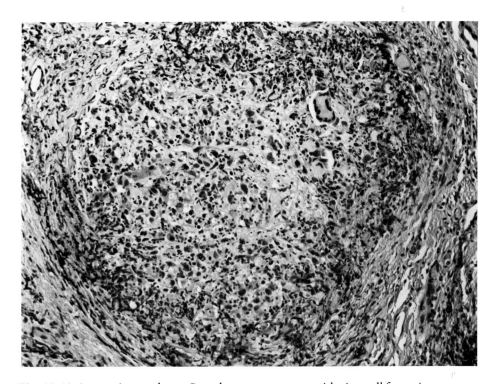

Fig. 28-19 Spermatic granuloma. Granulomatous response, with giant cell formation, to sperm extravasated into the fibrous tissue. Some sperm are still perceptible in the center. ×188.

40 percent of cases of renal tuberculosis. This underlines the role of urinary reflux along the vas deferens, which frequently shows microscopic lesions. Spread by the hematogenous route, more frequent among children, is expressed by lesions that are initially interstitial, extending later to the epididymal tubules and to the testes. In such a situation, the vas deferens would be relatively spared, as opposed to its involvement in reflux. In general, however, tuberculous epididymitis is not a disease of children, but attacks young adults and middle-aged individuals who have genitourinary or pulmonary tuberculosis.

Clinically, tuberculous epididymitis, which is bilateral in at least one-third of cases, may present as a large painless scrotal mass or as a hydrocele, or may rarely mimic an acute epididymitis. Alternatively, it may pass entirely unnoticed and be discovered during workup for infertility.[113]

Signs of tuberculous epididymitis are an indolent scrotal fistula; marked increase in epididymal volume, frequently with areas of variable consistency; a hard knot of the head, with or without beading of the vas deferens; and thickening of the ipsilateral seminal vesicle.

Grossly, the epididymis is dilated, thickened, and sausagelike and adheres to adjacent structures. Involvement of the vas deferens, a hydrocele, or fistulas may also be noted. On cut section, the walls are thickened and the tubular lumens contain soft caseous material, or there may be numerous foci of caseous material (Fig. 28-20). In other instances the architecture is destroyed by fibrocaseous nodules or even more extensive caseation.[125]

An associated tuberculous orchitis may be recognized by an increase in the size of the testes or by peripheral foci of caseation or fibrosis.

Microscopically, in the initial stages, the tubules contain desquamated epithelial cells, polymorphs, and numerous bacilli (Fig. 28-21). This is followed by variable necrosis of the tubules, associated with a tuberculoid inflammatory response often commencing in the epithelium. Caseation extends into the interstitial tissue to produce the typical appearance of tuberculous epididymitis, with lesions at various stages, that is, exudative, granulomatous, and fibrous. This occurs against a fibrous or edematous background, destroying the normal architecture. There may also be small hemorrhages as well as spermatic granulomas. Much more rarely, the appearance is that of a

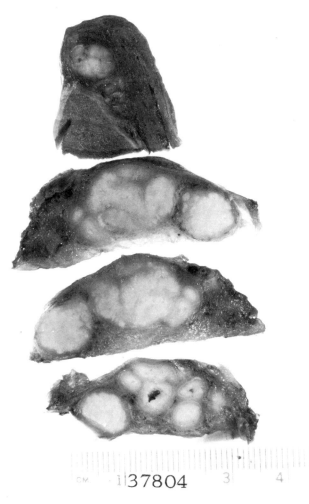

Fig. 28-20 Tuberculous epididymitis. Gross specimen showing numerous, sometimes confluent, caseating granulomas. Portion of testis (in upper slice) is uninvolved.

miliary spread, with small tuberculoid granulomas all at the same stage.

Difficulty in diagnosis arises either from minimal lesions such as hard, noncaseating granulomas resembling sarcoidosis or from atypical lesions such as recent caseous necrosis with cellular debris bounded by a nonspecific infiltrate. Other agents may also produce the appearance of necrotizing tuberculoid inflammation. To make the diagnosis, other fungi and bacteria should be ruled out with special stains and a patient search should be made for tubercle bacilli. The auramine–rhodamine stain for acid-fast bacteria, examined under fluorescence, is probably more reli-

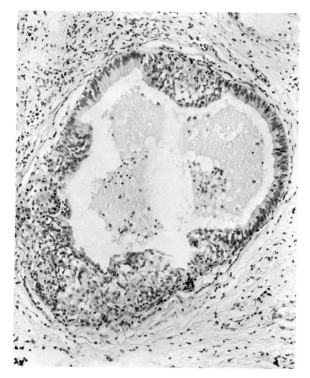

Fig. 28-21 Tuberculous epididymitis. Tubule showing early involvement, with granulomas forming in epithelium in at least three sites, a pattern suggesting dissemination by reflux along the vas deferens rather than hematogenous spread. ×107.

able and certainly much easier to scan than the traditional Ziehl–Neelsen stain.

The course is generally toward extensive caseation, which may necessitate surgical excision. At the favorable end of the spectrum, walling off with fibrosis and/or calcification may sometimes occur, whereas at the unfavorable end fistulas may form. In cases of moderate severity, the scarring down of granulomata and destroyed tubules produces foci of concentric hyaline sclerosis, sometimes infiltrated by lymphocytes and plasma cells.

SARCOIDOSIS

Genital involvement by sarcoidosis[3,45,57,127,147] is symptomatic in 0.5 percent of cases and is found in 5 percent of autopsies of patients with this malady. It involves, in decreasing frequency, the epididymis or testis, prostate, penis, scrotal skin, seminal vesicles, and spermatic cord. Sarcoidosis is generally already recognized, and genital lesions are only rarely the presenting sign. The response to steroid treatment is variable.

Clinically, there are single or multiple firm painful or painless masses, which are bilateral in about one-third of cases.

Histologically, the normal interstitial and tubular tissue is replaced by small noncaseating epithelioid granulomas, which are somtimes confluent. The Langhans' giant cells frequently contain asteroid bodies or calcified inclusions (Schaumann bodies). Also occasionally noted are small central foci of granular or fibrinoid necrosis. Special stains and cultures for acid-fast bacilli and fungi are negative. No causal agent can be recognized by electron microscopy. Differential diagnosis from noncaseating tuberculosis depends principally on the clinical setting. Spermatic granulomas are easier to differentiate from sarcoid granulomas, as the sperm are generally readily recognizable.

LEPROSY

Lepromatous orchiepididymitis[37,105,146] is common in the lepromatous or borderline forms of leprosy. It is generally bilateral, beginning in the testis, and extending later to the epididymis. Involvement of the dartos is fairly frequent, but that of the vas deferens is rare.

Clinically, the testicles are swollen and painful. The epididymides are also large and painful, with markedly thickened walls.

Histologically, the epididymis contains an interstitial lepromatous infiltrate, with perivascular lymphocytes and the classical Virchow lepra cells (vacuolated macrophages containing myriads of acid-fast Hansen's bacilli). The lumens are empty in severe orchitis. It is the orchitis rather than epididymitis that leads to sterility in lepers.

The dartos muscle presents a generalized infiltrate, diffuse or localized between the smooth muscle fibers, with different degrees of leprous myositis. The most frequent type of nerve involvement is an infiltration with histiocytes and lymphocytes, but there may be simply a collagenous sclerosis. The bacilli, which may be numerous, are primarily localized in the Schwann cells.

SYPHILIS

Syphilis of the epididymis or vas deferens is rare, secondary to orchitis.[118] It has no characteristics to distinguish it from the orchitis, and it evolves toward interstitial fibrosis or the formation of isolated gummas.

RARER BACTERIAL, FUNGAL, AND PARASITIC INFECTIONS

In rare cases, epididymitis is secondary to systemic infection by fungi, parasites, or other microorganisms. These are sometimes difficult to see on routine H&E stains and often require a Gomori methenamine–silver stain or other special methods for their recognition. Among these organisms are the following.

In its pseudotubercular form, *Histoplasma capsulatum* may produce abscesses filled with thick, creamy material, which on histology have an appearance of caseous tubercles. In other cases, there may be a macroscopic and microscopic process similar to that seen with spermatic granulomas or sarcoid.[67,95] The methenamine–silver stain permits recognition of the characteristic intracellular yeastlike organisms measuring 2 μm to 4 μm and often surrounded by a clear halo. These may be found in macrophages or free, often clumped, and can be specifically identified by immunofluorescence.

Coccidioides immitis is responsible for hydroceles, prostatitis, and epididymitis.[50] Histologically, it causes caseating and noncaseating granulomas containing endosporulant spherules 30 μm to 80 μm in diameter, readily recognized on methenamine–silver stains.

Paraccoccidioides brasilienis[42] and *Blastomyces dermatitidis*[35] involve the epididymis and prostate. Blastomyces epididymitis is present in 20 percent to 30 percent of cases with systemic involvement. Microabscesses and a granulomatous response are observed. The budding yeastlike organisms lie free or in giant cells. They are large, measuring 5 μm to 15 μm, and have a thick, doubly refractile capsule readily identifiable on Gomori methenamine–silver stains.

Sporothrix schenckii is also responsible for abscesses. The necrotic center harbors the cigar-shaped yeast cell and is surrounded by an epitheloid and giant cell reaction.[130]

Schistosomes are easily recognizable on standard stains.[60,68] They may give rise to tuberculoid granulomas or may be surrounded by an eosinophilic necrotic material, which is itself walled in by a nonspecific inflammatory response, often with calcification. (See also Ch. 9.)

Actinomyces[69] produces an epididymitis that is nearly always unilateral, with microabscesses containing the characteristic sulfur granules. As elsewhere in the body, actinomycotic epididymitis leads typically to fistula formation. Histologically, the sulfur granules or bacterial colonies are found in the microabscesses and consist of clumped radiating filaments (rays) capped by eosinophilic hyaline material (clubs), creating a sunburst pattern. They are surrounded by numerous polymorphs, which are in turn surrounded by foamy macrophages and plasma cells and walled in by relatively avascular fibrous tissue.

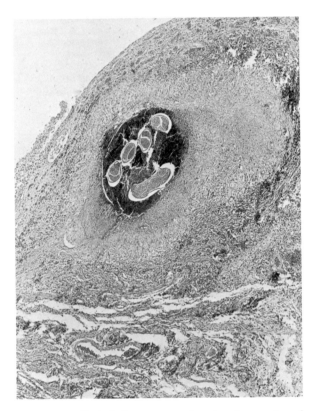

Fig. 28-22 Filariasis. Low-power view showing portion of a necrotic filaria obstructing a periepididymal lymphatic, with extensive necrosis and inflammation in surrounding tissue. ×32.

Wuchereria bancrofti filaria, sometimes found in the epididymis, produce an epithelioid response centered about the necrotic worms that is associated with an eosinophilic pseudoabscess or a foreign body reaction (Fig. 28-22). Fibrosis and calcification represent the end result of these inflammatory reactions. *Wuchereria bancrofti* also gives rise to inflammation of the spermatic cord, orchitis, hydrocele, chylocele and to scrotal and penile elephantiasis.[114,125] These latter are secondary to lymphatic obstruction by the worm and eventual obliteration by the subsequent inflammatory reaction.

Hydatid cysts may also be found in the epididymis, the seminal vesicles, or the prostate.[28,53]

Other Causes

Epididymitis may be found also in certain cases of brucellosis, typhoid, and rickettsial disease. In these situations, it is very much secondary to the systemic problem and does not necessitate a biopsy.

MALAKOPLAKIA

Malakoplakia only rarely involves the epididymis, generally in the setting of an orchiepididymitis or after trauma.[52,85,109] Clinically, it may be asymptomatic or may produce a constantly painful enlargement of the epididymis. Occasionally, it is associated with a hydrocele. Grossly, the epididymis is swollen and shows softened brownish areas measuring up to several millimeters in diameter and other associated signs of infection. The histologic features have previously been described. (See Ch. 8.)

Vasitis and Funiculitis

Vasitis, or deferentitis,[10,125] often accompanies an epididymitis, but represents in some cases the sole manifestation of a posterior urethritis. Inflammation of the cord, or funiculitis, occurs by direct extension of vasitis or by hematogenous routes, leading to one or several areas of painful swelling of the cord.

Among the various causes of acute nonspecific inflammation of the cord, two are noteworthy, although rare: (1) thrombosis of the pampiniform sinus, secondary to a funiculitis, with suppuration and even gangrene of the cord;[125] (2) unusual foreign body granulomas directed toward vegetable fibers, frag-

ments of bone, and other fecal residue. These result generally from a perforation of an inguinal hernia followed by spontaneous healing.[11]

Tuberculosis of the spermatic cord rarely occurs as an isolated lesion. Often there are one of several masses several centimeters in diameter that may or may not be separated from the vas deferens. The masses correspond to fibrocaseous nodules.[33] A more diffuse involvement leads to indurated thickening of the entire vas deferens.[125] In such cases, the cord is firm and rubbery, with a whitish and shiny surface, and cut section reveals yellowish streaks or caseation. The histologic appearance is as discussed above.

VASITIS NODOSA

Vasitis nodosa[10,73,145] is so named because of its gross appearance producing a nodular or fusiform thickening of the vas deferens, and the histologic resemblance of the irregularly proliferating ductules in the wall to those seen in salpingitis isthmica nodosa. This lesion has the same etiology and the same clinical presentation as the spermatic granuloma. Despite its sometimes ominous appearance, vasitis nodosa is strictly benign.

Its exact frequency is not known. In one series, it was identified in 12 of 210 previously vasectomized men,[153] up to 20 years after surgery. Some evidence of ductule proliferation, inflammation, and sperm granulomas can be recognized in the majority of vas deferens specimens examined at the time of reanastomosis.[139] Indeed, this process of ductule proliferation may be so vigorous as to result in effective recanalization of the vas, with resulting normal sperm counts.[112] However, vasitis nodosa has also been seen in 2 of 40 nonvasectomized men,[21,153] so vasectomy is clearly not the only responsible factor.

Grossly, the vas deferens is thickened in a diffuse or nodular fashion. Its diameter varies from the normal of approximately 4 mm to greater than 1 cm. On cut section the nodule is grayish, pale, and firm, and its surface is sometimes dotted with small holes. Associated spermatic granulomas appear as little whitish nodules.

Histologically, in vasitis nodosa, chronic inflammation with interstitial fibrosis involves the muscularis and surrounding tissue, but the key element is epithelial proliferation of variable severity (Fig. 28-23). In approximately 50 percent of cases, sperm

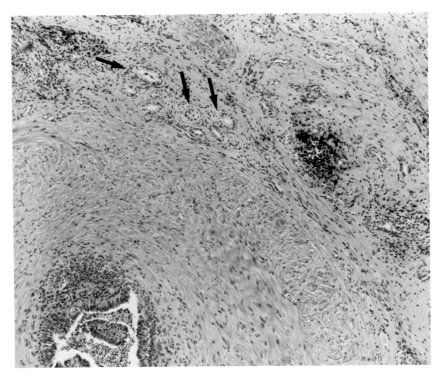

Fig. 28-23 Vasitis nodosa. The epithelium and muscularis at this level are intact, but numerous tubular profiles are apparent in the adventitia (arrows), with associated chronic inflammation. ×74.

granulomas are also present. The muscularis of the vas is thickened by fibrous tissue that may totally replace the smooth muscle. Muscle hyperplasia or proliferation is sometimes seen. The lumen of the vas deferens varies considerably, even within a given specimen, and may be normal, dilated, or compressed; it may be empty or contain sperm, and may even be obliterated by a marked inflammatory response. Inflammation also involves the surrounding connective tissue, with sperm granulomas and interstitial infiltration of epithelioid cells, voluminous macrophages, and lymphocytes.

The epithelial proliferation is haphazard and may be quite aggressive in the areas where it is associated with an inflammatory exudate. However, in less inflamed areas it produces cords and glandlike structures (Fig. 28-23) that are isolated or grouped into small clusters. These cords or ductules are irregular or sinuous, resulting in a somewhat plexiform pattern. They may contain sperm, and serial sections reveal that they have some connection with the lumen of the vas.

They are sometimes difficult to differentiate from vessels with swollen endothelium. The cells of the ductular structures are cuboidal, with lightly basophilic, finely granular cytoplasm, and are occasionally ciliated. Their centrally located nucleus is large and round, with a sharp nuclear membrane, regular chromatin, and a punctate nucleolus. The cells in the epithelial cords are more elongated, with oval nuclei.

Importantly, individual epithelial cells and sometimes entire ductular structures may be found in or around nerve bundles (Fig. 28-24), the appearance superficially resembling invasive adenocarcinoma.[76,153] Nerve involvement is actually fairly common and does not imply malignancy, nor does the worrisome, somewhat bizarre appearance of the more reactive ductules.

Ceroid granulomas are sometimes present (the ceroids are brown pigments resulting from degradation of lipids derived from spermatozoa)[107] According to Civantos et al.,[21] their number increases as the sperm granulomas decrease in frequency, and they may per-

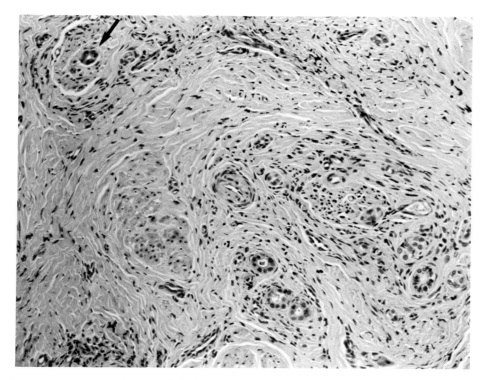

Fig. 28-24 Vasitis nodosa. Epithelial tubules penetrate the muscular and fibrous tissue in a pseudoinfiltrative pattern. A tubular profile is seen in the middle of a peripheral nerve (arrow, upper left). ×160.

sist for many years after sperm granulomas are no longer detectable. Finally, there may be foreign body granulomas surrounding suture threads in previously vasectomized patients.

Pathogenesis

The pathogenesis of vasitis nodosa is poorly understood. It is apparent that rupture of the epithelium with extravasation of sperm and resulting inflammation and epithelial proliferation must be the immediate events leading to vasitis nodosa. The epithelial proliferation attempting recanalization of the vas deferens would occur along the paths of least resistance, ending up as a branched ductular structure. Complete recanalization is rarely observed, although it was unequivocally demonstrated in one of eight cases described by Civantos et al.[21]

Trauma related to vasectomy would provide a sufficient explanation for the initial rupture of the epithelium. What about those cases occurring in the ab-

sence of trauma? A common supposition is that increased pressure in the vas deferens linked to lower genitourinary tract obstruction would produce such ruptures in the epithelium. In fact, this theory of increased pressure leading to rupture and inflammatory reaction must be taken with a grain of salt, as no inflammation or epithelial proliferation is observed in the epididymis in congenital absence of the vas deferens,[86] in which the pressure in the epididymal tubules would theoretically be increased.

Seminal Vesiculitis

Inflammation of the seminal vesicles is often secondary to a regional infection, usually prostatic or vesical, with frequent involvement of the ejaculatory ducts, the vas deferens, or the epididymis as well. Calculi, urethral stenosis, and injury, particularly surgical procedures and retrograde instrumentation, all predispose to seminal vesicle infection and inflammation. It may also represent a metastatic localization of

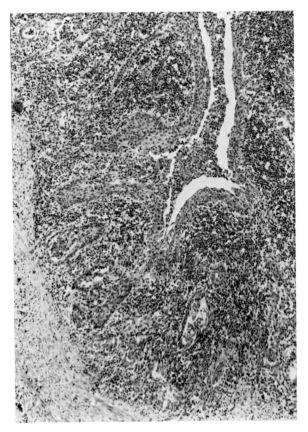

Fig. 28-25 Seminal vesiculitis. Extensive chronic inflammation centered about the seminal vesicle lumen. Much of the epithelium has undergone squamous metaplasia. ×122.

a generalized infection, either bacterial or viral.[117] Rarely, abscesses may develop in the absence of any obvious precipitating cause.[41a]

The complications of such infections are abscess formation and stricture, and there is a tendency to chronicity.

The acute inflammatory phase is comparable to that of the epididymis, with a diffuse leucocytic exudate, and it may be accompanied by squamous metaplasia of the epithelium (Fig. 28-25). Chronic inflammation shows the expected interstitial fibrosis and a mononuclear infiltrate. More importantly, it may result in marked atrophy of the gland or obstruction of the ejaculatory ducts.

Tuberculosis of the seminal vesicles is generally bilateral. There may be massive caseation obliterating the architecture, leading in some instances to perineal fistulas. In other cases, there are areas of fibrous indu-

ration containing obsolescent, often calcified caseous nodules, occasionally with fibrous adhesions to the perirectal tissue.[125] (See also Tuberculosis of Epididymis, above.)

MISCELLANEOUS CONDITIONS

Epithelial Metaplasia of Tunica

Foci of epithelial metaplasia of the tunica or other serosal linings were found in 17 percent of the case studied by Sundarasivarao.[136] These foci are isolated, unassociated with inflammation or hydroceles, and primarily found in the serosa of the testicle and of the epididymis, predominantly near the base of the appendix testis and over the head of the epididymis.

Such foci are sometimes visible as small cysts or plaques, but are often found only on microscopic examination. In rare instances, the cysts may attain a diameter of 0.5 cm to 4.0 cm, particularly in older patients, at which point they are dignified with the title of *tunica albuginea cyst*.[90,106] The plaques on the surface of the serosa may be several millimeters long with sharp margins. These plaques send fingerlike extensions down into the tissue. Cavitation of these epithelial protrusions leads to formation of the cysts so often seen, a process analogous to formation of cystitis cystica from Brunn's nests. (See Ch. 16.) The basal cells in these cystic cavities are flattened, and those of the three or four layers above are polyhedral in shape with a faintly eosinophilic cytoplasm and poorly defined cytoplasmic borders. These pseudoglandular or cystic structures sometimes contain a mucoid, palely eosinophilic material. Rarely, squamous metaplasia of the surface of the tunica has been reported.[70]

It would make sense that most of these epithelial lesions are derived from metaplasia of the mesothelium. However, ciliated cells have been reported in some, suggesting an origin from efferent ductules of the müllerian system.[90] In some instances, these solid masses and cystic structures are labeled as Walthard's rests because of their resemblance to their ovarian or tubal counterparts.[136,141] Their origin is debated, with an origin from müllerian derivatives or from metaplasia from overlying mesothelium being favored. Characteristic of these cells is the longitudinal groove or fold in the nucleus, giving them the so-called coffee bean appearance. For the most part, Walthard's rests are pathologic curiosities, but at least three instances of Brenner tumors of the testicular tunics have been described, presumably arising in just such rests.[47,98,123]

Reactive Mesothelial Proliferation

Reactive mesothelial hyperplasia, often florid, is seen in some hydroceles of inguinal hernias, apparently secondary to local irritation. It is generally asymptomatic.[122] This hyperplasia produces small nodules or whitish papillary structures on the surface of the tunica vaginalis or of the hernia sac (see Fig. 28-13). They may be difficult to distinguish from true mesotheliomas, a distinction that is in any event arbitrary. (Some clinicians would distinguish between them simply on the basis of size, with those visible only under the microscope designated as hyperplasias, and those grossly visible designated as benign mesotheliomas.)

Histologically, the proliferation forms papillary or tubular structures or cellular nests in a poorly developed fibrous matrix (Fig. 28-26). The surface is covered by one to several layers of mesothelial cells, which may detach individually or in clumps. The cells are rather large, cuboidal or low columnar, their upper surfaces often bulging outward. The cells of the tubular or glandular structures have a pseudoepithelial appearance.

The round or oval mesothelial nuclei of mesothelial cells have sharp margins and occupy a central or basal position. They may show a certain degree of nuclear irregularity, with small infoldings or even lobulation, but this always counterbalanced by regularity of the chromatin network, and the inconspicuous appearance of the nucleolus. Sometimes the cells are binucleated.

The mesothelial cell cytoplasm is often pale eosinophilic or lightly basophilic, sometimes vacuolated, and contains glycogen stainable with PAS. More importantly, intracytoplasmic hyalurionic acid is present, although in much smaller amounts than in mesotheliomas. The hyaluronic acid is stained blue by alcian blue at pH 2.6 and disappears after hyaluronidase digestion. Sometimes lipids are also present. Silver stains demonstrate the absence of a true basement membrane and cytoplasmic inclusions of unknown nature.[122]

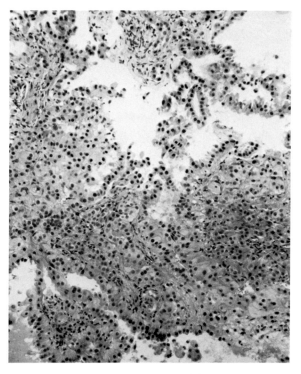

Fig. 28-26 Reactive mesothelial proliferation. Polygonal mesothelial cells arranged in sheets and papillary formations. ×116.

Despite the benign character of reactive mesothelial proliferation, atypical cells may be seen.[122] Most notable are giant cells, sometimes multinucleated, with abundant acidophilic or amphophilic cytoplasm and containing large hyperchromatic nuclei with prominent nucleoli. Also seen are fusiform cells with elongated nuclei resembling the strap cells of rhabdomyosarcoma. The setting in which these atypical cells occur suggests a mesothelial origin. The supporting connective tissue may contain rare psammoma bodies, congestion with or without hemorrhage, and/or a moderate inflammatory infiltrate composed of lymphocytes and a few eosinophils.

The distinction between reactive mesothelial proliferation and a malignant tumor is sometimes quite difficult. However, regular chromatin, unimpressive nucleoli, the continuity between the mesothelial proliferation and the surrounding normal mesothelial lining, together with its staining reactions, usually permit mesothelial proliferation to be distinguished from a well-differentiated carcinoma. Distinction between this lesion and a malignant mesothelioma, however, is more difficult. This distinction depends on the size of the lesion, the cellular differentiation, and the presence or absence of prominent nucleoli, abnormal mitoses, and invasion of vessels or surrounding structures. (See Ch. 29.)

Spermatocele

The spermatocele,[49,101,125] defined as an accumulation of sperm in a pre-existing cavity, occurs principally among middle-aged subjects. It is usually unilateral and is found most frequently in the head of the epididymis. It generally develops from an epididymal duct, but may occur in an embryonal remnant or in the tunica vaginalis, indicating that a communication exists between these structures and the spermatic passages.

Clinically, the scrotum is enlarged, and a small, round, nontender ball of variable size can be palpated. This mass is separated from the testicle and usually attached to the globus major, but may also be situated above the testicle or behind it. It transilluminates reasonably well. When it occurs in the tunica vaginalis, it may present all the features of a hydrocele; however, aspiration of fluid will distinguish between the two, the spermatocele containing sperm and the hydrocele containing none.

Macroscopically, the spermatocele may be unilocular or multilocular, with a fibrous wall and containing a milky or cloudy fluid.

Microscopically, in the epididymis the spermatocele is seen as a cyst containing sperm in varying stages of degeneration, lined by columnar-to-flat epididymal epithelium (Fig. 28-27). The underlying tissue is fibrous and devoid of smooth muscle. In some cases, the epithelium is desquamated or interrupted by an inflammatory reaction that leads to dense hyaline sclerosis, walling in masses of sperm. Rarely, there may be papillary proliferation of the lining cells to form a *mural papilloma.*[59,98] These papillary structures are lined by a single layer of columnar epithelium, often with some cytoplasmic vacuolation. They are

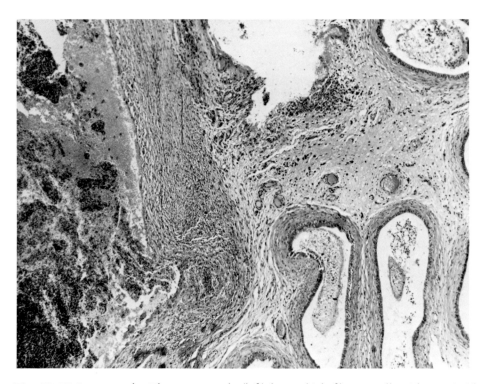

Fig. 28-27 Spermatocele. The spermatocele (left) has a thick fibrous wall, with associated inflammation. It is filled with dark masses of intact and degenerating spermatozoa. There is some scarring of the epididymis (right) with dilatation of tubules. ×53.

thought to be akin to papillary cystadenomas of the epididymis (see Ch. 29.)

Formation of spermatoceles is said to be due to obstruction of the efferent ducts, secondary to chronic epididymitis or to traumatic factors. Spermatocele of the tunica vaginalis, still called spermatic hydrocele, implies for certain clinicians prior rupture of an epididymal spermatocele in the scrotal sac.[49,125]

Vascular Lesions

VASCULITIS

The testicular and epididymal vessels may be involved during the course of polyarteritis nodosa, rheumatoid arthritis, or Henoch–Schönlein purpura.[110] Symptoms, if present, are confined to infrequent pain, testiculoepididymal swelling, or hydrocele.[124]

Histologic lesions are present in 80 percent of autopsies of patients having polyarteritis nodosa, even though their clinical expression is rare. Occasionally, however, pain is the presenting feature of the disease.[22] Extremely rarely, a necrotizing vasculitis involving only the epididymis remains isolated and has an excellent prognosis.[88]

VARICOCELE

Varicoceles are discussed in Chapter 25.

HEMATOCELE

Hematocele is defined as a hemorrhage into the tunica vaginalis and is generally due to a lesion of the spermatic vessels, usually surgical in origin. However, it may occur spontaneously in arteriosclerosis, diabetes, syphilis, cancer, scurvy, or inflammation of the surrounding tissues, as well as in coagulation abnormalities.

REFERENCES

1. Adams DO: The granulomatous inflammatory response. Am J Pathol 84:164, 1976
2. Allan FD: Essentials of Human Embryology. Oxford University Press, New York, 1960
3. Amenta PS, Gonick P, Katz SM: Sarcoidosis of testis and epididymis. Urology 17:616, 1981
4. Ayano Y, Omori K, Ogata J, Ikegami K: Retroperitoneal epididymal structures in adult male. Eur Urol 8:52, 1982
5. Beccia DJ, Krane RJ, Olsson CA: Clinical management of non-testicular intrascrotal tumors. J Urol 116:476, 1976
6. Beeby DI: Seminal vesicle cyst associated with ipsilateral renal agenesis: case report and review of literature. J Urol 112:120, 1974
7. Berg JW: Differential staining of spermatozoa in sections of testis. Arch Pathol 57:115, 1954
8. Berger RE, Alexander ER, Harnisch JP et al: Etiology, manifestations and therapy of acute epididymitis: prospective study of 50 cases. J Urol 121:750, 1979
9. Berger RE, Alexander ER, Monda GD et al.: *Chlamydia trachomatis* as a cause of an "idiopathic" epididymitis. N Engl J Med 238:301, 1978
10. Bissada NK, Redman JF: Unusual masses in the spermatic cord: report of six cases and review of the literature. South Med J 69:1410, 1976
11. Bissada NK, Finkbeiner AE, Rountree GA, Redman JF: Foreign bodies in the spermatic cord. J Urol 118:1010, 1977
12. Boyd W: A Textbook of Pathology. Lea & Febiger, Philadelphia, 1970
13. Brannen GE, Eggleston JC, Adams JS, et al: The effects of immunosuppression on sperm granulomas in vasectomized rats. J Urol 112:733, 1974
14. Bursell S: Beitrag zur Kenntnis der Para-amyloidose im urogenitalen System unter besonderer Berucksichtigung der sog. Senilen Amyloidose in den Samenbläschen und ihres Verhaltnisses zum Samenbläschenpigment. Ups Läkaref Förh 47:313, 1942
15. Byne PD, May RE: Aspiration and injection treatment of hydroceles and epididymal cysts. Br J Clin Pract 32:256, 1978
16. Cabanne F, Bonenfant JC: Anatomie Pathologique. Principes de Pathologie Générale et Spéciale. Librarie Maloine, Paris, 1982
17. Carris CK, McLaughlin AP, III, Gittes RF: Amyloidosis of the lower genitourinary tract. J Urol 115:423, 1976
18. Chapman ES, Heidger PM, Jr: Spermatic granuloma of vas deferens after vasectomy in rhesus monkeys and men: light and electron microscopic study. Urology 13:629, 1979
19. Charny CW, Meranze DR: Pathology of mumps orchitis. J Urol 60:140, 1948
20. Chatterjee AC: A rare complication of hydrocele. Br J Surg 62:891, 1975
21. Civantos F, Lubin J, Rwylin AM: Vasitis nodosa. Arch Pathol 94:355, 1972
22. Crémault A, Goust D, Lemaire M, et al: Funiculite

aiguë bilatérale révélatrice d'une peri-artérite noueuse chez un adolescent. Nouv Presse Med 11:2850, 1982

23. Currie JS, Ngaei G: A papilloma of epididymis of Müllerian vestigial origin. Br J Urol 49:331, 1977

24. Dahl EV, Bahn RC: Aberrant adrenal cortical tissue near the testis in human infants. Am J Pathol 40: 587, 1962

25. Damjanov I, Apic R: Cystadenoma of seminal vesicles. J Urol 111:808, 1974

26. Das S, Amar AD: Ureteral ectopia into cystic seminal vesicle with ipsilateral renal dysgenesis and monorchia. J Urol 24:574, 1980

27. Dehner LP, Scott D, Stocker JT: Meconium periorchitis: a clinicopathologic study of four cases with a review of the literature. Hum Pathol 17:807, 1986

28. Deklotz RJ: Echinococcal cyst involving the prostate and seminal vesicles: a case report. J Urol 115:116, 1976

29. Donohue RE, Greenslade NF: Seminal vesicle cyst and ipsilateral renal agenesis. Urology 2:66, 1973

30. Doremieux J, Reziciner S, Grinenwald P, Batzenschlager A: Une cause rare de rétention aiguë d'urine: un volumineux kyste de la vésicule séminale gauche. Revue de littérature. J Urol Nephrol (Paris) 81:848, 1975

31. Drach GW: Urinary lithiasis. p. 856. In Harrison JH, Gittes RF, Perlmutter AD et al (eds): Campbell's Urology. Vol 1, 4th Ed. Saunders, Philadelphia, 1978

32. Drosse M, Voeth C: Cytologic features of seminal vesicle epithelium in aspiration biopsy smears of the prostate. Acta Cytol 20:120, 1976

33. Duchek M, Winblad B: Tuberculosis of the spermatic cord. Case report. Scand J Urol Nephrol 8:65, 1974

34. Dunner PS, Lipsit ER, Nockomovitz LE: Epididymal sperm granuloma simulating a testicular neoplasm. JCU 10:353, 1982

35. Eickenberg HU, Amin M, Lich R, Jr: Blastomyocosis of the genitourinary tract. J Urol 113:650, 1975

36. Elder JS, Jeffs RD: Suprainguinal ectopic scrotum and associated anomalies. J Urol 127:336, 1982

37. El-Shiemy S, El-Hefnawi H, Abdel-Fattah A et al: Testicular and epididymal involvement in leprosy patients with special reference to gynecomastia. Int J Dermatol 15:52, 1976

38. Eusebi V, Masserilli G: Pheochromocytoma of the spermatic cord: report of a case. J Pathol 105:283, 1971

39. Feldman AE, Rosenthal RS, Shaw JL: Aberrant adrenal tissue: an incidental finding during orchiopexy. J Urol 113:706, 1975

40. Fitzpatrick RJ: Torsion of the appendix testis. J Urol 79:521, 1958

41. Fiumara NJ: The sexually transmissable diseases. DM 24:2, 1978

41a. Fox CW Jr, Vaccaro JA, Kiesling VJ Jr, Belville WD: Seminal vesicle abscess: the use of computerized coaxial tomography for diagnosis and therapy. J Urol 139:384, 1988

42. Frias FS, Nascimento SP, Pasian S et al: South American blastomycosis of epididymis. Urology 14:85, 1979

43. Fuselier HA, Jr, Peters DH: Cyst of seminal vesicle with ipsilateral renal agenesis and ectopic ureter: case report. J Urol 116:833, 1976

44. Gall AE: The histopathology of mumps orchitis. Am J Pathol 23:637, 1947

45. Gerstenhaber BJ, Green ZR, Sachs LL: Epididymal sarcoidosis: a report of two cases and a review of the literature. Yale J Biol Med 50:669, 1977

46. Glassy FJ, Mostofi FK: Spermatic granulomas of the epididymis. Am J Clin Pathol 26:1303, 1956

47. Goldman RL: A Brenner tumor of the testis. Cancer 26:853, 1970

48. Goodson JM, Fruchtman B: Spermatic granulomas of epididymis. Urology 5:278, 1975

49. Gott LJ: Common scrotal pathology. Am Fam Physician 15:165, 1977

50. Gottesman JE: Coccidioidomycosis of prostate and epididymis, with urethrocutaneous fistula. Urology 4:311, 1974

51. Gray H: The urogenital system. p. 1518. In Clemente CD (ed): Anatomy of the Human Body. 13th Ed. Lea & Febiger, Philadelphia, 1985

52. Guccion JG, Thorgeirson VP, Smith BH: Malacoplakia of the epididymis. Urology 12:713, 1978

53. Halim A, Vaezzadeh K: Hydatid disease of the genitourinary tract. Br J Urol 52:75, 1980

54. Handelsman DJ, Conway J, Boylan LM, Turtle JR: Young's syndrome: destructive azoospermia and chronic sinopulmonary infections. N Engl J Med 310:3, 1984

55. Hanid TK: Letter: Infectious mononucleosis complicated by hydrocele. Br Med J 2:706, 1977

56. Healey GB, McDonald GF: Talc granuloma presenting as a testicular mass. J Urol 118:122, 1977

57. Heffernan JC, Blenkinsopp WK: Epididymal sarcoidosis. Br J Urol 50:211, 1978

58. Heydenrych JJ, Marcus PB: Meconium granulomas of the tunica vaginalis. J Urol 115:596, 1976

59. Hill RB, Jr: Bilateral papillary, hyperplastic nodules of epididymis. J Urol 87:155, 1962

60. Honore LH, Coleman GU: Solitary epididymal schistosomiasis. Can J Surg 18:479, 1975

61. Honore LH: Uncommon benign scrotal masses. A report of ten cases. Practitioner 221:632, 1978

62. Hublet D, Kaechenbeek B, DeBacker J et al: Kyste dysgénétique de la prostate et duplication bilatérale des vésicules séminales avec duplication unilatérale du canal déférent, de l'épididyme et dysplasie rénale—à propos d'un cas et revue de la littérature. Acta Urol Belg 48:424, 1980

63. Isaacs AJ, Havard CW: Myxoedema and hydrocele. Br Med J 1:322, 1976

64. Japko L, Horta AA, Schreiber K et al: Malignant mesothelium of the tunica vaginalis testis: report of first case with preoperative diagnosis. Cancer 49:119, 1982

65. Kaplan E, Shwachman H, Perlmutter AD et al: Reproductive failure in males with cystic fibrosis. N Engl J Med 279:65, 1968

66. Karamcheti A, Berg G: Seminal vesicle cyst associated with ipsilateral renal agenesis. Urology 12:572, 1978

67. Kauffman CA, Slama TG, Wheat LJ: Histoplasma capsulatum epididymitis. J Urol 125:434, 1981

68. Kazzaz BA, Salmo NA: Epididymitis due to *Schistosoma haematobium* infection. Trop Geogr Med 26:333, 1974

69. Kernbaum S, Vilde JL: Actinomycose cervico-ganglionnaire et épididymo-testiculaire. Semin Hop Paris 50:363, 1974

70. Kirk D, Gingell JC, Feneley RC: Infarction of the testis: a complication of epididymitis. Br J Urol 54:311, 1982

71. Kissane JM (ed): Anderson's Pathology. 8th Ed. Mosby, St. Louis, 1985

72. Koivuniemi A, Tyrkko J: Seminal vesicle epithelium in fine-needle aspiration biopsies of the prostate as a pitfall in the cytologic diagnosis of carcinoma. Acta Cytol (Baltimore) 20:116, 1976

73. Kovi J, Agbata A: Letter: Benign neural invasion in vasitis nodosa. JAMA 228:1519, 1974

74. Krane RJ, Klugo RC, Olsson CA: Seminal vesicle amyloidosis. Urology 2:70, 1973

75. Kuo T, Gomez LG: Monstrous epithelial cells in human epididymis and seminal vesicles. A pseudomalignant change. Am J Surg Pathol 5:483, 1981

76. Kupfer M, Buschmann G: Spermienvasion und -granulome des Nebenhodens. Frankfurter Z Pathol 74:742, 1965

77. Lambrecht W, Kortmann KB: Häufigkeit und Bedeutung akzessorischen Nebennierengewebes in der kindlichen Inguinalregion. Chirurg 54:39, 1983

78. Lazarus JA, Marks MS: Anomalies associated with undescended testis. J Urol 57:567, 1947

79. Lingardh G, Domello JL, Eriksson S, Fahroens B: Dysplasia of the testis and epididymis. Scand J Urol Nephrol 9:1, 1975

80. Lowenthal SB, Goldstein AM, Terry R: Cholesterol granuloma of tunica vaginalis simulating testicular tumor. Urology 18:89, 1981

81. Lyon RP, Bruyn HB: Mumps epididymo-orchitis. Treatment by anesthetic block of the spermatic cord. JAMA 136:736, 1966

82. Madara JL, Haggitt RC, Federman M: Intranuclear inclusions of the human vas deferens. Arch Pathol Lab Med 102:648, 1978

83. Mares AJ, Shkolnik A, Sacks M, Feuchtwanger MM: Aberrant (ectopic) adrenocortical tissue along the spermatic cord. J Pediatr Surg 15:289, 1980

84. May JE, Bourne CW: Ectopic spleen in the scrotum: report of 2 cases. J Urol 111:120, 1974

85. McClure JJ: A case of malacoplakia of the epididymis associated with trauma. J Urol 124:934, 1980

86. McConnell EM: The histopathology of the epididymis in a group of cases of azoospermia with normal testicular function. Br J Urol 53:173, 1981

87. McDonald JH, Heckel NJ: Primary amyloidosis of the lower genitourinary tract. J Urol 75:122, 1956

88. McLean NR, Burnett RA: Polyarteritis nodosa of epididymis. Urology 21:70, 1983

89. Meisels A, Ayotte D: Cells from the seminal vesicles: contaminants of the V-C-E smear. Acta Cytol (Baltimore) 20:211, 1976

89a. Melekos MD, Asbach HW: Epididymitis: aspects concerning etiology and treatment. J Urol 138:83, 1987

90. Mennemeyer RP, Mason JT: Non-neoplastic cystic lesions of the tunica albuginea: an electron microscopic and clinical study of 2 cases. J Urol 121:373, 1979

91. Mikuz G, Damjanov I: Inflammation of the testis, epididymis, peritesticular membranes and scrotum. Pathol Annu 17:101, 1982

92. Miller RA, Kiviat MD, Graves J: Glove-starch granuloma in congenital hydrocele. Urology 3:610, 1974

93. Mittemeyer BT, Lennox KW, Borski AA: Epididymitis: a review of 610 cases. J Urol 95:390, 1966

94. Mohr W, Kesenhiemer M, Beneke G: Altersabhängige Polyploidisierung der Zellkerne menschlicher Samenbläsenepithelien. Beitr Pathol 151:331, 1974

95. Monroe M: Granulomatous orchitis due to *Histoplasma capsulatum* and masquerading as a sperm granuloma. J Clin Pathol 27:929, 1974

96. Morehead RP: Human Pathology. p. 812. McGraw-Hill, New York, 1905

97. Mostofi FK, Davis CJ: Male reproductive system and prostate. p. 791. In Kissane JM (ed): Anderson's Pathology. 8th Ed. Mosby, St. Louis, 1985

98. Mostofi FK, Price EB: Tumors of the male genital system. In Atlas of Tumor Pathology. Fascicle 8, 2nd Series. AFIP, Washington, DC, 1973

99. Murphy GP, Gaeta JF: Tumors of testicular adnexal structures and seminal vesicles. p. 1607. In Harrison JH, Gittes RF, Perlmutter AD et al (eds): Campbell's Urology. Vol. 2, 5th Ed. Saunders, Philadelphia, 1986

100. Nelson AA: Accessory adrenal cortical tissue. Arch Pathol 27:955, 1939

101. Netter FH, Oppenheimer E: Reproductive system. p. 62. The CIBA Collection of Medical Illustrations. Vol. 2. CIBA, 1954

102. Orecklin JF: Testicular tumor occurring with hydrocele and positive cytologic fluid. Urology 3:232, 1974

103. Orlowski JP, Levin HS, Dyment PG: Intrascrotal Wilms' tumor developing in a heterotopic renal anlage of probable mesonephric origin. J Pediatr Surg 15:679, 1980

104. Ostermayer H, Frei A: Nebenhoden und Samenbläse als Mündungsort ektoper Harnleiter. Urologe 20:389, 1981

105. Pandya NJ: Skin, dartos, and nerve biopsies as aids to diagnosis in leprosy. Plast Reconstr Surg 54:70, 1974

106. Petersen RO: Urologic Pathology. Lippincott, Philadelphia, 1986

107. Phillips DEH: Lipid granulomata of the testis and epididymis. Br J Urol 33:448, 1961

108. Pitkänen P, Westermark P, Cornwell GG, III, Murdock W: Amyloid of the seminal vesicles. A distinctive and common localized form of senile amyloidosis. Am J Pathol 110:64, 1983

109. Povysil C: Extravesical malakoplakia. Arch Pathol 97:273, 1974

110. Prebble JJ: Scrotal involvement in Henoch Schönlein syndrome. Aust Paediatr J 16:63, 1980

111. Priebe CJ, Holahan JA, Ziring PR: Abnormalities of the vas deferens and epididymis in cryptorchid boys with congenital rubella. J Pediatr Surg 14:834, 1979

112. Pugh RCB, Hanley HG: Spontaneous recanalization of the divided vas deferens. Br J Urol 41:340, 1969

113. Raghavaiah NV: Epididymal tuberculosis: an unusual presentation. Aust NZ J Surg 44:149, 1974

114. Raghavaiah NV: Epididymal calcification in genital filariasis. Urology 18:78, 1981

115. Redman JF, Jacks DC, Golladay ES: Vasal vesical communication. Urology 22:59, 1983

116. Reeve HR, Weinerth JL, Peterson LJ: Tuberculosis of epididymis and testicle presenting as hydrocele. Urology 4:329, 1974

117. Reichert CM, O'Leary TJ, Levens DL et al.: Autopsy pathology in the acquired immune deficiency syndrome. Am J Pathol 112:357, 1983

118. Robbins SL, Cotran RS, Kumar V: Pathologic Basis of Disease. 3rd Ed. p. 1081. Saunders, Philadelphia, 1984

119. Rodriguez WC, Rodriquez DD, Tortuno RF: The operative treatment of hydrocele: a comparison of 4 basic techniques. J Urol 125:804, 1981

120. Rolnick D, Kawanoue S, Szanto P et al: Anatomical incidence of testicular appendages. J Urol 100:755, 1968

121. Rosai J: Reproductive system. p. 866. In Ackerman's Surgical Pathology. Vol. 1. Mosby, St. Louis, 1981

122. Rosai J, Dehner LP: Mesothelial hyperplasia in hernia sacs. Cancer 35:165, 1975

123. Ross L: Paratesticular Brenner-like tumor. Cancer 21:722, 1968

124. Roy JB, Hamblin DW, Brown CH: Periarteritis nodosa of epididymis. Urology 10:62, 1977

125. Saphir O: A Text on Systemic Pathology. Vol. I. p. 719. Grune & Stratton, New York, 1958

126. Sarma DP, Hanemann MS: Ossification of the vas deferens. J La State Med Soc 135:30, 1983

127. Schaeffer J, Nussbaum M, Meyersfield S: Paratesicular mass as a presenting sign of sarcoidosis. Pediatrics 66:462, 1980

128. Schellen TM, van Straaten A: Autosomal recessive hereditary congenital aplasia of the vasa deferentia in four siblings. Fertil Steril 34:401, 1980

129. Schmidt SS, Morris RR: Spermatic granuloma: the complication of vasectomy. Fertil Steril 24:941, 1973

130. Selman SH, Hampel N: Systemic sporotrichosis: diagnosis through biopsy of epididymal mass. Urology 20:620, 1982

130a. Sigel A, Snyder H, Duckett JW: Epididymitis in infants and boys: underlying urogenital anomalies and efficacy of imaging modalities. J Urol 138:1100, 1987

131. Silber SJ: Sperm granuloma and reversibility of vasectomy. Lancet 2:588, 1977

132. Simon GL, Worthington MG: An unusual case of pleural, epididymal and sternoclavicular tuberculosis. J Infect 4:259, 1982

133. Skoglund RW, McRoberts JW, Ragde H: Torsion of testicular appendages: presentation of 43 new cases and a collective review. J Urol 104:598, 1970

134. Soejima H, Ogawa O, Nomura Y, Ogata J: Pheochromocytoma of the spermatic cord: a case report. J Urol 118:495, 1977

135. Steinhauser K, Wurster K: Die Nebenhodentuberkulose im Wandel der Zeit. Urologe 14:6, 1975

136. Sundarasivarao D: Müllerian vestiges and benign epithelial tumors of the epididymis. J Pathol Bacteriol 66:417, 1953

137. Tannenbaum M: Differential diagnosis in uropathology. I. Carcinoma of prostate versus seminal vesicle. Urology 4:354, 1974

138. Taussig LM, Lobeck CC, diSant'Agnese PA et al: Fer-

tility in males with cystic fibrosis. N Engl J Med 287:586, 1972

139. Taxy JB, Marshall FB, Erlichman RJ: Vasectomy: subclinical pathologic changes. Am J Surg Pathol 5:767, 1981

140. Taylor WF, Myers M, Taylor WR: Letter: Extrarenal Wilms' tumour in an infant exposed to intrauterine phenytoin. Lancet 2:481, 1980

140a. Tejada E, Eble JN: Simple cyst of the rete testis. J Urol 139:376, 1988

141. Teoh TB: The structure and development of Walthard nests. J Pathol Bacteriol 66:433, 1953

142. Thomas D, Simpson K, Ostojioc H et al: Bacteremic epididymo-orchitis due to Hemophilus influenzae type B. J Urol 126:832, 1981

143. Vassilakos P, Cox JN: Filariasis diagnosed by cytologic examination of hydrocele fluid. Acta Cytol (Baltimore) 18:62, 1974

144. Walker AW, Mills SE: Glandular inclusions in inguinal hernial sacs and spermatic cords: Müllerian-like remnants confused with functional reproductive structures. Am J Clin Pathol 82:85, 1984

145. Warner JJ, Kirchner FK, Jr, Wong SW, Dao AH: Vasitis nodosa presenting as a mass of the spermatic cord. J Urol 129:380, 1983

146. Watson RA, Gangai MP, Skinsnes OK: Genitourinary leprosy. Urol Int 29:312, 1974

147. Weinberg A, Ginsburg CM: Epididymal sarcoidosis in a prepubertal child. Am J Dis Child 136:71, 1982

148. Weitzenfeld MB, Brown BT, Marillo G, Block NL: Scrotal kidney and ureter: an unusual hernia. J Urol 123:437, 1980

149. Wick MR, Rife CC: Paratesticular accessory spleen. Mayo Clin Proc 56:455, 1981

149a. Wiener LB, Richl PA, Baum N: Xanthogranulomatous epididymitis: a case report. J Urol 138:621, 1987

150. Williams CB, Litvak AS, McRoberts JW: Epididymitis in infancy. J Urol 121:125, 1979

151. Winblad B: Male genital tuberculosis—the possibility of lymphatic spread. A case report. Acta Pathol Microbiol Scand 83:425, 1975

152. Winkler B, Reumann W, Metao M et al: Chlamydial endometritis. A histological and immunohistochemical analysis. Am J Surg Pathol 8:771, 1984

152a. Wallin M, Marshall FF, Fink MP, et al: Aberrant epididymal tissue: a significant clinical entity. J Urol 138:1247, 1987

152b. Wood TW, Mangelson N: Urological accessory splenic tissue. J Urol 137:1219, 1987

153. Zimmerman KG, Johnson PC, Paplanus SH: Nerve invasion by benign proliferating ductules in vasitis nodosa. Cancer 51:2066, 1983

154. Zivkovic SM, Janjic G: Traumatic rupture of the testis and epididymis. J Pediatr Surg 15:287, 1980

29

Paratesticular Structures: Tumors

Gary S. Hill
Claire Billey-Kijner

According to Altaffer and Steele,[2] the most common initial diagnoses in cases of paratesticular tumors are epididymo-orchitis and hydrocele, with as many as 25 percent to 50 percent initial diagnostic errors. Fortunately, pathologists do not have the same difficulties as clinicians, but they will have to decide whether a mesothelial proliferation is benign or malignant or whether a poorly differentiated tumor is a fibrous mesothelioma, fibrosarcoma, or leiomyosarcoma.

Neoplasms of the testicular adnexa are rare. Beccia and colleagues[8] found only 91 nontesticular intrascrotal tumors in 10 years at the Boston University Medical Center and the Veterans Administration Hospital in Boston. Of those 91 cases, the overwhelming majority were spermatic cord lipomas (77 percent). Of the remaining 21 cases, the majority (16 of 21 or 76 percent) were epididymal neoplasms, 12 of which were adenomatoid tumors. The last five cases studied by Beccia and co-workers consisted of three spermatic cord tumors followed by two cases of scrotal tunic tumors.

Adenomatoid tumors and mesotheliomas excepted, most of the paratesticular neoplasms are of mesodermal origin. Among the truly rare paratesticular tumors are serous or mucinous papillary tumors resembling their ovarian counterparts.[25,153]

This chapter is divided into five parts — tumors of the rete testis, testicular tunics, epididymis, spermatic cord, and seminal vesicles. However, this division has the disadvantage of separating the discussions of benign and malignant mesothelial lesions. The benign adenomatoid tumor, thought to be of mesothelial origin (although there is some doubt on this score), is most frequent in the epididymis, whereas the malignant mesothelioma is most frequent in the testicular tunics.

TUMORS OF THE RETE TESTIS

Primary neoplasms of the rete testis are exceedingly rare. The majority are carcinomas,[55,66a,140] and only occasional cases of adenomas have been reported.[150]

Carcinoma

Most carcinomas of the rete testis occur during the 4th and 5th decades of life[55,140] and present as testicular masses, sometimes associated with hydrocele.

To be diagnosed as such, a primary carcinoma of the rete testis should involve primarily the rete, and there should be no other primary carcinoma elsewhere. Thus, only small tumors will be diagnosed as primary neoplasms of the rete testis, and larger tumors are likely to be misdiagnosed as carcinoma of the testis or of the epididymis. Other criteria, such as transition between normal epithelial cells of the rete and tumor cells,[57] a histologic pattern consistent with a papillary adenocarcinoma[140] or with an origin from the rete epithelium,[153] and growth outside the testis into the sac of the tunica vaginalis but not outside the parietal layer of the tunica[48] have all been proposed.

GROSS APPEARANCE

The tumors consist of a main mass, sometimes surrounded by satellite confluent nodules, that may involve the testicular tunics.[57,66a,112] They are whitish to reddish, often papillary, and may show necrotic and cystic areas.[148]

HISTOLOGY

Primary carcinomas of the rete testis are often papillary (Fig. 29-1), but they may show glandular[112] or tubular[57] differentiation (Fig. 29-2). The neoplastic epithelium is cuboidal to columnar, with ovoid nuclei showing moderate atypia. Mitoses are rather frequent. Occasional tumors show evidence of secretion[145,148] with supranuclear vacuolation. Such an appearance raises the possibility of an epididymal origin, however.

PROGNOSIS AND TREATMENT

Primary carcinoma of the rete testis metastasizes frequently to the regional lymph nodes[57,148] and, in decreasing order, to the lung, skin, liver, bones,[57] and retroperitoneum.[145]

Treatment consists of radical orchiectomy with or without lymphadenectomy. Adjuvant radiation or

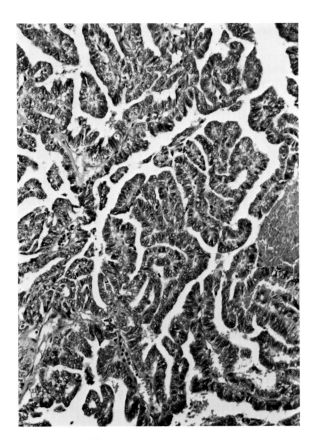

Fig. 29-1 Papillary carcinoma, rete testis. In this cystic area, the papillary configuration is well seen. Cells lining the papillae are small and dark, with rather prominent nuclei. ×135.

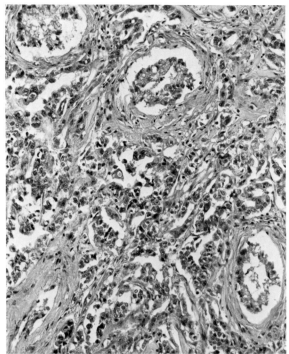

Fig. 29-2 Papillary carcinoma, rete testis. Solid area from same tumor as Figure 29-1. Pattern is one of infiltration by columnar glandlike elements, reminiscent of breast carcinomas. ×132.

chemotherapy or both have been used with variable results, probably depending on the spread of tumor at the time of discovery, as many of the patients who died have had advanced disease at the time of diagnosis.[153,154] Reported follow-up is usually too short to allow a good estimation of the prognosis. However, approximately one-half of the patients described since 1945 have died, usually within 1 year.[55] Extension outside the tunica albuginea has invariably been associated with a poor prognosis, regardless of the therapy employed.[66a] Follow-up for the other patients has ranged from 4 months to 3.5 years.

TUMORS OF THE TESTICULAR TUNICS

The testicular tunics include the tunica albuginea immediately surrounding the testicular parenchyma and the tunica vaginalis, which derives from the peritoneum and covers the lateral and anterior surface of the testis.[35]

According to Beccia et al.,[8] 59 percent of scrotal tunic tumors are malignant and 41 percent are benign (Table 29-1). The most common tumor is rhabdomyosarcoma. The most common benign tumor is the fibroma or fibrous pseudotumor. The rare Brenner tumor is mainly found in the epididymotesticular groove. It is benign and may originate from Walthard's nests.[131] (See Ch. 28.)

Fibrous Pseudotumor

Fibromas or fibrous pseudotumors have also been called *chronic (proliferative) periorchitis,*[62] *pseudofibromatous periorchitis,* and *paratesticular pseudotumor.*[93,118] These names reflect the shift in thinking about this lesion away from the earlier notion that it represented a neoplasm toward the notion that it represents a reactive, inflammatory process. *Fibrous pseudotumor,* termed by Mostofi and Price,[93] is currently the name in widest usage. Two-thirds of these lesions, found mostly in patients older than 20 years of age,[8] involve the testicular tunics; the others are seen in the proximal portion of the spermatic cord, and rarely in the epididymis.[111] They present as painless masses measuring up to 8 cm, are nodular and firm to hard, and are often multiple. They are associated with hydroceles in almost 50 percent of cases.[93] Sometimes, the

Table 29-1 Tumors of the Scrotal Tunics (156 Cases)

Benign (64 cases) 41%	Fibromas (57)	89%
	Others (7): Paratesticular Brenner tumor (4) Leiomyoma (1) Neurofibroma (1) Lymphangioma (1)	11%
Malignant (92 cases) 59%	Rhabdomyosarcomas (74)	80%
	Undifferentiated (18)	20%

(Modified from Beccia DJ et al.,[8] with permission.)

tunica vaginalis is transformed into an irregular sheet of dense fibrous tissue, from which arise many white to greyish, often coalescent nodules ranging from 0.1 cm to 2 cm in diameter.[62,93] Those nodules have a fibrillar, sometimes slightly bulging cut surface and tend to peel away from the surrounding tissue.[62,82] Diffuse fibrous thickening of the tunica vaginalis can also occur (Fig. 29-3) and is considered as a variant of this process.

Microscopically, nodules of dense fibrous tissue are seen, often with interlacing bundles of collagen. The proportion of fibroblasts is variable, perhaps as a function of the age of the lesion. In older lesions, hyalinization or calcifications may be present and are sometimes prominent. Scattered or clumped lymphocytes, plasma cells, and macrophages in many apparently younger lesions raise the possibility of an inflammatory origin. This notion is supported by the presence of organizing nodules of fibrin (Fig. 29-4), as described by Goodwin and Vermooten[62] in a case of multiple fibromas, and by the fact that half of the fibrous pseudotumors of the cord have features of fibroxanthoma or sclerosing lipogranuloma.[93] Also in favor of an inflammatory origin is the frequent history of prior trauma or epididymo-orchitis. There is no evidence of invasion of underlying structures.

Mesothelioma

Mesotheliomas[53,72,102] represent one of the greatest challenges to the pathologist in the area of paratesticular tumors, as much in their identification as in their precise origin (tunica or cord).

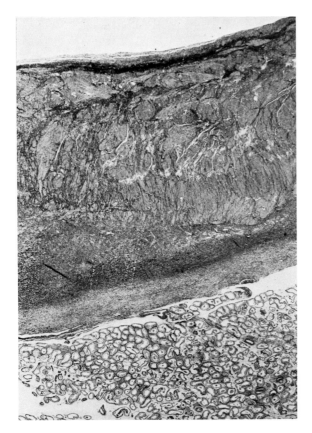

Fig. 29-3 Fibrous pseudotumor of testicular tunics. Size of testicular tubules (below) gives an indication of the massiveness of tunic thickening by fibrous tissue, in this instance with some smooth muscle admixed. Masson trichrome, ×13.

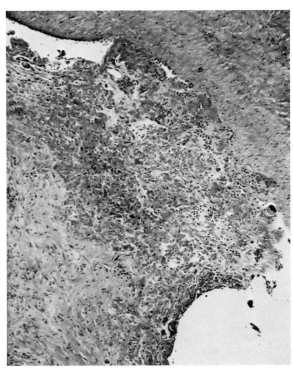

Fig. 29-4 Fibrous pseudotumor of testicular tunics. Surface of lesion with organizing fibrinous exudate, supporting the contention that these lesions may have an inflammatory origin. ×45.

The mesothelioma is considered to be the malignant counterpart of the benign adenomatoid tumor (see below). It is also distinguished from the florid reactive mesothelial proliferation (see Ch. 28).

Mesotheliomas are relatively rare tumors, tending to occur in older adults, although some patients present in their 20s. They present as a firm painless mass of variable growth rate (from a few weeks to several years), as a scrotal induration, or as a relapsing hydrocele. The fluid is clear or sometimes serosanguinous, and cytologic examination may lead to the diagnosis, as with pleural mesotheliomas.[72]

GROSS APPEARANCE

The tumor is usually solitary and consists of a poorly delimited mass that may infiltrate the entire wall or of a papillary proliferation in which are mixed solid and cystic areas. It is white to brown and is frequently friable but may be smooth, and its consistency varies from firm to soft.[93]

HISTOLOGY

Mesotheliomas are divided into three types: (1) epithelial, the most frequent type in the testicular appendages as well as in the pleura and peritoneum; (2) fibrous, mostly found in the pleura; and (3) mixed, with both fibrous and epithelial elements.

Epithelial Type

The architecture is composed of papillary formations, tubular or tubuloacinar areas, slitlike spaces, compact masses of cells, and individual cells (Fig. 29-5). The fibrous stroma is of variable abundance. There may be psammoma bodies in the papillary areas.[93]

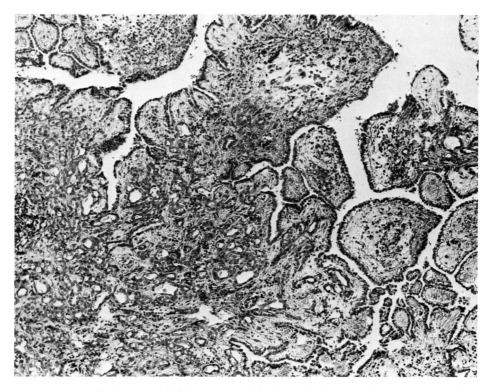

Fig. 29-5 Mesothelioma, epithelial type. Epithelial mesothelioma with prominent papillary configuration covered by a uniform, single-cell-thick epithelium. In its interior (lower left), it takes on a tubular character, closely resembling an adenomatoid tumor. ×67.

The cells lining the papillary formations are columnar or cuboidal and regular and eosinophilic, or they may resemble polygonal epithelial cells, with very eosinophilic, often finely vacuolated cytoplasm and pleomorphic, sometimes bizarre nuclei. The tubular structures are lined by a layer of regular cuboidal cells with vesicular nuclei and prominent nucleoli. Endothelial-like areas are also observed, as well as poorly differentiated foci where large cells with ground-glass cytoplasm and large central vesicular nuclei group themselves into masses resembling those in melanomas. More rarely found are esterase-negative pseudohistiocytic cells. The pseudoepithelial cells invade the surrounding tissues in clumps denuded of stroma or blood vessels and propagate along the vessels and in the perineural spaces.

The mesothelial origin of the epithelial-type mesothelioma is recognized by morphologic and histochemical criteria: (1) The continuity and the resemblance between the normal adjacent mesothelial cells and tumor cells. (2) The existence of a reticulin network around the pseudoepithelial cells, but without true basement membranes.[53] (3) The intracellular presence of glycogen and hyaluronic acid, both found in reactive mesothelial hyperplasia. Glycogen is recognized by its periodic acid-Schiff (PAS) positivity, which can be eliminated by pretreatment with diastase. Hyaluronic acid similarly stains blue with Alcian blue at pH 2.5, and this reactivity can be removed by prior incubation with hyaluronidase. However, these compounds are not entirely specific, as both are present in rare adenocarcinomas and glycogenic squamous carcinomas. (4) An important negative is the absence of true epithelial mucins stainable by mucicarmine. (5) Mesotheliomas are generally positive for cytokeratin[15] and are inconstantly positive for carcinoembryonic antigen (CEA).[22,69] They are usually negative for desmin and α-fetoprotein. Formalin-fixed mesotheliomas give variable results when stained for vimentin.[15] Alcohol (rather than Formalin) fixation increases the rate of positivity of mesotheliomas for vimentin, with 100 percent positivity in the cases studied by Churg.[19] The identification of specific mesothelial antigens, which would be the ideal means to make a definite diagnosis, has been achieved experimentally,[72,120] but this technique is not yet available commercially.

Electron microscopy is of only modest interest. The pseudoepithelial mesothelial cells do not possess any unique features that would permit their distinction from carcinomatous cells. However, if true cilia or endocrine secretion are demonstrated, the mesothelial origin is eliminated.

The difficulty with most mesotheliomas is, not in deciding whether the lesion is benign or malignant, for pleomorphism and mitoses are often prominent, but rather deciding whether the lesion represents a mesothelioma or an adenocarcinoma. Japko and colleagues believe that a suspicious tumor should meet the following criteria[72] to be acceptable as a mesothelioma: (1) no evidence of adenocarcinoma elsewhere, (2) no mucicarmine positivity, (3) in situ changes in the lining of the tunica adjacent to the tumor.

Fibrous and Mixed Forms

The fibrous form of mesothelioma is rarely described in pure form about the testicular appendages, but is perhaps less rare than it appears, for it can easily masquerade as a fibroma, a fibrosarcoma, or a leiomyosarcoma.[10] However, fibrous or pseudosarcomatous areas are seen in many solid epithelial-type mesotheliomas of the tunica (Fig. 29-6).[97]

The rare paratesticular fibrous or mixed forms[10,38] are seen as whitish, circumscribed but nonencapsulated masses. They are sometimes invasive and have a whorled, firm cut section.

Microscopically, the fibrous form is composed of interlacing bundles of spindle cells, with intercellular mature collagen. These may be associated with larger polygonal cells, sometimes multinucleated, with eosinophilic cytoplasm. The spindle cells have vesicular nuclei with prominent nucleoli, and transitional forms between the two types of cells may be seen. The stroma varies from loose myxoid to fascicular to dense and hyalinized. At the periphery one may occasionally see foci of adenomatoidlike differentiation of the tumor. However, there are no glandular or cleftlike spaces. PAS and mucicarmine stains are negative in these tumors, but the tumor cells contain demonstrable hyaluronic acid.

The diagnosis may rely on electron microscopy, which demonstrates fibroblastoid elements containing, in addition to intracytoplasmic microfilaments, microvilli, rudimentary desmosomes, and tight junctions that would not be anticipated in true fibroblasts.

The mixed or biphasic form admixes clefts and tubuloglandular structures in a monomorphous or polymorphous fibrous tissue that is rich in fibroblasts and histiocytes. The presence of forms transitional between the epithelial and fibrous forms, as well as transition between the tumor cells and normal mesothelial cells at the border of the tumor, is suggestive of the diagnosis. Once again, special stains and electron microscopy are quite helpful in diagnosis.

PATHOGENESIS

The different patterns in this tumor might be explained by the assumption that the mesothelial cells are derived from primitive mesenchymal elements of the tunica that retain the possibility of dual differentiation, that is, mesothelial and fibroblastic. Another hypothesis suggests that the mesothelial cells behave as facultative fibroblasts.

An association with scrotal trauma, prior scrotal procedures, or hydrocele has been found in some cases. Prior exposure to asbestos, well recognized as a major carcinogen in pleural and peritoneal mesotheliomas, appears to be more frequent than trauma.[4] Experimentally, intraperitoneal injection of nitrosamines in rats causes more mesothelial lesions of the tunica vaginalis than of the peritoneum.[90] However, the relationship of this observation to human genitourinary mesotheliomas is speculative.

PROGNOSIS AND TREATMENT

According to McDonald et al.,[90] the criteria in favor of malignancy are: pleomorphism and a significant mitotic activity (although even well-differentiated tumors can also behave in an aggressive fashion); the presence of vascular invasion or invasion of neighboring organs; a size equal to or greater than 2 cm; or a rapidly relapsing hydrocele. They also consider papillary configurations as an additional sign of potential malignancy (although these are quite frequent in benign reactive mesothelial proliferation). When the tumor is aggressive, it is characterized by

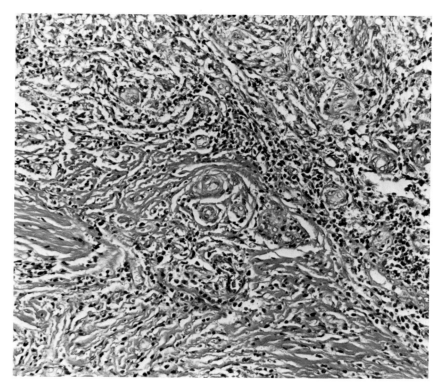

Fig. 29-6 Mesothelioma, fibrous type. The tumor is composed of small, irregular spindled cells lying in a whorled fibrous matrix. (This fibrous area was present in an otherwise predominantly epithelial mesothelioma.) ×66.

multiple recurrences, often with peritoneal spread. Lymph node and eventual pulmonary metastases are less frequent. Its prognosis, however, is better than that of pleural or peritoneal mesotheliomas.

McDonald and colleagues recommend that any mass not unequivocally benign by clinical examination be approached through an inguinal incision, followed by orchiectomy to include the spermatic cord.[90]

Evaluation includes thoracic radiographs, lymphangiography, or a computed tomography (CT) scan and exploratory laparotomy to rule out the possibility of a primary peritoneal tumor. Inguinal pelvic and retroperitoneal lymphadenectomy have been recommended in addition to the surgical resection of tumor. Chemotherapy with doxorubicin and alkylating agents has been tried as well as radiotherapy. However, too few cases are available to allow comparison of the different modalities.

Rhabdomyosarcoma

The most frequent cancer of the scrotal tunics or spermatic cord is rhabdomyosarcoma.[5,8,16,75,122,138] This tumor is also found in other parts of the urogenital system, in particular the bladder and prostate, and more rarely the penis and epididymis. (See Ch. 20) Its origin is debated, and the theory most commonly accepted is that it derives from immature muscular tissue or from undifferentiated mesenchyme.[5,68,100]

Rhabdomyosarcomas occur most frequently during the first 20 years of life with two peaks at 4 and at 16 to 19 years of age. Blacks appear to be less affected than whites and Asiatics.[93] Clinically, it presents as a solid unilateral scrotal mass, which does not transilluminate unless it is associated with a hydrocele. It is generally painless, but may be tender or cause a feeling of discomfort.[66]

Its size varies between 1 cm and 20 cm in diameter

at diagnosis. It is not associated with cryptorchidism, and most often arises from the tunica or from the lower part of the spermatic cord. It seems to be 2.5 times more frequent on the left in children aged less than 10 years.[87,100]

GROSS APPEARANCE

The tumor is nodular, sometimes bosselated, with a smooth surface, but is only rarely encapsulated (Fig. 29-7). It compresses the epididymis and the testicle and on occasion invades the epididymis and tunics. On cut section it has a yellowish or grayish appearance, sometimes mixed with zones of necrosis or hemorrhage. Its fish-flesh appearance and consistency vary according to the constituent elements: hard or firm in fibrous areas and soft in necrotic or myxoid areas.

MICROSCOPIC APPEARANCE

Rhabdomyosarcomas are classified by their histologic appearance into alveolar rhabdomyosarcoma, embryonal rhabdomyosarcoma, and pleomorphic rhabdomyosarcoma. Over 95 percent of the genitourinary rhabdomyosarcomas are of the embryonal type, with only occasional alveolar-type tumors.[41]

The diagnosis, which is sometimes extremely difficult, usually requires special stains, including a Masson's trichrome (staining the cytoplasm of muscle cells bright red) or a phosphotungstic acid-hematoxylin (PTAH) stain to demonstrate the striations. Only the best-differentiated cases will have recognizable striations by light microscopy, but the finding of deeply eosinophilic, fibrillar cells is quite suggestive of myogenic differentiation. Since glycogen in substantial quantity is characteristic of rhabdomyosarcomas, PAS with and without diastase may be valuable. In addition, a silver stain for demonstration of the existence of basement membrane and an oil-red-0 stain to eliminate the possibility of liposarcoma may be helpful.

Immunohistochemical studies[107] for myoglobin may confirm the diagnosis. However, other tumors may give false-positives related to skeletal muscle invasion with trapping of atrophic muscle fibers, which may even be phagocytosed by the cells of various tumors. All cases studied by Eusebi et al.[43] were posi-

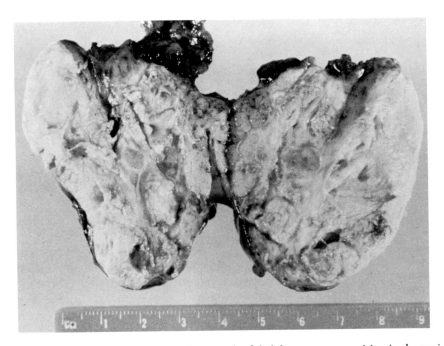

Fig. 29-7 Rhabdomyosarcoma. Gross photograph of rhabdomyosarcoma arising in the testicular tunics of a 5-year-old boy and filling the entire scrotum at operation. Note the bulging cut surface and the white, fish-flesh appearance.

tive for desmin. Electron microscopy may also be helpful in identifying thin (actin) and thick (myosin) filaments, which in the more differentiated cells may be aggregated into parallel bundles, and Z bands may even form.[41] Other authors have demonstrated the presence of intracellular laminin and type IV collagen in all three types of rhabdomyosarcoma.[4a]

Embryonal Type

The embryonal type, which occurs mainly in infants,[8,41,42,61,138] arises also in the prostate and bladder, the uterine cervix, the head, and rarely in other locations. Its macroscopic variant, the *sarcoma botryoides* (so called because of its appearance resembling a bunch of grapes), is submucosal and arises most frequently in the cervix and bladder (see Ch. 20). Rarely, it takes origin beneath the mesothelium of a body cavity. Three such cases of the botryoid subtype were recorded by Olney and associates in a study of 47 paratesticular rhabdomyosarcomas.[100]

Histologically, the embryonal type and its botryoid variant are composed of a proliferation of small undifferentiated cells resembling lymphocytes and spindle or stellate rhabdomyoblasts, set in a scant and sometimes myxoid background (Figs. 29-8, 29-9, 29-10). Rhabdomyoblasts with recognizable cross-striations may be rare; in other cases, particularly the botryoid variant, cross-striations may be present in most of the larger cells (Fig. 29-9). There may be more differentiated, round or oblong, straplike sarcoblasts,[61] with a brightly eosinophilic and distinctly fibrillar cytoplasm. In some tumors, the arrangement of myofilaments at the periphery of the cytoplasm confers a tubular appearance that resembles that of the tubular stage of fetal muscle development. Some rhabdomyoblasts contain large vacuoles of intracytoplasmic glycogen. The absence of lipoblasts is against the possibility of myxoid liposarcoma.

Alveolar Type

The alveolar type is classically described as a pseudoalveolar or pseudoglandular arrangement of moderately sized cells in a fibrous, fairly prominent stroma arranged in trabecular fashion (Fig. 29-11). The tumor cells range from the size of lymphocytes to three or four times larger (15 μm – 30 μm). The larger

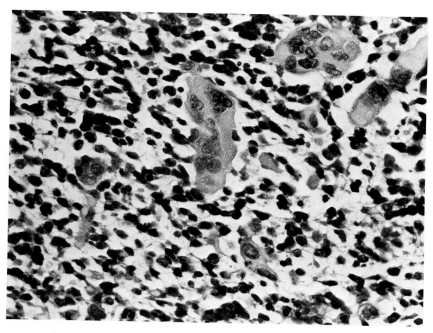

Fig. 29-8 Embryonal rhabdomyosarcoma. In the midst of a background of small round cells are several tumor giant cells, the one at the center bearing recognizable striations. Compare with Figure 29-9. $\times$250.

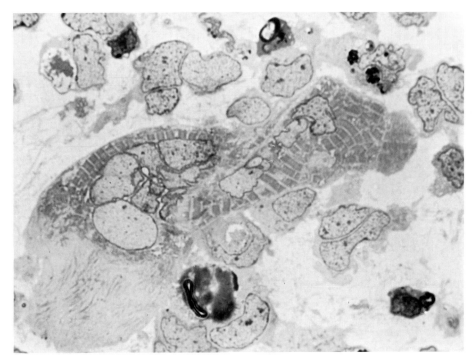

Fig. 29-9 Giant cell with striations, embryonal rhabodmyosarcoma. In this thick section prepared for electron microscopy, a giant cell with multiple nuclei and several rows of irregularly arranged striations indicating skeletal muscle origin is seen. Note also the markedly irregular contours of the nuclei of the small cells that are seen simply as round cells in routine histologic sections. Toluidine blue, ×1,400.

ones may contain small hyaline globules. The nuclei are often grooved or lobulated. The tumor cells are poorly cohesive, and only those immediately adjacent to trabeculae are attached through a tapered end, their nucleus lying at the opposite end.[61] The remainder lie free in the centers of the alveolar spaces and are often round. In about 30 percent of cases there are cells with more abundant cytoplasm, multinucleated giant cells of variable form containing striations, and other bizarre cells.

Pleomorphic Type

The pleomorphic rhabdomyosarcoma is quite rare in the genitourinary tract and occurs primarily in adults. It involves mostly the lower part of the spermatic cord[8] and is composed of a haphazard proliferation of bizarre cells of all sizes and shapes with numerous mitoses and occasionally areas of myxomatous degeneration of the stroma.[78,138] Fibrosarcomatous areas with a proliferation of fusiform cells may be

present. Positive diagnosis is established by identifying cells of rhabdomyoblastic origin, that is, cells with recognizable striations, racket cells, straplike cells, and pleomorphic cells.[93] Cells with identifiable striations are inconstant and are found in the zones of pleomorphic and straplike cells. The racket cell has one end elongated, while the other end is rounded up by an accumulation of eosinophilic cytoplasm about the nucleus. The large straplike cells are elongated or ovoid, may have several nuclei, and have very eosinophilic cytoplasm stained bright red by Masson trichrome. Finally, there may be bizarre pleomorphic cells with vacuolar cytoplasm containing glycogen.

PROGNOSIS AND TREATMENT

The prognosis depends on how early the lesion is recognized and treated, the age of the patient (younger patients have a better prognosis), and the type of treatment. The Intergroup Rhabdomyosarcoma Study Protocol proposes a staging of this

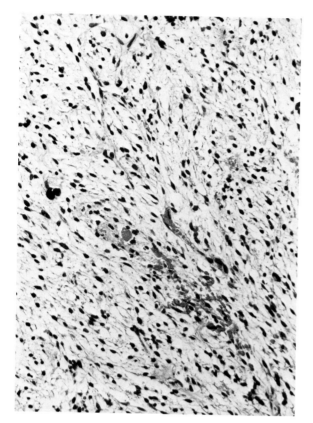

Fig. 29-10 Rhabdomyosarcoma, myxoid area. This area of myxoid appearance with small spindle and stellate cells in a loose matrix is from the embryonal rhabdomyosarcoma in Figure 29-7. ×124.

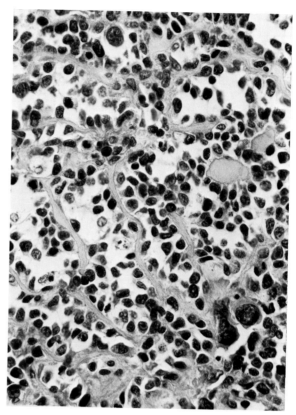

Fig. 29-11 Alveolar rhabdomyosarcoma. This tumor arose from the spermatic cord. Small, dark, somewhat pleomorphic cells are seen attached to an alveolar arrangement of connective tissue septae. Those cells not attached to the septae seem to lie free in the middle of the alveolae. Occasional larger pleomorphic cells are also present; these may sometimes show typical striations. ×292.

tumor[52,89] (Table 29-2) that requires evaluation including chest radiograph, intravenous urography, lymphangiography, sonography, and scans, with dissection and study of the resected lymph nodes.

Treatment

Current treatment[7,8,14,68,75,109,127] begins with an inguinal orchiectomy with high ligation of the inguinal cord. For involvement of the tunics or the skin, the procedure includes a hemiscrotectomy and inguinal lymphadenectomy. These procedures are followed by a retroperitoneal lymphadenectomy that is performed even in the absence of recognizable spread from the primary tumor. Preoperative radiotherapy is often used for tumors that are large or nonresectable, or it is used postoperatively for residual tumor. Chemotherapy is now employed in almost all pa-

tients, regardless of whether radiotherapy is administered.[81a] The protocol generally used combines vinblastine, cyclophosphamide, and actinomycin D or doxorubicin hydrochloride. The actinomycin and doxorubicin potentiate the effects of the radiotherapy. Immunotherapy and treatment by interferon have been proposed but remain investigational.[121]

Prognosis

Numerous studies describing various different therapies have been performed. Alveolar or pleomorphic types have a generally less favorable prognosis than the embryonal form.[81a] Local recurrence occurs in about 10 percent of cases, and nodal metastases are

Table 29-2 Staging from the Intergroup Rhabdomyosarcoma Study

Group I: Localized tumor, completely resected, with no microscopic evidence of residual disease. Regional lymph nodes negative. No other organs involved.

Group II: (a) Grossly resected tumor with microscopic residual disease (nodes negative)
(b) Regional disease, completely resected (nodes positive or negative)
(c) Regional disease with involved nodes, grossly resected but with evidence of microscopic residual disease

Group III: Incomplete resection of biopsy with gross residual disease

Group IV: Metastatic disease present at onset

(Revised from Maurer HM: The Intergroup Rhabdomyosarcoma Study (N.I.H.)—objectives and clinical staging of classification. J Pediatr Surg 10:977, 1975.)

Table 29-3 Tumors of the Epididymis (341 Cases)

Benign (257 cases) 75%	Adenomatoid Tumors (188)	73%
	Leiomyomas (28)	11%
	Papillary Cystadenomas (23)	9%
	Others:	7%
	Angiomas	
	Cystic embryoma	
	Fibroma	
	Cholesteatoma	
	Teratoma	
	Lipoma	
	Hamartoma	
	Dermoid Cysts	
Malignant (84 cases) 25%	Sarcomas (37)	44%
	Metastases (23)	27%
	Primary Carcinomas (20)	24%
	Others (4)	5%

(Modified from Beccia DJ, et al.,[8] with permission.)

present in about 20 percent of cases at the time of operation, with 15 percent having hematogenous metastases. These appear between 2 weeks and 2.5 years after surgery. They involve the retroperitoneal nodes, the pleura, peritoneum, lungs, liver, pelvis, bones, ribs, adrenals, and vertebra.[100] Olney and colleagues,[100] in their excellent study of 140 cases of rhabdomyosarcomas in 1979, found that overall survival at 1 year was 68 percent (with or without disease); 47 percent at 2 years; and 30 percent at 5 years. The prognosis at 5 years seemed to be better if the patient was less than 11 years old (67 percent survival) or more than 21 years old (38 percent survival) at diagnosis. These trends still apply, but overall survivals are now better. Current 2-year survival rates by group include group I, 83 to 90 percent; group II, 75 to 85 percent; group III, 65 to 75 percent; and group IV, 28 to 35 percent.[81a] The combination of several therapeutic modalities seems promising and allows hope for a better prognosis in the future.

TUMORS OF THE EPIDIDYMIS

Most of the epididymal tumors are benign, and of these the most frequent is the adenomatoid tumor, followed by leiomyomas.[8] (Table 29-3).

Sarcomas account for 44 percent of the malignant tumors, and the average survival of patients is 1.5 years.[86] The average age is 40 years,[86] although rhabdomyosarcomas affect a younger population. The most frequent sarcoma is fibrosarcoma. Tumors metastatic to the epididymis originate from the stomach,[94] prostate,[1,105,129,130,132] pancreas,[47] kidney,[114] colon,[18,94] skin,[3] and other sites.[8]

The clinical approach to epididymal masses is outlined in Fig. 29-12.

Adenomatoid Tumor

The adenomatoid tumor[8,86,95,124,141,152] (also called *benign mesothelioma, lymphangioma, adenomyoma,* and *grade 1 adenocarcinoma*) is by far the most common epididymal benign neoplasm. It is also found in the retroperitoneum[93] and in the female genital tract (uterus and, less frequently, vagina, ovaries, fallopian tubes, and broad ligament).[99]

Adenomatoid tumors mostly occur in persons between 30 and 50 years of age and appear to be more common in whites.[93] They are almost always unilateral. Most of the scrotal adenomatoid tumors are attached to the epididymis (80 percent) and involve the globus minor three to four times more frequently than the head of the epididymis. Rare adenomatoid tumors involve the spermatic cord[99] or the tunica vag-

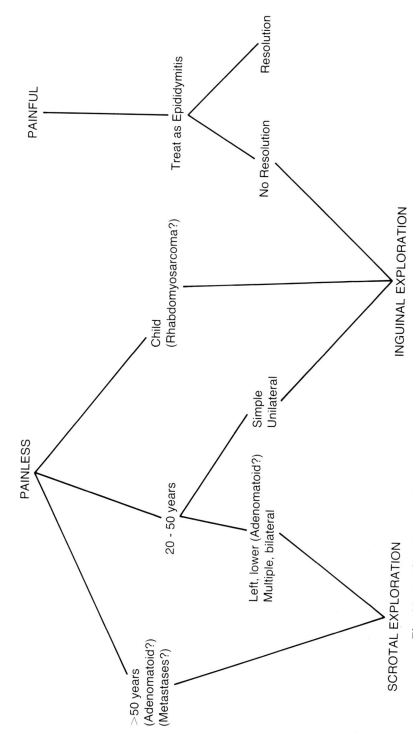

Fig. 29-12 Clinical approach to epididymal masses. (Modified from Beccia DJ et al.,[8] with permission.)

inalis.[58] They are generally painless but may be tender or cause discomfort when located near the testis or within the epididymis. Tumors in this last location may clinically mimic an epididymitis. They grow very slowly and usually measure less than 5 cm in their greatest dimension (80 percent of the tumors in the 55 cases reviewed by Longo et al. measured less than 2.5 cm[86]). In 20 percent of patients, they are associated with a hydrocele.

GROSS APPEARANCE

The tumor is whitish to gray, homogeneous, and firm, and on sectioning shows a whorled appearance. It is usually well delineated and has a pseudocapsule formed from compressed adjacent tissue.[58] Occasionally, yellowish areas or tiny cysts are also seen.

MICROSCOPIC APPEARANCE

Histologically, the tumor is composed of cords and rows of cells admixed with tubular and angiomatoid structures in a fibrous stroma (Figs. 29-13, 29-14, 29-15). The rows and cords have a plexiform pattern and are composed of cuboidal, often vacuolated, epitheliumlike cells. The cell boundaries are often poorly discernible. The cytoplasm is palely eosinophilic and finely granular and generally contains one or several clear vacuoles of variable size. Large vacuoles compressing and displacing the nucleus to one pole are common. The nuclei are inconspicuous, with regular chromatin. Oval or round, they are central or peripheral, may be vacuolated, and often contain a small nucleolus. The tubular formations consist of irregular glandlike spaces, lined by the same epitheliumlike cells, which sometimes present a brush border (Fig. 29-14). Larger spaces of various sizes and irregular shapes that are lined by flat cells result in an angiomatoid pattern (Fig. 29-13). Rarely, small canaliculi are identified between the cells, and these are best seen on electron microscopy.[124] The neoplastic cells are stained blue by Alcian blue, with decrease or absence of positivity after hyaluronidase treatment; they contain glycogen but not lipids. They are positive for keratin and epithelial membrane antigen[141] and negative for CEA. Mitoses and nuclear atypia are absent.

A reticulin network surrounds the canaliculi, cell nests, and sometimes even individual cells. It is similar to the reticulin fibers surrounding the epithelial ducts.

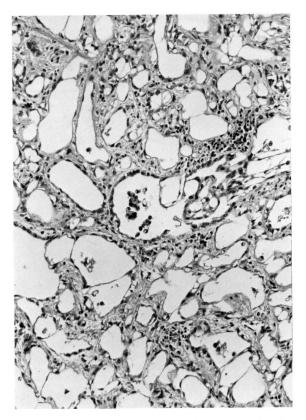

Fig. 29-13 Adenomatoid tumor. This is a typical region from an epididymal adenomatoid tumor, with irregular angiomatoid structures intermixed with smaller vessels and some lymphocytes. Some spaces (center) are lined by cuboidal epithelium-like cells. ×136.

The stroma varies in amount and consists of loose to dense, sometimes hyalinized connective tissue containing collagen and sometimes elastic fibers.[99] Also seen are interlaced bundles of smooth muscle cells, often at the periphery of the lesion, thought by Sidhu and Fresko[119] to be trapped non-neoplastic cells. They may be a prominent feature, justifying the designation of *adenomatoid leiomyoma*. Foci of inflammatory cells, mainly lymphocytes, may also be noted, mostly at the periphery. Rarely, there are areas of ischemic necrosis and acute inflammatory exudate. The tumor may extend into the rete testis and/or testicular parenchyma (Fig. 29-15). This invasion does not modify the prognosis of this benign condition, which does not exhibit recurrences or metastases. Two ostensibly malignant adenomatoid tumors have been described,[51,125] but the

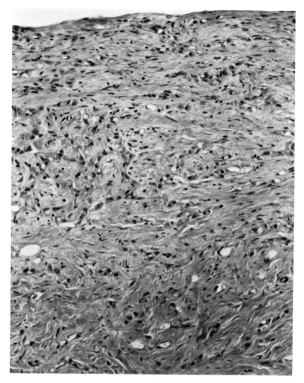

Fig. 29-14 Adenomatoid tumor. Another region from the tumor in Figure 29-13 shows a somewhat denser area with small tubular structures and individual epitheliumlike cells enmeshed in dense fibrous stroma. Masson trichrome. ×69.

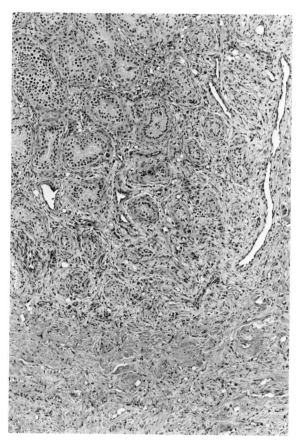

Fig. 29-15 Adenomatoid tumor involving testis. At its periphery this epididymal adenomatoid tumor is penetrating into the testis, with strands of tumor insinuating themselves between seminiferous tubules that are undergoing resultant atrophy. This "invasion" has no ominous significance. ×65.

diagnosis in these cases was open to question in that there was no transition to benign areas identifiable as adenomatoid. All other adenomatoid tumors have had a benign course.

Treatment consists of transcrotal excision or epididymectomy.[8]

HISTOGENESIS

Most clinicians now accept a mesothelial origin for adenomatoid tumors, but there is still room for reasonable debate on this subject. Some researchers have suggested an endothelial origin. Their hypothesis is supported by the fact that rare histologically typical adenomatoid tumors were found to contain Weibel-Palade bodies or were factor VIII positive.[31,133] However, most adenomatoid tumors are factor VIII negative and have ultrastructural or immunohistochemical properties of mesothelium or epithelium.

The most commonly suggested origin, originally raised in 1942 by Masson and colleagues,[88] is mesothelium, on the basis that mesotheliomas may contain adenomatoidlike areas (see Fig. 29-5). This hypothesis is also supported by the fact that continuity was noted between normal mesothelial cells and tumor cells of a fallopian adenomatoid tumor, and by the histochemical and ultrastructural characteristics of the tumor cells. Like mesothelial cells, they contain acid mucopolysaccharides and microfilaments and have junctional complexes and numerous microvilli. As with pleural mesotheliomas, adenomatoid tumors have intracytoplasmic spaces lined by microvilli.[49,99] They have also recently been reported to be positive for an unspecified "antimesothelial cell" antigen and cytokeratin[96] (although this observation has not yet been confirmed by other workers).

However, many of these features, such as desmosomes, microvilli, and microfilaments, are also present in epithelial cells. Other criticisms of the mesothelial theory are that many adenomatoid tumors have no evident connections with the surface, for they tend to grow deep toward the testis;[35] that in the uterus, their geographic center lies within the myometrium; that no papillary formations, such as expected in mesotheliomas are found; and that adenomatoid tumors are exclusively located in genital areas.

This location raised the hypothesis of müllerian[71,98,152] or wolffian[134] origin, but no one has been able to demonstrate this satisfactorily. Moreover, the cells of müllerian and wolffian vestigial structures do not resemble those of the adenomatoid tumor.

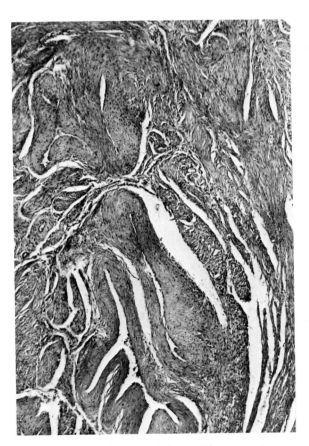

Fig. 29-16 Leiomyoma, epididymis. The tumor is composed of whorled bundles of smooth muscle, often centered about large vessels. ×48.

The possibility of an epithelial origin was raised in the past[59] because of the similarities between epididymal cells and tumor cells: presence of glycogen in the epididymal cells and inconstantly in tumor cells; reticulin network; intercellular canaliculi; intracytoplasmic vacuoles; microvilli and desmosomes. But it is then difficult to explain why the tumor cells are alcian blue positive, whereas the müllerian, mesonephric, and epididymal epithelial cells are not,[95] and why the adenomatoid tumor is found in the female genital tract. Noting the similarities between epithelial, mesothelial, and adenomatoid cells, Elsasser[40] and Soderstrom[124] suggested that this tumor is derived from bipotent coelomic epithelium (which differentiates into genital tract epithelium and mesothelium). This explanation brings us back to the mesothelium, which remains the most widely accepted origin.

Leiomyoma

Far less frequent that the adenomatoid tumors, the epididymal leiomyoma[70,85,93,135] appears as a painless mass. It is associated with a hydrocele in 50 percent of the cases and is bilateral in 15 percent of the cases.[86] The peak age of occurrence is 50 years. Morphologically, leiomyomas are quite similar to their counterparts elsewhere (Fig. 29-16). Adenomatoid leiomyomas are described with the adenomatoid tumors.

Papillary Cystadenoma

These benign tumors[8,20,23,67,80,84,139] are interesting because of their histologic appearance and the association in 50 percent of cases[8] with the neuroectodermal dysplasia (von Hippel-Lindau) syndrome. This syndrome, defined by the association of cerebellar and retinal hemangioblastomas, also includes a combination of visceral cysts or neoplasms (adenoma of the liver, cysts of the kidney and/or pancreas; renal cell carcinoma, pancreatic adenocarcinoma, and pheochromocytoma).[65,84] This syndrome is transmitted in autosomal dominant fashion with variable penetrance, such that the tumor may often be found in several members of a family.[139] The tumor is generally unilateral, but is bilateral in 15 percent of the patients,[63] and it has been suggested that those with bilateral lesions are more likely to develop the stigmata of von Hippel-Lindau disease.[103] The tumor generally grows slowly and painlessly, may be multiple, and occurs after puberty, slightly more often in the 2nd and 3rd decades.[93]

GROSS APPEARANCE

The papillary cystadenoma involves the head of the epididymis, commencing in the efferent ducts. Like the adenomatoid tumor, it is of small size (1 cm to 5 cm) and is well circumscribed, but without a true capsule. Its surface is grayish or reddish brown. Of firm consistency, it has a mottled cut section; may have cystic areas containing a clear yellow, rarely hemorrhagic fluid; or may be yellow and round, resembling an adrenal rest.

HISTOLOGIC APPEARANCE

Histologically, the tumor has a papillary and tubular architecture associated with a fibrous stroma (Fig. 29-17). Hyalinized areas and rare psammoma bodies may be present.[80] The tubules and papillae are lined by a single layer of cuboidal to columnar, clear epithe-

lium composed of two types of cell.[139] These cells, by both light and electron microscopy, resemble the normal epithelium lining the efferent ductules.[117,139] The first type of cell has pale, PAS-positive, finely granular cytoplasm, and its round nucleus lies toward the basal pole (Fig. 29-18). The second type is an oval cell with pale vacuolar cytoplasm containing numerous lipid droplets toward the luminal surface and a round nucleus remaining in the center of the cell. Foci of necrosis or hemorrhage may be visible. Hyaline, PAS-positive, and mucicarmine-negative amorphous material lies in the lumens. In focal areas, the cells may grow in solid masses that encroach on the cyst wall, although true invasion is absent. There is nothing to distinguish those tumors associated with von Hippel-Lindau disease from those which are not.

In strictly morphologic terms, the differential diagnostic possibilities are papillary cystadenocarcinoma of the thyroid and renal cell carcinoma. However, metastasis from a papillary cystadenocarcinoma of the thyroid would be extremely rare in the epididymis. Renal cell carcinomas in general have more pleo-

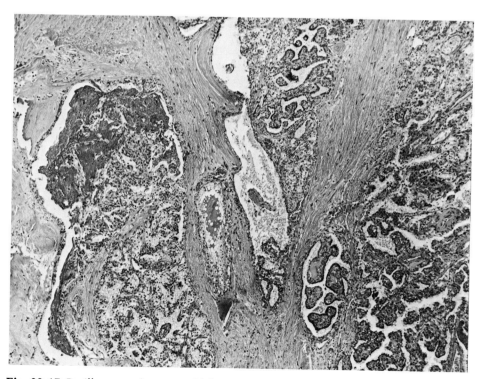

Fig. 29-17 Papillary cystadenoma, epididymis. Typical example from a patient with von Hippel-Lindau syndrome. The arborizing papillae are well seen. ×53.

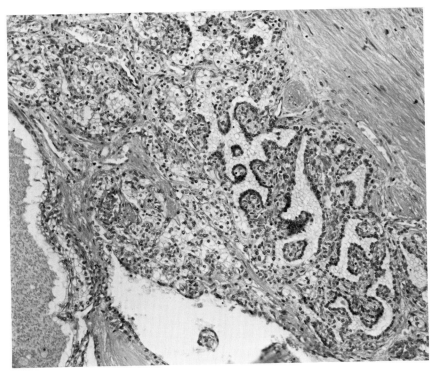

Fig. 29-18 Papillary cystadenoma, epididymis. Higher magnification of tumor in Figure 29-17. Papillae are lined principally with small dark cuboidal cells, interior cells are clear polygonal cells resembling those in renal cell carcinoma. ×128.

morphic nuclei, will have areas that are solid rather than papillary or glandular in appearance, and will have no or only spotty areas in which a colloidlike material is found in cystic or pseudoglandular spaces. (Papillary cystadenoma of the epididymis was sometimes designated in the past as mesonephroma, perhaps because of this resemblance to hypernephromas. Some investigators consider it to be a hamartoma of mesonephric origin.[93])

Retinal Anlage Tumor

Also called *melanotic hamartoma, melanotic progonoma, retinoblastic teratoma,* or *neuroectodermal tumor of infancy,* this very rare tumor usually arises in the maxilla of infants. The epididymal lesions are also confined to infancy.[26,76,153] In the epididymis, these tumors are round to oval and cream, gray, or more often brown to black because of their melanin content. They do not invade the testis. They are composed of two cell types: cuboidal cells and round to oval, smaller cells. The cuboidal cells contain melanin

and surround dark-staining smaller cells, which contain a hyperchromatic, sometimes vesicular nucleus and resemble the cells of a neuroblastoma.[153] These are often clumped together in a glomeruloid structure.[93] The stroma is fibrous and sometimes prominent. The course is said to be benign, although one patient presented with lymph node metastases.[153]

Carcinoma of the Epididymis

Carcinoma of the epididymis is quite rare compared with other epididymal tumors.[110] The patients have often been relatively young, with 50 percent 20 to 40 years old, and the lesions are associated with hydroceles in about one-half of the cases, a fact that may delay diagnosis.

The patterns reported have been truly heterogeneous with papillary adenocarcinomas, other adenocarcinomas, undifferentiated carcinomas, and even squamous cell carcinomas.[110] The diagnosis of carcinoma should be one of exclusion here, for adenomatoid tumors, papillary cystadenomas, and mesotheliomas with an adenocarcinomatous growth pattern are all much more frequent in this site than are primary carcinomas.

The lesion tends to behave in an aggressive fashion, with 8 of the 10 patients in one series dying of their tumors within 45 months of diagnosis.[110]

TUMORS OF THE SPERMATIC CORD

Primary tumors[8,13,39,126,151] of the spermatic cord are rare and basically of connective tissue origin (Table 29-4). The most frequent is the lipoma, which alone constitutes 45 percent of all the tumors of the spermatic cord and 66 percent of the benign tumors or pseudotumors.[8] Malignant tumors form 31 percent of the tumors of the spermatic cord and are divided between sarcomas (91 percent) and carcinomas and others (9 percent). Table 29-4 represents the spermatic cord lesions in the extensive series collected by Beccia et al.[8] Other, even rarer malignant tumors reported in the spermatic cord include teratocarcinomas, seminomas, mesotheliomas, neurofibrosarcomas, embryonal carcinoma, malignant angioendothelioma, angiosarcoma,[91] dysembryomas, and malignant fibrous histiocytomas.[8,33,113,123,147] The clinical approach to spermatic cord tumors is summarized in Figure 29-19.

Table 29-4 Tumors of the Spermatic Cord (636 Cases)

Benign (439 cases) 69%	Lipoma and Lipomatosis (287)	66%
	Fibroma (36)	20%
	Wolffian Duct Tumor (19)	
	Dermoid Cyst (16)	
	Lymphangioma (9)	
	Adrenal Rest Tumors (4)	
	Others:	14%
	Leiomyoma, myxoid tumor, angioma, mixed benign tumors, teratoma, embryoma, neurofibroma, cystadenoma, osteoma, histiocytofibroma, interstitial cell tumor, pheochromocytoma	
Malignant (197 cases) 31%	Sarcomas (179):	91%
	Unspecified type (51)	
	Rhabdomyosarcoma (46)	
	Leiomyosarcoma (29)	
	Fibrosarcoma (21)	
	Other Sarcomas (26):	
	Liposarcoma	
	Fibromyxosarcoma	
	Rhabdomyxofibrosarcoma	
	Lipoosteofibrosarcoma	
	Other Malignancies (18)	9%

(Modified from Beccia DJ, et al.,[8] with permission.)

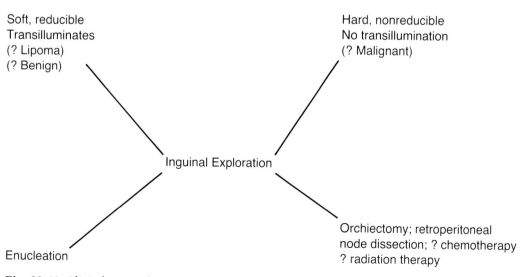

Soft, reducible
Transilluminates
(? Lipoma)
(? Benign)

Hard, nonreducible
No transillumination
(? Malignant)

Inguinal Exploration

Enucleation

Orchiectomy; retroperitoneal node dissection; ? chemotherapy ? radiation therapy

Fig. 29-19 Clinical approach to tumors of the spermatic cord. (Modified from Beccia DJ et al.,[8] with permission.)

Benign Spermatic Cord Tumors

These tumors are characterized by slow and indolent growth and may be confused clinically with chronic epididymitis or inguinal hernia. They do not transilluminate.

LIPOMA

Lipomas of the cord occur predominantly in adults aged 30 to 70 years.[54] The nature of these lesions is somewhat controversial, and a question has been raised whether these are true neoplasms or simply localized collections of adult adipose tissue. The true lipoma is a benign tumor that develops from the adipose tissue of the internal spermatic fascia. It presents clinically as an inguinal hernia.[8] It is generally covered by the tunica vaginalis, and its vessels are derived from the vessels of the spermatic cord. More frequently, "lipomas" originate from peritoneal fat that has infiltrated the inguinal canal and should more properly be called scrotal lipomatosis.[108,116] They may extend along the upper part of the spermatic cord and are situated outside the tunica vaginalis, and their vessels are derived from properitoneal fat.[35]

Grossly, lipomas vary considerably in size between different patients. The tumor is encapsulated, lobulated, and of elastic consistency, and cut section reveals soft yellowish-white lobules.

Microscopically, the tumor is composed of mature adipose tissue, separated by fibrous bands. It sometimes shows areas of focal alteration, such as myxoid degeneration, but atypical, or pleomorphic, lipomas, which have been described in the neck, shoulder and back, have not yet been described in the testicular adnexa.

DERMOID AND EPIDERMOID CYSTS

These cystic lesions[15a,37,52a,56] have the clinical distinction of being frequently fluctuant, resembling a hydrocele, but do not transmit light. They are situated in the inguinal portion of the spermatic cord. The cysts have a smooth whitish outer surface and are filled with dense creamy to grumous yellowish material, admixed with hair in dermoid cysts. Histologically, the dermoid cysts and epidermoid cysts of the cord are similar to their testicular counterparts. Both are lined by keratinizing squamous epithelium, and the dermoid cyst is distinguished from the epidermoid cyst by having hair and sweat glands as well. Epidermoid cysts are much more common than the dermoid variety, and both are more frequent in the testis than the cord. (Fig. 29-20). It has been suggested that the dermoid cysts of the cord are derived from abnormal ectodermal cells of the embryo displaced with the wolffian body from the lumbar area.[37]

Malignant Spermatic Cord Tumors

Except for liposarcomas, the prognosis of malignant tumors[127] of the cord is very poor, marked by local recurrences and dissemination via hematogenous and lymphatic channels.[6,81] Clinically, these are painless scrotal masses increasing in size at variable speeds. They are often taken for a hernia, hydrocele, spermatocele, chronic epididymitis, or even a testicular tumor. Initially, they are confined to the cord, the sarcomas characteristically beginning just below the external inguinal ring.[81] Once they invade surrounding tissues, determination of their origin becomes difficult if not impossible.

RHABDOMYOSARCOMA

Rhabdomyosarcomas of the spermatic cord have been described above with those of the testicular tunics.

LEIOMYOSARCOMA

Leiomyosarcomas[5,17,30,32,46,77,142-144] affect mainly adults, especially those over 50 years. They constituted approximately 10 percent of 101 spermatic cord tumors studied by Banowsky and Shultz.[6] Clinically, leiomyosarcomas present as a mass that is frequently separated from the testicle and extends upward toward the inguinal canal. The tumor may resemble a hydrocele of the cord. It is painless and hard with smooth contours and borders. The evolution of the lesion may be slow or very rapid.

Gross Appearance

The specimen is firm, lobulated, and well circumscribed with a whitish gray fasciculated appearance on cut section.

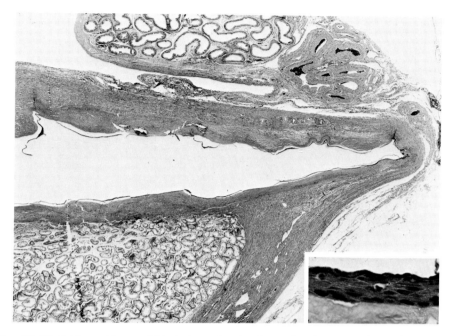

Fig. 29-20 Epidermoid cyst. This lesion arises in the testis adjacent to the epididymis and extends into the base of the spermatic cord. It is lined by a bland, low squamous epithelium. ×6.

Histologic Appearance

The diagnosis is usually easy, but may be problematic when the tumor is very well or very poorly differentiated. The histologic appearance in the well-differentiated areas consists of interlacing or intersecting bundles of smooth muscle cells. These are typically elongated, spindle-shaped, or ribbonlike and show a long blunt-ended (cigar-shaped) nucleus that is often surrounded by a perinuclear halo. They tend to align in tandem arrangement, with palisading. The cytoplasm is pale and eosinophilic and is stained red by Masson trichrome. Myofibrils parallel to the long axis of the cell are sometimes seen on hematoxylin and eosin sections and stain red-purple with phosphotungstic acid-hematoxylin (PTAH). Anisocytosis, poikilocytosis, and bizarre, multinucleated giant cells, sometimes anaplastic, may be also present. Abnormal mitoses and areas of necrosis or hemorrhage may be found. (The microscopic appearance of leiomyosarcomas is well illustrated in Ch. 20.)

The main differential diagnosis for the well-differentiated tumors is leiomyoma, which may be associated with leiomyosarcoma.[12,24,87,144] In trying to establish criteria for malignancy of superficial smooth muscle tumors, Stout and Hill[128] found that the most valuable criterion for benignity was absence of mitoses. The number of mitoses present in leiomyosarcomas varied from 1 in 10 or more high-power fields (with at least 50 fields inspected) in a minority of cases, to more than 1 per high-power field in many of them. They concluded that a tumor with an average of one or more mitoses per five high-power fields was almost certainly malignant. Malignancy was also suggested by tumors larger than 2.5 cm or the presence of anaplastic or bizarre cells, although both these features may on occasion be found in clearly benign leiomyomas. On the contrary, in this setting, nuclear hyperchromasia and pleomorphism carry little weight as criteria for malignancy. However, in their study of subcutaneous and cutaneous leiomyosarcomas (which unfortunately excluded tumors of the genital area), Fields and Helwig[50] found that the mitotic count could not predict the behavior (i.e., recurrence or metastasis) of subcutaneous leiomyosarcomas. It is not known whether this holds true for leiomyosarcomas of the cord as well. Other, less frequent lesions in the differential diagnosis include fibrosarcoma, neurofibrosarcoma, and malignant mesothelioma in its pseudosarcomatous pattern.

Pathogenesis

Occasional leiomyosarcomas[32,73,81,87] have a benign component, so that a hypothetical malignant transformation of leiomyoma could be suggested.[32,81] However, this does not necessarily mean that all leiomyosarcomas arise from leiomyomas. The most common theories are that this malignant tumor originates from smooth muscle cells of vessel walls or the smooth muscle of the vas deferens[142,143] or, as rhabdomyosarcoma, from undifferentiated mesenchymal tissue.

Treatment and Prognosis

Leiomyosarcomas are prone to local recurrences and show relatively little tendency to metastasize to lymph nodes.[24,142] When they metastasize, it is essentially by the vascular route,[81] and they seem not to be sensitive to radiotherapy. Thus, treatment combines radical orchiectomy with high ligature of the cord and chemotherapy, the efficacy of which is doubtful.[13,14,32,127]

The small series available do not permit analysis of the survival in the various modalities of therapy. On the average, the prognosis is 50 percent survival at 2 years, with a 25 percent to 30 percent 5-year survival rate reported by Jenkins and Subbuswamy.[73]

FIBROSARCOMA AND FIBROMATOSIS

According to Sogani et al.,[127] only 30 cases of paratesticular fibrosarcomas have been described. They generally occur in adults, often in their later years.[87,127,137] Their slow development, local extension with multiple recurrences, and few metastases have led some to regard them as a fibromatosis. Microscopically, fibrosarcomas have a great variety of appearances with a proliferation of spindle cells in a variable background. The diagnosis of fibrosarcoma is essentially one of exclusion. To be diagnosed as such, a spindle cell tumor must elaborate collagen (although the presence of collagen is certainly not specific for fibrosarcoma) and must lack other differentiation, such as myomatous or mesothelial. Therefore, special stains, immunohistochemistry, or electron microscopy may be necessary for the diagnosis (see Leiomyosarcoma and Mesothelioma). The treatment is surgical.[127]

LIPOSARCOMA

This rare tumor[9,106,115] develops slowly and behaves generally as a low-grade, attenuated malignancy, with local recurrences. It may attain gigantic dimensions,[27,34,136] with one tumor reported as weighing 13.5 kg.[27] It affects primarily men from 40 years to 80 years of age and clinically is a voluminous, firm mass located in the scrotum or in the inguinal canal.

Gross Appearance

Its appearance depends on the constituent elements and the quantity of fat contained in it. When it is well differentiated, it resembles a lipoma and is frequently lobular or nodular, with a smooth and rubbery surface, but is sometimes unencapsulated and infiltrating. In myxoid areas, it may have a gelatinous appearance and texture. Cut section reveals fibrous septae. Liposarcomas are classically firmer than lipomas.[93] When the tumor contains only a little fat, it may be whitish and soft or like fish flesh in character. Areas of necrosis or hemorrhage may be seen.

Histologic Appearance

One distinguishes between *well-differentiated, myxoid, pleomorphic,* and *round cell liposarcomas.* The well-differentiated and myxoid variants (Figs. 29-21, 29-22, 29-23) are the most frequent in the spermatic cord, and both are characterized by local recurrences, whereas the latter two variants metastasize more frequently.[74] The histologic appearance varies according to the type and the diagnosis.

A constant element is the lipoblast (Fig. 29-22), smaller than adult fat cells or lipocytes. Lipoblasts have round or oval peripheral nuclei, and their cytoplasm contains one or more lipid-filled vacuoles stained red by oil-red-O. Other, more variable components are undifferentiated round cells, precursors of lipoblasts, found primarily in the round cell liposarcoma variant; bizarre cells, some of them giant, with dark and often multiple nuclei (pleomorphic liposarcoma); fusiform or stellate cells in a myxoid stroma (Figs. 29-21 and 29-22) suggesting primitive mesenchyme (myxoid liposarcoma); and finally lipocytes (well-differentiated liposarcoma). Fibrous or myxomatous areas with plexiform vessels associated with pleomorphic giant cells are suggestive of a liposar-

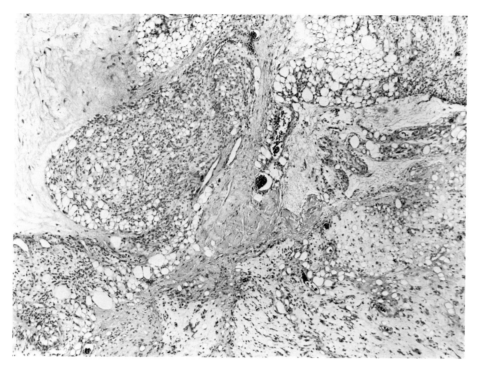

Fig. 29-21 Liposarcoma. Areas of well-differentiated liposarcoma (above and left), with some portions approaching the appearance of normal adipose tissue, abut on region of myxoid differentiation (lower right). ×58.

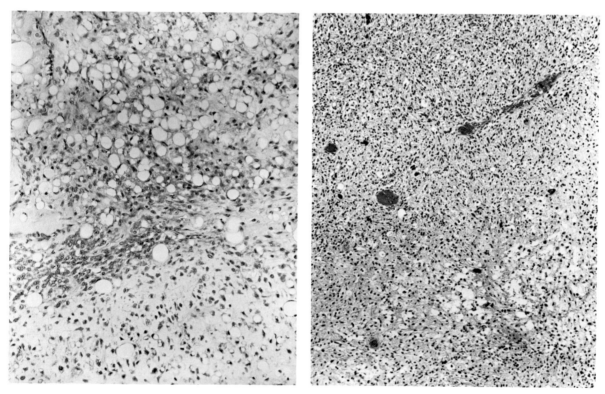

Fig. 29-22 Liposarcoma. Junction between well differentiated (above) and myxoid variants (below). Typical lipoblasts with small nuclei compressed to edge of cell by fat globule. Lipoblasts are also admixed among the stellate cells in the myxoid portion. ×112.

Fig. 29-23 Liposarcoma. Above, tumor is a spindle and round cell lesion with only minimal differentiation, with some lipoblastic differentiation below. ×47.

coma (Fig. 29-23). However, some lesions diagnosed as well-differentiated sarcomas of slow and benign evolution may in fact have been atypical lipomas.

Histogenesis

As with the muscular tumors, the origin of this sarcoma is debatable. There is little clinical or morphologic evidence to suggest that they arise from preexisting lipomas. Direct origin from mesenchymal elements seems more probable.

Treatment and Prognosis

The treatment consists of radical orchiectomy with emphasis on wide local excision because of the problem of local recurrences, with ligation of the cord at the deep inguinal ring. Radiotherapy is added if the tumor has been incompletely removed or if it is locally extensive. Because of the slow growth, re-excision of recurrences may be rewarded with prolonged survival.[74,87,127] Although only 10 percent of liposarcomas have lymph node metastasis at the time of surgery, the role and efficacy of lymphadenectomy and chemotherapy are debatable.[127] The prognosis in 1978 was 35 percent survival at 5 years.[9]

RARER MALIGNANT NEOPLASMS

As might be expected, a variety of primary malignant neoplasms have been reported on a sporadic basis in the spermatic cord, including angiosarcomas,[104] myxosarcomas,[6] malignant fibrous histiocytomas,[21,45,113,123] malignant mixed tumors,[36,64] and pheochromocytomas.[44,126] All of these are sufficiently rare that no generalizations can be made about their occurrence or prognosis. Morphologically, they generally resemble their namesakes occurring elsewhere in the body.

In the older literature, there remains a group of sarcomas occurring in the paratesticular tissues, composed of dark rounded cells with scant cytoplasm and stellate mesenchymal elements, with a loose and myxomatous stroma.[93] At the time, these were diagnosed simply as undifferentiated sarcomas. They behaved clinically as embryonal rhabdomyosarcomas, although light microscopy failed to reveal any rhabdomyoblastic differentiation. It seems likely that modern immunohistochemical and electron micro-

scopic techniques would enable such tumors to be classified as rhabdomyosarcoma, extraosseous Ewing's sarcoma, or other malignant mesenchymal tumor.

SECONDARY MALIGNANT TUMORS

Most secondary tumors of the spermatic cord result from direct extension from testicular or prostatic tumors, and metastases are much rarer. They are usually discovered at autopsy or orchiectomy for primary testicular tumor. For some reason, the stomach is by far the most frequent site of origin, accounting for 10 of 15 cases in one series.[92] Other primary sites include the colon[92] and the kidney,[149] prostate, and lung. Most are believed to be secondary to retrograde lymphatic spread.[92]

TUMORS OF THE SEMINAL VESICLES

Carcinoma

Benign tumors of the seminal vesicles are quite rare, with only occasional reports in the world literature.[29] Thirty-four cases of primary carcinoma were found to be acceptable by Goldstein and Wilson[60] in their study of the world literature up to 1973; but only 9 of them were considered as true primary epithelial neoplasms by Benson and associates[11] in 1984. At least one definite case has since been added,[132a] and a cystic epithelial-stromal tumor of probable low-grade malignancy has also recently been described, with a pelvic recurrence.[89a] The criteria set by Dalgaard and Giertsen[28] and modified by Benson et al.[11] are the following:

1. The tumor should involve primarily the seminal vesicle and should preferably be papillary.

2. An anaplastic carcinoma localized primarily to a seminal vesicle must demonstrate some degree of mucin secretion to be distinguished from an anaplastic prostatic carcinoma.

3. Similarly, the tumor must be negative for prostatic acid phosphatase and prostate-specific antigen.

4. There must be no other primary carcinoma.

Primary adenocarcinoma of the seminal vesicle occurs mostly in elderly patients. The mean age is 62 years. This tumor seldom attracts attention before it measures several centimeters and causes hematospermia[83] and urinary symptoms (hematuria, dysuria, and urinary tract obstruction). It may cause groin pain and may invade the prostate and rectum.

Grossly, the tumor has usually reached significant size by the time of discovery, for example, 50 g for the neoplasm described by Kindblom and Petterson.[79] It is grayish, generally friable, and may have a gritty appearance.

Microscopically, the tumor is often papillary (this being a criterion in favor of the diagnosis of primary adenocarcinoma of the seminal vesicle). However, poorly differentiated tumors may exist. The tumor cells are columnar to polygonal, rather clear,[79] and may even contain lipofuscin.[93]

These tumors are negative for prostate-specific antigen and prostatic acid phosphatase. However, it should be pointed out that lipofuscins may be present in prostatic carcinomas,[93] and that negativity for prostatic acid phosphatase does not completely rule out a prostatic tumor. The neoplasm described by Benson and colleagues[11] was positive for CEA, which they considered as suggestive of a seminal vesicle rather than a prostatic origin. The surgical treatment consists of a prostatovesiculectomy, often with cystectomy.[101] Surgery alone or associated with radiation and/or chemotherapy is not successful, often with rapid death of the patient.

Estrogen therapy, suggested because of the hormone dependency of seminal vesicle[146] and associated with the other modalities of therapy, is more promising, with extended survival of patients.[79]

Secondary carcinomas of the seminal vesicles are most commonly of prostatic or rectal origin. However, bladder carcinoma may involve the seminal vesicle as well, either by mucosal spread, or more banally by direct extension by muscle-invasive tumors.[107a] The frequency of mucosal spread is not known, however.

REFERENCES

1. Addonizio JC, Thelmo W: Epididymal metastasis from prostatic carcinoma. Urology 18:490, 1981
2. Altaffer LF, Steele SM, Jr: Scrotal explorations negative for malignancy. J Urol 124:617, 1980
3. Anselmo G, Rizzotti A, Gramegna V: A metastatic melanoma in the spermatic cord. Br J Urol 51:416, 1979
4. Antman K, Cohen S, Dimitrove NV et al: Malignant mesothelioma of the tunica vaginalis testis. J Clin Oncol 2:447, 1984
4a. Autio-Harmainen H, Apaja-Sarkkinen M, Martikainen J et al: Production of basement membrane laminin and type IV collagen by tumors of striated muscle: an immunohistochemical study of rhabdomyosarcomas of different histologic types and a benign vaginal rhabdomyoma. Hum Pathol 17:1218, 1986
5. Banik S, Guha PK: Paratesticular rhabdomyosarcomas and leiomyosarcomas: a clinicopathological review. J Urol 121:823, 1979
6. Banowsky LH, Shultz GN: Sarcoma of the spermatic cord and tunics: review of the literature, case report and discussion of the role of retroperitoneal lymph node dissection. J Urol 103:628, 1970
7. Beall ME, Young IS: Spermatic cord rhabdomyosarcoma: case report. J Urol 117:807, 1977
8. Beccia DJ, Krane RJ, Olsson CA: Clinical management of non-testicular intrascrotal tumors. J Urol 116:476, 1976
9. Bellinger MF, Gibbons MD, Koontz WW, Jr., Graff M: Paratesticular liposarcoma. Urology 11:285, 1978
10. Benisch B, Peison B, Sobel HJ, Marquet E: Fibrous mesotheliomas (pseudofibroma) of the scrotal sac: a light and ultrastructural study. Cancer 47:731, 1981
11. Benson RC, Jr, Clark WR, Farrow GM: Carcinoma of the seminal vesicle. J Urol 132:483, 1984
12. Bevan PG: Malignant leiomyosarcoma of the spermatic cord. Br J Surg 42:101, 1954
13. Bissada NK, Finkbeiner AE, Redman JF: Paratesticular sarcomas: review of management. J Urol 116:198, 1976
14. Blitzer PH, Dosoretz DE, Proppe KH, Shipley WV: Treatment of malignant tumors of the spermatic cord: a study of 10 cases and a review of the literature. J Urol 126:611, 1981
15. Blobel GA, Moll R, Franke WW et al: The intermediate filament cytoskeleton of malignant mesothelioma and its diagnostic significance. Am J Pathol 121:235, 1985
15a. Bloom DA, Dipietro MA, Gikas PW, McGuire EJ: Extratesticular dermoid cyst and fibrous dysplasia of epididymis. J Urol 137:89, 1987
16. Brenez J, Rettmann R: Rhabdomyosarcome du cordon spermatique. Présentation d'un cas et revue de la littérature. Acta Urol Belg 41:609, 1973
17. Buckley PM, Tolley DA: Leiomyosarcoma of the spermatic cord. Br J Urol 53:193, 1981

18. Burger R, Guthrie TH: Metastatic colonic carcinoma to epididymis. Urology 2:566, 1973

19. Churg A: Immunohistochemical staining for vimentin and keratin in malignant mesothelioma. Am J Surg Pathol 9:360, 1985

20. Civil ID, Hackett AH: Papillary cystadenoma of the epididymis: a case report. Aust NZ J Surg 51:304, 1981

21. Cole AT, Straus FH, Gill WB: Malignant fibrous histiocytoma: an unusual tumor. J Urol 107:1005, 1972

22. Corson JM, Pinkus G: Mesothelioma: profile of keratin proteins and carcinoembryonic antigen: an immunoperoxidase study of 29 cases and comparison with pulmonary adenocarcinomas. Am J Pathol 108:80, 1982

23. Crisp JC, Roberts PF: A case of bilateral cystadenomas of the epididymides presenting as infertility. Br J Urol 47:682, 1975

24. Cruze K: Leiomyosarcoma of the spermatic cord. Arch Surg 76:151, 1958

25. Currie JS, Ngaei G: A papilloma of epididymis of Müllerian vestigial origin. Br J Urol 49:331, 1977

26. Cutler LS, Chaudry AP, Topazian R: Melanotic neuroectodermal tumor of infancy: An ultrastructural study, literature review, and reevaluation. Cancer 48:257, 1981

27. D'Abrera VS, Burfitt-Williams W: A giant scrotal liposarcoma. Med J Aust 2:854, 1973

28. Dalgaard JB, Giertsen JC: Primary carcinoma of the seminal vesicle; case and survey. Acta Pathol Microbiol Scand 39:255, 1956

29. Damjanov I, Apic R: Cystadenoma of seminal vesicles. J Urol 111:808, 1974

30. Davides KC, King LM, Paat F: Primary leiomyosarcoma of the epididymis. J Urol 114:642, 1975

31. Davy CL, Tang CK: Are all adenomatoid tumors adenomatoid mesotheliomas? Hum Pathol 12:360, 1981

32. Deluise VP, Draper JW, Gray CF, Jr: Smooth muscle tumors of the testicular adnexa. J Urol 115:685, 1976

33. Dias R, Fernandes M, Gaetz HP: Malignant fibrous histiocytoma of spermatic cord. Urology 12:365, 1978

34. Dimacopoulos DG: Paratesticular liposarcoma. Br J Urol 46:347, 1974

35. Dixon FJ, Moore RA: Tumors of the testicular appendages and of the seminal vesicles. p. 127. In Tumors of the Male Sex Organs. Armed Forces Institute of Pathology, Washington, D.C., 1952

36. Dreyfuss ML, Lubash S: Malignant mixed tumor of the spermatic cord (lipo-osteofibrosarcoma). J Urol 44:314, 1940

37. Eason AA, Spaulding JT: Dermoid cyst arising in testicular tunics. J Urol 117:539, 1977

38. Eimoto T, Inoue I: Malignant fibrous mesothelioma of tunica vaginalis, a histologic and ultrastructural study. Cancer 39:2059, 1977

39. El Badawi AA, Al Ghorab MM: Tumors of the spermatic cord: a review of the literature and report of a case of lymphangioma. J Urol 94:445, 1965

40. Elsasser E: Tumors of the epididymis. Recent Results Cancer Res 60:163, 1977

41. Enzinger FM, Weiss SW: Soft Tissue Tumors. p. 338. Mosby, St. Louis, 1983

42. Enzinger FM, Shiraki M: Alveolar rhabdomyosarcoma. An analysis of 110 cases. Cancer 24:18, 1969

43. Eusebi V, Ceccarelli C, Gorza L et al: Immunocytochemistry of rhabdomyosarcoma: the use of four different markers. Am J Surg Pathol 10:293, 1986

44. Eusebi V, Massarelli G: Pheochromocytoma of the spermatic cord: report of a case. J Pathol 105:283, 1971

45. Farah RN, Bohne AW: Malignant fibrous histiocytoma of spermatic cord. Urology 3:782, 1974

46. Farrell MA, Donnelly BJ: Malignant smooth muscle tumors of the epididymis. J Urol 124:151, 1980

47. Faysal MH, Strefling A, Kosek JC: Epididymal neoplasms: a case report and review. J Urol 129:843, 1983

48. Feek JD, Hunter WC: Papillary carcinoma arising from rete testis. Arch Pathol 40:399, 1945

49. Ferenczy A, Fenoglio J, Richart RM: Observations on benign mesothelioma of the genital tract (adenomatoid tumor). A comparative ultrastructural study. Cancer 30:244, 1972

50. Fields JP, Helwig EB: Leiomyosarcoma of the skin and subcutaneous tissue. Cancer 47:156, 1981

51. Fisher ER, Klieger H: Epididymal carcinoma (malignant adenomatoid tumor, mesonephric mesodermal carcinoma of the epididymis). J Urol 95:568, 1966

52. Fleischmann J, Perinetti EP, Catalona WJ: Embryonal rhabdomyosarcoma of the genito-urinary organs. J Urol 126:389, 1981

52a. Ford J Jr, Singh S: Paratesticular dermoid cyst in 6-month-old infant. J Urol 139:89, 1988

53. Frea B, Tizzani A, Tasso M: Mésothéliome du cordon spermatique. J Urol (Paris) 87:291, 1981

54. Fujimura N, Kurokawa K: Primary lipoma of the scrotum. Eur Urol 5:182, 1979

55. Fukunaga M, Aizawa S, Furusato M: Papillary adenocarcinoma of the rete testis. A case report. Cancer 50:134, 1982

56. Ghosh DP: Dermoid cyst of the spermatic cord. J Indian Med Assoc 74:18, 1980

57. Gisser SD, Nayak S, Kaneko M, Tchertkoff V: Adenocarcinoma of the rete testis: a review of the literature and presentation of a case with associated asbestosis. Hum Pathol 8:219, 1977

58. Glover L, Frensilli FJ, Derrick FC, Jr: Simultaneous

adenomatoid tumors of epididymis and tunica vaginalis. Urology 2:192, 1973

59. Golden A, Ash JE: Adenomatoid tumors of the genital tract. Am J Pathol 21:63, 1945

60. Goldstein AG, Wilson ES: Carcinoma of the seminal vesicle with particular reference to the angiographic appearances. Br J Urol 45:211, 1973

61. Gonzalez-Crussi F, Black-Schaffer S: Rhabdomyosarcoma of infancy and childhood. Problems of morphologic classification. Am J Surg Pathol 73:157, 1979

62. Goodwin WE, Vermooten V: Multiple fibromata of tunica vaginalis testis or a proliferative type of chronic periorchitis. A report of 2 cases. J Urol 56:430, 1946

63. Grant SM, Hoffman EF: Bilateral papillary adenomas of the epididymes. Arch Pathol 76:620, 1963

64. Graves RC, Kickham CJE: Teratoma of the spermatic cord. Case report with a consideration of the prolan test. Am J Surg 47:116, 1940

65. Gruber MB, Healey GB, Toguri AG, Warren MM: Papillary cystadenoma of epididymis: component of von Hippel-Lindau syndrome. Urology 16:305, 1980

66. Gulati SM, Sharma RC, Iyengar B, Thusoo TK: Rhabdomyosarcoma of the spermatic cord. Indian J Cancer 15:81, 1978

66a. Haas GP, Ohorodnik JM, Farah RN: Cystadenocarcinoma of the rete testis. J Urol 137:210, 1987

67. Hesp WL, Debruyne FM, Bogman MJ: Papillary cystadenoma of the epididymis. Neth J Surg 35:97, 1983

68. Hoekstra HJ, Wobbes T, Brouwers TM et al: Embryonal rhabdomyosarcoma of spermatic cord. Urology 16:360, 1980

69. Holden J, Churg A: Immunohistochemical staining for keratin and carcinoembryonic antigen in the diagnosis of malignant mesothelioma. Am J Surg Pathol 8:277, 1984

70. Iloreta AT, Bekirov H, Newman HR: Leiomyoma of scrotum. Urology 10:48, 1977

71. Jackson JR: The histogenesis of the adenomatoid tumor of the genital tract. Cancer 11:337, 1958

72. Japko L, Horta AA, Schreiber K et al: Malignant mesothelioma of the tunica vaginalis testis: report of first case with preoperative diagnosis. Cancer 49:119, 1982

73. Jenkins DG, Subbuswamy SG: Leiomyosarcoma of the spermatic cord. A case report. Br J Surg 59:408, 1972

74. Johnson DE, Harris JD, Ayala AG: Liposarcoma of spermatic cord. Urology 11:190, 1978

75. Johnson DE, McHugh TA, Jaffe N: Paratesticular rhabdomyosarcoma in childhood. J Urol 128:1275, 1982

76. Johnson RE, Scheithauer BW, Dahlin DC: Melanotic neuroectodermal tumor of infancy. A review of seven cases. Cancer 52:661, 1983

77. Johnson S, Rundell M, Platt W: Leiomyosarcoma of the scrotum: a case report with electron microscopy. Cancer 41:1830, 1978

78. Kaneti J, Inbas IJ, Sober I, Smailowitz Z: Paratesticular rhabdomyosarcoma in an adult. Urology 16:614, 1980

79. Kindblom LG, Petterson G: Primary carcinoma of the seminal vesicle. Case report. Acta Pathol Microbiol Scand 84:301, 1976

80. Küchemann K: Papillary cystadenoma of the epididymis with psammoma bodies. Beitr Pathol 153:406, 1974

81. Kyle VN: Leiomyosarcoma of the spermatic cord: a review of the literature and report of an additional case. J Urol 96:795, 1966

81a. Lacey JR, Jewett TC Jr, Karp JE et al: Advances in the treatment of rhabdomyosarcoma. Sem Surg Oncol 2:139, 1986

82. Laky D, Mihailescu E, Stefanescu D: Fibrome géant de la vaginale scrotale. Morphol Embryol (Bucur) 23:203, 1977

83. Lathem JE: Carcinoma of seminal vesicle. South Med J 68:473, 1975

84. Lister IS, Vanreenen RM: Lindau's disease. Proc R Soc Med 68:520, 1975

85. Livne PM, Nobel M, Savir A et al: Leiomyoma of the scrotum. Arch Dermatol 119:358, 1983

86. Longo V, McDonald JR, Thompson G: Primary neoplasms of the epididymis. Special reference to adenomatoid tumors. JAMA 147:937, 1951

87. Malek RS, Utz DC, Farrow GM: Malignant tumors of the spermatic cord. Cancer 29:1108, 1972

88. Masson P, Riopelle JL, Simard LC: Le mésothéliome bénin de la sphère génitale. Rev Can Biol Exp 1:720, 1942

89. Maurer HM: Recent advances in management of childhood rhabdomyosarcoma. Va Med Mon 102:476, 1975

89a. Mazur MT, Myers JL, Maddox WA: Cystic epithelial-stromal tumor of the seminal vesicle. Am J Surg Pathol 11:210, 1987

90. McDonald RE, Sago AL, Novicki DE, Bagnall JW: Paratesticular mesotheliomas. J Urol 130:360, 1983

91. Millstein DI, Tang CK, Campbell EW, Jr: Angiosarcoma developing in a patient with neurofibromatosis (von Recklinghausen's disease). Cancer 47:950, 1981

92. Monn I, Poticha SM: Metastatic tumors of spermatic cord. Urology 5:821, 1975

93. Mostofi FK, Price EB: Tumors of the male genital system. In Atlas of Tumor Pathology. 2nd Series, Fascicle 8. Armed Forces Institute of Pathology, Washington, D.C., 1973

94. Mouchet A, Marquand J, Barbagelatta M: Métastases juxtaépididymaires bilatérales révélant un adénocarcinome gastrique. Chirurgie 102:209, 1976

95. Mucientes F: Adenomatoid tumor of the epididymis. Ultrastructural study of three cases. Pathol Res Pract 176:258, 1983

96. Mucientes F, Govindarajan S, Burroto S: Immunoperoxidase study of the adenomatoid tumor of the epididymis using antimesothelial serum. Cancer 55:363, 1985

97. Murphy GP, Gaeta JF: Tumors of testicular adnexal structures and seminal vesicles. p. 1607. In Harrison JH, Gittes RF, Perlmutter AD et al (eds): Campbell's Urology. Vol. 2. 5th Ed. Saunders, Philadelphia, 1986

98. Naegeli T: Ein Mischtumor des Sammenstranges. Virchows Arch 208:364, 1912

99. Nistal M, Contreras F, Paniagua R: Adenomatoid tumour of the epididymis: histochemical and ultrastructural study of 2 cases. Br J Urol 50:121, 1978

100. Olney LE, Narayana A, Loening S, Culp DA: Intrascrotal rhabdomyosarcoma. Urology 14:113, 1979

101. Palmer JM: Surgery of the seminal vesicles. p. 2846. In Harrison JH, Gittes RF, Perlmutter AD et al (eds): Campbell's Urology. Vol. 3. 5th Ed. Saunders, Philadelphia, 1986

102. Pizzolato P, Lamberty J: Mesothelioma of spermatic cord: electron microscopic and histochemical characteristics of its mucopolysaccharides. Urology 8:403, 1976

103. Price EB, Jr: Papillary cystadenoma of the epididymis. A clinicopathologic analysis of 20 cases. Arch Pathol 91:456, 1971

104. Prince CL: Malignant tumors of the spermatic cord: a brief review with presentation of a case of angioendothelioma. J Urol 47:793, 1942

105. Puigvert A: Metastasis of prostatic carcinoma in the epididymis. Eur Urol 4:220, 1978

106. Reyes CV: Spermatic cord liposarcoma. Urology 15:416, 1980

107. Riehle RA, Jr, Venkatachalam H: Electron microscopy in diagnosis of adult paratesticular rhabdomyosarcoma. Urology 19:658, 1982

107a. Ro JY, Ayala AG, el-Naggar A, Wishnow KI: Seminal vesicle involvement by in situ and invasive transitional cell carcinoma of the bladder. Am J Surg Pathol 11:951, 1987

108. Rosenberg N: Letter: "Lipoma" of the spermatic cord: potential relationship to indirect inguinal hernia in adults. Arch Surg 114:549, 1979

109. Sago AL, Novicki DE: Rhabdomyosarcoma of spermatic cord. Urology 19:606, 1982

110. Salm R: Papillary carcinoma of the epididymis. J Pathol 97:253, 1969

111. Sarlis T, Yakoymakis S, Rebelakos AG: Fibrous pseudotumor of the scrotum. J Urol 124:742, 1980

112. Schapira HE, Engel M: Adenocarcinoma of rete testis. NY State J Med 72:1283, 1972

113. Sclama AO, Berger BW, Cherry JM et al.: Malignant fibrous histiocytoma of the spermatic cord: the role of retroperitoneal lymphadenectomy in management. J Urol 130:577, 1983

114. Selli C, Woodard BH, Paulson DF: Late intrascrotal metastases from renal cell carcinoma. Urology 20:423, 1982

115. Senoh K, Osada Y, Kawachi J: Spermatic cord liposarcoma. Br J Urol 50:429, 1978

116. Shafik A, Olfat A: Lipectomy in the treatment of scrotal lipomatosis. Br J Urol 53:55, 1981

117. Sherrick JC: Papillary cystadenoma of the epididymis. Cancer 9:403, 1956

118. Shindelman L, Marchevsky AM: Paratesticular pseudotumor following herniorraphy. Urology 21:72, 1983

119. Sidhu GS, Fresko O: Adenomatoid tumor of the epididymis: ultrastructural evidence of its biphasic nature. Ultrastruct Pathol 1:39, 1980

120. Singh G, Whiteside TL, Dekker A: Immunodiagnosis of mesothelioma: use of antimesothelial cell serum in an indirect immunofluorescence assay. Cancer 43:2288, 1979

121. Sinkovics JG, Plager C, von Eschenbach A, Johnson DE: Sarcomas of the genitourinary tract: case histories. p. 284. In Johnson DE, Saumels ML (eds): Cancer of the Genitourinary Tract. Raven Press, New York, 1979

122. Skeel DA, Drinker HR, Jr, Witherington R: Rhabdomyosarcoma of the spermatic cord: report of 3 cases with review of the literature. J Urol 113:279, 1975

123. Smailowitz Z, Kaneti J, Sober I et al: Malignant fibrous histiocytoma of the spermatic cord. J Urol 130:150, 1983

124. Soderstrom KO: Origin of adenomatoid tumor: a comparison between the structure of adenomatoid tumor and epididymal duct cells. Cancer 49:2349, 1982

125. Soderstrom J, Liedberg CF: Malignant "adenomatoid" tumor of the epididymis. Acta Pathol Microbiol Scand 67:165, 1966

126. Soejima H, Ogawa O, Nomura Y et al.: Pheochromocytoma of the spermatic cord. A case report. J Urol 118:495, 1977

127. Sogani PC, Grabstald H, Whitmore WF, Jr: Spermatic cord sarcoma in adults. J Urol 120:301, 1978

128. Stout AP, Hill WT: Leiomyosarcoma of the superficial soft tissues. Cancer 11:844, 1958

129. Suhler A, Blanchard J: Un cas de métastase épididymaire prévalente. J Urol (Paris) 86:301, 1980

130. Suhler A, Blanchard J: Un nouveau cas curieux de métastase épididymaire. J Urol (Paris) 86:574, 1980

131. Sundarasivarao D: Müllerian vestiges and benign epithelial tumors of the epididymis. J Pathol Bacteriol 66:417, 1953

132. Talbot RW, McCann BG: Secondary prostatic tumour of the spermatic cord and epididymis 5 years after prostatectomy and vasectomy. Br J Urol 51:48, 1979

132a. Tanaka T, Takeuchi T, Oguchi K. et al: Primary adenocarcinoma of the seminal vesicle. Hum Pathol 18:200, 1987

133. Taxy JB, Battifora H, Oyasu R: Adenomatoid tumors: a light microscopic, histochemical and ultrastructural study. Cancer 34:306, 1974

134. Teilum G: Histogenesis and classification of mesonephric tumors of the female and male genital system and relationship to benign so-called adenomatoid tumors (mesotheliomas): a comparative histological study. Acta Pathol Microbiol Immunol Scand 34:431, 1954

135. Tomera KM, Gaffey TA, Goldstein IS, Zincke H: Leiomyoma of scrotum. Urology 18:388, 1982

136. Treadwell T, Treadwell MA, Owen M, McConnell TH: Giant liposarcoma of the spermatic cord. South Med J 74:753, 1981

137. Tripàthi VNP, Dic VS: Primary sarcoma of the urogenital system in adults. J Urol 101:898, 1969

138. Trippitelli A, Rosi P, Selli C et al: Rhabdomyosarcoma of spermatic cord in adult. Urology 19:533, 1982

139. Tsuda H, Tukushima S, Takahashi M et al: Familial bilateral papillary cystadenoma of the epididymis: report of three cases in siblings. Cancer 37:1831, 1976

140. Turner RW, Williamson J: Adenocarcinoma of the rete testis. J Urol 109:850, 1973

141. Urialdes-Viedma M, Martos-Padilla S, Caballero-Morales T: Adenomatoid tumors: immunohistochemical study and histogenesis. Arch Pathol Lab Med 109:636, 1986

142. Weitzner S: Leiomyosarcoma of spermatic cord: report of a case and summary of the literature. Rocky Mountain Med J 64:73, 1967

143. Weitzner S: Leiomyosarcoma of spermatic cord and retroperitoneal lymph node dissection. Am Surg 39:352, 1973

144. Wessel HN: Leiomyosarcoma of the spermatic cord. J Urol 69:823, 1953

145. Whitehead ED, Valensi OJ, Brown JS: Adenocarcinoma of the rete testis. J Urol 107:992, 1972

146. Williamson RC, Slade N, Fenelay RC: Seminal vesicle tumours. J R Soc Med 71:286, 1978

147. Williamson JC, Johnson JD, Lamm DL et al: Malignant fibrous histiocytoma of the spermatic cord. J Urol 123:785, 1980

148. Winter CL, Puente E, Lai DY, Sharma HM: Papillary carcinoma of rete testis. Urology 18:168, 1981

149. Yadav K, Pathak IC: Wilms tumour with left cord metastasis. Br J Urol 49:536, 1977

150. Yadav SB, Patil PN, Karkhanis RB: Primary tumors of the spermatic cord, epididymis and rete testis. J Postgrad Med 15:49, 1969

151. Yamamoto M, Miyaka K, Mitsuya H: Intrascrotal extratesticular neurofibroma. Urology 20:200, 1982

152. Yasuma T, Saito S: Adenomatoid tumor of the male genital tract—a pathological study of eight cases and review of the literature. Acta Pathol Jpn 30:883, 1980

153. Young RH, Scully RE: Miscellaneous neoplasms and nonneoplastic lesions. p. 93. In Talerman A, Roth LM (eds): Pathology of the Testis and Its Adnexa. Churchill Livingstone, New York, 1986

154. Young RH, Scully RE: Testicular and paratesticular tumors and tumor-like lesions of ovarian, common epithelial and Müllerian types. Am J Clin Pathol 86:146, 1986

30

Prostate Gland: Embryology, Anatomy, and Histology

David Brandes

EMBRYOLOGY, ANATOMY, AND PHYSIOLOGY OF THE PROSTATE

Over 10 percent of admissions to general hospitals are for urologic problems, and diseases of the prostate represent a major part of the clinical cases.

The prostate completely surrounds the bladder neck and the urethra, creating a potential threat of urinary obstruction. Benign prostatic hyperplasia, a noninvasive, expansile, focal growth within the organ, may create life-threatening situations through urinary obstruction, with dilatation of the excretory system, mechanical atrophy of renal parenchyma, and serious infections.

The development and growth of the prostate are under an elaborate hormonal control exercised through the hypothalamic, pituitary gonadal-adrenal axis. Not only the normal gland but benign hyperplastic and malignant growths are also under such hormonal influences, although malignant prostatic tissues may escape such control and assume autonomous growth. The understanding of the mechanism of action of these hormones, particularly at the level of the target organ interaction, may in the future enable the exogenous regulation of prostatic abnormal growth.

Anatomically and functionally, as well as pathologically, the prostate gland is not a homogeneous structure. The main diseases that affect the prostate, such as carcinoma, benign prostatic hyperplasia, and infections, arise with greater frequency in different anatomic regions of this organ. Such different prostatic zones may be endowed with particular features in regard to their embryologic origin, histologic appearance, and responsiveness to various steriod hormones.

DEVELOPMENTAL ANATOMY

In embryos about 16 mm long from crown to rump, the descending portion of the urorectal septum reaches the cloacal membrane. This establishes the separation of the cloaca into the dorsally placed rectum and the ventrally located primitive urogenital sinus, both of which are lined by endoderm (Fig. 30-1).[2,33,64] The opening of the mesonephric ducts into the primitive urogenital sinus divides this structure into a cranial portion, the *vesicourethral canal*, and a caudal portion, the *definitive urogenital* sinus. The fused caudal tip of the paramesonephric (müllerian) duct and the mesonephric (wolffian) duct on each side penetrates dorsally the wall of the future urethra, at the junction of the vesicourethral canal and the uro-

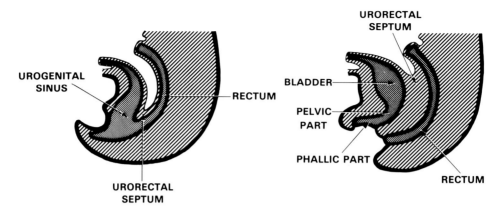

Fig. 30-1 Cloacal region: Formation of the urogenital, sinus and rectum. Proliferation of the mesoderm gives rise to the urorectal septum that divides the cloaca into the anteriorly located urogenital sinus and rectum. The urogenital sinus then differentiates into an upper bladder portion, an intermediate pelvic part, and a lower phallic part.

genital sinus. They produce an elevation known as the müllerian tubercule (Fig. 30-2), which is subsequently overgrown by epithelium derived from the wolffian duct orifices.[26] The müllerian tubercule gives rise to the seminal colliculus (verumontanum), and the remnant of the distal part of the fused müllerian ducts gives rise to the prostatic utricle[20] (Fig. 30-3), although this structure may arise solely from urogenital entodermal mucosa.[2,26,33,49,50,64]

The opening of the mesonephric ducts into the

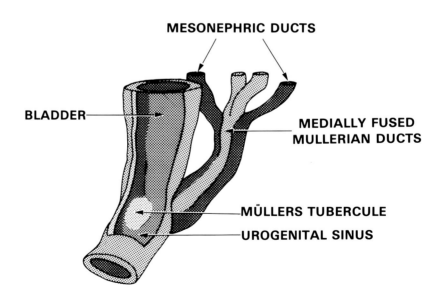

Fig. 30-2 Vesicourethral canal. At the junction of the vesicourethral canal, the fused caudal tips of the paramesonephric (müllerian) ducts and the mesonephric (wolffian) ducts form the müllerian tubercle.

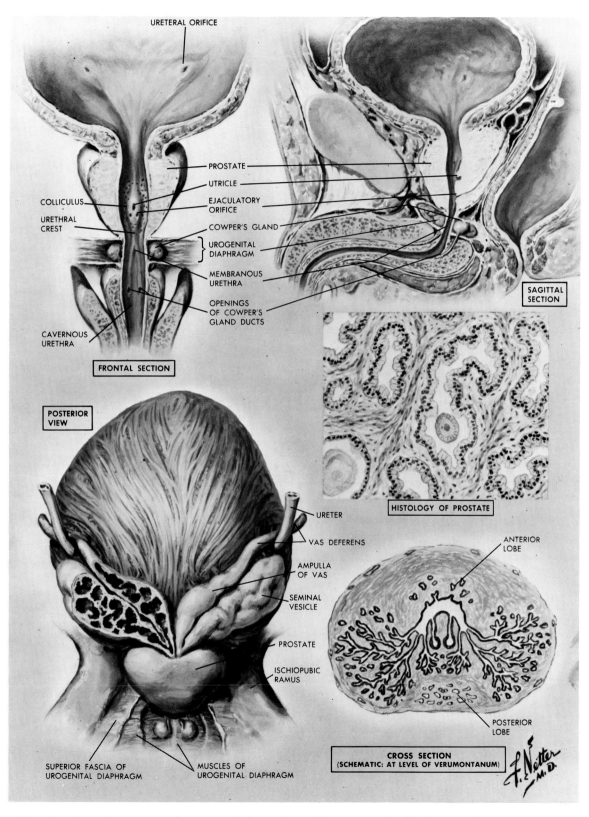

Fig. 30-3 Normal anatomy and anatomical relationships of the prostate gland (schematic). (© Copyright 1953, CIBA Pharmaceutical Company, Division of CIBA-GEIGY Corporation. Reprinted with permission from The CIBA Collection of Medical Illustrations, illustrated by Frank H. Netter, M.D. All rights reserved.)

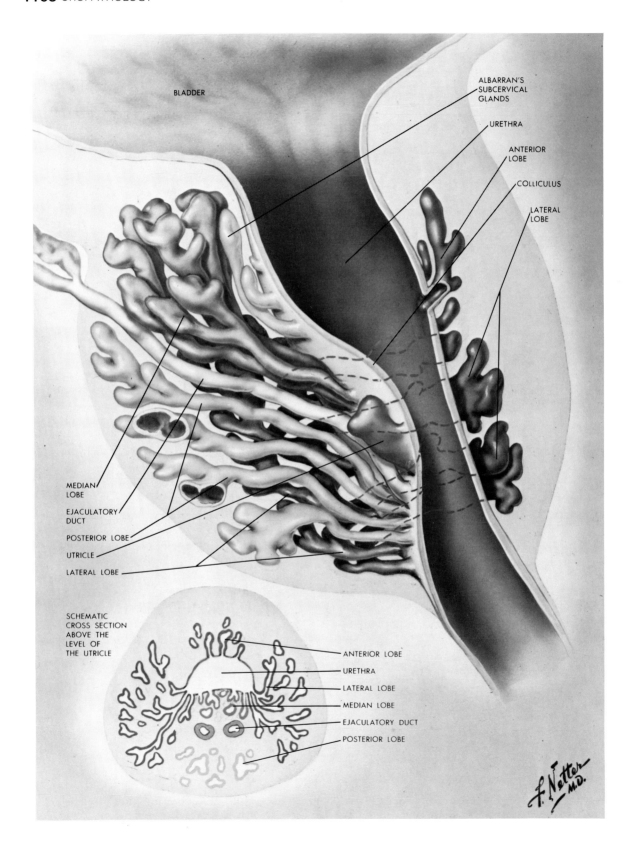

BLADDER

ALBARRAN'S SUBCERVICAL GLANDS

URETHRA

ANTERIOR LOBE

COLLICULUS

LATERAL LOBE

MEDIAN LOBE

EJACULATORY DUCT

POSTERIOR LOBE

UTRICLE

LATERAL LOBE

SCHEMATIC CROSS SECTION ABOVE THE LEVEL OF THE UTRICLE

ANTERIOR LOBE

URETHRA

LATERAL LOBE

MEDIAN LOBE

EJACULATORY DUCT

POSTERIOR LOBE

F. Netter M.D.

primitive urogenital sinus divides this structure into a cranial portion, the vesicourethral canal, and a caudal portion, the definitive urogenital sinus. As development proceeds, the upper (cranial) part of the vesicourethral canal becomes dilated and forms the bladder, and the narrow lower portion will constitute the *primitive urethra*[33] (Fig. 30-1). The definitive urogenital sinus is also divided into an upper pelvic portion (pelvic part) and a lower portion (phallic part) (Fig. 30-1). The pelvic portion of the sinus becomes the lower part of the prostatic urethra and the membranous urethra, whereas the phallic portion forms the cavernous urethra (Figs. 30-1 and 30-2). The uppermost portion of the prostatic urethra is formed by that part of the primitive urethra extending from the bladder neck to the müllerian tubercle[2] (Figs. 30-2 and 30-3).

The prostatic gland arises from a series of buds growing out from the endodermal urethral epithelium, at the level of both the primitive urethra and the pelvic portion of the urogenital sinus.[2,20,33,48–50] The buds grow into the surrounding mesenchymal tissue which then differentiates into the fibromuscular stroma characteristic of the prostate gland.

The concept of a lobar arrangement of glandular elements within the prostate was based on the embryologic studies of Lowsley,[48] who described five prostatic lobes derived from the cephalic portion of the urogenital sinus (Fig. 30-4). The paired lateral lobes originate from the lateral walls of the primitive urethra and extend upward and anteriorly to form most of the lateral lobes as well as the anterior commissure of the adult prostate. The median lobe develops from the portion of the floor of the urethra proximal to the ejaculatory duct and occupies a dorsocranial position at the angle between the posterior wall of the urethra and the ejaculatory ducts. The glands of the posterior lobe arise from the portion of the floor of the urethra distal to the verumontanum and grow backward to occupy the area behind the ejaculatory ducts. The posterior lobe remains separated from the median and lateral lobes by fibromuscular tissue which persists in adult life. The glands of the anterior lobe, although large with abundant branching in the embryo, undergo early atrophy and are reduced to negligible size in the newborn. The clinical significance of this subdivision of the prostate resides in Lowsley's assertion that the posterior lobe was the favored site for the development of carcinoma.[48]

DEVELOPMENTAL HISTOLOGY

The prostate, during the fetal and neonatal periods, undergoes metaplastic and hyperplastic changes which relate to the process of maturation but also reflect fluctuations in the hormonal environment of the host.

Up to approximately 24 weeks of gestation, the prostatic glands are scarce and consist mostly of solid cords, but from then up to term the number of acini increases and they develop lumina.[1,9,62] Near birth, some of the acini are lined by tall columnar epithelium and reveal focal hyperplastic changes, which subside at about 4 weeks to 6 weeks after birth.[9,62]

Squamous metaplasia is a striking histologic feature in the prostate of the fetus and newborn.[1,9,49,50,62,76] It can be detected as early as the fifth month of gestation and regresses after birth, but traces may still be present at about 2 months of age.[1,9,76] Squamous metaplasia occurs particularly in the prostatic utriculus, the terminal portions of the prostatic ducts, especially the uppermost ducts in the area of the medial lobe, and in the posterior urethral wall, partly in the area of the colliculus seminalis.[1,62,63,76] The squamous metaplasia and hyperplasia in the fetal and newborn prostate result from the effects of maternal estrogens.[1,63,76] Experimental data in animals subjected to prolonged estrogenic stimulation and observations on adult males and children treated with estrogens support the contention of a sustained estrogenic stimulus as the cause of such metaplastic and hyperplastic changes.[26,63,76] The squamous metaplastic changes described in the fetal prostates are more prominent in what will later correspond to the inner zone, in the estrogen-sensitive or "female" portion of the prostate, implicated as the site of the development of nodular hyperplasia in the elderly.[1,24–27,33,63,68]

POSTNATAL GROWTH AND DEVELOPMENT OF THE PROSTATE

There is very little growth of the prostate during the first 5 years of life, so that up to that age the prostate is only slightly larger than that of the newborn. Average measurements of the prostate during the first 5 years showed a length of 1.2 cm, a width of 1.5 cm, and a thickness of 0.9 cm. There is a great increase in the size of the prostate after the 12th year of age. Between 15 years and 20 years of age the length averages 3.0 cm, the width 3.8 cm, and the thickness 2.1 cm. The prostate gland reaches adult size during the third decade, the average figure for the length being 3.3 cm, for the width 4.1 cm, and for the thickness 2.4 cm.[49,50,61]

During childhood, there is a gradual increase in the number of acini, and by ten years of age these have developed more definite lumina and appear lined by tall cuboidal cells, although the epithelium remains pseudostratified until full maturation at puberty.[62]

STRUCTURE OF THE PROSTATE IN THE ADULT

The lobe boundaries cannot be readily identified in the adult prostate,[24,25] and the studies of LeDuc[45] of prostates injected with opaque material did not show the existence of the posterior lobe described in the fetus by Lowsley.[48]

In transverse sections of the adult prostate, the glands are arranged in concentric groups of inner mucosal glands, intermediate submucosal glands, and external (main or outer) glands[24,25] (Fig. 30-5). The true prostatic glands of the outer zone seem to correspond to the lateral and posterior lobes of Lowsley[48] (Fig. 30-4). Embryologically, the glands of the outer zone derive from the endodermal lining of the pelvic part

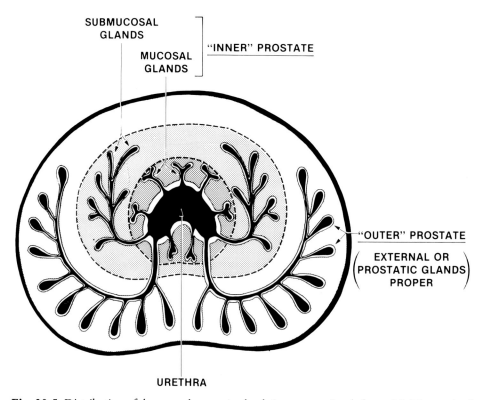

Fig. 30-5 Distribution of the normal prostatic glands in cross-section (schematic). The urethral (mucosal) and submucosal glands together form the inner group, which is separated from the outer gland group by an inconstant capsule.

of the definitive urogenital sinus (future prostatic urethra)[26,33] (Fig. 30-1). They are formed around the 12th week as buds from the wall of the urethra, lateral to the verumontanum. The inner prostatic zone includes the colliculus seminalis, derived from the müllerian tubercle, the prostatic utricle, and the glands of the median lobe (Figs. 30-2 and 30-3) and develops later than the outer zone. All these structures develop in an area of composite epithelial origin, including admixture of endodermal urogenital sinus cells and mesodermal mesonephric (wolffian) and paramesonephric (müllerian) cells. This region has been described as the estrogen-sensitive zone of the urogenital sinus in the human male.[12,76,93] The selective sensitivity of the inner groups of glands to estrogens suggests that this "female" area is probably derived from the müllerian system.

The dual origin of the epithelial glandular elements of the prostate may account for the differences in sensitivity to estrogenic stimulus.[41] Beckman et al.[3] have stressed the histogenic potential of this area of the urethral crest as a source of differentiated estrogen-sensitive müllerian tissue, describing foci of endometriosis in the area of the internal urethral orifice and adjacent prostate in a man after a long-term course of estrogen treatment.

McNeil[58,59] described four basic anatomic zones in the prostate: peripheral, central, transitional, and anterior. The *peripheral* zone comprises approximately 75 percent of the glandular tissue and derives from duct buds arising from the lateral recesses of the posterior urethral wall. These ducts radiate laterally from the portion of the urethra distal to the verumontanum. The *central* zone derives from ducts originating in the convexity of the verumontanum around the ejaculatory ducts. The acini arising from these ducts are oriented proximally and laterally around the ejaculatory ducts. The central zone is conically shaped and surrounds the ejaculatory ducts, whereas the peripheral zone is at first located laterally and posteriorly to the central zone but expands anteriorly at the level of the verumontanum. The *transition* zone develops from the periurethral duct system originating at the junction of the proximal and distal urethra. After clearing the lower border of the smooth muscle sphincter that surrounds the proximal urethra, the ducts progress anteriorly and upward toward the bladder neck, nearly parallel to the periurethral glands that remain encased between the urethral wall and

smooth muscle sphincter. The *anterior* muscular stroma is virtually devoid of glands, but nevertheless constitutes approximately one-third of the bulk of the prostate and is responsible for the characteristic convexity of the anterior surface of the organ.

There are clinicoanatomic correlations in McNeil's zonal subdivisions. The smallest benign prostatic hyperplasia nodules arise either in the transition zone or in the periurethral submucosal glandular region. Pathologic processes rarely originate in the central zone, whereas the vast majority of prostatic carcinomas arise in the peripheral zone.

ANATOMIC RELATIONS OF THE PROSTATE

These are schematically illustrated in Figure 30-3. The pointed lower extremity, or apex, and the inferolateral surfaces of the prostate rest against the fascia of the levator ani. There is considerable variation in the prostatic apex.[63a] Some prostates have only a small anterior commissure and an apical notch below where the urethra and its external (skeletal muscles) sphincter lie. In others the commissure is large and extends to the apex, with the sphincteric fibers spreading out over the capsule at the point where the urethra penetrates the apex. Preservation of this external sphincter as high up as possible is one of the keys to ensuring continence post-prostatectomy.

The base or upper end of the prostate is partly embedded in and continuous with the base of the bladder. The anterior surface faces the pubis and is attached to it by puboprostatic ligaments. The posterior surface is in contact with the lower ends of the vas deferens and seminal vesicles, which in conjunction with the rectovesical septum (Denonvilliers' fascia) and the rectal fascia separate the prostate from the rectum.[36,37,49,50]

Externally, the fibromuscular stroma of the prostate condenses into a capsule (true capsule) from which strands of connective tissue extend into the gland proper.[49,50] The capsule of the prostate is surrounded, particularly laterally and anteriorly, by a connective tissue fascia or sheath. At all surfaces of the prostate this fascia blends or becomes continuous with other fascia or ligaments, such as the puboprostatic ligaments, the fascial sheath of the bladder, and the rectovesical septum. The rectovesical septum is applied to the posterior surface of the bladder, seminal vesicles, and prostate and is attached above to the peritoneum of the rectovesical pouch, laterally to the walls and floor of the pelvis, and inferiorly also to the levator ani behind the prostate. The rectovesical septum has also been designated as the prostatoperitoneal membrane and Denonvilliers' fascia.[36,37,49,50]

The surgical or false capsule of the prostate is a band of newly formed connective tissue arising between hyperplastic nodules and compressed peripheral tissue. The glands of the true prostate compressed by the hyperplastic nodules may undergo atrophy, inhibition of secretion, and focal degradation.[8] It has been suggested that these atrophic, compressed glands are the favorite site for the origin of carcinoma in the prostate,[8,60,70] based on the assumption that the initiation of malignant growth in general may be preceded by a phase of cellular inhibition.[31]

INNERVATION OF THE PROSTATE

The autonomic innervation of the pelvic organs, including the bladder, prostate, seminal vesicles, ejaculatory ducts, and corpora cavernosa, is derived from the pelvic plexus (inferior hypogastric plexus), from which the vesical, prostatic, and cavernous plexus originate.[36,37]

The pelvic plexus is formed by sympathetic fibers arising from the thoracolumbar center (T11–L2) and parasympathetic visceral efferent preganglionic fibers derived from the sacral center (S2–S4).[46]

The sympathetic nerves from the prostatic plexus to the prostate gland have a motor function and produce the contraction of the smooth muscle fibers surrounding the acini, necessary for the release of the prostatic secretion into the urethra. Pain fibers emanating from the prostate run along parasympathetic fibers from sacral nerves S2 to S4.[36,37,65] The branches of the pelvic plexus that innervate the corpora cavernosa (cavernous nerves) are first contained within the prostatic plexus and reach the corpora cavernosa after penetration of the urogenital diaphragm, near the muscular wall of the urethra.[46,89] The pathway of the cavernous nerves from the pelvic plexus to the point of the penetration of the urogenital diaphragm includes a passage located dorsolaterally between the rectum and prostate,[46,51,89] and through this itinerary the cavernous nerves are topographically related to

the urethra, the capsule of the prostate, and the fascia of Denonvilliers. These nerves need to be spared during urologic pelvic procedures to prevent iatrogenic impotence.[46,51,89]

HISTOLOGY

Histologically, the prostate is composed of tubuloalveolar glands lined by columnar or cuboidal cells (Fig. 30-6). On reaching the urethral outlet, the epithelial lining acquires transitional features similar to those seen in the lining of the urethra and the urinary bladder. The ducts of the mucosal glands open at various points in the urethra, whereas the ducts of the submucosal and main, external glands open into the posterolateral urethral grooves or sinuses (Figs. 30-3 and 30-5).

Two layers of cells line the alveoli (Fig. 30-6). The flat basal cells are applied against the basement membrane, and their scanty cytoplasm appears interspersed between the cuboidal or columnar cells, without reaching the luminal border of the alveolus. The cuboidal or columnar secretory cells may rest on the basement membrane or on top of the basal cells, and their apical borders reach the lumen of the alveolus. The nuclei of the secretory cells are located basally, toward the periphery of the acini, indicating their functional polarity. Their contour is regular, and the chromatin is finely dispersed. Nucleoli are very rarely seen. The nuclei of the basal cells are elongated and oriented parallel to the basement membrane (Fig. 30-6) and have a markedly condensed chromatin network. The collagen fibers and smooth muscle cells of the stroma follow the contour of the alveoli.

There are variations in the histologic appearance of the stroma and the glandular elements in the different anatomic regions of the prostate.[24,25,58,59,73] In the peripheral zone, the ducts originate from the prostatic sinus in the area lateral and distal to the verumontanum (Fig. 30-3) and they are long and narrow and branch into small regular acini with rounded profiles devoid of papillary projections. The cells in these glands are simple columnar and reveal basally located small nuclei with a condensed uniform chromatin pattern. The glands of the central zone, which originate mainly from the area of the convexity of the verumontanum immediately surrounding the ejaculatory duct orifices (Fig. 30-3), reveal a system of

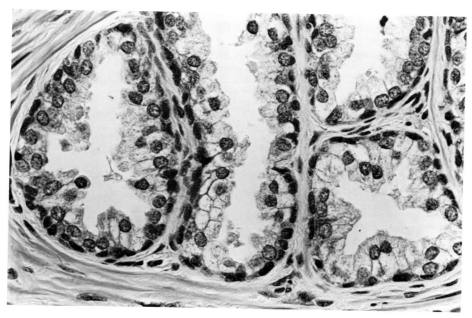

Fig. 30-6 Normal prostate. Two cell layers seen in normal acini. Basal cells and secretory cells. ×450.

ducts with elaborate and expanded terminal acini and prominent papillary intraacinar infoldings.

The stroma of the prostate consists of connective tissue and smooth muscle fibers, some of which extend from the condensed fibromuscular stroma surrounding the urethra.[49,50] The fibromuscular stroma in the central zone is prominent and thick, but it is more delicate in the peripheral zone. In both zones, the ducts and acini are surrounded by slender smooth muscle fibers, which upon contraction may contribute to the expression of their secretion into the urethra.[4,23,49,50] This periglandular layer of smooth muscle fibers is absent in the periurethral group of glands. Salander et al.[73] divided the prostate into medial, dorsal, and lateral lobes and found increased arborization of the acini and prominent papillary infoldings in the medial lobes, whereas the stroma was less dense than in the lateral and dorsal lobes.

The relevant markings in the prostatic urethra are best observed by cutting away the anterior wall including the isthmus of the gland (Fig. 30-3). There is an elevation of the posterior wall, the urethral crest, that is continuous above with the neck of the bladder and widens in the lower part of the urethra to form the more prominent verumontanum or colliculus semin-

alis. In the midline of the verumontanum and somewhat distal to the center is the slitlike opening of the prostatic utricle (uterus masculinus). The ejaculatory ducts also open on the verumontanum near the opening of the utricle. At each side of the crest and the verumontanum there is a linear depression, the prostatic sinus, that nests the openings of the prostatic ducts (Fig. 30-3).

PHYSIOLOGY

The exocrine secretion of the prostate contributes considerably to the volume of the seminal plasma,[55,57,92] but the specific role of the various substances produced by the prostate gland in the biology of spermatoza and the fertilization process are not thoroughly clarified.[13,23,92]

Mann[55,57] extensively investigated the biochemical components of prostatic fluid and its contribution to the composition of semen, as well as the effect of nutritional status on the quantitative and qualitative characteristic of prostatic fluid.[56] Prostatic secretion is under hormonal and pharmacologic control,[23,39,55,57,69] and the basal rate of flow of the secretion may relate to the development of prostatic concretions and the incidence of cancer.[42]

There is a continued basal flow of prostatic fluid, even in the absence of ejaculation.[42] This was demonstrated by the work of Scott and Huggins,[75] who showed a net increase of acid phosphatase in the urine of postpubertal males compared with that in prepubertal males or age-matched females. Huggins and colleagues[39,40] estimated that the 20 hour basal fluid output of the prostate in humans was 0.5 ml to 2.0 ml/day, and according to Lundquist,[52] the output during active ejaculation was 0.5 ml to 1.0 ml.

The mechanism of secretion in the human prostate is partly apocrine,[6,7,35] and this may explain the remarkably high content in the seminal plasma of material normally found within intact cells and tissues such as flavoproteins and various oxidizing enzymes.[55] This is best illustrated by the presence of transaminases, dehydrogenases, and intermediary enzymes of glycolysis in the seminal plasma.[55,57] Acid phosphatase and citric acid are among the most characteristic components of prostatic fluid and seminal plasma, and their production and secretion are under androgenic control.[57] At its optimal pH level below 6, acid phosphatase is capable of catalyzing the hydrolysis of many phosphoproteins and polynucleotides of low molecular weight.[23]

Several proteolytic enzymes in the prostatic secretion, including fibrinolysin, fibrinogenase, and aminopeptidase, may act synergistically in the liquifaction of coagulated human semen,[23,55,80] and the release of these enzymes into the blood stream in patients with metastatic prostatic carcinoma may cause serious bleeding problems. Prostatic fibrinolysis has been described as a syndrome[80] in some patients with advanced cancer of the prostate and consists of hypofibrinogenemia and bleeding. Tissue fibrinolysin decreased in prostatic cancer patients treated with estrogens; although it remained unchanged in orchiectomized patients and increased significantly in those treated with cyproterone acetate.[83] There may also be depression of serum antithrombin III activity, which may be further reduced by estrogen therapy.[82,83] The reduction in fibrinolytic activity and the depression of antithrombin III activity in prostatic cancer patients treated with estrogens may contribute to increased risk of thromboembolic phenomena in these patients.[82,83]

Acid phosphatase activity in seminal plasma correlates with the secretory activity of the glandular tissue. It is very low in newborn infants and increases considerably in adults. Citric acid is another prominent component of the secretion, in which it is equal in concentration to sodium, and serves to lower the pH to about 6.5.[23] The ability to produce citric acid is preserved in metastatic prostatic cancer tissue.[53] Seminal fluid also contains prostaglandins derived from the seminal vesicles (PGE_2) and from the prostate gland ($PGF_2\alpha$). $PGF_2\alpha$ increases the binding of testosterone in vitro, stimulates the cyclic AMP-dependent secretion of some intracellular materials, and increases the motility of the fibromuscular stroma to facilitate the transport of secretory products from storage in the acini into the pool of seminal fluid.[23]

Many factors are involved in prostatic secretion, including parasympathetic and sympathetic stimulation resulting in contraction of the stromal smooth muscle fibers with gradual progression of the secretion as ejaculate.[23] Cyclic AMP and a sodium pump apparatus, which is stimulated and appears to be completely under the control of androgens, are also important factors in the production and propulsion of prostatic secretion into the ejaculate.[23]

ZINC

There is a high concentration of zinc in the human prostate, as well as in the testes and other accessory male organs.[14] The content of zinc in the prostate is about 70 mg/100 g (dry weight).[55,57] The metal appears to be associated with a zinc-binding protein.[30] Localization of administered [65]Zn in the glandular epithelium has been demonstrated by autoradiography.[19] The localization of zinc in prostatic glandular epithelium has also been shown by histochemical staining techniques and by atomic absorption spectrophotometry.[29]

Zinc uptake, content, and excretion appear to be under hormonal control, but species differences have been noted experimentally.[28] Estrogens and castration produced a decrease in uptake of zinc, which in the castrate could be restored by administration of testosterone. Hypophysectomy also lowered zinc uptake, which could be restored by testosterone administration.[28] Pituitary hormones, particularly prolactin, growth hormone, and human chorionic gonadotropin, affect ^{65}Zn uptake by the prostate.[14,28,71] Atomic absorption spectrophotometry studies[29] have indicated a decrease of Zn content in human prostatic carcinoma, but thus far, there is no definitive evidence as to whether the uptake of ^{65}Zn is decreased in human prostate cancer.[14] In contrast, zinc levels are increased in benign prostatic hyperplasia.[14] Clinical trials with dithizone (diphenylcarbazone), a chelating agent with affinity for zinc, have been conducted in patients with prostate cancer without clear-cut evidence of any beneficial effects.[14] Toxic effects on the lungs and brain have been reported in dogs after the administration of dithizone, presumably owing to the high contents of zinc in such organs.[14] Clinical studies in humans receiving ^{65}Zn revealed a low absorption in prostatic cancer patients in the active phase of the disease. Absorption of ^{65}Zn became normal during estrogen-induced remission, but no change occurred in prostatic cancer patients who failed to respond to estrogen therapy.[78]

HORMONAL CONTROL OF PROSTATIC GROWTH

Hormonal interactions that integrate the hypothalamic-hypophysial-testicular axis in the control of prostatic structure and function are represented schematically in Figure 30-7. Normal and abnormal growth of prostatic tissue is dependent on testicular hormones, and it is believed that prepubertal orchiectomy may prevent the development of prostatic hyperplasia.[85,88,90]

Clinical and experimental animal studies have attempted to establish whether hormonal changes in the course of aging might be responsible for the development of abnormal stromal-glandular nodularity in the prostate of the elderly.[15,87,88,90,91]

Testicular androgens control the differentiation of the prostate during embryogenesis and its maturation at puberty and are responsible for the preservation of functional and structural integrity in the adult. The principal circulating androgen is testosterone, produced by the testes under the control of pituitary luteinizing hormone (LH) (Fig. 30-7) and circulating either bound to a protein or as free testosterone. In the castrated male,[17] androgen produced by the adrenal gland may represent the primary source of androgen. Upon entering the prostatic epithelial cells, approximately 90 percent of the free testosterone is metabolized to dihydrotestosterone (DHT)[10,11,90] by the action of the enzyme 5-alpha-reductase, which is located in the endoplasmic reticulum and the nuclear membrane.[10,11,16-18,90] DHT is regarded as the active androgen that mediates intracellular action of androgens,[10,11,90,91] and it can undergo reversible metabolism to 3-α-androstanediol. Testosterone can also be converted to 17-β-estradiol in many tissues, especially adipose tissue. After binding to a specific high-affinity androgen receptor protein in the cytosol, DHT is transported to the nucleus, where the DHT-receptor complex interacts with a nuclear acceptor and results in messenger and ribosomal RNA synthesis, protein synthesis, and cell replication.[10,11,16-18,21]

Significant changes occur in the endocrine status of the male and in the functional properties of prostatic tissues during aging.[70,85,90] LH levels may be increased in 62 percent of men above the age of 70.[5,17,18,79] LH levels, in several studies, have shown increments of the following magnitude: means LH levels of 9.0 mU/ml in men 20 years to 60 years old, increased to 13.1 mU/ml in men 60 years to 90 years old[66]; 13.0 mU/ml in men below the age of 50, compared with 24.1 mU/ml after the age of 65 years.[72] When men between the ages of 16 years and 40 years were compared with those above 41 years of age, a significant increase in LH levels was detected during each decade after the age of 41.[43]

Changes in sex hormone levels occur during aging, in benign prostatic hyperplasia, and in prostatic carcinoma.[17,18,22,38,43,72,84,85,90,91] Plasma testosterone levels reach a plateau after puberty, with individual values between 280 ng and 1,000 ng/dl and a mean of 600 ng/dl.[17,18,84,85] Testosterone is largely bound to plasma proteins. Approximately 2 percent is free, and only a fraction not specifically bound is biologically active.[17,18,84,85] After the sixth decade, a gradual decrease in plasma testosterone level takes place, but this decrease shows broad individual variations.[84,85,90] Owing to a gradual increase of testosterone estradiol-binding globulin (Te BG) with aging, free testosterone levels have already begun to decline in the fifth decade, and the concomitant decrease in total levels of testosterone results in a steeper decline of free testosterone.[84,85] Other hormones of testicular or adrenal

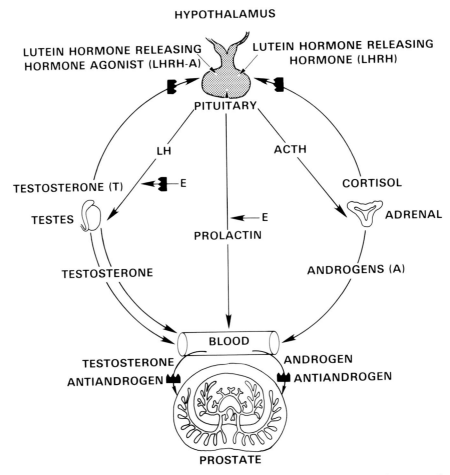

Fig. 30-7 Hypothalamic-pituitary-gonadal-prostatic axis: hormonal control of prostatic function and growth (schematic). Lutein hormone releasing hormone (LHRH) controls the synthesis and release of luteinizing hormone (LH), which in turn controls the synthesis of testosterone (T) by the testes. Prostatic growth is stimulated by prolactin. Estrogens (E) stimulate prolactin production, but inhibit LH production and hence testosterone output by the testes. Testosterone inhibits LH secretion. Sustained exposure to LHRH-A interferes with the pulsatile pattern of LHRH necessary for stimulating LH release. Antiandrogens block the effects of androgens at the level of target tissue. Stimulation: ⟶ ; inhibition-suppression: ▲ .

origin that decrease with aging include 5-androstane-3,17β-diol, 17-hydroxyprogesterone, 17-hydroxypregnenolone, and pregnenolone.[67,84,85] There is no clear-cut evidence as to whether DHT levels in plasma also decrease with age.[32,67,84–86,90]

The decreased production of testosterone by the testis with aging, particularly after the age of 60,[44,84] may relate to an age-dependent structural alteration of the testes, such as changes in cytochemical properties[54] and reduction in Leydig cell mass.[34,81] These testicular changes and the increase in both LH and follicle-stimulating hormone (FSH) levels in plasma in the aging male[43,66,74,79,84] might indicate a testicular origin of decreased testosterone secretion, but administration of human chorionic gonadotropin produces an increase in levels of plasma testosterone.[47,77,84] Stimulation with gonadotropin-releasing hormone, in turn, induces an increase of LH and FSH output, but such response might be somewhat weaker in older individuals.[77,84]

Estradiol levels in the male, on the other hand, do not decrease during aging, but appear to be slightly, but significantly, higher in elderly individuals.[67,72,84] The concomitant rise in Te BG with aging provokes a further fall in free testosterone concentration and results in a relative increment of the ratio of free estradiol to free testosterone levels. These alterations in sex hormone production, particularly in the estrogen/androgen balance in the elderly male, may be implicated in the development of benign prostatic hyperplasia.

REFERENCES

1. Andrews GS: The histology of the human fetal and prepubertal prostates. J Anat 85:44, 1951
2. Arey LB: Developmental Anatomy. 7th Ed. WB Saunders, Philadelphia, 1965
3. Beckman EN, Leonard GL, Pintado SO, Sternberg WH: Endometriosis of the prostate. Am J Surg Pathol 9:374, 1985
4. Blacklock NJ: Surgical Anatomy. p. 473. In Chisholm GD, Williams DI (eds): Scientific Foundations of Urology. Year Book Medical Publishers, Chicago, 1982
5. Boyar RM, Hellman LD: Hypothalamus-pituitary function: LH changes with age. p. 153. In Grayhack JT, Wilson JD, Scherbenske MJ (eds): Benign Prostatic Hyperplasia. Department of Health, Education and Welfare (NIH) Publication no. 76-1113, 1976
6. Brandes D: The fine structure and histochemistry of prostatic glands in relation to sex hormones. Int Rev Cytol 20:207, 1966
7. Brandes D: Fine structure and cytochemistry of male sex accessory organs. p. 18. In Brandes D (ed): Male Accessory Sex Organs: Structure and Function in Mammals. Academic Press, Orlando, 1974
8. Brandes D, Kirchheim D, Scott WW: Ultrastructure of the human prostate: normal and neoplastic. Lab Invest 13:1541, 1964
9. Brody H, Goldman SF: Metaplasia of the epithelium of the prostate glands, utricle and urethra of the fetus and newborn infant. Arch Pathol 29:494, 1940
10. Bruchovsky N, Wilson JD: The conversion of testosterone to 5-α-androstan-17β-ol-3-one by rat prostate in vivo and in vitro. J Biol Chem 243:2012, 1968
11. Bruchovsky N, Wilson JD: The intranuclear binding of testosterone and 5-α-androstan-17β-ol-3-one by rat prostate. J Biol Chem 243:5953, 1968
12. Bulmer D: The epithelium of the urogenital sinus in female human foetuses. J Anat 93:491, 1959
13. Burgos MH: Biochemical and functional properties related to sperm metabolism and fertility. p. 151. In Brandes D (ed): Male Accessory Sex Organs: Structure and Function in Mammals. Academic Press, Orlando, 1974
14. Byar DP: Zinc in male sex accessory organs: distribution and hormonal response. p. 161. In Brandes D (ed): Male Accessory Sex Organs: Structure and Function in Mammals. Academic Press, Orlando, 1974
15. Chesterman FC, Franks LM, Williams PC: Effects of age, castration and stilbestrol treatment on the guinea pig prostate and associated structures. p. 223. In Grayhack JT, Wilson JD, Scherbenske MJ (eds): Benign Prostatic Hyperplasia. Department of Health, Education and Welfare (NIH) Publication no. 76-1113, 1976
16. Coffey DS: The effects of androgens on DNA and RNA synthesis in sex accessory tissue. p. 307. In Brandes D (ed): Male Accessory Sex Organs: Structure and Function in Mammals. Academic Press, Orlando, 1974
17. Coffey DS: Physiological control of prostatic growth: an overview. p. 4. In Coffey DS, Isaacs JT (eds): Prostate Cancer. Vol. 48. UICC Technical Report Series, Geneva, 1979
18. Coffey DS: The biochemistry and physiology of the prostate and seminal vesicles. p. 161. In Harrison JH, Gittes RF, Perlmutter AD et al (eds): Campbell's Urology. Vol. 1. WB Saunders, Philadelphia, 1985
19. Daniel O, Haddad F, Prout G, Whitmore WF, Jr.: Some observations on distribution of radioactive zinc in prostate and other human tissues. Br J Urol 28:271, 1956
20. Davies J: Human Developmental Anatomy. Ronald Press, New York, 1963
21. DeKlerk DP, Heston WDW, Coffey DS: Studies on the role of macromolecular synthesis in the growth of the prostate. p. 43. In Grayhack JT, Wilson JD, Scherbenske MJ (eds): Benign Prostatic Hyperplasia. Department of Health, Education and Welfare (NIH) Publication no. 76-1113, 1976
22. Ewing LL: Testis: changes with age. p. 195. In Grayhack JT, Wilson JD, Scherbenske MJ (eds): Benign Prostatic Hyperplasia. Department of Health, Education and Welfare (NIH) Publication no. 76-1113, 1976
23. Farnsworth WE: Physiology and biochemistry of prostatic secretion. p. 485. In Chisholm GD, Williams DI (eds): Scientific Foundations of Urology. 2nd Ed. W. Heineman Medical Book Publications, Portsmouth, NH, 1982
24. Franks LM: Benign nodular hyperplasia of the prostate: a review. Ann R Coll Surg Engl 14:92, 1954

25. Franks LM: Benign prostatic hyperplasia: gross and microscopic anatomy. p. 63. In Grayhack JT, Wilson JD, Scherbenske MJ (eds): Benign Prostatic Hyperplasia. Department of Health, Education and Welfare (NIH) Publication no. 76-1113, 1976

26. Glenister TW: The developement of the utricle and of the so-called "middle" or "median" lobe of the human prostate. J Anat 96:443, 1962

27. Gray SW, Skandalakis JE: Embryology for Surgeons. p. 596. WB Saunders, Philadelphia, 1972

28. Gunn SA, Gould TC, Anderson WAD: The effect of growth hormone and prolactin preparations on the control of intestinal cell-stimulating hormone of uptake of ^{65}Zn by the rat dorsolateral prostate. J Endocrinol 32:205, 1965

29. Gyorkey F, Kyung-Whan M, Huff JA, Gyorkey P: Zinc and magnesium in human prostate gland: normal, hyperplastic and neoplastic. Cancer Res 27:1348, 1967

30. Habib FK, Stitch SR: The interrelationship of the metal and androgen binding proteins in normal and cancerous human prostatic tissues. Acta Endocrinol, suppl., 199:129, 1975

31. Haddow A: Cellular inhibition and the origin of cancer. Acta Un Int Contr Cancer 3:342, 1938

32. Hallberg MC, Wieland RG, Zorn EM et al : Impaired Leydig cell reserve and altered serum androgen binding in the aging male. Fertil Steril 27:812, 1976

33. Hamilton WJ, Boyd JD, Mossman HW: Human Embryology. 3rd Ed. Williams & Wilkins, Baltimore, 1962

34. Harbitz TB: Morphometric studies of the Leydig cells in elderly men with special reference to the histology of the prostate. An analysis in an autopsy series. Acta Pathol Microbiol Scand Sect A 81:301, 1973

35. Heidger PM, Jr., Feuchter FA, Hawtrey CE: Scanning and transmission electron microscopy of human prostatic carcinoma. p. 185. In Yates R, Gordon M (eds): Male Reproductive System. Masson, New York, 1977

36. Hollinshead WH: Anatomy for Surgeons. Vol. 2, 2nd Ed. Harper & Row, New York, 1971

37. Hollinshead WH: Textbook of Anatomy, 3rd Ed. Harper & Row, Hagerstown, Maryland, 1974

38. Horton RJ: Androgen hormones and prehormones in young and elderly men. p. 183. In Grayhack JT, Wilson JD, Scherbenske MF (eds): Benign Prostatic Hyperplasia. Department of Health, Education and Welfare (NIH) Publication no. 76-1113, 1976

39. Huggins C: The prostatic secretions. Harvey Lecture 42:148, 1946–47

40. Huggins C, Scott WW, Heimen JH: Chemical composition of human semen and of the secretions of the prostate and seminal vesicle. Am J Physiol 136:467, 1941

41. Huggins C, Webster WO: Duality of the human prostate in response to estrogen. J Urol 59:258, 1948

42. Isaacs JT: Prostatic structure and function in relation to the etiology of prostatic cancer. Prostate 4:351, 1983

43. Isurugi K, Fukutani K., Takayasu H et al : Age-related changes in serum luteinizing hormone (LH) and follicle-stimulating hormone (FSH) levels in normal men. J Clin Endocrinol 39:955, 1974

44. Kent J, Acone A: Testosterone metabolic clearance in elderly men. p. 31. In Vermeulen A (ed): Androgens. Vol. 101. Excerpta Medica, Amsterdam, 1966

45. LeDuc IE: The anatomy of the prostate and the pathology of early benign hypertrophy. J Urol 42:1217, 1939

46. Lepor H, Gregerman M, Crosby R et al: Precise localization of the autonomic nerves from the pelvic plexus to the corpora cavernosa: a detailed anatomical study of the adult male pelvis. J Urol 133:207, 1985

47. Longcope C: The effect of human chorionic gonadotropin on plasma steroid levels in young and old men. Steroids 21:583, 1973

48. Lowsley OS: The development of the human prostate gland with reference to the development of other structures at the neck of the urinary bladder. Am J Anat 13:299, 1912

49. Lowsley OS: The prostate gland. In Lowsley OS, Hinman F, Smith DR, Gutierrez R (eds): The Sexual Glands of the Male. Oxford University Press, New York, 1942

50. Lowlsey OS, Kirwin TJ: Embryology, anatomy, anomalies and physiology of the prostate gland. p. 787. In Clinical Urology. 3rd Ed. Williams & Wilkins, Baltimore, 1956

51. Lue TF, Zeineh SJ, Schmidt RA, Tanagho EA: Neuroanatomy of penile erection: its relevance to iatrogenic impotence. J Urol 131:273, 1984

52. Lundquist F: Aspects of the biochemistry of human semen. Acta Physiol Scand, suppl., 19:66, 1949

53. Lutwak-Mann C: Citric acid in metastasizing carcinoma of the prostate gland. NCI Monogr 12:307, 1963

54. Lynch KM, Jr, Scott WW: The lipid content of the Leydig cell and Sertoli cell in the human testis as related to age, benign prostatic hyperplasia and prostatic cancer. J Urol 64:767, 1950

55. Mann T: Biochemistry of the prostate gland and its secretion. NCI Monogr 12:235, 1963

56. Mann T: Effects of nutrition on male accessory organs. p. 173. In Brandes D (ed): Male Accessory Sex Organs: Structure and Function in Mammals. Academic Press, Orlando, 1974

57. Mann T: Biochemistry of semen. p. 461. In Greep RO, Astwood EB (eds): Handbook of Physiology. Male Reproductive System. Vol. 5. Williams & Wilkins, Baltimore, 1975

58. McNeal JE: The zonal anatomy of the prostate. Prostate 2:35, 1981
59. McNeal JE: Normal and pathologic anatomy of prostate. Urology, suppl., 17:11, 1981
60. Moore RA: The morphology of small prostatic carcinoma. J Urol 33:224, 1935
61. Moore RA: The evolution and involution of the prostate gland. Am J Pathol 12:599, 1936
62. Moore RA: The histology of the newborn and prepubertal prostate gland. Anat Rec 66:1, 1936
63. Moore RA, McLellan AM: A histological study of the effect of sex hormones on the human prostate. J Urol 40:641, 1938
63a. Myers RP, Goellner, JP, Cahill, DR: Prostate shape, external striated urethral sphincter and radical prostatectomy: the apical dissection. J Urol 138:543, 1987
64. Narbaitz R: Embryology, anatomy, and histology of the male sex accessory glands. p. 3. In Brandes D (ed): Male Accessory Sex Organs: Structure and Function in Mammals. Academic Press, Orlando, 1974
65. Netter F: The Ciba Collection of Medical Illustrations—Reproductive System. p. 18. Ciba, Summit NJ, 1961
66. Nieschlag E, Kley KH, Wilgelmann W: Age dependence of the endocrine testicular function in adult men. Acta Endocrinol, suppl., 177:122, 1973 (Abstract)
67. Pirke KM, Doerr P: Age related changes in free plasma testosterone, dihydrotestosterone and oestradiol. Acta Endocrinol 89:171, 1975
68. Raynaud A: The histogenesis of urogenital and mammary tissues sensitive to estrogens. p. 179. In Zuckerman S (ed): The Ovary. Vol. 2. Academic Press, Orlando, 1961
69. Reeves DS: Pharmacology of the prostate. p. 514. In Chisholm GD, Williams DI (eds): Scientific Foundations of Urology. 2nd Ed. Year Book Medical Publishers, Chicago, 1982
70. Rich AR: On the frequency of occurrence of occult carcinoma of the prostate. J Urol 33:215, 1935
71. Rosoff B, Martin CR: Effect of gonadotropins and of testosterone on organ weights and zinc-65 uptake in the male rat. Gen Comp Endocrinol 10:75, 1968
72. Rubens R, Dhont M, Vermeulen A: Further studies on Leydig cell function in old ages. J Clin Endocr 39:40, 1974
73. Salander H, Johansson S, Tissell LE: The histology of dorsal, lateral and medial prostatic lobes in man. Invest Urol 18:479, 1981
74. Schalch DS, Parlow AF, Boon RC, Reichlein S: Measurement of human luteinizing hormone in plasma by radioimmunoassay. J Clin Invest 47:665, 1968
75. Scott WW, Huggins C: The acid phosphatase activity of human urine, an index of prostatic secretion. Endocrinology 30:106, 1942
76. Sharpey-Schaefer EP, Zuckerman S: The effect of estrogenic stimulation on the human prostate at birth. J Endocrinol 2:431, 1940
77. Snyder PJ: Effect of age on the serum LH and FSH responses to gonadotropin-releasing hormone. p. 161. In Grayhack JT, Wilson JD, Scherbenske MJ (eds): Benign Prostatic Hyperplasia. Department of Health, Education and Welfare (NIH) Publication no. 76-1113, 1976
78. Spencer H, Kramer L, Osis D et al : Zinc^{65} absorption in patients with carcinoma of the prostate. Prostate 1:239, 1980
79. Stearns EL, MacDonnell SA, Kaufman BJ et al : Declining testicular function with age. Hormonal and clinical correlates. Am J Med 57:761, 1974
80. Tagnon HJ, Steens-Lievens A: Studies of fibrinolysis and acid phosphatase in cancer of the prostate. NCI Monogr 12:297, 1963
81. Tillinger K-G: Testicular morphology. Acta Endocrinol, suppl., 30:192, 1957
82. Varenhorst E: Metabolic changes during endocrine treatment in carcinoma of the prostate. A prospective study in man with special reference to cardiovascular complications during treatment with oestrogens or cyproterone acetate or after orchiectomy. Linkoping University of Medicine, Med Dissertation no. 103, 1980
83. Varenhost E, Risberg B: Effect of estrogen, orchiectomy and cyproterone acetate on tissue fibrinolysis in patients with carcinoma of the prostate. Invest Urol 18:355, 1981
84. Vermeulen A: Testicular hormonal secretion and aging in males. p. 177. In Grayhack JT, Wilson JD, Scherbenske MJ (eds): Benign Prostatic Hyperplasia. Department of Health, Education and Welfare (NIH) Publication no. 76-1113, 1976
85. Vermeulen A, Van Camp A, Mattelaer J, DeSy W: Hormonal factors related to abnormal growth of the prostate. p. 81. In Coffey DS, Isaacs JT (eds): Prostate Cancer. Vol. 48. UICC Technical Report Series, Geneva, 1979
86. Vermeulen A, Verdonck L: Radioimmunoassay of 17β-hydroxy-5α-androstan-3-one, 4-androstene-3, 17-dione, dehydroepiandrosterone, 17-hydroxyprogesterone and progesterone and its application to human male plasma. J Steroid Biochem 7:1, 1976
87. Walsh PC: Experimental approaches to benign prostatic hypertrophy: animal models utilizing the dog, rat and mouse. p. 215. In Grayhack JT, Wilson JD, Scherbenske MJ (eds): Benign Prostatic Hyperplasia. Department of Health, Education and Welfare (NIH) Publication no. 76-1113, 1976
88. Walsh PC: Benign prostatic hyperplasia. p. 949. In

Harrison JH, Gittes RF, Perlmutter AD, Stamey TA, Walsh PC (eds): Campbell's Urology. Vol. 2. WB Saunders, Philadelphia, 1985

89. Walsh PC, Donker PJ: Impotence following radical prostatectomy: insight into etiology and prevention. J Urol 128:492, 1982

90. Wilson JD: The pathogenesis of benign prostatic hyperplasia. Am J Med 68:745, 1980

91. Wilson JC, Walsh PC, Siiteri PK: Studies on the pathogenesis of benign prostatic hypertrophy in the dog. p. 205. In Grayhack JT, Wilson JD, Scherbenske MJ (eds): Benign Prostatic Hyperplasia. Department of Health, Education and Welfare (NIH) Publication no. 76-1113, Washington, DC 1976

92. Zaneveld LJD, Tauber PF: Contribution of prostatic fluid components to the ejaculation. p. 265. In Murphy GP, Sandberg AA, Karr JP (eds): The Prostatic Cell: Structure and Function. Part A. Alan R Liss, New York, 1981

93. Zuckerman S: The histogenesis of tissue sensitive to oestrogens. Biol Rev 15:231, 1971

31

Non-neoplastic Lesions of the Prostate and Benign Prostatic Hyperplasia

David Brandes

PROSTATIC INFLAMMATORY PROCESSES

Prostatitis is a common condition, but the etiology of the inflammatory processes and the pathogenic role of the organisms cultured from prostatic secretion and tissues remain uncertain.[14,69,70]

Inflammatory processes are preferentially localized in the periurethral glands and in the peripheral zone glands[65] that drain through the ducts that terminate at the sulci lateral to the verumontanum.[14]

Diagnostic Procedures

In the presence of clinical symptomatology of prostatitis, such as urinary frequency and urgency, nocturia and terminal dysuria, urethral discharge, and prostatic tenderness, bacteriologic analysis of voided urine and expressed prostatic secretions may identify the causative agent. When justified, cultures and histologic examination of biopsy specimens may contribute to the diagnosis. Divided urinary specimens and prostatic secretions, expressed by prostatic massage, yield urethral, bladder, and prostatic specimens that on culture may serve to localize the source of lower genitourinary infection. Leukocytes in

the prostatic fluids may also be of diagnostic value,[12,14,69,70] particularly if increased numbers of lipid-laden macrophages (oval fat bodies) are seen in the prostatic expressate.[1,68] Compared with normal, the content of these macrophages in the prostatic fluid is increased in patients with nonbacterial prostatitis, and still more in instances of bacterial prostatitis. The presence of these macrophages in the expressate localizes the site of infection to the prostate, since they are not detected in exudates derived from the urethra.[1,68] Elevated pH in prostatic fluid has been reported in patients with prostatitis, with a return to normal after the infection has been controlled.[20] The content of zinc appears decreased in patients with prostatitis and often returns to normal levels after successful therapy.[21] The presence of antibody-coated bacteria in the expressed prostatic fluid[46,90] and the demonstration in the serum and prostatic secretion-expressate of antigen-specific antibodies to infecting prostatic organisms[22,23,68,114] have also been used for diagnosis and to monitor effectiveness of therapy.

The values of isoenzymes of lactate dehydrogenase (LDH) in prostatic fluid are altered in prostatitis. The ratio of isoenzymes LDH-5/LDH-1, usually <2 in the absence of prostatic disease, may reach values of 3 or more in the presence of prostatitis, but even more accentuated predominance of LDH-5 is seen in prostatic cancer patients.[33,94] Elevated white blood cell counts and LDH-5/LDH-1 ratios in prostatic fluid are prevalent in patients with bacterial prostatitis.[33,94]

Classification of Prostatitis

Nonbacterial prostatitis, acute and chronic bacterial prostatitis, and prostatodynia are the prevalent clinical forms of prostatitis.[70] Various special forms, such as those produced by gonococcus, tubercle bacillus, fungi, viruses, *Trichomonas vaginalis*, T mycoplasma, and various types of granulomatous prostatitis occur less frequently.[4,5,14,15,69,70]

NONBACTERIAL PROSTATITIS

This is the most common type of prostatic inflammation[12,14,69] and has clinical symptoms of prostatitis. The prostatic expressate may contain elevated numbers of white blood cells and lipid-laden macrophages, but bacteriologic tests almost invariably are negative[14,69,70] except for some gram-positive bacteria in prostatic fluid regarded merely as commensals.[69]

Chlamydia, mycoplasma, or ureaplasma and viruses have been suggested as possible pathogenic organisms in the etiology of nonbacterial prostatitis.[12,14,69,70] *Chlamydia trachomatis* is implicated in the etiology of male nongonococcal urethritis and in acute epididymitis. Although *C. trachomatis* has been isolated from the urine of men with histories suggestive of chronic prostatitis, neither localization of the organisms to the prostate nor development of serum or prostatic antibodies to *C. trachomatis* have been demonstrated.[69,70]

Ureaplasma urealyticum has been isolated from the urethra of patients with chronic prostatitis more frequently than from normal controls,[111] and a 10-fold increase in quantitative counts of *U. urealyticum* was found in prostatic cultures as compared with urethral cultures of patients with chronic prostatitis.[11] These bacteriologic findings and the favorable response to tetracycline therapy suggest that ureaplasmas occasionally are true pathogens in patients with apparent nonbacterial prostatitis.[69]

Trichomonas vaginalis has been implicated as an etiologic agent in prostatitis and urethritis[30] and has been reported as present in the prostatic secretion and semen of about 23 percent of men with chronic non-gonorrheal prostatitis.[30] Moreover, by immunoperoxidase methods, *T. vaginalis* has been identified in the prostatic urethra, within the lumen of glands, and in the submucosa and stroma. These findings associated with intraepithelial vacuolization and acute and chronic inflammation suggest a possible role of this organism in nonspecific prostatitis.[30]

Histopatholic changes in the prostate of patients with nonbacterial prostatitis cannot be established because patients are not subjected to biopsy. In surgically resected hyperplastic prostates, the incidence of inflammation has been reported as 98.1 percent without significant morphologic differences among groups with positive or negative bacterial cultures.[54] The most common pattern is that of segregated glandular inflammation, with dilated glands filled with intraluminal neutrophils and foamy macrophages and chronic inflammatory cells in the surrounding stroma.[54] Other, less frequent forms of inflammation include periglandular or diffuse stromal inflammation, isolated lymphoid nodules, and acute necrotizing or localized granulomatous lesions.

BACTERIAL PROSTATITIS

Acute and chronic bacterial prostatitis are characterized by a white blood cell count greater than 20 per high-power field and the presence of significant pathogenic bacteria in the prostatic fluid or prostatic secretion expressate.[70] Gram-negative bacteria prevail as causative agents, and the infections are predominantly caused by *Escherichia coli* strains.[70] With lesser frequency, infections may be due to *Klebsiella, Enterobacter, Proteus, Pseudomonas,* and other less common gram-negative bacteria. Infections due to gram-positive bacteria, with the exception of enterococci (*Streptococcus faecalis*), appear to be less common and of less clinical significance than gram-negative infections.[69,70] However, *Staphylococcus epidermidis* may also be a causative pathogen in prostatitis.[12]

ACUTE BACTERIAL PROSTATITIS

The acute form of bacterial prostatitis is characterized by a sudden onset, with fever, chills, low back pain, and perineal pain. Urinary symptoms include frequency and urgency, nocturia and dysuria, and some degree of bladder outlet obstruction. Rectal palpation may reveal a tender, swollen prostate. The prostatic secretion reveals the presence of leukocytes and oval fat bodies, and considerable bacterial growth occurs on culture. The pathology of acute bacterial prostatitis may show focal or diffuse aggregates of neutrophils, both within and around the acini. Lymphocytes, plasma cells, and macrophages may also be present.

PROSTATIC ABSCESS

Most prostatic abscesses develop as a complication of acute bacterial prostatitis. Microabscesses may be noted early, but larger abscesses occur later in the course of the disease.[69] Pai and Bhat[86] reported that most of the cases are due to infections with coliform bacilli (particularly *E. coli*) frequently associated with anaerobic bacteria, such as *Bacteroides fragilis*.[87] Rarely, anaerobic bacteria alone may be the causative organisms. The majority occur in men in the fifth or sixth decade of life, and diabetics are particularly susceptible to develop prostatic abscesses.

Clinically, this condition may be accompanied by fever, acute retention frequency, and dysuria, and the gland may be focally enlarged and tender. Fluctuation may be also detected.

CHRONIC BACTERIAL PROSTATITIS

Most patients do not give a history of a preceding acute prostatitis and in some cases may present with a totally asymptomatic bacteriuria. In most patients, however, there is increased urinary frequency, dysuria, and nocturia with low back and perineal discomfort. Except when prostatic hyperplasia or prostatic calculi are present, rectal examination is usually negative. In the pathologic specimen, the inflammation is generally less intense and more focal than that observed in the acute form. Plasma cells and macrophages are present within and around acini, and interstitial infiltration by lymphocytes is also detected.[69]

UNCOMMON FORMS OF PROSTATITIS

Tuberculous Prostatitis

Tuberculous prostatitis may develop in patients with tuberculous cystitis when bacilli from the urinary bladder colonize the prostatic ducts that empty into the urethra. Occasionally, prostatic involvement may occur in the form of miliary spread from distant pulmonary tuberculosis.[55] Tuberculous lesions in the prostate are usually fibrocaseous in nature.[78] Epstein and Hutchins[16] found 9 cases of tuberculosis of a total of 62 cases of granulomatous prostatitis, and the lesions showed typical caseous necrosis. Nowadays, the so-called nonspecific granulomatous prostatitis of nontuberculous, perhaps noninfectious etiology is much more common than the tuberculous form (see below).

Gonococcal Prostatitis

Gonococcal prostatitis occurs very rarely. However, gonocci are capable of invading the male accessory sex organs during acute urethral infection, and it is possible that goncocci may persist in the prostatic fluid of infected men after the conventional short-term therapy. It has been suggested that patients with a previous history of gonorrhea may develop symptomatic prostatitis even though the cultures for *Neisseria gonorrhoeae* are negative.[69]

Fungal Infections

Fungal infections of the prostate are extremely rare and are almost invariably associated with disseminated disease. Prostatic involvement in patients with disseminated blastomycosis and coccidioidomycosis has been reported.[4,5,14,15,99b]

Most cases of cryptococcosis of the prostate have been incidental autopsy findings, although about 10 cases of cryptococcal prostatitis diagnosed histologically during life have been reported.[40,41,57] More recently, cryptococcal prostatitis was diagnosed after cystoscopy biopsy in a patient with acquired immune deficiency syndrome.[57]

NONSPECIFIC GRANULOMATOUS PROSTATITIS

The first comprehensive study of this condition was that of Tanner and McDonald,[104] who described 34 cases of granulomatous prostatitis in 1,028 surgical specimens from patients with inflammatory lesions of the prostate. In all the cases, tuberculous prostatitis could be ruled out by laboratory and clinical data. Subsequently, several other reports described the occurrence of granulomatous prostatitis in large series of surgically removed specimens.[50,84,95,101] The incidence ranged from 2 in 450 (0.44 percent) consecutive routine prostatectomies[101] to as high as 70 histologically documented cases among 1,100 patients (6.4 percent) treated surgically for prostatic inflammatory lesions.[50]

Histologically, the areas affected are infiltrated with an admixture of lymphocytes, plasma cells, and large, pale-staining mononuclear cells with vacuolated or eosinophilic cytoplasm, in a background of damaged ducts and acini.[80,102] When pale histiocytic infiltrates predominate (Fig. 31-1), distinction from poorly differentiated solid prostatic carcinomas of the vacuolated clear-cell variety must be made.[50,80,102]

Factors in the development of granulomatous prostatitis include nodular hyperplasia with ductal obstruction, ectasia, and extravasation of luminal con-

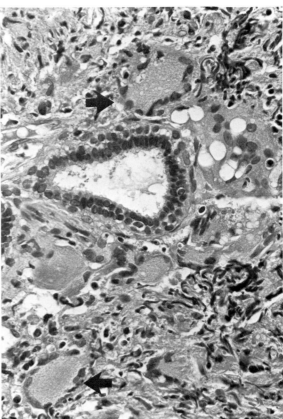

Fig. 31-2 Noncaseating granulomatous prostatitis. Area with abundant multinucleated giant cells (arrows). ×340.

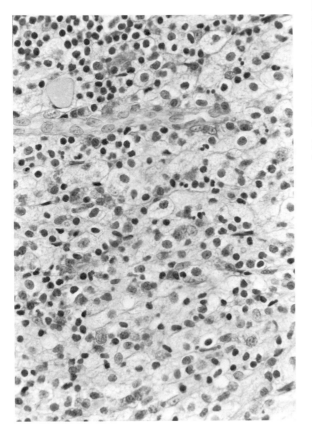

Fig. 31-1 Histiocytic granuloma. Closely packed foamy histiocytes and focal aggregates of lymphocytes. This lesion must be distinguished from undifferentiated infiltrating carcinoma. ×310.

tents into the adjacent stroma, followed by a foreign body-type inflammatory reaction (Fig. 31-2). In other instances, granulomas develop as a sequela to previous transurethral resection. Granulomas with foci of fibrinoid necrosis, surrounded by epitheloid cells, and containing giant cells were described in post-transurethral resection specimens in the study of Hedelin et al.[37] A lesion with the appearance of a rheumatoid nodule with central fibrinoid necrosis surrounded by palisading histiocytes was seen in association with prior prostatic surgery.[19]

Epstein and Hutchins[16] have reviewed 62 cases of granulomatous prostatitis that occurred from 1950 to 1982. Nonspecific granulomatous prostatitis was the most frequently encountered variety (31 cases). Pathologically, it consisted of large, nodular, granulomatous infiltrates with frequent liquefaction necrosis of the center and surrounded by infiltrates of epithelioid histiocytes, lymphocytes, and plasma cells, as well as multinucleated histiocytes. Three of the 31 cases showed significant numbers of eosinophils in the infiltrate, but none of these cases had any history of asthma or allergy nor was there any systemic involvement with a granulomatous process. The second largest group (13 cases) was that of focal granulomas after transurethral resection that were typically composed of central fibrinoid necrosis and palisading epithelioid histiocytes, surrounded by lymphocyte and plasma cells, with scattered eosinophils. A rare histologic variant of granulomatous prostatitis, described as nodular histiocytic prostatitis,[24] was characterized by the presence of well-demarcated cellular nodules, composed exclusively of histiocytes with foamy cytoplasm, resembling the cells seen in xanthogranulomatous pyelonephritis.

Helpap and Vogel[39] examined a series of 2,850 cases of prostatitis, histologically classified as (1) acute (12 percent); (2) nonspecific chronic, including periductal-periglandular with hyperplasia (84.3 percent), relapsing (4.2 percent), granulomatous (3.1 percent), and specific tuberculosis prostatitis (7.1 percent).

Post-transurethral resection changes at 8 to 14 days after primary transurethral resection were mainly of the inflammatory type around the areas of necrosis. Transurethral resection specimens obtained 4 weeks to 8 weeks after primary transurethral resection showed a variety of lesions, including granulomas with multinucleated cells and palisadelike macrophages with or without central necrosis. Granulomas of the typical tuberculoid type with central necrosis and palisadelike macrophages could also be seen. The granulomatous reactions were proved in 70 percent of secondary resectates.

Granulomatous prostatitis, with vasculitic lesions, has been reported in patients with systemic manifestations of Wegener's granulomatosis.[99a]

Eosinophilic and Allergic Granulomas

Prostatic granulomas showing a predominance of eosinophilic cell infiltrates may or may not be accompanied by allergic and hypersensitivity phenomena such as bronchial asthma and vasculitis. Melicow[71] described a case of granulomatous prostatitis in which the lesions showed areas of fibrinoid necrosis, surrounded by eosinophilic cells with a very scanty giant cell component. Autopsy findings in that case revealed a generalized multisystem allergic vasculitis. Similar cases of eosinophilic granulomas, with fibrinoid necrosis and a fatal outcome, apparently related to a systemic allergic or hypersensitive condition, have been reported.[36,82,99b,105] Among the reported cases of eosinophilic granulomatous prostatitis that followed a benign course, some of the patients were afflicted with asthma or other allergic manifestations, and the histopathology ranged from simple eosinophilic infiltrates in the prostate to more complex lesions, particularly foci of fibrinoid necrosis.[51,106] Responses to antihistamines[77] or steroids[51] have been reported in some cases of eosinophilic prostatitis.

Epstein and Hutchins[16] have recently called attention to the distinguishing clinical and pathologic features among nonspecific, allergic, and post-transurethral resection granulomatous prostatitis. They and others[99b] consider that nonspecific granulomatous prostatitis and post-transurethral resection granulomas are the most frequent prostatic granulomatous lesions and that the presence of abundant eosinophils must not be attributed to allergic reactions. Allergic granulomatous prostatitis is an exceedingly rare condition and can be diagnosed in the setting of a generalized allergic reaction, most commonly asthma, in the patient.[16]

Prostatodynia (Prostatosis)

This condition affects younger adults, 20 years to 40 years old, and is characterized by pain referred to the pelvis, without evidence of primary neurologic disorder or neurogenic bladder dysfunction.[70] Patients with prostatodynia may have some of the symptoms seen in prostatitis and typically show a picture of functional obstruction affecting the bladder neck and prostatic urethra. Bacteriologic localization cultures invariably prove negative, and microscopic examination of the prostatic expressate fails to reveal an increased white blood cell count as seen in nonbacterial prostatitis.[12,14,70]

Miscellaneous Processes

MALAKOPLAKIA

Malakoplakia is a granulomatous inflammatory process. Although it occurs most frequently in organs of the genitourinary tract, there have been case reports with similar or identical lesions in a variety of other organs, including skin, bone, lungs, lymph nodes, gastrointestinal tract, and brain.

Malakoplakia of the prostate is rare, only 22 cases having been reported.[49,53,96] All patients had symptoms consistent with urinary tract infection and prostatic enlargement and hardening that prompted biopsy for tissue diagnosis.

Grossly, the lesions are yellowish brown plaques with soft consistency that on histologic examination reveal a predominantly histiocytic granulomatous inflammatory response with the characteristic von Hansemann histiocytes. Many of the histiocytes contain intracytoplasmic inclusions, the Michaelis-Gutmann bodies, generally rounded or oval and measuring 2 μm to 10 μm in diameter. These structures are basophilic and usually show some degree of concentric lamination as well as positive reactivity with the periodic acid-schiff (PAS) stain (after diastase digestion) and Von Kossa's stain for calcium.[58] They may also react positively for iron on Prussian blue stain. (The pathogenesis of malakoplakia is discussed in Chapter 8.)

CORPORA AMYLACEA AND PROSTATIC CALCULI

Corpora amylacea appear as intraductal and intra-acinar spherical concretions that form characteristic concentric rims. As they mature, they reveal increased calcification in the form of hydroxyapatite deposits that resemble those seen in bone. The laminar appearance of corpora amylacea indicates that expansion and calcification is an intermittent process, since it requires fluctuation in composition that would increase the calcium phosphate saturation and thus favor calcification.[42] The number and calcification of corpora amylacea increases markedly with age, and a significantly higher frequency of prostatic calcification with age has been demonstrated in populations with a high incidence of prostatic cancer.[42]

Frequently, corpora amylacea compress and cause the atrophy and destruction of the glandular epithelium, which may be replaced by multinucleated cells (Fig. 31-3). Similar multinucleated giant cells are seen within the lumen of the acini and produce images suggestive of an "osteoclastic" type of resorption of corpora amylacea (Fig. 31-3).

Minute calculi are very frequently present in pros-

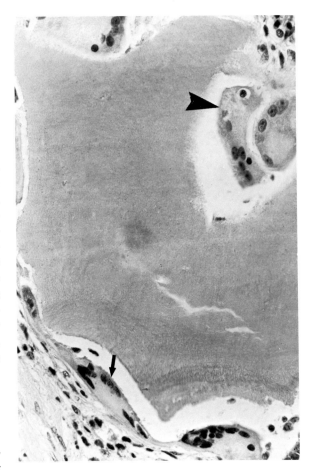

Fig. 31-3 Multinucleated giant cell reaction to corpora amylacea. Giant cells (arrows) replace the epithelial lining of the acinus and are also aligned along scalloped areas in the contour of the corpora amylacea (arrowhead). ×340.

tates of men over 50 years of age and may be associated with urinary tract infection and prostatitis.[18,25,67,69] Prostatic calculi seem to develop by deposition of calcium salts (calcium phosphate trihydrate and carbonate) on corpora amylacea.[13] Both corpora amylacea and true prostatic calculi prevail in the posterior segment of the prostate. Some prostatic calculi may arise from the precipitation of calcium and magnesium phosphates present in normal prostatic fluid, and infection may contribute to the development of calculi. Prostatic calculi may be associated with nodular hyperplasia, carcinoma, and urethral strictures. Any condition producing mechanical obstruction and stasis of prostatic fluid may contribute to the development of calculi.[52] Prostatic stones are usually harmless and asymptomatic, but they may harbor bacterial pathogens responsible for persistent relapsing bacteriuria.[18,69] Prostatic calculi may be single or multiple and may vary in size from millimeters to centimeters in diameter. When multiple and contained within a single cavity, the stones may be faceted. When single and small, their surface tends to be smooth. Hematuria and abscess formation, although very rare, may be associated with prostatic calculi.

MELANOSIS OF THE PROSTATE GLAND

Benign melanotic lesions in the prostate have been observed in the stroma (blue nevus) and in the glandular epithelium.[102] Dendritic stromal cells possess melanogenic capabilities as judged by the presence of promelanosomes and melanosomes demonstrated by electron microscopy.[44]

Rios and Wright[91] described a case of melanosis of the prostate gland with melanin present in the stromal cells and glandular epithelium, as well as in the epithelial component of a well-differentiated prostatic carcinoma present in their material. They reviewed the literature and pointed out that in their own case and in most of the cases they reviewed, the melanin in the epithelial cells appeared to have been transferred from adjacent stromal melanocytes. They concluded that the melanogenic potential of prostatic epithelial cells has yet to be proved conclusively.

DEVELOPMENTAL, HYPERPLASTIC, ATROPHIC, AND DYSPLASTIC LESIONS

Developmental Anomalies

Derivatives of the müllerian duct in the male are found in the testes (appendix testes) and in the prostate gland (prostatic utricle). During development, the hollow müllerian distal remnant present in the müllerian tubercle (the verumontanum) forms an epithelial-lined sinus approximately 4 mm to 6 mm long. This opens into the prostatic urethra between the orifices of the ejaculatory ducts. Occasionally, the cavity of the prostatic utricle becomes dilated and forms a cyst that extends between the seminal vesicles,

beyond the bladder wall. Such cysts represent diverticuli that reproduce the uterine tubes, and their size may be variable. A large utriculus is found in 4 percent of newborn male infants and in 1 percent of adult males.[99] The sizes of utricular cavities vary, but symptomatic cystically dilated utricles rarely occur.

Anomalies of the prostate gland proper are rare. They include cases of partial or complete absence of the prostate, invariably accompanied by pituitary insufficiency, infantile genitalia, and eunuchoid habitus. It is possible that some of these cases that were generally diagnosed by rectal palpation were due to atrophy rather than agenesis.[32]

In rare instances, the anterior lobes of the prostate may fail to regress in fetal life and persist and even undergo hypertrophy in adult life.[61] Although usually asymptomatic, the hypertrophied anterior lobes may contribute to the obstructive symptoms of benign prostatic hyperplasia (BPH).

Marion's disease is a fibrous dysplasia of the prostate gland producing obstruction of the bladder neck in infants.[32] A pathologic study of five infants who died from this disease[6] revealed an elongated prostate with an increase in fibrous and elastic tissue throughout the gland, as well as hypertrophy of the colliculus seminalis.

Atrophy and Hyperplasia

As early as the third decade,[29a] and particularly from the fifth decade onward, a number of alterations that involve both the epithelial structures and the stroma occur in the outer prostate. These hyperplastic, atrophic, and dysplastic lesions may affect small groups of acini or may extend to whole lobes or the entire outer gland. Contrary to what is seen in the inner prostate during the development of benign nodular hyperplasia, the alterations in the outer prostate as a rule are not nodular in nature. Recognition of these hyperplastic, atrophic, and dysplastic changes in the outer prostate is of interest from the viewpoint that some of them may represent preneoplastic lesions with potential to evolve into frank malignancy.

Hyperplastic and atrophic changes appear interrelated. Moore[73] described a presenile period extending approximately between 40 and 60 years of age in which hyperplastic changes such as pseudostratification and new acinar formation occurred concurrently with atrophy. The atrophic changes presented as simple epithelial atrophy; simple acinar atrophy, usually involving an entire lobule (lobular atrophy); and sclerotic atrophy, in which continued production and hyalinization of the collagen led finally to the obliteration of the acinar structures. These changes progressed but at a slower pace during the senile period that extended from 60 years onward.

In the studies of Franks[27] hyperplastic processes in the outer prostate appeared to develop in relation to pre-existing atrophy. The atrophic changes that result in focal or diffuse epithelial atrophy and interstitial fibrosis affected primarily the outer or true prostate and have been implicated as the site of origin of prostatic carcinoma. Simple atrophy was characterized by flattened epithelium and sometimes cystic-dilated glands, while in sclerotic atrophy the atrophic epithelium eventually becomes obliterated by fibrous hyalinized connective tissue.[27]

Since prostatic carcinoma occurs predominantly in the later decades, attempts have been made to correlate age-linked involution changes with hyperplastic and neoplastic processes. Franks[27] classified *hyperplastic* lesions into postatrophic and secondary types. *Postatrophic hyperplasia* includes the following: (1) *Lobular hyperplasia* is related to simple atrophy and is characterized histologically by the proliferation of newly formed, closely packed acini around a central duct or alveolus. (2) *Postsclerotic hyperplasia* has hyperplastic buds, originating from a central atrophic acinus, that penetrate the surrounding connective tissue and may develop luminae or remain as solid structures. *Secondary hyperplasia* is observed in areas of stromal atrophy, but the epithelial lining may form papillae and have signs of secretion.

Development of carcinoma in relation to those various types of hyperplasia was only apparent in the postsclerotic group, since areas of small acinar carcinoma appeared to arise in the vicinity of the hyperplastic areas within a sclerotic stroma.[27,28]

McNeal[62] distinguished an involutional type of atrophy with acini lined by cuboidal cells with clear cytoplasm and distinct borders; a preatrophic type with acini lined by pseudostratified epithelium, indistinct cell boundaries, and scanty cytoplasm; and advanced atrophy with acini lined by a single layer of flattened cells.

Mostofi and Davis[78] have separated a group of benign epithelial abnormalities characterized by various types of atypical hyperplastic activities, including *lobular hyperplasia, postatrophic hyperplasia* (atrophy-associated hyperplasia), *focal intra-acinar hyperplasia* (secondary hyperplasia), and *basal cell hyperplasia*. In the glands, intra-acinar epithelial proliferation may assume a cribriform pattern,[3] which can be differentiated from carcinoma by the lack of atypia and the presence of slender fibrovascular cores. Acinar proliferation in lobular hyperplasia is characterized by the presence of newly formed acini, of uniform size, around a centrally located duct or acinus. In postatrophic hyperplasia, proliferation occurs around ducts with atrophic epithelium, and the newly formed acini are small and irregular. This type of hyperplasia is considered as precancerous and is often associated with small acinar carcinoma. Focal intra-acinar hyperplasia (secondary hyperplasia) also develops in relation to ducts or acini showing cystic dilation and flattened atrophic epithelium, and proliferative activity is in the form of focal intra-acinar plaques and papillary fronds. This histologic appearance of proliferative activity in a background of epithelial atrophy suggests renewed (secondary) postinvolution hyperplastic growth. The hyperplastic process may on occasion affect predominantly the basal cell layers, to such an extent that it may result in the obliteration of the lumen of the acinus.[78,81]

Atypia and Dysplastic Lesions

For many years there have been continuous attempts to establish whether some changes that occur with aging, such as the hyperplastic and atrophic lesions described in the previous section, are associated with the development of cancer. Also, there is the question of whether atypical and dysplastic alterations that may represent preneoplastic lesions with the potential to evolve into frank malignancy occur in the prostates of aging individuals.[8,27,72] Gardner and Culberson[29a] have recently documented such lesions in men in their 20's. The hyperplastic changes described in the previous section occur in the outer prostate and appear to be associated, at least topographically, with the development of malignancy. Franks[27] described the presence of small foci of clear cell acinar carcinoma at the margins of postsclerotic hyperplastic lesions. Brandes,[8] Moore,[72,75] and Rich[89] referred to the frequent association between sclerotic atrophic changes and the occurrence of latent carcinoma. Mostofi and Davis[78] have also pointed to the association between post atrophic hyperplasia and the development of small acinar carcinoma.

McNeal[62] has expressed the belief that tubular-scirrhous prostatic carcinomas develop in relation to glands that have preserved an active, "youthful" epithelial lining, through a sequence of alterations ranging from progressively anaplastic changes to frank carcinoma in situ and finally invasive carcinoma. A second variety, the alveolar medullary carcinoma, appears to be related to prostatic ducts with involutional epithelial changes.[62]

Glandular proliferative disorders in the prostate that may represent atypical or dysplastic lesions with neoplastic potentials have been recognized by terms such as marked atypia, atypical epithelial hyperplasia, atypical glandular hyperplasia, atypical adenomatous hyperplasia, and dysplasia.[9,47,48] Dysplastic lesions of the prostate[47,48] are divided into atypical primary hyperplasia, unrelated to atrophy, and atypical postatrophic hyperplasia on the basis of cytologic atypia, irregular glandular arrangement, and disorganization of the epithelial stromal architecture. In a series of 118 total prostatectomies for carcinoma, atypical primary hyperplasia was present in 58.9 percent of all cases, and the association was still more evident (83.3 percent) when considering only the early stages. In the group of 524 cases of prostatic cancer reviewed by Helpap,[38] atypical hyperplasia was present in approximately 50 percent of the cases.

Prostatic adenosis is considered a dysplastic glandular proliferation characterized by nuclear pleomorphism, the presence of nucleoli, or an infiltrative growth pattern of the prostatic glands. Brawn[9] described three levels of dysplasia, mild, moderate, and severe. The grade of the dysplasia relates to either the degree of nuclear pleomorphism and atypia or the extent of the infiltrating patterns of the prostatic glands. The latter range from mild to severe adenosis and are determined by an increasing infiltrative pattern of the glands but with a preservation of benign nuclear appearance.

McNeal and Bostwick[66] included 100 benign and 100 cancerous prostates in a study intended to correlate the relation between dysplastic lesions and carcinoma. Dysplastic lesions were graded 1 to 3 according to cell crowding, nuclear irregularity, chromatin distribution, and the presence of nucleoli. Chromatin condensation beneath the nuclear membrane and the presence of prominent acidophilic nucleoli were the salient features of grade 3 dysplasia.[66] In prostates with carcinoma, the frequency of dysplastic foci was 82 percent, with a 33 percent incidence of grade 3 dysplasia. Corresponding figures for benign prostates showed an overall frequency of dysplasia of 43 percent with only 4 percent incidence of grade 3 dysplasia, suggesting dysplastic lesions as precursors of carci-

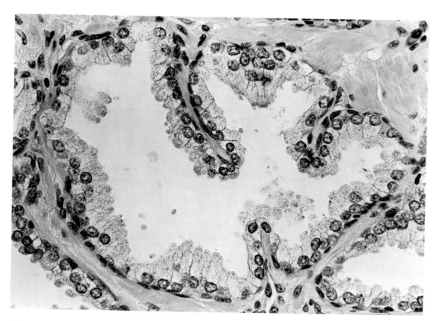

Fig. 31-4 Benign intra-acinar papillary hyperplasia. Preservation of two-cell layer. Basal cells and secretory cells; a fibrovascular core is present in the papillary projections. ×360.

noma.[66] Oyasu et al.[85] also reported increased frequency of dysplastic lesions in prostate cancer (48 of 51) with a predominancy of severe dysplasia (42 of 48), whereas the frequency of dysplastic lesions in autopsy prostates was 14 of 37, with only 3 cases of 14 showing severe dysplastic changes.

It is uncertain whether atypical hyperplastic lesions and adenosis are forerunners of prostatic carcinoma. It is possible that patients with atypical hyperplasia or adenosis of the prostate develop carcinoma from the same source as do all males over 50 years of age, that is, the reservoir of latent carcinoma present in 25 percent of men over the age of 50.[9] Figures 31-4 through 31-6 are intended to illustrate apparent histologic differences between benign intra-acinar papillary proliferation, epithelial dysplasia, and early cribriform in situ carcinoma.

BENIGN PROSTATIC HYPERPLASIA

Prostatic hyperplasia is apparently a manifestation of the aging process. Although the clinical symptomatology becomes manifest late in life, with the highest frequency in men 60 to 70 years of age,[10,93] the onset of the pathologic alterations that give rise to the symptoms may have occurred years earlier, as early as the third decade.[29a,107,112,113]

Benign prostatic hyperplasia (BPH) seems to occur solely in the aging man and dog.[43,109] In both species, the presence of intact testicular function is required for the development of BPH (although rarely BPH may be stimulated by nontesticular androgens, as seen in female pseudohermaphrodites)[39a]; and in the dog, but not as much in man, orchiectomy or administra-

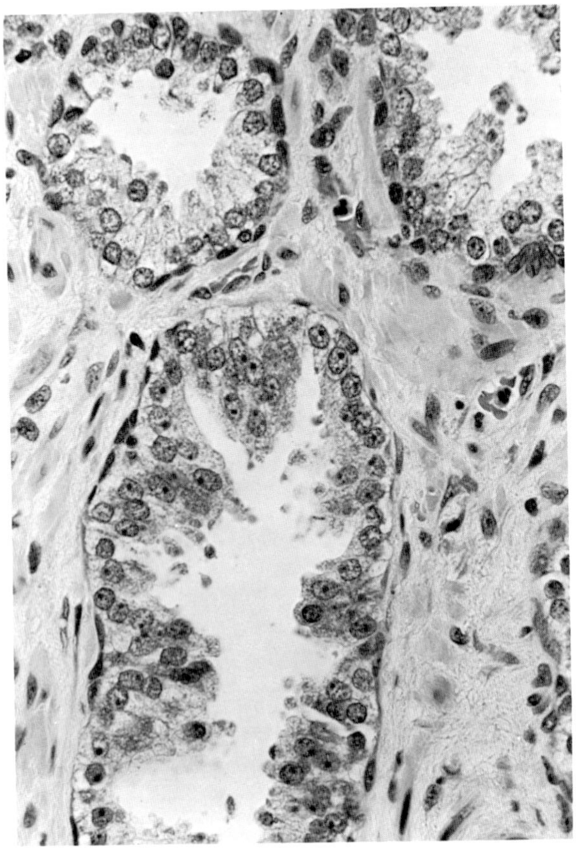

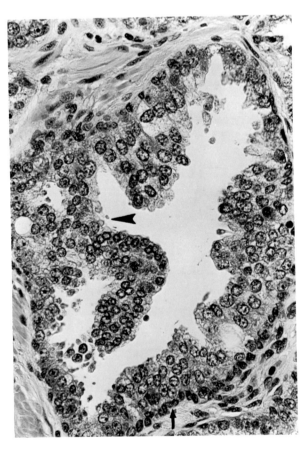

Fig. 31-5 Intra-acinar proliferation with moderate atypia. Basal layer still present. Nuclear irregularity, open chromatin, and occasional nucleoli are seen in the hyperplastic atypical secretory cells. ×340.

Fig. 31-6 Atypical intra-acinar proliferation with incipient cribriform pattern. Some basal cells still present (arrow); solid cell bridging with cribriform pattern (arrowheads). ×360.

tion of antiandrogenic compounds may result in regression of the hyperplastic changes.

Epidemiology and Etiology

INCIDENCE, PREVALENCE, AND MORTALITY

There is very little growth of the prostate during the first 5 years of life,[100] but there is a great increase in the size of the prostate after the 12th year of age, and the gland reaches adult size during the third decade. The size of the prostate remains constant until approximately the age of 45 years, although the earliest stages of atrophy and hyperplasia may occur during this period.[29a] In the absence of BPH or cancer, the prostate begins to involute and progressively decreases in size. Beginning at approximately age 45, the prostate may undergo BPH in which case there is a rapid increase of volume that may continue until death.[109] The risk of developing BPH increases with age, particularly after the age of 40. The overall incidence of prostatic hyperplasia at autopsy may reach the figure of 80.1 percent,[35] with a maximum of 95.5 percent in the eighth decade of life.[109] The mean age at detection by race is about 65 years for whites and approximately 5 years earlier for blacks.[93,109] Mortality rates from BPH show variations by geography and race. They are very high in Iceland and in most European populations. In the United States, Canada, and some European and South American countries, mortality is low to average, whereas the lowest mortality occurs in countries with oriental popluations, such as Philippines, Singapore, China, Hong Kong, and Japan.[93,109] The same populations have an extremely low death rate from prostatic cancer. Some of the factors examined that may be associated with higher risk of BPH include cirrhosis of the liver, coronary heart disease, prostatitis, hypertension, and diabetes mellitus, but only in relation with the latter condition has there been any likelihood of a positive correlation.[7,92]

The relation between BPH and cancer has been a controversial issue. In a study of 290 prostatic cancer cases against 290 age-matched controls, the association of prostatic cancer with BPH was considered significant and the death rate from prostatic cancer was 3.7 times higher in BPH patients, with a relative risk of 5 for the development of prostatic cancer in patients previously treated for BPH.[2] In the study of

Greenwald et al.,[34] which included 838 patients with BPH and 802 age-matched controls, the number of patients developing prostatic cancer was similar in both groups. It would be unlikely that prostatic hypertrophy, which occurs late in life, might represent a precursor to a solid cancer, such as prostatic carcinoma, which is known to have an extended latent period. Furthermore, latent carcinomas are found in young men and also in men at low risk of developing clinical cancer, such as orientals, and BPH is seldom found in men under the age of 40.[93] The relationships and sequence of events in the development of prostatic cancer and BPH have been theoretically analyzed by Rotkin,[93] who considers the possibility that development of BPH represents a separate condition, a precursor to onset of prostatic cancer, or a sequel to an already established carcinoma.

Such chains of events could lead to (1) formation of hyperplastic lesions evolving independently; (2) development of a stationary neoplasm, with the characteristics of latent carcinoma, stage A; (3) possibly normal or hyperplastic tissue evolving into nonstationary, latent tumor with potential to progression into invasive stage. (4) BPH might also derive from an established cancer, or (5) it might be possible that cancer and BPH share a common origin. Such events require the existence of two stage A cancers, one stationary and one progressive, or the occurrence of early cellular changes producing BPH and then developing into cancer.

CLINICAL MANIFESTATION OF BPH

The symptomatology derives from the degree of urethral or bladder neck obstruction that will ultimately affect the bladder, ureters, and kidneys. Bladder neck obstruction causes at first minimal symptoms, but with progressive obstruction the patient develops prostatism, with reduction in the caliber and strength of the urinary stream and ability to terminate micturition abruptly, postvoiding dribbling, and remnant residual urine in the bladder that predisposes to recurrent urinary tract infections. The muscle wall of the bladder undergoes gradual hypertrophy producing a trabeculated appearance of the bladder wall, with troughlike depressions in the bladder mucosa between interlacing bands of hypertrophic muscle. These depressions may develop into true acquired diverticula. Persistence of the bladder neck obstruction by prostatic hyperplasia may eventually lead to an obstructive atrophy of the kidney (hydronephrosis) (see Chapter 11).

In BPH, enlargement is invariably nodular and originates in the inner prostate, proximal to the verumontanum. Although the prostatic lobes described by Lowsley in the fetus[59] are no longer discernible in the adult, the zonal distribution of hyperplastic nodules is sometimes referred to the various lobes, including the lateral lobes and the median lobes. When the median lobe is enlarged, it may remain contained by the internal urethral sphincter, in which case it expands into the subtrigonal area producing an elevation of the base of the bladder. The internal urethral orifice thus becomes displaced anteriorly. With less frequency, the enlarged medial lobe slides through the inner surface of the central sphincter and protrudes into the lumen of the bladder. This type of medial expansion is referred to as a subcervical lobe. It protrudes into the

bladder in a relatively small space that confines its mobility, permitting the expanded lobe to obstruct the internal urethral orifice in a valvelike fashion.[26,60,75,103]

Figures 31-7 through 31-10 illustrate the appearance of the normal gland and changes that occur with increased extent of benign hyperplastic nodularity.

SECONDARY CHANGES AND COMPLICATIONS OF PROSTATIC HYPERPLASIA

Prostatic Infarction

In approximately 25 percent of the cases, hyperplastic glands reveal recent or healed infarcts. Urinary retention appears to be the single most common symptom in patients with a prostatic infarct. It has

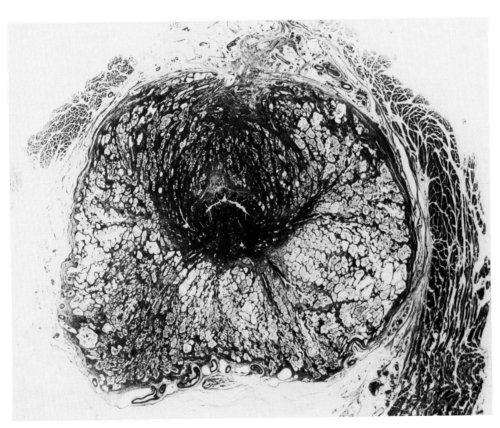

Fig. 31-7 Normal prostate. Transverse section of normal prostate showing mucosal, submucosal, and outer glands. ×2. (Obtained through the courtesy of L. M. Franks, Imperial Cancer Research Fund Laboratories, London, England.)

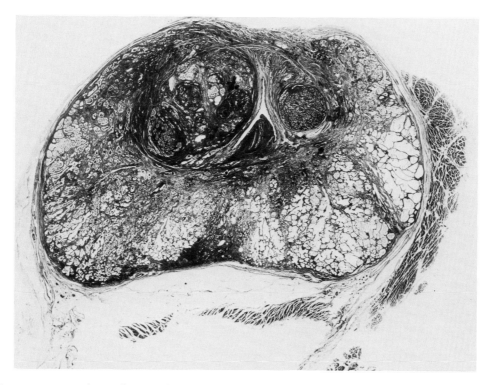

Fig. 31-8 Benign hyperplastic nodules. Benign hyperplastic nodules evolving in the area of the inner group of glands in transverse section. Outer glands are not involved. ×2. (Obtained through the courtesy of L. M. Franks, Imperial Cancer Research Fund Laboratories, London, England.)

been elicited in about one-half of the cases.[78,79] Histologically, recent infarcts reveal coagulation necrosis with or without the presence of marginal or diffuse hemorrhage. Squamous metaplasia was observed in 47 of 50 cases of prostatic infarct. These squamous metaplastic changes occur near the areas of infarct where hyperplastic and regenerating glands may also be present. There is no evidence that prostatic infarcts are due to thrombosis or occlusion in the arteries of the organ. Infarction may also occur in hyperplastic nodules.[78,79]

Prostatic infarction may cause transient elevation of serum prostate-specific acid phosphatase. Silber et al.[98] measured the catalytic activity of the enzyme and found it to be elevated in 30 percent of patients with prostatic infarcts. Vihko and Kontturi[108] found a transient elevation of serum prostate-specific acid phosphatase, measured by radioimmunoassay, in a patient with prostatic infarction associated with prostatic hyperplasia.

Infections

Ascending duct infection with formation of microabscesses, foci of regenerating hyperplasia with some atypia, and squamous metaplasia may also be seen in association with benign hyperplasia, particularly in the presence of infarcts and necrosis.[78,103] Foci of granulomatous prostatitis and acinar squamous metaplasia are also frequently observed in association with infarctions occurring in hyperplastic glands.[102,103,109]

Pathogenesis

The likelihood that hormonal factors may be implicated in the development of benign nodular hyperplasia in humans stems from the following: (1) BPH occurs late in life, concomitant with the occurrence of alteration in the hormonal milieu of the host, and does not seem to develop in individuals castrated be-

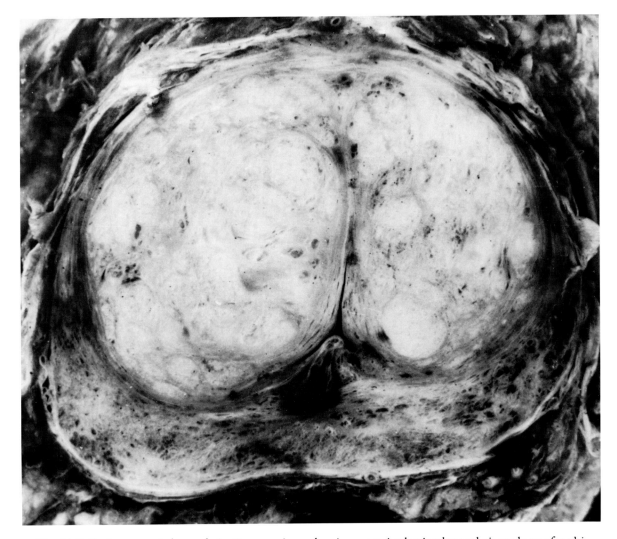

Fig. 31-9 Benign prostatic hyperplasia. Gross specimen showing extensive benign hyperplasia made up of multitude of nodules in inner prostate (BPH). The outer prostate is compressed around the edges of the specimen. A thin false capsule has formed between the two zones. ×2. (Obtained through the courtesy of L. M. Franks, Imperial Cancer Research Fund Laboratories, London, England.)

fore puberty. (2) Established BPH may regress after castration. (3) The accumulation of the potent androgen dihydrotestosterone (DHT) is increased in the hyperplastic areas of prostatic glands,[97,112,113] Wilson and colleagues[112,113] suggested that the accumulation of DHT in the prostate and the age-related increase in the ratio of the concentation of free estradiol to free testosterone are the most relevant hormonal changes in the etiology of prostatic hyperplasia.

Studies on the dog prostatic hyperplasia model re-

vealed an increase in DHT concentration in the hyperplastic glands,[31] and in early periurethral hyperplasia the concentration of DHT is higher than in normal areas of the same gland. The factors that may lead to the accumulation of DHT in prostatic hyperplastic tissues[112,113] include increased transport from the plasma, more substrate available for synthesis within the gland, increased rate of synthesis, and decreased catabolism or enhanced intracellular binding. From clinical data and experimental studies on the

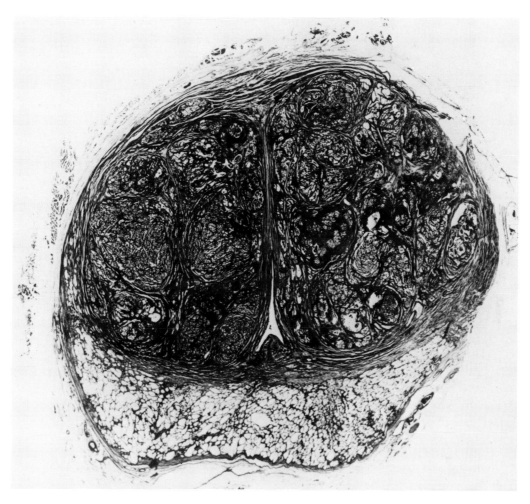

Fig. 31-10 Benign prostatic hyperplasia. Transverse histologic section with changes similar to those in gross specimen (Fig. 31-9). Extensive nodularity in inner prostate (BPH) with compression of outer group of glands, particularly at edges. False capsule between inner hyperplastic nodules and outerprostatic glands. Original magnification ×2. (Obtained through the courtesy of L. M. Franks, Imperial Cancer Research Fund Laboratories, London, England.)

dog, it appears that a net decrease in the catabolism of DHT, and partly an increase in the receptor for this hormone, are most likely responsible for the DHT accumulation.[112,113]

The role of DHT accumulation in the production of BPH was later questioned as a result of studies by Walsh and his collaborators.[110] Assays for DHT concentration in normal and hyperplastic prostatic tissues were almost identical (normal tissue, 5.1 ± 0.4 ng/g

of tissue; BPH tissue, 5.0 ± 0.4 ng/g of tissue) when performed on fresh surgical material.[110] Similarly, Bartsch, et al.[3b] were unable to find any signifant difference in testosterone or DHT concentrations between normal and hyperplastic prostate tissue.

From the data in the literature (see Table 27 in reference 96), it appears that the approximately two to fivefold increase of DHT content in BPH tissue over that of normal prostatic tissue may have represented an artifact. In all the reports showing such a difference, levels of DHT in "normal" tissues were performed in autopsy materials, whereas DHT content in BPH was determined on fresh material obtained at surgery. The results from the studies of Walsh and collaborators[109,110] would indicate that the assayed DHT in prostatic tissues procured at autopsy are factitiously low.

The studies in dogs, which appeared to support the role of DHT in the etiology of BPH, such as the increased DHT concentration in hyperplastic tissue[31] and the concurrent induction of prostatic growth and increased DHT concentration by some steroids,[76] were also later questioned.[110] In age-matched dogs, DHT contents in normal and spontaneous BPH tissue did not show significant differences, and although administration of some steroid compounds produced a positive correlation between increased prostate weight and DHT contents, other steroid regimens enhanced the content of DHT without an equivalent increment in prostate weight. Moreover, incidence of BPH in beagles increases with aging despite a decrease of prostatic DHT that is apparent at the age of 4 years.[17]

Data derived from studies in the castrated dog indicate that the increase in the ratio of 17β-estradiol to testosterone during aging has a synergistic effect in the accumulation of DHT, since estrogens appear to enhance the level of androgen receptors in prostatic tissue.[112,113] The question as to whether a synergism between estrogens and androgens plays a role in the development of BPH has been critically analyzed by Walsh.[109] Apparent substantiation of the role of estrogens is based on (1) the syngerism of estrogen and 5α-reduced androgens in induction of BPH in dogs; (2) the induction of androgen receptor in canine prostate by estrogen; (3) the increase in the value for the ratio of free estradiol/free testosterone with aging; and (4) the presence of estrogen receptor and increased nuclear androgen levels in BPH in man.

Factors that fail to support a role of estrogen in the development of BPH include the late onset and the minuteness of the alteration of the estrogen-androgen production; the lower than normal values of nuclear and cytoplasmic estrogen receptor concentrations in BPH; and the similarity of cytosolic progesterone receptor concentrations in normal and BPH tissue. In the dog, estrogens appear to sensitize the prostate toward development of BPH, but it remains to be determined whether estrogenic synergism has a role in the development of BPH in man. It must also be taken into consideration that in many animal experiments stimulatory and synergistic effects are obtained with the use of pharmacologic rather than physiologic doses. A human prostatic growth factor (hPGF) extracted from BPH tissues,[45,83] which is capable of stimulating fibroblastic growth in vitro and DNA synthesis, has been suggested as having a role in the induction of BPH.[45]

Site of Origin and Morphological Aspects

Benign hyperplasia of the prostate is characteristically nodular, with participation of epithelial and fibromuscular stromal components, but without involvement of elastic elements.[29] As early as 1894, Jores (as quoted by Franks[29]) detected the presence of groups of glands in the submucosa of the trigone, in the vesical neck, and in the urethral wall, immediately below the bladder neck, and described submucosal and median enlargements of the prostate arising from these glands. In the 1940s, Moore[74] stated that BPH nodules appeared to originate in the lateral and middle lobes of the true prostate as described by Lowsley.[59] However, other researchers concur that the site of origin of BPH is resticted to the immediate periurethral tissues, as well as a special group of adjacent inner prostatic glands.[26,29,56]

McNeal[63-65] has more precisely defined the area of benign nodular formation. According to his studies, benign hyperplastic nodules originate exclusively in periurethral glands and particularly in an area designated as the transition zone of the prostate, located between the base of the veramontanum and the bladder neck. The glands in the transition zone derive from periurethral ducts that emerge laterally at the lower border of the cylindrical smooth muscle sphincter that surrounds the urethra from the base of the verumontanum to the bladder neck. Branching and acinar proliferation from such ducts expands mainly toward the bladder neck, where they lie in apposition to the external fibers of the smooth muscle sphincter.[64]

Whether benign hyperplastic nodules derive from focal glandular proliferation or from initial stromal nodules with subsequent glandular involvement is still a matter of controversy. Reischauer (quoted by

Franks[29]) maintained that the initial formation of fibrous nodules in periglandular stroma next to the urethra stimulated proliferation of epithelial elements from neighboring glands, which then penetrated the nodules from the periphery. Although this assumption has been supported in a number of studies,[26,56,88] the issue remains unresolved. Hyperplasia in the dog appears to be primarily glandular;[3a] in man, although nodules vary considerably in composition, (see below), on balance there is an absolute increase in stromal, but not glandular elements in BPH.[3b]

There are differences in the size and composition of hyperplastic nodules in relation to age groups and also to their location in the transition zone or in the periurethral stroma.[63-65] In the younger group (median age, 58 years), the total nodule cross-sectional area was 20 mm² or less, and the nodules in the transitional zone were predominantly glandular, whereas those in the periurethral tissue were mostly stromal. In the next age group (median age, 70 years), the total nodular cross-sectional area was 20 mm² to 100 mm². The majority of the nodules in the transition zone were glandular, and those in the periurethral areas were predominantly stromal. In the oldest age group (median age, 79 years), the total nodular cross-sectional area was more than 100 mm². Most nodules were located in the transition zone and were predominantly glandular in nature, and glandular periurethral nodules became apparent in this age group.[63,64] Taking into consideration the relation of stromal and epithelial elements present in the hyperplastic nodules, Franks[29] has described fibrous nodules that consist predominantly of a meshwork of fine reticulin fibers, some collagen fibers, and numerous spindle and stellate fibroblasts with few, if any, elastic fibers. Fibromuscular nodules reveal a mixed composition of fibrous tissue and smooth muscle elements, whereas in some rare cases smooth muscle cells predominate producing pure muscular nodules. The admixture of epithelial and stromal elements in the proliferative process may give rise to two types of hyperplastic nodule. In the fibroadenomatous nodules, the acini are lined by low cuboidal epithelium and the connective tissue is of the loose variety, resembling the periacinar stroma in breast lobules. The second variety, the fibromyoadenomatous nodule, represents the common type of large hyperplastic nodules seen in surgically removed prostates and shows a predominance of epithelial over stromal fibromuscular proliferation.

They may be small or large and are lined by tall columnar epithelium with prominent basal cells or by low cuboidal epithelium with a rather inconspicuous basal cell layer. Proliferative patterns may assume the form of intra-acinar papillary hyperplasia or, less frequently, a pseudocribriform or solid trabecular arrangement.

The morphology of early and late extensive prostatic nodularity is illustrated in Figures 31-7 through 31-10.

Regressive changes are commonly seen in hyperplastic nodules, including epithelial atrophy, cystic dilation of the acini, and infarcts with subsequent scarring. Chronic inflammatory changes are also frequent and consist of focal or diffuse lymphocytic infiltrates; acute and chronic abscesses may also be seen. Distended acini may rupture, and their inspissated content extruded into the surrounding stroma may elicit a chronic inflammatory reaction including foreign body-type granulomas containing multinucleated giant cells and histiocytes.

REFERENCES

1. Anderson RW, Weller C: Prostatic secretion leukocyte studies in nonbacterial prostatitis (prostatosis). J Urol 121:292, 1979
2. Armenian HK, Lilienfeld AM, Diamond EL, Bross LDJ: Relationship between benign prostatic hyperplasia and cancer of the prostate: a prospective and retrospective study. Lancet 2:115, 1974
3. Ayala AG, Srigley JR, Ro JY et al : Clear cell cribriform hyperplasia of prostate. Am J Surg Pathol 10:665, 1986
3a. Bartsch G, Bruennger A, Deklerk DP, et al: Light-microscopic stereologic analysis of spontaneous and steroid-induced canine prostatic hyperplasia. J Urol 137:552, 1987
3b. Bartsch G, Keen F, Daxenbichler G, et al: Correlation of biochemical (receptors, endogenous tissue hormones) and quantitative morphologic (stereologic) findings in normal and hyperplastic human prostates. J Urol 137:559, 1987
4. Bergner DM, Kraus SD, Duck GB, Lewis R: Systemic blastomycosis presenting with acute prostatic abscess. J Urol 126:132, 1981
5. Bissada NK, Finkbeiner AE, Redman JF: Prostatic mycosis: nonsurgical diagnosis and management. Urology 9:327, 1977
6. Bodian M: Some observations on pathology of con-

genital idiopathic bladder neck obstruction. Br J Urol 29:393, 1957

7. Bourke JB, Griffin JP: Diabetes mellitus in patients with benign prostatic hyperplasia. Br Med J 4:492, 1968

8. Brandes D, Kirchheim D, Scott WW: Ultrastructure of the human prostate: normal and neoplastic. Lab Invest 13:1541, 1964

8a. Brawer MK, Stamey TA: Prostatic abscess owing to anaerobic bacteria. J Urol 138:1254, 1987

9. Brawn PN: Interpretation of prostate biopsies. Biopsy Interpretation Series. Raven Press, New York, 1983

10. Brendler H: Benign prostatic hyperplasia: natural history. p. 101. In Grayhack JT, Wilson JD, Scherbenske MJ (eds): Benign Prostatic Hyperplasia. Department of Health, Education and Welfare (NIH) Publication no. 76-1113, 1976

11. Brunner H, Weidner W, Schiefer HG: Studies of the role of *Ureaplasma, Urealyticum* and *Mycoplasma hominis* in prostatitis. J Infect Dis 147:807, 1983

12. Drach GW: Prostatitis and prostatodynia. Their relationship to benign prostatic hypertrophy. Urol Clin North Am 7:79, 1980

13. Drach GW: Urinary lithiasis. p. 1093. In Walsh PC, Gittes RF, Perlmutter AD, Stamey TA (eds): Campbell's Urology. Vol. 1, 5th Ed. WB Saunders, Philadelphia, 1986

14. Drach GW, Kohnen PW: Prostatitis. p. 157. In Tannenbaum M (ed): Urologic Pathology: The Prostate. Lea & Febiger, Philadelphia, 1977

15. Eickenberg H-U, Amin M, Lich R, Jr : Blastomycosis of the genitourinary tract. J Urol 113:650, 1975

16. Epstein JI, Hutchins GM: Granulomatous prostatitis: distinction among allergic, nonspecific and posttransurethral resection lesions. Hum Pathol 15:818, 1984

17. Ewing LL, Berry SJ, Higginbottom EG: Dihydrotestosterone content of beagle prostatic tissue: effects of age and hyperplasia. Endocrinology 113:2004, 1983

18. Eykyn S, Bultitude MJ, Mayo ME, Lloyd-Davies RW: Prostatic calculi as a source of recurrent bacteriuria in the male. Br J Urol 46:527, 1974

19. Eyre RC, Aaronson AG, Weinstein BJ: Palisading granulomas of the prostate associated with prostatic surgery. J Urol 136:121, 1986

20. Fair WR, Cordonnier JJ: The pH of prostatic fluid: a reappraisal and therapeutic implications. J Urol 120:695, 1978

21. Fair WR, Couch J, Wehner N: Prostatic antibacterial factor: identity and significance. Urology 7:169, 1976

22. Fowler JE, Jr., Kaiser DL, Mariano M: Immunologic response of the prostate to bacteriuria and bacterial prostatitis. I. Immunoglobulin concentrations in prostatic fluid. J Urol 128:158, 1982

23. Fowler JE, Jr., Mariano M: Immunologic response of the prostate to bacteriuria and bacterial prostatitis. II. Antigen-specific immunoglobulin in prostatic fluid. J Urol 128:165, 1982

24. Fox H: Nodular histiocytic prostatitis. J Urol 96:372, 1966

25. Fox M: The natural history and significance of stone formation in the prostate gland. J Urol 89:716, 1963

26. Franks LM: Benign nodular hyperplasia of the prostate: a review. Ann R Coll Surg Engl 14:92, 1954

27. Franks LM: Atrophy and hyperplasia in the prostate proper. J Pathol Bacteriol 68:627, 1954

28. Franks LM: Etiology, epidemiology, and pathology of prostatic cancer. Cancer 32:1092, 1973

29. Franks LM: Benign prostatic hyperplasia: gross and microscopic anatomy. p. 63. In Grayhack JT, Wilson JD, Scherbenske MJ (eds): Benign Prostatic Hyperplasia. Department of Health, Education and Welfare (NIH) Publication no. 76-1113, 1976

29a. Gardner WA, Jr., Culberson, DE: Atrophy and proliferation in the young adult prostate. J Urol 137:57, 1987

30. Gardner WA, Jr., Culberson DE, Bennett BD: *Trichomonas vaginalis* in the prostate gland. Arch Pathol Lab Med 110:430, 1986

31. Gloyna RE, Siiteri PK, Wilson JD: Dihydrotestosterone in prostatic hypertrophy. II. The formation and content of dihydrotestosterone in the hypertrophic canine prostate and the effect of dihydrotestostrone on prostate growth in the dog. J Clin Invest 49:1746, 1970

32. Gray SW, Skandalakis JE: Embryology for Surgeons. p. 596. WB Saunders, Philadelphia, 1972

33. Grayhack JT, Lee CH, Oliver L et al : Biochemical profiles of prostatic fluid from normal and diseased prostate glands. Prostate 1:227, 1980

34. Greenwald P, Kirmss V, Polan AK, Dick VS: Cancer of the prostate among men with benign prostatic hyperplasia. J Natl Cancer Inst 53:335, 1974

35. Harbitz TB, Haugen OA: Histology of the prostate in elderly men. Acta Pathol Microbiol Scand (A) 80:756, 1972

36. Harrison FG, Neander DG: Allergic granuloma of prostate. J Urol 72:1218, 1954

37. Hedelin H, Johansson S, Nilsson S: Focal prostatic granulomas. A sequel to transurethral resection. Scand J Urol Nephrol 15:193, 1981

38. Helpap B: The biological significance of atypical hyperplasia of the prostate. Virchows Arch (A) 387:307, 1980

39. Helpap B, Vogel J: TUR-prostatitis: histological and immunohistochemical observations on a special type of granulomatous prostatitis. Pathol Res Pract 181:301, 1986

39a. Heyns CF, Rimington PD, Kruger TF, Falck VG: Benign prostatic hyperplasia and uterine leiomyomas in a female pseudohermaphrodite: a case report. J Urol 137:1245, 1987

40. Hinchey WW, Someren A: Cryptococcal prostatitis. Am J Clin Pathol 75:257, 1981

41. Huynh MT, Reyes CV: Prostatic cryptococcosis. Urology 20:622, 1982

42. Isaacs JT: Prostatic structure and function in relation to the etiology of prostatic cancer. Prostate 4:351, 1983

43. Isaacs JT, Coffey DS: Animal models in the study of prostatic growth. p. 743. In Chisholm GD, Williams DI (eds): Scientific Foundations of Urology. Year Book Medical Publishers, Chicago 1982

44. Jao W, Fretzin DF, Christ ML, Prinz LM: Blue nevus of the prostate gland. Arch Pathol 91:187, 1971

45. Jinno H, Ueda K, Otaguro K et al : Prostate growth factor in the extracts of benign prostatic hypertrophy. Eur Urol 12:41, 1986

46. Jones SR, Smith JW, Sanford JP: Localization of urinary tract infections by detection of antibody-coated bacteria in urine sediment. N Engl J Med 290:591, 1974

47. Kastendieck H: Correlations between atypical primary hyperplasia and carcinoma. Pathol Res Pract 169:366, 1980

48. Kastendieck H, Altenahr E, Husselmann H, Bressel M: Carcinoma and dysplastic lesions of the prostate. A histomorphological analysis of 50 total prostatectomies by step-section technique. Z Krebsforsch 88:33, 1976

49. Kawamura N, Murakami Y, Okada K: Three cases of malakoplakia of prostate Urology XV(1):77, 1980

50. Kelalis PP, Greene LF, Harrison EG, Jr : Granulomatous prostatitis. A mimic of carcinoma of the prostate. JAMA 191:287, 1965

51. Kelalis PP, Harrison EG, Jr., Utz DC: Allergic granulomas of the prostate: treatment with steroids. J Urol 96:573, 1966

52. Klimas R, Bennett B, Gardner WA, Jr : Prostatic calculi, a review. Prostate 7:91, 1985

53. Koga S, Arakaki Y, Matsuoka M, Ohyama C: Malakoplakia of prostate. Urology 27:160, 1986

54. Kohnen PW, Drach GW: Patterns of inflammation in prostatic hyperplasia. A histologic and bacteriologic study. J Urol 121:755, 1979

55. Lattimer JK, Wechsler M: Genitourinary tuberculosis. p. 557. In Harrison JH, Gittes RF, Perlmutter AD et al (eds): Campbell's Urology. Vol. 1. WB Saunders, Philadelphia, 1978

56. LeDuc IE: The anatomy of the prostate and the pathology of early benign hypertrophy. J Urol 42:1217, 1939

57. Lief M, Sarfarazi F: Prostatic cryptococcosis in acquired immune deficiency syndrome. Urology 28:318, 1986

58. Lou TY, Teplitz C: Malakoplakia: pathogenesis and ultrastructural morphogenesis: a problem of altered macrophage (phagolysosomal) response. Hum Pathol 5:191, 1974

59. Lowsley OS: The development of the human prostate gland with reference to the development of other structures at the neck of the urinary bladder. Am J Anat 13:299, 1912

60. Lowsley OS, Kirwin TJ: Textbook of Urology. Lea & Febiger, Philadelphia, 1926

61. Lowsley OS, Venero AP: Persistent anterior lobe of the prostate gland. J Urol 71:469, 1954

62. McNeal JE: Morphogenesis of prostatic carcinoma. Cancer 18:1659, 1965

63. McNeal JE: Origin and evolution of benign prostatic enlargement. Invest Urol 15:340, 1977

64. McNeal JE: The zonal anatomy of the prostate. Prostate 2:35, 1981

65. McNeal JE: Normal and pathologic anatomy of prostate. Urology Suppl 17:11, 1981

66. McNeal JE, Bostwick DG: Intraductal dysplasia: a premalignant lesion of the prostate. Hum Pathol 17:64, 1986

67. Meares EM: Prostatitis. Kidney Int 20:289, 1981

68. Meares EM, Jr.: Prostatitis syndromes: new perspectives about old woes. J Urol 123:141, 1980

69. Meares EM, Jr.: Prostatitis and related disorders. p. 868. In Walsh PC, Gittes RF, Perlmutter AD, Stamey TA (eds): Campbell's Urology. Vol. 1, 5th Ed. WB Saunders, Philadelphia, 1986

70. Meares EM, Jr., Barbalias GA: Prostatitis: bacterial, nonbacterial and prostatodynia. Sem Urol 1:46, 1983

71. Melicow MM: Allergic granulomas of the prostate gland. J Urol 65:288, 1951

72. Moore RA: The morphology of small prostatic carcinoma. J Urol 33:224, 1935

73. Moore RA: The evolution and involution of the prostate gland. Am J Pathol 12:599, 1936

74. Moore RA: Benign hypertrophy of the prostate. A morphological study. J Urol 50:680, 1943

75. Moore RA: Benign hypertrophy and carcinoma of the prostate. p. 194. In Twombly GH, Pack GT (eds): Endocrinology of Neoplastic Diseases. Oxford University Press, New York, 1947

76. Moore RJ, Gazak JM, Quebbeman JF, Wilson JD: Concentration of dehydrotestosterone and 3- androstanediolin naturally occurring and androgen induced prostatic hyperplasia in the dog. J Clin Invest 64;1003, 1979

77. Morton WJ: Allergic prostatosis. J Urol 118:123, 1977

78. Mostofi FK, Davis CJ, Jr.: Male reproductive system and prostate. p. 791. In Kissane JM (ed): Anderson's Pathology. Vol. 1., 8th Ed. CV Mosby, St. Louis, 1985

79. Mostofi FK, Morse WH: Epithelial metaplasia in "prostatic infarction." Arch Pathol 51:340, 1951

80. Mostofi FK, Price EB, Jr.: Malignant tumors of the prostate. p. 253. In Firminger HI (ed): Tumors of the Male Genital System: Atlas of Tumor Pathology. Second Series, Fascicle 8. Armed Forces Institute of Pathology, Washington, DC, 1973

81. Mostofi FK, Sesterhenn I, Sobin LH: Histological Typing of Prostate Tumours. World Health Organization, Geneva, 1980

82. Nickey WM, Montgomery POB: Eosinophilic granulomatous prostatitis. J Urol 75:730, 1956

83. Nishi N, Matuo Y, Muguruma Y et al : A human prostatic growth factor (hPGF): partial purification and characterization. Biochem Biophys Res Commun 132:1103, 1985

84. O'Dea MJ, Hunting DB, Greene LF: Non-specific granulomatous prostatitis. J Urol 118:58, 1977

85. Oyasu R, Bahnson RR, Nowels K, Garnett JE: Cytological atypia in the prostate gland: frequency, distribution and possible relevance to carcinoma. J Urol 135:959, 1986

86. Pai MG, Bhat HS: Prostatic abscess. J Urol 108:599, 1972

87. Pfau A: Prostatitis: a continuing enigma. Urol Clin North Am 13:695, 1986

88. Pradham BK, Chandra K: Morphogenesis of nodular hyperplasia—prostate. J Urol 113:210, 1975

89. Rich AR: On the frequency of occurrence of occult carcinoma of the prostate. J Urol 33:215, 1935

90. Riedasch G, Ritz E, Mohring K et al : Antibody-coated bacteria in the ejaculate: a possible test for prostatitis. J Urol 118:787, 1977

91. Rios CN, Wright JR: Melanosis of the prostate gland: report of a case with neoplastic epithelium involvement. J Urol 115:616, 1976

92. Roberts HJ: Pathogenesis of prostatic hyperplasia and neoplasia. Geriatrics 22:85, 1967

93. Rotkin ID: Epidemiology of benign prostatic hypertrophy: review and speculations. p. 105. In Grayhack JT, Wilson JD, Scherbenske MJ (eds): Benign Prostatic Hyperplasia. Department of Health, Education and Welfare (NIH) Publication no. 76-1113, 1976

94. Schaeffer AJ, Wendel EF, Dunn JK, Grayhack JT: Prevalence and significance of prostatic inflammation. J Urol 125:215, 1981

95. Schmidt JD: Non-specific granulomatous prostatitis: classification, review and report of cases. J Urol 94:607, 1965

96. Shimizu S, Takimoto Y, Niimura T et al : A case of prostatic malacoplakia. J Urol 126:277, 1981

97. Siiter PK, Wilson JD: Dihydrosterone in prostatic hypertrophy. I. The formation and content of dihydrosterone in the hypertrophic prostate of man. J Clin Invest 49:1737, 1970

98. Silber I, Rosai J, Cordonnier FJ: The incidence of elevated acid phosphatase in prostatic infarction. J Urol 103:765, 1970

99. Slocum RC: Müllerian duct cysts. Trans South East Sect Am Urol Assoc 18:26, 1954

99a. Stillwell TJ, DeRemee RA, McDonald TJ, et al: Prostatic involvement in Wegener's granulomatosis. J Urol 138:1251, 1987

99b. Stillwell TJ, Eugen DE, Farrow GM: The clinical spectrum of granulomatous prostatitis: a report of 200 cases. J Urol 138:320, 1987

100. Swyer GIM: Post-natal growth changes in the human prostate. J Anat 78:130, 1944

101. Symmers W: Nonspecific granulomatous prostatitis. Br J Urol 22:6, 1950

102. Tannenbaum M: Histopathology of the prostate gland. p. 303. In Tannenbaum M (ed): Urologic Pathology: The Prostate. Lea & Febiger, Philadelphia, 1977

103. Tannenbaum M, Romas N: The prostate gland. p. 1189. In Silverberg SG (ed): Principles and Practice of Surgical Pathology, Vol. 2. Wiley Medical Publications, New York, 1983

104. Tanner FH, McDonald JR: Granulomatous prostatitis. A histologic study of a group of granulomatous lesions collected from prostate glands. Arch Pathol 36:358, 1943

105. Thompson GJ, Albers DD: Granulomatous prostatitis: a condition which clinically may be confused with carcinoma of the prostate. J Urol 69:530, 1953

106. Toweighi J, Sadeghee S, Wheeler JE, Enterline HT: Granulomatous prostatitis with emphasis on the eosinophilic variety. Am J Clin Pathol 58:630, 1972

107. Vermeulen A, Van Camp A, Mattelaer J, DeSy W: Hormonal factors related to abnormal growth of the prostate. p. 81. In Coffey DS, Isaacs JT (eds): Prostate Cancer. Vol. 48. UICC Technical Report Series, Geneva, 1979

108. Vihko P, Kontturi M: Transient high serum prostate-specific acid phosphatase measured by radioimmunoassay in prostatic infarction. Scand J Urol Nephrol 15:213, 1981

109. Walsh PC: Benign prostatic hyperplasia. p. 1248. In Walsh PC, Gittes RF, Perlmutter AD, Stamey TA, (eds): Campbell's Urology Vol. 1, 5th Ed. WB Saunders, Philadelphia, 1986

110. Walsh PC, Hutchins GM, Ewing LL: The tissue con-

tent of dihydrotestosterone in human prostatic hyperplasia is not supranormal. J Clin Invest 72:1772, 1983

111. Weidner W, Brunner H, Krause W: Quantitative culture of *Ureaplasma urealyticum* in patients with chronic prostatitis or prostatosis. J Urol 124:622, 1980

112. Wilson JD: The pathogenesis of benign prostatic hyperplasia. Am J Med 68:745, 1980

113. Wilson JC, Walsh PC, Siiteri PK: Studies on the pathogenesis of benign prostatic hypertrophy in the dog. p. 205. In Grayhack JT, Wilson JD, Scherbenske MJ (eds): Benign Prostatic Hyperplasia. Department of Health Education and Welfare (NIH) Publication no. 76-1113, 1976

114. Wishow KI, Wehner N, Stamey TA: The diagnostic value of the immunologic response in bacterial and nonbacterial prostatitis. J Urol 127:689, 1982

32

Prostate Carcinoma

David Brandes

There is a cumulation of unique, if not exclusive, features in prostate cancer that is unequaled by any other tumor in humans. Statistically, cancer of the prostate is second only to lung cancer in terms of frequency in males. If incidental cancer found at prostectomy or latent carcinomas discovered at autopsy are included, prostate carcinoma becomes the most prevalent cancer in the male.

The majority of prostate carcinomas never become clinically apparent through the lifetime of the patient. This intriguing latent type of malignant neoplasia constitutes an enigma in terms of biologic behavior of tumors.

The discovery in the 1930s that metastatic prostate cancer could be detected by measuring the increase of the enzyme acid phosphatase in the blood was the cornerstone for the subsequent development of the concept of tumor markers, both in cells and in the blood of cancer patients.

Treatment of prostate cancer by orchiectomy or by estrogen was instrumental in the development of the concept of control of tumor growth by alterations in the hormonal environment of the host. The highly sophisticated mechanisms that control normal and neoplastic growth of the prostate through the hypothalamic-hypophyseal-gonadal-target tissue axis are providing a model for prospective multimodal hormal therapy. Thus (see Fig. 30-7) prostate cancer growth may be inhibited or restrained by concerted interference with several of the key mechanisms that control prostate cell growth and function.

EPIDEMIOLOGY

Prostate cancer death rates in the United States in 1981 per 100,000 population ranged from 0.1 for the 35 to 39 age group to 605.1 for men in the 85 + age group. The death rate for all ages in 1981 was 21.0 per 100,000 population.[115]

It was estimated that in 1986, 90,000 new cases of prostate cancer would be diagnosed in the United States and that 24,100 men would ultimately die from this disease.[204] If incidental and latent carcinomas were included, prostate carcinoma would be the most prevalent malignant tumor in males.[44] Prostate cancer incidence and mortality rates in the United States are higher for black males. For example, the death rate in 1981 per 100,000 nonwhite male population was 2.9 for the 45 to 49 age group, 845.3 for the 85 + age group, and 25.5 for all ages. In the same year, the figures for white males were 1.0 for the 45 to 49 age group, 580.1 for the 85 + age group, and 20.2 for all ages.[115]

For 1985, it is estimated that prostate carcinoma will represent 19 percent of all malignancies developing in men and that 10 percent of all deaths from cancer in men will be due to prostate carcinoma (25,000 prostate cancer deaths of a total of 230,000 cancer deaths in men). Demographic information regarding prostate cancer in the United States and other nations and statistics regarding prostate cancer incidence and mortality are listed in accompanying Tables 32-1 to 32-5.[195,201-204]

Table 32-1 Cancer Around the World, 1978 to 1979
(Age-Adjusted Death Rates per 100,000 Population
for All Sites and Prostate for 48 Countries)

Country	All Sites (Male)	Prostate
United States*	216.9 (18)	22.9 (13)
Argentina*	215.9 (19)	18.9 (24)
Australia	212.4 (21)	22.2 (16)
Austria	247.3 (9)	22.5 (15)
Barbados**	179.0 (30)	41.0 (1)
Bulgaria	156.3 (38)	9.0 (38)
Canada*	214.9 (20)	21.9 (18)
Chile	191.3 (26)	16.5 (29)
Costa Rica	178.6 (31)	14.8 (31)
Cuba*	172.1 (34)	23.3 (11)
Denmark	233.3 (13	23.2 (12)
Dominican Republic*	53.7 (45)	8.6 (39)
Ecuador*	87.3 (42)	10.5 (37)
Egypt*	39.0 (47)	1.5 (46)
England and Wales	248.7 (8)	18.3 (25)
Fiji*	54.0 (44)	3.3 (45)
Finland*	243.9 (10)	24.0 (8)
France*	255.7 (6)	22.0 (17)
Germany, Federal Republic	242.0 (11)	23.9 (9)
Greece	188.3 (28)	11.0 (36)
Guatemala*	68.6 (43)	4.9 (41)
Hong Kong	235.2 (12)	3.7 (44)
Hungary	269.3 (3)	24.2 (7)

Continued

ETIOLOGY

Many etiologic factors have been considered in relation to the development of prostatic cancer, including alterations of structure and function that may predispose to the initiation or promotion of carcinogenesis in this organ.[44,118]

A possible role of genetic factors is suggested by an apparently higher incidence of prostate cancer in blood relatives of prostate cancer patients[193a] and by racial differences in incidence and mortality. These appear higher in American blacks,[25,70] whereas lower mortality rates from prostate cancer are found among American Indians,[56] Orientals,[83] and Hispanics.[158] Of particular interest are racial and national differences in the incidence of clinically manifest carcinoma versus incidental or latent carcinoma found at autopsy. The occurrence of incidental or latent prostatic cancer found at autopsy is similar in most countries,[2,38,117] whereas age-adjusted mortality rates from cancer of

the prostate per 100,000 in 44 nations ranged from 0.0 in Honduras to 22.3 in the United States and 32.3 in Sweden.[201-204]

Meikle and Stanish[154] observed a familial effect on the risk of development of cancer of the prostate and the plasma levels of androgens. The probability of developing cancer by the age of 85 years was about four times higher for brothers of their index cases, diagnosed as having prostate cancer before age 62. This increased risk for developing prostatic cancer was accompanied by significantly lower mean plasma testosterone levels in probands and their brothers than those in the control group of comparable age. Similarly, mean levels of testosterone and dihydrotestosterone (DHT) in the sons of the patients were significantly lower than those in control groups of similar age.

Incidence and mortality differ with migration, particularly the prevalence of the infiltrative type of latent carcinoma over the noninfiltrative variant of

Table 32-1 Cancer Around the World, 1978 to 1979
(Age-Adjusted Death Rates per 100,000 Population
for All Sites and Prostate for 48 Countries) *Continued*

Country	All Sites (Male)	Prostate
Iceland	150.7 (39)	14.0 (33)
Ireland*	219.0 (17)	23.9 (9)
Israel	174.7 (32)	13.1 (34)
Italy	228.5 (15)	15.8 (30)
Japan	190.0 (27)	3.9 (42)
Luxembourg	269.0 (4)	20.7 (20)
Mauritius	100.0 (41)	5.4 (40)
Netherlands	266.2 (5)	24.3 (6)
New Zealand	172.0 (35)	22.7 (14)
Nicaragua*	22.9 (48)	0.0 (48)
Northern Ireland*	226.0 (16)	19.3 (23)
Norway	193.8 (25)	31.1 (3)
Poland	214.2 (22)	12.2 (35)
Portugal	180.1 (29)	21.8 (19)
Puerto Rico**	157.3 (37)	17.6 (26)
Romania*	161.7 (36)	20.2 (21)
Scotland	275.0 (1)	17.4 (27)
Singapore	249.6 (7)	3.9 (42)
Spain*	194.9 (24)	19.4 (22)
Sweden	198.0 (23)	31.8 (2)
Switzerland	230.3 (14)	27.7 (4)
Thailand	46.2 (46)	0.2 (47)
Uruguay*	271.8 (2)	27.6 (5)
Venezuela*	135.0 (40)	16.8 (28)
Yugoslavia*	172.7 (33)	14.7 (32)

* 1978 only.
** 1979 only.
Note: Figures in parentheses are order of rank within site and sex group.
(Based on data from Silverberg E: Cancer statistics 1985. CA 35:19, 1985.)

prostatic cancer in Japanese migrants to Hawaii, and similar results have been found among Polish immigrants to the United States.[2,104,216,237] This suggests that environmental factors, in addition to genetic predisposition, influence the development of prostate cancer, particularly the induction of proliferative changes in latent cancers.[44]

Extended interaction between prostatic fluid components and the lining acinar epithelium, particularly in species with low basal prostatic output, may influence the onset of prostate carcinogenesis, particularly when modulation of the basal prostatic fluid leads to the formation of corpora amylacea.[118] It is interesting in this respect that the rat, which has the highest ratio of basal prostatic fluid output per organ weight, rarely develops corpora amylacea or cancer of the prostate.[118] The opposite is true of the human prostate, which has the lowest ratio of basal prostatic fluid output per organ weight, and the highest incidence of both prostatic concretions and cancer.

The increased time for modulation/interaction between components of prostatic fluid and acinar epithelium in the human prostate is of interest since the prostate secretes a series of proteases, including plasminogen activator, that may be actively involved in carcinogenesis.[118]

Attempts have been made to establish correlations between prostate cancer and other prostatic condi-

Table 32-2 Prostate Cancer Death Rates Per 100,000 Population by Race and Age, 1979 to 1981

	White Males				Nonwhite Males		
Age	1979	1980	1981	Age	1979	1980	1981
−5				−5			
5–9	0.0		0.0	5–9			
10–14	0.0		0.0	10–14			
15–19	0.1	0.0	0.0	15–19		0.1	
20–24		0.0	0.0	20–24	0.7		
25–29		0.0		25–29			
30–34		0.0	0.0	30–34		0.0	
35–39	0.0	0.0	0.1	35–39		0.2	
40–44	0.0	0.2	0.2	40–44	0.4	0.3	
45–49	0.6	1.1	1.0	45–49	3.7	2.2	2.9
50–54	3.5	3.6	3.7	50–54	9.0	10.4	10.5
55–59	11.2	11.2	10.8	55–59	26.9	28.1	27.8
60–64	28.8	30.0	29.7	60–64	75.3	71.4	78.3
65–69	65.1	67.9	66.6	65–69	153.7	166.1	166.2
70–74	136.9	130.2	132.0	70–74	277.3	270.5	278.9
75–79	239.3	240.2	234.9	75–79	406.6	402.8	412.8
80–84	390.4	382.0	383.4	80–84	629.1	664.0	645.7
85+	563.0	576.6	580.1	85+	722.0	829.0	845.3
All Ages	19.7	20.1	20.2	All Ages	24.5	24.9	25.5

(Based on data from Horm JW, Asire AJ, Young JL, Pollack ES (eds): SEER Program: Cancer Incidence and Mortality in the United States, 1973–81. NIH Publication no. 85-1837. National Cancer Institute Bethesda, MD, 1984.)

tions, such as prostatic atrophy[138,185] and benign prostatic hypertrophy (BPH),[9] but such correlations were not confirmed.[98,153]

Catalona[44] has summarized the conflicting results on the possible role of sexually transmitted viral infections in the etiology of prostate cancer. Several studies have implicated specific viral infections in the etiology of prostate carcinoma. These include in vitro transformation of prostate cells by simian virus 40;[180] detection of herpes simplex virus type 2 particles by electron microscopy;[45] detection of antibodies against herpesvirus;[111] demonstration of tissue-associated herpes simplex virus type 2 antigen in 5 percent of prostate cancer;[14] finding of cytomegaloviruses (CMV) in human semen[136] and CMV antigen in a genital strain of virus.[190] There appears to be no definite correlation between increasing number of sexual partners, history of venereal diseases, sexual activities particularly with prostitutes, early or late age of onset of sexual activity, marital status, and number of chil-

Table 32-3 Probability at Birth of Eventually Developing Prostate Cancer Relative to All Cancer (Including Carcinoma In Situ), by Race and Sex, United States 1975, 1980, and 1985

	White Males %			Black Males %		
Site	1975	1980	1985	1975	1980	1985
All cancer	30.3	33.6	36.9	28.0	31.6	35.2
Prostate	6.1	7.4	8.7	7.2	8.3	9.4

Note: Exclusive of epidermoid skin cancer.
(Based on data from Seidman H, Mushinski MH, Gelb SK, Silverberg E: Probabilities of eventually developing or dying of cancer—United States 1985. CA 35:36, 1985.)

Table 32-4 Probability at Birth of Eventually Dying of Prostate Cancer Relative to All Cancer by Race and Sex, United States 1975, 1980, and 1985

	White Males %			Black Males %		
Site	1975	1980	1985	1975	1980	1985
All cancer	18.9	21.1	23.2	18.4	21.5	24.6
Prostate	2.0	2.3	2.6	2.6	3.4	4.3

Note: Exclusive of epidermoid skin cancer.
(Based on data from Seidman H, Mushinski MH, Gelb SK, Silverberg E: Probabilities of eventually developing or dying of cancer—United States, 1985. CA 35:36, 1985.)

Table 32-5 Trends in Survival: Prostate Cancer by Race (Cases Diagnosed
in 1960 to 1963, 1970 to 1973, 1973 to 1975, and 1976 to 1981

| | Relative 5-Year Survival Rate (Percent) | | | | | | | |
| | 1960–63[a] | | 1970–73[a] | | 1973–75[b] | | 1976–81[b] | |
Cancer	White	Black	White	Black	White	Black	White	Black
Prostate	50	35	63	55	65	56	71	61

[a] Rates are based on data from a series of hospital registries and one population-based registry.
[b] Rates are from SEER program and include patients diagnosed through 1981 and follow-up on all patients through 1982.
They are based from population-based registries in Connecticut, New Mexico, Utah, Iowa, Hawaii, Atlanta, Detroit,
Seattle-Puget Sound, and San Francisco-Oakland. Source: Biometry Branch, National Cancer Institute, Bethesda, MD.
(Based on data from Horm JW, Asire AJ, Young JL, Pollack ES (eds): SEER Program: Cancer Incidence and Mortality in
the United States, 1973–81. NIH Publication no. 85-1837. National Cancer Institute, Bethesda, MD, 1984.)

dren and an increased risk of developing cancer of the prostate.[193a,217]

Endocrine Setting in Patients with Prostate Cancer

Although sex steroid metabolism is not altered in any particular pattern in cancer patients, changes have been described in the binding, metabolism, and circulating levels of sex steroid hormones in patients with prostate cancer. However, the role that these changes may play with respect to pathogenesis and hormonal responsiveness of cancer of the prostate is not known.[52,53,101,133,135,239]

Circulating levels of androgens do not appear to be significantly increased in patients with prostate cancer. No differences in the circulating levels of testosterone are detected between BPH patients and prostate cancer patients[102] or between BPH patients and normal subjects.[108] There are no significant differences in the blood levels of 5α-DHT between normal, BPH, and prostate cancer patients[101,102] The blood levels of the adrenal androgen androstenedione were reported as elevated in prostatic cancer patients,[194] but others have indicated that mean values for peripheral plasma androstenedione were essentially of the same order in normal, BPH, and prostate cancer subjects.[102]

Despite the lack of changes of circulating androgens in patients with prostate cancer, an increased concentration of testosterone, DHT, and androstenedione has been reported in prostate cancer tissues when compared with the normal tissues.[100,133]

Contrary to what has been observed with testosterone and its precursors, concentrations of estradiol in the serum of males are not reduced as a function of age

and may even increase.[181] This increase in estradiol levels and the decrease in the ratio of free androgen to free estrogen as a function of aging does not appear to be related to the development of prostatic disease since estrogen levels in patients with BPH and carcinoma of the prostate are similar to those in normal age-matched subjects.[108]

In prostate carcinoma, less testosterone is metabolized than in BPH and normal prostate, and the amount of formed DHT plus 5α-androstanediols is decreased by approximately 15 percent in prostate cancer. The metabolism of DHT is also decreased in prostate cancer, reflected in a lower amount of formed 5α-androstanediols in comparison with the amounts formed in BPH and normal prostates.[133] Comparable differences have also been noted in the metabolism of testosterone between BPH and poorly differentiated carcinoma tissue, which showed a marked reduction in the formation of 5α-DHT and androstanediol, accompanied by significant increase in the formation of androstenedione.[100,101]

The concentration of assayable DHT receptor in the cytosol of prostate cancer cells is significantly higher than in BPH or normal prostatic cell cytosol.[133-135] In addition, the assayable DHT receptor concentration is significantly higher in cribriform and in poorly differentiated prostate tumors than in well-differentiated adenocarcinoma. In a comparative study of BPH and prostate carcinoma specimens, the highest DHT receptor concentration was also found in poorly differentiated carcinomas.[212]

Nuclear binding sites for androgens are also more abundant in prostate carcinoma than in BPH and normal prostate.[139] Androgen receptor in prostatic tissues was subsequently localized in three subcellular compartments, including the cytosol fraction, the salt-resistant nuclear matrix fraction, and the salt-extractable nuclear fraction.[16] Androgen receptors were quantitated by an in vitro exchange assay[17,112] with tritiated methyltrienolone (R1881),[159] which has high affinity for androgen receptor. Under maximally controlled conditions of incubation including temperature, time, buffers, etc., it has been possible to study the compartmentalization of androgen receptors in the cell and also to determine the number of unoccupied sites and the total number of receptor sites.[88,89] It appears, however, that even when incubation is performed at 0°C certain proportions of the occupied site may be exchanged with ^{3}H-ligands in the incubation medium, owing to partial exchange of bound radioinert steroids with ^{3}H-labeled ligands.[178] Barrack et al.[16] have demonstrated that compared with normal prostate tissue, the nuclear salt-extractable receptors are significantly elevated in both BPH and cancer, whereas nuclear salt-resistant receptors are only elevated in BPH and not in cancer.

Zumoff et al.[239] have reported significant differences in the endogenous hormonal patterns of prostate cancer patients younger than 65 and patients 65 years or older. Testosterone decreased with age, but DHT showed no change with age in normal men. Prostate cancer patients under the age of 65 had significantly subnormal levels of both hormones, whereas in patients 65 years or older the values for the two hormones appeared normal. The concentration of cortisol was age invariant in normal men, but fell sharply with age in prostate cancer patients. Plasma estrone levels were age invariant in controls and in prostate cancer patients, but the mean level in the latter was markedly elevated. This dichotomy in the endogenous hormonal patterns between patients older and younger than 65 concurs with a significantly poorer prognosis and possibly a more definite genetic risk in younger patients, suggesting a two-disease theory of prostate cancer.[239]

NATURAL HISTORY OF PROSTATE CARCINOMA

The natural history of prostate tumors has been defined as "the evolution of the clinical and pathological manifestations of the neoplasm from inception until death in the untreated host."[235] This natural history is variable and unpredictable. Wide dissemi-

nation may occur before local symptoms become apparent, as for occult carcinoma.[185] Or prostate tumors may have an indolent course, remain localized, and produce few if any symptoms. They may be discovered at autopsy (latent tumors).[79] If found during transurethral resection or prostatectomy for benign obstructive disease, they are incidental findings. The variability and unpredictability of the course of the disease depends on host factors that will influence the quality and duration of life and on tumor-related factors that will determine the biologic malignant potential of the neoplasia.

The age of the host appears to influence the natural history of prostate cancer. Owing to the increase of life expectancy, more men reach the age of 50 and more live to the age of 75. This results in an increased risk of developing and dying from prostate cancer, since this is a disease prevalent in men over 50 years of age. Although over 20,000 deaths from cancer of the prostate have been projected to have occurred in the United States during each of the past 10 years, this figure represents less than 1 percent of the males estimated to have histologic evidence of cancer of the prostate.[10] Such a difference between latent and clinically manifest prostatic cancer may result from the rather advanced age of the host when this disease develops and death from other causes becomes increasingly competitive.[186,189] Patients under 50 years of age may present in a more advanced stage of their disease at the time of diagnosis, because stage A tumors, reflecting the occurrence of latent carcinoma, are less likely to be incidentally detected in subjects below 50 years of age, since surgical procedures for outlet obstruction are less frequent in this age range.[116] Also, younger patients have fewer competing causes of death, and they may remain at risk longer for cancer progression, thus appearing to have a higher prostate cancer mortality than older patients.[44] Benson, et al,[22a] however, feel that age at presentation is not as important a variable as clinical stage, histologic grade, or treatment modality in determining the ultimate outcome.

STAGING

In the staging system introduced by Whitmore,[234,235] patients with prostate carcinoma fall into four broad clinicopathologic categories, designated as

A, B, C, and D. In stage A, no tumor is detected by rectal examination and there are no clinical manifestations. The tumor is found microscopically during examination of prostatic tissue removed for apparently benign conditions. Stage B presents with a palpable nodule confined to the prostate. In stage C, the tumors have extended through the prostatic capsule into adjacent organs, such as seminal vesicles, bladder neck, or to the lateral side wall of the pelvis, but without metastases. In stage D, metastatic spread has occurred to lymph nodes or to other organs, such as liver, lungs, and bone.

(The traditional conception implies that stage A lesions are the precursors of stage B lesions, stage A lesions simply being smaller and thus impalpable. However, McNeal et al.[153b] have recently presented evidence that the distinction between stage A and stage B carcinomas is more one of location than of size. In their studies stage A lesions were auterior, reachable by transurethral resection, and stage B lesions were posterior and thus palpable rectally. However, measurement revealed that stage A and stage B lesions were basically coextensive both in volume and grade. As had been previously described,[153a] the larger lesions (of both stages) were usually higher grade and more invasive.)

The staging system has been modified by Jewett[120] as new series of treated cases were examined and survival results were re-evaluated. Stage A tumors were separated into A1, with focal limited tumor infiltration, and A2, with diffuse and extensive infiltration or when tumors are poorly differentiated. Stage B tumors were separated into two subclasses: B1 when less than one lobe had been involved, and B2 when a complete lobe and part of the second lobe of the prostate were involved. Stage D carcinomas were in turn separated into D1, when pelvic lymph node metastasis remained confined to below the bifurcation of the aorta, and D2, reserved to cases in which lymph node or bone metastasis extended above the aortic bifurcation or when other organs such as the lung or liver are compromised.

The American Joint Committee for Cancer Staging and End Results Reporting Committee[7] recommended the use of Roman numerals I, II, III, and IV to designate the four recognized stages (A, B, C, D) of prostate cancer, and this system was adopted by the Veterans Administration Cooperative Urological Research Group (VACURG) in their studies.[40]

In the tumor-node-metastasis (TNM) system for staging prostate carcinoma,[7,44,47,173] T0 to T4 categorize the local extension ranging from a nonpalpable tumor (T0) to a fixed tumor extending beyond the capsule into neighboring structures (T4). Similarly, N0 to N4 and M0 to M1 are used to categorize the presence and extension of regional and distant lymph node, visceral, and bone metastasis. The TNM system is only partially comparable to the A–D system that is used prevalently in the United States.

CLINICAL PRESENTATION

Mostofi and Davis[168] have delineated the various types of presentation of prostate carcinoma:

Clinical carcinoma. Cases in which diagnosis is made clinically and confirmed by histology.

Incidental (subclinical) carcinoma. Cases detected during microscopic examination of the tissues surgically removed for nonmalignant disease, particularly BPH.

Occult carcinoma. Metastases are detected before the identification of a primary prostatic tumor.

Latent carcinoma. Tumors of the prostate detected during autopsy in patients that showed no clinical evidence of prostate cancer.

Reports on the relative prevalence of these various forms of presentation of cancer of the prostate fluctuate widely, particularly since the various terms have been indiscriminantly interchanged. Thus, incidental carcinomas detected in surgical specimens removed for benign hyperplasia have been refered to as "occult," "latent," "unsuspected," "early," or "Stage A."[15,20,56,114,198] Routine screening by digital rectal examination will substantially lower the average clinical stage at diagnosis by increasing the percentage of clinically silent stage A and B lesions.[224a]

The frequency of latent carcinoma of the prostate in autopsies has been estimated to be 6.6 to 66.7 percent,[23] and most clinicians find a significant increase with aging,[23,79,105,144,185] whereas the overall frequency of occurrence of incidental carcinoma is about 10 percent and its prognosis may be influenced by the extent or volume of the tumor and histologic grade.[42,198]

Several studies have addressed the problem of the amount of sampling adequate for the detection of all clinically significant prostate cancers.[87,174,227] Garborg and Eide[87] indicate that the probability of 100 percent detection in patients with a clinical diagnosis of malignancy is attained by processing one block, but at least eight blocks are required to attain the probability of 98 percent detection when the clinical diagnosis is benign. Vollmer[227] considers that five-block sampling of transurethral prostatectomy (TURP) specimens will detect 90 percent of cancers, particularly high grade (Gleason patterns 4 and 5), all progressive tumors, and clinically stage 3 and 4 carcinomas. Detection of all focal cancers would require examination of all tissue, but may not be important for the prognosis. All stage A2 prostate carcinomas were detected by microscopic observation of 6 g of chips selected at random.[174] Sampling of 12 g of chips detected approximately 90 percent of incidental carcinomas including all those of clinical significance.[174] In a similar study Rohr[188a] found that 8 blocks (12.8g) of chips detected all A2 carcinomas and 90 percent of A1 carcinomas.

Probability formulations express the likelihood that in randomly selected fragments from a given TURP specimen at least one fragment containing cancer will be found.[165] If only one fragment of the specimen should contain carcinoma, a minimum of 95 percent of the specimen needs to be examined to achieve 95 percent probability of detection. Ninety-five percent probability can be detected examining 63.1 percent of the specimen, if 3 chips contain tumor, and the figure is reduced to 25 percent of the specimen if 10 fragments contain carcinoma.

SIGNS AND SYMPTOMS

The first objective sign, which corresponds to stage B tumors, is a discovery of a small prostatic nodule by digital rectal examination. Early nodules will become stony during the course of the disease, and in time the tumor may extend through the entire prostate gland and into neighboring sectors such as the seminal vesicles. Symptoms of bladder outlet obstruction, irritation of the prostatic urethra, incomplete bladder emptying, and occasional hematuria may lead to complete urinary retention and eventually to decreased renal function. With the onset of stage D, the symptomatology is dominated by the occurrence of metastasis and will depend on the organs or structures invaded. Pelvic lymph node invasion may cause no symptoms. Bone metastases are not painful when small but may become painful with extensive growth of the tumor. Increased blood and bone marrow acid phosphatase levels are almost pathognomonic of prostatic metastatic disease. Osteoblastic metastases, particularly in the vertebral column, also strongly suggest prostate carcinoma.

Rarely, the prostate carcinoma may manifest either initially or later in the course with a paraneoplastic syndrome.[149a] Most of these syndromes, including ectopic hormone production by the tumor (Cushing's syndrome due to adrenocorticotrophic hormone, inappropriate antidiuretic hormone secretion, human chorionic gonadotrophin secretion) or neuromuscular disorders (carcinomatous neuropathy, dermatomyositis) have been reported but are extremely rare.[149a] However, chronic disseminated intravascular coagulation (DIC) and the related nonbacterial thrombotic endocarditis are reasonably common, prostate carcinoma accounting for as much as 18% of malignancy-related cases. Chronic DIC may manifest as a hemorrhagic diathesis or may be recognized only by abnormal coagulation studies. Thrombotic (or marantic) endocarditis may be responsible for systemic emboli, particularly to the central nervous system.[149a]

HISTOPATHOLOGY OF PROSTATE TUMORS

Tissue Diagnosis

In stage A tumors, tissue diagnosis is incidentally obtained during transurethral resection or prostatectomy for BPH. Presumptive stage B tumors, suspected from rectal palpation of an indurated prostatic nodule, are traditionally diagnosed by transrectal core biopsy. Thin-needle aspiration biopsy may be possible in lieu of the routine core biopsy.

Thin-Needle Aspiration Biopsy of the Prostate

Various researchers[71,129,130,141] have examined in detail the advantages of thin-needle aspiration biopsy. Complications of core biopsy include hematuria, hemorrhage, infection, sepsis, seeding through the needle tract, fever, and urinary retention. Complications from fine-needle aspiration, in contrast, are very rare[129] and include transient pyrexia, hematospermia, transient hematuria, and epididymitis.[130] Acute or subacute prostatitis is the principal contraindication to the aspiration procedure.[130] In general, needle aspiration biopsy is obtained through the rectum with the Franzen instrument[130,141] or with a disposable 80-mm spinal needle, gauge 18 to 20.[129] The sensitivity of fine-needle aspiration biopsy in cases of biopsy-verified carcinomas has ranged from 68 percent to 91 percent,[129] and unsatisfactory results have ranged from 2 percent to 10 percent. Kline [129] reported a sensitivity of 85 percent and a specificity of 91 percent in a series of 540 cases with 158 proven carcinomas, 158 biopsy-verified benign lesions, and 224 cases devoid of pathologic alterations.

Ljung et al.[142] reported a sensitivity of 95 percent, a specificity of 97 percent, and an efficiency of 87 percent in fine-needle aspiration as compared with a 76 percent sensitivity, 100 percent specificity, and 71 percent efficiency attained by core needle biopsy. Chodak et al.[48] also found better sensitivity by fine-needle aspiration (98 percent) as compared with only 81 percent sensitivity by core biopsy.

The needle aspirate may contain a variety of benign cells, such as cells from prostatic glands, columnar cells from the rectal mucosa, epithelial cells from the seminal vesicle, and occasionally urothelial cells from the urethral lining.[130] In the aspirate from areas of benign hyperplasia, the cells form cohesive, monolayered, sometimes honeycombed sheets. The cell membranes are distinct and well demarcated, and the nuclei are regular with evenly distributed finely granular chromatin.[129,130,141] In prostate carcinoma, the cellularity of the needle aspirate is increased, and the cohesiveness and polarity of the cells is reduced. The loss of cohesiveness, crowding, nuclear atypia, and the occurrence of prominent nucleoli are accentuated with the loss of differentiation in the tumor.[129,130,141]

Classification of Prostate Tumors

Classification of Prostate tumors is based partly on the various designations proposed by Mostofi and colleagues.[169,170] Most prostate cancers are acinar adenocarcinomas, originating in the peripheral[153] or outer prostatic regions. Nonacinic carcinomas are relatively

Table 32-6 Classification of Prostate Tumors

Malignant Epithelial Tumors
Acinic carcinomas
Nonacinic carcinomas
Periurethral duct carcinoma
Transitional cell carcinoma
Papillary duct carcinoma
Endometrial carcinoma
Carcinomas with unusual features
Prostatic mucinous carcinoma
Primary prostatic carcinoid and oat cell carcinoma
Salivary gland-type tumors
Adenoid cystic carcinoma
Malignant mixed salivary tumors
Carcinosarcomas
Nonepithelial Tumors
Leiomyosarcomas
Rhabdomyosarcomas
Lymphomas

rare tumors, apparently arising either from prostatic ducts in the vicinity of the urethra or from the prostatic utricle.[169] A simplified delineation of prostate tumors is found in Table 32-6.

ACINAR ADENOCARCINOMA

Gross Morphology

In prostates removed for suspected carcinoma, foci of carcinoma tend to be located in the outer prostate or peripheral zone (see Fig. 30-5) and appear gritty and firm. The tumors usually protrude posteriorly toward the rectum and appear contained by Denonvilliers' fascia. In stage B cases, the cut sections will reveal one or more undefined, small hard nodules, slightly elevated. Early nodules of stage A prostate carcinoma are usually located in the inner gland and/or anteriorly.[153b] As the tumor grows, the malignant tissue extends to the inner zone and may penetrate into the hyperplastic nodules in that area. Laterally, the tumor may infiltrate around the urethra and anteriorly toward the trigone of the bladder. Posteriorly and upward, it may infiltrate the seminal vesicles and eventually the posterior wall of the bladder and the anterior wall of the rectum.

Histologic Typing of Prostate Adenocarcinoma

On the basis of their growth patterns and degrees of differentiation, Mostofi et al.[170] have described the following histologic types of epithelial malignant tumors of the prostate:

Small acinar. Closely packed small glands, lined by single layers of cuboidal cells with homogeneous lightly basophilic cytoplasm (dark cells).

Large acinar. Glands approximately the same size or slightly smaller than normal glands, lined by single layers of cuboidal or columnar cells.

Cribriform. Distended acinar structures with intraluminal epithelial proliferation. Small round spaces in between the cells produce a gland-in-gland pattern. Staining variability is reflected by the presence of cells with clear, dark, or granular-eosinophilic cytoplasm.

Solid/trabecular. Instead of glandular structures, the cells are arranged in sheets or trabeculae. Dark, clear, or eosinophilic cells or admixtures of them are seen in this type of tumor.

(As will be seen, however, most investigators tend to think more in terms of tumor grade than of the histologic type.)

GRADING OF PROSTATE CARCINOMA

The great variation in the natural history of prostate cancer has stimulated many investigators to search for systems of grading that would provide an accurate prognostic indicator for the individual patient, by correlating the grade of the tumor with available patient survival data for tumors of comparable grade. Most of the systems are based on the degree of glandular differentiation, that is, to what extent the tumor is forming glands that resemble or differ from the normal prostatic acinar elements. Tumors in which the glands deviate minimally from normal acini have been classified as well differentiated, and at the other end of the spectrum those lacking recognizable glandular formation have been designated as undifferentiated or anaplastic. Several other architectural parameters, the scoring of cytologic features, and sophisticated quantitative analytical techniques have

been progressively incorporated into grading systems, intended to predict more accurately the clinical progression of the disease as well as the metastatic potentials of the tumors.

Older Systems for Grading Prostate Carcinoma

The Gleason System[94-96] currently has wide acceptance and will be discussed in some detail, following a brief review of earlier systems.

Mostofi[166,167] discussed early attempts to grade carcinoma of the prostate and to establish correlations between the histologic appearance and clinical course and indicated that Broders[39] was likely the first to formalize a system of grading by establishing four categories ranging from well-differentiated to undifferentiated tumors (grades I to IV). The need to keep separate the terms "differentiation" and "anaplasia" was also emphasized by Mostofi.[166,167] Differentiation, in prostate cancer, relates to the extent that the tumor forms recognizable glands, whereas anaplasia should be reserved to departure from the normal appearance of the nuclei in prostatic acini and ducts.

Evans et al.[73] graded prostatic tumors from grade I to grade IV by glandular architecture and cell morphology. Low grade tumors (grade I), formed large acini with papillary intra-acinar growth, and the lining cells were tall columnar. With increasing grade, the acini became smaller (grade II), incomplete or abortive (grade III), or glandular formation was absent (grade IV). Nuclear atypia was graded from I to IV, according to size: 5 or less microns to more than 10 μm. Mitotic figures and nucleoli were graded from I to IV, according to whether they were absent or present in less than one-tenth, one-tenth to one-half, or in more than one-half the fields examined.

Shelley et al.[199] arranged their cases in four classes, roughly paralleling those of Evans et al.[73]

In the system proposed by Utz and Farrow,[225] low-grade tumors show well-developed acini, lined by low cuboidal cells with enlarged dark nuclei and prominent nucleoli. Mitotic figures are rare, and invasion at the margins is minimal. With increasing tumor grade, the acini tend to become smaller and the nuclei irregular. In grade 4 tumors, glandular differentiation is lost, and the neoplastic cells are arranged in solid masses. Invasion at the margin is markedly conspicuous, and mitotic figures are numerous.

The Gleason System of Grading

The Gleason system was developed by reviewing 270 cases of prostatic carcinomas from the Minneapolis Veterans Administration Hospital, which were randomized in a cancer chemotherapy study by the VA Cooperative Urological Research Group (VA-CURG).[93,157] Based on the degree of glandular differentiation and patterns of growth, including infiltration of adjacent stromal and normal glandular elements, the tumors were classified into five patterns, without taking into account the cytologic characteristics of the tumors. Since most tumors showed more than one pattern, the grading included a predominant primary pattern and a secondary pattern, usually but not always more malignant.[94] Both grades were recorded as digits, (e.g., 3 and 4) and pure single-grade tumors were also assigned two digits, (e.g. 3 and 3). The sum of the digits gives the histologic score, which is reported as Gleason 3 + 4 = 7, etc.

In addition to the above histoarchitectural criteria employed in the Gleason original grading, I have attempted to characterize distinctively the cytologic features that prevail in each of the Gleason patterns.*

Grade 1 (Very well differentiated): Prevailing glands are of medium size, round and uniform in shape and diameter, and closely packed (back to back) (Figs. 32-1 and 32-2). Margins of tumor areas are well defined (Fig. 32-1*).

Cytologically, in grade 1 tumors (Fig. 32-3), the acini are lined by tall cuboidal cells with clear cytoplasm, and the basally located nuclei contain uniformly dense chromatin. Nucleoli and mitotic figures are rare. The basal layer of cells seen in normal glands is absent.

---

* Figures 32-1 to 32-18 describe the Gleason histologic grading system, expressed as Gleason grades 1 to 5. The illustrations are based on cases from the Johns Hopkins and Francis Scott Key Medical institutions. Cytologic details assigned to the various Gleason grades represent the sole interpretation of the author.

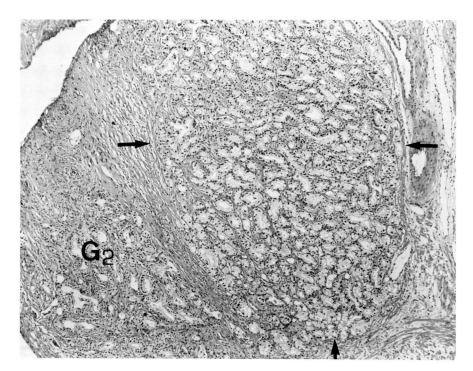

Fig. 32-1 Gleason grade 1 (histology). Well-defined margins of tumor area (arrows). Closely packed single, round, separate glands, with little variation in size or shape. A small tumor, Gleason grade 2, is seen to the left. ×60.

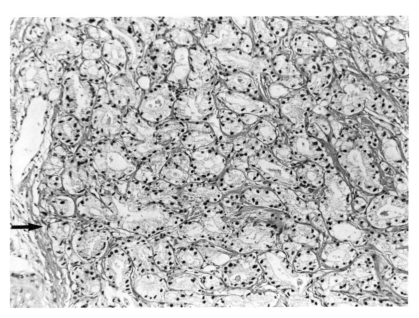

Fig. 32-2 Gleason grade 1 (histology). Higher power view of area indicated by left arrow in Fig. 32-1. ×155.

Grade 2 (Well differentiated): Glands are still well differentiated but show variations in size and shape (Figs. 32-4 and 32-5). Spacing between glands is more noticeable and variable, usually up to one gland diameter (Figs. 32-4 and 32-5). Glandular epithelium may be piled up in more than one layer, and mild cribriform pattern may be present. Margins are less defined than in grade 1, with neoplastic glands surrounding or replacing adjacent normal lobules, but there is no penetration of surrounding stroma by abortive glands or single cells.

Cytologically, the acini in grade 2 are also lined by tall cuboidal cells with clear cytoplasm (Figs. 32-5 and 32-6). The nuclei are basally located, and the chromatin network is uniformly dense. Nucleoli and mitotic figures are only rarely seen. The distinguishing features between grade 1 and 2 tumors are strictly architectural and glandular, rather than cytologic.

Grade 3 (Moderately differentiated): The architecture is markedly variable and may consist of well-differentiated glands, or a variety of cribriform structures, or may show occa-sional cords and masses of cells with some glandular differentiation. Grade 3 is characterized (Fig. 32-7) by the presence of ragged borders with diffuse penetration of the adjacent stroma by small abortive glands and single cells (Figs. 32-7, 32-8, and 32-9). There is marked variation in the shape and size of glands (Fig. 32-8), with small, medium, and large glandular elements prevailing in different areas, and the spacing between glands is also markedly irregular (Figs. 32-7, 32-8, and 32-9). Grade 3 also includes tumors with prevailing cribriform pattern (Fig. 32-10).

Cytologically, in grade 3 tumors (Fig. 32-9) the acinar cells are low cuboidal and the cytoplasm is granular. As opposed to the dense, evenly distributed chromatin network seen in grades 1 and 2, the chromatin network in grade 3 tumors is open and irregularly distributed and nucleoli are frequently present (Fig. 32-9). In some acini the nuclei display a vesicular appearance and contain nucleoli with basophilic staining properties. Similar cytologic appearances may be seen in the cribriform structures.

Grade 4 (Poorly differentiated): The tumors in this

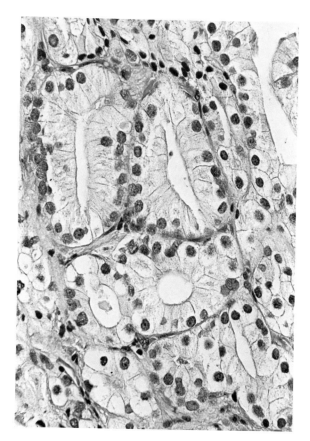

Fig. 32-3 Gleason grade 1 (cytologic detail). Single layer of tall cuboidal epithelium, with clear cytoplasm. Nuclei located toward the base, with uniformly dispersed, dense chromatin. Nucleoli are very infrequent. Glands are arranged back-to-back. ×430.

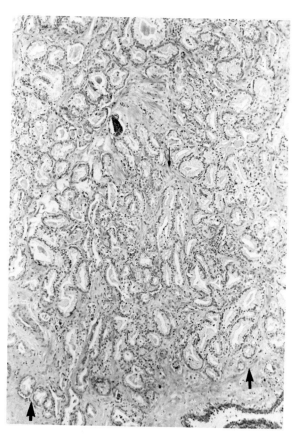

Fig. 32-4 Gleason grade 2 (histology). Tumor margins somewhat irregular, slightly infiltrative, with smaller glands at the periphery (arrow); glands are irregularly spaced, with some variation in size and shape. Stromal plane invasion is seen (thin arrows). ×60.

group either are characterized by masses of apparently fused glands (Figs. 32-11 and 32-12) or may consist of closely packed, large, polygonal, clear "hypernephroid" cells resembling clear cell carcinoma of the kidney (Figs. 32-13 and 32-14). Tumors are assigned to this group when the clear cell pattern is extensive and well developed. The growth pattern through the stroma is diffuse, and the margins are ragged and infiltrative.

Grade 5 (Very poorly differentiated): Glandular differentiation is minimal or absent, and cells grow either in an infiltrative trabecular arrangement (Figs. 32-15 and 32-16), or as nonglandular masses (Figs. 32-17 and

32-18). Although the margins of these masses are usually well defined and expansile in appearance (Fig. 32-17), areas of infiltration of the surrounding stroma by single cells or groups of cells can ordinarily be detected (Fig. 32-18).

There is considerable diversity in the cytologic appearance in grades 4 and 5. Nuclear pleomorphism with variation in size and shape is frequent. Many nuclei reveal an open chromatin network and prominent nucleoli (Figs. 32-16 and 31-18), and vesicular nuclei with acidophilic nucleoli are not infrequent (Figs. 32-16 and 32-18). The main features of Gleason's grading system are summarized in Table 32-7. The cytologic characteristics are shown in Table 32-8.

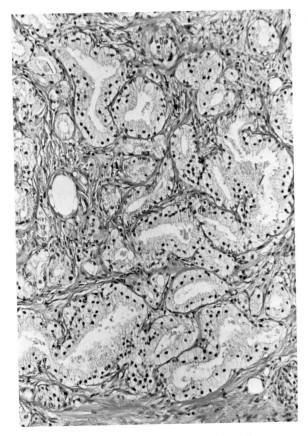

Fig. 32-5 Gleason grade 2 (histology). Higher power view; features as described in Fig. 32-4. ×155.

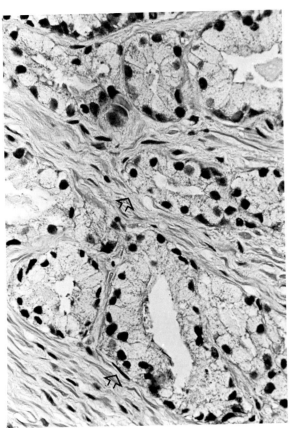

Fig. 32-6 Gleason grade 2 (cytologic detail). Tall cuboidal epithelium, clear cytoplasm. Single layer of cells; basally located nuclei; uniformly dispersed dense chromatin. Stromal plane invasion is seen (open arrows). ×430.

Because the Gleason system has gained such wide acceptance, the Subcommittee on Diagnostic Nomenclature of the Prostate Cancer Working Group has issued a plea that it be the reference standard in pathologic grading, and that clinical and pathologic studies use this system only, or at the least provide a translation of the grading system used into Gleason terminology and grading.[219a]

Other Recent Grading Systems

Gaeta[84,85] developed a four-grade system based on glandular and nuclear cytologic features of the tumor. Grade I carcinomas have closely packed glands lined by a single layer of cuboidal cells with basally located nuclei containing dense, evenly distributed chromatin. Grade II carcinomas retain the glandular architec-ture. Stromal infiltration is present, and the nuclei reveal moderate pleomorphism as well as prominent basophilic nucleoli. In grade III tumors, poorly developed, abortive glands blend with scirrhous areas and clusters of cribriform glands. Vesicular nuclei with prominent acidophilic nucleoli predominate. In grade IV carcinomas there is complete loss of glandular differentiation, and growth takes place in a diffusely infiltrating pattern, or as masses of closely packed cells with expansile edges. Nuclear anaplasia and high mitotic activity (average, > 3 per high-power field) were used as criteria to include in this grade some tumors that might have been included in lower-grade categories.

A recent modification of the Gaeta system from the National Prostatic Cancer Treatment Group

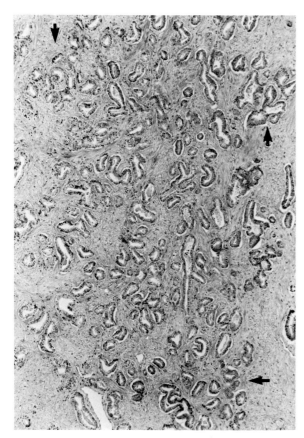

Fig. 32-7 Gleason grade 3 (histology). Tumor margins are poorly defined and infiltrative (arrows). Glands are single, usually widely separate, with marked variations in size and shape. ×60.

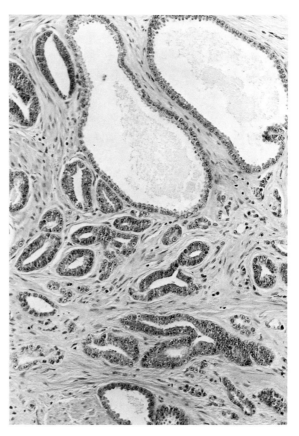

Fig. 32-8 Gleason grade 3. Variations in glandular size and shape, including large, medium-size, and small glands. Spacing between glands is usually wide and variable. ×127.

(NPCTG) incorporates the NPCTG score, which is the sum of the glandular and nuclear grades of previous studies,[84-86] and this was compared with the Gleason grading system based on the score sum of primary and secondary patterns.[94,95] An analysis based on progression-free survival (minimum of time to progression or death)[86] indicated some degree of superiority for the Gleason score over the new NPCTG score, particularly in relation to the primary tumor.

Table 32-9 summarizes the distinguishing features of Gaeta's grading system. Table 32-10 compares the features of Gleason's and Gaeta's grading systems.

Schroeder et al.[191,192] extensively analyzed the prognostic influence of single or multiple architectural patterns (single or multiple formations). In patients with tumors consisting of a single type of for-

mation,[191] only the tumor architecture (in terms of gland formation) and nuclear anaplasia (as judged by variation in size and shape) appeared to influence overall survival and intercurrent death-corrected survival. Of adjuvant value were other parameters such as amount of tumor, presence of large cells, and mitoses.

In tumors with multiple architectural formations, the prognosis of the "worst" part of the tumor is affected by the presence of more benign formations.[192] In exclusively grade III tumors, survival is very poor (70 percent of 18 patients died from prostate carcinoma within 9 years),[192] but the prognosis of grade III tumors improve in when they were admixed with better differentiated portions.[192] The difference in corrected survival is significant in favor of tumors with gland formation (small, intermediate, large),

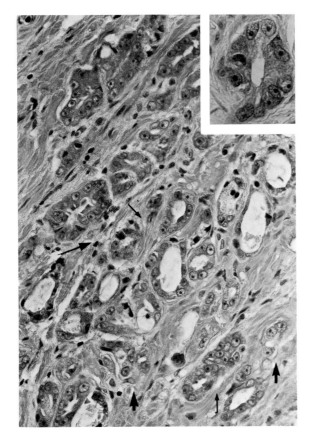

Fig. 32-9 Gleason grade 3. Infiltrative nature of the glands and loss of differentiation with formation of abortive, incomplete glands at periphery (arrows). Stromal plane invasion (thin arrows). ×270. **Insert:** Cytologic detail. Low cuboidal epithelium, open nuclei and prominent nucleoli. ×316.

followed by combined gland and cribriform or solid formations, with the worst survival for homogeneously cribriform or solid tumors.[192]

From these various comprehensive studies[191-193] it appears that tumor architecture, nuclear anaplasia, and presence or absence of mitoses may represent truly significant parameters for grading prostatic cancer into prognostically different subgroups.

Brawn et al.[36,37] describe a grading system based on the percentage of the tumor that shows differentiated (gland-forming) or undifferentiated (non-gland-forming) components: gland formation in grade 1, 75 percent to 100 percent; in grade 2, 50 percent to 75 percent; in grade 3, 25 percent to 50 percent; and in grade 4, 0 percent to 25 percent.

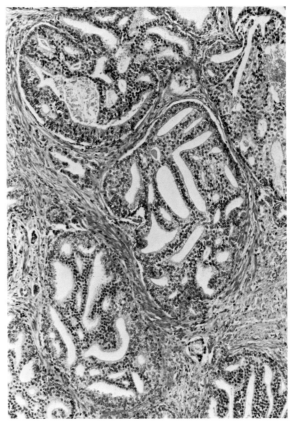

Fig. 32-10 Gleason grade 3. Expansile masses of cribriform structures. ×84.

Muller et al.[171] graded the tumors histologically as highly differentiated, poorly differentiated, cribriform, and solid (scored as 0, 1, 2, 3, respectively), and nuclear anaplasia was graded as mild, moderate, or marked and scored as 0, 1, and 2, respectively. The sum of the score assigned to glandular differentiation and nuclear anaplasia determined the degree of malignancy. A score sum of 0 to 1 was designated as grade I, 2 to 3 as grade II, and 4 to 5 as grade III.

A scoring system for prognostic purposes developed by Bocking[28] assigns a 1 to 3 score to nuclear and nucleolar characteristics such as area, regularity, and size, as well as the extent of dissociation of tumor cells.

The various grading systems of prostate cancer are useful when applied to large groups of patients, but it is not certain that they will serve as prognostic indicators for individual patients.[57,58] Because of variations

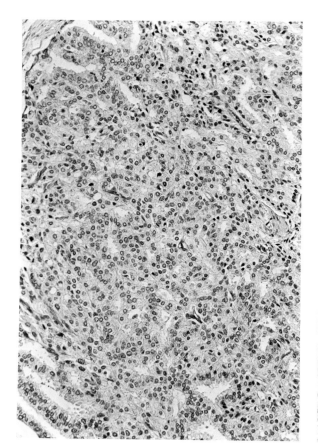

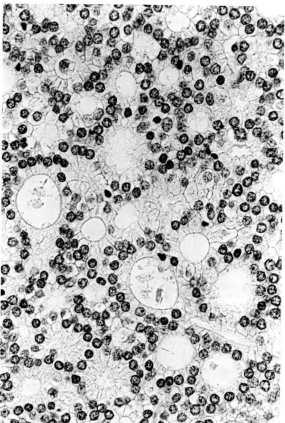

Fig. 32-11 Gleason grade 4. "Fused glandular" arrangement of the tumor cells. Low power showing apparent conglomerate of "fused" glands. ×140.

Fig. 32-12 Gleason grade 4. "Fused glandular"; at higher power the cells appear arranged in sheets with intervening pseudoluminal spaces. True glands and lumina are not seen. ×360.

in the natural history of prostate cancer,[80,235] any system that would predict the course of the disease on an individual basis might also facilitate categorizing the patients for clinical therapeutic modalities intended to demonstrate differences in response to various procedures or agents. With such purposes in mind, many investigators have embarked in developing highly sophisticated quantitative, rather than subjective, grading systems for cancer of the prostate.

Quantitative Methods of Grading

Recent studies have focused on quantitative analysis of nuclear and nucleolar areas and shape as predictors of the biologic behavior of an individual tumor, particularly in relation to metastatic potential and clinical course.

Diamond et al.[57,58] and Epstein et al.[65] have analyzed nuclear area and shape in prostatic tissue from radical prostatectomy specimens for stage B1 and B2 prostatic disease. In the study, 7-μm-thick sections at two to three different levels of the total surgical specimen were stained with hematoxylin and eosin (H&E), graded by the Gleason system and then subjected to computer-assisted image analysis at a magnification of ×1,250. Tracings of the perimeter of the nucleus and calculation of nuclear shape (circumference, area, and a roundness factor calculated from these data) were thus obtained, and the perimeters of 300 normal and 300 malignant nuclei were traced for each tumor. Follow-up data in the 27 patients up to 14 years to 15 years after prostatectomy of stage B1 and Stage B2 carcinomas made it possible to evaluate and compare

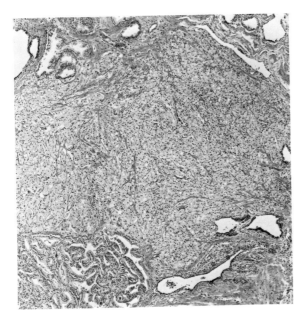

Fig. 32-13 Gleason grade 4. Clear cell, hypernephroid appearance. Non-gland-forming masses of clear cells. Papillary cribriform expansile masses are also visible at lower left. ×36.

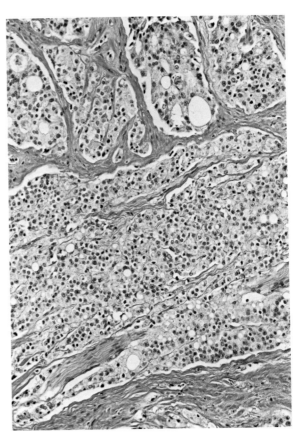

Fig. 32-15 Gleason grade 5. Sheets and cords of anaplastic carcinoma, infiltrating and disrupting the collagen and smooth muscle fibers. Cribriform structures are seen above. ×135.

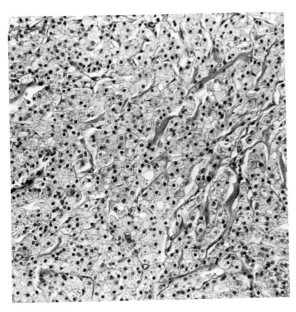

Fig. 32-14 Gleason grade 4. Sheets of polyhedral cells with pale cytoplasm and intervening fibrovascular stalks. The presence of fibrous septa accentuates the hypernephroid appearance. ×135.

the reliability of nuclear roundness and nuclear area measurements with Gleason's grading as prognosticators of development of metastatic disease. Computerized image analysis of the relative or absolute nuclear roundness in prostate tumors could separate accurately the stage B prostatic cancer patients into two distinct groups, one with high lethal metastatic potential and one with a more benign clinical course. By comparison, the Gleason grading system could not separate the metastatic and nonmetastatic groups without significant overlap.

Tannenbaum and co-workers[224] assessed the value of nucleolar surface area measurements (NSAM) as objective parameters for prognosticating the biologic behavior of prostate tumors. Methenamine–silver-stained sections were examined in a scanning electron

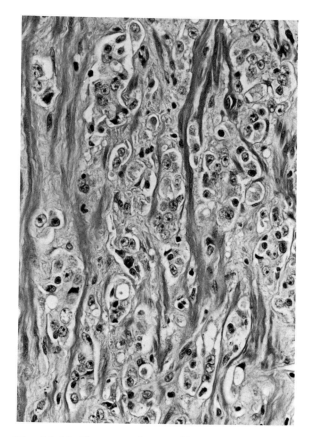

Fig. 32-16 Gleason grade 5. Infiltration through major and minor stromal planes with fragmentation and fraying of smooth muscle fibers and collagen. Marked nuclear pleomorphism and atypia are seen. Mostly open nuclei with nucleoli. ×265.

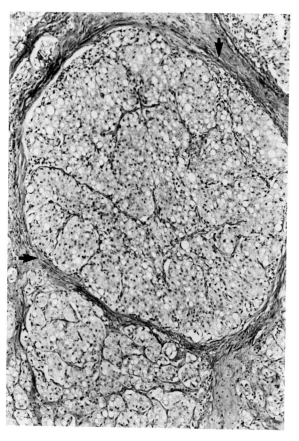

Fig. 32-17 Gleason grade 5. Ragged masses of undifferentiated, almost solid tumor. Tumor masses appear expansile and may have a thick fibrous envelope (arrows), but are invariably surrounded by infiltration. ×160.

microscope, and a minimum of 100 nucleoli in each specimen were measured. The study included the initial biopsy and the prostatectomy specimen from 40 stage B and 12 stage D patients, and only in 30 percent of the cases was there a difference of more than 30 percent in the NSAM between the initial biopsy and the surgical specimen. In contrast, nearly 70 percent of the patients showed a difference of more than 30 percent variation between the initial biopsy specimens and the prostatectomy specimen when Gleason grading was used.

Nucleolar surface area appeared to correlate with the biologic behavior of the tumor. Values ranged from 0.82 μm^2 to 3.40 μm^2 in the 40 stage B patients who had no evidence of disease for 3 or more years. In those dying of prostatic cancer or developing metastasis after radical prostatectomy, values ranged from 4.1 μm^2 to 5.64 μm^2. In patients with stage D disease, NSAM ranged from about 3 μm^2 to slightly over 10 μm^2 with an average of 5.36 μm^2. The correlation between Gleason's histologic grading and disease progression was less accurate. In 4 of 40 prostatectomy patients who developed metastasis or died of prostatic cancer between 36 months and 72 months after surgery, the histologic pattern scores were 5, 6, 6, and 8 respectively, whereas 6 additional patients with Gleason scores of 8 remained free of disease between 6 years and 16 years after prostatectomy. In NSAM studies, there appears to be a better correlation between the initial biopsy and the prostatectomy speci-

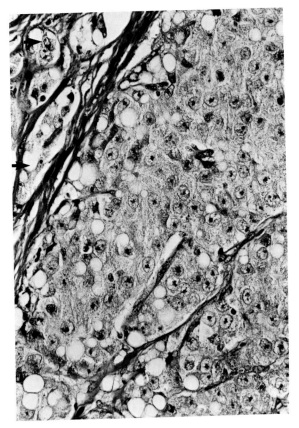

Fig. 32-18 Gleason grade 5 (cytologic detail). Solid masses of highly undifferentiated, anaplastic cells, many with open vesicular nuclei. Prominent acidophilic nucleoli are seen in many cells. The margins, although rounded and apparently expansile, are infiltrative (arrows). ×265.

men and a more accurate correlation with disease progression.

Using a much simpler "eyeball" approach, Meyers and collaborators[161] tried to correlate nucleolar prominence with disease progression in 13 patients who were treated by radical prostatectomy. Within each of the primary and secondary Gleason patterns, the nucleoli were assigned grade 3 when they were large and prominent in virtually every cell, grade 2 when they had an intermediate appearance, and grade 1 when they were tiny and difficult to find. Regardless of the Gleason grade, the mean interval to progression of the disease was shorter in the patients having tumors with nucleoli designated as prominent or intermediate than in those with tumor nucleoli graded as nonprominent.

CORRELATION AMONG TUMOR GRADE, VOLUME, AND STAGE

The natural history of prostate cancer is also influenced by the biologic behavior of the tumors, in particular their potential with respect to growth rate and metastatic capabilities. It would appear that there is a correlation between growth rate, tumor grade, and propensity to metastasize. Tumor grade combined with tumor stage may serve to estimate the likelihood of spread to the pelvic lymph nodes,[132] and tumor grade determined by assessment of the relative nuclear roundness of the tumor cells may have predictive value for survival in patients with clinical stage B prostatic cancer treated by radical prostatectomy.[57,58,65]

Neither tumor grade nor tumor volume alone are good predictors of the metastatic potential of prostatic cancer. Grade and volume, in combination with stage, have a greater value for predicting growth rate and metastatic potential.[94,95,211] Small tumors tend to be well differentiated and have a low incidence of lymph node and bone metastases. Larger tumors, on the contrary, are generally less differentiated, and their incidence of lymph node and bone metastases is more prevalent. Lymph node metastases were found in approximately one-third of patients with small (stage B), poorly differentiated tumors, but occurred in almost all the patients with poorly differentiated tumors that were of large volume (stage C).[211]

Tumor progression rate and cancer death rate are probably the most relevant parameters in the natural history of prostate carcinoma, influenced by the tumor grade and the age and health status of the patient.[44] Stage A prostate cancer generally has a long natural history, and its incidence increases progressively after the age of 50.[235] Recognition of its presence in the patient derives from an incidental finding in prostatic tissue removed for the relief of bladder neck obstruction resulting from benign hypertrophy. The prevalence of incidental stage A prostatic cancer is one-half of that anticipated from autopsy findings of latent carcinoma of the prostate.[77] This discrepancy can be attributed to the peripheral location, extent of the resection, or percentage of tissue examined microscopically.[235] The prevalence of stage A carcinoma of the prostate, including incidental findings at prostatectomy and latent carcinoma found at autopsy, far

Table 32-7 Gleason System of Grading Prostrate Carcinoma

	Glandular-Architectural Differentiation	Tumor-Stromal Relation	
	Distinctive Gland Formation	**Boundary of Tumor Mass**	**Stromal Infiltration**
Grade 1	Distinct glands; uniform size and shape; closely packed	Sharply defined, rounded	Negligible
Grade 2	Distinct glands; irregularities in size and shape; varying interglandular spacing	Defined, but less sharp than grade 1	Bland along major stromal planes
Grade 3A	Distinct glands; accentuated irregularities in size and shape; interglandular spacing	Ill defined, ragged	Along major and smaller fiber planes
3B	Abortive, minute glands and cell clusters	Ill defined, ragged	Along major and smaller fiber planes
	Conglomerate and Uncohesive Growth		
3C	Rounded masses, cribriform or papillary	Sharply defined, rounded	Expansile
Grade 4A	Apparently fused glandular tumor	Ill defined, ragged	Severe, across smaller fiber planes
4B	Conglomerates of pale cells with hyper-nephroid appearance	Ill defined, ragged	Severe, across smaller fiber planes
Grade 5A	Solid tumor masses	Sharply defined	Expansile
5B	Diffusely infiltrating anaplastic carcinoma	Poorly defined, ragged	Severe, across stromal fibers

(Based on the studies of Gleason DF: Histologic grading and clinical staging of prostatic carcinoma. p. 171. In Tannenbaum M (ed): Urologic Pathology: The Prostate. Lea & Febiger, Philadelphia, 1977, and Gleason DF: The pathologist's contribution to the clinical management of adenocarcinoma of the prostate. p. 73. In Skinner DG (ed): Urological Cancer. Grune & Stratton, New York, 1983.)

Table 32-8 Cytologic Features in the Various Tumor Grades

Tumor Grade	Cytoplasmic	Nuclear	Nucleolar
Very well differentiated	Columnar cells; clear cytoplasm	Basal location; condensed, uniform chromatin	Very rarely present
Well differentiated	Columnar cells; clear cytoplasm	Basal location; condensed, uniform chromatin	Very rarely present
Moderate differentiated	Cuboidal cells; granular, nonclear cytoplasm	Central location; "open" chromatin network	Frequent, prominent, basophilic
Poorly differentiated	Cuboidal, polygonal, pleomorphic cells	No polarization; pleomorphic, hyperchromatic or vesicular	Frequent, prominent, often acidophilic
Very poorly differentiated	Cuboidal, polygonal, pleomorphic cells	No polarization; pleomorphic, hyperchromatic or vesicular	Frequent, prominent, often acidophilic

Table 32-9 Histologic Grades of Prostate Cancer (Gaeta System)

Grade	Glands	Cells
I	Well defined and separated by scant stroma	Uniform and normal size; nucleoli conspicuous; chromatin dark and dense
II	Medium and small, scattered and infiltrating prostatic stroma	Slightly pleomorphic; nucleoli conspicuous and small; basophilic
III	Small, irregular, or poorly formed acini combined with areas devoid of organization; includes also cribriform patterns	Significant pleomorphism; nuclei vesicular and show large, often acidophilic nucleoli
IV	Round and solid masses of cells or diffuse infiltration of small cells with no glands	Small or large, uniform or pleomorphic with significant mitotic activity (>3 per high-power field)

(Data from Gaeta JF, Asirwatham JE: Prostate cancer grading: the NPCP system. p. 193. In Vaughan ED, Jr. (ed): Seminars in Virology. Grune & Stratton, New York, 1983.)

exceeds the clinical incidence and mortality from prostatic carcinoma,[10] suggesting that a great number of stage A tumors do not evolve into clinically manifest disease, even though it appears that stage A tumors are the ultimate source of all prostate cancers that become clinically manifest.

Taking into consideration the grade and the percentage of tumor mass within the resected specimen, stage A tumors have been subdivided into A1 (low grade or less than 5 percent tumor in the specimen) and A2 (high grade or greater bulk of tumor mass).[42] In 47 stage A1 untreated patients followed for 5 years to 10 years, cancer progression occurred in 2 percent, with no cancer deaths. The corresponding figures for 23 A2 untreated patients was 48 percent progression and 22 percent cancer deaths.[42]

The Johns Hopkins study of stage A1 carcinomas has been expanded to include 94 patients and to encompass a follow-up period of up to 18 years.[68] Stage A1 tumors included clinically unsuspected adenocarcinomas, which occupied 5 percent or less of the specimen and were histologically not high grade (combined Gleason grade < 8). Some of the patients had

Table 32-10 Comparison of Gleason and Gaeta Systems of Grading Prostate Carcinoma

Distinct Gland Formation		Fused, Indistinct Glands, or No Gland Formation	
Gleason 1	Gaeta I	Gleason 4	Gaeta IV
Gleason 2	Gaeta II	Gleason 5	
Gleason 3	Gaeta III		

follow-up periods extending to 18 years from diagnosis. Twenty-six (approximately 27 percent) of the 94 patients died without progression, of unrelated causes, less than 4 years after diagnosis, and 18 patients died a later time, between 4 years and 8 years after diagnosis, without evidence of progression. Of the 50 remaining patients, 42 (84 percent) remained free of progression at 8 years to 18 years after diagnosis, and 8 (16 percent) showed progression of prostatic cancer at 3.5 years to 8 years after diagnosis.

The occurrence of progression in 16 percent of the patients remaining at risk for 8 years or longer indicates that stage A1 disease is not entirely free of risk from progression.[68] Results reported for stage A1 by Correa et al.[55] showed 8 percent progression and no deaths, and for stage A2 the figures were 63 percent progression and 25 percent cancer deaths. (One possible reason for progression of the seemingly small A1 lesions has been suggested by McNeal et al.[153b] They found that a small amount of tumor in the transurethral resection (TUR) did not necessarily imply a small tumor in the prostatectomy specimen. In one case they found that only 1 percent of the total tumor was present in the TUR specimen. Thus, in many instances of progression a substantial amount of tumor may have been missed by the TUR.)

Because of longer life expectancy, incidental carcinoma of the prostate in younger persons with Stage A1 disease implies increased risk for local or systemic progression of the disease.[27] To achieve more accurate staging, in this study A1 tumors are those smaller than 1 cm³ in volume and histologically well differentiated, and tumors more than 1 cm³ in volume or of higher histologic grade (3,4) are considered as stage A2. From a series of 23 stage A cases in patients less than 60 years old, 2 of 8 patients reclassified as A2 had progression of the disease and 1 died of metastatic prostatic carcinoma.[27] Of the 15 patients that remained as stage A1, disease progression occurred in 4.

A 20 percent 5-year survival rate has been reported in patients with stage B prostatic carcinoma who were treated solely by transurethral resection.[107] Separate data for stage B1 indicates that approximately one-third of patients developed metastasis within 5 years and that death from prostatic cancer was about 20 percent.[54] With stage B2, however, within 5 years to 10 years, up to 80 percent of patients developed metastasis, and about 70 percent died of cancer of the prostate.[107]

Stage C cancer is often associated with regional lymph node metastasis.[235] Within a 5-year period, metastasis developed in approximately 50 percent of patients, with a 75 percent mortality from prostate cancer within 9 years.[24] Stage D prostate disease is more or less consistently lethal.[235] In a series of 231 patients with metastases who were not receiving endocrine treatment, survival rates were 47 percent for 1 year, 11 percent for 3 years, and 6 percent for 5 years.[176] Bone metastases are the dominant clinical and autopsy finding.[234,235]

In the studies of Gleason,[94,95] it was noted that in about one-half of the patients the tumors presented two grades: a predominant, primary grade, and a secondary grade (comprising a lesser area of the tumor). The sum of the two grades assigned to the tumor creates the histologic score, and the sum of the stage (I to IV) plus the histologic score creates the category score.

It appears that there are strong correlations between the histologic score and death rates, the incidence of lymph node and bone metastases, levels of serum prostatic acid phospatase, and clinical stage.[94,95] In patients with tumors composed of two different grades, death rates were intermediate between those of patients with tumors of the pure forms of such grades, rather than corresponding to the highest-grade component.

In the VACURG studies,[96] cancer deaths were nonexistent in patients with tumors of histologic score 2 (1 + 1), but reached about 25 percent per year in patients with tumors of a histologic score of 10 (pure 5 + 5).[94,96] Kramer et al.[132] found strong corre-

lation between histologic scores and incidence of lymph node metastasis during staging lymphadenectomy. The histologic score also correlates with the clinical stage, with more low-grade tumors found in stages I and II, and high grade tumors being prevalent in stages III and IV.[94-96]

Grayhack and Assimos[97] evaluated the reproducibility of grade and stage assessments and the significance of grade and stage in prostate cancer, using representative current staging systems. Grade and stage alone or in combination were analyzed in connection with tumor persistence or progression, survival, and patient death. The exhaustive data presented by these investigators show that the reproducibility of grading in tumors classified as well differentiated oscillates between 3.5 percent and 50 percent according to reports from various institutions. Concurrence between biopsy and prostatectomy specimens is influenced by grade of tumor and is more accurate in midrange histologic score than in low- and high-grade tumors.[97] Conformity in grades between biopsy and excised specimens has been reported to be as low as 28 percent[171] but other researchers have reported 51 percent,[162] 59 percent,[44] and 76 percent[131] conformity.

When results of the biopsy were compared with those of the corresponding prostatectomy specimen,[162] the Gleason score of the biopsy specimens was less than that of the prostatectomy in 45 percent of cases and greater in 4 percent, but no correlation was found between clinical understaging of the primary tumor and histologic undergrading of the prostatectomy specimen.[162] If the true Gleason score may influence management decisions, repeat biopsies may be advisable for low Gleason scores based on a scanty initial biopsy.[162]

Tumor progression including local spread and metastasis is higher in patients with high-grade tumors, but local spread of 34.5 percent and 12.3 percent metastasis occurred in patients with Gleason grades 2 and 3,[94] and progression of tumor and death from malignancy have been observed in patients with low-grade tumor.[97,120] Approximately 10 percent of patients with well-differentiated tumors treated with ^{125}I implantation developed metastatic disease.[18] Clearly, tumor grade alone is not an adequate prognosticator of tumor progression. Stage and grade considered jointly provide a more adequate assessment of this risk. Pelvic lymph node metastases have not been detected in patients with histologically well-differentiated A2 tumors, whereas they occurred in nearly 80 percent of patients with A2 moderately or poorly differentiated tumors.[60]

Similarly, progression of stage B tumors is influenced by the extent and grade of tumor. Prout et al.[183] and Kramer[132] failed to detect pelvic lymph node metastasis in well-differentiated or in Gleason grade 2 to 4 stage B tumors, whereas Donohue et al.[60] and Fowler and Whitmore[77] reported, respectively, an incidence of 16 percent and 19 percent of nodal metastasis in patients with well-differentiated stage B tumors. Stage was an important determining factor since the incidence of pelvic nodal metastasis in well-differentiated stage B1 tumors was 6 percent to 9 percent, but raised to 37 percent to 39 percent in well-differentiated stage B2 tumors. Additional data pertaining to the probable predictive validity of grade-stage correlates in relation to progression and prospective biologic behavior of prostatic cancer are shown in Tables 32-11 to 32-14.

NONACINAR CARCINOMAS

These are relatively rare tumors, apparently originating from either prostatic ducts in the vicinity of the urethra or from the prostatic utricle, rather than from the tubuloalveolar glands in the outer or peripheral prostatic zone.

Periurethral Duct Carcinoma: Transitional Cell Carcinomas and Papillary Duct Carcinomas

Histologically, tumors originating from periurethral prostatic ducts are either transitional cell[46,63,81,121,232] or papillary[19,61,63]carcinomas. Transi-

Table 32-11 Correlation between Tumor Grade and Nodal Metastasis in Prostate Carcinoma

Tumor Grade	No. of Positive Patients	Nodal Metastasis (%)	Reference
Well differentiated	1/6	13	McCullough et al.[151a]
Moderately differentiated	9/20	50	
Poorly differentiated	27/35	64	
Well differentiated (Gleason Sum 2 & 3)	3/19	16	Barzel et al.[18]
Moderately differentiated (Gleason Sum 5, 6 & 7)	18/46	39	
Poorly differentiated (Gleason Sum 8, 9 & 10)	9/15	60	
Well differentiated	0/16	0	Prout et al.[183]
Moderately differentiated	18/51	35.2	
Poorly differentiated	14/25	64	
Gleason Sum 2–4	0/31	0	Kramer et al.[132]
Gleason Sum 5–7	26/84	31	
Gleason Sum 8–10	27/29	93	
Gleason Sum 2–5	5/36	13.9	Paulson et al.[180a]
Gleason Sum 6	11/34	32.4	
Gleason Sum 7	10/21	49.9	
Gleason Sum 8	9/11	75	
Gleason Sum 9–10	7/7	100	

Table 32-12 Correlation between Clinical Stage and Nodal Metastasis in Prostate Carcinoma

Clinical Stage	No. of Positive Patients	% Patients with Node Metastasis	Reference
B	1/4	25	McCullough et al.[151a]
B[1]	5/75	7	Fowler & Whitmore[77]
	4/19	21	McLaughlin et al.[152a]
B$_2$	56/129	43	Fowler & Whitmore[77]
	5/17	30	McLaughlin et al.[152a]
C	18/35	51	McCullough et al.[151a]
	58/96	60	Fowler & Whitmore[77]
	12/24	50	McLaughlin et al.[152a]
C$_1$	9/11	82	McCullough et al.[151a]
D	9/11	82	McCullough et al.[151a]

tional cell carcinomas arise in the periurethral primary prostatic ducts in the junctional area of columnar and transitional epithelium,[63] and the histologic pattern may correspond to that of in situ grade I papillary transitional cell carcinoma[121] or may show overt invasiveness.[221] Subtle histologic differences have been noted between papillary carcinomas arising from primary prostatic ducts and those originating in secondary ducts.[61] Primary duct papillary tumors show intraluminal papillary fronds consisting of fibrovascular cores lined by tall columnar or cuboidal epithelium (Fig. 32-19), whereas those tumors arising in secondary ducts contain smaller papillary projections lined by single or multilayered columnar cells or appear as solid islets of cells, many of which reveal clear, apocrine-type cytoplasm (Fig. 32-20).

Although these tumors originate in the more centrally located periurethral primary or secondary ducts, and their histologic configuration is different from that of acinic tumors, their prostatic, rather than transitional, origin is supported by histochemical studies that reveal positive acid phosphatase and negative aminopeptidase reactions described as typical for the usual acinic prostatic carcinomas.[61,126,127]

Endometrial Carcinomas

These tumors are believed to originate in the prostatic utricle at the level of the verumontanum[43,156,169,222] and most cases are associated with

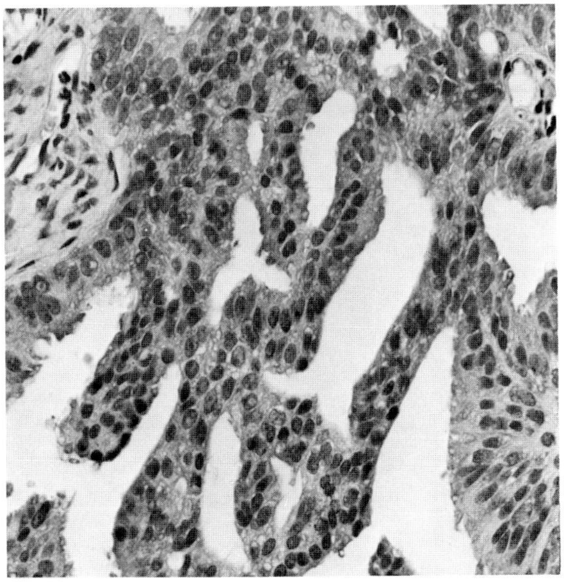

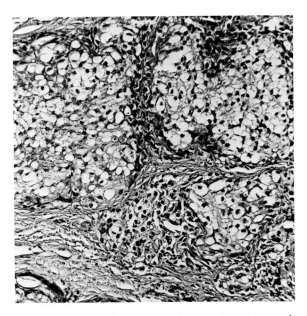

Fig. 32-19 Papillary duct carcinoma arising in primary duct. Papillary fronds and cribriform pattern composed of tall cuboidal cells. ×235.

Fig. 32-20 Periurethral duct carcinoma arising in secondary ducts. The tumors consist of solid islets of cells with clear, apocrine-type cytoplasm. ×160.

Table 32-13 Correlation between Tumor Grade, Clinical Stage, and Incidence of Nodal Metastasis in Prostate Carcinoma

Stage	Tumor Grade	No. of Positive Patients	% Nodal Metastasis	Reference
A_2	Well differentiated	0/24	0	Donohue[60]
	Moderately differentiated	6/12	50	
	Poorly differentiated	4/8	50	
B_1	Well differentiated	5/53	9	
	Moderately differentiated	8/32	25	
	Poorly differentiated	4/10	40	
B_2	Well differentiated	6/16	37	
	Moderately differentiated	13/21	62	
	Poorly differentiated	10/19	53	
A_2	Well differentiated (Gleason Sum 2-4)	0/7	0	Smith & Middleton[211]
	Moderately differentiated (Gleason Sum 5-7)	5/19	21	
	Poorly differentiated (Gleason Sum 8–10)	3/7	30	
B_1	Well differentiated	2/53	4	
B_1	Well differentiated	2/33	6	Fowler et al.[77]
	Moderately differentiated	2/28	7	
	Poorly differentiated	—	—	
B_2	Well differentiated	12/39	31	
	Moderately differentiated	32/68	47	
	Poorly differentiated	4/5	80	
C	Well differentiated	9/14	64	
	Moderately differentiated	33/53	62	
	Poorly differentiated	3/5	60	
B	Well differentiated	1/40	3	Catalona et al.[44a]
	Moderately differentiated	6/17	35	
	Poorly differentiated	5/9	56	
B+	Well differentiated	6/45	13	
	Moderately differentiated	11/22	50	
	Poorly differentiated	7/11	64	

Table 32-14 Grade, Stage, and Survival in Prostate Carcinoma

Stage	Grade	Treatment	Survival	Reference
Incidental	Well differentiated	Suprapubic prostatectomy	75% (5 years)	Bauer et al.[20]
			47% (10 years)	
	Less-well differentiated		33% (5 years)	
			14% (10 years)	
B pathologic		Radical prostatectomy	27% (≥ 15 years)	Jewett[120]
B₁ clinical		Radical prostatectomy	33% (≥ 15 years)	
A	Lower grade (I, II)	Transurethral resection & endocrine treatment	61% (5 years)	Barnes et al.[15]
			44% (10 years)	
			32% (15 years)	
	High grade (II, III)		60% (5 years)	
			44% (10 years)	
			25% (15 years)	
B	Lower grade (I, II)		81% (5 years)	
			70% (10 years)	
			42% (15 years)	
	High grade (II, III)		53% (5 years)	
			43% (10 years)	
			15% (15 years)	
I	Well differentiated	Radical prostatectomy	90.5% (5 years)	Vickery & Kerr[225a]
			50.5% (10 years)	
	Poorly differentiated		(One patient only)	
II	Well differentiated	Radical prostatectomy	80.5% (5 years)	
			58.5% (10 years)	
	Poorly differentiated	Radical prostatectomy	56.5% (5 years)	
			15.0% (10 years)	
III	Well differentiated	Radical prostatectomy	65.6% (5 years)	
			26.9% (10 years)	
	Poorly differentiated	Radical prostatectomy	45.8% (5 years)	
			10.0% (10 years)	

invasive carcinoma of the prostate of the usual microacinar type.[168,223] Grossly, they may appear as papillary, exophytic masses. They are composed of glands arranged as filamentous infoldings with fibrovascular stalks. Endometrial carcinomas may also assume a frankly infiltrative growth pattern (Fig. 32-21). The glands may be partially lined by columnar cells with dense granular cytoplasm and interspersed with ciliated cells, resembling endometrial glandualr epithelium (Fig. 32-21). In other areas, the lining epithelium consists of one or two layers of columnar cells arranged in palisades, possessing predominantly clear, vacuolated cytoplasm and resembling endocervical glands (Fig. 32-22). The presence of two distinct cytological patterns in tumors apparently originating from the prostatic utricle suggests that this müllerian structure gives rise to two separate neoplasms. On the one hand, there are uterine rest elements, exemplified by solid infiltrative tumors with cells characterized by dark granular cytoplasm and occasional ciliated cells, and on the other hand, there are cervical rest elements consisting of tall columnar cells with clear vacuolated cytoplasm.[155,156]

Epstein and Woodruff[69] were able to identify 10 carcinomas with predominantly endometroid features from a review of histologic slides of 2,600 cases of prostate carcinomas seen at Memorial Hospital (New York). In many of these cases, the tumors with

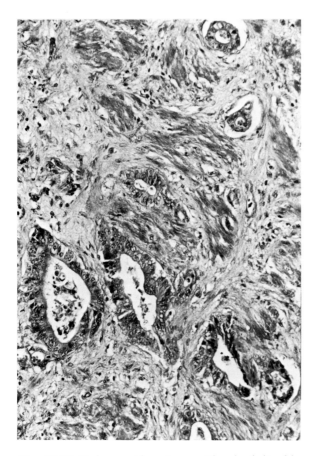

Fig. 32-21 Endometroid carcinoma. The glands lined by endometrial-type columnar epithelium reveal frank infiltrative pattern. ×140.

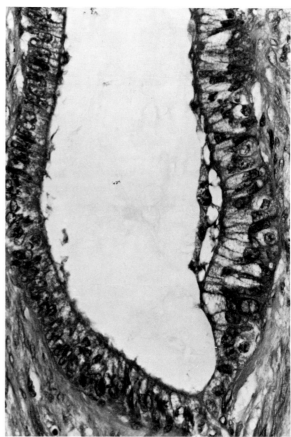

Fig. 32-22 Endometroid carcinoma. The tall columnar, partly ciliated, lining cells on left of the duct show a frank endometroid appearance. The cells on the right resemble mucoid endocervical glands. ×350.

endometroid features coexisted with microacinar prostatic carcinomas. Since all these tumors with endometroid features showed prostate-specific antigen and prostate-specific acid phosphatase immunoreactivity and since some of the treated cases responded to diethylstilbestrol treatment, the authors believe that they should be classified and treated as variants of duct carcinomas.

Bostwick et al.[29] reviewed 13 cases of prostatic adenocarcinoma with endometroid features, all of which exhibited exophytic growth into the prostatic urethra and involved the verumontanum. As in the cases reported by Epstein and Woodruff,[69] cytoplasmic immunoreactivity for prostatic acid phosphatase and prostate-specific antigen were present. Coexistent acinar adenocarcinoma was present in 77 percent of their cases. The endometroid tumors exhibited a

complex glandular pattern simulating endometrial carcinoma, and electron microscopic observations revealed ultrastructural features of acinar adenocarcinoma. Follow-up of the 13 tumors revealed an aggressive behavior, since 7 patients died from metastatic disease 49 months to 70 months after diagnosis, and the other 6 had local recurrence of metastatic spread.[29]

Sufrin et al.[220] presented six cases of endometrial prostatic carcinoma. These tumors also originated in the area of the verumontanum, particularly at the prostatic utricle. Paradoxically, serum prostatic acid phosphatase was not elevated in the cases of metastatic spread, although immunoreactivity for prostatic acid phosphatase and prostate-specific antigen have been proven histochemically in the tumor cells.[220]

Thus, in all of the tumors so tested,[29,69,220] prostate specific antigen and prostatic acid phosphatase have been positive. This challenges the concept that these tumors derive from müllerian remnants at the utriculus masculinus and therefore may display estrogen dependency. In fact, Sufrin, et al.[220] think that the müllerian epithelium is replaced by that of the urogenital sinus, so that in the adult the utricular epithelium is of endodermal origin. If the prostatic utricle is indeed of müllerian origin and is estrogen rather than androgen dependent,[155,156] orchiectomy or estrogen may be ineffective therapy in endometrial carcinoma.[43,155,156] However, objective tumor regression after orchiectomy has been reported in one case of carcinoma of the prostatic utricle.[238] This issue continues to be strongly disputed.

Prostate Carcinomas with Unusual Features

This group comprises tumors likely related to the tubuloalveolar elements in the outer prostate, but differing from ordinary acinic peripheral adenocarci-

nomas by unique histologic and histochemical features, as well as by their biologic behavior and response to routine hormonal treatment. These tumors may occur concurrently with the usual types of acinar carcinoma.

Prostatic Mucinous Carcinoma

Mucin-containing cells can be detected in the non-neoplastic prostate, particularly within prostatic ducts and periurethral glands, and neutral and sulfated mucins have been detected in some clinical as well as latent prostatic carcinomas.[62,82] Mucicarmine stain may react positively with intracellular substances that do not represent true mucin secretory products and it should not be used as the sole method to demonstrate mucin. Elbadawi et al.[62] defined the criteria for establishing the valid diagnosis of mucinous prostatic carcinoma. The tumor should originate in the outer prostate, as does the corresponding non-mucus-secreting acinar carcinoma, and true mucin production, including acidic sulphomucins and sialomucins as well as neutral mucins, must be demonstrated within

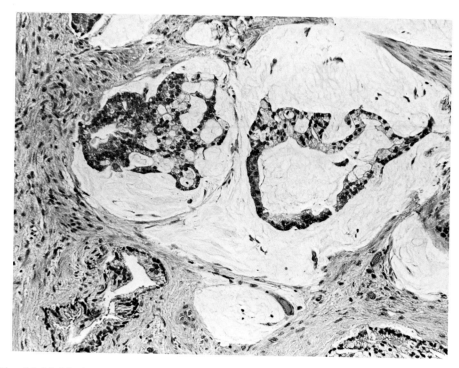

Fig. 32-23 Mucinous carcinoma of prostate. The neoplastic acini appear suspended within mucous pools. ×165.

tumor cells. The neutral mucins contain vicinal 1,2-glycol-reactive groups demonstrable by the periodic acid-Schiff (PAS) stain. Alcian blue staining at different pHs and in combination with PAS will help distinguish sialo from sulfated mucins. In these tumors, signet-ring cells are conspicuously absent. Periurethral duct carcinomas, endometrial carcinomas of the prostatic utricle, and mucus-producing urothelial tumors invading the prostate, although they may contain mucin-secreting cells, should not be included within this distinctive group.

Eighteen tumors that fulfilled the criteria of mucinous prostatic carcinomas have been reported in the literature.[62] Histologically, all proved to be predominantly colloid carcinomas, acinic in nature, since they originated in the outer prostate in relation to tubuloalveolar glands. Typical non-mucus-producing acinar carcinoma occurred concurrently in most of the cases.

Epstein and Liberman[67] found 6 cases of mucinous adenocarcinomas among 2,600 prostatic carcinomas available for review. Criteria for inclusion was that at least 25 percent of the tumor resected during a single procedure contained lakes of extracellular mucin and that an extraprostatic tumor site could be ruled out. All the mucinous carcinomas described by these investigators had positive immunoreactivity for prostate-specific acid phosphatase and prostate-specific antigen.

The histologic appearance of colloid mucinous carcinoma of the prostate is illustrated in Figure 32-23. Although signet-ring cells are said to be conspicuously absent from mucinous prostatic carcinomas,[62] a case of prostatic carcinoma consisting predominantly of signet-ring cells has been described.[92] The prostatic origin was confirmed at autopsy, which revealed an enlarged, hard gland diffusely infiltrated by tumor, without evidence of a primary elsewhere in the body.

Primary Carcinoid and Oat Cell Tumors

Several cases of carcinoid tumors, documented by histologic, histochemical, or electron microscopic studies, have been reported.[8,164,230,231] The histologic appearance is that of sheets and columns of cells of uniform size, with rounded nuclei and small nucleoli and with very infrequent mitotic figures. The cells usually show argyrophilic or argentaffin granules[164,231] and contain intracytoplasmic dense-core granules when examined by electron microscopy.[230] Strong argyrophilia, membrane-bound dense-core granules, and positive immunoperoxidase stain for prostate-specific antigen and prostatic acid phosphatase have been documented in a primary prostatic carcinoid tumor.[12]

Sixty-seven percent of carcinoids of the rectum and 15 percent of carcinoids in other segments of the gastrointestinal tract have shown positive immunohistochemical reactivity for prostatic acid phosphatase, and this should be taken into consideration in differential diagnosis.[214]

A small number of cases of prostatic carcinomas have been associated with the ectopic production of adrenocorticotropic hormone ACTH and the development of Cushing's syndrome.[143,177,228,233] Histologically, some of the tumors had a small cell anaplastic component[177,228,233] (Fig. 32-24) that also showed argyrophilia and contained dense-core granules revealed by electron microscopy. ACTH was demonstrated in the tumor cells by immunofluorescence or immunoperoxidase techniques and in tissue extracts

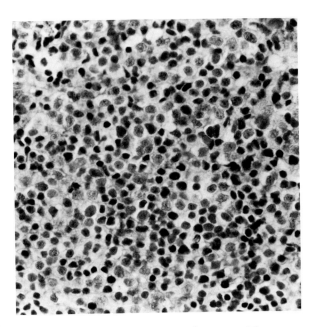

Fig. 32-24 Small cell carcinoma of prostate. The tumor cells show nuclei with dark, condensed chromatin and very scanty cytoplasm. There is a background of necrotic tumor cells. ×350. (Courtesy of Dr. F. Vuitch.)

by bioassay[177] or radioimmunoassay[143,233] methods. Inappropriate antidiuretic hormone secretion by a prostate carcinoma has been described in a patient with hyponatremia and hemodilution.[196] Inappropriate ACTH secretion has been found in association with a carcinoid tumor of the prostate gland.[209]

Bleichner et al.[26] described a case of pure small cell carcinoma of the prostate with metastasis to the liver, but immunocytochemical stains for carcinoembryonic antigen, calcitonin, serotonin, ACTH, and prostate-specific acid phosphatase and prostate-specific antigen were negative. Electron microscopy failed to reveal dense-core neurosecretory granules.

Ghandur-Mnaymneh et al.[90] described the occurrence in the prostate of two separate tumors, one with characteristics of prostate adenocarcinoma that showed positive immunoreactivity for prostate-specific antigen, but reacted negatively for carcinoembryonic antigen and neuron-specific enolase.

Argentaffin and argyrophilic cells may be present in the normal prostate as well as in acinic prostatic carcinomas[13] and may represent the source of the tumors with carcinoid or oat cell features as described above. DiSantagnese and Jensen[57a] have found that 47 percent of prostate carcinomas had immunohistochemical evidence (staining for serotonin, neuron-specific enolase or chromogranin) of neuroendocrine differentiation. It has been postulated that in prostate tumors the APUD cells arise by divergent differentiation, rather than being derived from neural crest progenitor cells.[12,228]

Salivary Gland-Type Tumors

Two variants of tumor indigenous to the salivary glands, adenoid cystic carcinoma and a malignant mixed tumor of the salivary gland type, have been reported as primary prostatic cancers.[78,91,147] Adenoid cystic carcinoma showed a pleomorphic histologic pattern, including the characteristic cribriform, cord-like, and basaloid components with the basaloid cells arranged in solid or glandular islands surrounded by a hyaline sheath. Both the content of the lumina and the sheaths surrounding the islands showed PAS–diastase-resistant positivity.[78] A primary malignant mixed salivary gland-type carcinoma described in the prostate[147] included the usual cell types in this tumor, such as basaloid cells, tubular and cribriform struc-

tures, and myxoid and chondroid elements, as well as areas of frank epidermoid carcinoma.

Squamous Cell Carcinomas

These occur rarely in the prostate gland and usually arise from large ducts or from the urethra.[169] However, secondary transformation of adenocarcinomas to adenosquamous carcinomas has been described in the wake of irradiation in three cases.[170a]

Carcinomas Associated with Schistosomiasis

Association of schistosomiasis with bladder cancer is well documented in the literature, but association with prostate cancer is of rare occurrence. The adult worm usually resides in the vesical venous plexus, and sometimes they may lodge in the prostatic venous plexus, which communicates with the plexus in the bladder.[3,4]

Al Adnani[3] reported two cases of prostatic squamous cell carcinoma associated with schistosomiasis in which prostatic origin could be demonstrated by positive immunoreactivity with prostate-specific antigen. Positive staining for keratin was also present, but immunoreactivity to prostatic acid phosphatase was absent.

Alexis and Domingo[4] described a case of adenocarcinoma of the prostate associated with schistosomiasis. *Schistosoma mansoni* eggs were found in the prostatic chips including the tumor, and the prostatic origin of the carcinoma was documented by positive immunoreactivity to prostate-specific antigen.

Carcinosarcomas

Carcinosarcomas of the prostate are extremely rare tumors. Some of the tumors reported as primary carcinosarcomas may have represented epithelial tumors with foci of spindle-shaped anaplastic elements with sarcomatoid features.[223] Quay and Proppe[184] reported a case of carcinosarcoma in which the carcinomatous component was a poorly differentiated adencarcinoma and the sarcomatous elements consisted of osteogenic sarcoma and foci of chondrosarcoma. Haddad and Reyes[103] reported a case of carcinosarcoma containing poorly differentiated adenocarcinoma and rhabdomyosarcoma. A combination of adenocarcinoma and chondrosarcoma was reported by Hamlin and Lund.[106]

NONEPITHELIAL TUMORS

Despite their rarity, a significant number of non-epithelial tumors, particularly sarcomas, may occur as primary prostatic malignancies, including leiomyosarcomas, rhabdomyosarcomas, and osteosarcomas. Rhabdomyosarcomas, particularly the embryonal variety, are more prevalent in children,[109,150-152] and the tumors may involve both prostate and bladder. Leiomyosarcomas in contrast, show a peak incidence in middle and old age.[41,50,172]

Sarcomas represent approximately 0.1 percent of all primary prostatic malignant neoplasms, and although they may occur at any age, about 30 percent develop during the first decade of life and 75 percent occur before the age of 40.[169] Their potential for rapid growth exceeds that of the prevailing acinar carcinomas. This is particularly true for the rhabdomyosarcomas, whereas fibrosarcomas and leiomyosarcomas grow less rapidly.[169] Sarcomas produce early compression of the prostatic urethra and invade the periprostatic and perivesical tissue. In 75 percent of the cases there is extension to the bladder, abdominal wall, rectum, and perineum. Lymphatic and vascular permeation is followed by metastasis to regional lymph nodes, liver, and lung and to the bones, where the metastases are osteolytic.[41,169]

Leiomyosarcomas follow a prolonged course with multiple recurrences.[41,210] Grossly, leiomyosarcomas are red-gray and of dense consistency, and histologically, the elongated and fusiform smooth muscle cells are arranged in interlacing whorls and fasicles. Cellular atypia with nuclear hyperchromasia, pleomorphism, and mitoses indicates the malignant nature of these tumors.

Embryonal rhabdomyosarcomas are the most common type among the various categories of rhabdomyosarcomas. These tumors bear a close resemblance to various stages in the development of normal muscle tissue, and their histologic appearance ranges from poorly differentiated tumors with very scanty rhabdomyoblasts to very well differentiated tumors formed almost exclusively of rhabdomyoblasts with cross striations.[64] At the Armed Forces Institute of Pathology the overall incidence of rhabdomyosarcoma of the genitourinary tract and retroperitoneum over 10 years was 558 cases, 15 of which occurred in the prostate. In this location the majority of the tumors were of the embryonal variety and affected mostly children between birth and 15 years of age. In the prostate, embryonal rhabdomyosarcomas are deep-seated tumors, not well defined, and almost invariably they infiltrate the surrounding tissue. On manual examination, the tumors are firm and rubbery. They often reveal a bulging surface and are grayish to pink-tan. Histologically, these tumors show variation in cellularity, with hypercellular areas alternating with areas of scanty cellularity. In many of the cases, there are scattered cells with hyperchromatic nuclei and eosinophilic cytoplasm that is characteristic of rhabdomyoblasts.[64] The degree of differentiation is variable and ranges from poorly differentiated tumors that are difficult or nearly impossible to diagnose to very well differentiated tumors in which the cells have the appearance of striated muscle tissue. The course of the disease on patients with rhabdomyosarcoma depends on the stage at the time of presentation.

The disease has been staged as stage I when the tumor is confined to the prostate and stage II when it extends to adjacent structures. Stage III implies regional lymph node metastasis, and stage IV implies distant metastasis.[109,150-152,213] The Intergroup Rhabdomyosarcoma Study (IRS) clinical grouping classification is based on the resectability of the tumor and lymph node involvement.[151,152]

Group I includes localized disease confined to organ site (A) or extending outside the organ of origin (B).

Group II includes a subgroup (A) with microscopic residual disease but no regional node involvement and a subgroup (B) with regional node involvement.

Group III includes cases with gross residual disease.

Group IV includes cases with distant metastatic disease observed at onset.

These tumors have been treated by radical surgery, alone or in combination with chemotherapy and x-ray therapy. Chemotherapy includes monthly courses of vincristine, actinomycin, and cyclophosphamide with pathologic evaluations of surgically resected tumor and additional x-ray therapy for residual disease. Results thus far obtained with intense chemotherapy indicate that with chemotherapy alone, relapse-free survival was achieved by approximately 10 percent of the patients.[213] Approximately three-fourths of the bladder and prostate tumors required radiotherapy. Two-thirds of these patients were alive and relapse-free with a median follow-up of 2.7 years.[213]

Malignant lymphomas of the prostate may occur as primary extranodal tumors or as secondary involvement from previously documented lymphoma at other sites. The patients with prostatic lymphomas usually develop symptoms of urinary obstruction, whereas systemic symptoms, such as fever, weight loss, night sweats, and chills rarely occur. Bostwick and Mann[30] identified 13 cases of lymphoma of the prostate, including 7 primary extranodal prostatic lymphomas and 6 cases of secondary involvement. These tumors appear to have a very poor prognosis as 12 of the 13 patients died within 2 years after diagnosis, despite a variety of therapeutic approaches including radiation therapy, chemotherapy, or surgery, in many cases in a combined modality.

Ben-Ezra et al.[21] reported the incidental finding of an angiotropic large cell lymphoma of the prostate gland in a patient with prostatic carcinoma, and immunohistochemical studies showed it to be a lymphoma of B-cell origin.

The prostate may also be the site of infiltration in leukemic patients,[160] especially in the cases of lymphatic leukemia, and involvement of this organ has also been seen in two patients with multiple myeloma.[72]

Manivel et al.[146] described two cases of cystosarcoma phyllodes of the prostate, in one of which the stromal elements appeared frankly sarcomatous. Immunohistochemical stains showed positive reaction for vimentin, whereas reactivity for desmin was positive only in the benign-appearing stromal cells. The epithelial component in both cases showed positive reactivity for epithelial membrane antigen, low- and high-molecular-weight keratin, and prostate-specific antigen.[146]

TUMOR MARKERS FOR PROSTATE CANCER

The characterization of tumor cell markers, unique to a specific organ or tissue site, is presently a major goal in cancer research. In the prostate gland, identification of some of these markers may serve to establish the prostatic nature of a metastatic tumor and provide significant predictive information on biologic behavior of prostate cancer. The substances that constitute these markers may be present exclusively in the tumor cells, in the blood of the patient, or in both.

In general, these markers have contributed to diagnosis, detection of metastases, and staging and may serve as parameters for prediction of therapeutic response and for monitoring the course of the disease.[51]

Acid Phosphatase: Catalytic Methods

The acid phosphatases hydrolyze esters of orthophosphoric acid, most reactions being measured at an acid pH, in the range of 4.8 to 6.0. Using a variety of substrates, including glycerophosphate, *para*-nitrophenyl phosphate, and naphthol AS phosphate, acid phosphatase reaction products are visualized in the acinar cells as minute intracytoplasmic granules. Some of these represent secretory granules; others indicate the presence of lysosomal bodies.[31,32,110,125] Secretory acid phosphatase is released into the prostatic fluid, where it may participate in the metabolism of spermatozoa by catalyzing transfer of phosphates.[145] Lysosomal acid phosphatase is part of the acid hydrolase complement of lysosomal enzymes, which are concerned with catabolic and digestive intracellular events.[33]

Numerous substrates and inhibitors have been tried for the specific localization of prostatic acid phosphatase. Tartrate greatly inhibits catalytic activity of secretory acid phosphatase,[1] but this substance depresses lysosomal phosphatase activity as well. Phosphorylcholine and D-ephedrine phosphate (DEP) were extensively investigated as to their validity for demonstration of prostatic acid phosphatase in tissue sections.[179,197] However, other tissues (pancreas, epididymis, thyroid, and preputial glands) react positively when incubated with DEP. Happily, these methods are now largely of historical interest, having been supplanted by more sensitive and specific immunohistochemical techniques.

Acid Phosphatase: Immunohistochemical Methods

Immunohistochemical methods for prostatic acid phosphatase (PAP) are now widely applied to investigative and diagnostic problems and include a wide range of conventional and monoclonal antibodies for immunofluorescence and immunoperoxidase techniques.

Pontes et al.,[182] using the indirect immunofluorescence method with an antibody against acid phosphatase, showed specific fluorescence in benign prostatic epithelium as well as in the epithelium of carcinoma cells. Later, Choe et al.[49] prepared specific antiphosphatase antisera from a purified PAP obtained from prostatic tissue and from a lysosomal acid phosphatase obtained from diploid fibroblasts (WI 38). By direct immunofluorescence and by the unlabeled antibody method, lysosomal acid phosphatase was recognized as granules in all the epithelial cells, fibroblasts, and peripheral blood cells examined, whereas PAP was only detected in prostatic epithelial cells.

The immunoperoxidase method for the histochemical demonstration of PAP in tissue sections is a highly specific and sensitive technique. Of particular interest has been the application of immunoperoxidase techniques to the identification of the prostatic origin in metastatic disease of undetermined primary site, such as in occult prostate carcinoma, and in the resolution of the identity of collision tumors, such as coexisting prostate and rectal carcinomas.[75,137,175,236] This method can also be applied to the differential diagnosis of rare prostate tumors, such as periurethral duct carcinomas, endometroid carcinomas, carcinoids, and transitional cell tumors.

Immunocytochemical staining of material from fine-needle aspiration biopsy for prostate-specific antigen and prostate-specific acid phosphatase revealed positive reactivity in 93 percent of the cases stained for prostate-specific acid phosphatase and in 81 percent of cases investigated for prostate-specific antigen reactivity.[123] There was good correlation between cytologic and histologic specimens regarding prostate-specific antigen and acid phosphatase immunoreactivity, but not as regards tumor grade and the percentage of cells showing positive immunoreactivity.[123]

Immunoultrastructural studies have demonstrated the presence of secretory acid phosphatase in the rough endoplasmic reticulum, in the Golgi complex, and in secretory vacuoles and vesicles.[11,140,215] Acid phosphatase may be seen in lysosomes, dense bodies, and leucocyte granule lysosomes.[11]

The varied localization of prostatic acid phosphatase indicates that enzyme synthesis occurs at the bound ribosomes, from where it is discharged into the cisternae of the rough endoplasmic reticulum to be transported to the Golgi complex and Golgi complex-associated vesicles.[11,140,215] It has been also noted that vesicles and vacuoles from the Golgi complex may fuse with the plasma membrane and discharge their content, including acid phosphatase, into the lumen of the gland as well as into the interstitial space and lymphatic channels.[11] The latter may explain the elevation of acid phosphatase in the serum of some patients with prostatic cancer.[11]

Prostate-Specific Antigen: Immunohistochemical Localization

Several studies have documented the specificity and sensitivity of the immunoperoxidase staining method for prostate-specific antigen for the identification of

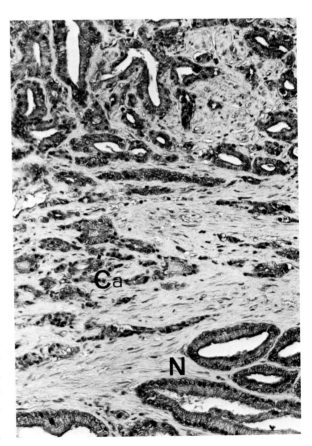

Fig. 32-25 Prostatic acid phosphatase—immunoperoxidase technique. There is intense reactivity in normal (N) and carcinoma (Ca) glands. ×174.

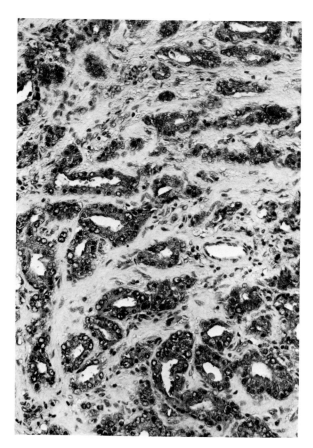

Fig. 32-26 Prostate-specific antigen—immunoperoxidase technique. There is intense reactivity in the cytoplasm of this moderately differentiated carcinoma. ×174.

all but one of which were positive for prostatic acid phosphatase. Keidlor and Aterman[123a] obtained similar results in a group of 20 patients. All of the above evidence indicates that prostate-specific antigen is reliably found only in well differentiated lesions, and its absence may well have negative import for the prognosis.

Figure 32-25 illustrates the immunohistologic localization of PAP, and Figure 32-26 demonstrates the localization of prostate-specific antigen in normal prostate glands and in moderately differentiated and

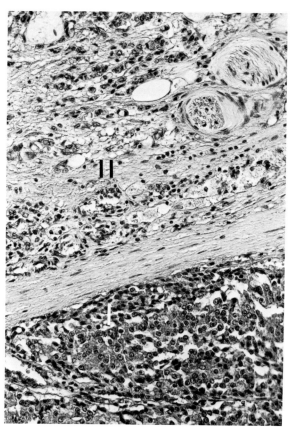

Fig. 32-27 Collision tumors in the pouch of Douglas. There are two separate areas of undifferentiated carcinoma (I and II). Tumor area designated as I (below) reveals intense reactivity for prostatic acid phosphatase. Identical staining obtained also with prostate-specific antigen, identifying it as prostatic cancer. From autopsy studies, this patient had prostate and colon carcinomas that had infiltrated in the pouch of Douglas. Area I, positive for PAP and prostate-specific antigen, corresponds to the area of prostate carcinoma. Area II, (above) which remained negative, corresponds to the colon cancer and stained positive for carcinoembryonic antigen and mucin. ×174.

primary and metastatic prostatic tumors.[5,218] Attempts have also been made to correlate prostate-specific antigen reactivity with tumor differentiation and clinical outcome.

Stein[218] noted that in high-grade tumors, such as Gleason grade 10, there was a prevalence of focal rather than diffuse staining with the prostate-specific antigen method when compared with that of low-grade tumors. In a study correlating prostate-specific antigen reactivity with the biologic behavior of prostate tumors, Epstein et al.[66] were able to demonstrate that patients with tumors that expressed weak or negative prostate-specific antigen immunoreactive staining showed a greater tendency toward tumor progression than those with tumors that showed moderate or intense staining. Feiner and Gonzalez[73b] have described a group of 7 poorly differentiated prostate carcinomas all negative for prostate-specific antigen,

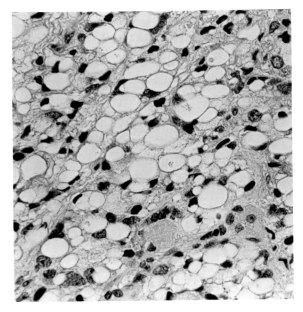

Fig. 32-28 Metastatic carcinoma. Metastatic carcinoma with signet-ring type cells. ×350.

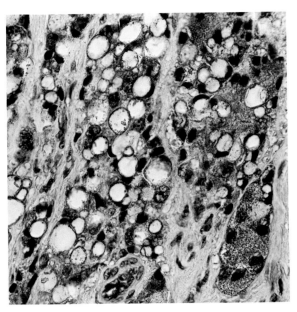

Fig. 32-29 Prostatic acid phosphatase. Immunoperoxidase stain of tumor in Fig. 32-28, showing intense reactivity in many of the tumor cells, thus establishing the prostatic origin of the neoplasm. ×350.

poorly differentiated prostate carcinoma. Application of these techniques in distinguishing collision carcinomas, that is, prostate and rectal carcinomas invading the pouch of Douglas, is illustrated in Figure 32-27. Positive reactivity to PAP in the lower part of this illustration (Fig 32-27) identifies the area with a poorly differentiated prostatic adenocarcinoma, separated by a band of connective tissue from unstained cells that correspond to a rectal adenocarcinoma invading also the pouch of Douglas. Results are similar to those observed when the tissues were stained for prostate-specific antigen (not shown). Figures 32-28 and 32-29 dramatize the role of PAP in establishing the diagnosis of a metastatic mucus-secreting carcinoma (Fig. 32-28, routine H&E stain) as prostatic in origin by demonstration of PAP immunoreactive staining (Fig. 32-29).

ras Oncogene p21 in Prostate Cancer

The expression of the *ras* p21 antigen in prostate carcinoma represents a biologic marker that correlates with tumor grade and may have predictive value in relation to behavior of the tumor.[226] Immunoperoxidase staining of formalin-fixed paraffin-embedded sections revealed positive staining of the antigen in prostate carcinomas, particularly in less differentiated cases. Tissues from normal or BPH prostates failed to reveal immunoreactivity for *ras* p21 antigen. Intensity of staining of the p21 antigen strongly correlated to nuclear anaplasia, but inversely correlated to glandular differentiation of the tumor. Immunoreactivity was demonstrated in 2 of 6 grade I prostate carcinomas and 4 of 6 grade II tumors, whereas all 17 tumors higher than grade II were invariably positive.[226]

Fan[73a] analyzed a case of prostate carcinoma and found that although only 25 percent of the cells from the primary lesion expressed the *ras* p21 protein, almost 90 percent of the cells from a vertebral metastasis did so. He suggested that only certain subpopulations of tumor cells have metastatic potential, and that the *ras* p21 protein may be a marker for these cells.

Prostatic Crystalloids

The intra-acinar crystalloids identified in prostate carcinoma[113,119] may also be found, but with less frequency, in tissues from BPH.[22] Holmes[113] proposed that these crystalloids were closely related, if not identical, to Bence Jones crystals. She also speculated that in normal prostates corpora amylacea are enzymatically split from Bence Jones-like protein, whereas malignant cells lack the splitting enzyme system, which results in accumulation of crystalloids. Recently, Ro et al.[188] identified intraluminal crystalloids in 10.2 percent of sections from 343 cases of prostate adenocarcinomas. Contrary to the assertion of Holmes,[113] their immunohistochemical and ultrastructural studies indicate that these prostatic crystalloids are different from Bence Jones crystals as well as from corpora amylacea.[187]

OTHER POTENTIAL MARKERS

Immunoreactive Inhibinlike Material

Immunoreactive inhibinlike material (ILM) has been detected in prostatic tissues by immunohistochemical methods.[59,200] Immunoreactive ILM in BPH was strictly localized to the epithelial glandular cells.[200] In a comparative study,[59] the intensity of immunoreactivity to ILM decreased from hyperplastic to normal to well-differentiated, to poorly differentiated prostate carcinoma. Tissues with metaplasia or from granulomatous prostatitis as well as nonprostatic tissues were unreactive to ILM, which suggested the potential use of ILM as a marker for prostatic tissues.[59]

Monoclonal Antibody (Anti-Leu 7)

The reactivity was demonstrated by the immunoperoxidase method on formalin-fixed prostatic tissue.[229] Anti-Leu 7 immunoreactivity in prostatic epithelial cells was localized in the supranuclear region, but the stromal cells remained unstained. This antibody specifically identified metastatic prostate tumors (5 of 5). The intensity of staining was somewhat enhanced in BPH and carcinoma cells, and the percentage of positive cells was also higher in BPH and cancer cells, but decreased in poorly differentiated carcinomas.[229] Anti-Leu 7 has been suggested as a useful marker of prostate cancer tissue.[229]

c-myc Proto-oncogene as Marker

Fleming et al.[76] observed a higher level of c-myc transcripts in prostatic tissues from patients with adenocarcinoma that in those with BPH and suggested that such elevated levels of c-myc expression have prognostic value.

Other Enzymatic and Nonenzymatic Products

Normal and cancer prostate cells differ considerably in their concentration of various enzymes. Naphthol-soluble esterases appear to be reduced in prostate carcinoma.[34] Patterns of glycosidase distribution are altered in prostate cancer cells. Gyorkey[99] noted an overall increase in β-glucuronidase activity, but according to Sinowatz et al.[208] only the undifferentiated portions of the tumors reveal increased β-glucuronidase and N-acetylglucosaminidase activity, possibly related to invasive properties. A striking decrease, or perhaps deletion, of the enzyme leucine aminopeptidase has been noted in prostatic cancer cells.[35,125] An increase in lipid droplets in cancer cells has been demonstrated by several histochemical procedures.[34]

The distribution of mucins in normal prostatic tissue and in prostate carcinomas has been described by Franks et al.[82] Normal prostatic epithelium produces only neutral mucins, whereas prostate cancer cells from well-differentiated small acinar and cribriform tumors, and particularly colloid cancers, may produce mucins containing sulfated sialic acid residues. Colloid carcinomas and tumors with extensive mucin secretion may contain a nonsulfated acid mucin.

Cytokeratins occur in human normal, BPH, and carcinoma tissues in which they have been localized immunohistochemically.[128,163] Positive staining was seen in basal and columnar cells.[128,163] Both normal and cancerous columnar cells showed a specialized labeling in the luminal portion,[128] and basal cells in malignant tumors appeared to retain strong staining characteristics for cytokeratin.[128]

ELECTRON MICROSCOPY

Normal Cells

In normal glands[32,33,125] prostatic acini are lined by columnar secretory cells (Fig. 32-30). Small, irregularly shaped basal cells are interposed between the basal portion of the columnar cells and the basement membrane of the acinus. The nuclei of the columnar cells are generally located toward the periphery of the acinus and contain finely dispersed chromatin. The secretory nature of the columnar cells and functional apical polarization of organelles, characteristic of differentiated prostatic epithelium, are appreciated by the presence of abundant electron-lucent vacuoles and occasional secretory granules, by a well-developed Golgi apparatus, and by the abundance of small vesicles. The cytoplasm is studded with free ribosomes arranged as polyribosomes and with irregularly distributed cisternae of the rough endoplasmic reticulum. Mitochondria and occasional lysosomes are also present. The apposing plasma membranes of adjacent cells show usually irregular infoldings and contain desmosomes with attached tonofibrils. Thin filaments are also irregularly dispersed in the cytoplasm. There are marked variations in the appearance of the free surface at the luminal border since some cells have microvilli of many sizes and various densities and others show a ruffled surface.[219] The acinar basement membrane is a band of amorphous material interposed between the acinus and the periacinar connective tissue that contains collagen fibers, fibroblasts, smooth muscle fibers, and capillaries.

The cytoplasm of the basal cells contains very few secretory vacuoles, and the Golgi apparatus, when present, is poorly developed. The question as to

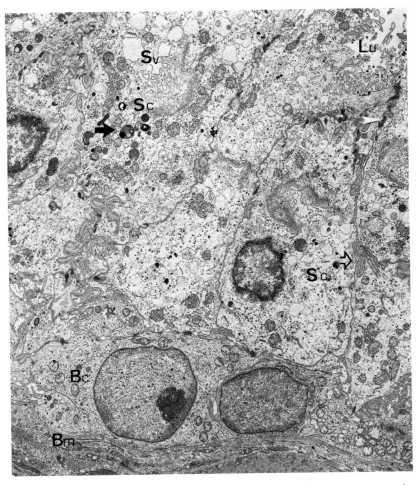

Fig. 32-30 Normal prostatic acinus. Secretory cells (Sc) with abundant secretory vacuoles (Sv) and microvilli at the luminal border (Lu). Basal cells (Bc) lack secretory vacuoles. Infoldings of plasma membranes of adjacent cells (open arrows). Bm, basement membrane; arrowhead, junctional complex; solid arrows, lysosomes. ×3,500.

whether the basal cells represent myoepithelium or reserve elements is still controversial. They do contain actinlike filaments but seem to lack some of the enzymes described in myoepithelial cells in salivary glands and the breast.[148]

The mechanism of secretion of prostatic columnar cells is both merocrine and apocrine.[31,149,219] Secretory vacuoles may open into the lumen and extrude their contents, whereas in other cells apical, homogeneous cytoplasmic blebs are pinched off into the lumen. Microvilli, ruffled, and bared cell surfaces are present in normal, BPH, and neoplastic acini, without any sig-

nificant qualitative or quantitative differences in surface morphology by scanning and transmission electron microscopy.[219]

Prostate Carcinoma

Fine structural changes in prostate malignancies become accentuated with loss of histologic differentiation of the tumor.[6,35,74,122,124,125] The acini in well-differentiated tumors, such as those corresponding to Gleason patterns 1 and 2, are lined by tall columnar cells, which differ minimally from normal cells.[35,125]

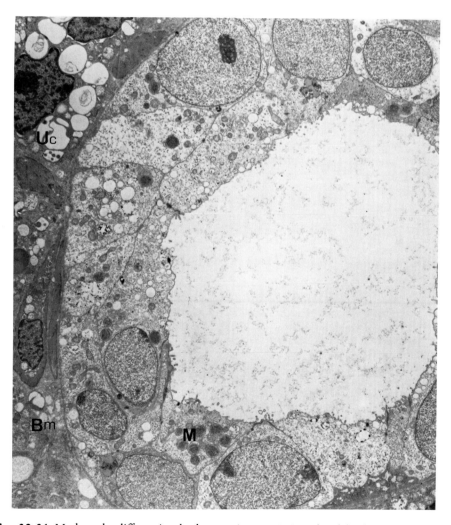

Fig. 32-31 Moderately differentiated adenocarcinoma. Acinus lined by low cuboidal cells (Gleason grade 3). Open nuclei with finely dispersed chromatin and nucleolus. Clusters of altered mitochondria (M). The acinus is surrounded by infiltrating, undifferentiated cells (Uc) with anaplastic nuclei. The basement membrane (Bm) is still intact.

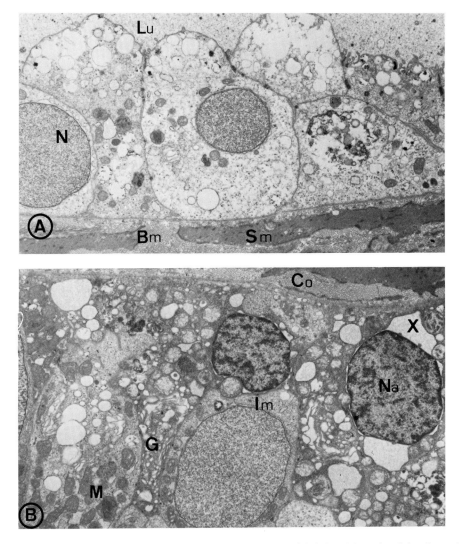

Fig. 32-32 Two "back-to-back" acini. Acinus in upper half **(A)** lined by cuboidal cells with scanty organelles (immature cells) and low-grade nuclei (N), with regular contour and finely distributed chromatin; Lu, lumen. The basement membrane (Bm), although thin, is still intact. Sm, stromal smooth muscle; Co, collagen. **(B)** Intra-acinar proliferation and loss of differentiation. Some cells show anaplastic nuclei (Na), dilation of nuclear envelope (X), and cytoplasmic vacuolization. Immature type cell (Im) with scanty organelles. Other cells are overloaded with mitochondria (M) and have a prominent Golgi complex (G). ×5,500.

Higher-grade tumors reveal architectural and nuclear changes and alterations in the distribution and morphology of cytoplasmic organelles. The overall cytoarchitecture is still preserved in moderately differentiated, Gleason pattern 3 tumors (Fig. 32-31). The acini are generally fully developed and lined by cuboidal cells. The nuclei are uniform in size and shape, and the chromatin is finely distributed and nucleoli are frequently observed.

The acini in these moderately differentiated tumors (Gleason pattern 3) may be lined by cells that show a reduction in the distribution of cytoplasmic organelles, particularly secretory vacuoles, endoplasmic reticulum, and mitochondria. Alterations in mitochondrial morphology are frequent (Figs. 32-31 and 32-32). Other acini are lined by immature cells, characterized by marked paucity of cytoplasmic organelles. The basement membrane in moderately differentiated, Gleason pattern 3 tumors, however, usually remains intact (Figs. 32-31, 32-32).

Transition from Gleason pattern 3 to poorly differentiated pattern 4 and 5 tumors includes intra-acinar proliferation, the formation of abortive acini, cribriforming, development of markedly atypical, disorganized cell types, and finally the appearance of frankly invasive anaplastic cells.

Various types of cells participate in the process of intra-acinar proliferation, including cells with clear cytoplasm and relatively scanty organelles, such as immature cells, deranged cells with an overload of cytoplasmic organelles, particularly mitochondria and abundant electrolucent vacuoles, and cells with marked nuclear atypia (Figs. 32-32 to 32-34). In Figure 32-32, the acinus at the top is lined by immature cells with scanty cytoplasmic organelles. In the acinus at the bottom, intra-acinar proliferation includes cells with an overload of cytoplasmic organelles, nuclear atypia, and dilated perinuclear spaces. In Figure

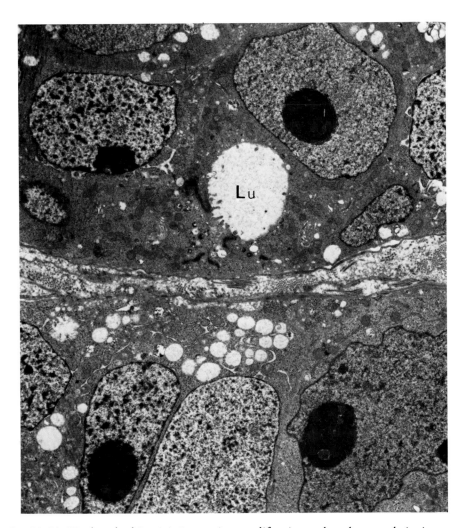

Fig. 32-33 "Back-to-back" acini. Intra-acinar proliferation and nuclear anaplasia, increased nuclear/cytoplasmic ratio, thickened and irregular nuclear membranes, prominent nucleoli, coarser chromatin granules. One cell shows an intracytoplasmic lumen (Lu). ×5,600.

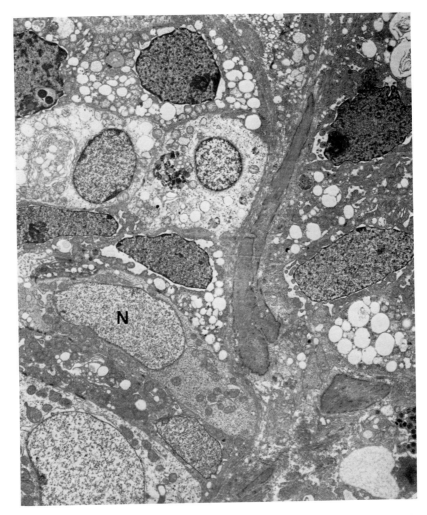

Fig. 32-34 "Back-to-back" acini. Advanced loss of differentiation, intra-acinar proliferation, and early fusion of contiguous acini. The basement membrane appears replaced by fibrillar strands. There are moderately differentiated cells with relatively scanty organelles and bland nuclei (N) with finely dispersed chromatin. Undifferentiated cells have anaplastic nuclei and extensive cytoplasmic vacuolization. ×3,500.

32-33, the acini are being crowded with cells displaying severe nuclear anaplasia and very prominent nucleoli, and intracytoplasmic lumina are seen in individual cells.

In the two contiguous acini in Figure 32-34, the lumina have been obliterated by the intra-acinar proliferation. The basement membranes have been disrupted, and the intervening smooth muscle fibers are fragmented. These fused, solid acini give rise to poorly differentiated tumor masses as seen in Gleason

grades 4 and 5. The acini are crowded by immature cells with scanty cytoplasmic organelles and by more anaplastic elements, overcrowded with cytoplasmic vacuoles and atypical nuclei.

Intra-acinar proliferation may result not only in the formation of Gleason grade 4 or 5 solid structures, but may also give rise to development of cribriform (Gleason 3) or fused gland (Gleason 4) patterns.

Abortive acini are formed by the lateral apposition of very few cells (Fig. 32-35), and in some instances

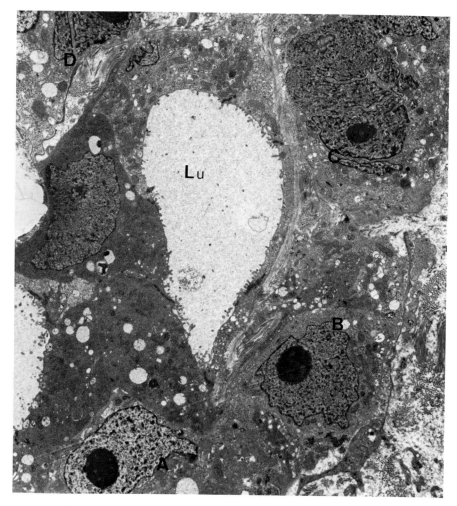

Fig. 32-35 Infiltrative margin of tumor. Abortive acini (Lu, lumen) surrounded by markedly anaplastic invasive single cells (A, B, C, D), with markedly atypical nuclei and prominent nucleoli. ×2,100.

the acinar structures appear to be replaced by individual cells with intracytoplasmic lumen. Development of the cribriform pattern results from the formation of contiguous abortive acini, with little or no interposition of stromal elements, but may also result from intra-acinar proliferation.

Cytoplasmic and nuclear alterations become accentuated in poorly differentiated tumors, as well as in the infiltrative components seen in the moderately differentiated tumors, such as abortive glands and single cell(s) infiltration at the periphery (Figs. 32-31 and 32-35).

Frankly invasive cells, whether at the infiltrative margins of moderately differentiated tumors or when present in poorly differentiated tumors, reveal distinguishing architectural and cytologic features. Nuclei are irregular, with condensed chromatin and a markedly expanded nuclear envelope (Fig. 32-36) or extremely irregular "stretched" multilobular nuclei (Fig. 32-37). In both cell types, the cytoplasm is filled with electrolucent vacuoles (Figs. 32-36 and 32-37).

In areas of diffuse infiltration as seen in poorly differentiated tumors, these cell types assume syncytial growth (Figs. 32-36 and 32-37). The cytoplasm of

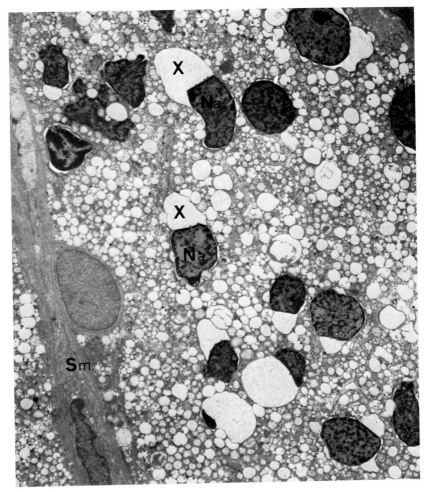

Fig. 32-36 Syncytial infiltrative growth. Syncytial infiltrative growth of undifferentiated cells with highly anaplastic nuclei (Na) and markedly dilated nuclear envelope (X). The cytoplasm is studded with vacuoles. Tumor cells invade along smooth muscle fibers (Sm). ×3,500.

these syncytial masses is crowded predominantly by electrolucent vacuoles. The nuclei may be irregularly ovoid and show marked dilatation of the nuclear envelope (Fig. 32-36), or they may appear as multilobular, markedly elongated structures.

The invasive and destructive capability of these syncytial undifferentiated cells is apparent in Figure 32-38. The plasma membranes of the tumor cells in the areas of contact with stromal smooth muscle fibers are indistinct or absent, and the fragmented muscle fibrils are in direct contact with the cytoplasm of the tumor cells.

It is possible that these alterations in the plasma membrane of the prostatic invasive cells facilitate release of lytic enzymes capable of destroying stromal components and producing the space required for local tumor progression. The morphology of mitochondria is markedly altered in prostate cancer cells, in both differentiated (Fig. 32-31) and poorly differentiated invasive cells (Fig. 32-37). Possibly these morphologic changes relate to the biochemical abnormalities described in tumor cell mitochondria.[35]

Altenahr and Kastendieck[6,122] have described five cell types with distinctive ultrastructural features: un-

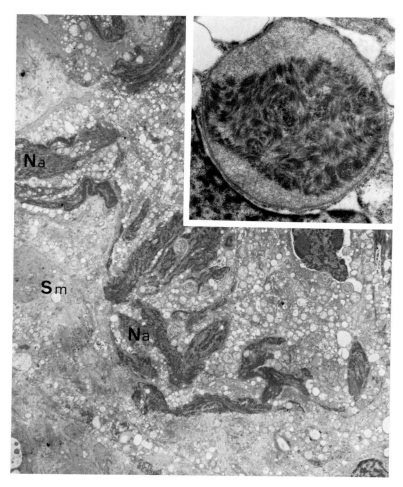

Fig. 32-37 Syncytial infiltrative growth. The nuclei (Na) are markedly anaplastic and deformed with the appearance of "ameboid"-like stretching during infiltration through fibromuscular planes. Fragmented smooth muscle fibers (Sm) are seen at the tumor front. ×2,100. **Insert:** Detail of deranged mitochondria. ×14,000.

differentiated embryonic cells with large nuclei, prominent nucleoli, and scanty cytoplasm lacking signs of secretory activity; immature cells revealing evidence of incipient secretory activity; highly differentiated glandular cells similar in appearance to normal prostatic secretory cells; functionally deranged tumor cells containing heterochromatic nuclei, some loss of polarity, and superabundance of cytoplasmic organelles, many with vacuolar degeneration; and degenerative cells, which show loss of polarity, marked cytoplasmic vacuolization, and heterochromatic or pyknotic nuclei. These various cell types appear to be correlated with tumor differentiation and infiltrative growth patterns[122] (Figs. 32-35 to 32-38).

Sinha et al.[205-207] described light and dark basal cells in human prostate cancer and postulated that these two cell types, rather than the columnar cells, represented the invasive elements within the tumor. These two cell types, particularly those designated as dark cells, appeared to be unresponsive to endocrine procedures and hence responsible for recurrence of disease after endocrine therapy.[205-207] Cells with markedly anaplastic dark nuclei, resembling those described by Sinha et al.,[205-207] appear to represent the

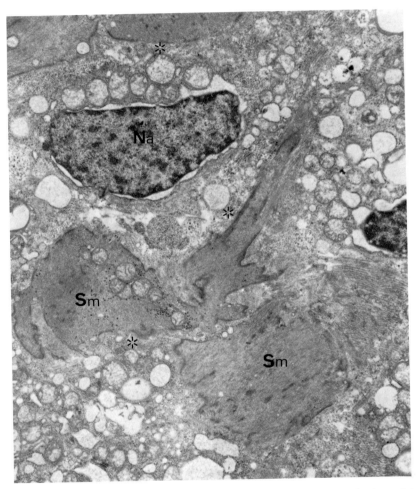

Fig. 32-38 Invasive undifferentiated syncytial cells. Syncytial cells, with anaplastic nuclei (Na) and dilated nuclear envelope. There are no apparent plasma membrane boundaries between the neoplastic cells and the breaking down stromal smooth muscle (Sm). Asterisks indicate areas of direct contact between tumor cell cytoplasm and smooth muscle fragment.

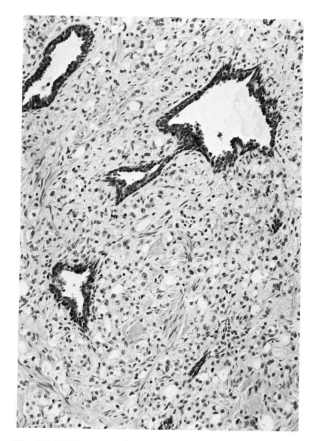

Fig. 32-39 Prostate adenocarcinoma. Low-power view of extremely poorly differentiated prostate adenocarcinoma simulating histocytic prostatitis (compare with Fig. 31-1, Ch. 31). ×180.

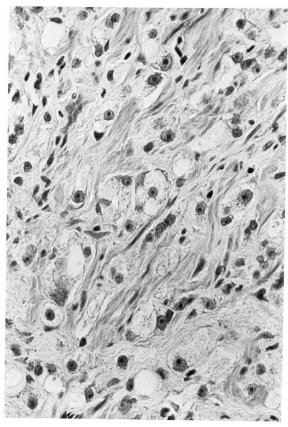

Fig. 32-40 Prostate adenocarcinoma. High-power view of tissue as shown in Fig. 32-39, showing the malignant nature of this anaplastic carcinoma. ×336.

population of the tumor capable of infiltrating and causing destruction of stromal elements, required for the creation of space for tumor progression.

HISTOPATHOLOGIC DIAGNOSTIC PROBLEMS: UROLOGIC AND TISSUE-PROCESSING ARTIFACTS

The microscopic analysis of sections for tissue diagnoses may be hindered because of distortion artifacts during tissue procurement or during histologic processing.

Tannenbaum[222] described in much detail the problems derived from such circumstances. These include cauterization and crushing artifacts, distortion by concurrent inflammatory processes, changes in the vicinity of prostatic infarcts, and various types of dysplastic lesion that may simulate carcinoma. Inflammatory processes with an infiltrate comprising predominantly histiocytic cells (see Fig. 31-1) may be erroneously considered as poorly differentiated carcinoma. Conversely, what appears on low-power view to be a diffuse histiocytelike infiltrate may in fact be an undifferentiated, high-grade carcinoma (Figs. 32-38 and 32-39). When tissue from the seminal vesicle is

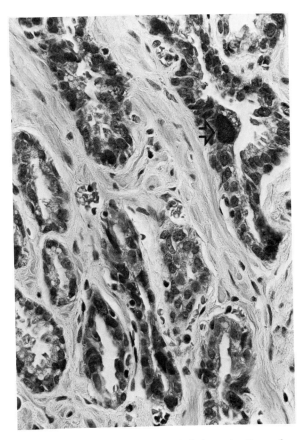

Fig. 32-41 Seminal vesicle epithelial atypia. From fragments of seminal vesicles, sometimes included within the needle biopsy core. Note the pseudo-infiltrative appearance and the marked nuclear atypia (open arrow) seen in seminal vesicle epithelium of older individuals. ×308.

included in the needle biopsy of the prostate, this may give rise to an erroneous diagnosis of prostate carcinoma. As seen in Figure 32-40, the seminal vesicle fronds may assume the architectural conformation of an infiltrating prostate carcinoma, particularly since the epithelial cell nuclei develop age-associated atypical changes (Fig. 32-41). (See also Ch. 28.)

REFERENCES

1. Abul-Fadl MAM, King EJ: The inhibition of acid phosphatase by D-tartrate. Biochem J 42:28, 1948
2. Akazaki K, Stemmermann GN: Comparative study of latent carcinoma of the prostate among Japanese in Japan and Hawaii. J Natl Cancer Inst 50:1137, 1973
3. Al Adnani MS: Schistosomiasis, metaplasia and squamous cell carcinoma of the prostate: histogenesis of the squamous cancer cells determined by localization of specific markers. Neoplasma 32:613, 1985
4. Alexis R, Domingo J: Schistosomiasis and adenocarcinoma of prostate: a morphologic study. Hum Pathol 17:757, 1986
5. Allhoff EP, Proppe KH, Chapman CM et al : Evaluation of prostate specific acid phosphatase and prostate specific antigen in identification of prostatic cancer. J Urol 129:315, 1983
6. Altenahr E, Kastendieck H: Proliferative patterns in prostatic carcinoma. p. 437. In Spring-Mills E, Hafez ESE (eds): Male Accessory Sex Glands: Biology and Pathology. Elsevier/North Holland Biomedical Press, Amsterdam, 1980
7. American Joint Committee for Cancer Staging and End Results Reporting. p. 123. Committee: Beahrs OH, Carr DT, Rubin P. Manual for Staging of Cancer. Whiting Press, New Jersey, 1978
8. Ansari MA, Pintozzi RL, Choi YS, Ladove RF: Diagnosis of carcinoid-like metastatic prostatic carcinoma by an immunoperoxidase method. Am J Clin Pathol 76:94, 1981
9. Armenian HK, Lilienfeld AM, Diamond EL, Bross LDJ: Relationship between benign prostatic hyperplasia and cancer of the prostate: a prospective and retrospective study. Lancet 2:115, 1974
10. Ashley DJB: On the incidence of carcinoma of the prostate. J Pathol 90:217, 1965
11. Aumuller G, Seitz J: Cytochemistry and biochemistry of acid phosphatases: VI. Immunoelectron microscopic studies on human prostatic and leukocytic acid phosphatases. Prostate 7:161, 1985
12. Azumi N, Shibreya H, Ishikura M: Primary prostatic carcinoid tumor with intracytoplasmic prostatic acid phosphatase and prostate-specific antigen. Am J Surg Pathol 8:545, 1984
13. Azzopardi JG, Evans DJ: Argentaffin cells in prostatic carcinoma: differentiation from lipofuscin and melanin in prostatic epithelium. J Pathol 104:247, 1971
14. Baker LH, Mebust WK, Chin TDY et al : The relationship of herpesvirus to carcinoma of the prostate. J Urol 125:370, 1981
15. Barnes R, Hirst A, Rosenquist R: Early carcinoma of the prostate: comparison of stages A and B. J Urol 115:404, 1976
16. Barrack ER, Bujnoszky P, Walsh PC: Subcellular distribution of androgen receptors in human normal, benign hyperplastic and malignant prostatic tissue: characterization of nuclear salt-resistant receptors. Cancer Res 43:1107, 1983

17. Barrack ER, Coffey DS: The specific binding of estrogens and androgens to the nuclear matrix of sex hormone responsive tissues. J Biol Chem 255:7265, 1980

18. Barzell W, Bean MA, Hilaris BS, Whitmore WF, Jr.: Prostatic adenocarcinoma: relationship of grade and local extent to the pattern of metastases. J Urol 118:278, 1977

19. Bates HR, Thornton JC: Carcinoma of the prostatic ducts. Am J Clin Pathol 45:96, 1966

20. Bauer WC, McGavran MH, Carlin MR: Unsuspected carcinoma of the prostate in suprapubic prostatectomy specimens. A clinicopathological study of 55 consecutive cases. Cancer 13:370, 1960

21. Ben-Ezra J, Sheibani K, Kendrick FE et al : Angiotropic large cell lymphoma of the prostate gland: an immunohistochemical study. Hum Pathol 17:964, 1986

22. Bennett B, Gardner WA: Crystalloids in prostatic hyperplasia. Prostate 1:31, 1980

22a. Benson MC, Kaplan SA, Olsson CA: Prostate cancer in men less than 45 years old: influence of stage, grade and therapy. J Urol 137:888, 1987

23. Billis A: Latent carcinoma and atypical lesions of prostate: an autopsy study. Urology 28:324, 1986

24. Blackard CE, Byar DP, Jordan WP, Jr.: Veterans Administration Cooperative Urological Research Groups: orchiectomy for advanced prostatic carcinoma: a reevaluation. Urology 1:553, 1973

25. Blair A, Fraumeni JF, Jr.: Geographic patterns of prostate cancer in the United States. J Natl Cancer Inst 61:1379, 1978

26. Bleichner JC, Chun B, Klappenbach RS: Pure small-cell carcinoma of the prostate with fatal liver metastasis. Arch Pathol Lab Med 110:1041, 1986

27. Blute ML, Zincke H, Farrow GM: Long-term followup of young patients with stage A adenocarcinoma of the prostate. J Urol 136:840, 1986

28. Bocking A: Reproducible grading of prostatic carcinoma based on cytological criteria of malignancy. Akt Urol 12:240, 1981

29. Bostwick DG, Kindrachuk RW, Rouse RV: Prostatic adenocarcinoma with endometroid features. Am J Surg Pathol 9:595, 1985

30. Bostwick DG, Mann RB: Malignant lymphomas involving the prostate. Cancer 56:2932, 1985

31. Brandes D: The fine structure and histochemistry of prostatic glands in relation to sex hormones. Int Rev Cytol 20:207, 1966

32. Brandes D: Fine structure and cytochemistry of male sex accessory organs. p. 18. In Brandes D (ed): Male Accessory Sex Organs: Structure and Function in Mammals. Academic Press, Orlando, 1974

33. Brandes D: Hormonal regulation of fine structure. p. 183. In Brandes D (ed): Male Accessory Sex Organs: Structure and Function in Mammals. Academic Press, Orlando, 1974

34. Brandes D, Bourne G: Histochemistry of the human prostate: normal and neoplastic. J Pathol Bacteriol 71:33, 1956

35. Brandes D, Kirchheim D: Histochemistry of the prostate. p. 99. In Tannenbaum, M (ed): Urologic Pathology: The Prostate. Lea and Febiger, Philadelphia, 1977

36. Brawn PN: Interpretation of prostate biopsies. Biopsy Interpretation Series. Raven Press, New York, 1983

37. Brawn PN, Ayala AG, Von Eschenbach AC et al : Histologic grading study of prostate adenocarcinoma: the development of a new system and comparison with other methods—a preliminary study. Cancer 49:525, 1982

38. Breslow N, Chan CW, Dhom G et al : Latent carcinoma of prostate of autopsy in seven areas. Int J Cancer 20:680, 1977

39. Broders AC: Carcinoma: grading and practical application. Arch Pathol 2:376, 1926

40. Byar DP: VACURG studies on prostate cancer and its treatment. p. 241. In Tannenbaum M (ed): Urologic Pathology: The Prostate. Lea & Febiger, Philadelphia, 1977

41. Camuzzi FA, Block NL, Charyulu K et al : Leiomyosarcoma of prostate gland. Urology 18:295, 1981

42. Cantrell BB, deKlerk DP, Eggleston JC et al : Pathologic factors that influence prognosis in stage A prostatic cancer: the influence of extent versus grade. J Urol 125:516, 1981

43. Carney JA, Kelalis PP: Endometrial carcinoma of the prostatic utricle. Am J Clin Pathol 60:565, 1973

44. Catalona WJ: Prostate Cancer. Grune & Stratton, Orlando, 1984

44a. Catalona WJ, Stein AJ, Fair WR: Grading errors in prostatic needle biopsies: relation to the accuracy of tumor grade in predicting lymph node metastasis. J Urol 127:919, 1982

45. Centifano YM, Kaufman HE, Zam ZS et al : Herpesvirus particles in prostatic carcinoma cells. J Virol 12:1608, 1973

46. Chibber PJ, McIntyre MA, Hindmarsh JR et al : Transitional cell carcinoma involving the prostate. Br J Urol 53:605, 1981

47. Chisholm GD: The TNM classification of prostatic cancer and activities of British prostate groups. p. 117. In Jacobi GH, Hohenfellner R (eds): Prostate Cancer. International Perspectives in Urology. Vol. 3. Williams & Wilkins, Baltimore, 1982

48. Chodak GW, Steinberg GD, Bibbo M et al : The role of transrectal aspiration biopsy in the diagnosis of prostatic cancer. J Urol 135:299, 1986

49. Choe BK, Pontes JE, Lillehoj HS, Rose NR: Immunohistological approaches to human prostatic epithelial cells. Prostate 1:383, 1980

50. Christoffersen J: Leiomyosarcoma of the prostate. Acta Chir Scand suppl., 433:75, 1973

51. Chu TM, Murphy GP: What's new in tumor markers for prostate cancer? Urology 27:487, 1986

52. Coffey DS: Physiological control of prostatic growth: an overview. p. 4. In Coffey DS, Isaacs JT (eds): Prostate Cancer. Vol. 48. UICC Technical Report Series, Geneva, 1979

53. Coffey DS: The biochemistry and physiology of the prostate and seminal vesicles. p. 233. In Walsh PC, Gittes RF, Perlmutter AD, Stamey TA (eds): Campbell's Urology. Vol. 1, 5th Ed. WB Saunders, Philadelphia, 1986

54. Cook GB, Watson FR: A comparison by age of death rates due to prostate cancer alone. J Urol 100:669, 1968

55. Correa RJ, Jr., Anderson RG, Gibbons RP, Mason JT: Latent carcinoma of the prostate — why the controversy? J Urol 111:644, 1974

56. Creagan ET, Fraumeni JF, Jr: Cancer mortality among American Indians. 1950–1967. J Natl Cancer Inst 49:959, 1972

57. Diamond DA, Berry SJ, Jewett HJ et al: A new method to assess metastatic potential of human prostate cancer: relative nuclear roundness. J Urol 128:729, 1982

57a. di Sant'Agnese PA, de Mesy Jensen KL: Neuroendocrine differentiation in prostatic carcinoma. Hum Pathol 18:849, 1987

58. Diamond DA, Berry SJ, Umbrecht C et al: Computerized image analysis of nuclear shape as a prognostic factor for prostatic cancer. Prostate 3:321, 1982

59. Doctor VM, Sheth AR, Simha MM et al: Studies on immunocytochemical localization of inhibin-like material in human prostatic tissue: comparison of its distribution in normal, benign and malignant prostates. Br J Cancer 53:547, 1986

60. Donohue RE, Fauver HE, Whitesel JA et al: Prostatic carcinoma: influence of tumor grade on results of pelvic lymphadenectomy. Urology 17:435, 1981

61. Dube VE, Farrow GM, Greene LF: Prostatic adenocarcinoma of ductal origin. Cancer 32:402, 1973

62. Elbadawi A, Craig W, Linke CA, Cooper RA, Jr.: Prostatic mucinous carcinoma. Urology 13:658, 1979

63. Ende N, Woods LP, Shelley HS: Carcinoma originating in ducts surrounding the prostatic urethra. Am J Clin Pathol 40:183, 1963

64. Enzinger FM, Weiss SW: Soft Tissue Tumors. CV Mosby, St. Louis, 1983

65. Epstein JI, Berry SJ, Eggleston JC: Nuclear roundness factor: a predictor of progression in untreated state A_2 prostate cancer. Cancer 54:1966, 1984

66. Epstein JI, Eggleston JC: Immunohistochemical localization of prostate-specific acid phosphatase and prostate-specific antigen in stage A_2 adenocarcinoma of prostate. Prognostic implications. Hum Pathol 15:853, 1984

67. Epstein JI, Lieberman PH: Mucinous adenocarcinoma of the prostate gland. Am J Surg Pathol 9:299, 1985

68. Epstein JI, Paull G, Eggleston JC, Walsh PC: Prognosis of untreated state A_1 prostate carcinoma: a study of 94 cases with extended follow up. J Urol 136:837, 1986

69. Epstein JI, Woodruff JM: Adenocarcinoma of the prostate with endometrioid features: a light microscopic and immunohistochemical study of ten cases. Cancer 57:111, 1986

70. Ernster VL, Selvin S, Sacks ST et al: Prostatic cancer: mortality and incidence rates by race and social class. Am J Epidemiol 107:311, 1978

71. Esposti PL: Aspiration biopsy and cytological evaluation for primary diagnosis and follow up. p. 71. In Jacobi GH, Hohenfellner R (eds): International Perspectives in Urology. Vol. 3. Prostate Cancer. Williams & Wilkins, Baltimore, 1982

72. Estrada PC, Scardino PL: Myeloma of the prostate: a case report. J Urol 106:586, 1971

73. Evans N, Barnes RW, Brown AF: Carcinoma of the prostate. Correlation between the histologic observations and the clinical course. Arch Pathol 34:473, 1942

73a. Fan K: Heterogeneous subpopulations of human prostatic adenocarcinoma cells: potential usefulness of P21 protein as a predictor for bone metastasis. J Urol 139:318, 1988

73b. Feiner HD, Gonzalez R: Carcinoma of the prostate with atypical immunohistological features. Am J Surg Pathol 10:765, 1986

74. Fisher ER, Sieracki JC: Ultrastructure of human normal and neoplastic prostate. Pathol Ann 5:1, 1970

75. Fishleder A, Tubbs RR, Levin HS: An immunoperoxidase technique to aid in the differential diagnosis of prostatic carcinoma. Cleve Clin Q 48:331, 1981

76. Fleming WH, Hamel A, MacDonald R et al: Expression of the c-myc protooncogene in human prostatic carcinoma and benign prostatic hyperplasia. Cancer Res 46:1535, 1986

77. Fowler JE, Jr., Whitmore WF, Jr.: The incidence and extent of pelvic lymph node netastases in apparently localized prostatic cancer. Cancer 47:2941, 1981

78. Frankel K, Craig JF: Adenoid cystic carcinoma of the prostate. Am J Clin Pathol 62:639, 1974

79. Franks LM: Latent carcinoma of the prostate. J Pathol Bacteriol 68:603, 1954

80. Franks LM: Latency and progressions in human tumors: natural history of prostatic cancers. Lancet 2:1037, 1956

81. Franks LM, Chesterman FC: Intraepithelial carcinoma of prostatic urethra, periurethral glands and prostatic ducts (Bowen's disease of urinary epithelium). Br J Cancer 10:223, 1956

82. Franks LM, O'Shea JD, Thomson AER: Mucin in the prostate: a histochemical study in normal glands, latent, clinical and colloid cancers. Cancer 17:983, 1964

83. Fraumeni JF, Jr., Mason TJ: Cancer mortality among Chinese-Americans. 1950-1969. J Natl Cancer Inst 52:659, 1974

84. Gaeta JF: Glandular profiles and cellular patterns in prostatic cancer grading. Urology, suppl., 17:33, 1981

85. Gaeta JF, Asirwatham JE: Prostate cancer grading: the NPCP system. p. 193. In Vaughan ED, JR (ed): Seminars in Virology. Grune & Stratton, Orlando, 1983

86. Gaeta JF, Englander LC, Murphy GP: Comparative evaluation of National Prostatic Cancer Treatment Group and Gleason systems for pathologic grading of primary prostatic cancer. Urology 23:306, 1986

87. Garborg I, Eide TJ: The probability of overlooking prostatic cancer in transurethrally resected material when different embedding practices are followed. Acta Pathol Microbiol Immunol Scand 93:205, 1985

88. Ghanadian R: Mechanism of action of androgens. p. 491. In Chisholm GD, Williams DI (eds): Scientific Foundations of Urology. Year Book Medical Publishers, Chicago, 1982

89. Ghanadian R, Auf G: Receptor proteins for androgens in benign prostatic hypertrophy and carcinoma of the prostate. p. 110. In Schroder FH, de Voogt HJ (eds): Steroid Receptors, Metabolism and Prostatic Cancer. Excerpta Medica, Amsterdam, 1980

90. Ghandur-Mnaymneh L, Satterfield S, Block NL: Small cell carcinoma of the prostate gland with inappropriate antidiuretic hormone secretion: morphological, immunohistochemical and clinical expressions. J Urol 135:1263, 1986

91. Gilmour AM, Bell TJ: Adenoid cystic carcinoma of the prostate. Br J Urol 58:105, 1986

92. Giltman LI: Signet ring adenocarcinoma of the prostate. J Urol 126:134, 1981

93. Gleason DF: Classification of prostatic carcinomas. Cancer Chemother Rep 50:125, 1966

94. Gleason DF: Histologic grading and clinical staging of prostatic carcinoma. p. 171. In Tannenbaum M (ed): Urologic Pathology: The Prostate. Lea & Febiger, Philadelphia, 1977

95. Gleason DF: The pathologist's contribution to the clinical management of adenocarcinoma of the prostate. p. 73. In Skinner DG (ed): Urological Cancer. Grune & Stratton, Orlando, 1983

96. Gleason DF, Mellinger GT, VACURG: Prediction of prognosis for prostatic adenocarcinoma by combined histological grading and clinical staging. J Urol 111:58, 1974

97. Grayhack JT, Assimos DG: Prognostic significance of tumor grade and stage in the patient with carcinoma of the prostate. Prostate 4:13, 1983

98. Greenwald P, Kirmss V, Polan AK, Dick VS: Cancer of the prostate among men with benign prostatic hyperplasia. J Natl Cancer Inst 53:335, 1974

99. Gyorkey F: Some aspects of cancer of the prostate gland. In Busch H (ed): Methods in Cancer Research. Academic Press, Orlando, 1973

100. Habib FK: Studies on the in vitro binding and metabolism of testosterone in benign prostatic hypertrophy and carcinoma of the prostate: a correlation with endogenous androgen levels. p. 157. In Schroder FJ, de Voogt HJ (eds): Steroid Receptors, Metabolism and Prostatic Cancer. Excerpta Medica, Amsterdam, 1980

101. Habib FK: Factors controling abnormal growth. p. 499. In Chisholm GD, Williams DI (eds): Scientific Foundation of Urology. Year Book Medical Publishers, Chicago, 1982

102. Habib FK, Lee IR, Stitch SR, Smith PH: Androgen levels in the plasma and prostatic tissue of patients with benign hypertrophy and carcinoma of the prostate. J Endocrinol 71:99, 1976

103. Haddad JR, Reyes EC: Carcinosarcoma of the prostate with metastasis of both elements: case report. J Urol 103:80, 1970

104. Haenszel W, Kurihara M: Studies of Japanese migrants: I. Mortality from cancer and other diseases among Japanese in the United States. J Natl Cancer Inst 40:43, 1968

105. Halpert B, Schmalhorst WR: Carcinoma of the prostate on patients 70 to 79 years old. Cancer 19:695, 1966

106. Hamlin WB, Lund PK: Carcinosarcoma of the prostate: a case report. J Urol 97:518, 1967

107. Hanash KA, Utz DC, Cook EN et al : Carcinoma of the prostate: a 15-year follow-up. J Urol 107:450, 1972

108. Harper ME, Peeling WB, Cowley T et al : Plasma steroid and protein hormone concentrations in patients with prostatic carcinoma, before and during oestrogen therapy. Acta Endocrinol 81:409, 1976

109. Hays DM, Raney RB, Lawrence W, Jr, et al : Bladder

and prostatic tumors in the intergroup rhabdomyosarcoma study (IRS-1). Results of therapy. Cancer 50:1472, 1982

110. Helminen HJ, Ericsson JLE: On the mechanism of lysosomal enzyme secretion. Electron microscopic and histochemical studies on the epithelial cells of the rat's ventral prostate lobe. J Ultrastruct Res 33:528, 1970

111. Herbert JT, Birkuff JD, Feorino PM, Caldwell GG: Herpes simplex virus type 2 and cancer of the prostate. J Urol 116:611, 1976

112. Hicks LL, Walsh PC: A microassay for the measurement of androgen receptors in human prostatic tissue. Steroids 33:389, 1979

113. Holmes EJ: Crystalloids of prostatic carcinoma: relationship to Bence-Jones crystals. Cancer 39:2073, 1977

114. Holund B: Latent prostatic cancer in a consecutive autopsy series. Scand J Urol Nephrol 14:29, 1980

115. Horm JW, Asire AJ, Young JL, Jr, Pollack ES (eds): SEER Program: Cancer Incidence and Mortality in the United States, 1973–81. NIH Publication no. 85-1837. National Cancer Institute, Bethesda, Md., 1984

116. Huben R, Mettlin C, Natarajan N et al : Carcinoma of prostate in men less than fifty years old: data from American College of Surgeons' National Surgery. Urology 20:585, 1982

117. Hutchison GB: Incidence and etiology of prostate cancer. Urology, suppl., 17:4, 1981

118. Isaacs JT: Prostatic structure and function in relation to the etiology of prostatic cancer. Prostate 4:351, 1983

119. Jensen PE, Gardner WA, Piserchia PV: Prostatic crystalloids: association with adenocarcinoma. Prostate 1:25, 1980

120. Jewett HJ: The present status of radical prostatectomy for stages A and B prostatic cancer. Urol Clin North Am 2:105, 1975

121. Karpas CM, Moumgis B: Primary transitional cell carcinoma of the prostate gland: possible pathogenesis and relationship to reverse cell hyperplasia of the prostatic periurethral ducts. J Urol 101:201, 1969

122. Kastendieck H, Altenahr E: Cyto- and histomorphogenesis of the prostate carcinoma. A comparative light- and electron-microscopic study. Virchows Arch (A) 370:207, 1976

123. Katz RL, Raval P, Brooks TE, Ordonez NG: Role of immunocytochemistry in diagnosis of prostatic neoplasia by fine needle aspiration biopsy. Diagn Cytopathol 1:28, 1985

123a. Keillor JS, Aterman K: The response of poorly differentiated prostatic tumors to staining for prostate

specific antigen and prostatic acid phosphatase: a comparative study. J Urol 137:894, 1987

124. Kirchheim D, Bacon RL: Ultrastructural studies of carcinoma of the human prostatic gland. Invest Urol 6:611, 1969

125. Kirchheim D, Brandes D, Bacon RL: Fine structure and cytochemistry of human prostatic carcinoma. p. 397. In Brandes D (ed): Male Accessory Sex Organs: Structure and Function in Mammals. Academic Press, Orlando, 1974

126. Kirchheim D, Gyorkey F, Brandes D, Scott WW: Histochemistry of the normal, hyperplastic and neoplastic human prostatic gland. Invest Urol 1:403, 1964

127. Kirchheim D, Niles NR, Frankus E, Hodges CV: Correlative histochemical and histological studies on thirty radical prostatectomy specimens. Cancer 19:1683, 1966

128. Kitajima K, Tokes ZA: Immunohistochemical localization of keratin in human prostate. Prostate 9:183, 1986

129. Kline TS: Guides to Clinical Aspiration Biopsy: Prostate. Igaku-Shoin New York, Tokyo, 1985

130. Koss LG, Woyke S, Schreiber K et al : Thin-needle aspiration biopsy of the prostate. Urol Clin North Am 11:237, 1984

131. Kramer SA, Farnham R, Glenn JF, Paulson DF: Comparative morphology of primary and secondary deposits of prostatic adenocarcinoma. Cancer 48:271, 1981

132. Kramer SA, Spahr J, Brendler CB et al : Experience with Gleason histopathologic grading in prostatic cancer. J Urol 124:223, 1980

133. Krieg M, Bartsch W, Janssen W, Voigt KD: A comparative study of binding, metabolism and endogenous levels of androgens in normal, hyperplastic and carcinomatous human prostate. p. 93. In Coffey DS, Isaacs FT (eds): Prostate Cancer. Vol. 48. UICC Technical Report Series, Geneva, 1979

134. Krieg M, Bartsch W, Janssen W, Voigt KD: A comparative study of binding, metabolism and endogenous levels of androgens in normal, hyperplastic and carcinomatous human prostate. J Steroid Biochem 11:615, 1979

135. Krieg M, Grobe I, Voigt KD et al: Human prostatic carcinoma: significant differences in its androgen binding and metabolism compared to the human benign prostatic hypertrophy. Acta Endocrinol 88:397, 1978

136. Lang DJ, Kummer JF, Hartley DP: Cytomegalovirus in semen: persistence and demonstration in extracellular fluids. N Engl J Med 291:121, 1974

137. Li CY, Lam KW, Yam LT: Immunohistochemical

diagnosis of prostatic cancer with metastasis. Cancer 46:706, 1980

138. Liavag I: Atrophy and regeneration in the pathogenesis of prostatic carcinoma. Acta Pathol Microbiol Scand 73:338, 1968

139. Lieskovsky G, Bruchovsky N: Assay of nuclear receptor in human prostate. J Urol 121:54, 1979

140. Lin CT, Liu JW, Song GX et al: Immunoultrastructural demonstration of prostatic acid phosphatase isoenzyme 2 in prostatic carcinoma. J Urol 136:173, 1986

141. Linsk JA, Franzen S: Aspiration biopsy cytology of the prostate gland. p. 243. In Linsk JA, Franzen S (eds): Clinical Aspiration Cytology. JB Lippincott, St. Louis, 1983

142. Ljung B-M, Cherrie R, Kaufman JJ: Fine needle aspiration biopsy of the prostate gland: a study of 103 cases with histological followup. J Urol 135:955, 1986

143. Lovern WJ, Fariss BL, Wittlanfer JN, Hane S: Ectopic ACTH production in disseminated prostatic adenocarcinoma. Urology 5:817, 1975

144. Lundberg S, Berge T: Prostatic carcinoma: an autopsy study. Scand J Urol Nephrol 4:93, 1970

145. Lundquist F: Function of prostatic phosphatase. Nature, 158:710, 1946

146. Manivel C, Shenoy BV, Wick MP, Dehner LP: Cystosarcoma phyllodes of the prostate. Arch Pathol Lab Med 110:534, 1986

147. Manrique JJ, Albores-Saavedra J, Orantes A, Brandt H: Malignant mixed tumor of the salivary-gland type, primary in the prostate. Am J Clin Pathol 70:932, 1978

148. Mao P, Angrist A: The fine structure of the basal cell of human prostate. Lab Invest 15:1768, 1966

149. Mao P, Nakao K, Bora R, Geller J: Human benign prostatic hyperplasia. Arch Pathol 79:270, 1965

149a. Matzkin H, Braf Z: Paraneoplastic syndromes associated with prostatic carcinoma. J Urol 138:1129, 1987

150. Maurer HM, Donaldson M, Gehan EA et al : Rhabdomyosarcoma in childhood and adolescence. Curr Probl Cancer 11:9, 1978

151. Maurer HM, Moon T, Donaldson M: The intergroup rhabdomyosarcoma study: a preliminary report. Cancer 40:2015, 1977

151a. McCullough DL, Prout GR, Daly JJ: Carcinoma of the prostate and lymphatic metastasis. J Urol 111:65, 1974

152. McDougal WS, Persky L: Rhabdomyosarcoma of the bladder and prostate in children. J Urol 124:882, 1980

152a. McLaughlin AP, Saltzstein SL, McCullough DL, Gittes RF: Prostatic carcinoma: incidence and location of unsuspected lymphatic metastases. J Urol 115:89, 1976

153. McNeal JE: New morphologic findings relevant to the origin and evolution of carcinoma of the prostate and BPH. p. 24. In Coffey DS, Isaacs JT (eds): Prostate Cancer. Vol. 48. UICC Technical Report Series, Geneva, 1979

153a. McNeal JE, Bostwick DG, Kindrachuk RA, et al: Patterns of progression in prostate cancer. Lancet 1:60, 1986

153b. McNeal JE, et al: Stage A versus stage B adenocarcinoma of the prostate: morphological comparison and biological significance. J Urol 139;61, 1988

154. Meikle AW, Stanish WM: Familial prostatic cancer risk and low testosterone. J Clin Endocrinol Metab 54:1104, 1982

155. Melicow MM, Pachter MR: Endometrial carcinoma of prostatic utricle (uterus masculinus). Cancer 20:1715, 1967

156. Melicow MM, Tannenbaum M: Endometrial carcinoma of uterus masculinus (prostatic utricle). Report of six cases. J Urol 106:892, 1971

157. Mellinger GT, Gleason D, Bailer J, III: The histology and prognosis of prostatic cancer. J Urol 97:331, 1967

158. Menck HR, Handerson BE, Pike MC et al : Cancer incidence in the Mexican-American. J Natl Cancer Inst 55:531, 1975

159. Menon M, Tananis CE, Hicks LL et al : Characterization of the binding of a potent synthetic androgen, methyltrienolone, to human tissue. J Clin Invest 61:150, 1978

160. Merimsky E, Baratz M, Kahn Y: Leukemic infiltration of the prostate. Br J Urol 53:150, 1981

161. Meyers RP, Neves RJ, Farrow GM, Utz DC: Nucleolar grading of prostatic adenocarcinoma. Light microscopic correlation with disease progression. Prostate 3:432, 1982

162. Mills SE, Fowler JE: Gleason histologic grading of prostatic carcinoma: correlations between biopsy and prostatectomy specimens. Cancer 57:346, 1986

163. Molinolo AA, Meiss RP, Leo P, Sens AI: Demonstration of cytokeratins by immunoperoxidase staining in prostatic tissue. J Urol 134:1037, 1985

164. Montasser AY, Ong MG, Mehta UT: Carcinoid tumor of the prostate associated with adenocarcinoma. Cancer 44:307, 1979

165. Moore GH, Lawshe B, Murphy J: Diagnosis of adenocarcinoma in transurethral resectates of the prostate gland. Am J Surg Pathol 10:165, 1986

166. Mostofi FK: Grading of prostatic carcinoma. Cancer Chemother Rep 59:111, 1975

167. Mostofi FK: Problems of grading carcinoma of prostate. Semin Oncol 3:161, 1976

168. Mostofi FK, Davis CJ, Jr.: Male reproductive system and prostate. p. 791. In Kissane JM (ed): Anderson's Pathology. Vol. 1., 8th Ed. CV Mosby, St. Louis, 1985

169. Mostofi FK, PRice EB, Jr.: Malignant tumors of the prostate. p. 253. In Firminger HI (ed): Tumors of the Male Genital System: Atlas of Tumor Pathology. Second Series, Fasicle 8. Armed Forces Institute of Pathology, Washington, DC, 1973

170. Mostofi FK, Sesterhenn I, Sobin LH: Histological Typing of Prostate Tumours. Workd Health Organization, Geneva, 1980

170a. Moyana TN: Adenosquamous carcinoma of the prostate. Am J Surg Pathol 11:403, 1987

171. Muller H-A, Ackerman R, Frohmuller HGW: The value of perineal punch biopsy in estimating histological grade of carcinoma of the prostate. Prostate 1:303, 1980

172. Muller H-A, Wunsch PH: Features of prostatic sarcomas in combined aspiration and punch biopsies. Acta Cytol, (suppl.) 25:480, 1981

173. Murphy GP, Gaeta JF, Pickren J, Wajsman Z: Current status of classification and staging of prostate cancer. Cancer 45:1889, 1980

174. Murphy WM, Dean PJ, Brasfield JA, Tatum L: Incidental carcinoma of the prostate: how much sampling is adequate? Am J Surg Pathol 10:170, 1986

175. Nadji M, Tabei SZ, Castro A et al : Prostatic origin of tumors: an immunohistochemical study. Am J Clin Pathol 73:735, 1980

176. Nesbit RM, Baum WC: Endocrine control of prostatic carcinoma. JAMA 143:1317, 1950

177. Newmark SR, Dluhy RG, Bennett AH: Ectopic adrenocorticotropin syndrome with prostatic carcinoma. Urology 2:666, 1973

178. Onoyama S, Ichi S: Nuclear binding sites in the liver of dexamethasone and in the ventral prostate for R1881. Endocrinol Jpn 29:349, 1982

179. Paul BD, Serrano JA, Wasserkrug HL et al : D-Ephidrine-phosphate, Dep: a new substrate with specificity for prostatic acid phosphatase (PAP). Histochemistry 56:133, 1978

180. Paulson DF, Rabson AS, Fraley EE: Viral neoplasmic transformation of hamster prostate tissue in vitro. Science 159:200, 1968

180a. Paulson DF: Assessment of anatomic extent and biologic hazard of prostatic adenocarcinoma. Urology 15:537, 1980

181. Pirke KM, Doerr P: Age related changes in free plasma testosterone, dihydrotestosterone and oestradiol. Acta Endocrinol 89:171, 1975

182. Pontes JE, Choe B, Rose N, Pierce JM, Jr.: Indirect immunofluorescence for identification of prostatic epithelial cells. J Urol 117:459, 1977

183. Prout GR, Heaney JA, Griffin PP et al : Nodal involvement as a prognostic indicator in patients with prostatic carcinoma. J Urol 124:226, 1980

184. Quay SC, Proppe KH: Carcinosarcoma of the prostate: case report and review of the literature. J Urol 125:436, 1981

185. Rich AR: On the frequency of occurrence of occult carcinoma of the prostate. J Urol 33:215, 1935

186. Riley MW: Cancer and the life course. In Yanick R (ed): Perspectives on Prevention and Treatment of Cancer in the Elderly. Raven Press, New York, 1983

187. Ro J, Ayala A, Ordonez N et al : Intraluminal crystalloids in prostatic adenocarcinoma: immunohistochemical electron microscopic and x-ray microanalytic studies. Cancer 57:2397, 1986

188. Ro J, Ayala A, Ordonez N et al : Intraluminal crystalloids in prostatic adenocarcinoma: immunohistochemical electron microscopic and x-ray microanalytic studies. Lab Invest 54:315, 1986 (Abstract)

188a. Rohr LR: Incidental adenocarcinoma in transurethral resections of the prostate: partial versus complete microscopic examination. Am J Surg Pathol 11:53, 1987

189. Rowe JW, Bradley EC: The elderly cancer patient: pathophysiological considerations. In Yancik R (ed): Perspectives on Prevention and Treatment of Cancer in the Elderly. Raven Press, New York, 1983

190. Sanford EJ, Geder L, Laychock A et al : Evidence for the association of cytomegalovirus with carcinoma of the prostate. J Urol 118:789, 1977

191. Schroeder FH, Blom JHM, Hop WCJ, Mostofi FK: Grading of prostatic cancer: I. An analysis of the prognostic significance of single characteristics. Prostate 6:81, 1985

192. Schroeder FH, Blom JHM, Hop WCJ, Mostofi FK: Grading of prostatic cancer: II. The prognostic significance of the presence of multiple architectural patterns. Prostate 6:403, 1985

193. Schroeder FH, Hop WCJ, Blom JHM, Mostofi FK: Grading of prostatic cancer: III. Multivariate analysis of prognostic parameters. Prostate 7:13, 1985

193a. Schuman LM, Mandel J, Blackard C, et al : Epidemiologic study of prostatic cancer: preliminary report. Cancer Treatment 61:181, 1977

194. Sciarra F, Sorcini G, DiSilverio F, Gagliardi V: Testosterone and 4-androstenedione concentration in peripheral and spermatic venous blood of patients with prostatic adenocarcinoma. Effects of diethylstilbestrol and cyproterone acetate therapy. J Steroid Biochem 2:313, 1971

195. Seidman H, Mushinski MH, Gelb SK, Silverberg E: Probabilities of eventually developing or dying of cancer — United States, 1985. CA 35:36, 1985

196. Sellwood RA, Spencer J, Azzopardi JG et al : Inappropriate secretion of ADH by carcinoma of the prostate. Br J Surg 56:933, 1969

197. Serrano JA, Wasserkrug HL, Serrano AA et al : The histochemical demonstration of human prostatic acid phosphatase with phosphorylcholine. Invest Urol 15:123, 1977

198. Sheldon CA, Williams RD, Fraley EE: Incidental carcinoma of the prostate: a review of the literature and critical reappraisal of classification. J Urol 124:626, 1980

199. Shelley HS, Auerbach SH, Classen KL et al : Carcinoma of the prostate. Arch Surg 77:751, 1958

200. Sheth NA, Doctor VM, Sheth AR: Cellular immunolocalization of inhibinlike peptide in human benign prostatic hyperplasia. Arch Androl 14:155, 1985

201. Silverberg E: Cancer statistics, 1984. CA 34:7, 1984

202. Silverberg E: Cancer statistics, 1985. CA 35:19, 1985

203. Silverberg E, Lubera JA: A review of American Cancer Society estimates of cancer cases and deaths. CA 33:2, 1983

204. Silverberg E, Lubera JA: Cancer statistics 1986. CA 36:9, 1986

205. Sinha AA, Blackard CE: Ultrastructure of prostatic benign hyperplasia and carcinoma. Urology 2:114, 1973

206. Sinha AA, Blackard CE, Doe RP et al : The in vitro localization of ^{3}H-estradiol in human prostatic carcinoma. Cancer 31:682, 1973

207. Sinha AA, Blackard CE, Seal US: A critical analysis of tumor morphology and hormone treatments in the untreated and estrogen-treated responsive and refractory human prostatic carcinoma. Cancer 40:2836, 1977

208. Sinowatz F, Weber P, Gasser G et al : A histochemical study of glycosidases in benign prostatic hyperplasia and in prostatic carcinoma in the human. Urol Res 6:103, 1978

209. Slater D: Carcinoid tumour of the prostate associated with inappropriate ACTH secretion. Br J Urol 57, 591, 1985

210. Smith BH, Dehner LP: Sarcoma of the prostate gland. Am J Clin Pathol 58:43, 1972

211. Smith JA, Jr., Middleton RG: Pelvic lymph node metastasis from prostatic cancer: influence of tumor grade and stage. Am Urol Assoc Program Abstract no. 238, 1982

212. Snochowski M, Pousette A, Akam P et al : Characterization and measurement of the androgen receptor in human benign prostatic hyperplasia and prostatic carcinoma. J Clin Endocrinol Metab 45:920, 1977

213. Snyder HM, III, D'angio GJ, Evans AE, Raney RB: Pediatric oncology. p. 2244. In Walsh PC, Gittes RF, Perlmutter AD, Stamey TA (eds): Campbell's Urology. Vol. 2. WB Saunders, Philadelphia, 1986

214. Sobin LH, Hjermstad BM, Sesterhenn IA, Helwig EB: Prostatic acid phosphatase activity in carcinoid tumors. Cancer 58:136, 1986

215. Song GX, Lin CT, Wu JY et al : Immunoelectron microscopic demonstration of prostatic acid phosphatase in human hyperplastic prostate. Prostate 7:63, 1985

216. Staszewski J, Haenszel W: Cancer mortality among the Polish-born in the United States. J Natl Cancer Inst 35:291, 1965

217. Steele J, Lees REM, Kraus AS, Rao C: Sexual factors in the epidemiology of cancer of the prostate. J Chronic Dis 24:19, 1971

218. Stein BS, Petersen RO, Vangore S, Kendall AR: Immunoperoxidase localization of prostate-specific antigen. Am J Surg Pathol 6:553, 1982

219. Stone MP, Stone KR, Ingram P et al : Scanning and transmission electron microscopy of human prostatic acinar cells. Urol Res 5:185, 1977

219a. Subcommittee on Diagnostic Nomenclature, Prostate Cancer Working Group, Organ Systems Program, Gardner WA, Jr, et al: A uniform histopathologic grading system for prostate cancer. Hum Pathol 19:120, 1988

220. Sufrin G, Gaeta J, Staubitz WJ et al : Endometrial carcinoma of prostate. Urology 23:18, 1986

221. Tannenbaum M: Transitional cell carcinoma of prostate. Urology 5:674, 1975

222. Tannenbaum M: Histopathology of the prostate gland. p. 303. In Tannenbaum M (ed): Urologic Pathology: The Prostate. Lea & Febiger, Philadelphia, 1977

223. Tannenbaum M, Romas N: The prostate gland. p. 1189. In Silverberg SG (ed): Principles and Practice of Surgical Pathology. Vol. 2. Wiley Medical Publications, New York, 1983

224. Tannenbaum M, Tannenbaum S, DeSanctis PN, Olsson CA: Prognostic significance of nucleolar surface area in prostatic cancer. Urology 19:546, 1982

224a. Thompson IM, Rounder JB, Teague JL, et al: Impact of routine screening for adenocarcinoma of the prostate on stage distribution. J Urol 137:424, 1987

225. Utz DC, Farrow GM: Pathologic differentiation and prognosis of prostatic carcinoma. JAMA 209:1701, 1969

225a. Vickery AL Jr, Kerr WS: Carcinoma of the prostate

treated by radical prostatectomy. A clinicopathological survey of 187 cases followed for 5 years and 148 cases followed for 10 years. Cancer 16:1598, 1963

226. Viola MV, Fromowitz F, Oravez S et al : Expression of *ras* oncogene p21 in prostate cancer. N Engl J Med 314:133, 1986.

227. Vollmer RT: Prostate cancer and chip specimens: complete versus partial sampling. Hum Pathol 17:285, 1986

228. Vuitch MF, Mendelsohn G: Relationship of ectopic ACTH production to tumor differentiation: a morphologic and immunohistochemical study of prostatic carcinoma with Cushing's syndrome. Cancer 47:296, 1981

229. Wahab ZA, Wright GL: Monoclonal antibody (anti-Leu 7) directed against natural killer cells reacts with normal, benign and malignant prostate tissues. Int J Cancer 36:677, 1985

230. Wasserstein PW, Goldman RL: Primary carcinoid of prostate. Urology 13:318, 1979

231. Wasserstein PW, Goldman RL: Diffuse carcinoid of prostate. Urology 18:407, 1981

232. Wendelken JR, Schellhammer PF, Ladaga LE, El-Mahdi AM: Transitional cell carcinoma: cause of refractory cancer of prostate. Urology 13:557, 1979

233. Wenk RE, Bhagavan BS, Levy R et al : Ectopic ACTH, prostatic oat cell carcinoma, and marked hypernatremia. Cancer 40:773, 1977

234. Whitmore WF, Jr.: Hormone therapy in prostatic cancer. Am J Med 21:697, 1956

235. Whitmore WF, Jr.: Natural history and staging of prostate cancer. Urol Clin North Am 2:205, 1984

236. Yam T, Winkler CF, Janckila AJ et al : Prostatic cancer presenting as metastatic adenocarcinoma of undetermined origin. Immunodiagnosis by prostatic acid phosphatase. Cancer 51:283, 1983

237. Yantani R, Chigusa L, Akazaki K et al : Geographic pathology of latent prostatic carcinoma. Int J Cancer 29:611, 1982

238. Young BW, Lagios MD: Endometrial (papillary) carcinoma of the prostatic utricle-response to orchiectomy. A case report. Cancer 32:1293, 1973

239. Zumoff B, Levin J, Strain GW et al : Abnormal levels of plasma hormones in men with prostate cancer: evidence toward a "two-disease" theory. Prostate 3:579, 1982

33

Biologic Characteristics of Prostate Carcinoma

David Brandes

METASTASIS

Prostate carcinoma may remain confined within the prostate gland, as evidenced by the relatively large number of patients with stage A and B disease at the time of diagnosis, the incidental finding of malignancy in prostate chips removed transurethrally for benign prostatic hypertrophy (BPH), and the not infrequent occurrence of latent caraicnoma at autopsy. However, 35 percent to 40 percent of patients with prostate carcinoma have pelvic lymph node metastases at the time of diagnosis (stage D disease). Extraprostatic lymphatic plexuses through which tumor cells may reach the pelvic lymph nodes are described in textbooks of anatomy[89] and have been reviewed recently.[141] The periprostatic plexuses at the surface of the prostate can terminate (1) in the external iliac group of lymph nodes, (2) in the internal iliac group, (3) in the internal iliac group opposite the 2nd and 3rd sacral foramen, with the larger internal trunks terminating in the common iliac group on the promontory of the sacrum. From this location they may proceed to the abdominal aortic nodes.[141]

Considerable divergence of opinions exists on how tumor cells in the prostate reach these periprostatic plexuses. Although some clinicians have claimed to have visualized intraprostatic lymphatics with India ink particles,[47] others have reported negative results in studies with injections of radioisotopes,[73] vital dyes,[209] or iodinated emulsions into the prostate gland. Indirect evidence for the existence of intraprostatic lymphatics in dogs[161] and in man[182] was obtained by injection of radioactive gold[161] or Ethiodol[182] into the prostate and subsequent demonstration of direct spread of those substances into regional lymph nodes. Lymphatic channels in the prostatic stroma, as demonstrated by electron microscopy,[80] are lined by thin attenuated endothelium, are attached to the muscle cells by anchoring filaments and microfibrils, and can be distinguished from capillaries by the absence of endothelial fenestrations, marginal folds, or pericytes.

Site of Metastasis

Lymph nodes and bones are the major site of metastasis in patients with prostate cancer.[62,78] Pelvic lymph nodes are most frequently involved, followed by periaortic, mediastinal, and bronchial lymph nodes. Visceral metastasis includes the lungs, liver, adrenal gland, and kidneys in decreasing order of frequency. The incidence and distribution of metastasis in prostate cancer are illustrated in Figure 33-1.

PERINEURAL INVASION

Invasion of the perineural space by tumor cells is frequently observed in prostatic carcinoma (Fig. 33-2). Invasion of the endoneural compartment (Fig.

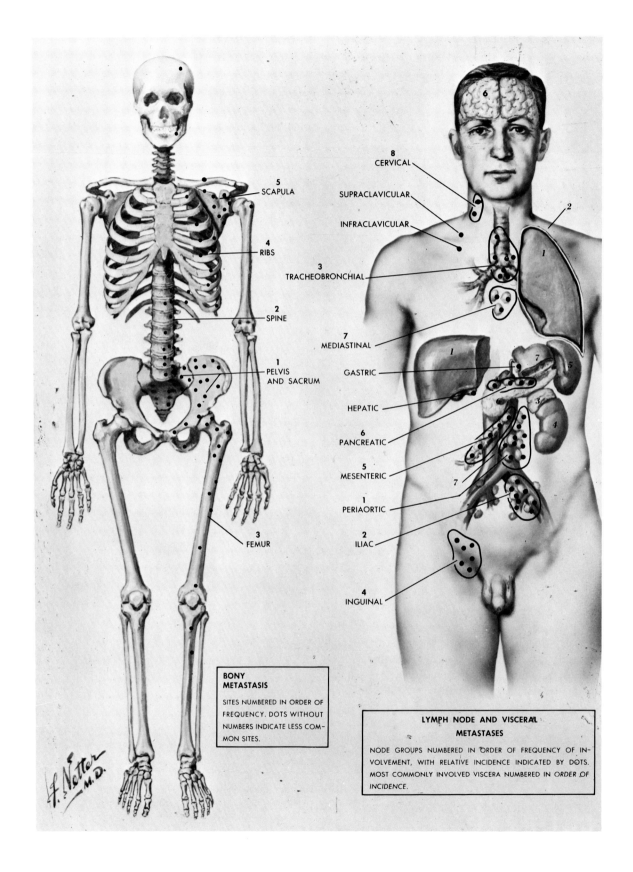

5
SCAPULA

4
RIBS

2
SPINE

1
PELVIS
AND SACRUM

3
FEMUR

8
CERVICAL

SUPRACLAVICULAR

INFRACLAVICULAR

3
TRACHEOBRONCHIAL

7
MEDIASTINAL

GASTRIC

HEPATIC

6
PANCREATIC

5
MESENTERIC

1
PERIAORTIC

2
ILIAC

4
INGUINAL

**BONY
METASTASIS**

SITES NUMBERED IN ORDER OF
FREQUENCY. DOTS WITHOUT
NUMBERS INDICATE LESS COM-
MON SITES.

**LYMPH NODE AND VISCERAL
METASTASES**

NODE GROUPS NUMBERED IN ORDER OF FREQUENCY OF IN-
VOLVEMENT, WITH RELATIVE INCIDENCE INDICATED BY DOTS.
MOST COMMONLY INVOLVED VISCERA NUMBERED IN *ORDER OF
INCIDENCE.*

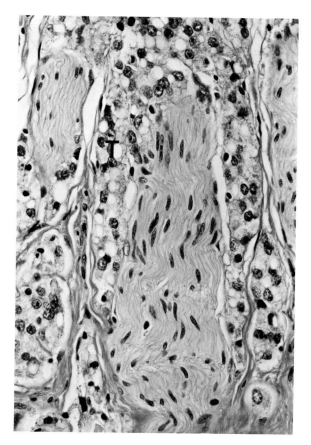

Fig. 33-2 Perineural invasion. Tumor cells (T) along the perineural space. ×280.

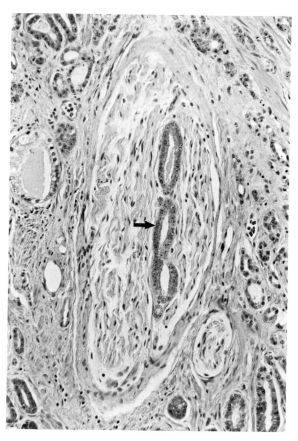

Fig. 33-3 Endoneural invasion. Well-differentiated prostate cancer acini (arrow). ×150.

33-3) and intramural ganglia occur less frequently. Perineural spaces were formerly considered to be lymphatic channels, through which tumor cells spread to extraprostatic plexuses and eventually reached regional lymph nodes. The marked incidence of metastasis of prostate cancer to the lower lumbar vertebrae and pelvic bones was attributed to spread of tumors along perineural lymphatics.[227]

However, electron microscopic studies by Rodin et al.[189] and Hassan and Maksem[106] failed to demonstrate structures lined by endothelium that could be interpreted as lymphatics in the perineural space. The perineurium appeared as several layers of flattened cells, arranged concentrically around the nerve fascicle. Tumor cells found in the perineural area might occupy the perineural space, but more frequently were located outside the perineural sheath, and in no instance were they within endothelium-lined spaces of lymphatic nature.[106] The tendency of tumor cells to spread along the perineurium spaces suggests that they constitute anatomic areas of less resistance to tumor growth.[106,189]

LYMPH NODE METASTASIS

Correlation between Tumor Grade, Clinical Stage, and Nodal Metastasis

Clinically silent and unsuspected pelvic lymph node metastasis may be discovered in patients otherwise diagnosed as having clinically stage A to stage C disease. When three or less microscopic foci of well-differentiated carcinoma are present in transurethral or enucleation specimens for BPH, the incidence of positive nodes will be approximately zero.[156]

Correlating tumor grade with the incidence of lymph node involvement reveals that poorly differentiated tumors tend to metastasize with more frequency than well-differentiated tumors.[39,133,156,157] In various series, the incidence of lymph node metastasis was two to three times more frequent in undifferentiated tumors than in differentiated tumors.[11,157,160]

Kramer et al.[133] correlated the histologic grade of tumors, according to Gleason's patterns, with the incidence of nodal metastasis. Pelvic lymphadenectomy specimens revealed the absence of metastasis in patients with Gleason's patterns 2 to 4. With Gleason's patterns 5 to 7, the percentage of positive lymph nodes was 31 percent, and increased to 93 percent for tumors with patterns 8 to 10.

Detection of lymph node metastases in grossly uninvolved pelvic lymph nodes by frozen section is important because even microscopic metastasis may identify patients in whom radical prostatectomy may not be curative.[64] Epstein et al.[64] reviewed the frozen section experience in 310 pelvic lymphadenectomy specimens. Intraoperative evaluation of lymph nodes was correct in 95 percent of cases (299 patients), including the identification of microscopic metastasis in 67.6 percent of cases (23 of 34 patients).[64]

Luciani et al.[146] compared the accuracy of lymphography versus aspiration cytology in the detection of node metastasis in patients with prostate carcinoma in a series of 35 patients. By lymphography, sensitivity was 67 percent, false-negative rate was 34 percent, false-positive rate was 43 percent, specificity was 47 percent, and accuracy was 57 percent. By aspiration cytology, the corresponding values were as follows: sensitivity, 83 percent; false-negative, 17 percent; false-positive, 0 percent; specificity, 100 percent; accuracy, 91 percent.

In patients with early stage prostate carcinoma and negative pedal lymphogram, percutaneous transperitoneal fine-needle aspiration on 10 pelvic lymph nodes in each patient yielded 20 percent micrometastases detected cytologically, a procedure that could serve to exclude such patients from elective surgery.[90]

Nodal metastases present outside the pelvis more frequently than is generally recognized. Cho and Epstein[40a] have reviewed 26 biopsies of supradiaphragmatic (usually supraclavicular) lymph nodes with metastatic prostate carcinoma. Only 7 patients had a history of prostate carcinoma; the remaining 19 presented with solitary nodes, some with concomitant urinary obstruction. They found that 22 of the 26 cases were high grade and not particularly suggestive of prostate. Only immunoperoxidase staining for PSA and/or PAP confirmed the diagnosis.

EXTRANODAL SPREAD

Bone Metastasis

Bone metastasis is the most common form of extranodal spread.[8,62,91,203] This fact has long been recognized, and figures in early papers range from 30 percent to over 70 percent.[227] Most early researchers accepted the hematogenous route, comprising the regional veins, vena cava, lungs, and arterial circulation as a means by which prostate tumor cells might reach the skeleton. It was long contended that osseous metastases from prostate carcinoma are preferentially located in the pelvic bones, lumbar spine, and sacrum and that dissemination to these bones occurs through the system of vertebral veins described by Batson.[15,16]

However, more recently, Dodds et al.[55] reviewed this generally accepted contention. Bone scans and radiographs from 136 patients over the age of 40, with histologically documented primary tumors (prostate, 73 cases; lung, 35 cases; bladder, 7 cases; kidney, 6 cases; head and neck, 6 cases; colon, 5 cases; esophagus, 2 cases; duodenum, 1 case; breast, 1 case), were analyzed, and the results were subjected to statistical treatment. The rank order of osseous metastasis revealed that the various bony regions were involved in the following order of decreasing frequency: spine, ribs, pelvis, femurs, shoulders, sternum, skull, humeri. The order of skeletal involvement in early stages did not appear to change significantly with the progression of the disease and was similar to that encountered in patients with solitary metastases from a variety of tumors.[55] Prostate carcinoma is not associated with a unique pattern of osseous metastasis, as was believed previously, since the distribution of skeletal metastasis and the rank order of metastatic involvement in age- and sex-matched patients with prostate and nonprostate carcinoma appear to be virtually identical.[55] Twenty-five percent of all patients with prostate carcinoma that had metastasized to the bone did not reveal involvement of the pelvis, lumbar spine, or sacrum, suggesting that metastasis from prostatic carcinoma does not necessarily occur through the vertebral veins. More likely prostate carcinoma cells enter the vena cava, pass through the lungs, and reach the skeletal system through the arterial circulation.[55] Among osseous metastases from prostate carcinoma, involvement of the bones of the skull occurs with relative frequency,[55,130] and occasionally occult carcinoma of the prostate may first present as an intracranial tumor

with multiple cranial nerve palsies.[183] Isolated cases of subdural metastasis from prostate carcinoma, without evidence of direct extension from underlying bone lesions,[173] and orbital metastasis with or without accompanying skull metastasis[214] have been described.

Metabolic Alterations in Patients with Bone Metastases

Bone metastasis may be accompanied by either hypercalcemia or hypocalcemia according to the osteolytic or osteoblastic nature of the disease.[52,184,191,208] Hypocalcemia may be more common than hypercalcemia in patients with metastatic bone involvement. Osseous metastasis from prostate carcinomas is generally osteoblastic, but osteomalacia has also been reported.[52] Hypocalcemia has been reported in 31 percent to 45 percent of patients with metastatic prostate carcinoma,[184,191] whereas in cases of breast or lung cancer it occurs in only approximately 13 percent of patients.[184] Calcium levels in patients with hypocalcemia and osteoblastic metastatic prostatic tumors

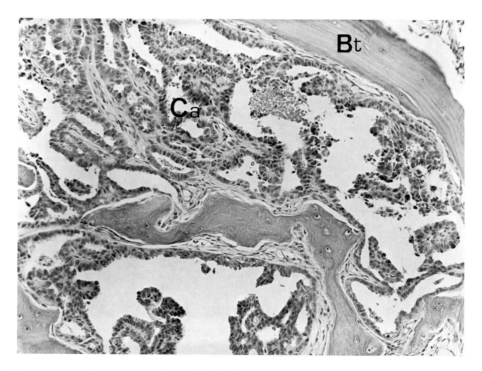

Fig. 33-4 Bone invasion. Papillary and cribriform prostate cancer (Ca) in bone marrow spaces. Note thickened bone trabeculae (Bt). ×125.

have oscillated from 4.1 mg to 8.0 mg/dl of serum. Metabolic alterations in patients with hypocalcemia and osteoblastic metastasis may include hypoparathyroidism, secondary hyperparathyroidism, alterations in vitamin D metabolism, hypomagnesemia, and a refractoriness to parathyroid hormone of renal origin, but the common denominator in all patients appears to be increased calcium in the bones.[208] The almost unique tendency of prostate carcinoma to produce osteoblastic bone metastasis could be explained on the basis of the identification in prostatic tissue of a substance with mitogenic activity for osteoblasts.[132] A representative section illustrating prostatic bone metastasis is seen in Figure 33-4.

Hydroxyproline is released from bone matrix when it is destroyed, and thence metabolized by the liver or excreted in the urine. Increased excretion of hydroxyproline has been shown to be an early index of bony metastases in other malignancies.[168a] However, studies of hydroxyproline excretion in prostate carcinoma do not show any consistent pattern, either in stable patients or in those whose disease is clearly progressing, so it is of no use as a clinical marker.[168a]

Lung Metastasis

The rank order of metastatic involvement of different organs[8,62,78] places the lung and liver in third order of frequency in comparison with lymph nodes and bone metastasis. Metastasis to the lungs has been reported at autopsy in 25 percent to 38 percent of patients with prostate carcinoma.[24,62] Microscopic pulmonary embolization by prostate carcinoma as a cause of respiratory insufficiency has been described in a recent case report.[163] Embolization of pulmonary venules and lymphatics is illustrated in Figure 33-5.

Skin and Subcutaneous Metastasis

Skin and subcutaneous metastasis from prostate carcinoma are infrequent. They constituted between 0.7 percent and 1.7 percent of skin metastases from a variety of tumors[32,81] and were found in 3 of 1,300 autopsies reviewed.[185] In a review of 21,718 charts, Arnheim[8] found 4 cases of cutaneous metastasis of prostatic origin. Katske et al.[121] thoroughly reviewed this subject and added 2 cases of their own and found

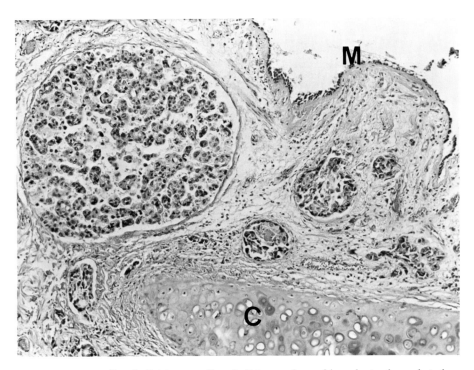

Fig. 33-5 Tumor cell emboli. Tumor cell emboli in venules and lymphatic channels in bronchial wall (M, mucosal lining; C, cartilage). ×80.

18 previously published cases of skin and subcutaneous metastasis of prostatic origin. In 16 of those cases and in their own 2 cases, the histology of the cutaneous lesion revealed poorly differentiated tumors.

ACID PHOSPHATASE: DIAGNOSTIC AND PREDICTIVE ROLE

The finding of elevated acid phosphatase in the serum of patients with prostate carcinoma[98,100] was among the first tumor markers detected in the blood of cancer patients. Serum and bone marrow acid phosphatase determinations have potential value for early diagnosis and may serve to monitor the course of the disease during therapeutically induced regression, as well as during the almost inevitable recurrence and progression seen in the patient with metastatic prostate carcinoma. (However, prostate specific antigen is rapidly replacing acid phosphatase in the monitoring of patients after prostatectomy (see below).)

PRODUCTION AND RELEASE OF ACID PHOSPHATASE

In the secretory cells, the enzyme acid phosphatase is synthesized in the rough endoplasmic reticulum, transported to the Golgi complex, and packed into lysosomes or into secretory granules[26,107,142] that are then secreted into the prostatic fluid forming part of the ejaculate. Apparently the function of acid phosphatase in the semen is to hydrolyze phosphorylcholine esters and thus provide material required for the metabolism of spermatozoa.[147] A certain proportion of the enzyme enters the blood stream, since measurable levels can be detected in the normal adult male. Serum acid phosphatase in healthy subjects may also be derived from platelets and erythrocytes.[23,240]

Acid phosphatase is considered as a secondary sex marker in men, since demonstrable levels both in prostatic tissue and in the serum are reached during puberty, coincidental with the onset of androgen production by testicular Leydig cells.[99] In addition, the levels of acid phosphatase in serum decrease after orchiectomy or antiandrogen treatment, and after the use of estrogens,[111] pointing to the dependence of prostatic cells on androgens for the synthesis of this enzyme.

It should not be surprising that the content of the enzyme is decreased in prostatic cancer cells,[231,232] since malignant transformation is amost invariably accompanied by some loss of functional and structural differentiation. Elevation of serum acid phosphatase in patients with prostate carcinoma, particularly in the presence of metastasis, would seem paradoxical in view of the decrease of enzyme activity per unit of malignant prostatic tissue. However, acid phosphatase in normal glands is released into the lumen of the acini and then conveyed to the major ducts and into the urethra during ejaculation. In prostate cancer most of the newly formed acini, especially in poorly differentiated tumors as well as metastases, are not connected with ductal systems, resulting in enzyme leakage into the interstitium, lymph spaces, and finally to the bloodstream.[142]

Methods for Acid Phosphatase Determination

ENZYMATIC PROCEDURES

A variety of substrates have been used to measure serum acid phosphatase in an attempt to distinguish selectively the enzyme originating from prostatic tissue from that derived from pathologic conditions in other organs or from platelets and red blood cells.[148,178] Gutman and colleagues[100] had originally used phenyl phosphate as a substrate, but subsequently with β-glycerophosphate[23] there was a lower incidence of elevated acid phosphatase in nonprostatic disease. Numerous other substrates were subsequently tested,[71] but they did not appear specific for a particular acid phosphatase isoenzyme.[138]

L-(+)-tartrate and formaldehyde[5,6] inhibit prostatic acid phosphatase (PAP) by approximately 95 percent but have no effect on erythrocyte acid phosphatase.[23] Tartrate inhibition may increase the specificity of measuring serum acid phosphatase of prostatic origin, but tartrate also inhibits acid phosphatase derived from other tissues: 75 percent for liver, 80 percent for kidney, and 70 percent for spleen.[23] The method of Fishman et al.[71] distinguished "total" acid phosphatase, determined in the absence of L-(+)-tartrate, from tartrate-labile acid phosphatase considered as prostatic in origin.

IMMUNOCHEMICAL METHODS

There are many immunochemical methods of high specificity for the detection of PAP in serum, bone marrow, and tissue sections. Prostatic tissue, sperm-free ejaculates, and prostatic fluid obtained by rectal massage have been used as enzyme sources for subsequent purification by filtration on Sephadex, ion-exchange chromatography, affinity chromatography, immunoabsorbent column chromatography, salt or acid precipitation, or isoelectric focusing. Antisera to purified PAP were raised in rabbits, monkeys, and goats,[19,42,76,151,190,199,220,221] and monoclonal antibodies to human PAP were produced by the hybridoma technique.[139]

Immunochemical assays for the determination of serum and bone PAP levels have included gel diffusion, immunoelectrophoresis, solid-phase radioimmunoassay, double-antibody radioimmunoassay, counterimmunoelectrophoresis, and various types of enzyme immunoassay[19,42,76,151,199,220,221]

Serum Acid Phosphatase Elevations and Clinical Stage

The percentage of elevated serum acid phosphatase as measured by modern immunochemical assays in patients with stage A prostate carcinoma have been reported as 0 percent,[41] 10 percent,[57] 13 percent,[151] and 33 percent.[75] Since in some of these patients clinical staging was not followed by surgical staging, extraprostatic extension or lymph node metastasis (stage C to D) may have been present at the time of serum acid phosphatase determination. Bahnson and Catalona[8b] found a 6 percent incidence of PAP elevations among 102 surgically staged patients, with 5 of 6 having extraprostatic extension of tumor. More importantly, they found that serum PAP values in the upper half of the normal range were associated with an 84 percent incidence of extraprostatic extension.

Studies on the frequency of elevation of serum acid phosphatase in more advanced stages (B through D) yield variable results. The proportion of patients with elevated serum PAP significantly rises with increasing stage. In stage B, percentages of patients with elevated serum PAP range between 21 percent,[33] 26 percent,[151] and 79 percent;[75] in stage C between 30 percent,[151] 37 percent,[33] and 71 percent;[75] and in stage D between 74 percent,[33] 92 percent,[75] and 94 percent.[151]

Serum acid phosphatase may be elevated in other prostatic conditions. Up to 42 percent of patients with retention from BPH may have elevated serum acid phosphatase levels.[151] Increased levels have also been detected in patients with prostatitis[215a,216] and in prostatic infarction.[204,219]

Bone Marrow Acid Phosphatase Determinations

These have been widely used in the staging of prostate carcinoma and in searching for occult osseous metastasis. As with serum stage-related acid phosphatase determinations, wide variations are found in the figures of different investigators. Percentages of patients with elevated bone marrow acid phosphatase levels in different stages have ranged as follows: stage A to B, 6.5 percent,[34] 33 percent,[43] and 50 percent;[238] stage C, 6.7 percent,[43] 20 percent,[115] 71 percent,[124] and 100 percent[43,238] stage D, 52 percent,[115] 54.5 percent[34] 72 percent,[124] and 100 percent.[43,238] In contrast, by catalytic methods, only 35 percent of patients with stage D prostate cancer showed increased tartrate-labile acid phosphatase in the bone marrow.[115]

There is no definite pattern in bone marrow acid phosphatase changes that would permit discrimination between benign conditions, such as BPH, and metastatic prostatic disease.[19] Levels of bone marrow acid phosphatase may be elevated in patients with nonprostatic disease, including hematologic disorders, leukemias, lymphomas, and various types of malignancy such as lung, breast, and gastrointestinal carcinomas, and melanoma.[34,54,144,162,192,237] High levels of bone marrow acid phosphatase activity, measured catalytically, may result from the lysis and release of enzyme from platelets and erythrocytes that are known to contain acid phosphatases.[178] Free hemoglobin, if present in the bone marrow homogenate, may also interfere in the determination of total and tartrate-labile acid phosphatases.[231]

Despite these drawbacks, some studies have concluded that determinations of bone marrow acid phosphatase values were more sensitive than other staging procedures, such as serum acid phosphatase assays, bone biopsies, and scanning, in detecting metastatic spread in patients with carcinoma of the prostate.[43,95,218,237,238]

When the acid phosphatase levels in serum and bone marrow of prostate cancer patients with bone metastases were compared by radioimmunoassay, increased levels were noted in both serum and bone marrow in approximately 95 percent of the cases.[34] In parallel assays by enzymatic methods with various substrates, elevated serum levels were detected in 67 percent to 82 percent of the patients, whereas bone marrow assays were positive in only 50 percent to 67 percent of the patients.[34]

Studies have recently been reported utilizing radio-labelled antibodies to PAP for visualization of osseous metastases on bone scan.[8a] There was no reported toxicity and results, though preliminary, were promising.

Serum Acid Phosphatase Levels: Association with Therapeutic Response and Survival

A relationship between serum acid phosphatase levels and the effect of treatment was first noted by Huggins and Hodges[111] and later by other researchers,[72,228] who reported a fall in serum acid phosphatase levels after orchiectomy or estrogen therapy. Studies by enzymatic methods have indicated an inverse relationship between initial serum levels of acid phosphatase and length of survival after hormonal[35] or chemotherapeutic treatments.[21,118] Fluctuations of serum acid phosphatase levels during treatment may also have predictive value, since increases have been associated with a shortened survival, and decreases predict an extended survival.[35] Reduction of tumor size and pain relief have also been correlated with normalization of serum acid phosphatase levels,[118] but this was observed in only approximately one-half of the patients with objective tumor response. There are some questions about the validity of catalytic determinations of serum acid phosphatase levels as the sole index for monitoring the course of the disease.[58,118]

The improvement of radioimmunoassay procedures over enzymatic methods for the detection of elevated serum acid phosphatase in patients with untreated prostate carcinoma and for monitoring fluctuations during and after various treatments has been documented by Vihko et al.[220] Before therapy, enzymatic methods depicted elevated serum acid phosphatase in 24 percent of the patients, whereas by radioimmunoassay the enzyme activity was elevated in 80 percent of the patients. Favorable effects of endocrine treatment were detected more clearly by radioimmunoassay. After therapy, there was a significant decrease in radioimmunoassayable acid phosphatase in 6 of 12 patients with nonmetastatic disease and in 6 of 8 patients with metastases. With the enzyme assay, acid phosphatase was decreased in 1 of 12 patients in the nonmetastatic group and in 3 of 8 in the group of patients with metastases.

Changes in serum PAP determined by radioimmunoassay were also noted after transurethral resection for benign and malignant prostatic disease, after radical prostatectomy, and after orchiectomy, diethylstilbestrol therapy, or supervoltage therapy.[48] Surgical procedures were followed by a transient rise in acid phosphatase of short duration, with a rapid decrease to normal levels within 24 hours to 72 hours thereafter. The pre-existing high levels of radioimmunoassayed serum PAP decreased more slowly and eventually reached normal values in responsive tumors treated by orchiectomy, diethylstilbestrol therapy, or supervoltage radiation.[48]

Overall, the changes detected by radioimmunoassays are more valuable as objective parameters in monitoring response to therapy and progression of the disease than those by the enzymatic methods.[220]

Serum Acid Phosphatase Levels: Tumor Grade

There are some discrepancies regarding the relationship between the degree of differentiation of the primary prostate tumor and the release of acid phosphatase into the blood. Enzyme-based assays have indicated elevated total serum PAP levels in a greater percentage of patients with differentiated tumors, in all the clinical stages of the disease.[164,166] In contrast, immunochemical assays indicate that there is a greater percentage of elevations of serum acid phosphatase in patients with poorly differentiated, as opposed to well-differentiated, carcinomas.[33,151] Percentages of elevations of serum prostatic acid phosphatase have ranged as follows: well-differentiated tumors, 5 percent to 14 percent; moderately differentiated, 34 percent to 41 percent; and poorly differentiated, 54 percent to 65 percent.[33,151]

Tissue Content of Acid Phosphatase: Tumor Grade

The overall content of acid phosphatase in prostate carcinoma determined biochemically or by histochemistry[14,33,34,56,128,231,232] is less than that present in normal and hyperplastic glands, and the staining of cancer cells is not only less intense but also less uniform than in normal tissue. Biochemical assays of tissue homogenates by enzymatic assays[231,232] or by immunochemistry[77] have indicated a decreased concentration of acid phosphatase in poorly differentiated tumors when compared with those that are well differentiated. There has been less agreement in establishing a correlation between tumor grade and reactivity for acid phosphatase in tissue sections when using either enzyme histochemistry or immunohistochemistry methods.

Poorly differentiated prostate tumors stained catalytically for acid phosphatase showed a less intense and uniform reaction than the well-differentiated prostate tumors.[56,127,128,172] There was a discrepancy when the correlation between tumor grade and acid phosphatase reactivity was re-examined by immunohistochemical methods. The data presented by Bates et al.,[14] Yam et al.,[234] and Griffiths[92,93] supported the findings previously obtained with enzyme catalytic methods showing decreased immunoreactivity for acid phosphatase in poorly differentiated tumors. In the hands of other investigators,[20,33,117,142,143,150,167] application of comparable immunohistochemical methods failed to detect a consistent pattern of decreased acid phosphatase reactivity with loss of histologic differentiation of prostate tumors.

Epstein and Eggleston[63] were not able to establish a statistically significant correlation between the presence of poor acid phosphatase immunoreactivity and a prediction of the progression of prostate tumors.

PROSTATE-SPECIFIC ANTIGEN

Prostate-specific antigen (PSA) is a serine protease whose natural substrate is the predominant protein of the seminal vesicle coagulum.[161a] It is found exclusively in prostatic ductal and acinar epithelial cells, and is present in normal, hyperplastic, and malignant prostate cells, but not in any other cell of the body, nor in females or, to date, any other tumor.[85a]

Immunoperoxidase studies consistently identify PSA in sections of normal and hyperplastic prostate.[63,170,212] It is present in most carcinomas as well, although in the more undifferentiated tumors staining tends to be weak and is sometimes absent altogether. (See Ch. 32.)

The PSA in prostatic tissue is immunologically identical to that found in the serum.[171] Two different assays have been developed to measure serum PSA,

one a solid-phase test using monoclonal antibodies, the other a competitive radioimmunoassay involving displacement of radiolabelled PSA from polyclonal antibodies.[109a] These two assays, although quite reproducible, yield very different values, the competitive radioimmunoassay values averaging 1.85 times those of the solid-phase, so that the normal ranges are entirely different.[109a] Thus, in evaluating PSA studies it is crucial to know which assay was employed. It should also be noted that PSA spills readily into the circulation, with substantial elevations following prostatic massage, needle or other biopsy.[111a,209a]

Clinically, serum determinations of PSA are rapidly replacing acid phosphatase as the most important tumor marker for following patients after radical prostatectomy.[47a,168b,209a] PSA has a half-life in the range of 2.2 to 3.15 days,[168b,209a] and will fall to near zero within two to three weeks if all antigen-bearing tissue has been removed. Any residual PSA (above the test's upper limit for females) is very strong evidence that tumor persists.[126a,168b,209a] Killian et al.[126a] found that 24 of 26 patients with recurrences had an elevated serum PSA concentration for at least 12 months before clinical manifestations of recurrence. Stamey et al.[209a] treat presumptively for recurrence on the basis of elevation with pelvic irradiation and have been rewarded with a fall of PSA to zero levels.

Moreover, it is generally agreed that PSA is more sensitive than prostatic acid phosphatase (PAP) in following patients following prostatectomy. For example, in one study, only 4 to 8 patients with documented recurrence had elevated PAP's but all had elevated PSA's.[168b] That experience has been universal in other studies addressing this issue.[126,126a,135,209a] Ahmann and Schifman[6a] found that among men with known stage D disease 76 percent had elevated PSAs versus only 49 percent elevated PAPs. The same approximate ratio of positivity is maintained in bone marrow evaluation of these enzymes.[165a]

It was hoped that serum PSA would aid in the detection of prostate carcinoma. However, this was not to be. PSA levels are elevated above the normal range in 55 to 83 percent of patients with BPH, sometimes very substantially.[209a] Oesterling et al.[168b] found that the PSA levels in BPH were statistically indistinguishable from those of patients with carcinoma confined to the prostate (Fig. 33-6). Because of this, no matter what cutoff value of PSA was used to separate benign from malignant, there was a prohibitively high level of false-positives, 59 percent even at the highest cutoff. Thus, all agree that PSA cannot function as a single, stand-alone test in detection of carcinoma.

However, Stamey et al.[209a] demonstrated that there is a broad correlation between serum PSA levels and tumor volume, and generally with stage. Oesterling et al.[168b] have considerably refined these observations, demonstrating that PSA levels increase progressively from those in patients with tumor confined to the prostate, to those with capsular penetration, to those with seminal vesicle involvement, to those, finally, with lymph node metastases (Fig. 33-6). Unfortunately, these correlations, although highly significant

statistically for the group as a whole, do not allow prediction of pathologic stage from the serum PSA in the individual patient.

IMMUNOLOGY OF PROSTATE CARCINOMA

Immunologic studies related to prostate carcinoma primarily ask whether this tumor expresses antigenic capabilities that could result in immune responses in the host. Reviews by Catalona[36] and Ablin and Bhatti[1-3] reveal that studies in this field, although sparse, include a wide spectrum of serologic as well as cellular immunologic investigations.

Humoral Immunology

Indirect immunofluorescence staining has shown that sera of patients with prostate carcinoma react positively with the plasma membrane of prostatic cells.[3] As judged by these indirect immunofluorescence methods, prostatic antibodies are present in 54 percent of prostate cancer patients, compared with an incidence of 10 percent in subjects without this type of tumor. The incidence of positive reactions and higher antibody titers was 92 percent in stage D patients compared with only 20 percent in stage B patients. Sera of 38 percent of prostate cancer patients with antibodies to prostate reacted also with normal stratified squamous epithelium, suggesting a lack of tumor as well as tissue specificity to these antibodies. The sera of the other 62 percent of prostate cancer patients, however, reacted only with prostatic epithelium, and thus it would appear that at least in some patients with prostate cancer the serum contains prostate tumor-associated antibodies.[3]

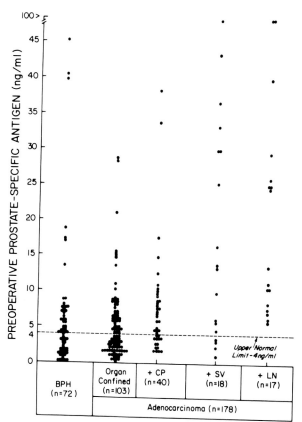

Fig. 33-6 Prostate-specific antigen. Plot of individual preoperative PSA values with respect to pathology of the prostate. BPH, benign prostatic hyperplasia, CP, capsular penetration, SV, seminal vesicle involvement, LN, lymph node involvement. (From Oesterling et al.,[168b] with permission.)

Cell-Mediated Immunity

Cell-mediated immunity in prostate cancer patients has been investigated by (1) the assessment of T-lymphocyte function by the phytohemagglutinin (PHA) stimulation test; (2) the skin test response to dinitrochlorobenzene (DCNB); (3) the inhibition of leukocyte migration tests; (4) the leukocyte adherence inhibition test; and (5) the spontaneous and antibody-dependent cell-mediated cytotoxicity properties of peripheral blood leukocytes. The monocyte chemotactic response, the in vitro macrophage-mediated cytotoxicity test, the cytolytic functions of killer (K) cells, and the role of suppressor cells in patients with prostatic cancer have been reviewed by a number of investigators.[1-3,36,66]

MITOGEN-INDUCED LYMPHOCYTIC BLASTOGENESIS

Studies by Robinson et al.[186] indicated that the lymphocyte proliferative responses to PHA were markedly reduced in patients with advanced metastatic carcinoma of the prostate, as compared with patients with BPH. However, in patients with small foci of cancer, the response was not significantly different from that of the normals, whereas some patients with focal carcinomas exhibiting lymphocytic infiltration actually had reactivity above that of normal controls. Patients with a lymphocyte transformation response to PHA stimulation with a ratio to control greater than 200 (test/control [T/C] > 200) generally had a better 3-year survival rate than those with T/C ratios below 200.[186] Reduced lymphocyte responsiveness to stimulation with PHA in prostate cancer patients was noted by other researchers,[40,158,159] and the results suggested a lack of correlation between the clinical stage of the disease and the blastogenic response to PHA.[40,159]

Comparative studies with autologous versus homologous serum in the incubation procedure indicate that both an intrinsic alteration of lymphocytic function and the presence of inhibitory factors of lymphocytic blastogenic reactivity in the serum of prostate cancer patients may be responsible for observed impairment of mitogen-induced lymphocytic blastogenesis.[2,36,159] Further studies have implicated an elevation of serum α-2-globulin and other serum inhibitors in the impairment of lymphocytic reactivity in prostate cancer patients as well as some degree of deficiency of lymphocytes in the peripheral circulation.[36]

Lymphocytic blastogenesis, induced by mitogens, may be affected by alterations in the hormonal status of the host. In vitro studies indicate that the responsiveness of peripheral blood lymphocytes from normal adult men to PHA stimulation may be significantly reduced in the presence of exogenous steroids and synthetic estrogens added to the culture medium.[4]

In prostate cancer patients, a decrease in lymphocyte responsiveness to PHA stimulation was observed when lymphocytes were collected after estrogen administration to the patient, as compared with the response before the estrogen treatment.[4,105] After cryosurgery, PHA responsiveness increased when lymphocytes were cultured in homologous serum, but was reduced in autologous serum.[4]

ASSESSMENT OF GENERAL DELAYED-TYPE SKIN TEST RESPONSE

Examination of T-cell function by the skin test response to dinitrochlorobenzene (DNCB) revealed impaired DNCB response in patients with prostate carcinoma. Some clinicians have found no correlation between the stage of the disease and the degree of impairment of DNCB reactivity.[36,37,60] In contrast, others have found that the degree of impairment of DNCB reactivity was greater in patients with metastatic disease.[51]

LEUKOCYTE MIGRATION INHIBITION TESTS

Migration of leukocytes from patients with malignant tumors may be inhibited when the leukocytes are cultured in the presence of tumor extracts to which the cells are sensitized. Specific reactivity to malignant prostatic antigens has been seen in patients with prostate carcinoma by direct inhibition of leukocyte migration.[2,61,66] In addition, inhibition of migration has been observed with both autogenous and allogeneic prostatic tumor extracts, suggesting that cell-mediated immunity to common prostatic tissue-associated antigens may be present in prostate cancer patients.[2] Specific reactivity of leukocytes from patients with prostate carcinoma to allogeneic malignant prostatic tumors was observed in patients with localized and disseminated disease, but the degree of reactivity was greater in patients with localized disease, low-grade tumor, and inactive clinical states than it was in patients with widespread disease, high-grade tumor, and active clinical disease.[2] In a comparable study, inhibition of the migration of autogenous leukocytes was noted in patients with localized prostate cancer, but was not apparent in patients with hematogenous metastasis or widespread disease.[61]

LEUKOCYTE ADHERENCE INHIBITION TEST

Leukocytes from patients with various types of malignancy may react with extracts of the autologous tumor or with extracts of allogeneic tumors of the same organ site.[66,104] This reactivity can be assessed by the leukocyte adherence inhibition technique, which measures the percentage of leukocytes adhering to nylon fibers packed into small plastic tubes or adhering directly to the wall of Pyrex test tubes.[66,104] The inhibition of adherence can be expressed as percent leukocyte adherence or as a nonadherence index calculated on the number of nonadherent cells.[66,104]

Inhibition of adherance has been noted in leukocytes from patients with prostate cancer toward extracts of autologous and allogeneic prostatic carcinomas.[2,22] The reactivity or inhibition of adherence toward allogeneic malignant prostatic tissue is noted when the test is performed with homologous or autologous serum. Reactivity toward autologous malignant prostate, however, takes place only with homologous serum. This lack of reactivity with autologous serum has been attributed to the presence of blocking factors and possibly to sensitization of peripheral blood leukocytes by the autologous serum.[3] Application of the leukocyte adherence inhibition test in 342 patients with prostate adenocarcinoma and in 192 normal subjects and patients with other types of cancer revealed reactivity to prostate tumor-associated antigens in 276 prostate cancer patients, with an overall sensitivity of 81 percent and specificity of 56 percent. There is, however, no apparent correlation between the clinical stage of the disease and the in vitro reactivity to prostate tumor-associated antigens.[22]

SPONTANEOUS AND ANTIBODY-DEPENDENT CELL-MEDIATED CYTOTOXICITY

Spontaneous cell-mediated cytotoxicity (SCMC) and antibody-dependent cell-mediated cytotoxicity (ADCC) have been investigated in cancer patients, including cases of prostate carcinoma,[38] by using peripheral blood leukocytes from the cancer patients as effector cells and Chang human liver cells or chicken erythrocytes as the target cells. Cancer patients showed a significantly depressed ADCC against Chang liver cells. No significant difference in ADCC directed against chicken erythrocyte target cells could be detected between cancer patients and controls.[38] In cancer patients, SCMC was significantly depressed against Chang liver cell targets, but it was markedly enhanced against chicken erythrocyte targets.[38] Since Chang human liver cell targets are susceptible to both ADCC and SCMC, facilitated only by K cells or K cell-like lymphocytes, these results and data from studies with effector cell fractions indicate that cancer patients have elevation of macrophage cytotoxic activity concomitantly with a depressed K-cell activity.[38]

HORMONE RECEPTORS AND OTHER BINDING SUBSTANCES

Prostatic cells contain steroid receptors for androgens, estrogens, and progesterone; binding protein for estramustine phosphate; and binding sites for prolactin. The interaction between these compounds and their respective receptors, binding proteins, or membrane binding sites influences the physiologic activities, growth, and differentiation of prostatic tissues.

Androgen Receptors

The growth and function of normal prostatic tissue and to a certain extent prostate carcinoma are dependent primarily on androgenic stimulation, which follows uptake and retention by the prostatic cells of testosterone and its metabolites, dihydrotestosterone (DHT) and androstanediols. The various steps in the formation of the DHT–receptor complex and its activation of the events that lead to macromolecular synthesis and cell replication have been described in detail in Chapters 30 to 32.

Estrogen and Progesterone Receptors

The presence of estrogenic and progestenic steroids in the plasma of men and the occurrence of specific receptors for these compounds in prostatic tissues suggested a role of estrogen and progesterone in regulation of prostatic function and growth. In healthy men, plasma levels of 17 β-estradiol [estra-1,3,5(10)-

triene-3,17 β-diol] are approximately 1.5 ng/100 ml. The levels of estrone [3-hydroxy-1,3,5(10)-estratriene-17-one] are approximately 4.6 ng/100 ml, and the levels of progesterone (4-pregnene-3,20-dione) in plasma are approximately 2.5 ng/100 ml.[44,45]

Several investigators have been able to demonstrate the presence of a specific receptor protein for 17 β-estradiol in prostate carcinoma.[12,13,239] Significant concentrations of 17 β-estradiol receptor protein (more than 3.5 fmol/mg of protein) were detected in 8 of 10 patients with prostate carcinoma, and in 50 percent the receptor content surpassed 25 fmol/mg of cytosol protein.

A high-affinity, low-capacity progesterone receptor was demonstrated in prostatic cytosol of 17 patients with BPH and 3 with prostate carcinoma.[96] In six patients with prostate carcinoma, the concentration of progesterone receptor in prostatic tissue cytosol oscillated between 6.4 fmol and 89.4 fmol/mg of protein.[239]

Prolactin-Binding Sites

Prolactin-binding sites that have high affinity and are saturable and displaceable have been detected in animal and human prostatic tissues.[7,131,230]

Localization of prolactin-binding sites in rat and human prostatic epithelial cells has been demonstrated by the immunoperoxidase method[7,230] with rat or human prolactin. The reaction products are confined to the cytoplasm of the acinar epithelium. The pattern of staining is diffuse in human normal and cancerous prostate. Normal, hyperplastic, and malignant prostatic cells contain specific high-affinity receptors for prolactin.[7,131] Quantitative assays with radiolabeled hormone (125-iodine–prolactin) have shown specific binding to membrane-rich particulate fractions of prostatic tissues, and these assays revealed high-affinity, saturable, and displaceable binding properties.[122]

Retinoic Acid-Binding Protein

A cytoplasmic protein that binds retinoic acid specifically — retinoic acid-binding protein (cRABP) — has been detected in various fetal and a few adult tissues. The ability of retinoic acid to maintain the differentiated state of epithelial structures is mediated by this binding protein.[145] In many instances, cRABP is present in fetal tissues and becomes undetectable in postnatal life, and some malignant tumors arising from cRABP-negative tissues may reveal re-expression of this binding protein.[30,85,145] Although cRABP cannot be detected in adult rat and human prostates, the binding protein for retinoic acid has been shown to be present in human prostate cancer and in the R-3327 rat prostate carcinoma.[27,85] These findings suggest that growth and differentiation of prostate cancer cells are modulated through the interaction of retinoic acid with its binding protein, in a fashion comparable to the interaction between steroid hormones and their receptors.[145,215]

HORMONAL TREATMENT FOR PROSTATE CARCINOMA

In many patients with prostate carcinoma, temporary remission can be obtained during the early endocrine-dependent phase by interfering with the hormonal stimulation required for the maintenance of the structural and functional integrity of the neoplastic cells. The mechanisms by which male sex hormones control the growth and function of prostatic cells are shown in Figure 30-7 (Chapter 30). Any compound that interferes with this chain of biologic events will deprive the neoplastic cells of the required endocrine stimulus and cause a temporary restraint of tumor cell growth.

Hormone manipulation for the treatment of prostate carcinoma includes orchiectomy, administration of estrogenic compounds, and the use of substances with antiandrogenic properties. 5 α-reductase inhibitors and luteinizing hormone releasing hormone (LHRH) agonists[136,137] also have therapeutic potentialities. These and other advances in hormonal treatment are discussed in a recent excellent review by Smith.[208a]

Orchiectomy and Adrenalectomy

Bilateral orchiectomy reduces plasma testosterone levels approximately 93 percent, since approximately 95 percent of the hormone in men is produced by the testes. The average value for plasma testosterone after bilateral orchiectomy is 43 ± 32 ng/100 ml compared with 611 ng/100 ml in the intact normal adult.[45] Several studies have demonstrated that plasma testosterone remains suppressed uniformly for up to 2 years after orchiectomy,[188,198,200] without significant elevation in orchiectomized men who have reactivation of prostate cancer.[198,225]

Since the postcastration levels of testosterone (43 ± 32 ng/100 ml) are still approximately sixfold higher than those present in prepubertal males (6.6 ng/100 ml) it was presumed that at least part of the circulating androgens were produced by the adrenal gland, and adrenalectomy was performed as a palliative treatment in patients with progressing prostate carcinoma.[9,187,197]

Results of adrenalectomy in patients who had relapsed after orchiectomy and estrogen therapy have indicated subjective improvement in 81 percent of patients but an objective response in only 36 percent.[152] Criteria for objective response included reduced tumor mass and decreased calcium excretion and acid phosphatase serum levels. When relapse occurs after primary adequate hormonal treatment, it is likely that regrowth of the tumor consists of mainly androgen-independent cells, and the elimination of the small amount of adrenal androgens by adrenalectomy does not serve any practical purpose in control of tumor growth.

Pharmacologic suppression of sex steroid production by the adrenal gland in patients who had become refractory to orchiectomy was also attempted by using such drugs as spironolactone[45,225] and aminoglutethimide.[45,233] In patients treated with aminoglutethimide and hydrocortisone, complete response was seen in 4 percent, partial response in 16 percent, and objective stabilization in 24 percent. Twenty percent of patients treated with spironolactone experienced relief from bone metastases.[233]

More recently an attempt was made to produce androgen stimulation of prostate tumors refractory to orchiectomy, before chemotherapy.[153,154] The underlying hypothesis was to attempt to temporarily increase tumor growth by androgen priming and therefore enhance sensitivity to the chemotherapeutic agents. Results, however, suggest that in patients with advanced prostate disease androgen priming did not enhance the antitumor effects of the drugs employed and was associated with significant toxicity.[154] Such negative results could be accounted for by the prevalence of hormone-resistant cells in tumors that have become refractory to orchiectomy.[153,154] In line with these results in the experimental observation that in-

termittent or late therapy does not have any effect on the growth of the Dunning R3327H prostate carcinoma.[214a]

Estrogen Therapy

In hormone-sensitive prostate carcinoma, response to estrogens is mediated through the hypothalamic-pituitary-testicular axis and results in the blocking of testicular synthesis of testosterone and a concomitant drop in plasma testosterone levels (see Fig. 30-7).[17,45,198] In the intact male, the action of estrogens consists primarily in a suppression of the release of LH from the pituitary, but estrogens may also act directly on the Leydig cells and produce an inhibition of their steroidogenic response.[17,45,110,119,198] Moreover, there is some evidence that estrogens may have a direct effect on prostatic cells, particularly on those that contain estrogen receptors.[17,201,236] Estrogens may inhibit deoxyribonucleic acid (DNA) polymerase as well as 5 α-reductase activity, which could lead to direct inhibition at the level of the nucleus.[119,201,202]

Some prostate cancer patients with relapse after conventional primary androgen withdrawal therapy have been treated with high-dose intravenous diethylstilbestrol diphosphate.[37] It was hypothesized that this compound concentrates in the prostate, where hydrolysis of the phosphate group by PAP would release the uncoupled estrogen.[28] Treatment with high-dose diethylstilbestrol diphosphate in a small number of patients with stage D disease, who had failed to respond to therapy with conventional doses of estrogens, produced subjective and objective response. However, the available clinical data are not sufficient for evaluating response to high-dose diethylstilbestrol phosphate. Previous studies had shown that a variety of phosphatases from tissue other than prostate can dephosphorylate this and other estrogen phosphates.[28]

Varenhorst[216] has described the metabolic changes occurring during endocrine treatment of prostate carcinoma, particularly in relation to cardiovascular complications secondary to treatment with estrogens or cyproterone acetate.

Antiandrogens

Orchiectomy removes the primary source of androgen production, and estrogens exert their major effect at the level of the hypothalamus by inhibiting the release of LHRH factors. Subsequent suppression of the release of LH by the pituitary leads to the reduction of testosterone production by the testes.[45,193] Antiandrogens, on the other hand, act at the target level, by inhibiting formation of the DHT–receptor complex. They thus interfere with the binding of this complex to nuclear acceptors, a necessary step for the initiation of macromolecular synthesis and cell replication in the prostate.[94,116,224] Cyprotrone acetate is one of the antiandrogens that has received wide clinical attention, but other substances with antiandrogenic activity, such as flutamide,[83] anandron, and the progestational antiandrogen, megestrol acetate,[84] have also been tried clinically.

Cyproterone acetate competitively inhibits the binding of androgens to the cytoplasmic receptor. This interferes with the translocation of the DHT–receptor complex into the nucleus resulting in decreased concentration of free and bound DHT in the nucleus.[116,140,168] In patients with advanced prostate carcinoma, both subjective and objective parameters are more favorably influenced by cyproterone acetate than by estradiol treatment, although suppression of plasma testosterone levels is more pronounced in the estrogen-treated patients.[116] Relative temporary remission, including reduction of the local tumor, has been observed after exclusive treatment with cyproterone either in previously untreated patients or after unsuccessful treatment with other modalities.[114,116,217] Overall, cyproterone acetate appears superior to estradiol treatment in regard to avoidance of side effects, such as gynecomastia, thrombophlebitis, coronary heart disease, and temporary impairment of liver function.[114] As for estrogen treatment, prolactin levels in plasma are increased during cyproterone treatment, but the effect is far less pronounced.[114]

Repeat biopsy in patients who had been treated for 6 months with cyproterone acetate revealed changes in the tumor cells similar to those seen after estrogen therapy. They were characterized by cytoplasmic vacuolization and condensation of chromatin in the tumor cells as well as marked acinar atrophy and stromal reaction.[114]

A blocker of testosterone synthesis, ketoconazole, has been tried in stage D disease, with relief of pain and normalization of acid phosphatase levels.[175a] Side effects, mainly nausea, were unacceptably high, but the study did demonstate that the process may be attached at the level of testosterone synthesis, not just at the receptor level.

Luteinizing Hormone Releasing Hormone Agonists

LHRH agonists, administered by nasal spray or subcutaneously, at doses ranging from 50 ng to 500 ng daily induce a maximal inhibition of testicular androgen secretion and a corresponding decrease in serum testosterone levels (see Fig. 30-7).[136,137,196a] Medical castration with LHRH agonists inhibits almost completely the biosynthesis of androgens with no secondary effects such as those produced by estrogens or the psychologic limitation of surgical castration.[136,137,196a] In men, inhibition of the steroidogenic pathway by LHRH agonists appears to occur at the level of 17-hydroxylase and 17,20-desmolase activity.

Serum levels of LH measured by radioimmunoassay have remained normal or have been only slightly decreased in monkeys. In men, treatment with LHRH agonists induced more than 95 percent inhibition of testosterone and DHT levels.[68] Similarly, in men at 1 month after treatment with LHRH, radioimmunoassaysable LH was reduced by only 40 percent to 50 percent, whereas LH bioactivity was only approximately 5 percent of the control, which indicates that the inhibition of testicular steroidogenesis during chronic treatment with LHRH is most likely due to loss of bioactivity rather than testicular desensitization.[123]

Patients treated exclusively with LHRH agonists suffer an initial transient deterioration (the flare) related to an increase in serum androgens, likely induced by the agonist, and a relatively large proportion of the patients relapse within 1 year or more after initiation of treatment. Attempts have been made to overcome these adverse effects, attributed to continued stimulation of prostate tumor cells by adrenal androgens, by the combined use of an LHRH agonist and pure antiandrogens to attain complete androgen blockade.[136,137]

In patients with prostate carcinoma treated with a LHRH agonist combined with the pure antiandrogen flutamide,[210,211] bioactive LH was markedly reduced and this was accompanied by a decrease of serum testosterone levels. The parallel between drop of serum testosterone and bioactive LH levels indicates that loss of the biologic activity of LH is mostly responsible for the inhibition of androgen secretion by the testes during chronic treatment with LHRH agonists.[210,211]

The rate of objective response in stage C and stage D2 previously untreated patients receiving complete androgen blockade (LHRH agonist plus pure antiandrogen) compared most favorably with that of those who had been treated with diethylstilbestrol or were previously orchiectomized. At 1 month after combined treatment with LHRH agonist plus pure antiandrogen, serum testosterone level decreased from 5.4 ± 0.4 ng/ml to 0.26 ± 0.09 ng/ml, and serum DHT levels were reduced from 0.40 ± 0.06 ng/ml to 0.03 ± 0.008 ng/ml. Antiandrogens, given by themselves, lead to a progressive increase in gonadotropin and androgen secretion by their interference with the inhibitory feedback action of androgens at the level of the hypothalamus-adenohypophysis. This unwanted effect can be prevented by the LHRH agonist.

Prolactins and Antiprolactins

Experimental studies in animals and clinical investigations in humans have indicated that prolactin may play a role in the hormonal regulatory process of growth and function of normal and neoplastic prostatic cells. Prolactin binding to both prostatic tissue membrane and cytosol is androgen dependent.[131] Castration and estrogens reduce specific prolactin binding in prostatic tissues, and testosterone administration can restore prolactin-binding activity to precastration levels.[131] The mechanism of action of prolactin on the prostate may be indirect and mediated through the testes. The sensitivity of Leydig cells to LH stimulation is enhanced by prolactin, which increases their ability to bind LH.[10,229] The synergism between prolactin and LH results indirectly in stimulation of testosterone production by the testes.[10,229] In the prostate, prolactin may act synergistically with testosterone,[229] by increasing testosterone uptake and conversion to 5α-dihydrotestosterone through potentiation of 5α-reductase activity.[67,87,229,235] Estradiol (E2) levels in males may increase as a function of age,[175,217] and an increment in the ratio of the concentration of available free estradiol to available free testosterone may occur with aging.[217] This increase of estrogen levels in elderly men may result in increased production of prolactin, through suppression of the release of prolactin-inhibiting factors from the hypothalamus.[229] The increased release of prolactin induced by estrogens, and the occurrence of higher levels of peripheral prolactin during long-term treatment with estrogens or with antiandrogens, raised the question as to whether prolactin was implicated in the

development of the so-called estrogen escape phenomenon, characterized by the recurrence and progression of prostate cancer after an initial favorable response to hormone therapy.[112,113,194,213] Prolactin may also influence the development and progression of prostate carcinoma by modulating the uptake, intracellular metabolism, and utilization of androgens by the prostate. Since the prostate has a high number of prolactin-binding sites[7] the intraprostatic action of androgens may be mediated by interaction of prolactin and the steroid hormone receptor mechanisms.

Clinical data have shown that the increase in prolactin plasma levels after estradiol or diethylstilbestrol diphosphate treatment could be prevented by bromocriptine, a prolactin-inhibiting substance,[112] and other compounds.[207] The above-mentioned data have led to speculations whether high prolactin levels in patients treated with estrogens represent a risk factor, possibly associated with a poorer prognosis. To counteract such risks, therapeutic protocols in which estrogens are combined with antiprolactins have been designed for treating patients with prostate carcinoma. Compounds with antiprolactin activity that have been tried either clinically or in experimental studies include levodopa, bromocriptine, and lisuride.[112,113]

Estramustine Phosphate (Estracyt)

Estramustine phosphate is a non-nitrogen mustard carbamate derivative of 17β-estradiol esterified with phosphoric acid that displays an estrogenic effect approximately 100 times weaker than that of estradiol.[59,174] Experimental studies have indicated that estramustine phosphate decreases the 5α-reductase activity and reduces the incorporation of thymidine into DNA in prostatic tissues.[109,129] In experimental animals, there is a significant concentration of estramustine in the prostate gland resulting from binding to estramustine-binding protein, a cytosol protein with high affinity for estramustine.[74,174] Estramustine-binding protein is also present in the cytosol of human normal prostate, BPH, and prostatic carcinoma. Estramustine-binding protein is androgen dependent since its concentration in the prostate is markedly reduced after castration and after hypophysectomy and can be restored to precastration or to prehypophysectomy levels by treatment with testosterone.[176,177] Various studies have shown that unresponsive or secondary refractory prostate carcinoma patients experienced subjective and objective response to treatment with estramustine phosphate.[59]

Correlation between Steroid Hormone Receptor and Hormone Content, Tumor Grade, and Clinical Hormonal Responsiveness

Since approximately one-third of the patients with metastatic carcinoma do not respond to hormonal therapy, many investigators have tried to determine whether prostate tumors contain either biochemical or morphologic markers characteristic of hormone dependence. There is evidence indicating that histologic differentiation of the tumor (tumor grade) correlates with patient response to endocrine therapy. Hormone responsiveness in estrogen-treated patients decreases in relation to the loss of histologic differentiation.[46,65,196] As reported by Schirmer et al.,[196] the 5-year survival rate of estrogen-treated patients was 90 percent for grade I, 71 percent for grade II, 65 percent for grade III, and 52 percent for grade IV prostate carcinomas. Similar correlations between tumor grade and survival after estrogen treatment have been noted by various other researchers.[18,46,65] In contrast, Stone et al.[213] have found considerable variations in the duration of hormonal responsiveness and noted a lack of correlation with the histologic grade of the tumor.

The content of steroid hormones in prostate cancer tissues, including DHT, 17β-estradiol, estrone, and progesterone, have been correlated with response to hormonal therapy, such as estrogen treatment or orchiectomy. The content of DHT in the neoplastic tissue correlates with the response to hormone therapy and the degree of histologic differentiation. The tissue content of DHT falls within the higher values in well-differentiated low-grade carcinomas, whereas in poorly differentiated and anaplastic high-grade tumors, DHT content falls within the lower values.[18,82] Prostate cancer tissue DHT content and tumor grading may represent promising methods for predicting initial response to hormonal therapy.[18,82]

As suggested from the correlation with DHT content, tumor grade seems also to correlate with the rate of testosterone conversion to 5α-DHT.[165] In BPH and well-differentiated prostate carcinomas, ^{3}H-testosterone was actively metabolized to 5α-reduced 17β-hydroxy-C19-radiosteroids, particularly 5α-DHT. The majority of poorly differentiated carcinomas showed decreased transformation to 5α-DHT, whereas conversion to 17-oxosteroid radiometabolites remained unchanged or greatly enhanced.[165]

As might be anticipated from the correlation between tumor grade and DHT tissue content, studies have indicated that patients with tumors containing significant amounts of androgen receptor respond more favorably to hormone therapy.[18,46,82,97,155] DHT receptor concentration in prostate cancer tissues represents a marker for the prediction of clinical response to therapy and also tumor grade, since well-differentiated tumors contain higher concentrations of DHT receptor.

Habib et al.,[103] however, found no correlation between histologic grade of the tumor and either cytosolic or nuclear androgen receptor in the cancer cells, and presented data suggesting that hormone dependence of the malignant tissue is proportional to the bulk of the tumor.[103]

Determination of nuclear receptor content in prostate cancer cells showed an apparent correlation between concentration of nuclear receptor with the duration of response and survival after hormonal therapy. Gonor et al.[88] found that extractable and matrix-bound nuclear androgen receptor contents were significantly higher in patients who responded to hormonal treatment, but there was no correlation with concentrations of cytoplasmic receptor. More recently, however, with the use of a selected threshold concentration of receptors,[69] it appears that it is the cytosolic, nuclear KCl-extractable, and total cellular receptor content that serve as pedictors of hormonal response, particularly in the differentiation between long-term and short-term survivors.

Wagner and co-workers[222] were unable to detect any correlation between androgen receptor content and response to hormonal treatment. Young et al.[239] found that prostate cancer tissues from patients who failed to show objective response to hormonal treatment had higher concentrations of DHT receptors than 17-β-estradiol receptors. High contents of DHT receptors have been reported in poorly differentiated prostate carcinomas in patients with clinical evidence of progressive metastatic disease.[134,223] Conversely, Young et al.[239] noted a significantly higher estrogen receptor content in tumors from prostate cancer patients who had a favorable response to hormone therapy.

Haapiainen et al.[101] found higher levels of 17β-estradiol in patients with lower-grade, lower-stage prostate carcinomas. In patients treated by orchiectomy or with estrogens, survival was significantly longer in subjects with high pretreatment plasma levels of 17β-estradiol, as compared with those with low E2 values.[101] The authors concluded that endogenous pretreatment levels of 17β-estradiol may have inhibitory effect on growth, metastasizing capabilities, and may influence the degree of differentiation of the prostate tumor.[101]

Brendler et al.[31] measured multiple biochemical and histologic variables, including six enzymes and androgen receptor and steroid content, as possible predictors of hormonal response in patients with prostate cancer. An index based on multiple enzyme activities and nuclear androgen receptor values served to partially, but not completely, separate two categories of patients who differed significantly in hormonal response and survival. This index was developed on the basis of the measurements of relative activities of the enzymes 3β-hydroxysteroid oxidoreductase, 17β-hydroxysteroid oxidoreductase, 5α-reductase, and acid phosphatase and served to distinguish a group of poor responders from a group of good responders. Including the values obtained from measuring salt-extractable nuclear androgen receptor in this index enabled the least overlap of individual patients between the two groups to be seen.[31]

The findings of Habib et al.[102] indicate that high enzyme activity for 5α-reductase was associated with well-differentiated tumors (Gleason score 1), whereas the capacity of the enzyme to metabolize testosterone appeared markedly depressed in poorly differentiated tumors (Gleason score 4).[102]

de Larminat et al.[50] were able to increase the recovery of androgen receptors from human prostate tissue by using mersalyl to dissociate endogenously bound hormone receptor complexes. Normal prostate contains the highest receptor values, significantly different from those of hyperplastic tissues but not from those of carcinoma. Normal prostate had the highest absolute and relative total specific nuclear binding values, and the lowest was found in carcinoma.

A correlation could be established between androgen receptor content and clinical response to hormone therapy (orchiectomy and 2 mg of diethylstilbestrol per day for several months). The population was divided into AR(+), with androgen receptor levels higher or equal to 2 pmol/g of tissue, and AR(−), with androgen receptor levels below 2 pmol/g of tissue. Results indicate that seven of eight AR(+) patients responded favorably, whereas four of five AR(−) patients failed to respond.

Radwan et al.[181] found that androgen receptor complexes of prostate carcinomas had different sedimentation profiles compared with normal as well as a different dissociation rate constant in nuclei. The androgen receptor complexes prepared from normal tissues sedimented mainly in the 8S to 9S area of the sucrose density gradient. For malignant tissues, 50 percent were sedimented in the 8S to 9S area and 50 percent in the 4S area. Androgen receptors were increased in the nuclei of human prostate cancer cells when compared with normal prostatic tissues.

Bowman et al.[25] tried to determine differences in the distribution of androgen receptor in relation to the well-established zonal heterogeneity of the prostate gland. Androgen receptor was more often found in the peripheral zone (71 percent positive). The receptor was found in 39 percent of the periurethral region and in only 24 percent of the tissues obtained from the peripheral limits of resection. Androgen receptor was detected in 16 percent more specimens from carcinomatous glands than from benign prostates, and receptor levels were consistently lower in benign than in malignant specimens.[25]

HISTOPATHOLOGIC AND ULTRASTRUCTURAL PATTERNS OF REGRESSION AFTER THERAPY

Estrogen Therapy

Early histologic changes produced in prostate cancer cells by estrogen treatment include cytoplasmic vacuolization and condensation of nuclear chromatin that may terminate in pyknosis.[53,79,120,195] In later stages, the cell membranes rupture, and the contents of the cells, including pyknotic nuclei, are extruded into the lumen. In other areas, the acinar lining undergoes squamous metaplasia under the influence of estrogens. Many of the neoplastic acinar structures end up as empty spaces containing nuclear and cyto-

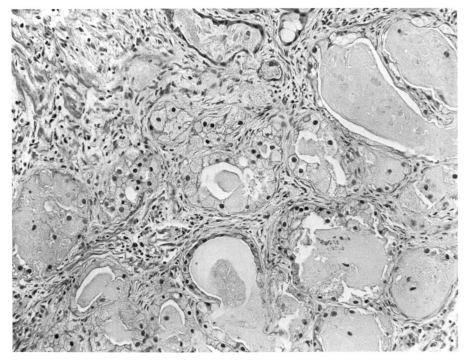

Fig. 33-7 Prostate carcinoma, estrogen effect. Survey picture: architectural disorganization, widespread nuclear pyknosis, ballooning degeneration, necrosis, and shedding of the epithelium. ×140.

plasmic debris. These changes are illustrated in Figures 33-7 through 33-9.

Histochemical studies have shown that the intensity of staining for acid phosphatase is reduced after estrogen treatment.[70] Sinha et al.[206] described two types of basal cell in prostate carcinoma: light cells with round, euchromatic nuclei and large nucleoli, and dark cells with irregular nuclei containing aggregates of heterochromatin and large pleomorphic nucleoli. Both basal cell types appear as the early invasive elements, breaking through the basement membrane. In patients with recurrent prostate cancer, after various periods of hormonal response, the tumors appear to consist mostly of basal cells with a predominance of the dark-cell variety.[206] The same researchers[205] had noted that in vitro incorporation of ³H-estradiol occurred almost exclusively in a certain subpopulation of the basal and invasive cells. It is possible, as they suggest, that the basal cells that bind ³H-estradiol represent the hormone-sensitive component of the tumor, whereas those that fail to bind the hormone may constitute the nonsensitive component, responsible for recurrence and development of a refractory state.[205,206]

Franks[79] described the histologic appearance of prostates obtained at autopsy from patients who had received full estrogen treatment for prostate cancer for up to 9 years. The primary tumors and their metastases were grouped according to histologic appearance. In some cases the histology revealed no estrogenic effect, whereas in a second group, the tumor cells in both the primary and metastatic sites appeared inactive, and many revealed early and late estrogen-induced cytologic changes. In the third group, the primary tumor appeared inactive, whereas metastatic deposits showed evidence of active growth. In the fourth group, both the primary tumors and metastases, when present, showed evidence of active growth, although cytologic evidence of previous estrogenic effect could still be recognized.[79] Response of tumor cells to treatment differed from tumor to tumor as well as within separate areas of the same

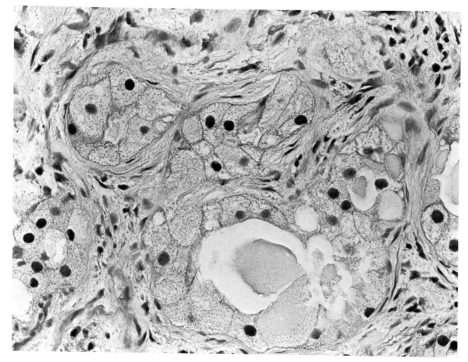

Fig. 33-8 Prostate carcinoma, estrogen effect. Detail of the ballooning degenerative changes and nuclear pyknosis. ×350.

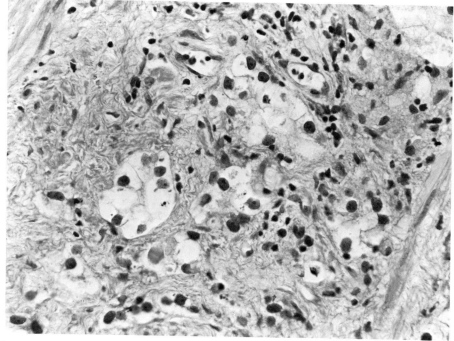

Fig. 33-9 Prostate carcinoma, estrogen effect. Areas of frank necrosis in estrogen-treated prostate cancer. ×350.

tumor, suggesting the presence of subpopulations of cells differing in their hormonal sensitivity or dependence.

Prout et al.[180] described the histologic changes in prostate tumors and functional changes of the pituitary-gonadal axis in patients with prostate carcinoma treated with diethylstilbestrol. Follow-up biopsies at 3 months after initiation of treatment with diethylstilbestrol revealed either focal squamous metaplasia or mild cytotoxic effects, such as cytoplasmic clearing and nuclear condensation.[179,180] Alterations reflecting the effect of diethylstilbestrol on the pituitary-gonadal axis were dose dependent.

Gittes et al.[86] have commented on the possibility that occult carcinoma of the prostate may represent an oversight of immune surveillance.

Orchiectomy

Heterogeneity in the cellular response to hormonal alterations was noted in acinar prostate cancer cells after orchiectomy.[29] The apparently hormone-sensitive cells experienced a loss of many of their cytoplasmic organelles, particularly endoplasmic reticulum, secretory vacuoles, and mitochondria, whereas other cells, probably belonging to a less hormone-sensitive subpopulation, were not affected.[29]

Cytologic and correlative biochemical changes produced by removal of androgenic stimulus (orchiectomy) or estrogen treatment have been investigated in the rat and in the dog.[26,169] After orchiectomy in the rat there is a marked depletion of cytoplasmic organelles in prostatic tissue. Mitochondria and portions of the endoplasmic reticulum become segregated within autophagic vacuoles, where they undergo degradation, presumably through the activities of lysosomal hydrolases.

Radiation Therapy

Prostatic follow-up biopsies obtained months or even years after radiation therapy have shown persistent carcinoma in about one-half of the patients.[108,149] The negative or positive results of prostatic biopsies after radiation therapy may or may not relate to the frequency of metastasis or to the length of survival,

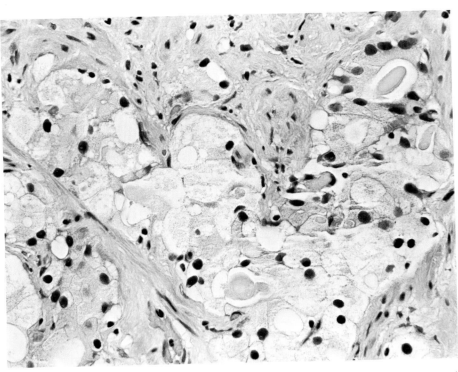

Fig. 33-10 Prostate carcinoma, x-irradiation effect. Ballooning degeneration and nuclear pyknosis, similar to that seen in estrogen-treated carcinomas of the prostate. ×300.

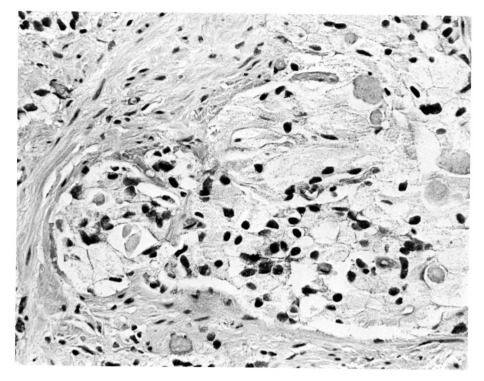

Fig. 33-11 Prostate carcinoma, x-irradiation effect. More severe effect of x-irradiation results in frank necrosis of tumor cells. ×300.

according to different investigators. Schellhammer et al.[194a] found that 65 percent of patients with positive biopsies at 18 months after radiation had eventual recurrent disease compared with only 21 percent of patients with negative biopsies.

The interval after radiotherapy when the biopsies are taken has an inverse relation to the proportion of positive cases. The figures reported by Cox and Stoffel[49] at various intervals after radiotherapy were 60 percent at 6 months, 37 percent at 1 year, 30 percent at 18 months, and 19 percent at 36 and 42 months.

Factors influencing tumor destruction include direct delivery of energy into cell components and a secondary effect resulting from damage to blood vessel walls and interference with blood supply.

Cytologic changes are similar to those described after estrogen therapy and include cytoplasmic vacuolization and pyknosis.[149] (See Figs. 33-10 and 33-11 and compare with Figs. 33-7 to 33-9).

The viability and biologic potential of residual tumor after radiation therapy cannot be thoroughly assessed by the histologic appearance. Immunohisto-

chemical evaluation of PAP in biopsies obtained after radiotherapy showed persistent acid phosphatase activity in the tumor cells, suggesting maintenance of metabolic activity possibly related to potential growth and metastasis.[150] Kiesling et al.[125] examined tissues of irradiated prostate cancer by electron microscopy and noted the persistence of cells with malignant characteristics, such as loss of polarization, paucity of secretory material, nuclear abnormalities, and abortive acinar formation.

REFERENCES

1. Ablin RJ: Immunologic properties of sex accessory tissue components. p. 434. In Brandes D (ed): Male Accessory Sex Organs: Structure and Function in Mammals. Academic Press, Orlando, FL, 1974
2. Ablin RJ: Immunobiology of the prostate. p. 33. In Tannenbaum M (ed): Urologic Pathology: The Prostate. Lea & Febiger, Philadelphia, 1977
3. Ablin RJ, Bhatti RA: Tumor-associated immunity in

prostatic cancer. p. 183. In Ablin RJ (ed): Prostatic Cancer. Marcel Dekker, New York, 1981

4. Ablin RJ, Bruns GR, Guinan PD et al: Hormonal therapy and alteration of lymphocyte proliferation. J Lab Clin Med 87:227, 1976

5. Abul-Fadl MAM, King EJ: The inhibition of acid phosphatase by D-tartrate. Proc Biochem Soc Biochem J 42, xxviii, 1948

6. Abul-Fadl MAM, King EJ: Inhibition of acid phosphatases by formaldehyde and its clinical application for determination of serum acid phosphatases. J Clin Pathol 1:80, 1948

6a. Ahmann FR, Schifman RB: Prospective comparison between serum monoclonal prostate specific antigen and acid phosphatase measurements in metastatic prostate cancer. J Urol 137:431, 1987

7. Aragona C, Bohnet HG, Friesin HG: Localization of prolactin binding on prostate and testis. The role of serum prolactin concentration on the testicular LH receptor. Acta Endocrinol 84:402, 1977

8. Arnheim FK: Carcinoma of the prostate: a study of the postmortem findings in one hundred and seventy-six cases. J Urol 60:599, 1948

8a. Babaian RJ, Murray JL, Lamki LM, et al: Radioimmunological imaging of metastatic prostatic cancer with 111indium-labeled monoclonal antibody pay 276. J Urol 137:439, 1987

8b. Bahnson RR, Catalona WJ: Adverse implications of acid phosphatase levels in the upper range of normal. J Urol 137:427, 1987

9. Banalaph T, Varkarakis MS, Murphy CP: Current status of bilateral adrenalectomy for advanced prostatic carcinoma. Ann Surg 179:17, 1974

10. Bartke A: Role of prolactin in reproduction in male mammals. Fed Proc 39:2577, 1980

11. Barzell W, Bean MA, Hilaris BS, Whitmore WF, Jr.: Prostatic adenocarcinoma: relationship of grade and local extent to the pattern of metastases. J Urol 118:278, 1977

12. Bashirelahi N, Armstrong EG: 17β-Estradiol binding by human prostate. p. 632. In Golan M (ed): Normal and Abnormal Growth of the Prostate. Charles C Thomas, Springfield, IL, 1975

13. Bashirelahi N, Young JD: Specific binding protein for 17β-estradiol in prostate with adenocarcinoma. Urology 8:553, 1976

14. Bates RJ, Chapman CM, Prout GR, Jr., Lin CW: Immunohistochemical identification of prostatic acid phosphatase: correlation of tumor grade with acid phosphatase distribution. J Urol 127:574, 1982

15. Batson OV: The function of the vertebral veins and their role in the spread of metastases. Ann Surg 112:138, 1940

16. Batson OV: The role of the vertebral veins in metastatic processes. Ann Intern Med 16:38, 1942

17. Beach PD: Hormonal therapy for prostatic carcinoma. p. 273. In Johnson DE, Samuels ML (eds): Cancer of the Genitourinary Tract. Raven Press, New York, 1979

18. Belis JA, Tarry WF: Radioimmunoassay of tissue steroids in adenocarcinoma of the prostate. Cancer 48:2416, 1981

19. Belville WD, Cox HD, Mahan DE et al : Bone marrow acid phosphatase by radioimmunoassay. Cancer 41:2286, 1978

20. Bentz MS, Cohen C, Demers LM et al : Immunohistochemical acid phosphatase level and tumor grade in prostatic carcinoma. Arch Pathol Lab Med 106:476, 1982

21. Berry WR, Laszlo J, Cox E et al : Prognostic factors in metastasis and hormonally-unresponsive carcinoma of the prostate. Cancer 44:763, 1979

22. Bhatti RA, Ablin RJ, Guinan PD: Evaluation of leukocyte adherence inhibition in prostate cancer. p. 185. In Thompson DMP (ed): Leukocyte Adherence Inhibition Assays. Academic Press, Orlando, FL, 1982

23. Bodansky O: Acid phosphatase. p. 43. In Bodansky O, Latner AL (eds): Advances in Clinical Chemistry. Vol. 15. Academic Press, Orlando, FL, 1972

24. Bolton BH: Pulmonary metastases from carcinoma of the prostate: incidence and case report of a long remission. J Urol 94:73, 1965

25. Bowman SP, Barnes DM, Blacklock NJ, Sullivan PJ: Regional variation of cytosol androgen receptors throughout the diseased human prostate gland. Prostate 8:167, 1986

26. Brandes D: Fine structure and cytochemistry of male sex accessory organs. p. 18. In Brandes D (ed): Male Accessory Sex Organs: Structure and Function in Mammals. Academic Press, Orlando, FL, 1974

27. Brandes D: Retinoic acid receptor and surface markers: models for the study of prostatic cancer cells. p. 207. In Murphy GP, Sandberg AA, Karr JP (eds): The Prostatic Cell: Structure and Function. Part B: Prolactin, Carcinogenesis, and Clinical Aspects. Alan R Liss, New York, 1981

28. Brandes M, Bourne GH: Stilbestrol phosphatase and prostatic carcinoma. Lancet 1:481, 1955

29. Brandes D, Kirchheim D: Histochemistry of the prostate. p. 99. In Tannenbaum M (ed): Urologic Pathology: The Prostate. Lea Febiger, Philadelphia, 1977

30. Brandes M, Gesell MS, Ueda H et al : Retinoic acid binding protein in human and experimental pancreatic carcinomas in hamsters. Ann Clin Lab Sci 13:400, 1983

31. Brendler CB, Isaacs JT, Follanasbee AL, Walsh PC:

The use of multiple variables to predict response to endocrine therapy in carcinoma of the prostate: a preliminary report. J Urol 131:694, 1984

32. Brownstein MH, Helwig EB: Metastatic tumors of the skin. Cancer 29:1278, 1972

33. Bruce AW, Mahan DE: The role of prostatic acid phosphatase in the investigation and treatment of adenocarcinoma of the prostate. Ann NY Acad Sci 390:110, 1982

34. Bruce AW, Mahan DE, Morales A et al : An objective look at acid phosphatase determinations. BR J Urol 59:213, 1979

35. Byar DP: VACURG studies on prostate cancer and its treatment. p. 241. In Tannenbaum M (ed): Urologist Pathology: The Prostate. Lea & Febiger, Philadelphia, 1977

36. Catalona WJ: Immunobiology of carcinoma of the prostate. Invest Urol 17:373, 1980

37. Catalona WJ: Prostate Cancer. Grune & Stratton, Orlando, FL, 1984

38. Catalona WJ, Ratliff TL, McCool RE: Discordance among cell-mediated cytolytic mechanisms in cancer patients: Importance of the assay system. J Immunol 122:1009, 1979

39. Catalona WJ, Stein AJ: Staging errors in clinically localized prostatic cancer. J Urol 127:452, 1982

40. Catalona WJ, Tarpley JL, Chretien PB, Castle JR: Lymphocyte stimulation in urologic cancer patients. J Urol 112:373, 1974

40a. Cho KR, Epstein JI: Metastatic prostatic carcinoma to supradiaphragmatic lymph nodes: a clinicopathologic and immunohistochemical study. Am J Surg Pathol 11(6):457, 1987

41. Choe BK Pontes JE, McDonald I, Rose NR: Immunochemical studies of prostatic acid phosphatase. Cancer Treat Rep 61:201, 1977

42. Choe BK Rose NR, Korol M, Pontes JE: Immunoenzyme assay for human prostatic phosphatase. Proc Soc Exp Biol Med 162:396, 1979

43. Chua DT, Veenema RJ Muggia F, Graff A: Acid phosphatase levels in bone marrow: value in detecting early bone metastases from carcinoma of the prostate. J Urol 103:462, 1970

44. Coffey DS: The biochemistry and physiology of the prostate and seminal vesiclea. p. 233. In Walsh PC, Gittes RF, Perlmutter AD, Stamey TA (eds): Campbell's Urology. Vol. 1, 5th Ed. WB Saunders Philadelphia, 1986

45. Coffey DS: Physiological control of prostatic growth: an overview. p. 4. In Coffey DS, Isaacs JT (eds): Prostate Cancer. Vol. 48. UICC Technical Report Series, Geneva, 1979

46. Concolino G, Marocchi A, Margiotta G et al : Steroid receptors and hormone responsiveness of human prostatic carcinoma. Prostate 3:475, 1982

47. Connolly JG, Thomson A, Jewett et al : Intraprostatic lymphatics. Invest Urol 5:371, 1968

47a. Cooner WH, Mosley BR, Rutherford CL Jr, et al: Clinical application of transrectal ultrasonography and prostate specific antigen in the search for prostate cancer. J Urol 139:758, 1988

48. Cooper JF, Foti AG, Herschman H: Combined serum and bone marrow radioimmunoassay for prostatic acid phosphatase. J Urol 122:498, 1979

49. Cox JD, Stoffel TJ: The significance of needle biopsy after irradiation for stage C adenocarcinoma of the prostate. Cancer 40:156, 1977

50. de Larminat MA, Pasik L, Bellora O et al : Increased recovery of androgen receptors from human prostate through the use of mersalyl: evidence for androgen regulation of the binding sites in carcinomatous prostate. Prostate 9:97, 1986

51. Decenzo JM, Allison R, Leadbetter GW, Jr.: Skin testing in genitourinary carcinoma: 2-year follow up. J Urol 114:271, 1975

52. Delbarre F, Ghozlan R, Amor B: Métastases osseuses avec osteomalacie au cours du cancer de la prostate. Nouv Presse Med 4:1277, 1975

53. Dhom G, Degro S: Therapy of prostatic cancer and histopathologic follow-up, Prostate 3:531, 1982

54. Dias SM, Barnett RN: Elevated bone marrow acid phosphatase: the problem of false positives. J Urol 117:749, 1977

55. Dodds PR, Caride VJ, Lytton B: The role of vertebral veins in the dissemination of prostatic carcinoma. J Urol 126:753, 1981

56. Downey M, Hickey BB, Sharp ME: The acid phosphatase content of the enlarged and malignant prostate gland with some observations on histopathology as revealed by Gomori's staining. Br J Urol 26:160, 1954

57. Drucker JR, Moncure CW, Johnson CL et al : Immunologic staging of prostatic carcinoma: three years of experience. J Urol 119:94, 1978

58. Eagan RT, Hahn RG, Meyers RP: Adriamycin (NSC-123127) versus 5-fluorouracil (NSC-19893) and cyclophosphamide (NSC-24271) in the treatment of metastatic prostate cancer. Cancer Treat Rep 60:115,1976

59. Edsmyr F, Andersson L, Konyves I: Estramustine phosphate (Estracyt): experimental studies and clinical experience. p. 253. In Jacobi GH, Hohenfellner R (eds): Prostate Cancer. Williams & Wilkins, Baltimore, 1982

60. Elhilali MM, Brosman SA, Vescera C et al : The effects of treatment on delayed cutaneous hypersen-

sitivity with genitourinary cancer. Cancer 41:1765, 1978

61. Elias EG, Elias LS: Autogenous leukocyte migration in human malignancies. Cancer 36:1393, 1975
62. Elkin M, Mueller HP: Metastases from cancer of the prostate. Cancer 7:1246, 1954
63. Epstein JI, Eggleston JC: Immunohistochemical localization of prostate-specific acid phosphatase and prostate-specific antigen in stage A_2 adenocarcinoma of prostate. Prognostic implications. Hum Pathol 15:853, 1984
64. Epstein JI, Oesterling JE, Eggleston JC, Walsh PC: Frozen section detection of lymph node metastases in prostatic carcinoma: accuracy in grossly uninvolved pelvic lymphadenectomy specimens. J Urol 136:1234, 1986
65. Esposti PL: Cytologic malignancy grading of prostatic carcinoma by transrectal aspiration biopsy. A 5-year follow up study of 469 hormone-treated patients. Scand J Urol Nephrol 5:199, 1971
66. Evans CM, Bowen JG: Immunologic tests in carcinoma of the prostate. Proc R Soc Med 70:417, 1977
67. Farnsworth WE: Prolactin on androgen mobilization. p. 502. In Goland M (ed): Normal and abnormal growth of the prostate. Charles C Thomas, Springfield, IL, 1975
68. Faure N, Labrie F, Lemay A, et al: Inhibition of serum androgen levels by chronic intranasal and subcutaneous administration of a potent luteining hormone-releasing hormone (LHRH) agonist in adult men. Fertil Steril 37:416, 1982
69. Fentile DD, Lakey WH, McBlain WA: Applicability of nuclear androgen receptor quantification to human prostatic adenocarcinoma. J Urol 135:167, 1986
70. Fergusson JD, Pagel W: Some observations on carcinoma of prostate treated with oestrogens — as demonstrated by serial biopsies. Br J Surg 33:122, 1945
71. Fishman WH, Bonner CD, Homburger F: Serum "Prostatic" acid phosphatase and cancer of he prostate. N Engl J Med 255:925, 1956
72. Fishman WH, Dast RM, Bonner CD et al : A new method for estimating serum acid phosphatase of prostatic origin applied to the clinical investigation of cancer of the prostate. J Clin Invest 32:1034, 1953
73. Flocks RH, Culp D, Porter R: Lymphatic spread from prostatic cancer. J Urol 81:194, 1959
74. Forsgren B, Gustafsson J-A, Pousette A, Hogberg B: Binding characteristics of a major protein in rat ventral prostate cytosol that interacts with estramustine, a nitrogen mustard derivative of estradiol-17β. Cancer Res 39:5155, 1979
75. Foti AG, Cooper JF, Herschman H, Malvaez RR: Detection of prostatic cancer by solid-phase radioimmu-

noassay of serum prostatic acid phosphatase. N Engl J Med 297:1357, 1977
76. Foti AG, Cooper JF, Herschman H, Sapon SR: The detection of prostatic cancer by radioimmunoassay: a review. Hum Pathol 9:618, 1978
77. Foti AG, Herschman H, Cooper JF: Isoenzymes of acid phosphatase in normal and cancerous human prostatic tissue. Cancer Res 37:4120, 1977
78. Franks LM: The spread of prostatic cancer. J Pathol Bacteriol 72:603, 1956
79. Franks LM: Estrogen-treated prostatic cancer. The variation in responsiveness of tumor cells. Cancer 13:490, 1960
80. Furusato M, Mostofi FK: Intraprostatic lymphatics in man: light and ultrastructural observations. Prostate 1:15, 1980
81. Gates O: Cutaneous metastases of malignant disease. Am J Cancer 30:718, 1937
82. Geller J, Albert J, Loza D: Steroid levels in cancer of the prostate — markers of tumor differentiation and adequancy of anti androgen therapy. J Steroid Biochem 11:631, 1979
83. Geller J, Albert J, Nachtsheim DE et al : The effects of flutamide on total DHT and nuclear NHT levels in the human prostate. Prostate 2:309, 1981
84. Geller J, Albert J, Yen SSC et al : Medical castration of males with megestrol acetate and small doses of diethylstilbestrol. J Clin Endocrinol Metab 52:576, 1981
85. Gesell MS, Brandes MJ, Arnold EA et al : Retinoic acid binding protein in normal and neoplastic rat prostate. Prostate 3:131, 1982
85a. Gittes RF: Prostate-specific antigen. N Engl J Med 317:954, 1987
86. Gittes RF, McCullough DL: Occult carcinoma of the prostate: an oversight of immune surveillance — a working hypothesis. J Urol 112:241, 1974
87. Giuliani L, Pescatore D, Martorana G et al: Increased serum prolactin pituitary reserve in patients with prostatic neoplasms. Br J Urol 51:390, 1979
88. Gonor SE, Lakey WH, McBlain WA: Relationship between concentrations of extractable and matrix-bound nuclear androgen receptor and clinical response to endocrine therapy for prostatic adenocarcinoma. J Urol 131:1196, 1984
89. Goss CM (ed): Gray's Anatomy of the Human Body. 28th Ed. Lea & Febiger, Philadelphia, 1966
90. Gothin JH: Prostatic carcinoma: staging with percutaneous lymph node biopsy. Bull Cancer (Paris) 72:462, 1985
91. Graves RC, Militzer RE: Carcinoma of the prostate with metastases. J Urol 33:235, 1935
92. Griffiths J: Prostatic adenocarcinoma: a simultaneous

comparison of two enzyme markers: prostate specific acid phosphatase and creatine kinase isoenzyme. p. 74. In Burlina A, Galzigna L (eds): Clinical Enzymology Symposium. Vol. 3. Piccin Medical Books, Pauda, Italy, 1981

93. Griffiths J: The appropriate uses of prostatic acid phosphatase determination in the diagnosis of adenocarcinoma of he prostate. Ann NY Acad Sci 39:100, 1982

94. Gupta D: Prostate cancer: hormone profiles. p. 379. In Jacobi GH, Hohenfellner R (eds): Prostate Cancer. International Perspectives in Urology. Vol. 3. Williams & Wilkins, Baltimore, 1982

95. Gursel EO, Rezvan M, Sy FA, Veenema RJ: Comparative evaluation of bone marrow acid phosphatase and bone scanning in staging of prostatic cancer. J Urol 111:53, 1974

96. Gustaffson J, Ekman P, Pousette A et al : Demonstration of a progestin receptor in human benign prostatic hyperplasia and prostatic carcinoma. Invest Urol 15:361, 1978

97. Gustaffson JA, Ekman P, Snochowski M et al : Correlation between clinical response to hormone therapy and steroid receptor content in prostatic cancer. Cancer Res 38:4345, 1978

98. Gutman AB, Gutman EB: An "acid" phosphatase occurring in the serum of patients with metastasizing carcinoma of the prostate gland. J Clin Invest 17:473, 1938

99. Gutman AB, Gutman EB: Acid phosphatase levels in prepubertal rhesus prostate tissue after testosterone propionate. Pros Soc Exp Biol Med 41:277, 1939

100. Gutman EB, Sproul EE, Gutman AB: Significance of increased phosphatase activity of bone at the site of osteoplastic metastases secondary to carcinoma of the prostate gland. Am J Cancer 28:485, 1936

101. Haapiainen R, Rannikko S, Adlercreutz H, Alfthan O: Correlation of pretreatment plasma levels of estradiol and sex-hormone-binding globulin-binding capacity with clinical stage and survival of patients with prostatic cancer. Prostate 80:127, 1986

102. Habib FK, Busuttil A, Robinson RA, Chisholm GD: 5α-reductase activity in human prostate cancer is related to the histological differentiation of the tumour. Clin Endocrinol 23:431, 1985

103. Habib FK, Odoma S, Busuttil A, Chisholm GD: Androgen receptors in cancer of the prostate: Correlation with the stage and grade of the tumor. Cancer 57:2351, 1986

104. Halliday WJ, Maluish AE, Stephenson PM, Davis NC: An evaluation of leukocyte adherence inhibition in the immunodiagnosis of colorectal cancer. Cancer Res 37:1962, 1977

105. Harty JI, Catalona WJ, Gomolka DM: Modification of lymphocyte responsiveness by hormones used in the treatment of urologic malignancies. J Urol 116:484, 1976

106. Hassan MO, Maksem J: The prostatic perineural space and its relation to tumor spread-an ultrastructural study. Am J Surg Pathol 4:143, 1980

107. Helminen HJ, Ericsson JLE: On the mechanism of lysosomal enzyme secretion. Electron microscopic and histochemical studies on the epithelial cells of the rat's ventral prostate lobe. J Ultrastruct Res 33:528, 1970

108. Herr HW, Whitmore WF, Jr.: Significance of prostatic biopsies after radiation therapy for carcinoma of the prostate. Prostate 3:350, 1982

109. Hoisaeter PA: Incorporation of ^{3}H-thymidine into rat ventral prostate in organ culture. Invest Urol 12:479, 1975

109a. Hortin GL, Bahnson RR, Daft M, et al: Differences in values obtained with 2 assays of prostate specific antigen. J Urol 139:762, 1988

110. Hsueh AJW, Dufau ML, Catt KJ: Direct inhibitory effect of estrogen on Leydig cell function of hypophysectomized rats. Endocrinology 103:1096, 1978

111. Huggins C, Hodges CV: Studies on prostatic cancer. I. The effect of castration, of estrogen, and of androgen injection on serum phosphatases in metastatic carcinoma of the prostate. Cancer Res 1:293, 1941

111a. Hughes H, Penney MD, Ryan P, Peeling WB: Prostate-specific antigen in adenocarcinoma of the prostate (letter to the editor). N Engl J Med 318:993, 1988

112. Jacobi GH: Experimental rationale for the investigation of antiprolactins as palliative treatment for prostate cancer. p. 419. In Jacobi GH, Hohenfellner R (eds): Prostate Cancer. Williams & Wilkins, Baltimore, 1982

113. Jacobi GH, Altwein JE, Hohenfellner R: Adjunct bromocriptine treatment as palliation for prostate cancer: experimental and clinical evaluation. Scand J Urol Nephrol, suppl., 55:107, 1980

114. Jacobi GH, Altwein JE, Kurth KH et al : Treatment of advanced prostatic cancer with parenteral cyproterone acetate: a phase III randomized trial. Br J Urol 52:208, 1980

115. Jacobi GH, Kurth KH, Boos J, Dennebaum R: Stellenwert der Knochenmarkphosphatasen als "Staging" beim Prostatakarzinom. Verh Disch Ges Urol 395, 1979

116. Jacobi GH, Tunn U, Senge T: Clinical experience with cyproterone acetate for palliation of inoperable prostate cancer. p. 305. In Jacobi GH, Hohenfellner R (eds): Prostate Cancer. Williams & Wilkins, Baltimore, 1982

117. Jobsis AC, De Vries GP, Anholt RRH, Sanders GTB: Demonstration of the prostatic origin of metastases: an immunohistochemical method for Formalin-fixed embedded tissue. Cancer 41:1788, 1978

118. Johnson DE, Scott WW, Gibbons RP et al : Clinical significance of serum acid phosphatase levels in advanced prostatic carcinoma. Urology 8:123, 1976

119. Jones TM, Fang VS, Landau RL, Rosenfield R: Direct inhibition of Leydig cell function by estradiol. J Clin Endocrinol Metab 47:1368, 1978

120. Kahle PJ, Schencken JR, Burns EL: Clinical and pathologic effects of diethylstilbestrol and diethylstilbestrol dipropionate on carcinoma of the prostate gland: a continuing study. J Urol 50:911, 1945

121. Katske FA, Waisman J, Lupu AN: Cutaneous and subcutaneous metastases from carcinoma of prostate. Urology 19:373, 1982

122. Keenan EJ, Ramsey EE, Kemp ED: The role of prolactin in the growth of the prostate gland. p. 9. In Murphy GP, Sandberg AA, Karr JP (eds): The Prostatic Cell: Structure and Function. Part B. Prolactin, Carcinogenesis and Clinical Aspects. Alan R Liss, New York, 1981

123. Kelly S, Labrie F, Dupont A: Loss of LH bioactivity in men treated with an LHRH agonist and an antiandrogen. Proceedings of the 65th Annual Meeting of the Endocrine Society, p. 81, 1983

124. Khan R, Turner B, Edson M, Dolan M: Bone marrow acid phosphatase: another look. J Urol 117:79, 1977

125. Kiesling VJ, Friedman HI, McAnnich JW et al : The ultrastructural changes of prostate adenocarcinoma following external beam radiation therapy. J Urol 122:633, 1980

126. Killian CS, Emrich LJ, Vargas FP et al : Relative reliability of five serially measured markers for prognosis of progression in prostate cancer. Natl Cancer Inst 76:179, 1986

126a. Killian CS, Yang N, Emrich LJ, et al: Prognostic importance of prostate-specific antigen for monitoring patients with stages B_2 to D_1 prostate cancer. Cancer Res 45:886, 1985

127. Kirchheim D, Gyorkey F, Brandes D, Scott WW: Histochemistry of the normal, hyperplastic and neoplastic human prostate gland. Invest Urol 1:403, 1964

128. Kirchheim D, Niles NR, Frankus E, Hodges CV: Correlative histochemical and histological studies on thirty radical prostatectomy specimens. Cancer 19:1683, 1966

129. Kirdani RY, Muntzing J, Varkarakis JM et al : Studies on the antiprostatic action of Estracyt, a nitrogen mustard of estradiol. Cancer Res 34:1031, 1974

130. Kirkwood JR, Margolis MT, Newton TH: Prostatic metastases to the base of the skull stimulating meningioma en plaque. Am J Roentgenol Radium Ther 112:774, 1971

131. Kledzik GS, Marshall S, Campbell GA et al : Effects of castration, testosterone, estradiol and prolactin on specific prolactin-binding in ventral prostate of male rats. Endocrinology 98:373, 1976

132. Koutsilieris M, Rabbani SA, Goltzman D: Selective osteoblast mitogens can be extracted from prostatic tissue. Prostate 9:109, 1986

133. Kramer SA, Spahr J, Brendler CB et al : Experience with Gleason histopathologic grading in prostatic cancer. J Urol 124:223, 1980

134. Krieg M, Grobe I, Voigt KD et al : Human prostatic carcinoma: significant differences in its androgen binding and metabolism compared to the human benign prostatic hypertrophy. Acta Endocrinol 88:397, 1978

135. Kuriyama M, Wang MC, Lee C-L, et al : Use of human prostate-specific antigen in monitoring prostate cancer. Cancer Res 41:3874, 1981

136. Labrie F, Dupont A, Belanger A: Complete androgen blockade for the treatment of prostate cancer. p. 193. In Devita VT, Hellman S, Rosenberg SA (eds): Important Advances in Oncology. JB Lippincott, Philadelphia, 1985

137. Labrie F, Dupont A, Belanger A et al : Simultaneous administration of pure antiandrogens, a combination necessary for the use of luteinizing hormone-releasing hormone agonists in the treatment of prostate cancer. Proc Natl Acad Sci USA 81:3861, 1984

138. Lam KK, Li CY, Lung TY et al : Comparison of prostatic and non-prostatic acid phosphatase. Ann NY Acad Sci 390:1, 1982

139. Lee C-L, Li C-Y, Jou Y-H et al : Immunochemical characterization of prostatic acid phosphatase with monoclonal antibodies. Ann NY Acad Sci 390:52, 1982

140. Liao S, Fang S, Tymoczko JL, Liang T: Androgen receptors, antiandrogens, and uptake and retention of androgens in male sex accessory organs. p. 237. In Brandes D (eds): Male Accessory Sex Organs: Structure and Function in Mammals. Academic Press, Orlando, FL, 1974

141. Lich R, Jr., Howerton LW, Amin M: Anatomy and surgical approach to the urogenital tract in the male. p. 3. In Harrison JH, Gittes RF, Perlmutter AD et al (eds).: Campbell's Urology. 4th Ed., Vol. 1. WB Saunders, Philadelphia, 1978

141a. Lilja H: A kallikrein-like serine protease in prostatic fluid cleaves the predominant seminal vesicle protein. J Clin Invest 76:1899, 1985

142. Lin CT, Song GX, Wu FY et al : Studies of human

prostatic acid phosphatase in prostatic carcinoma by immunoelectronmicroscopy (meeting abstract). J Cell Biol 99: 304, 1984

143. Lippert MC, Bensinon H, Javadpour N: Immunoperoxidase staining of acid phosphatase in human prostatic tissue. J Urol 128:1114, 1982

144. Little C, Shojania AM, Green PP, Weinerman BH: Bone marrow acid phosphatase concentrations in individuals with prostatic carcinoma or other disorders. Can med Assoc J 119:259, 1978

145. Lotan R: Effects of vitamin A and its analogs (retinoids) on normal and neoplastic cells. Biochim Biophys Acta 605:33, 1980

146. Luciani L, Scappini P, Pusiol T, Piscioli F: Comparative study of lymphography and aspiration cytology in the staging of prostatic carcinoma. Urol Int 40:181, 1985

147. Lundquist F: Function of prostatic phosphatase. Nature 158:710, 1946

148. Lung TY: Clinical significance of the human acid phosphatases. Am J Med 56:604, 1974

149. Lytton B, Collins JT, Weiss RM et al : Results of biopsy after early stage prostatic cancer treatment by implantation of I-125 seeds. J Urol 121:306, 1979

150. Mahan DE, Bruce AW, Manley PN, Franchi L: Immunohistochemical evaluation of prostatic carcinoma before and after radiotherapy. J Urol 124:488, 1980

151. Mahan DE, Doctor BP: A radioimmune assay for human prostatic acid phosphatase-levels in prostatic disease. Clin Biochem 12:10, 1979

152. Mahoney EM, Harrison JH: Bilateral adrenalectomy for palliative treatment of prostatic cancer. J Urol 108:936, 1972

153. Manni A, Santen RJ, Boucher AE et al : Hormone stimulation and chemotherapy in advanced prostate cancer: interim analysis of an ongoing randomized trial. Anticancer Res 6:309, 1986

154. Manni A, Santen RJ, Boucher AE et al : Androgen priming and response to chemotherapy in advanced prostatic cancer. J Urol 136:1242, 1986

155. Martelli A, Soli M, Bercovich E et al : Correlation between clinical response to antiandrogenic therapy and occurrence of receptors in human prostatic cancer. Urology 16:245, 1980

156. McCullough DL: Surgical staging of carcinoma of the prostate. Cancer 45:1902, 1980

157. McCullough DL, Prout GR, Daly JJ: Carcinoma of the prostate and lymphatic metastases. J Urol 111:65, 1974

158. McLaughlin AP, III, Brooks JD: A plasma factor inhibiting lymphocyte reactivity in urologic cancer patients. J Urol 112:366, 1974

159. McLaughlin AP, III, Kessler WO, Triman K, Gittes RF: Immunologic competence in patients with urologic cancer. J Urol 111:233, 1974

160. McLaughlin AP, Saltzstein SL, McCullough DL, Gittes RF: Prostatic carcinoma: incidence and location of unsuspected lymphatic metastases. J Urol 115:89, 1976

161. Menon M, Menon S, Strauss W, Catalona WJ: Demonstration of the existence of canine prostatic lymphatics by radioisotope techniques. J Urol 118:274, 1977

162. Mercer DW: Acid phosphatase isoenzymes in Gaucher's disease. Clin Chem 23:631, 1977

163. Miedema EB, Redman JF: Microscopic pulmonary embolization by adenocarcinoma of prostate. Urology 18:399, 1981

164. Mobley TL, Frank SN: Influence of tumor grade on survival and on serum acid phosphatase levels in metastatic cancer of prostate. J Urol 99:321, 1968

165. Morfin RF, Leav I, Charles J-F et al : Correlative study of the morphology and C_{19}-steroid metabolism of benign and cancerous human prostatic tissue. Cancer 39:1517, 1977

165a. Morote J, Ruibal A, Pascual C, et al: Bone marrow prostatic specific antigen and prostatic acid phosphatase levels: are they helpful in staging prostatic cancer. J Urol 137:891, 1987

166. Murphy GP, Reynoso G, Kenny GM, Gaeta JF: Comparison of total and prostatic fraction serum acid phosphatase levels in patients with differentiated and undifferentiated prostatic carcinoma. Cancer 23:1309, 1969

167. Nadji M, Tabei SZ, Castro A et al : Prostatic origin of tumors: an immunohistochemical study. Am J Clin Pathol 73:735, 1980

168. Neuman F, Humpel M, Senge et al : Cyproterone acetate-biochemical and biological basis for treatment of prostatic cancer. p. 269. In Jacobi GH, Hohenfellner R (eds): Prostate Cancer. Williams & Wilkins, Baltimore, 1982

168a. O'Brien WM, Lynch JH: Hydroxyproline as a marker for following patients with metastatic prostate cancer. J Urol 139:66, 1988

168b. Oesterling JE, Chan DW, Epstein JI, et al: Prostate specific antigen in the preoperative and postoperative evaluation of localized prostatic cancer treated with radical prostatectomy. J Urol 139:766, 1988

169. Ofner P, Leav I, Cavazos LF: C-19 steroid metabolism in male accessory sex glands. Correlation of changes in fine structure and radiometabolite patterns in the prostate of the androgen-deprived dog. p. 267. In Brandes (ed): Male Accessory Sex Organs: Structure and Function in Mammals. Academic Press, Orlando, FL, 1974

170. Papsidero LD, Kuriyama M, Wang MC et al : Prostate antigen: a marker for human prostate epithelial cells. J Natl Cancer Inst 65:37, 1981

171. Papsidero LD, Wang MC, Valenzuela LA et al : A prostate antigen in sera of prostatic cancer patients. Cancer Res 40:2428, 1980

172. Parkin L, Bylsma G, Torres AV et al : Acid phosphatase in carcinoma of the prostate in man. J Histochem Cytochem 12:288, 1964

173. Penley MW, Kim YC, Pribram HFW: Subdural metastases from prostatic adenocarcinoma. Surg Neurol 16:131, 1981

174. Peterson C, Bjork P, Forsgren B, Hogberg B: Intracellular localization of estramustine in rat ventral prostate in vitro. Prostate 2:143, 1981

175. Pirke KM, Doerr P: Age related changes in free plasma testosterone, dihydrotestosterone and oestradiol. Acta Endocrinol 89:171, 1975

175a. Pont A: Long-term experience with high dose ketoconazole therapy in patients with stage D2 prostatic carcinoma. J Urol 137:902, 1987

176. Pousette A, Bjork P, Carlstrom K et al : Influence of sex hormones on prostatic secretion protein, a major protein rat prostate. Cancer Res 41:688, 1981

177. Pousette A, Bjork P, Carlstrom K et al : Influence of pituitary and adrenocortical hormones on prostatic secretion protein, a major protein in rat prostate. Prostate 3:109, 1982

178. Prellwitz W, Ehrenthal W: Serum and bone marrow acid phosphatase as a diagnostic marker in prostatic carcinoma patients. p. 129. In Jacobi GH, Hohenfellner R (eds): Prostate Cancer. Williams & Wilkins, Baltimore, 1982

179. Prout GR, Irwin RJ, Kliman B et al : Prostatic cancer and SCH-13521: II. Histological alterations and the pituitary gonadal axis. J Urol 113:834, 1975

180. Prout GR, Jr., Kliman B, Daly JJ et al : Endocrine changes after diethylstilbestrol therapy. Effects on prostatic neoplasm and pituitary-gonadal axis. Urology 7:148, 1976

181. Radwan F, Leger F, Carmel M et al: Characterization of androgen receptors in normal and malignant human prostatic tissues. Prostate 9:147, 1986

182. Raghavaiah NV, Jordan WP, Jr.: Prostatic lymphography. J Urol 121:178, 1979

183. Rao KG: Carcinoma of prostate presenting as intracranial tumor with multiple cranial nerve palsies. Urology 19:433, 1982

184. Raskin P, McClain CJ, Medsger TA, Jr.: Hypocalcemia associated with metastatic bone disease. Arch Intern Med 132:539, 1973

185. Reingold IM: Cutaneous metastases from internal carcinoma. Cancer 19:162, 1966

186. Robinson MR, Rigby CC, Nakhla LC, Shearer R: Prostate carcinoma: mitogenic stimulation of lymphocytes with phytohemagglutinen. p. 123. In Bonney WW (ed): Workshop on Genitourinary Cancer Immunology. Department of Health, Education and Welfare (NIH) Publication no. 78-1467, 1978

187. Robinson MR, Shearer RJ, Fergusson JD: Adrenal suppression in the treatment of carcinoma of the prostate. Br J Urol 46:555m 1974

188. Robinson MR, Thomas BS: Effect of hormonal therapy on plasma testosterone levels in prostatic carcinoma. Br Med J 4:391, 1971

189. Rodin AE, Larson DL, Roberts DK: Nature of the perineural space invaded by prostatic carcinoma. Cancer 20:1772, 1967

190. Romas NA, Shaw LM, Hsu KC et al : Clinical comparison of immunological assays for determining prostatic acid phosphatase. Ann NY Acad Sci 390:104, 1982

191. Rychewaert A, de Seze S, Lanham C et al : Troubles du métabolisme phosphocalcique au cours des cancers secondaires des os à forme condensante d'origine prostatique. Sem Hop Paris 42:1051, 1966

192. Sadlowski RW: Early stage prostatic cancer investigated by pelvic lymph node and bone marrow acid phosphatase. J Urol 119:89, 1978

193. Sandberg AA: Endocrine control and physiology of the prostate. Prostate 1:169, 1980

194. Saroff J, Kirdani RY, Chu TM et al : Measurements of prolactin and androgens in patients with prostatic disease. Oncology 37:46, 1980

194a. Schellhammer PF, El-Mahdi AM, Higgins EM, et al: Prostate biopsy after definitive treatment by interstitial ^{125}iodine implant or external beam radiation therapy. J Urol 137:897, 1987

195. Schenken JR, Burns EL, Kahle PF: The effect of diethylstilbestrol and diethylstilbestrol dipropionate on carcinoma of the prostate gland. II. Cytologic changes following treatment. J Urol 48:99, 1943

196. Schirmer HKA, Murphy GP, Scott WW: Hormonal therapy of prostatic cancer—a correlation between Broders' classification (and staging) and clinical course. Urol Digest 3:15, 1965

196a. Schroeder FH, Lock TMTW, Frans DRC, et el: Metastatic cancer of the prostate managed with buserelin versus buserelin plus cyproterone acetate. J Urol 912:137, 1987

197. Scott WW: Endocrine management of disseminated prostatic cancer, including bilateral adrenalectomy and hypophysectomy. Trans Am Assoc Genitourin Surg 44:101, 1952

198. Scott WW, Menon M, Walsh PC: Hormonal therapy of prostatic cancer. Cancer 45:1929, 1980

199. Shaw LM, Romas NA, Cohen H (eds): Prostatic acid phosphatase measurement: its role in detection and management of prostatic cancer. Ann NY Acad Sci 390:73, 1982

200. Shearer RJ, Hendry WF, Sommerville IF, Fergusson JD: Plasma testosterone: an accurate monitor of hormone treatment in prostate cancer. Br J Urol 45:668, 1973

201. Shimazaki J, Kurihara H, Ito Y, Shida K: Testosterone metabolism in prostate. Formation of androstane-17β-ol-3-one and androst-4-ene-3,17-dione, and inhibitory effect of natural and synthetic estrogens. Gunma J Med Sci 14:313, 1965

202. Shimazaki J, Kurihara H, Ito Y, Shida K: Metabolism of testosterine in prostate. Separation of prostatic 17β-ol-dihydrogenase and 5 alpha-reductase. Gunma J Med Sci 14:326, 1965

203. Shirazi PH, Rayudu GV, Fordham EW: Review of solitary 18F bone scan lesions. Radiology 112:369, 1974

204. Silber I, Rosai J, Cordonnier FJ: The incidence of elevated acid phosphatase in prostatic infarction. J Urol 103:765, 1970

205. Sinha AA, Blackhard CE, Doe RP et al : The *in vitro* localization of ^{3}H-estradiol in human prostatic carcinoma. Cancer 31:682, 1973

206. Sinha AA, Blackhard CE, Seal US: A critical analysis of tumor morphology and hormone treatments in the untreated and estrogen-treated responsive and refractory human prostatic carcinoma. Cancer 40:2836, 1977

207. Slaunwhite WR, Jr.: Inhibitors of prolactin secretion: a mini-review. p. 19. In Murphy GP, Sandberg AA, Karr JP (eds): The prostatic Cell: Structure and Function. Part B. Prolactin, Carcinogensis and Clinical Aspects. Alan R Liss New York, 1981

208. Smallridge RC, Wray HL, Schaaf M: Hypocalcemia with osteoblastic metastases in a patient with prostate carcinoma. A cause of secondary hyperparathyroidism. Am J Med 71:184, 1981

208a. Smith JA Jr: New methods of endocrine management of prostatic cancer. J Urol 137:1, 1987

209. Smith MJV: The lymphatics of the prostate. Invest Urol 3:439, 1966

209a. Stamey TF, Yang N, Hay AR, et al: Prostate-specific antigen as a serum marker for adenocarcinoma of the prostate. N Engl J Med 317:909, 1987

210. St. Arnaud R, Lachance R, Dupont A, Labrie F: Serum luteinizing hormone (LH) biological activity in castrated patients with cancer of the prostate receiving a pure antiandrogen and in estrogen-pretreated patients with an LH-releasing hormone agonist and antiandrogen. J Clin Endocrinol Metab 63:297, 1986

211. St. Arnaud R, Lachance R, Kelly SJ et al : Loss of luteinizing hormone bioactivity in patients with prostatic cancer treated with an LHRH agonist and a pure antiandrogen. Clin Endocrinol 24:21, 1986

212. Stein BS, Peterson RO, Vangore S, Kendall AR: Immunoperoxidase localization of prostate-specific antigen. Am J Surg Pathol 6:553, 1982

213. Stone AR, Hargreave TB, Chisholm GD: The diagnosis of oestrogen escape and the role of secondary orchiectomy in prostatic cancer. Br J Urol 52:535, 1980

214. Terzakian GM, Herr HW, Metha MB: Orbital metastases from prostatic carcinoma. Urology 19:427, 1982

214a. Trachtenberg J: Experimental treatment of prostatic cancer by intermittent hormonal therapy. J Urol 137:785, 1987

215. Ueda H, Takenawa T, Millan JC et al : The effects of retinoids on proliferative capacities and macromolecular synthesis in human breast cancer (MCF-7) cells. Cancer 46:2203, 1980.

215a. Van Cangh PJ, Opsomer R, DeNayer PH: Serum prostatic acid phosphatase determination in prostatic diseases: A critical comparison of an enzymatic and a radioimmunologic assay. J Urol 128, 1212, 1982

216. Varenhorst E: Metabolic changes during endocrine treatment in carcinoma of the prostate. A prospective study in man with special reference to cardiovascular complications during treatment with oestrogens or cyproterone acetate or after orchiectomy. Linkoping University of Medicine, Dissertation no. 103, 1980

217. Vermeulen A, Van Camp A, Mattelaer J, DeSy W: Hormonal factors related to abnormal growth of the prostate. p. 81. In Coffey DS, Isaac JT (eds): Prostate Cancer. Vol. 48. UICC Technical Report Series, Geneva, 1979

218. Vienema RJ, Gursel EO, Romas N et al : Bone marrow acid phosphatase: prognostic value in patients undergoing radical prostatectomy. J Urol 117:81, 1977

219. Vihko P, Kontturi M: Transient high serum prostate-specific acid phosphatase measured by radiommunoassay in prostatic infarction. Scand J Urol Nephrol 15:213, 1981

220. Vihko P, Lukkarienen O, Kontturi M, Vihko R: Effectiveness of radioimmunoassay of human prostate-specific acid phosphatase in the diagnosis and follow-up of therapy in prostate carcinoma. Cancer Res 41:1180, 1981

221. Vihko P, Sojanti E, Janne O et al : Serum prostate-specific acid phosphatase: development and validation of a specific radioimmunoassay. Clin Chem 24:1915, 1978

222. Wagner RK, Schulze KH, Jungblut PW: Estrogen

and androgen receptor in human prostate and prostatic tumor tissue. Acta Endocrinol (suppl) 193:52, 1975

223. Walsh PC, Greco JM, Tananis CE et al : The binding of a potent synthetic androgen-methyltrienolone (R1881)-to cytosol preparations of human prostatic cancer. Trans Am Assoc Genitourin Surg 69:78, 1977

224. Walsh PC, Korenman SG: Action of the antiandrogens: Preservation of 5 alpha-reductase activity and inhibition of chromatin-dihydrotestosterone complex formation. Clin Res 18:126, 1970

225. Walsh PC, Siiteri PK: Suppression of plasma androgens by spironolactone in castrated men with carcinoma of the prostate. J Urol 114:254, 1975

226. Wang MC, Papsidero m, Kuriyama LA et al : Prostate antigen: A new potential marker for prostatic cancer. Prostate 2:89, 1981

227. Warren S, Harris PN, Graves RC: Osseous metastasis of carcinoma of the prostate. With special reference to the perineural lymphatics. Arch Pathol 22:139, 1936

228. Watkinson JM, Delory GE, King EJ, Haddow A: Plasma acid phosphatase in carcinoma of prostate and effect of treatment with stilbestrol. Br Med J 2:491, 1944

229. Webber MM: Polypeptide hormones and the prostate. p. 63. In Murphy GP, Sandberg AA, Karr JP (eds): The Prostatic Cell: Structure and Function. Part B. Prolactin, Carcinogenesis and Clinical Aspects. Alan R Liss, New York, 1981

230. Witorsch RJ: Visualization of prolactin binding sites in prostate tissue. p. 89. In Murphy GP, Sandberg AA, Karr JP (eds): The Prostatic Cell: Structure and Function. Part B. Prolactin, Carcinogenesis & Clinical Aspects. Alan R Liss, New York, 1981

231. Woodard HQ: Factors leading to elevation in serum acid by glycerophosphatase. Cancer 5:236, 1952

232. Woodard HQ: Quantitative studies of beta-glycerophosphatase activity in normal and neoplastic tissues. Cancer 9:352, 1956

233. Worgul TJ, Santen RJ, Samojlik E et al : Clinical and biochemical effect of aminoglutethimide in the treatment of advanced prostatic cancer. J Urol 129:51, 1983

234. Yam LT, Janckila AJ, Lam KW et al : Immunohistochemistry of prostatic acid phosphatase. Prostate 2:97, 1981

235. Yamanaka H, Kirdani RY, Saroff J et al : Effects of testosterone and prolactin on rat prostatic weight, 5 alpha-reductase and arginase. Am J Physiol 229:1102, 1975

236. Yanihara T, Troen P: Studies of the human testis: III. Effect of estrogen on testosterone formation in human testis in vitro. J Clin Endocrinol 34:968, 1972

237. Yarrison G, Mertens BF, Mathies JC: New diagnostic use of bone marrow acid and alkaline phosphatase. Am J Clin Pathol 66:667, 1976

238. Yesus YW, Taylor HM: Diagnostic use of bone marrow acid and alkaline phosphatases. Am J Clin Pathol 67:92, 1977

239. Young JD, Jr., Sidh SM, Bashirelahi N: The role of estrogen, androgen and progesterone receptors in the managment of carcinoma of the prostate. Trans Am Assoc Genitourin Surg 71:23, 1979

240. Zucker MB, Borelli J: A survey of some platelet enzymes and functions. The platelets as the source of normal serum acid glycerophosphatase. Ann NY Acad Sci 75:203, 1958

34

Congenital Anomalies of the Penis

Robert S. Katz

CONGENITAL ANOMALIES OF THE PENIS

As is the case with virtually every other organ, the penis is subject to a variety of embryologic and developmental disorders. These represent a major problem in urologic management. The young boy with malformed genitalia may have serious difficulties in excretory function and profound psychologic and sexual difficulty.

A brief overview of these developmental disorders of the penis is presented here as a prelude to discussion of the range of acquired disease of the external male genitalia. The developmental anatomy of the normal male is illustrated for reference (Figs. 34-1 and 34-2).

MICROPENIS

A striking finding of multifactorial etiology is micropenis. As the term implies, micropenis is an abnormally short penis. The penis should be of sufficient length to permit urination while standing, penetration during intercourse, and the avoidance of embarrassment when viewed by others. Statistical data on penile length as a function of age are available and suggest that a penis with a length less than 2.5 standard deviations below the mean should be categorized

as a micropenis, as 99.4 percent of a normally distributed population will have a longer organ.[17]

In general, the penis appears relatively normal, although sometimes hard to find in pubic fat (Figs. 34-3 and 34-4). A careful examination of the penis should be made to exclude associated urogenital anomalies, which may include hypospadias and undescended testes.[10]

There are many causes of micropenis, most of which are hormonal in nature. Fetal androgens affect the development of the penis during gestation. As a result, abnormalities of hormonal secretion and function may result in penile malformation. Pituitary or hypothalamic disorders are a common finding (hypogonadotropic hypogonadism), with lower levels of luteinizing hormone (LH) and follicle-stimulating hormone (FSH) present.[11,12,18] Failures of testosterone secretion by the gonads themselves (primary hypogonadism) may result in micropenis, with high FSH levels seen.[19] Another cause of micropenis is end-organ failure, with either complete or partial androgen insensitivity.[6] A recent study investigated a mixed group of patients with sexual differentiation disorders.[10] Included were boys with epispadias, hypospadias, and micropenis. The patients manifested adequate levels of androgen receptors but subnormal binding to nuclei of androgen–androgen receptor complexes. This partial androgen insensitivity may

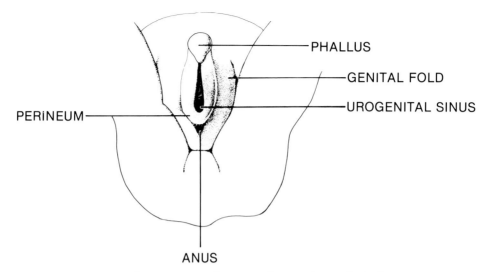

Fig. 34-1 Normal anatomy. Development of external genitalia in first trimester.

explain the pathogenesis of some cases of micropenis and other developmental disorders, although the authors do not speculate beyond this. Patients lacking cytoplasmic androgen receptors will experience complete androgen insensitivity and micropenis on this end-organ failure basis.[10]

EPISPADIAS

Epispadias is an abnormality of penile and urethral development in which the urethral meatus opens proximally on the dorsal aspect of the penis. The penis is short, and chordee, an upward bend of the penis, is present. The corpora are short, often rudimentary, and curved, causing the chordee.[28] A short penis also results from pubic bone separation and a short urethra. The embryologic origin of epispadias appears related to the failure of the precursors of the genital tubercle to meet dorsally in the midline. As a result, a small part of the cloacal membrane remains and eventually breaks down, leaving the abnormal urethral orifice.[21] In a more severe developmental anomaly, exstrophy of the bladder is also present.[7] (See also Ch. 6.) This represents failure of mesoderm from the caudal end of the primitive streak to reach the midline below the umbilicus. In the absence of mesoderm, the abdominal muscle does not extend fully, causing the exstrophy. The two halves of the pelvis are open but rotated downward.[28] If the mesodermal defect con-

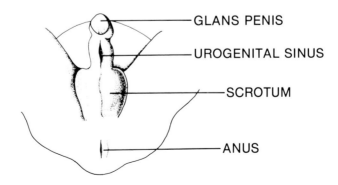

Fig. 34-2 Normal anatomy. Development of external genitalia in second trimester.

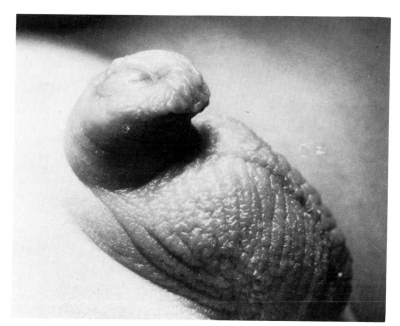

Fig. 34-3 Microphallus. Two examples of microphallus of hormonal etiology. (From Hinman,[11] with permission.)

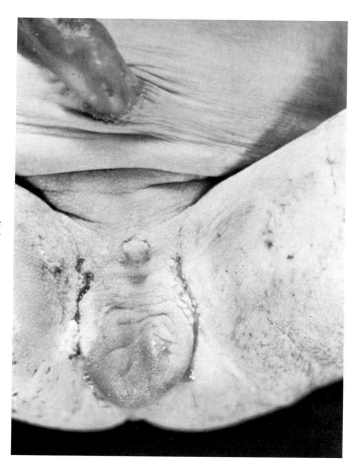

Fig. 34-4 Microphallus. In this case the penis is nearly absent. (Incidental autopsy finding.)

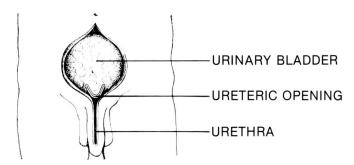

Fig. 34-5 Epispadias. In this instance, the dorsal urethral opening is associated with bladder exstrophy.

tinues downward so the genital tubercles fail to meet in the midline to form a single tubercle, the exstrophy will be associated with epispadias[21] (Fig. 34-5). To repair this anomaly, the urethra must be mobilized. The penis can be lengthened by partial detachment of the penile crura from the puboischial rami, bringing more corporal length into the shaft. The abnormal urethral orifice is closed, and a new orifice is constructed at the glans.[14]

HYPOSPADIAS

Hypospadias is another congenital anomaly of the penis, rather like a "mirror-image" of epispadias. The urethral meatus is situated on the ventral surface of the penis or in the perineum (Fig. 34-6).[2] The development of hypospadias is associated with defective production of androgen by the fetal testes. This inadequate production persists after birth, as well.[1]

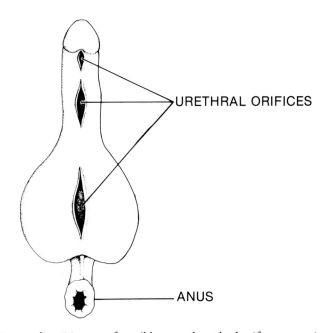

Fig. 34-6 Hypospadias. Diagram of possible ventral urethral orifices on penis and perineum.

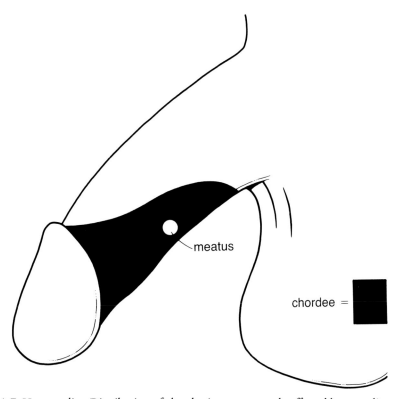

Fig. 34-7 Hypospadias. Distribution of chordee in more severely affected hypospadias patients. (From Page,[23] with permission.)

Masculinization of the genitalia is interrupted, with incomplete closure of the urethral groove.[21] Serious urinary and sexual function problems may result if repair is not performed. The patient may also have various degrees of chordee, usually lateral (Fig. 34-7). Although fibrous tissue has been presumed as the anatomic correlate of chordee, recent studies have found smooth muscle remnants within the excised tissues (Fig. 34-8).[23] This suggests that the chordee is really derived from the corpus spongiosum. The etiology of the chordee appears related to a failure of closure of the corpus spongiosum urethrae.[3] The spongiosum tissue extends laterally and irregularly, causing the chordee. With increasing age, the corpus spongiosum may become surrounded by collagen, probably secondary to mechanical insults (coital erection) or inflammation of the penile skin.[3]

In addition, other urogenital anomalies have been found in association with hypospadias, including cryptorchism, urethral valves, and upper urinary tract abnormalities (Fig. 34-9).[2] These should be considered when evaluating the patient with hypospadias. The study cited earlier on partial androgen insensitivity suggests that these disorders are various reflections of inadequate androgen secretion or uptake.[10] Intersex disorders are associated with the more severe forms of hypospadias, particularly when accompanied by undescended testes. These disorders include male pseudohermaphroditism, mixed gonadal dysgenesis, true hermaphroditism, 46XX male syndrome, and Klinefelter's syndrome.[24a]

DIPHALLUS

Diphallus, double penis, is a very rare developmental anomaly. The disorder may take three forms, bifid glans, bifid diphallia (partial separation), or complete diphallia (Fig. 34-10). Abnormalities of the bladder and kidney are often found. In bifid penis, there are

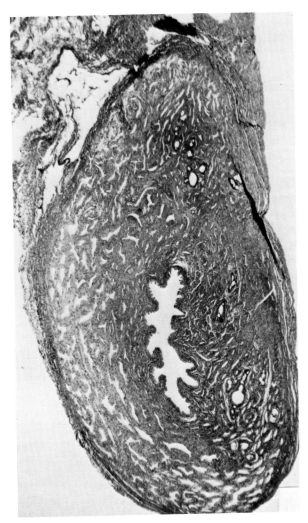

Fig. 34-8 Hypospadias. Transverse section of urethra showing lumen surrounded by oval-shaped corpus spongiosum. The corpus spongiosum is itself surrounded by thick, sclerotic connective tissue. (From Avellan,[2] with permission.)

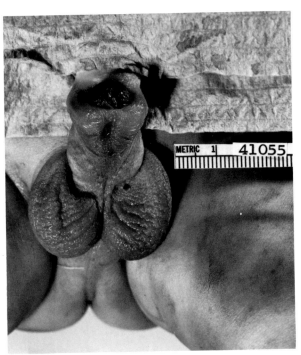

Fig. 34-9 Hypospadias. External genitalia in a case of hypospadias. This patient also had bifid scrotum.

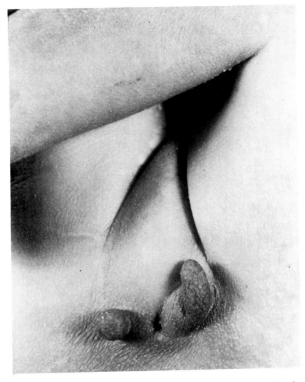

Fig. 34-10 Diphallus. A striking example. Note that both organs are quite malformed.

two sets of corpora cavernosa, with the urethra opening in the midline. In complete diphallus, there are two sets of corpora cavernosa along with corpora spongiosa and double urethrae.[9,20] The developmental anomaly may represent a split in the cloacal membrane (early genital tubercle) with separate segments formed.[24] The cloacal membrane extends from below the umbilicus to the caudal end of the embryo. The genital tubercles at the lower part of this membrane give rise to the scrotum, urethra, and penis. A split occurs in this region. The depth of the split deter-

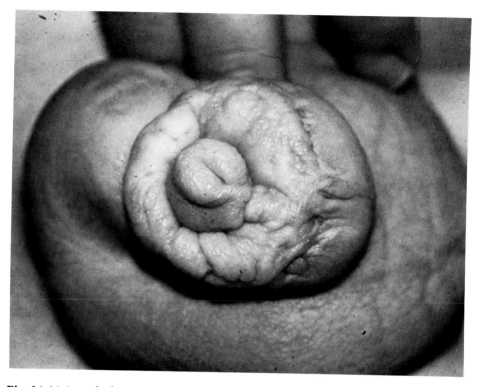

Fig. 34-11 Lymphedema. Severe penile and scrotal edema in a patient with congenital lymphedema. (From Tapper,[27] with permission.)

Fig. 34-12 Apenia. Total absence of penis in a child with normal scrotum and numerous anomalies of the kidneys. (From Roth,[25] with permission.)

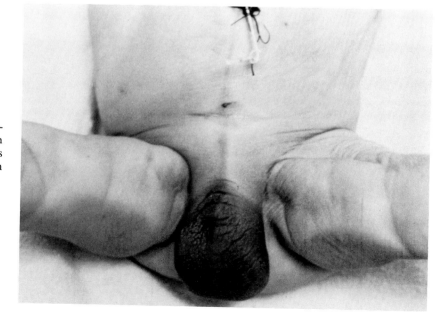

mines the amount of tissue involved and the extent of the deformity.[24] Abnormalities such as bifid scrotum and imperforate anus are often found as well, again owing to anomalous development of the cloacal membrane, from whose posterior portion the rectum also derives.[16,24]

Surgical repair of the region is usually necessary with reconstruction of a normal urogenital tract. The duplicate penis may have a separate bladder and a ureter draining one kidney that necessitates additional repair.

WEBBED PENIS

An unusual deformation of the penis is webbed penis. In this disorder, the penile and scrotal skin are fused together. The penis may be engulfed in this structure, or only partially fused, with a web of tissue connecting penis and scrotum.[4] The anomaly may be associated with hypospadias.[26]

CONGENITAL LYMPHEDEMA

Another rare penile deformity is congenital lymphedema. This disease generally involves the lower extremities, but it may affect the penis, with or without associated limb involvement. The lymphatics are generally dilated, and marked sluggishness of flow is seen in the vessels. The penis and scrotum demonstrate considerable swelling with a risk of urethral obstruction (Fig. 34-11). In addition, the psychologic trauma of this congenital disease is a serious problem. Operative repair with resection of skin and involved subcutaneous tissue and covering with skin grafts may help affected men. The resected tissue will demonstrate marked lymphatic ectasia with an extensive fibrous matrix between the dilated vessels.[27] An association with lymphangiosarcoma development has not been demonstrated, perhaps owing to the rarity of cases.[8]

CONGENITAL ABSENCE OF THE PENIS

Perhaps the most dramatic of congenital anomalies of the penis is congenital absence of the penis. This extremely rare condition occurs about once in 30 million male births. The child generally has a normal scrotum but no demonstrable penile shaft. There may, however, be a perineal appendage or elevation behind the scrotum. Beasley et al.[5] have found in one case that buried beneath this appendage was cavernous tissue through which the urethra ran. They suggested that this case, and perhaps others, represent posterior ectopia of the penis. If so, penile agenesis might represent a variant of transposition of the genitalia, in which a recognizable penis is found between the scrotum and rectum.[15a] The urethra ends in the perineum near the anus or in the rectum.[13] Many patients have other associated, often severe, congenital anomalies involving the urogenital system and additional organ systems (Fig. 34-12).[22,25] The disease results from failure of formation of the genital tubercule during gestation.[15]

In cases of apenia, the usual recommendation is to treat the child as a female since it is easier to construct female external genitalia.[22] The testes are resected, and an appropriate urethral orifice is prepared that avoids the bacterial contamination of the ano-rectal area.[13]

REFERENCES

1. Allen T, Griffin J: Endocrine studies in patients with advanced hypospadias. J Urol 131:310, 1984
2. Avellan L: Morphology of hypospadias. Scand J Plast Reconstr Surg 14:239, 1980
3. Avellan L, Knutsson F: Microscopic studies of curvature-causing structures in hypospadias. Scand J Plast Reconstr Surg 14:249, 1980
4. Azmy A: Webbed penis. Br J Urol 58:460, 1986
5. Beasley SW, Hutson JM, Kelly JH, Howat AJ: Re: testicular function in 12 cases of penile agenesis (letter to the editor). J Urol 137:317, 1987
6. Burstein S, Grumbach M, Kaplan S: Early determination of adrogen-responsiveness is important in the management of microphallus. Lancet 2:983, 1979
7. Devine C, Horton C, Scarff J: Epispadias. Urol Clin North Am 7:465, 1980
8. Fonkalsrud E: A syndrome of congenital lymphedema of the upper extremity and associated systemic lymphatic malformations. Surg Gynecol Obstet 145:228, 1977
9. Fujita K, Tamjima A, Suzuki K, Aso Y: Diphallia with a normal and a blind-ending urethra. Eur Urol 5:328, 1979

10. Gyorki S, Warne GL, Khalid B, Funder J: Defective nuclear accumulation of androgen receptors in disorders of sexual differentiation. J Clin Invest 72:819, 1983

11. Hinman F, Jr.: Microphallus: distinction between anomalous and endocrine types. J Urol 123:412, 1980

12. Johanson A: Abnormalities of sexual development. p. 373. In Devine C, Stecker J (eds): Urology in Practice. Little, Brown, Boston, 1978

13. Johnson W, Yeatman G, Weigel J: Congenital absence of the penis. J Urol 117:508, 1977

14. Johnston JH: Epispadias. p. 1663. In Harrison JH et al (eds): Campbell's Urology. Vol. 2, 4th Ed. WB Saunders, Philadelphia, 1979

15. Kumar A, Wakhlu AK, Chandra H: Congenital absence of penis. Indian Pediatr 23:303, 1986

15a. Lage JM, Driscoll SG, Bieber FR: Transposition of the external genitalia associated with caudal regression. J Urol 138:387, 1987

16. Landy B, Signer R, Oetjen L: A case of diphallia. Urology 28:48, 1986

17. Lee P, Mazur T, Danish R et al : Micropenis: I. Criteria, etiologies and classification. Johns Hopkins Med J 146:156, 1980

18. Lee P, Danish R, Mazur T et al : Micropenis: II. Hypogonadotropic hypogonadism. Johns Hopkins Med J 146:177, 1980

19. Lee P, Danish R, Mazur T et al: Micropenis: III. Hypogonadism, partial androgen insensitivity syndrome, and idiopathic disorders. Johns Hopkins Med J 147:175, 1980

20. Melekos MD, Barbalis GA, Asbach HW: Penile duplication. Urology 27:258, 1986

21. Moffat DB: Development abnormalities of the urogenital system. p. 357. In Chisolm GD, Williams DI (eds): Scientific Foundations of Urology. 2nd Ed. Year book Medical Publishers, Chicago, 1982

22. Oesch IL, Printer A, Ransley RG: Penile agenesis: a report of six cases. J Ped Surg 22:174, 1987

23. Page RE: Hypospadias revisited. Br J Plast Surg 34:149, 1981

24. Rao TV, Chandrasekharam V: Diphallus with duplication of cloacal derivatives: report of a rare case. J Urol 124:555, 1980

24a. Rohatgi M, Menon PSN, Verma IC, Iyengar JK: The presence of intersexuality in patients with advanced hypospadias and undescended gonads. J Urol 137:263, 1987

25. Roth JK, Marshall R, Angel J et al : Congenital absence of penis. Urology 17:579, 1981

26. Shepard G, Wilson C, Sallade R: Webbed penis. Plast Reconstr 53:453, 1980

27. Tapper D, Eraklis A, Colodny A et al : Congenital lymphedema of the penis: a method of reconstruction. J Pediatr Surg 15:481, 1980

28. Woodhouse CR, Kellett M: Anatomy of the penis and its deformities in extrophy and epispadias. J Urol 132:1122, 1984

35

Infections and Other Cutaneous Penile Lesions

Robert S. Katz

Because the penis is covered by skin, it is subject to the same array of cutaneous disorders as the other areas of the body. Some of these are generalized, but in addition, a variety of lesions unique to penile skin can develop. Finally, venereal infections deriving their portal of entry at the penis can produce characteristic changes.

The basic dermatologic anatomy of the skin begins at the penile fascia, elastic areolar tissue that both holds together the cavernous bodies and provides a flexible attachment for the skin itself. The epidermis of the penis is thinner than that of the trunk or extremities. The shaft and glans contain no hair follicles. The foreskin contains some elastic fibers to permit retraction and sebaceous glands to provide secretions that lubricate the passage of the foreskin over the glans.[21]

INFLAMMATORY CONDITIONS

Lichen Planus

Lichen planus is a common dermatologic disease of uncertain etiology. It can affect almost any area of the body, although the arms and mucous membranes are typical locations. The glans penis is a frequent site of occurrence.

The typical lesion of lichen planus is a papule that is shiny and violaceous. The papules are of various sizes but typically form an annular configuration on the glans. The cause of lichen planus is essentially unknown. No one theory has been proven, although psychogenic causes have been suggested frequently.[47]

Histologically, lichen planus is usually fairly easy to diagnose. A constellation of findings is usually noted. The keratin layer is markedly thickened (hyperkeratosis). In addition, the granular layer of the skin also shows thickening. These changes, however, are not present in all areas, leading to irregular acanthosis. The basal layer of the epidermis shows a liquefactive change at the dermal-epidermal border. A lymphohistiocytic infiltrate is found just below the dermal-epidermal junction. This infiltrate is quite well demarcated and forms a band hugging the junction. In addition, small, rounded, eosinophilic structures known as colloid bodies can be seen in the lower epidermis (Fig. 35-1). These represent degenerate epidermal cells.[27] The disorder is generally self-limiting and can respond well to local therapy.

Lichen Nitidus

Another disorder, perhaps a variant of lichen planus, is lichen nitidus. This rare lesion appears preferentially on the penis, although other skin regions

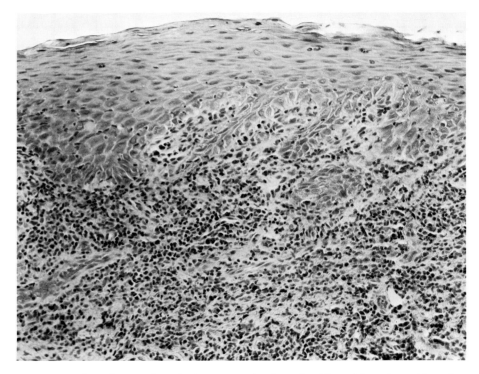

Fig. 35-1 Lichen planus. There is damage to the dermal-epidermal junction with a dense chronic inflammatory process at the junction. Some degenerate epithelial cells are also present at the junction. ×180.

may be involved. On gross inspection it consists of a group of small, shiny papules. They may appear anywhere along the shaft or glans, and may bear some similarity to the papules of lichen planus.

On histologic evaluation, lichen nitidis looks rather different from lichen planus. While there may be some basal layer degeneration as seen in lichen planus, the epidermis is thinned in lichen nitidis. In lichen planus there is usually acanthosis and hyperkeratosis. A well-defined, hugging, superficial dermal infiltrate is seen, lymphohistiocytic in nature but often containing a few giant cells. The rete ridges on either side of the inflammatory infiltrate may grow downward and then centrally, forming a collarlike appearance.[37] Colloid bodies are seldom seen. Lichen nitidis is also characterized by areas of parakeratosis, rare in lichen planus.[27]

Contact Dermatitis

A wide array of environmental agents can produce a pronounced skin reaction, often of intense discomfort. On the penis, lotions, contraceptive jellies, soaps (both personal and laundry types), and clothing bleaches may cause a profound skin irritation. Exposure to a contact allergen provokes a variety of immune responses via both cell- and antibody-mediated hypersensitivities. Lymphocyte transformation causes the release of lymphokines such as macrophage activating factor that can produce an inflammatory reaction. In addition to cell-mediated immunity, antibodies released at the site of contact may perpetuate the inflammatory response as well.[7] For a substance to function as a contact allergen, it generally must form a stable bond with skin proteins (keratin precursors, dermal collagen). The ensuing molecule then elicits the immune response through contact with macrophages and Langerhans cells.[7] Significant penile edema may develop along with erythema and scaling of the epidermis.[31] Microscopic examination of the skin in contact dermatitis may reveal a number of nonspecific patterns. An acute dermatitis, with erythema and vesicle formation, may appear. The skin will show spongiosis and intraepidermal vesicle formation (Fig. 35-2). A marked acute and chronic inflammatory infiltrate may be seen in the dermis and

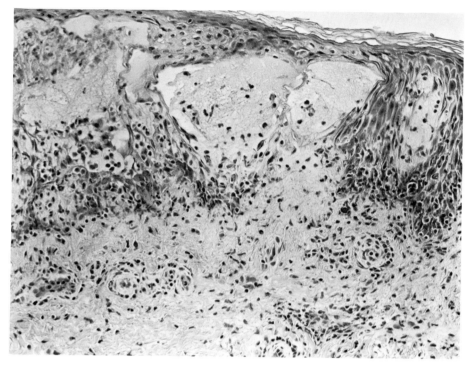

Fig. 35-2 Contact dermatitis. A typical intraepidermal vesicle is seen, showing extensive spongiosis of the epidermis. The basal layer here is not readily visible, but the intraepithelial nature of the lesions is visible at the sides of the epidermis. ×180.

epidermis. A more subacute dermatitis may also be seen in this syndrome. Again, blisters are present, although generally smaller, and some epidermal acanthosis is noted. A chronic dermatitis is the third pattern found in the contact dermatitis group. Scaling is common, and microscopic evaluation will reveal acanthosis, hyperkeratosis, and chronic perivascular inflammation.[27]

Local or systemic steroids, along with antihistamines, may be required to treat this disorder. Elimination of the inciting agent is the first priority in therapy. Careful clinical history is essential in this regard.

Psoriasis

Psoriasis has been well described as "chronic skin disease, characterized by epidermal hyperplasia and a greatly accelerated rate of epidermal turnover."[17] The process may affect almost any part of the skin, although the knees, elbows, and scalp are most typically affected.[17] On the penis, it often appears as a red pustule commonly enlarging to a large plaque. Any portion of the penis may be involved, along with the surrounding groin tissue. Although scaling is a hallmark of the disease elsewhere, this may not be so prominent on the penis, owing to the moistness of the area.[31]

The classic biopsy appearance of psoriasis is not seen in many cases, so a combination of clinical judgment and limited histologic correlation may be needed to establish a diagnosis. The fully formed case will show marked acanthosis and an elongation of the rete ridges. There is a loss of the epidermal granular layer, and the dermal papillae are edematous (Fig. 35-3). Extensive parakeratosis is present with localized microabscesses and collections of polymorphs in the epidermis (Kogoj's pustule) and parakeratotic scale (Munro microabscess).[20,27] The dermis shows edema and a scattered chronic inflammatory infiltrate.[35]

It is not unusual for major histologic features of psoriasis to be absent in a single punch or shave biopsy of skin; in particular, the Munro or Kogoj microabscesses are often not present. In these situations, the

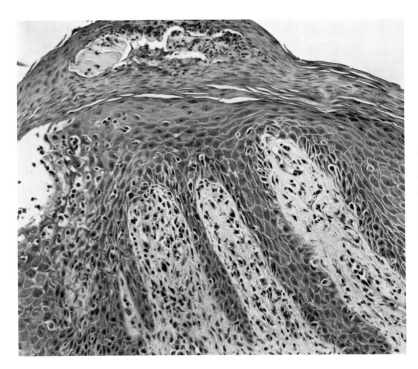

Fig. 35-3 Psoriasis. The marked acanthosis, elongation of rete ridges, and suprapapillary thinning are illustrated here. Munro microabscesses are present in the parakeratotic layer, as well as edema of dermal papillae and loss of the granular layer. ×180.

histologic diagnosis of psoriasiform dermatitis is a reasonable one, with appropriate microscopic description added.

In addition to skin manifestations, psoriasis has been associated with a form of arthritis. The percentage of patients with psoriasis and an arthritis has been estimated at anywhere from 1 percent to 30 percent of psoriatic patients depending on the definition of arthritis.[8] Skin lesions usually precede the development of arthritis by as much as 20 or 30 years. The arthritis is similar in clinical presentation to rheumatoid arthritis and is polyarticular, with preference for the small joints of the hands and feet. The patients are seronegative for the usual rheumatoid arthritis laboratory tests.[8]

A large number of local and systemic therapeutic measures have been attempted in this chronic condition with various degrees of success.

Pityriasis Rosea

Pityriasis rosea is a commonly seen disorder that sometimes involves the penis. The etiology of pityriasis rosea, as for many inflammatory skin conditions, is uncertain. However, the abrupt onset and self-limited nature of the process suggest a viral cause.

Pityriasis rosea generally becomes manifest with the appearance of a herald patch. This lesion, which appears in about 70 percent of cases, precedes the development of secondary lesions by approximately 7 days to 14 days. This patch may resemble that seen in psoriasis. However, psoriasis may progress relentlessly, whereas the herald patch of pityriasis rosea gives way to an erythematous, scaly, papular eruption typically involving the trunk, which will usually regress in a few weeks. The herald patch may manifest on the penile shaft, whereas the subsequent eruption may involve the shaft along with portions of the trunk.[9]

The histology of pityriasis rosea is nonspecific and is that of a chronic dermatitis. The biopsy shows some spongiosis and chronic inflammatory cells in the epidermis. A chronic inflammatory infiltrate is also seen scattered throughout the upper dermis. Small areas of parakeratosis are often seen. As the findings at microscopy are not definitive, clinical-histologic correlation is essential.

Erythema Multiforme

Erythema multiforme is a generalized skin disorder that may affect the penile skin. Although an inciting cause may never be found, the process has developed after exposure to infectious agents (particularly mycoplasma and herpes) or as a drug reaction, typically to penicillin or penicillinlike drugs. Immune complexes may be deposited around superficial dermal blood vessels, leading to vascular damage and leakage of plasma and cells, with edema.[16] Although erythema multiforme involves the skin alone, a variant of erythema multiforme, Stevens-Johnson syndrome, is characterized by extensive skin lesions and mucous membrane involvement. Stevens-Johnson syndrome is associated with high fever and a substantial mortality, owing to fluid loss from areas of epidermal sloughing similar to a severe burn.

Grossly, erythema multiforme, as would be expected from the name, has varied appearances. A characteristic lesion is the erythematous papule that evolves into a bulla. The target lesion is a macule or papule topped with a vesicle. Some lesions may be hemorrhagic.[22]

Microscopically, the lesions of erythema multiforme generally show a marked lymphohistiocytic perivascular infiltrate and a similar process at the dermal-epidermal junction. Eosinophilic necrosis of keratinocytes and damage to the base of the epidermis may lead to subepidermal blister formation (Fig. 35-4). More severe lesions, including the Stevens-Johnson syndrome, show extensive epidermal necrosis and separation of the epidermis from the dermis.[1]

The fixed drug eruption is essentially a variant of erythema multiforme. It is an allergic reaction that appears at the same location on the skin each time the drug is given. It may grossly resemble an individual lesion or group of lesions of erythema multiforme, with an erythematous papule becoming vesicular. The histologic appearance is the same as that of erythema multiforme. Many drugs can provoke the fixed drug eruption, but barbituates are frequently associated with this process.[27]

Behçet's Syndrome

Behçet's syndrome is an unusual disorder that often has genital involvement. This rare disease is diagnosed in individuals with recurring ulcers of the mouth, penis, and scrotum (vulva and vagina in women) and uveitis. In addition, arthritis and thrombophlebitis may occur.[10]

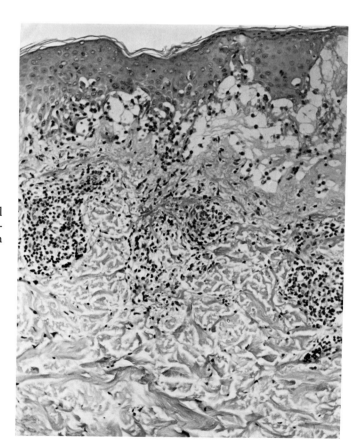

Fig. 35-4 Erythema multiforme. Subepidermal blisters, keratinocyte necrosis, and chronic inflammation at the dermal-epidermal junction are illustrated. ×128.

The etiology of Behçet's syndrome is quite uncertain. Viral infections, environmental agents, and autoimmune causes have been suggested, but recent studies appear inconclusive. An immunologic cause is suggested by reports of increased serum C9 levels, changes in T-cell function, and decreased to absent secretory IgA component.[4]

Young adult males are more commonly affected, and the disease may recur over years. Visual loss is perhaps the most serious complication, although thrombosis of the vena cava has been observed repeatedly.

On the penis, the patients may develop 2-mm to 10-mm ulcers with a necrotic base that are quite painful. The lesions often persist for 1 to 2 weeks, regress, and then reappear with exacerbations of the disease. The histopathology of the lesions is not specific, but biopsies of the skin or mouth in the early stages reveal the common microscopic picture of the disease—marked perivascular inflammation with lymphohistiocytic cells. Eventually, there is endothelial swelling and fibrinoid necrosis of blood vessels and more pronounced inflammation, a vasculitislike pattern. The ensuing necrosis of the epidermis and underlying tissue produces the clinical appearance of the deep, painful ulcer.[10]

No satisfactory treatment is available for this crippling disorder that often leads to blindness. Colchicine has shown some promise, but is still under investigation.[34]

Nonspecific Balanitis

Inflammation of the penile skin (glans and foreskin) is referred to as balanitis, or more specifically, balanoposthitis. This disorder has a multiplicity of causes in uncircumcised men. Poor hygiene, accumulation of smegma, and minor trauma can all lead to irritation of the skin in this area. Pemphigus vegetans, a rare variant of pemphigus, has been reported as a cause of chronic balanitis.[8a] The moist environment around the penis can provide an inviting field for the growth of numerous microbial agents. The application of ointments, harsh soaps, or other external

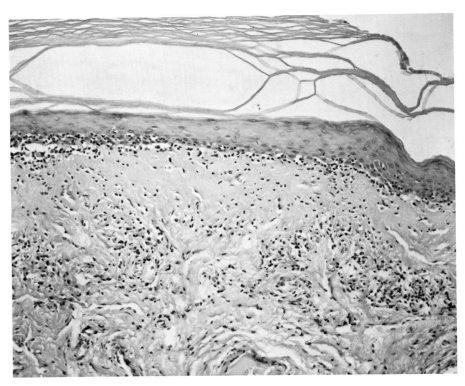

Fig. 35-5 Balanitis xerotica obliterans. The epidermal thinning is readily apparent. Eosinophilic change in the upper dermis and degeneration of the basal epidermal layer is also seen. ×128.

agents may further irritate the membrane. Histologic examination may reveal marked acute and chronic inflammation of the tissues. Ulceration is possible. Culture of exudate is helpful in characterizing the infective or superinfective organisms. Meticulous attention to hygiene in the uncircumcised man can alleviate or prevent nonspecific balanitis.

Balanitis Xerotica Obliterans

Balanitis xerotica obliterans is a chronic disease that may affect the prepuce, glans, and, rarely, the urethral meatus. It is of unknown etiology and may affect all age groups, although the incidence is increased after middle age. A few cases have been reported to cause stenosis of the urethral meatus in uncircumcised children.[19] When found in women, commonly in the vulvar region, it is known as lichen sclerosus et atrophicus.

The lesion first appears as a whitish plaque, causing a mottled appearance to the glans and/or prepuce.[24] Pruritis is often a symptom.

On microscopic examination, the picture is usually characteristic. There is often hyperkeratosis. The epidermis is thinned and atrophic in appearance, with thinning of the rete pegs. The most striking findings are in the dermis, as the papillary and reticular dermis develop a distinctive washed-out appearance. The dermal collagen becomes rather homogeneous, eosinophilic, and edematous, forming a smooth, continuous band along the dermal-epidermal junction, usually free of inflammation (Figs. 35-5 and 35-6). There is some capillary ectasia and a scattered chronic inflammatory infiltrate in the dermis below the band of smoothed-out homogeneous collagen. The basal layer of the epidermis may have undergone some degree of liquefactive degeneration.[22]

There is some controversy among both urologists and gynecologists as to the relationship of balanitis xerotica obliterans (lichen sclerosus et atrophicus) to the eventual development of squamous cell carcinoma.[22] Although a few cases have been reported anecdotally in the literature, a long-term study of many women with the disorder concluded that the cancer

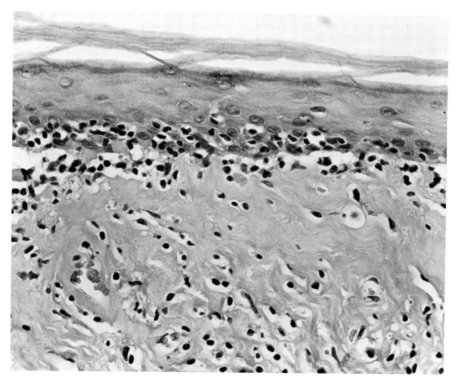

Fig. 35-6 Balanitis xerotica obliterans. The degeneration of the basal layer ("waxy") is more evident in this high-power photomicrograph. ×320.

risk was quite small.[22] In that series, only one patient developed genital squamous carcinoma, 12 years after the initial diagnosis of lichen sclerosus. A most unusual case of balanitis xerotica obliterans developed on the stump of a penis amputated for squamous cell carcinoma some 3.5 years earlier.[26]

Regardless of the questionable neoplastic potential of this lesion, most patients will require long-term follow-up care because of the symptomatic problems this slowly progressive process may produce. The collagenization of the upper dermis eventually results in wrinkling and retraction of tissues. The prepuce may become densely adherent to the glans. Pain and deterioration of sexual function may develop. If the lesion is at the urethral meatus, obstruction may develop because the sclerosing process may produce stenosis around the orifice.[24]

Zoon's Balanitis

Another type of balanitis that may often mimic a more serious genital lesion is chronic plasma cell balanitis of Zoon. This lesion appears as a shiny, sometimes velvety patch on the glans and prepuce. The plaque is generally well circumscribed (Fig. 35-7). On external examination, Zoon's balanitis may often resemble erythroplasia of Queyrat. However, the histologic appearance and clinical behavior of the two entities are quite different and indicate the need for biopsy of all suspicious genital sores.

Erythroplasia of Queyrat has an associated chronic inflammatory dermal infiltrate with associated plasma cells, but the major changes are in the thickened epidermis. That lesion, as discussed subsequently, represents an intraepithelial carcinoma (carcinoma in situ).

In balanitis of Zoon, by contrast, the epidermis is quite benign. It is thinned with a shortening of rete ridges. The epithelium shows maturation, and atypia and mitoses are not seen, as opposed to the picture of carcinoma in situ. The dermis is densely infiltrated with plasma cells. In addition, dermal blood vessels are prominent and dilated.[42]

The keratinocytes show a change characteristic of Zoon's balanitis in which the cells become diamond shaped, with the long axis horizontal (Fig. 35-8). There is also marked edema between keratinocytes that emphasizes the diamond-shaped cells.[46]

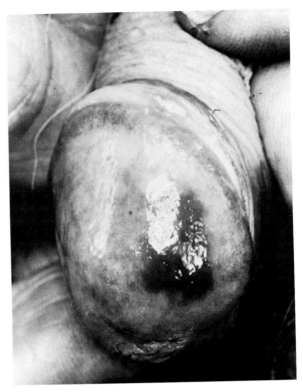

Fig. 35-7 Zoon's balanitis. Shiny, glazed macular erythema of the glans penis. (From MacDonald DM: Br J Dermatol 105:195, 1981.)

On external inspection balanitis of Zoon has been confused with syphilis. The surface of the lesion may bleed, which may suggest a variant of carcinoma. Histologic examination should demonstrate the benign nature of the epidermis.

Hidradenitis Suppurativa

Hidradenitis suppurativa is a chronic dermatologic disease that may be extremely uncomfortable and disfiguring. It does not affect the penile shaft (because it is hairless), but often involves the groin and scrotal regions in addition to the axillae. The chronic inflammatory process may cause skin breakdown, abscesses, and sinus tracts, along with the folliculitis that represents the basic pathology of the disorder.

On microscopic examination, one finds a destructive acute and chronic inflammatory process involving the hair follicles and apocrine glands. The earliest lesions develop around hair follicles. Polymorphs and

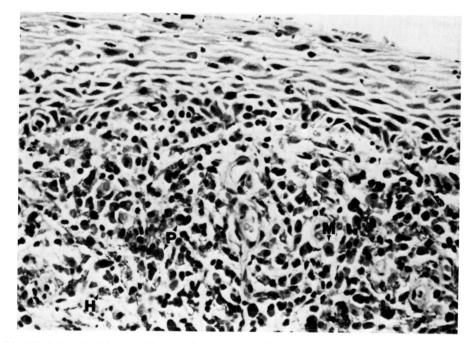

Fig. 35-8 Zoon's Balanitis. There are lozenge-shaped keratinocytes, along with loss of both the granular layer and the rete ridges. Plasma cells (P) are numerous, as well as hemosiderin-laden macrophages (H), and mast cells. ×280. (From MacDonald DM: Br J Dermatol 105:195, 1981.)

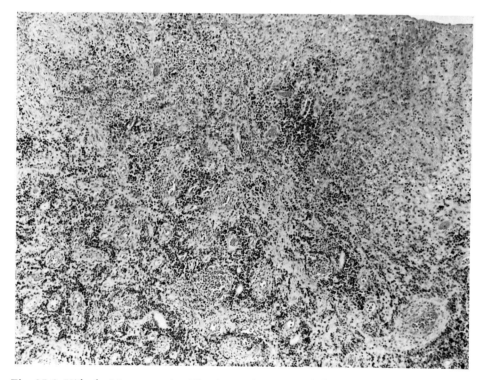

Fig. 35-9 Hidradenitis suppurativa. The destructive acute and chronic inflammatory process of hidradenitis suppurativa is illustrated here. The adnexal structures are virtually obliterated. ×72.

lymphocytes are seen, with confluent abscesses developing. These abscesses may obliterate the normal skin structure (Fig. 35-9). Chronic draining sinus tracts may form with time. Bacterial superinfection of the tissue is a frequent development, with *Staphylococcus aureus* a common pathogen. The lesions may heal with dense and disfiguring scarring. Foreign body giant cells surrounding incompletely digested hairs are observed in many cases.

Antibiotic therapy of secondary bacterial invaders may ameliorate the process. Many patients require surgery to remove the affected areas. The cause of hidradenitis suppurativa is not known with certainty. It is more common in diabetics. Although an autoimmune process directed at hair follicles has been proposed as an etiology, others have suggested a local defect in apocrine gland drainage, with obstruction of secretions leading to local inflammation and infec-

tion.[15] The good response to surgery and the limitation of the disease to the groin and axillae may support this concept.

Crohn's Disease

An unusual complication of a systemic disease has been reported to mimic hidradenitis suppurativa. A patient with extensive Crohn's disease of the gastrointestinal tract developed severe penile and scrotal edema with draining sinuses. Circumcision was performed because of severe phimosis, and the skin had the features of Crohn's disease — noncaseating granulomata, giant cells, and marked edema[11] (Fig. 35-10). These are extremely rare manifestations of the disorder, but again emphasize the need for biopsy of unusual penile lesions. Another patient had a penile ulcer, initially regarded as syphilis. Biopsy and clinical

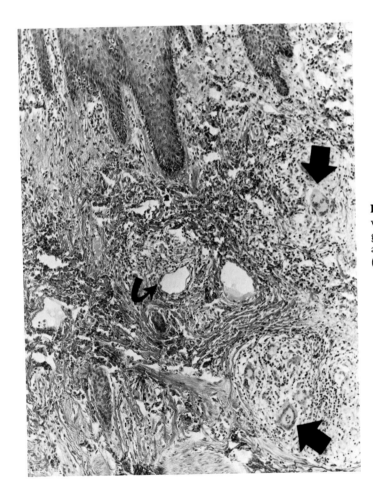

Fig. 35-10 Crohn's Disease. Microscopic view of scrotal skin showing noncaseating granulomata and giant cells (straight arrows) and dilated lymphatics (curved arrow). ×50. (From Cockburn et al.,[11] with permission.)

history showed changes consistent with Crohn's disease.[45] A young adult developed a urethropenile rectal fistula that was difficult to manage after a long history of Crohn's colitis.[3]

INFECTIONS

Syphilis

Perhaps the most famous of penile infections is syphilis. The protean manifestations of syphilis are well known. In addition, the story of the history of syphilis is among the most fascinating in the annals of medicine. Although such a discussion is beyond the scope of this work, it should be noted that the arrival of syphilis in Western Europe in all likelihood did coincide with the return of Columbus from the New World. Syphilis was, in the sixteenth century, a more virulent, acute process.[38] The organism has apparently developed a more benign symbiotic relationship with mankind.

Syphilis results from infection by the spirochete *Treponema pallidum*. The natural history of acquired syphilis can be divided into three major stages. First, after contact with an infected host and an incubation period of about 3 weeks, the primary lesion, the chancre, appears at the place of inoculation. Without treatment the chancre will heal in 3 to 6 weeks, with slight scarring remaining. Six to 8 weeks after the appearance of the chancre, secondary syphilis in its varying guises develops. The maculopapular eruption seen on the palms and soles is perhaps the best known of these. Others include papulosquamous lesions resembling psoriasis.[27] The genitalia, as will be seen shortly, may also be affected at this stage. After the lesions of secondary syphilis regress, about one-third of patients enter a period of latency that usually lasts 1 to 10 years but may be even longer before the development of tertiary syphilis. This stage is characterized by destructive, and sometimes fatal, lesions of the nervous system and cardiovascular system. The gumma, a destructive granulomatous process, may appear almost anywhere in the body.[40]

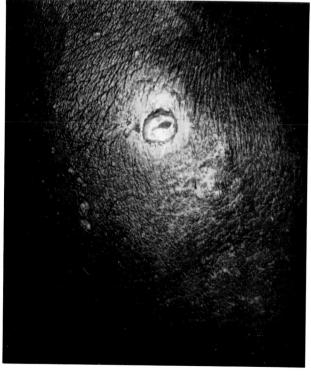

Fig. 35-11 Primary syphilis. A penile chancre is seen here, showing superficially eroded papules. (Courtesy of S. Lamberg.)

The traditional description of the lesion of primary syphilis, the chancre, is of an indurated, painless, superficially eroded papule.[27] It is located at the point of the entrance of the spirochete. The lesion may develop in the glans or along the shaft, and its entrance is faciliated by microscopic breaks in the integument (Fig. 35-11).

Review of the more recent literature indicates that atypical chancres are far more common than the traditional teaching suggests.[23] A large number of patients may present with multiple ulcers.[33] Some chancres are painful and soft instead of painless and indurated.[33] The problem with the atypical chancres is that they may be confused with herpes and other veneral infections.[49] Certainly the need for vigorous diagnostic evaluation of penile lesions, including dark-field microscopy, serology, and bacterial culture, is evident.[23]

On biopsy of the chancre, one sees a thinned epidermis with central erosion. Marked endothelial cell proliferation of the dermal vessels is a hallmark, with a dense surrounding lymphoplasmacytic infiltrate (Fig. 35-12). A variety of special stains for spirochetes, usually found in perivascular locations, have been developed including the Warthin–Starry stain, although the organisms are frequently difficult to find in fixed tissue. Positive control material is not often readily available. Dark-field microscopy of fluid from a fresh lesion may show the corkscrew movements of the spiral-shaped organism. When fresh fluid is avail-

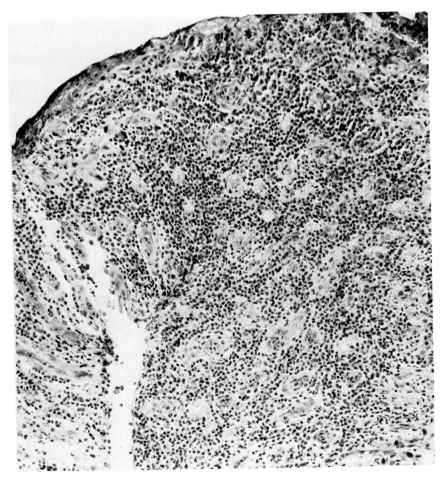

Fig. 35-12 Primary syphilis. Dense perivascular plasma cell infiltrate, superficial ulceration, and endothelial cell swelling are illustrated. ×120. (Courtesy of A. Hood.)

able, dark-field microscopy is a more reliable means of identifying the organism than the Warthin–Starry stain of histologic material.

In secondary syphilis, the glans penis may be covered with an elevated, flat papule (mucous patch). Histologically, the typical lesions are covered with an acanthotic epidermis (Fig. 35-13). Marked endothelial cell swelling and proliferation is again prominent, with extensive numbers of plasma cells surrounding the blood vessels.[27] These lesions are highly infective, and many spirochetes may be observed upon dark-field microscopy. Unfortunately, these dermatologic changes are not always pronounced, and diagnosis by histologic means alone may be difficult.

Similar secondary lesions in the groin (a moist, intertriginous area) can coalesce to form plaquelike lesions, the condyloma lata.

Tertiary syphilis, particularly of the gummatous variety, is extremely rare in Western civilization and usually does not involve the penis.

Chancroid

Chancroid is another veneral infection that commonly involves the penis. It is caused by *Hemophilus ducreyi*, a gram-negative rod that in culture grows in parallel groups like a "school of fish." The disease is rather rare in the United States and affects males much more commonly than females.

After sexual contact, the disease may become manifest within 5 days. The initial lesion is a small pustule that eventually develops into an ulceration. Autoinoculation via scratching may produce additional lesions. As with other veneral penile infections, the organism usually enters via a break in the integument.[25] The ulceration may appear on the glans or shaft (Fig. 35-14). The ulcer may bleed readily but may heal with scarring. However, lack of proper hygiene may lead to a more destructive ulceration. Lymphadenopathy in the inguinal area is common, with inflamed, tender, matted nodes. The overlying

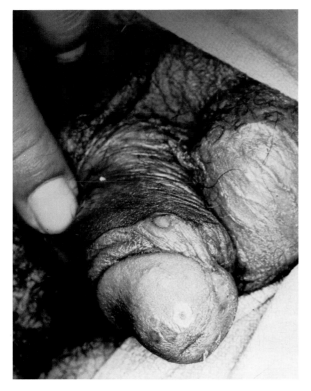

Fig. 35-13 Secondary syphilis. Flat papules of the mucous patch are evident on the glans penis. (Courtesy of S. Lamberg.)

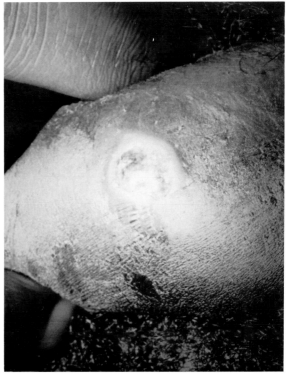

Fig. 35-14 Chandroid. Ulcerated penile pustule. (Courtesy of S. Lamberg.)

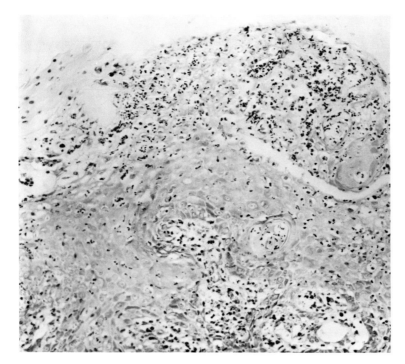

Fig. 35-15 Chancroid. Surface layer of the ulcer, with necrotic epidermis, polymorphs, and fibrin. ×144. (Courtesy of A. Hood.)

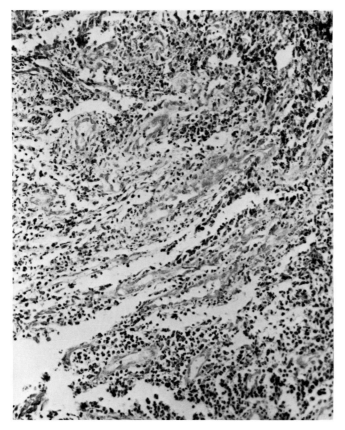

Fig. 35-16 Chancroid. Midzone of the ulcer, with endothelial cell proliferation, inflammation, and neovascularization. ×149. (Courtesy of A. Hood.)

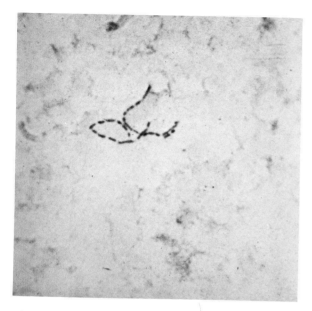

Fig. 35-17 Chancroid. Chain of short, gram-negative rods of *H. ducreyi.* (Courtesy of S. Lamberg.)

skin may break down and drain.[28] The inguinal lymphadenopathy is often rather characteristic.

Biopsy of the lesion of chancroid may reveal a multilayered process. The surface layer is the base of the ulcer. This is necrotic tissue with fibrin and polymorphonuclear leukocytes present (Fig. 35-15). The organism may be seen in this layer. The midzone of the lesion shows extensive endothelial cell proliferation (Fig. 35-16). The newly developed blood vessels grow in a palisading fashion relative to the ulcer base. The lower layer is filled with plasma cells and lymphocytes.[43] The syphilitic chancre is nontender, whereas that of chancroid is usually quite tender. In addition, the multilayered process of chancroid is rather distinctive and not seen in syphilis.[29] However, the diagnosis of chancroid is difficult to establish in many instances and is frequently made by exclusion or by therapeutic trial of sulfonamides. Penicillin, useful in syphilis, is ineffective in chancroid. The organisms, gram-negative rods forming short chains, may be demonstrated in the lesion upon smear of the exudate (Fig. 35-17), yet secondary infection may obscure the appearance of the organisms. The organism is fastidi-

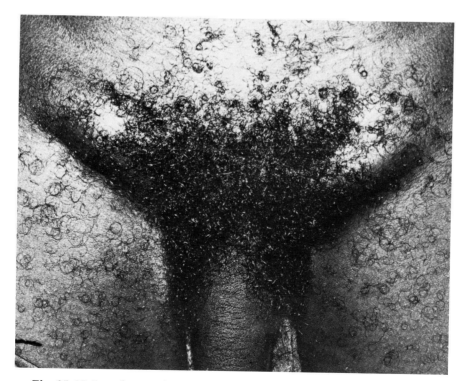

Fig. 35-18 Lymphogranuloma venereum. Prominent inguinal lymphadenopathy.

ous and does not easily grow on regular culture media. Careful biopsy should reveal the characteristic multi-layer ulcer. This, combined with clinicial evaluation and confirmatory culture or Gram stain, will contribute to accurate diagnosis.[29]

Lymphogranuloma Venereum

Lymphogranuloma venereum is a venereal infection caused by *Chlamydia trachomatis.* Asyptomatic carriers of the disease, especially women, may be a reservoir of the infection. A recent study indicates that as many as 10.6 percent of sexually active heterosexual men may be asymptomatic carriers.[25a] The disease first appears as a small red papule on the penile skin, usually around the coronal sulcus. The penile lesion is evanescent, heals promptly without scarring, and is commonly unseen by the patient. Then the patient develops inguinal lymphadenopathy with multiple fluctuant nodes attached to the overlying skin (Fig. 35-18). Multiple sinuses may form, as opposed to the picture in chancroid in which a single sinus is common. The lymphatic lesions of lymphogranuloma venereum are quite destructive and may leave permanent scarring. Eventually, deep lymphatic and rectal skin involvement may lead to rectal strictures with squamous cell carcinoma a possible sequel.[28]

The histopathology of the genital lesions of lymphogranuloma venereum is most interesting. The surface of the lesion is usually ulcerated with necrotic tissue and many polymorphonuclear leukocytes. Below this is an area of more chronic inflammation.

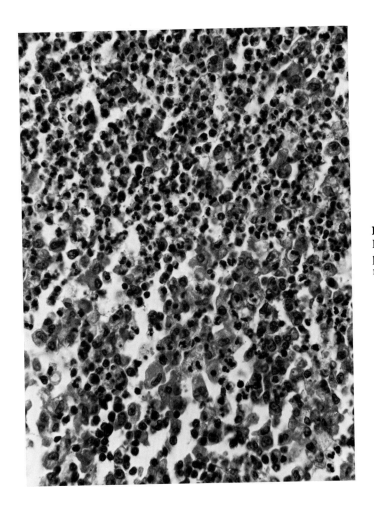

Fig. 35-19 Lymphogranuloma venereum. Large accumulations of necrotic tissue and polymorphs within the lymph node (stellate microabscess) are illustrated. ×420.

Mononuclear cells surround and invade the walls of blood vessels. These cells coalesce to form granulomalike structures with eventual compression and obliteration of the blood vessels. The tissue becomes necrotic, and acute inflammatory cells enter the area.[44]

A similar perivascular process takes place in the inguinal lymph nodes with necrosis of cortical tissue giving way to the formation of accumulations of acute inflammatory cells in a stellate pattern (Fig. 35-19). These stellate abscesses may lead to tissue breakdown and formation of sinus tracts. In opposition to the basic vascular processes seen in syphilis, endothelial cell proliferation and thrombosis are not seen in lymphogranuloma venereum.[44]

Granuloma Inguinale

Granuloma inguinale is a venereal disease caused by *Calymmatobacterium granulomatis,* the Donovan body. This is a gram-negative organism of the *Klebsiella* family. The disease appears as a raised ulcer with a serpiginous margin, usually on the glans or foreskin. The lesions may bleed but are generally painless.[27]

On biopsy, the ulcer is surrounded by keratinocytes with marked acanthosis (Fig. 35-20). Histiocytes and plasma cells are at the center of the ulcer (Fig. 35-21). On careful examination, Donovan bodies may be found inside the cytoplasm of some histiocytes.[18] Silver stain may reveal the small, intracellular structures that often have a saftey pin-like appearance.[27] A better method of diagnosis involves crushing a piece

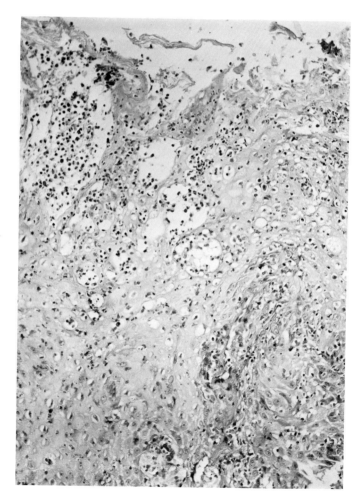

Fig. 35-20 Granuloma inguinale. Acanthosis and ulceration of surface. ✕ 140. (Courtesy of A. Hood.)

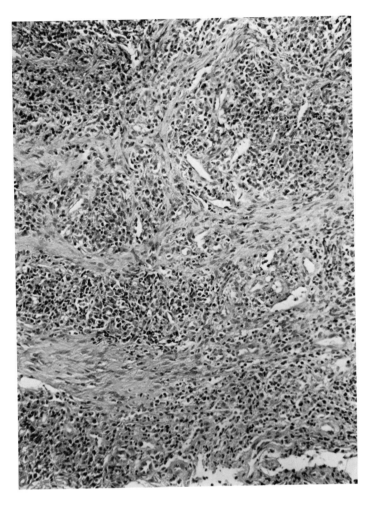

Fig. 35-21 Granuloma inguinale. Deeper into the ulcer are plasma cells and histiocytes. ×140. (Courtesy of A. Hood.)

of the lesion under a glass slide and staining with Wright stain, which reveals the rod-shaped organisms (Fig. 35-22). The lesions may become quite destructive and heal with scarring. Squamous cell carcinoma may develop at the edge of the ulcers.[28]

Candida Infections

The glans, particularly in uncircumcised men, may be affected by candida balanitis owing to the moist environment. The glans may show erythema (Fig. 35-23) and pustule formation with collections of polymorphs in the superficial epidermis (Fig. 35-24). The characteristic budding yeast forms may also be found in the uppermost layers of the epidermis. In addition, scraping and KOH preparation or culture may be used to establish the diagnosis.

Candida balanitis may be found in immunosuppressed patients. It is also seen in diabetics. The onset of candida balanitis in an otherwise normal-appearing male should arouse suspicion of latent or unsuspected diabetes or acquired immunodeficiency syndrome.

Scabies

Scabies is a very common generalized dermatologic infection that may involve the penis. It is usually transmitted through contaminated bedding. In general, scabies can be diagnosed upon external examination. The mite *Sarcoptes scabiei* is the causative agent and produces vesicles that later develop into tunnel-like lesions as the mite burrows through the skin. Eventually the intensely pruritic lesions become crusted (Fig. 35-25). The mite is extremely hard to

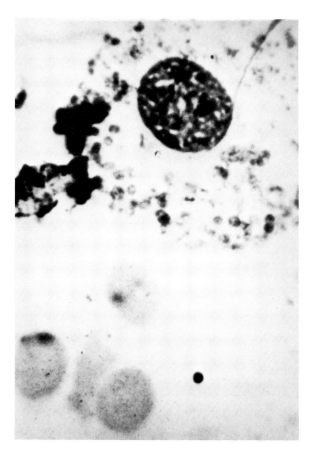

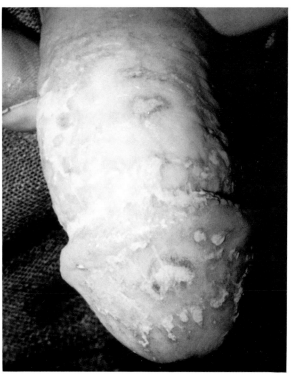

Fig. 35-23 Candida balanitis. Extensive pustule formation and crusting. (Courtesy of S. Lamberg.)

Fig. 35-22 Granuloma inguinale. Intracellular Donovan bodies, safety pin-like, within the cytoplasm of a histiocyte (left), much smaller than its dark, ovoid nucleus. (Courtesy of S. Lamberg.)

find in biopsy specimens because it digs into the keratinous layer. Routine sections often show only hyperkeratosis and dermal inflammation, along with edema of the epidermis.[35] A better way to attempt the diagnosis is to scrape some of the tunnels and examine the material directly under the microscope.

Herpesvirus Infections

Genital herpes simplex virus (HSV) infections of the genitalia have become medical and epidemiologic problems of immense magnitude. This painful, chronic disorder can produce disabling recurrences. In addition, the disease may be transmitted to the fetus with disastrous results. In the United States, herpes may be the most common venereal disease.

Although the lesions of genital herpes can be produced by either type of virus, HSV-1 or HSV-2, HSV-2 appears to be the more common type, causing approximately 90 percent of first episodes.[13] Herpes begins as a painful, vesiculated lesion. The blisters may rupture and produce extreme discomfort.[48] Multiple vesicles may affect large areas of the penile skin (Fig. 35-26). Vesicles, however, may not be present in immunosuppressed patients, as was seen in a patient treated for Hodgkin's disease.[41] In addition to pain, there may be fever, dysuria, and inguinal adenopathy.[12] Primary infections last between 2 and 3 weeks. As many as one-half of patients infected with HSV-1 will have recurrent infections, whereas nearly 90 percent of patients with HSV-2 will have recurrences. This may relate to a higher rate of involvement of the sacral ganglia, where the virus can reside, for HSV-2.[12] The virus passes via sensory nerves in the skin up to the sacral sensory ganglia.

There is still considerable uncertainty whether the rate of recurrence of genital herpes changes over time.

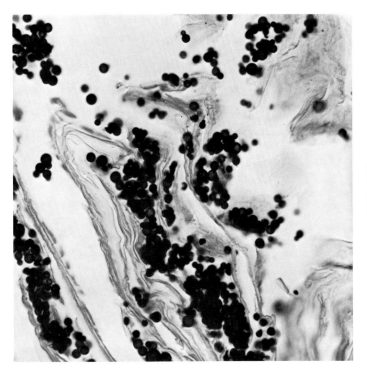

Fig. 35-24 Candida balanitis. Characteristic budding yeast forms are seen in the most superficial layer of the skin. Periodic acid-Schiff, ×510.

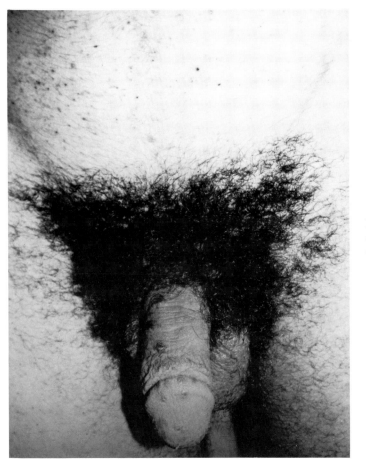

Fig. 35-25 Scabies. Generalized vesicular eruption affecting penis and surrounding areas. (Courtesy of S. Lamberg.)

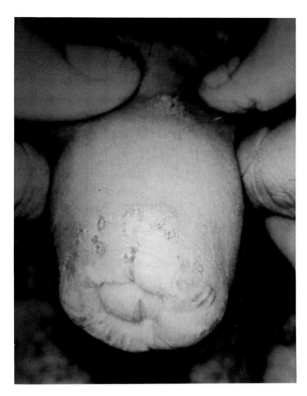

Fig. 35-26 Herpes. Multiple crusted vesicles of herpesvirus infection of the penis. (Courtesy of S. Lamberg.)

A recent survey suggests that, with time, the rate of recurrence diminishes. However, this was in a small study group.[12] As mentioned, HSV-2 recurs more frequently than HSV-1, owing to more extensive sacral ganglia involvement. This may be due to differences in the size of the inoculum, with the volume of the inoculum apparently related to the extent of involvement of the ganglia.[12] Specific inciting factors for recurrence of HSV-1 infections have been described and include psychologic stress, menstruation, exposure to sunlight (for lip lesions), and trauma.[27] The immune or biochemical processes leading to recurrence in the presence of one of the above phenomena are totally uncertain. The inciting factors noted above for HSV-1 do not appear to affect HSV-2.[27]

A rapid method of establishing the diagnosis is the Tzanck test. The vesicle is unroofed, and material from the base is smeared on a slide. It may be stained with Wright stain, or a cytology preparation may be made. Multinucleate giant cells may be seen and es-tablish the diagnosis (Fig. 35-27). Intranuclear inclusions are seen as a hyalinized ground-glass or hazy appearance in the central portion of the nucleus.

Culture techniques are also available. In fact, culture may be the most accurate means of diagnosis (85 percent), as opposed to immunoperoxidase visualization in tissues (50 percent) or direct scraping (40 percent). Electron microscopy may be done but is only rarely positive and probably not justified.[14]

On biopsy, an intraepithelial vesicle is the typical feature. The infected cells undergo ballooning degeneration. The cytoplasm in these cells undergoes intense swelling and manifests an eosinophilic appearance. This smooth, pinkish look may be viewed as a ground-glass cytoplasm.[27] A few multinucleate cells may be observed (Fig. 35-28). With swelling comes loss of intercellular bridges and cell separation or acantholysis. This separation is responsible for the formation of the vesicle in the central portion of the epidermis. Surrounding the vesicle itself, cells with intranuclear inclusions may be seen. These intranuclear inclusions are intensely eosinophilic round structures with a surrounding clear halo.[27] The dermis below the vesicle shows a mixed acute-chronic inflammatory infiltrate with occasional damage to the vascular walls.[27]

Electron microscopy reveals a spherical virus with a 40-nm core and a 100-nm virion. The virus is morphologically identical to the varicella-zoster agent.[27]

Candida superinfections of herpetic ulcers are not uncommon. The possibility of simultaneous herpes-candida infections should be considered when evaluating or treating gential herpes.[13]

Although the oncogenic potential of the herpesvirus in females has been discussed at length, no significant evidence has been presented for such a role in the male external genitalia.[6]

Although genital herpes, syphilis, chancroid, lymphogranuloma venereum, and granuloma inguinale all cause penile ulcers, there are significant histopathologic differences between them, as previously discussed. Serologic testing for syphilis is virtually mandatory in any patient with penile lesions. Serologic testing for herpes appears useful primarily for epidemiologic studies, rather than for routine clinical diagnosis.

The recent development of acyclovir, a purine analog antiviral agent, may offer some relief for patients affected by herpes. The drug may be given intra-

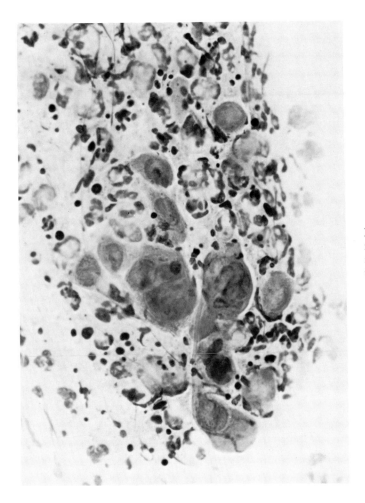

Fig. 35-27 Herpes. A Tzanck preparation reveals numerous multinucleate giant cells in material smeared from the base of a penile ulcer. Giemsa, ×510.

venously, orally, or topically. Although acyclovir reduces the severity and duration of attacks of both primary and recurrent herpes, it does not prevent recurrences.[14] In one recent study, the interval between primary attack and recurrence was shorter in the treated group, although the patients receiving acyclovir had less discomfort during the attacks.[30] The oral route of administration is the easiest and most effective. Acyclovir does not cure herpes. It just suppresses the virus. The natural history of the disease is softened but not really changed by its use.[30] Nevertheless, the herpesvirus produces such profound discomfort, sexual difficulty, and psychologic disturbance that medications of even partial effectiveness are to be welcomed.

Tuberculosis

A most unusual infection that may be spread by venereal contact is penile tuberculosis. The few reported cases have been found in underdeveloped countries. The lesions may be secondary to pulmonary tuberculosis or may be primary, after sexual contact with a woman with genital tuberculosis. The lesions develop as ulcerated masses on the glans penis in the primary cases. Biopsy shows the typical features of tuberculosis—caseation necrosis, giant cells, and epithelioid histiocytes.[2] Culture of the granulomas is advisable. Some of the lesions, called penis tuberculides, have shown the histologic features of tuberculosis but acid-fast organisms have not appeared on

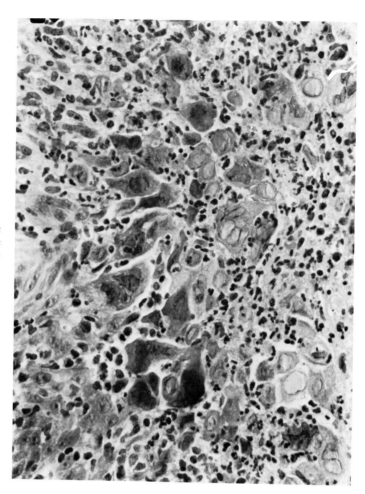

Fig. 35-28 Herpes. Biopsy of a herpetic ulcer reveals many nuclei with eosinophilic inclusions. A few giant cells are present at the bottom. ×320.

stain or culture. However, they have apparently responded to antituberculous therapy.[32,36]

To complicate diagnostic matters, sarcoidosis is an extremely rare, but reported, penile lesion. It presents with the typical noncaseating granulomas described in the disorder. However, the ultimate diagnosis was made only when the multisystem nature of the disease manifested.[39] This should be kept in mind when granulomatous lesions of the genitalia are evaluated.

REFERENCES

1. Ackerman AB: Histologic Diagnosis of Inflammatory Skin Disease. Lea & Febiger, Philadelphia, 1978
2. Agarwalla B, Mohanty G, Sahu L, Rath R: Tuberculosis of the penis: report of 2 cases. J Urol 124:927, 1980
3. Alperstein G, Daum F, Aiges H et al: Urethroperineal-rectal fistula in Crohn's disease. J Pediatr Surg 18:311, 1983
4. Ammann AJ, Johnson A, Fyfe GA et al: Behçet syndrome. J Pediatr 107:41, 1985
5. Anderson K: The painful, non-indurated chancre. Acta Derm Venereol 58:554, 1978
6. Aurelian L, Kessler I, Rosenshein N, Barbour G: Viruses and gynecologic cancers. Cancer 48:455, 1981
7. Baer RL, Gigli I: Allergic eczematous contact dermatitis. p. 512. In Fitzpatrick TB, Eisen AZ et al (eds): Dermatology in General Medicine. 2nd Ed. McGraw-Hill, New York, 1979
8. Black RL: Psoriatic arthritis. p. 248. In Fitzpatrick TB, Eisen AZ et al (eds): Dermatology in General Medicine. 2nd Ed. McGraw-Hill, New York, 1979

8a. Castle WN, Wentzell M, Schwartz BK, et al: Chronic balanitis owing to pemphigus vegetans. J Urol 137:289, 1987

9. Cavanaugh RM, Jr.: Pityriasis rosea in children. Clin Pediatr 22:200, 1983

10. Chajek T, Fainaru M: Behçet's disease: report of 41 cases and a review of the literature. Medicine 54:179, 1975

11. Cockburn A, Krolikowski J, Baloch K, Roth R: Crohn's disease of penile and scrotal skin. Urology 15:596, 1980

12. Corey L, Adams HG, Brown RA, Holmes KK: Genital herpes simplex virus infections: clinical manifestations, course, and complications. Ann Intern Med 198:958, 1983

13. Corey L, Vontver L, Brown Z: Genital herpes simplex infections. Semin Dermatol 3:89, 1984

14. Corey L, Holmes KK: Genital herpes simplex virus infections: current concepts in diagnosis, therapy, and prevention. Ann Intern Med 98:973, 1983

15. Dvorak V, Root R, MacGregor R: Host-defense mechanisms in hidraenitis suppurativa. Arch Dermatol 113:450, 1977

16. Elias PM, Fritsch PO: Erythema multiforme. p. 295. In Fitzpatrick TB, Eisen AZ et al (eds): Dermatology in General Medicine. 2nd Ed. McGraw-Hill, New York, 1979

17. Farber EM, VanScott EJ: Psoriasis. p. 233. In Fitzpatrick TB, Eisen AZ et al (eds): Dermatology in General Medicine. 2nd Ed. McGraw-Hill, New York, 1979

18. Fritz G, Hubler W, Dodson R, Rudolph A: Mutilating granuloma inguinale. Arch Dermatol 111:1464, 1975

19. Garat JM, Chechile G, Algaba F, Santaularia JM: Balanitis xerotica obliterans in children. J Urol 136:436, 1986

20. Gordon M, Johnson W: Histopathology and histochemistry of psoriasis. Arch Dermatol 95:402, 1967

21. Ham AW: Histology. 7th Ed. JB Lippincott, Philadelphia, 1974

22. Hart W, Norris H, Helwig E: Relation of lichen sclerosus et atrophicus of the vulva to the development of carcinoma. Obstet Gynecol 45:369, 1975

23. Headley J, Pilest N, Posnikoff J, Spence C: Nontypical syphilitic chancres. Arch Dermatol 117:2, 1981

24. Herschorn S, Colapinto V: Balanitis xerotica obliterans involving anterior urethra. Urology 14:592, 1979

25. Kampmeier R: Chancroid. p. 493. In Hoeprich P (ed): Infectious Diseases. 3rd Ed. Harper & Row, Philadelphia, 1983

25a. Karem GH, Martin DH, Flotte TR, et al: Asymptomatic Chlamydia trachomatis infections among sexually active men. J Infect Dis 154:900, 1986

26. Khezri AA: Balanitis xerotica obliterans on stump of amputated penis. Br J Urol 58:454, 1986

27. Lever W, Lever GS: Histopathology of the Skin. 6th Ed. JB Lippincott, Philadelphia, 1983

28. Lynch PJ: Sexually transmitted diseases: granuloma inguinale, lymphogranuloma venereum, chancroid, and infectious syphilis. Clin Obstet Gynecol 21:1041, 1978

29. Margolis RJ, Hood AF: Chancroid: diagnosis and treatment. J Am Acad Dermatol 6:493, 1982

30. Mertz G, Critchlow C, Benedetti J et al: Double-blind placebo-controlled trial of oral acyclovir in first-episode genital herpes infection. JAMA 252:1147, 1984

31. Nickel W, Plumb R: Other infections and inflammations of the external genitalia. p. 640. In Harrison JH et al (eds): Campbell's Urology. 4th Ed. Vol. 1. WB Saunders, Philadelphia, 1978

32. Nishigori C, Taniguchi , S, Hayakawa M, Imamura S: Penis tuberculides: papulonecrotic tuberculides on the glans penis. Dermatologica 172:93, 1986

33. Notowicz A, Menke H: Atypical urinary syphilitic lesions on the penis. Dermatologica 147:328, 1973

34. O'Duffy JD, Lehner T, Barnes C: Summary of the Third International Conference on Behçet's Disease. J Rheumatol 10:154, 1983

35. Okun M, Edelstein L: Gross and Microscopic Pathology of the Skin. Vol. 1. Dermatopathology Foundation Press, Boston, 1976

36. Ramesh V: Genital tuberculids — an appropriate term. Dermatologica 173:155, 1986

37. Rook A, Wilkinson D, Ebling F: Textbook of Dermatology. 3rd Ed. Vol. 2. Blackwell Scientific Publications, Oxford, 1979

38. Rosebury T: Microbes and Morals. Viking, New York, 1971

39. Rubenstein I, Baum GL, Hiss Y: Sarcoidosis of the penis: report of a case. J Urol 135:1016, 1986

40. Rudolph A: Syphilis. p. 611. In Hoeprich P (ed): Infectious Diseases. 3rd Ed. Harper & Row, Philadelphia, 1983

41. Schneiderman H, Robert NJ, Walker S, Memoli VA: Herpes without vesicles: limited, recurrent genital lesions in an immunodebilitated host. South Med J 79:368, 1986

42. Sehgal V, Rege V, Malik G: Chronic plasma cell balanitis of Zoon. Br J Vener Dis 49:86, 1973

43. Sheldon W, Heyman A: Studies on chancroid: I. Observations on the histology with an evaluation of biopsy as a diagnostic procedure. Am J Pathol 22:415, 1946

44. Sheldon W, Heyman A: Lymphogranuloma venereum. A histologic study of the primary lesion, bubonulus, and lymph nodes in cases proved by isolation of the virus. Am J Pathol 23:653, 1947

45. Slaney G, Muller S, Clay J et al: Crohn's disease involving the penis. Gut 27:329, 1986

46. Souteyrand P, Wong E, Macdonald D: Zoon's balanitis. B J Dermatol 105:195, 1981

47. Taafe A: Current concepts in lichen planus. Int J Dermatol 18:533, 1979

48. Tummon J, Dudley D, Walters J: Genital herpes simplex. Can Med Assoc J 125:23, 1981

49. Wade T, Huntley A: Multiple penile chancres. Arch Dermatol 115:227, 1979

36

Vascular Lesions and Other Conditions Affecting the Penis

Robert S. Katz

Owing to its extensive vascularity the penis is affected by a number of disorders involving the blood vessels. In addition, a wide variety of unusual, interesting, or hard-to-classify conditions may affect the penis. Some are traumatic in nature, others are inflammatory, and many are self-inflicted. The pathologic basis for a number of these disparate disorders is discussed in this chapter.

VASCULAR LESIONS

Atherosclerosis

Atherosclerotic disease of the infrarenal aorta with total occlusion (Leriche's syndrome) is an important cause of impotence. A large series of patients with this diagnosis underwent angiographic evaluation: 77 percent had aortic blockage in the infrarenal position, whereas 23 percent had obstruction below the inferior mesenteric artery. All patients had claudication, half had buttock pain, and half were impotent. The usual risk factors for atherosclerosis (hypertension and diabetes mellitus) were present in many of the patients. Of interest was the fact that all were heavy

smokers.[49] Impotence, perhaps, may be added to the long list of hazards of cigarette smoking.

As the penis derives its vascular supply from the internal pudenal artery, which in turn comes from the internal iliac, complete infrarenal aortic occlusion can clearly lead to impotence. Inadequate arterial flow prevents proper erection.[14] Patients with this type of occlusion who are not impotent have probably developed collaterals via the renal arteries and other arteries above the obstruction. Reconstructive procedures have been attempted with various degrees of success, but mortality in Leriche's syndrome is high owing to the generalized atherosclerosis affecting many of these patients.[10,49]

Recent work has shown that more distal vascular disease is also a penile problem. An interesting study in Czechoslovakia reported on postmortem analysis of the vascular system of the penises of men aged 19 years to 85 years.[37] Arteriosclerosis was noted in nearly all men older than 38 years. The involvement was greatest in the penis below and behind the symphysis pubis and decreased toward the glans.

Microscopic sections revealed the usual arteriosclerotic changes in penile arteries, with intimal proliferation, medial fibrosis, thrombosis and obliteration of vascular lumens, and calcium deposition in vessel

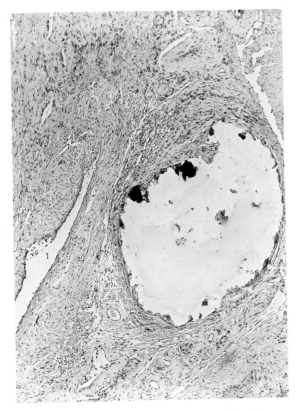

Fig. 36-1 Atherosclerosis. Atherosclerosis of penile vasculature. The large clear area filled with dark flecks of material represents extensive calcification (much of which has dissolved in processing). The vascular lumen is totally occluded. ×46. (See also Fig. 14-13.)

walls (Fig. 36-1). The changes were more pronounced and began at earlier ages in diabetic patients. This study shows a specific anatomic correlate for the increased incidence of erectile failure in older men, especially those with a history of diabetes.[37] Obstruction to distal penile blood flow is a factor in the progressive impotence seen in aging or diabetes.

Vasculitis

Although vasculitic diseases are common in the skin, respiratory tract, and kidney, they are extremely rare in the penis. One case of *Wegener's granulomatosis* has been reported. It was quite atypical in that the patient had swelling of the glans penis as the primary symptom. Biopsy revealed a granulomatous vasculitis with areas of necrosis. The necrosis eventually neces-

sitated partial penectomy. After some tine, the patient died of coronary artery disease, and autopsy revealed focal glomerulonephritis. The penile disease was the first sign of a limited form of Wegener's granulomatosis.[51]

There has been one report of another vasculitis, *polyarteritis nodosa*, to affecting the penis. The patient developed an ulcerative lesion initially believed to be cancer. Despite benign diagnoses, the patient was treated by radiotherapy for presumed tumor. The patient eventually died of uremia, and autopsy revealed fibrinoid necrosis of the penile vessels with a chronic inflammatory infiltrate in the vessel walls. Similar vascular lesions were found in the kidneys.[20]

Although vasculitic phenomena are obviously rare, the initial misdiagnosis of cancer in the second case should point out the need for care in the diagnosis of ulcerated penile lesions.

Fournier's Gangrene

The extensive vascularity of the penis permits the development of a number of circulatory problems. Perhaps the most dramatic of these disorders is Fournier's idiopathic penoscrotal gangrene. Furnier was a well-known French dermatologist and syphilologist in the nineteenth century who described a number of cases of unexplained gangrene of the external genitalia, especially the scrotum, in young men. Since then, all age groups, particularly young children, have been shown to be vulnerable to this disorder.

Although the older literature may refer to spontaneous or primary cases, as opposed to secondary cases, with a known etiology, this distinction is probably meaningless.

The unusal prodrome of the disease involves pain in the lower back and genital area. The scrotum and, possibly, penile skin become blackish yellow and necrotic and slough. Constitutional symptoms, including evidence of septicemia, may also appear.[3] The etiology of this disorder is open to some speculation. However, an infectious origin appears most reasonable. In a large number of cases reported from Africa, various bacterial organisms were cultured from the lesions,[3] including streptococcus, *Staphylococcus aureus,* and *Escherichia coli*. In addition, some cases showed the presence of *Onchocerca volvulus* and other microfilariae. Other cases were associated with the paraproteinemia of multiple myeloma. One other recent case was associated with the use of Pitressin (vasopressin) as a means of controlling bleeding.[7]

Patients with hematologic malignancies such as acute leukemia and non-Hodgkin's lymphoma under chemotherapy are also subject to Fournier's gangrene. Lesions have ranged from penile ulcerations to total penile and scrotal gangrene.[35,36] The infecting organisms have all been *Pseudomonas* species, with *Proteus rettgeri* as well in one case. Pathologic study where performed, showed extensive necrosis of the glans and bacterial invasion of the small penile blood vessels, with distal infarction.[35]

In a series of 20 patients, all had urologic disease (neurogenic bladder, urethral stricture) or colorectal disease (perirectal abscess), and many also were diabetic. Specimens from these primarily older patients all grew out multiple organisms from cultures of the scrotum, including *Bacteroides, Clostridia,* anaerobic gram-positive cocci, and *Pseudomonas.* The investigators suggested that the aerobes and anaerobes acted in synergism to seed the vascular space and cause thrombosis.[45]

The above cases offer much insight into the development of the syndrome. Gram-negative organisms, in particular, can grow into blood vessels and cause thrombosis and septic infarctions. The scrotal skin may easily become dry and excoriated, with ample opportunity for micropuncture and invasion by the mixed flora that live in the colonic and perineal area. The penis and scrotum possess an end-organ circulation, making them vulnerable to the effects of vascular damage in this area.

Vascular compromise was seen in those African cases that were associated with intravascular or peri-

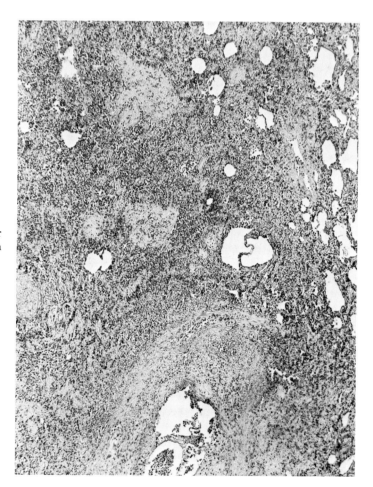

Fig. 36-2 Infective gangrene. Low-power view showing the extensive inflammation and necrosis of scrotal tissue. ×54.

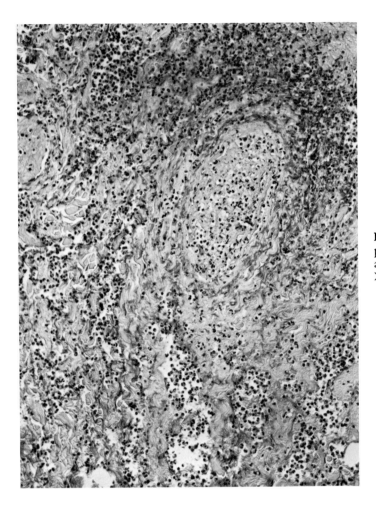

Fig. 36-3 Infective gangrene. Higher-power view illustrating vascular thrombosis and polymorphs in the blood vessel wall. ×136.

vascular parasites, in the patient receiving Pitressin, and in multiple myeloma, which may lead to hyperviscosity and vascular insufficiency.[6]

The patients with leukemia were subject to overwhelming bacteremia in their immunocompromised state. The development of Fournier's gangrene in this group suggests the need for cleanliness in the perineal area in patients undergoing chemotherapy. Finally, the series of older patients all had local infectious processes that provided a reservoir of bacteria.

The histopathology of Fournier's gangrene is similar to that seen in ecthyma gangrenosum, a necrotic ulceration of skin associated with *Pseudomonas* sepsis. The blood vessels show thrombosis with loss of vascular integrity. Red cells may extravasate into the surrounding tissue (Figs. 36-2 and 36-3). Gram stains (Brown–Brenn) may reveal bacteria in the vessel

walls (Fig. 36-4). Thrombosis develops, and the epidermis and underlying tissues become necrotic.[35] Healing proceeds via formation of granulation tissue and regeneration of scrotal skin from uninvolved tissue. The testes have a separate vascular supply and are usually spared necrosis.[45]

Vigorous debridement and antibiotic therapy may ameliorate the disease process and permit healing with little outward deformity. Scrotal skin has considerable regenerative ability, and good cosmetic results are obtainable, with help from skin grafts. The mortality, however, may be as high as 45 precent[18,45] owing to sepsis and shock. This probably reflects the underlying condition of the patient and his lack of ability to cope with a serious infection.[23]

This unusual and dramatic disease thus seems to be a direct complication of bacterial growth in the genital

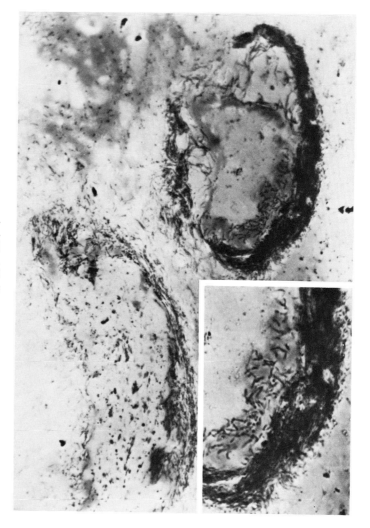

Fig. 36-4 Infective gangrene. Brown–Brenn bacterial stain demonstrating gram-negative rods lining distal penile corporeal vessels and invading adjacent tissue. ×720. Inset, high-power view of vessel wall filled with bacteria. ×1440. (From Rabinowitz et al.,[36] with permission.)

area. As one researcher suggests, the time may have come to drop the term "Fournier's idiopathic peno-scrotal gangrene" and substitute the more meaningful "infective gangrene of the penis and scrotum."[3]

Priapism

A problem of major clinical magnitude that, nevertheless, rarely produces tissue for pathologic evaluation is priapism. This is a painful, persistent penile erection, generally not associated with sexual activity. It is named after the Greek god Priapus, a symbol of fertility, who was often depicted with an erect penis of substantial dimensions.

The basic problem in priapism is failure of drainage of the corpora cavernosa. The penis becomes engorged with blood that cannot leave the vascular channels of the penis.[54] The glans and spongiosum are not involved. Then, stagnation of flow leads to loss of oxygen, local acidosis, and further sludging.

A valvular structure, the polster, has been postulated to be the means of controlling vascular outflow in the penis, permitting erection. Previous theories of the physiology of erection suggested that defects in autonomic stimulation of the polster were associated with the development of priapism. Some work, however, indicates that the polster was only an atherosclerotic plaque found in older men and had no physiologic role.[4] This concept remains a controversial one, as other groups suggest the presence of smooth muscle cushions whose contraction can lead to priapism.[15]

A variety of causes of priapism have been recorded (Table 36-1). Perhaps the most common is sickle cell disease. In younger children with sickle hemoglobin, priapism may occur. Older men with sickle cell trait may also suffer the problem. In this instance, the cells may be trapped in the penis during erection. The delayed penile emptying leads to the changes in oxygenation mentioned above, with increased sickling and further sludging of the blood flow. The penis fails to become flaccid, and priapism results.[25] Leukemia may produce priapism by causing obstruction to venous overflow by the sheer number and volume of cells. Metastatic neoplasms may also block venous outflow and cause priapism. Some neurologic diseases, including spinal trauma, may produce priapism as well. Recently, a number of drugs, including the phenothiazines, marijuana, and alcohol, have been implicated in the etiology of priapism, presumably by acting on the neural control of the outflow musculature.[56] Heparin may act paradoxically as a coagulant and cause priapism by a direct action on vascular smooth muscle. The use of intravenous fat solutions has produced penile thrombosis and priapism.[21] Finally, a number of cases have no readily apparent etiology, although excessive sexual stimulation has been cited in some instances. The pathophysiology in these situations is uncertain.

The pathology of priapism is difficult to describe since surgical pathology specimens are not submitted during the treatment process. However, prolonged thrombosis of the vascular channels seems to result in scarring of the erectile tissue. Repeated episodes of priapism may result in a fibrotic, deformed penis incapable of sexual function.[19]

Table 36-1. Etiologic Factors in Priapism

Sickle cell disorders
Medications (including phenothiazines, marijuana, antihypertensives, anticoagulants)
Solid tumors
Leukemia
Trauma
Prolonged sexual stimulation
Idiopathic

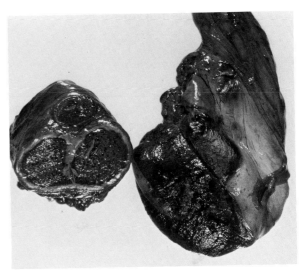

Fig. 36-5 Priapism. Note the marked engorgment of penile vessels.

Gangrene of the penis is a rare complication of priapism (Fig. 36-5). Necrosis of the penile tisue occurs in the presence of decreased venous drainage when other complications supervene. These include local infection, tight dressings, and catheterization. The combination of inadequate outflow and a second factor capable of producing edema or occulsion completely overwhelm the vascular supply and lead to penile necrosis.[19]

Priapism is a serious medical emergency and requires prompt treatment. A variety of remedies have been supplied with various degrees of success. Aspiration of the corpora cavernosa and surgical shunting and drainage procedures are used. However, at least 50 percent of patients with priapism never regain sexual potency after treatment regardless of the length of the episodes.[56]

Some success in patients with sickle cell disease has been achieved by exchange transfusion and hypertransfusion.[2] Automated techniques are available for accomplishing this.[53] The intent here is to reduce the amount of sickle hemoglobin present and to replace it with normal hemoglobin. This would not sickle and could then permit penile drainage. Certainly, a sickle cell preparation is mandatory in the evaluation of any black patient with priapism. Some cases of drug-related priapism have been managed with local therapy and spinal anaesthesia with apparently good results.[54]

Ischemic Injury

The direct obstruction of the penile circulation also may cause gangrene. A recent case describes the necrosis of the distal penis resulting from the presence of a tight condom catheter.[46] In most instances, penile strangulation causes pain. The patient seeks medical care before infarction can develop. However, the patient involved in this case was recovering from a stroke and may have been mentally incapacitated, with inability to draw attention to his plight (Fig. 36-6). Partial penectomy was performed as a result. The condom catheter may cause circulatory embarassment, and frequent inspection, especially in mentally depressed patients, is needed.

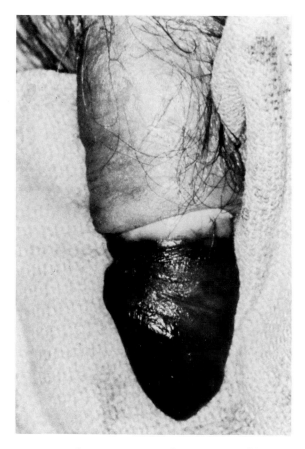

Fig. 36-6 Ischemic necrosis. Striking example of distal penile ischemic necrosis resulting from tightly constricting condom catheter. (From McRoberts JW, Steinhardt G: JAMA 244:1238. Copyright 1980, American Medical Association.)

One unusual case of penile gangrene was reported as a consequence of disseminated intravascular coagulation with thrombosis of the inferior vena cava. The patient also demonstrated occlusion of the right spermatic vein.[43] The patient progressed from penile edema to focal gangrene, probably resulting from local venous engorgement. Resolution of the underlying coagulopathy and restorative surgery left the patient with good cosmetic and functional results.

Penile vascular calcification and occlusion is an unusual manifestation of chronic renal failure. Metastatic calcification may involve penile vessels and produces gangrene of the glans penis secondary to extensive lumenal obliteration.[1]

Another phenomenon leading to penile gangrene has been described in intravenous heroin users. In their search for vascular access, some narcotics users have injected heroin into femoral vessels. Arterial injection may result in embolization of particulate matter with gangrene of portions of the penis and scrotum owing to end-organ circulation obstruction.[44]

INFLAMMATORY AND FIBROTIC LESIONS

Peyronie's Disease

Peyronie's disease is a progressive, fibrosing process involving the corpus cavernosum. Although all ages can be involved, most patients are in their mid-fifties.[57] The patients usually notice curvature of the erect penis, painful erection, and coital difficulty. A palable mass can be found on the penile shaft, usually on the dorsal aspect, and may cause a deformity in an upward direction.[41] One of the first systematic pathologic studies of Peyronie's disease was performed by Smith,[41] who made a careful review of the Armed Forces Institute of Pathology (AFIP) files on the disorder. Histologically, the site of the damage was in the junction zone between the corpus cavernosum and the covering tunica albuginea. In this area, a loose areolar connective tissue is found, with extensive numbers of small blood vessels. A chronic perivascular inflammatory infiltrate was noted, with some eventual damage to the small blood vessels. As the disorder progressed clinically, areas of perivascular scarring were seen, with the eventual formation of a plaque of fibrous tissue in this location (Figs. 36-7 and

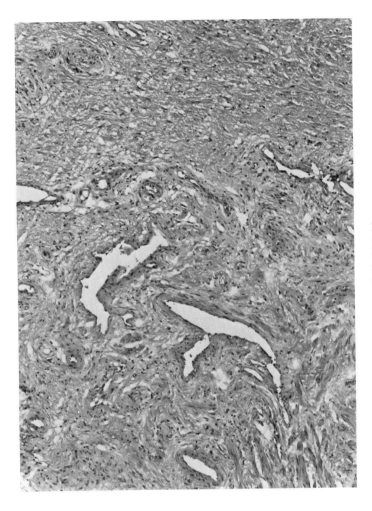

Fig. 36-7 Peyronie's disease. Low-power photomicrograph of typical plaque, showing thick fibrous plaque abutting on normal cavernous tissue. (From Hinman,[16] with permission.)

36.8). Inflammation persisted, and some patients developed foci of ossification, with islands of bone marrow.[41] The perivascular changes are evident in lesions of 2 or 3 years clinical duration, with later lesions showing the obliterative plaque.[50]

A further study by Smith on apparently normal penile tissue revealed cases showing small areas of inflammation in the junction zone.[42]

The etiology of this disease is open to question. There appears to be an association, in a few instances, with Dupuytren's contracture, which suggests a predisposition to fibrosis in some men. Trauma may be the common etiolgy. Repeated minor injury, perhaps during abnormal penile extension during coitus, might be the basic cause of the problem. Hinman[16] noted that patients had the plaque located in the dorsal aspect of the penis (Fig. 36-9). A majority of the patients had the plaque in the basal portion of the penis,

but some had a mid-shaft plaque and others had a distal plaque. The normally erect penis has a slight dorsal curvature owing to the greater extensibility of the lateral and ventral coverings. Forceful straightening could subject the dorsal attachment to undue stress, with production of a mild inflammatory response. The plaques eventually formed would produce the characteristic upward deformity.[16]

Smith added one other possible etiology.[42] In a number of the subclinical cases described, he noted a microscopic urethritis and suggested that infection plays a role in the process. An electron microscopic study noted the presence of bacteria in one case along with several mast cells, mediators of an inflammatory response.[50]

Although the complicating role of urethral inflammation remains a possibility in the development of Peyronie's disease, it should be noted that this was

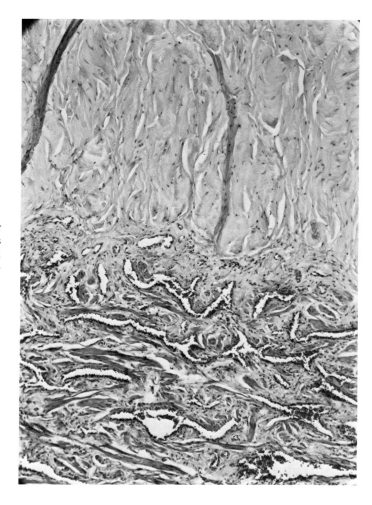

Fig. 36-8 Peyronie's disease. High-power view of same case as Figure 36-7 reveals dense fibrous tissue encroaching on normal erectile tissue. (From Hinman,[16] with permission.)

seen primarily in subclinical cases. The clinically apparent cases did not seem to manifest this process. Given the usual location of the lesions, the anatomic stress forces, and the characteristic histopathology, the basic cause of Peyronie's disease appears to be a mechanical one. It may develop in men with a disposition toward fibrosis, and it seems to reflect repeated mild trauma to the erect penis.

Gelbard[12a] has found radiologic evidence of dystrophic calcification in one-third of patients. Calcification corresponds generally to the distribution of plaques, predominantly dorsal, but occasionally involving the intercavernosal septum, and even extending to ventral plaques. He proposes that the calcification begins in areas of perivascular inflammation and plays a secondary role in perpetuating the inflammation.

The progression of pathologic changes in Peyronie's disease has been described earlier. In general, resection of penile plaques is performed in more advanced disease (see below). The specimen evaluated by the pathologist would, in all likelihood, consist of a rubbery scar, composed of thick collagen. Unless surgery were to be performed earlier in the disease process, the perivascular distribution of the lesions would not be readily apparent.

The therapy of Peyronie's disease is difficult owing to the problems of trying to dissolve or remove fibrous tissue. Intralesional cortisone has been attempted, with some controversy as to its utililty.[30] Recently dissatisfaction with medical approaches has led to more surgical treatments. As the lesions may progress to the point of making normal sexual activity impossible, resection of the plaques and grafting was first

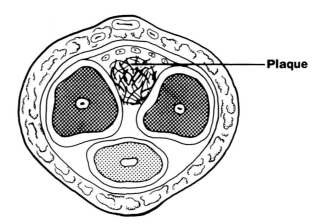

Fig. 36-9 Peyronie's disease. Diagrammatic representation of dorsal location of penile fibrous plaque.

undertaken. More recently, removal of plaques and insertion of a penile implant was tried. Correction of curvature seems achievable, with restoration of vaginal penetration ability.[48] In addition, the insertion of the prosthesis compensates for the penile shortening that accompanies the progressive fibrosis of Peyronie's disease.

Finally, a new approach to therapy involving the intralesional injection of collagenase to dissolve the plaques has been attempted. This treatment was followed by topical application of β-aminopronitride to prevent further cross-linking of collagen. Results appear comparable to those of surgery, and further study may yield promising data.[13]

Traumatic Injuries

Penile trauma is a problem that rarely provides material for the surgical pathologist, but it is an area of interest nonetheless. Injuries are uncommon but quite disabling, potentially deforming, and damaging to function. In civilian practice, most injuries are associated with intercourse or unusual sexual practices.

Perhaps the most dramatic of penile injuries is the rupture, or fracture, of the penis. This may occur during particularly athletic sexual intercourse when the erect penis is bent backwards.[11,17] The injury may also develop if a man rolls over upon the erect penis while in bed.[38] Urethrocavernous fistula is a rare form of penile injury, but one case was recently reported. A heavy blunt object fell upon the penis of the patient and caused damage to the erectile tissue and a traumatic communication between the corpus cavernosum and the urethra.[34]

Other types of penile trauma are even more unusual and often reflect underlying psychologic disorders or variant sexual practices. Patients have attached various instruments to the penis to heighten sexual pleasure. One recent case was that of a man who encircled his penis with five steel washers that had to be removed with a high-speed drill. The penis was quite swollen and painful, but long-term damage did not develop.[26]

Young boys may suffer zipper injury of the penis. The skin of the penis may become entrapped in the fly of the trousers and necessitate a trip to the emergency room. In some instances circumcision was necessary to free the entangled glans.[32] A final type of penile trauma is the vacuum cleaner injury. A number of men have stated they were vacuum cleaning while nude or scantily attired. The penis had "gotten caught" in the intake pipe of the duster with the fan blades lacerating the glans penis. The injuries have been surgically repaired, with good results.[8]

Prostheses, Complications

Recent developments in the therapy of impotence have involved the use of penile prostheses. These devices are designed to provide erectile strength to the penis. As any foreign body, they may cause complications after surgical insertion. The flexible silicone prostheses are inserted into the corpora cavernosa. They may cause erosions into the adjacent urethral tissue, local wound infections, and urinary retention.[12,22] In most instances, these complications are mangeable with local therapy. However, patients have developed distal penile necrosis after prosthesis insertion. The two patients reported were diabetic. After placement of the devices, infection and erythema of the glans penis developed. This was followed by necrosis of the glans penis and tissue in the corpora cavernosa.[27,40] Presumably, both patients had severe vascular disease, and in both instances, the prostheses may have been too tightly inserted.

Other complications of prostheses include extrusion of the device owing to erosion of the corpora or scrotum.[39] In patients with spinal cord injuries, gen-

tial ulcerations may result from vigorous intercourse involving a glans lacking in sensation.

MISCELLANEOUS PROBLEMS

Amyloid

Amyloid is quite rare in the penis. One recent case involved the dermis of the glans and some periurethral tissue. Pathologic examination showed the deposition of the acellular, hyaline material in perivascular areas in the corpus cavernosum. In addition, the periurethral tissues were surrounded by this material, which showed the characteristic green birefringence upon polarization of the Congo red stain.[5] A

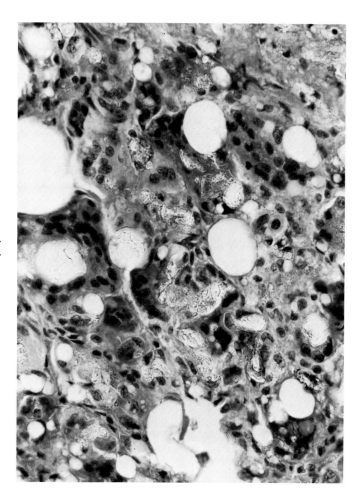

Fig. 36-10 Sclerosing lipogranuloma. Numerous multinucleate giant cells surrounding spaces containing mineral oil. ×340.

few of the patients reported had a history of gonococcal urethritis, so perhaps this represents an abnormal tissue response to the infectious agent.[33]

Histiocytosis X

A single case of histiocytosis X affecting the penis has been reported. This was an aggressive, destructive lesion of the glans penis in a young boy. Biopsy revealed the foamy histiocytes and eosinophils diagnostic of this lesion. Systemic treatment was eventually given, as the penile ulcer was but the first of a series of disseminated eosinophilic granulomata noted in the child.[28]

Sclerosing Lipogranuloma

To increase sexual potency, many men have applied or injected various substances into the penis and groin area. The pathologic sequel of this sort of behavior is sometimes seen as a tumorlike condition known as sclerosing lipogranuloma of the male genitalia. This condition was first described in the early 1950s.

The patient will often have a firm yellow-white mass on the penis, scrotum, or perineal area. The mass may be rather rubbery and on excision shows a fibrous network with interspersed cystic spaces.[25] Microscopically, the tissue shows marked disruption of the connective tissue stroma, with large droplets and vacuoles of fatty material present. Foreign-body giant cells can be seen easily, with collagenous bands traversing the lesion (Fig. 36-10). Inflammation of the adjacent tissue is noted along with many lipid-laden macrophages. Fat stains will demonstrate lipids. For some time there was uncertainty about the etiology of the entity. A panniculitis was suspected, although definite proof was not readily available.

A study from the AFIP[31] offered considerable insight into the cause of this problem. An extensive chemical analysis of cases of sclerosing lipogranuloma of the male genitalia showed that the lipid material is composed of paraffin hydrocarbon. The investigators speculated that the patients had injected paraffin oils into the penis to increase penile size, erectile ability, or potency.[31] (Indeed, in some cases baby oil and mineral oil application or injection have been admitted to by patients with these lesions.)[47,52,55] Some patients did have a history of penile trauma, so traumatic fat necrosis is a possible cause of some cases. Other patients had a history of psychiatric disorder. A more recent chemical evaluation of similar lesions confirmed their paraffin composition.[29]

The authors of this interesting analysis point out that this lesion should be differentiated from other, more serious entities including the sclerosing liposarcoma. The sclerosing lipogranulomas are distinguished by the variable size of the fat vacuoles, the lack of atypical cells, and the often patchy nature of the lesion. Wide areas may be uninvolved, with alternating sections of tissue showing the profound granulomatous response.[31]

A practice in the Far East may provoke the development of lesions somewhat like those of sclerosing lipogranuloma. In some areas, men will embed beads into the subcutaneous penile tissue. The resulting lumps are believed to provide greater stimulation to the female partner.[9]

REFERENCES

1. Ashouri OS, Perez RA: Vascular calcifications presenting as necrosis of penis in patient with chronic renal failure. Urology 28:420, 1986
2. Baron M, Leiter E: The management of priapism in sickle cell anemia. J Urol 119:610, 1978
3. Bejanga BI: Fournier's gangrene. Br J Urol 51:313, 1979
4. Benson GS, McConnel JA et al: Neuromorphology and neuropharmacology of the human penis. J Clin Invest 65:506, 1980
5. Bodner H, Retsky M, Brown G: Primary amyloidosis of glans penis and urethra: resection and reconstruction. J Urol 125:586, 1981
6. Buchanan DJ: Idiopathic scrotal gangrene. Br Med J 4:672, 1972
7. Chakravorty RC: Fournier's idiopathic penoscrotal gangrene. Va Med 108:188, 1981
8. Citron N, Wade P: Penile injuries from vacuum cleaners. Br Med J 3:26, 1980
9. Cohen E, Kim S: Subcutaneous artificial penile nodules. J Urol 127:135, 1982
10. Crespo E, Soltanik E, Bove P, Farrell G: Treatment of vasculogenic sexual impotence by revascularizing cavernous and/or dorsal arteries using microvascular techniques. Urology 20:271, 1982
11. Das S, Arjan DA: Fracture of the penis. J Fam Pract 23:71, 1986

12. Fuerst DE, Bendo JJ: An unusual complication of the inflatable penile prosthesis. J Urol 136:913, 1986

12a. Gelbard M: Dystrophic calcification in Peyronie's disease. J Urol 139:738, 1988

13. Gelbard M, Lindner A, Kaufman C: The use of collagenase in the treatment of Peyronie's disease. J Urol 134:280, 1985

14. Goldstein I, Siroky M, Nath R et al: Vasculogenic impotence: role of the pelvic steal test. J Urol 128:300, 1982

15. Hauri D, Spycher M, Bruhlmann W: Erection and priapism: a new physiopathologic concept. Urol Int 38:138, 1983

16. Hinman F: Etiologic factors in Peyronie's disease. Urol Int 35:407, 1980

17. Jallu A, Wani N, Rashid P: Fracture of the penis. J Urol 123:285, 1980

18. Kearney G, Carling P: Fournier's gangrene: an approach to its management. J Urol 130:695, 1983

19. Khoriaty N, Schick E: Penile gangrene: an unusual complication of priapism. Urology 16:280, 1980

20. Kinn A-C, Hedenborg L: Polyarteritis nodosa of the penis. Scand J Urol Nephrol 11:289, 1977

21. Klein E, Montague D, Steiger E: Priapism associated with the use of intravenous fat emulsion. J Urol 133:857, 1985

22. Kramer S, Anderson E, Bredael J et al: Complications of Small-Carrion penile prostheses. Urology 13:49, 1979

23. Lamb RC, Juler GL: Fournier's gangrene of the scrotum. Arch Surg 118:38, 1983

24. LaRocque M, Cosgrove M: Priapism: a review of 46 cases. J Urol 112:770, 1974

25. Marcial-Rojas R, Colon J, Figueroa J: Sclerosing lipogranulomas of the male genitalia: report of one case and review of the literature. J Urol 75:334, 1956

26. McCally D, Goldfarb M, Finelli R et al: Removal of a strangulating object from the penis. Urology 14:209, 1979

27. McClellan DS, Masih BK: Gangrene of the penis as a complication of penile prosthesis. J Urol 133:862, 1985

28. Myers D, Strandjord S, Marcus R et al: Histiocytosis X presenting as a primary penile lesion. J Urol 126:268, 1981

29. Nakamura M, Sakurai T, Yoshida K et al: Sclerosing lipogranuloma of the penis: chemical analysis of lipid from the lesional tissue. J Urol 133:1046, 1985

30. Nickel WR, Plumb RT: Other infections and inflammations of the external genitalia. p. 640. In Harrison JH et al (eds): Campbell's Urology. 4th Ed., Vol. 1. WB Saunders, Philadelphia, 1978

31. Oertel Y, Johnson F: Sclerosing lipogranuloma of male genitalia. Arch Pathol Lab Med 101:321, 1977

32. Oosterlinck W: Unbloody management of penile zipper injury. Eur Urol 7:365, 1981

33. Ordonez N, Atala A et al: Primary localized amyloidosis of male urethra (amyloidoma). Urology 14:617, 1979

34. Palaniswamy R, Rao M, Bapna B et al: Urethrocavernous fistula from blunt penile trauma. J Trauma 21:242, 1981

35. Rabinowitz R, Lewin E: Gangrene of the genitalia in children with pseudomonas sepsis. J Urol 124:431, 1980

36. Radaelli F, DellaVolpe A, Colombi M, et al: Acute gangrene of the scrotum and penis in four hematologic patients. The usefulness of hyperbaric oxygen therapy in one case. Cancer 60:1462, 1987

37. Ruzbarsky V, Michal V: Morphologic changes in the arterial bed of the penis with aging. Invest Urol 15:194, 1977

38. Sant GR: Rupture of the corpus cavernosum of the penis. Arch Surg 116:1176, 1981

39. Sawczuk I, Wechsler M: Erosion of the pump mechanism of an inflatable penile prosthesis through the scrotum in a diabetic patient. J Natl Med Assoc 78:577, 1985

40. Shelling R, Maxted W: Major complications of silicone penile prostheis. Urology 15:131, 1980

41. Smith B: Peyronie's disease. Am J Clin Pathol 45:670, 1965

42. Smith B: Subclinical Peyronie's disease. Am J Clin Pathol 52:385, 1969

43. Sodal G, Ly B, Borchgrevink H: Thrombosis of the inferior vena cava, disseminated intravascular coagulation and gangrene of the penis. Acta Med Scand 203:535, 1978

44. Somers WJ, Lowe FC: Localized gangrene of the scrotum and penis: a complication of heroin injection into the femoral vessels. J Urol 136:111, 1986

45. Spiranak JP, Resnick MI, Hampel N, Persky L: Fournier's gangrene: report of 20 patients. J Urol 131:289, 1984

46. Steinhardt G, McRoberts W: Total distal penile necrosis caused by condom catheter. JAMA 244:1238, 1980

47. Stewart R, Beason E, Hayes C: Granulomas of the penis from self-injections with oils. Plast Reconstr Surg 64:108, 1979

48. Subrini L: Surgical treatment of Peyronie's disease using penile implants: survey of 69 patients. J Urol 132:47, 1984

49. Traverso LW, Baker JD, Dainko EA, Machleder HI:

Infrarenal aortic occlusion. Ann Surg 187:397, 1977

50. Vande Berg J, Devine C, Horton C et al : Peyronie's disease: an electron microscopic study. J Urol 126:333, 1981

51. Vella E, Waller D: Granulomatous vasculitis of the penis with glomerulonephritis. Postgrad Med 57:262, 1981

52. Verret J-L, Hadet M, Barbin B, et al: Lipogranulome du penis et du scrotum. Ann Dermatol Venereol 112:915, 1985

53. Walker EM, Mitchum EN, Rous SN et al: Automated erythrocytopheresis for relief of priapism in sickle cell hemoglobinopathies. J Urol 130:912, 1983

54. Wasmer J, Carrion H, Mekras G et al: Evaluation and treatment of priapism. J Urol 125:204, 1981

55. Winslow P, Parks S, Whetstone C: Lipogranulomatosis of the genitalia caused by topical application of "baby oil." J Urol 123:127, 1980

56. Winter C: Priapism. Urol Surv 28:163, 1978

57. Yanagisawa Y, Nakamoto A, Ogawa A: Transverse septum-like plaque of Peyronie's disease in a young man. Int Urol Nephrol 18:85, 1986

37

Tumors of the Penis

Robert S. Katz

Although squamous cell carcinoma of the penis and its various precursor lesions are perhaps the most common and important of penile tumors, other neoplastic processes may also affect the external genitalia. This chapter reviews the different types of tumors and comments about their clinical behavior and the controversies of nomenclature and classification that have arisen over the years.

BENIGN TUMORS

Benign epithelial processes may arise on the penile skin. Epidermal inclusion cysts, small condylomata accuminata, and foreign body granulomata may all form masses around the penis. The soft tissues of the penis may also be the site of development of benign neoplasms. Dehner and Smith[18] made an extensive study of soft tissue tumors of the penis, as recorded in the files of the Armed Forces Institute of Pathology (AFIP) (Table 37-1). Essentially all the connective tissues in this area can give rise to both benign and malignant neoplasms. The benign neoplasms will be discussed in order of their relative frequency.

It should be noted that the "hirsutoid papilloma" is not a neoplasm but a frequent normal finding of the glans. It is a small excresscence of skin of no clinical significance.[93]

Angiomatous Lesions

Among benign soft tissue tumors of the penis, angiomatous lesions are perhaps the most common. Mortensen and Murphy[70] reported two cases of angiomatous lesions of the glans penis. In addition, their review of the early literature of the subject showed a number of similarities within this group. The angiomatous malformation, perhaps the best way to describe this process, is usually a circular, bluish-red, raspberry like lesion of the glans (Fig. 37-1). The lesion may fill and become painful during erection[53] and empty when compressed. Some years later, Senoh et al.[95] reviewed the subject and made similar observations about the process. In many cases, the tumors had been present since childhood and had enlarged during puberty.

Histologically, the lesions show the usual findings of hemangiomas, with dilated anastomosing vessels lined by endothelium and surrounded by a fibrous stroma (Fig. 37-2). They are usually classified as cavernous hemangiomas, although a number in the AFIP series were listed as capillary hemangiomas. These would show a more marked proliferation of small blood vessels, with considerably less dilatation. The response to surgical excision of these lesions has been excellent.[95]

The exact nature of these growths has been the subject of some discussion. In many cases, they may

Table 37-1 Benign Soft Tissue Tumors of Penis

Tumor Type	No. of Cases
Angiomatous	12
Neurogenous	8
Myogenous	3
Fibrous	1

(From Dehner et al.,[18] with permission.)

not represent true neoplasms. Mortensen and Murphy[70] suggested that the rapid filling and emptying of the tumors indicated a continuity with the corpus spongiosum. The enlargement of the tumor during erection would support this idea.[70] They concluded that herniation of the underlying corpus spon-

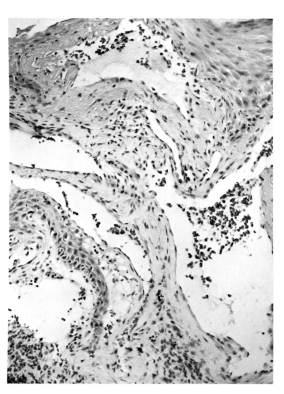

Fig. 37-2 Angiomatous lesion. High-power photomicrograph of a hemangioma, showing the dilated and anastomosing vessels. The endothelial lining of the spaces is evident. ×109.

giosum tissue during embryologic development may have been the true origin of the angioma of the glans. Puberty would make the tumor more evident. Senoh et al.[95] performed radiologic evaluation of one case and angiographically demonstrated a communication between the tumor and the spongiosum (Fig. 37-3). The precise mechanics of the formation of the angioma are still speculative. Perhaps it would be more appropriate to regard these lesions as vascular malformations, rather than as neoplastic processes.

Neural Tumors

Both the AFIP series and other reports[18,26] describe neurogenous tumors of the penis, although these are less common than angiomatous lesions. Both neurilemmomas and neurofibromas may develop and are similar in gross appearance. They are well to moder-

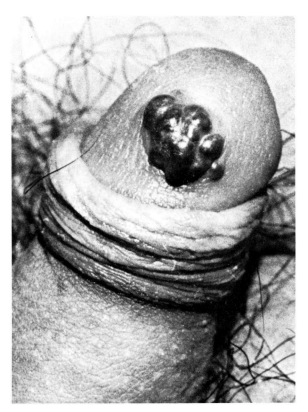

Fig. 37-1 Angiomatous lesion. Well-circumscribed, elevated angiomatous lesion on side of glans penis. (From Senoh K, et al.,[95] with permission.)

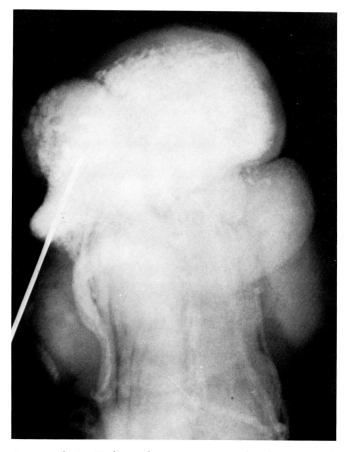

Fig. 37-3 Angiomatous lesion. Radiographic spongiosogram showing communication between penile tumor and corpus spongiosum.

ately circumscribed, rubbery lesions, sometimes bosselated in appearance, involving either the shaft or, more rarely, the glans.[18,26]

The neurilemmoma is often better encapsulated than the neurofibroma. The neurilemmoma shows a whorled pattern, with elongated cells of Schwannian origin forming two distinctive appearances. The Antoni A tissues are compact, with a palisading arrangement to the fibers (Verocay bodies). Palisading implies a growth process in which the nuclei are arranged in parallel rows, with their long axes pointing in the same direction. The Antoni B tissues are loose and often edematous or myxomatous in character, with stellate and occasionally giant cells.[5] As the neurilemmoma derives from the nerve sheath, nerve tissue itself is often not visible, being pushed to the side of the tumor or splayed over the capsule. The neurofibroma, by contrast, grows from within the nerve and may involve the perineurium.

The neurofibroma lacks the organized structure of the neurilemmoma, with more haphazardly arranged nerve and collagen fibers in bundles.[5] The cells of a neurofibroma are spindly, and although the fibers are often arranged in parallel, the palisading of the neurilemmoma is generally absent. Mast cells are frequently present, scattered about the tumor.

The response to resection of the solitary neural tumors, those not associated with von Recklinghausen's disease, has been excellent. A recent case in a child showed no recurrence after a short follow-up, although longer observation was recommended.[23] Neural tumors associated with von Recklinghausen's disease may recur or undergo malignant transformation.[75]

One patient with a history of neurofibromatosis developed an angiosarcoma of the external genitalia. However, this ultimately fatal tumor developed in a location that had been previously free of neurofibromas, suggesting a chance relationship or a genetic predisposition.[68]

The granular cell tumor (the granular cell myoblastoma) is extremely rare in this location. One case appears in the AFIP series,[18] and only a few others have been additionally reported.[100] This tumor, which has been seen at almost every anatomic site, is most common in the tongue. It is a solitary, hard, yellow nodule. The tumor probably is derived from the Schwann cell, perhaps from the fibroblasts of the peripheral nerve sheath.[5] On histologic examination there are groups of round cells with central nuclei and eosinophilic cytoplasm. The cells are filled with granules that will stain positively with the periodic acid-Schiff (PAS) reagent.[5] In most anatomic sites, including the few penile cases, complete surgical excision is sufficient.[100,101]

Leiomyoma

Leiomyomata are rare,[18] with only a few reported in the AFIP series, but may develop along the penis. These firm, white, nodular tumors develop from subcutaneous smooth muscle or the smooth muscle of the walls of blood vessels. The histologic appearance of the leiomyoma is one of interlacing bundles of spindly smooth muscle fibers, sometimes in a whorled arrangement. The nuclei are long, with blunt ends, and often palisade dramatically. Older lesions may become fibrotic, and special stains (trichrome) may demonstrate the smooth muscle.

The distinction between benign and malignant smooth muscle tumors revolves around the mitotic count. In leiomyomata of the uterus, criteria for malignancy have been defined.[39] Tumors with more than 10 mitoses per 10 high-power microscopic fields (HPF) are malignant. Those with less than 2 mitoses per 10 HPF are benign. Those with a mitotic count between 2 and 10 are of uncertain malignant potential, and the patients should be followed carefully. Nuclear atypia (enlargement) and cellular pleomorphism in themselves do not determine malignancy. However, their presence in conjunction with an intermediate mitotic count is a poor prognostic sign.

Smooth muscle tumors of the penis are too rare for criteria as clear-cut as those for the uterus to be established, but it seems likely they would parallel the uterine situation.

A single dermatofibroma has been reported and showed a circumscribed dermal collection of collagen fibers.[18]

In general, the benign tumors of the penis have responded well to therapy. Since malignant variants of soft tissue tumors may also affect this area, biopsy may be necessary.

Condyloma Acuminata

Condyloma acuminata are common lesions of the penis, often called venereal warts. The lesion appears sexually transmissible, with a 1-month to 2-month incubation period.

Extensive recent studies have established the human papillomavirus as the causative agent. There are a number of types of papillomavirus, although types 6 and 11 have most commonly been associated with condyloma.[62] A thorough study of lesions from both women and men revealed papillomavirus in the resected tumors and in some of the margins of resection. In the two penile condylomas, virus was left at the margins. Both patients had local recurrences.[27]

Careful examination of men who are the sexual partners of women with condylomas and cervical intraepithelial neoplasia reveals that the great majority have lesions bearing papilloma-virus.[5a,9a] A small percentage have macroscopically visible condylomas, but painting the surface of the penis with dilute acetic acid and examining with a colposcope reveals inapparent flat lesions as well as small macules and papules. The lesions found accord with the female-partner's lesions, nearly universally with the virus type, but also to a great extent with the histologic lesions as well. Partners of women with condyloma had HPV types 6, 11, or 42, and condylomatous histologic lesions, whereas partners of women with intraepithelial neoplasia, tended to have types 16 or 33, and their penile lesions also manifested intraepithelial neoplasia.[5a]

Although condylomas usually appear on the glans, the shaft may be involved as well. In addition, a few cases have been reported on the scrotum.[84] Younger adults are affected most frequently.

The condyloma is a raised, reddish, cauliflowerlike lesion with a circumscribed appearance. Multiple lesions may develop and then coalesce. They may

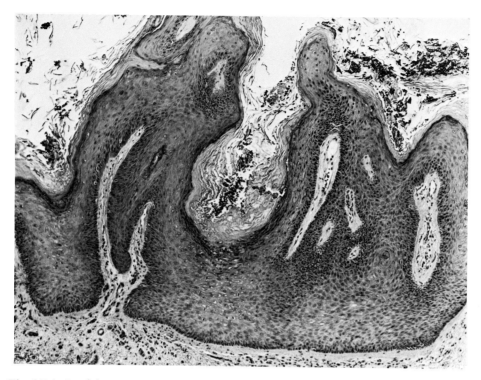

Fig. 37-4 Condyloma acuminatum. Papillomatous upward growth, smooth base, and minimal change in the dermis are seen. ×72.

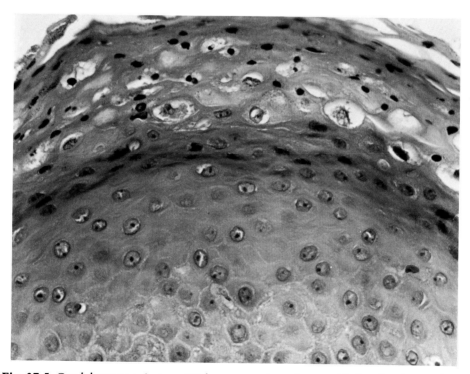

Fig. 37-5 Condyloma acuminatum. Higher-power view of a scrotal lesion showing parakeratosis and perinuclear clearing. ×320.

spread locally to involve wide areas in the anogenital region.

The biopsy of the condyloma shows a markedly acanthotic epithelium. Importantly, significant atypia is not seen. The lesion is papillomatous with considerable parakeratosis (Fig. 37-4). The upper epithelial cells may reveal a cytoplasmic clearing that gives prominence to the nuclei. The key observation is that the condyloma grows upward (Fig. 37-5). In other words, the base is generally smooth, the basement membrane is well preserved, and the lesion does not grow deeply into the dermis.[71] This differentiates it from the very destructive giant condyloma of Buschke-Loewenstein, which is better viewed as verrucous carcinoma and is discussed elsewhere in this chapter.

Although some condylomata may regress, many respond to surgery or pharmacologic therapy. A relationship between condyloma acuminata and cervical carcinoma has been suggested but is still under investigation.[62] Of additional interest is the finding of penile condylomata in a 17-month-old boy.[108] Papillomavirus has been demonstrated (types 6 and 11) in the foreskins of apparently normal newborns.[89] This case of condyloma suggests a maternal transmission, as the mother had an abnormal Papanicolaou (Pap) smear as well. Of greater concern is the fact that papillomavirus types 16 and 18, thought to be of greater malignant potential, have been seen in normal neonatal foreskins as well.[89]

IN SITU MALIGNANT TUMORS

Carcinoma In Situ

One of the major controversies in penile disease revolves around the in situ malignant states involving the penis. Bowen's disease and erythroplasia of Queyrat are entities that were described at the beginning of the twentieth century. Since then, there has been much discussion in the literature about their relationship and malignant potential.

There is agreement on one major issue. Any lesion with the features of carcinoma in situ (CIS) (intraepithelial neoplasia) should be treated promptly and thoroughly. The potential for development into invasive carcinoma is significant. With that in mind, a

discussion of the history and pathology of Bowen's disease and erythroplasia of Queyrat will be clearer.

Bowen[11] described a small series of *precancerous dermatoses* in 1912, although none of these lesions were on the penis. At about the same time, Queyrat[82] continued observations begun by Paget and Darier, among others, on a disorder involving the glans penis and prepuce. Eventually, cases diagnosed as either Bowen's disease of the penis or erythroplasia of Queyrat were described in the American literature, and some question about the malignant nature of the lesion developed. In 1955, Blau and Hyman[8] made an exhaustive survey of the available literature and reported on material from their own files. Their study greatly clarified many aspects of erythroplasia of Queyrat.[8]

Blau and Hyman[8] concluded that many of the cases classified as erythroplasia of Queyrat did, in fact, show carcinoma of the glans penis, which they took to represent Bowen's disease occurring on mucous membrane rather than skin. Unfortunately, these distinctions do not make the nomenclature any simpler. However, many of the other cases analyzed showed a variety of benign inflammatory conditions. Psoriasis, lichen planus, and other conditions without any malignant potential may have a gross appearance similar to that of erythroplasia of Queyrat. Blau and Hyman[8] excluded all those cases lacking intraepithelial neoplasia from the designation of erythroplasia of Queyrat. They noted the potential of the true lesions of erythroplasia of Queyrat to develop into invasive carcinoma.

Later, Anderson and colleagues[3] made another study of the problem and came to conclusions similar to those of Blau and Hyman.[8] They concluded that the histology of Bowen's disease of the skin was practically the same as that of erythroplasia of Queyrat. They believed that they could be regarded as the same disease but with different locations.

Graham and Helwig[32] then undertook a major study of material in the AFIP files and tried to clarify the matter. They demonstrated that there are some significant clinical differences between erythroplasia of Queyrat, as a disease limited to mucosal surfaces (glans and prepuce), and Bowen's disease. All 100 of their cases were found on the glans or prepuce. These were statistically compared with Bowen's disease elsewhere in the body. They noted that erythroplasia of Queyrat occurs in younger men than is the case with Bowen's disease. In addition, they commented on a higher rate of systemic malignancy for men with Bowen's disease, a sometimes generalized skin disorder.

The histologic similarities between the epithelial changes of erythroplasia of Queyrat and Bowen's disease are now basically agreed upon. Mostofi and Price[71] also noted the ability of both lesions to develop into invasive malignancies. They also commented that CIS may occur on shaft or scrotum (true skin) and that there it should be called Bowen's disease.

From the above, it is apparent that the use of either eponym serves only to obscure the basic nature of the process. Rosai[90] states that the entities are one and the same lesion. Coulson[15] views erythroplasia of Queyrat as the histologic homologue of Bowen's disease, or epidermoid CIS, on the glans or prepuce. Given the clinical differences, perhaps this is the best

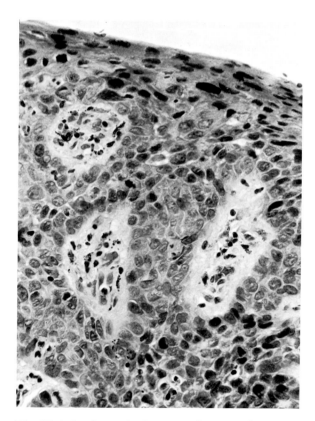

Fig. 37-6 Carcinoma in situ. Typical picture of squamous cell CIS. The orderly maturation of the nuclei is lacking. Large, atypical forms are seen at all levels, with mitosis apparent. ×290.

way to resolve the matter. The histology of CIS should be recognized and reported as such. This is the key point.

The etiology of CIS (erythroplasia of Queyrat) is similar to that of carcinoma of the penis in general and will be discussed in detail later. CIS (erythroplasia of Queyrat) does not occur in men circumcised in infancy, and cases in Jewish men are notably absent.[8]

Grossly, CIS (erythroplasia of Queyrat) affects the glans penis and prepuce. It appears as a smooth red plaque with a moist, glistening surface, sometimes described as red velvet. It is usually round and well demarcated from the surrounding normal tissue. The plaque is soft and level or only slightly raised and usually nontender.[8] The lesion may sometimes ulcerate. The urethral orifice may be involved.[3] In addition, the process may spread by continuity onto the surrounding skin.[45]

Microscopically, erythroplasia of Queyrat should meet the usual histologic criteria for squamous cell CIS. Specifically, it demonstrates an irregular acanthosis of the epidermis. The rete pegs show proliferation, more marked at the lower ends, giving rise to a bulbous appearance to the pegs. The normal polarity of cellular architecture is lost, and the usual basal-to-surface maturation is not apparent. The cells themselves show marked variation in size, nuclear atypia with hyperchromatism and large nucleoli, multinucleation, increased numbers of mitoses at various levels, and dyskeratosis with individual cell keratinization (Fig. 37-6).[8,71] Vacuolation of cells can occur. In addition, there is generally a bandlike inflammatory infiltrate, predominantly plasmacellular, beneath the epithelium. Submucosal blood vessels are often dilated. Some pigmentary incontinence may be noted, with melanin-laden macrophages seen in areas of inflammation.[32]

The border between epithelium and underlying tissue must be distinct, or microinvasion may have occurred.[3] Areas showing invasion of the submucosa should be described and diagnosed as squamous cell carcinoma arising in CIS (erythroplasia of Queyrat).

Between 5 percent and 10 percent of cases of CIS (erythroplasia of Queyrat) develop into invasive squamous cell carcinoma if untreated. In the series of Graham and Helwig,[32] 2 percent of their patients had not only invasive but metastatic lesions.

A variety of therapies are available for these lesions. If the neoplasm is confined to the foreskin, then circumcision may suffice.[86] An extensive case of erythroplasia of Queyrat was treated successfully with radiotherapy.[45] Fulguration may work, although considerable success has been achieved with the topical use of 5-fluorouracil.[93] The Mohs surgical technique has also been employed.[6]

If local therapy is to be applied, then it is essential that the diagnosis be properly established and the extent of the neoplasm determined. Biopsies of sufficient depth must be obtained to exclude areas of invasion. In addition, multiple biopsies may be needed to assure the diagnosis, since inflammatory changes so commonly associated with the in situ carcinomas may obscure it.[93]

Although the distinction in nomenclature is sometimes confusing, it must be remembered that the critical issue is the presence of intraepithelial neoplasia. As Schellhammer and Grabstald[93] conclude, "regardless of terminology, penile lesions with evidence of carcinoma-in-situ on histologic examination demand active treatment and close periodic follow-up."

Bowenoid Papulosis

Bowenoid papulosis of the penis has been recently discussed in a series of publications analyzing the external appearance, histology, and clinical behavior of the disease. Wade et al.[106] presented a considerable number of cases of bowenoid papulosis, which may develop as a result of penile infections, as noted below. The disorder generally involves the shaft of the penis, although the glans may be affected as well. It shows multiple, elevated, scaly papules, sometimes confluent, that are reddish. The lesions were an average of 4 mm in diameter (Fig. 37-7). In no instance was CIS suspected clinically, and prebiopsy diagnoses included lichen planus and psoriasis.

Microscopically, the lesions demonstrated many of the features of CIS. There was nuclear atypicality, with large bizarre cells present at all layers. Mitoses were frequent, along with an upper dermal infiltrate of chronic inflammatory cells and some blood vessel dilatation.[80,106] Again, the usual basal-to-surface layer maturation was lacking (Fig. 37-8). Invasive carcinoma was not described. In comparison with erythroplasia of Queyrat, bowenoid papulosis is a rather distinct phenomenon. Most of the patients are quite young (third and fourth decades), and many had a demonstrated history of viral genital infections

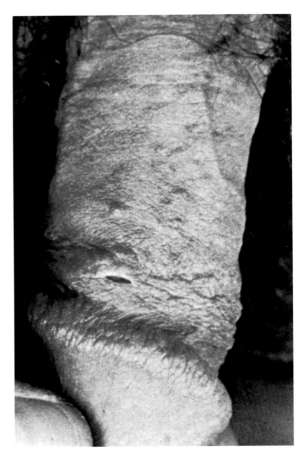

Fig. 37-7 Bowenoid papulosis. Bowenoid papulosis of the penis, showing the multiple flat-topped papules on the glans and penile shaft. (From Wade et al.,[106] with permission.)

(herpes and condyloma acuminata). Human papillomavirus was demonstrated in a number of these cases.[74] Type 16, thought to have neoplastic potential, has been identified, but type 18 has yet to be found. In addition, nearly all cases were in individuals circumcised in infancy.[51] The papules have all responded well to local therapy, including excision, dessication, and topical 5-fluorouracil.[51] However, long-term follow-up of these patients is lacking, since the disorder is so newly described. The potential invasiveness of bowenoid papulosis is uncertain, as is the ultimate fate of the patients. The relationship of antecedent viral infections of the penis and the development of this most atypical process is worrisome, as the incidence of herpetic and other viral genital infections increases. In

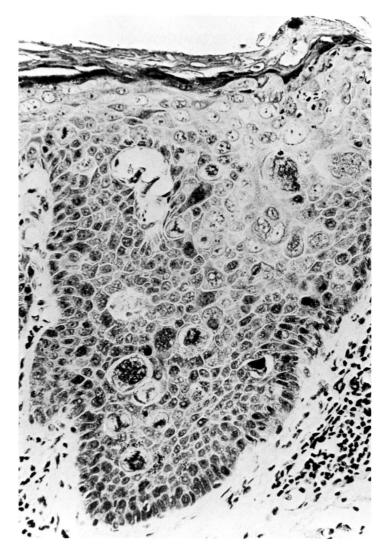

Fig. 37-8 Bowenoid papulosis. Photomicrograph of bowenoid papulosis, with full-thickness nuclear atypia, giant cells, and atypical mitoses. ×187. (From Wade et al.,[106] with permission.)

addition, the papillomavirus seems to be transmitted by infected males to female sexual partners, causing cervical dysplasia.[74] Whether bowenoid papulosis will become a more prevalent clinical problem remains to be seen, as well as its relation to invasive tumors of the penis.

In fact, one must wonder whether bowenoid papulosis is really a separate diagnostic entity. These lesions may just represent a variation on the theme of CIS of the penis. Again, the key point is to recognize the presence of intraepithelial carcinoma, communicate this effectively, and undertake vigorous therapy and follow-up.

MALIGNANT TUMORS

Verrucous Carcinoma

One of the most fascinating of penile disorders is the giant condyloma of Buschke and Loewenstein, perhaps more properly called verrucous carcinoma of the penis. A dramatic-appearing lesion, it has been the subject of some terminologic confusion and prognostic uncertainty over the years.

This lesion was first described in the German literature by Buschke alone in 1896, and then with Loewenstein in 1925, again in German. Loewenstein discussed the "carcinoma-like condyloma acuminata of the penis" in English in 1939.[58] Loewenstein stressed the histologic similarities of this lesion to the more typical condyloma acuminata of the penis, previously described. He noted, however, that in the Buschke-Loewenstein tumor the epithelium had a downward growth pattern. This, he thought, was due to the pressure of the epithelium above. The lower epithelial levels were displaced downward by the prolific growth of condyloma cells above. This caused compression of the corpus and connective tissue. His impression was that the giant condyloma was not a malignant entity.

Some years later, Ackerman[2] described the very well differentiated verrucous carcinoma of the oral cavity. Noting the similarities to the penile process, Kraus and Perez-Mesa[52] reviewed the entity more fully and defined it as a variant of epidermoid carcinoma. Their series included penile lesions, and they concluded that the verrucous carcinoma was the same as the giant condyloma of Buschke and Loewenstein.[52] With this history in mind, the clinical and histologic characteristics of the verrucous carcinoma of the penis can be discussed.

The tumor is almost always found in uncircumcised males and begins in the prepuce. It is often slow growing, but the process commonly destroys the glans and surrounding tissues. It may grow to immense size, forming a warty, cauliflowerlike mass (Fig. 37-9). The tumor is described almost universally as offensive, with a remarkable foul, putrid odor.[13] Surprisingly some patients do not present themselves for treatment until the odor becomes unbearable, despite the considerable size of the often painful, ulcerating tumor.[79,99] The urethral meatus may be destroyed, causing urinary difficulties and fistulas.[14] Inguinal lymph nodes may be palpable and tender.

The histology of the verrucous carcinoma of the penis has been quite well described by now. Yet, the use of the terms such as "condyloma" or "giant condyloma of Buschke-Loewenstein" may give the clinician an underestimated impression of the truly destructive capacity of this lesion.

Microscopically, the tumor shows tremendous acanthosis. There are large papillae growing upward, as seen in typical condylomata.[97] Hyperkeratosis may be seen overlying the papillary fronds. At the base of the lesion, there are bulbous rete ridges growing deeply into the underlying connective tissue. The epi-

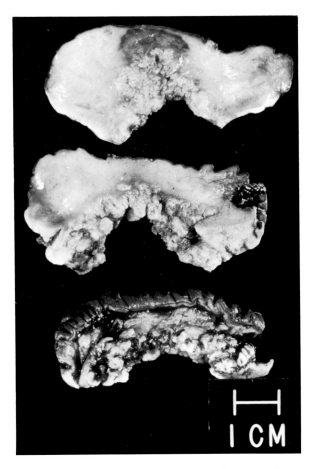

Fig. 37-9 Verrucous carcinoma. Resected prepuce showing the bulky, cauliflowerlike growth pattern of the verrucous carcinoma.

thelial cells are well oriented and not very atypical. The nuclei are uniform with an unremarkable nucleus/cytoplasm ratio. Mitoses are few or absent. Surface cells show evidence of maturation. Although the tumor compresses the submucosa, the epithelial margin remains well defined. Areas of true invasion of the underlying tissue are seldom seen until quite late in the disease. In addition, the growth lacks the fibroconnective tissue core seen in condyloma acuminata.[52] A chronic inflammatory infiltrate is often seen below the epithelium (Figs. 37-10, 37-11, and 37-12). The marked downgrowth of the epithelial process is responsible for the extensive penile destruction.

Perhaps the major problem in diagnosing this lesion is that of communication between clinician and

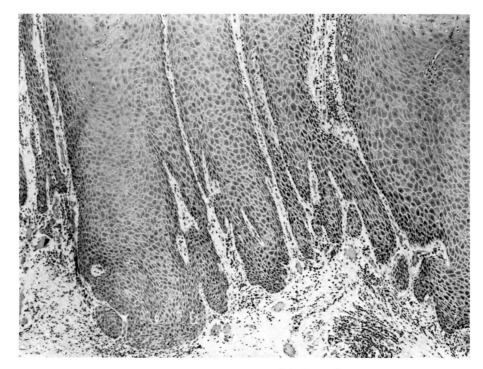

Fig. 37-10 Verrucous carcinoma. Low-power view of the base of a verrucous carcinoma. The bulbous rete ridges grow downward toward connective tissue. ×56.

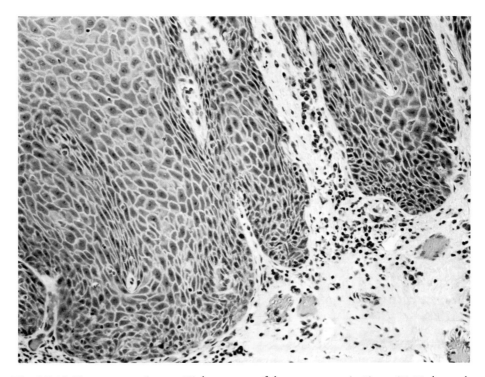

Fig. 37-11 Verrucous carcinoma. Higher-power of the same case as in Figure 37-10 shows the well-defined epithelial margin. ×140.

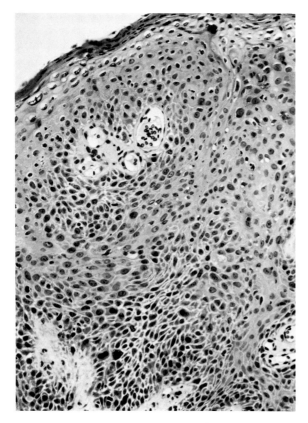

Fig. 37-12 Verrucous carcinoma. Surface of a verrucous carcinoma shows well-oriented epithelial cells with only rare foci of atypia. ×153.

pathologist. If the clinician suspects a verrucous carcinoma of the penis, it is essential that an adequate biopsy be obtained. Superficial samplings of the lesion may cause confusion when the diagnosis of condyloma or acanthosis is returned by the pathologist. The biopsy must include the base of the lesion, so that the characteristic bulbous, downgrowing rete pegs can be identified. In addition, the pathologist must be aware of the true gross appearance of the lesion. As the cellular morphology in verrucous carcinoma is quite bland, he may, as Kraus and Perez-Mesa caution, find himself making a totally benign diagnosis in a lesion that has destroyed the entire glans penis.[52]

In addition to obtaining an adequate biopsy of the lesion, thorough examination of resection specimens is necessary. Dawson and colleagues[17] report a case of Buschke-Loewenstein tumor that had been removed and showed a small area of invasive tumor. More ex-

tensive surgery may be required in these patients. The clinician dealing with verrucous carcinoma may also be misled by the often palpable inguinal lymph nodes, which reflect secondary infection of these ulcerated, grotesque tumors. The lymphadenectomy often regresses after the removal of the primary tumor.

Once the diagnosis of verrucous carcinoma of the penis has been made, surgical removal of the entire tumor is indicated.[13] Radiotherapy was given in some of the cases of oral verrucous carcinoma described by Kraus and Perez-Mesa,[52] and four of these cases underwent a histologic metaplasia to a highly anaplastic tumor, with metastases. Presumably the same might occur in penile verrucous carcinoma.[52] Attempts to treat the growth with topical therapy are also not successful. Usually, a resection of the primary lesion with clear margins is curative. Involvement of the urethra may require more complex procedures.[79]

The relationship between the benign condyloma and the verrucous carcinoma is speculative. Certainly, they share some histologic similarities. Many of the patients with verrucous carcinoma give a history of venereal infections, and nearly all are uncircumcised.[17] Perhaps the verrucous carcinoma represents a transition zone, in an area in which there may well be some relationship between venereal infections, hygiene, and the subsequent development of neoplasia.

Invasive Carcinoma

Penile carcinoma is an unusual disease in this country, forming only 0.3 percent to 0.4 percent of malignancies in men.[79] In other countries, penile cancer is much more common. In South America it occurs with greater frequency, and in Paraguay it is the fifth most common malignancy in men.[87] In certain regions of Africa, penile cancer accounts for 12 percent of all cancers in male patients.[21] In large part, these rates reflect differences in circumcision and penile hygiene among these groups.

ETIOLOGY

Penile carcinoma in persons circumcised at birth is extremely rare. Cases are still so unusual as to merit report,[9,57,89a] with less than a dozen cases recorded in the English literature. In those very few cases, some other factors appear operative. A few of the cases were in men who had undergone circumcision in infancy and had subsequent penile trauma with scarring. One of the patients had hygiene difficulties because of "incomplete" ritual circumcision.[55]

In carcinoma of the penis in other ethnic groups, a study in Africa noted that this lesion was a common problem in Uganda where circumcision is rarely practiced. However, in Kenya, the major tribe practices circumcision at puberty, and a low incidence of penile cancer is found.[21]

In India, penile carcinoma occurs almost exclusively in Hindus (98 percent of cases), who do not practice ritual circumcision. Moslem men (2 percent of cases) are circumcised between the ages of 4 and 9.[55]

A wide variety of causes for penile cancer have been suggested, although none have been proven. Penile hygiene is always mentioned as one factor. Some interesting research performed in the USSR by Shabad[96] points to smegma as a carcinogenic agent. Smegma begins to be secreted almost immediately after birth and consists of desquammated epithelial cells and the secretions of Tyson's glands.[96] It may be acted on by *Mycobacterium smegmatis* and converted into a more carcinogenic material. Shabad[96] suggests that the constant contact between epithelium and smegma, particulary in the phimotic penis, accounts for the development of carcinoma. He notes a higher incidence in men circumcised later in life.[96]

There may in fact be an cumulative risk to smegma exposure. Jews, circumsized at birth, rarely have penile cancer. Moslems, circumcised before puberty, have a low incidence of the lesion, but a higher one than Jews.[7] South African Bantus, circumcised at puberty, have a higher risk, and the uncircumcised have the greatest risk.[55]

Phimosis, with tight apposition of the prepuce to the foreskin, is a critical problem. In most series, more than one-half of the patients had phimosis at the time of diagnosis. Essentially all patients with penile cancer and phimosis in one series had phimosis from birth or of very long duration.[24] Clearly, there was prolonged contact between the penile epithelium and smegma.

The presence of a carcinogenic agent as the causative factor in penile carcinoma was given credence by the finding that the wives of men with penile carcinoma have a higher than usual incidence of cervical carcinoma. This pointed to the possibility of a venerally transmitted agent in penile cancer.[33] The relationship of viral infections, however, remains speculative. In fact, one recent review points out that neither venereal disease nor trauma or racial predilection are primary factors in the development of penile carcinoma. Only hygiene appears to be of etiologic importance.[73] One investigator points out that good penile hygiene in the uncircumcised, nonphimotic male could convey a level of protection comparable with that of infant circumcision.[50] One hopes that, at least in industrialized societies, this could be achieved. This is certainly a major factor in the development of penile cancer in the Third World.[85]

Recent work with human papillomavirus types 16 and 18 in Brazil, where penile carcinoma is more common than in America, suggests a substantial amount of viral infection in patients with penile carcinoma.[63,105] Most of the patients were of poor rural backgrounds. In light of the data mentioned earlier, one must wonder whether the combination of poor hygiene, foreskin presence, and viral infection provides a combination of circumstances conducive to the presence of invasive penile cancer. The patients with bowenoid papulosis, so far a noninvasive lesion, have generally been circumcised. The lack of a foreskin or good penile hygiene may provide a less favorable environment for virus-induced dysplasia to become invasive neoplasia. The development of penile carcinoma in Moslems circumcised at puberty[7] may reflect the long-term neoplastic effect of human papillomavirus type 16 or 18 transmitted from mother to child.

CLINICAL PICTURE

Squamous cell carcinoma of the penis is relatively rare. In America it comprises considerably less than 1 percent of all cancers in males. It is generally a disease of older men, with the usual age distribution between 40 and 70 years. The mean age at diagnosis is about 55 years.[20] Younger patients have been reported in studies from Asia.[76] The age distribution has not changed substantially during the past few decades.[56]

The usual clinical symptoms of penile carcinoma include a mass, ulceration, pain, discharge, or lymphadenopathy.[41] In many cases, the lymphadenopathy, like that of verrucous carcinoma (giant condyloma), is due to secondary infection. The discharge may be foul smelling, and the lesion may have attained considerable size before medical attention is sought.[67]

Many men, unfortunately, delay presentation for treatment until the disease is well advanced. In one

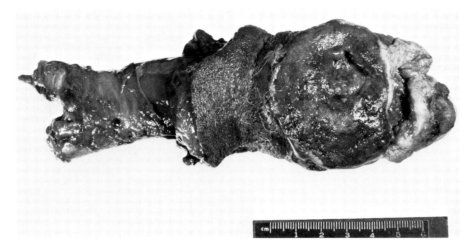

Fig. 37-13 Squamous cell carcinoma. Large, destructive squamous cell carcinoma with involvement of shaft and glans. The patient, interestingly, underwent circumcision 5 years earlier, for removal of a condyloma.

series, 25 percent of the patients admitted to a duration of symptoms of longer than 12 months.[73] This may be due to embarrassment, fear of surgical mutilation, or other psychologic factors.

MORPHOLOGY

Most tumors of the penis develop on the glans or prepuce.[102] The role of smegma in the formation of penile carcinomas has been discussed, and the usual location of penile carcinomas reflects the areas of exposure to this irritative agent. The tumors may be large, fungating masses associated with extensive destruction of the penile tissue (Fig. 37-13).[71] The entire glans may be obliterated, with extension of tumor into the shaft (Fig. 37-14).[102]

Histologically, the tumors are usually well-differentiated squamous cell carcinomas, manifesting the usual microscopic features of this lesion. There is extensive thickening and acanthosis of the squamous layer. The usual maturation of the squamous epithelium is disturbed. Instead of a progression from large basal-layer cells to flatter surface cells, there may be no maturation at all. Large cells may appear at the surface with open nuclei. There is often cellular pleomorphism and variation in cellular appearance (Fig. 37-15). In addition, the cells themselves are bizarre,

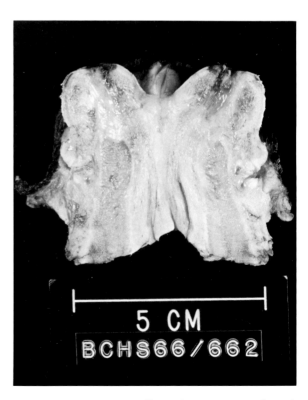

Fig. 37-14 Squamous cell carcinoma. Resected penis showing a tumor in the prepuce clearly growing into the connective tissue, as well as involving the urethra.

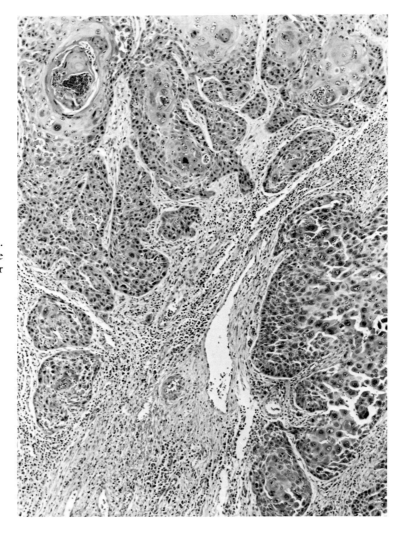

Fig. 37-15 Squamous cell carcinoma. Low-power view of a typical invasive squamous cell carcinoma. The tumor erodes deeply into the corpora. ×49.

with large nuclei and nucleoli evident. There is intercellular bridging, keratinization both within squamous pearls and intracellularly, and extensive invasion of the underlying tissue by the tumor cells (Figs. 37-16 and 37-17). It is this invasive behavior that separates the squamous cell carcinoma from the verrucous carcinoma and Buschke-Loewenstein giant condyloma. The verrucous carcinoma causes destruction by compression of the submucosal tissue. The squamous cell carcinoma invades deeply, destroying as it penetrates.[5,71] A small proportion (less than 10 percent) of penile cancers are poorly differentiated.[5] These may appear as tumors composed of large, bizarre sheets of cells not manifesting keratin or intercellular bridging by light microscopy. Immunoper-

oxidase staining for keratin may help demonstrate the cell of origin in these situations.

DISSEMINATION

Penile cancer usually spreads via lymphatic dissemination. Penetration of the fascia by tumor is associated with more extensive metastatic spread. The inguinal lymph nodes are generally the first involved, and hematogenous spread is possible, although surprisingly rare considering the vascularity of the corpus cavernosa.[37] Vascular spread is through the prostatic plexus, and local spread may cause bone and vascular damage.[67] Distant metastases may affect the lungs, liver, and brain.[72]

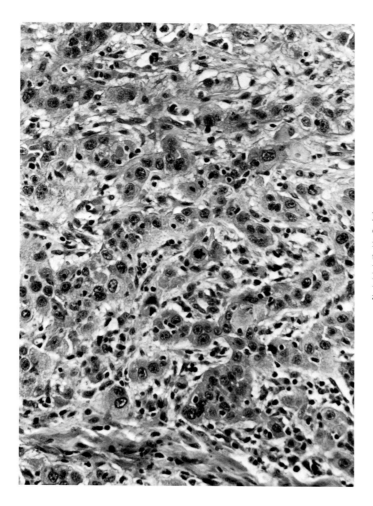

Fig. 37-16 Squamous cell carcinoma. A different case of squamous cell carcinoma, in this instance rather poorly differentiated. The tumor still grows in sheets. Intercellular bridges could be identified. However, bizarre mitoses and nuclear atypia are striking. ×230.

STAGING

For clinical purposes, penile carcinomas are staged based on the extent of penile involvement. Stage I is a superficial lesion of the glans penis or foreskin, stage II is a lesion that involves the corpora, stage III shows metastases to inguinal lymph nodes, and stage IV shows distant metastases.[19] In one recent series, 38 percent of patients could be classified as stage I and 25 percent as stage II. Thirty-one percent were in stage III, and 6 percent in stage IV.[19]

Some studies have suggested that a sentinel node, located just superior and medial to the saphenofemoral junction in each groin, can be identified. If this node is negative on biopsy, then inguinal or deep nodes will not be found. Twenty percent of patients with positive sentinel nodes will have more extensive nodal involvement.[78] This is a controversial area, however, as some researchers have identified patients with negative sentinel nodes in whom unresectable inguinal and iliac nodes developed within 1 year.[109]

Preoperative staging often differs from final pathologic staging because many patients have enlarged inguinal nodes. In some series, as many as one-half of the patients may have palpable adenopathy. However, of these, one-half may be free of inguinal node involvement on histologic examination.[19] The adenopathy is probably due to secondary enlargement as a result of infection of the primary tumor. Aspiration biopsy may simplify this evaluation.[92]

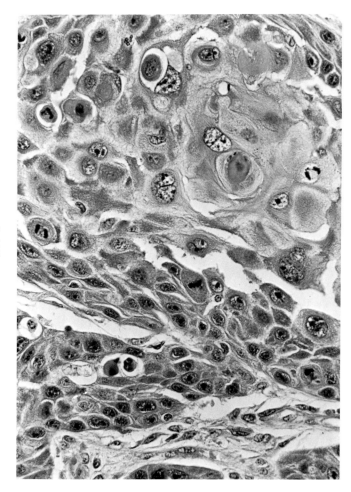

Fig. 37-17 Squamous cell carcinoma. High-power view of squamous cell carcinoma, demonstrating keratin pearls and intercellular bridges. ×340.

THERAPY AND PROGNOSIS

Stage I and II lesions are generally treated with partial penectomy, with average survivals of 7 years to 10 years. Stage III and IV lesions are usually treated by penectomy of a degree determined by the size of the tumor, and by lymphadenectomy. Survival is about 2 years to 3 years for stage III lesions, taken overall.[67] However, there is a marked difference in survival between patients with unilateral nodal involvement (56 percent 5-year survival) and those with bilaterally positive nodes (9 percent 5-year survival).[99a] Survival is only a matter of months for stage IV growths.[67]

A number of attempts have been made to relate histologic appearance (grade) of tumor to stage and, hence, survival. A large series found, after dividing tumors into low grade (well differentiated) and high grade (poorly differentiated), no statistically significant relationship with pathologic stage or survival.[107]

The survival statistics for patients with stage I and II tumors may reflect the fact that many die of causes unrelated to penile carcinoma. A substantial proportion of these men are 50 years of age or over and may have other medical disorders. Thus, the prognosis for these stages of penile cancer appears reasonably good. Of 129 patients with stage I tumors in one series, 111 died of causes other than carcinoma of the penis.[73] Some of the remaining patients had lymph node biopsies that showed metastatic disease, making them stage III patients by strict pathologic criteria. Of 24 patients with stage II disease, only 5 died of the carcinoma. One can only speculate on the effect on prognosis of the delay in seeking medical attention so commonly seen in this disorder.

The relationship of therapeutic modality to prognosis in stage I and II lesions is not an issue of controversy. Partial penectomy, with adequate margin of resection, is regarded as sufficient.[73] In patients with proven metastasis to lymph nodes, radiotherapy or radical inguinal node dissection are of no value in prolonging survival.[73] The prognosis in stage III disease is very poor and surgery or radiation of involved nodes adds no survival benefit.

Radiation therapy as a primary modality has been reported.[16] The data are difficult to evaluate, but they seem to show that patients with tumors of lower stages had a good survival percentage for up to 3 years. Long-term data were not presented.

Bleomycin as a chemotherapeutic agent has been used abroad in combination with radiation or surgery or as a sole modality. The number of patients in one series was nearly anecdotal. In a patient with a small tumor, "cure" was claimed but long-term follow-up was not clear. Other cases "failed" bleomycin, and conventional therapy was applied.[43] Studies utilizing significant numbers of patients in real comparisons with surgical approaches are not available.

Squamous cell carcinoma of the penis is a disorder with a good prognosis if treated early. Delay in seeking therapy is certainly lamentable as clinical stage is so closely related to survival.

Spindle Cell Carcinoma

Among the more unusual neoplasms, spindle cell carcinoma of the glans penis has been recently reported.[61] This tumor caused a mass on the glans and rapidly metastasized to the perineum, even after radical surgery. The patient died within 1 year of diagnosis. Histologically, the tumor showed a loose arrangement of spindle cells, with bundles and whorls of cells separated by collagen. There was marked nuclear atypia and mitotic activity. Electron microscopy showed desmosomes and other features of the epithelial origin of the tumor.[61] Although the spindle cells may resemble those seen in sarcomatous tumors, the electron microscopic data suggests that this is really a very poorly differentiated variant of squamous cell carcinoma.

Basal Cell Carcinoma

Despite its frequency on other areas of the skin, basal cell carcinoma of the penis is extremely rare. Less than 10 cases have been reported, a few occurring on the glans and a very few on the shaft.[36]

Basal cell carcinoma of the scrotum has also been reported as a rare entity. In one series of scrotal malignancies, a single case of basal cell carcinoma was discussed, with an additional two cases described in a later report from the same institution.[34,83]

Whether on the penis or on the scrotum, the basal cell carcinoma makes a very similar presentation. Grossly, it appears as a small, ulcerated mass. Upon excision, the microscopic examination shows rather small, uniform, dark cells, slightly spindled, forming nests and masses in the dermis. The peripheral nuclei in the nests commonly show palisading. Downgrowths of cells from the basal layer of the epidermis should be seen to establish the diagnosis definitively.[5] The response to surgical resection of these tumors has been good.

It should not be surprising that the basal cell carcinoma, although so frequently seen on other regions of the skin, is so rare in the penile area. The tumor may be induced by sun exposure and is a problem on the face and arms. In general, the opportunities for prolonged sun exposure of the penis and scrotum are rather limited.

Carcinoma of the Scrotum

Squamous cell carcinoma of the scrotum, originally described in the eighteenth century by Sir Percival Pott, among others, was associated with soot exposure in chimney sweeps. Since then, other occupational carcinogens leading to scrotal carcinoma have been noted, including some in the fabric industry. With improved industrial safety, the disorder has become extremely rare.[59]

The average age of patients with scrotal carcinoma is in the mid-fifties, with a general age distribution rather like that of penile carcinoma. The tumor may develop as an ulcerating mass of the scrotum, slow growing, and similar to penile lesions, sometimes foul smelling. It may grow locally to large size, but it rarely extends into the scrotal contents or penis.[83] The histology is that of a squamous cell carcinoma. Lymphatic spread usually first involves the inguinal nodes.[42]

A recent series provided criteria for staging the tumors, similar to those used for penile carcinomas.[83] Surgical excision with lymph node dissection was performed in cases showing involved nodes. Long-term survival was good in those patients in whom the tumor was confined to the scrotum, although a surprising number of patients later developed second neoplasms elsewhere.[83]

Extramammary Paget's Disease

Extramammary Paget's disease is an unusual disorder, particularly when it involves the penis, and represents a problem of classification. First described as a disorder of the breast, Paget's disease is usually associated with an underlying mammary cancer. It was subsequently described in extramammary sites, where again it appears associated with visceral tumors, particularly perianal Paget's disease and rectal tumors.[38] It may involve the penis and cause a reddish, scaly, crusted lesion. The relationship of penile Paget's disease to underlying malignancies is unclear. One series reports three cases, although long-term follow-up and presence of other neoplasms was lacking.[37] However, a more recent study reported one case of penile Paget's disease with an underlying prostate carcinoma.[66]

Histologically, Paget's disease of the penis meets the usual histologic criteria initially established for mammary Paget's disease. The epidermis is infiltrated by large, clear, vacuolated cells with small nuclei. The cells may be more numerous at the tips of the rete ridges. The cytoplasm, upon staining, is PAS positive and diastase resistant. Most cases stain with alcian blue and mucicarmine.[66] There is often pigmentary incontinence in the dermis and a chronic inflammatory infiltrate as well.[38] The microscopic differential diagnosis includes squamous cell CIS, which should show the typical bizarre cells, loss of epithelial polarity, and mitotic activity characteristic of this disorder. Malignant melanoma should also be kept in mind. In this instance, stains for melanin are useful, and the melanoma should be PAS and mucicarmine negative. The etiology of this disease in the penis is speculative. Little information is available regarding natural history. Follow-up data are limited, so it is difficult to determine whether patients initially having penile Paget's disease invariably develop carcinoma at any site, penile or visceral. Elsewhere, Paget's disease may represent a transformation of apocrine cells under stimulation, possibly of a neoplastic nature. Perhaps this is the multicentric malignant transformation of histogenetically similar cells that migrate together during embryonic life.[66] In view of the rarity of this disorder and the possible association with underlying neoplasia, patients with penile Paget's disease should be evaluated and followed carefully over time.

Malignant Melanoma

Malignant melanoma of the penis is also a rare tumor, with less than 40 cases in the literature. Most cases are in men between the ages of 50 and 60 years. The malignant melanoma usually appears as a lesion

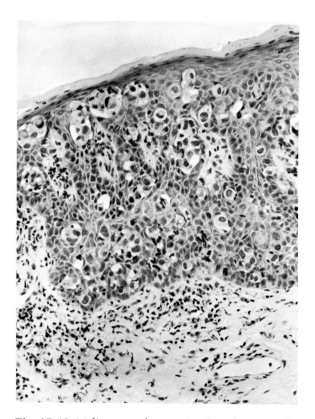

Fig. 37-18 Malignant melanoma. Penile malignant melanoma showing an area of intraepidermal growth. The pagetoid cells, with vesicular cytoplasm, are evident. ×140.

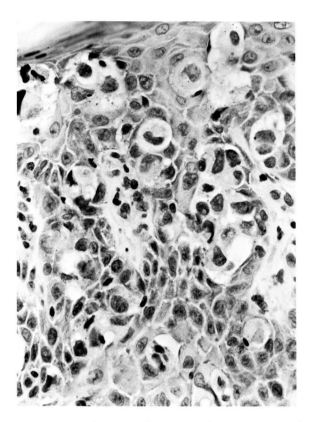

Fig. 37-19 Malignant melanoma. Higher-power view of the same melanoma, demonstrating the large cells and eosinophilic cytoplasm. Melanin is not visible on hematoxylin and eosin stain in this case. ×350.

of the glans, with the prepuce less commonly involved. It is often a red or black indurated ulcer.[28] The tumors have been staged as follows: stage I, localized melanoma without node involvement; stage II, one regional node area involved; stage III, disseminated melanoma.[12] Histologically, the malignant melanoma of the penis may show as much variation in appearance as its counterparts elsewhere in the skin. The tumor may demonstrate areas of junctional activity, with atypical cells at the border of the dermis and epidermis typically in nests of loosely arranged cells (Fig. 37-18). The cells may grow up into the epidermis and deeply down into the dermis. Often, the cells are quite large, with a substantial amount of eosinophilic cytoplasm (Fig. 37-19). The nuclei may be vesicular or otherwise pleomorphic. Nucleoli are typically prominent and large. Spindle cell formation is a not infrequent component of the tumors.[28] Melanin

may be readily apparent or not demonstrable except by special stain. The Fontana stain is commonly used and stains melanin black. In some cases, melanin is so abundant that it covers the cells, completely obscuring detail. Bleaching may be necessary to view cellular morphology.[5] There is usually marked chronic inflammation below the tumor. Melanin may be extruded from cells and lie free in the dermis or be engulfed by histiocytic cells (melanophages).[5]

The pathogenesis of malignant melanoma in this region is discussed in Chapter 38.

In general, this is an extremely aggressive neoplasm. Many of the reported patients have died very shortly after diagnosis. Metastases occur by inguinal lymph node involvement or by hematogenous dissemination to distant organs (lungs, brain, liver).[28] In the patients with Stage I disease, total penectomy, with possible lymphadenectomy, offers some chance of survival.[47]

Sarcomatous Neoplasms

The other family of primary malignant tumors of the penis are the sarcomas, which are much rarer than the carcinomas. Malignant neoplasms may arise from the supporting tissues of the penis, muscle, blood vessel, and nerve. As mentioned earlier, the best series of soft tissue tumors of the penis is that of Dehner and Smith from the files of the AFIP.[18] Other cases have been reported singly or in small groups. Vascular neoplasms appear to be the most common, with myogenous, fibrous, and neurogenous lesions of considerable rarity.

Because of the rarity of the lesions, it is difficult to generalize about their behavior. The gamut of clinical pictures may be seen, from a good response on resection, to local recurrence, to metastatic disease.

MALIGNANT VASCULAR NEOPLASMS

The blood vessels may give rise to malignant neoplasms of two main types: malignant hemangioendothelioma (angiosarcoma) and Kaposi's sarcoma. The angiosarcoma is a tumor of vascular endothelium, whereas the histogenesis of Kaposi's sarcoma is uncertain. It is a tumor of capillaries, but beyond that the cell of origin remains a subject of discussion.[5]

Hemangiosarcoma (angiosarcoma) is perhaps the more common of the two types. This tumor may be a penile mass, usually of the shaft. An extensive early series by Ashley and Edwards[4] mentions that painful erection was a feature of some cases, perhaps because of connection to the corpus cavernosum. There was a wide variety in ages of patients with these tumors, but middle-aged to older men were most frequently involved.

The tumors are either adjacent to or arising from the corpus cavernosum and show the histology of angiosarcoma seen elsewhere. The growth is that of an anastomosing network of blood vessels, lined by an atypical endothelium.[25] The endothelial nuclei may be hyperchromatic, pleomorphic, and large.[5] The tumor has a papillary appearance in some areas, caused by the presence of anastomosing channels, and forms more solid masses in others.[18] Mitoses are few, and the penile lesions are fairly circumscribed. Dehner and Smith[18] believed that these two factors explained the good outcome of the patients in their series after excision of the tumor. The older British series of Ashley and Edwards[4] reported numerous deaths, although many of the patients were treated at the turn of the century and are not comparable with patients cared for in this more recent era.

Recently, a case of angiosarcoma arising in a patient with von Recklinghausen's disease was described.[68] The patient succumbed to unknown causes, although recurrence of tumor was seen locally. The investigators suggest that this case may represent development of cancer in a patient with an abnormal genome.[68]

Another case was described in a patient with a history of exposure to vinyl chloride, a chemical well known for its effects in producing hepatic angiosarcoma. The tumor extensively involved the corpus cavernosum, and the patient died of metastatic disease.[29]

Kaposi's sarcoma may rarely affect the penis. The epidemiology of Kaposi's sarcoma has received intense study of late because of its association with the acquired immune deficiency syndrome (AIDS).[22] Kaposi's sarcoma may take several forms. The first type was originally described in elderly men of central European extraction. This was a rather indolent process with prolonged survivals. Many of the early cases of Kaposi's sarcoma of the penis, as reported in the literature, are probably in this group. This may well explain the good outcome of the cases.[4,18] A more aggressive form of Kaposi's sarcoma is seen in middle-aged Africans. A recently reported case on the penis of a 40-year-old Nigerian showed multiple lesions on the glans and was recurrent. There was some response to chemotherapy.[60]

The last type of Kaposi's sarcoma has been seen in patients with AIDS. The neoplasm is reported in a variety of skin and visceral locations with substantial mortality.[40] The lesion has been described on the penis in an AIDS patient as part of disseminated and ultimately fatal disease.[94] Kaposi's sarcoma develops as a blue-red lesion, single or multiple.[60] The tumors begin as circumscribed dermal nodules that may grow to ulcerate the epidermis. This tumor consists of sheets of spindle cells, with slitlike channels filled with blood (Fig. 37-20). There is often hemorrhage or hemosiderin in the midst of the tumor. The small vascular slits are lined by prominent endothelial cells, although the papillary tufts are not seen. Nuclei are hyperchromatic with few mitoses.[5,40]

NEUROGENIC SARCOMAS

Neurogenic sarcomas are exceedingly rare, with none in the British series,[4] and only two from the AFIP.[18] They show tight, whorled bundles of spindle cells with prominent mitoses. The tumors are often densely cellular with nuclear hyperchromatism and pleomorphism. Special stains may help assess the cell of origin of these lesions.[18] Both cases in the AFIP series occurred in patients with a history of von Recklinghausen's disease.

SARCOMAS OF MUSCLE

Leiomyosarcoma is another rare tumor, arising from smooth muscle. It is the malignant counterpart of the leiomyoma. These tumors are composed of whorled bundles of smooth muscle fibers. The basic histology is similar to that seen in the leiomyoma, with interlacing bundles of spindled, smooth muscle fibers. The nuclei usually have blunt ends. Again, distinction between fibrous and myogenous elements may require trichrome stain.

If one uses the criteria established in the uterus, tumors with less than two mitoses per 10 HPF will behave in a benign manner. Those with 2 to 10 mitoses per 10 HPF are more difficult to diagnose. The presence of nuclear atypia or bizarre (multipolar,

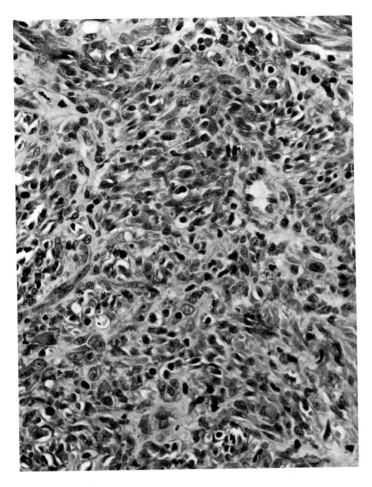

Fig. 37-20 Kaposi's sarcoma. Sheets of spindle cells, with slitlike channels filled with blood, are typical findings in this neoplasm. ×350.

pleomorphic) mitotic figures in one of these lesions would argue for a diagnosis of malignancy. Ten mitoses per 10 HPF is a sure sign of malignancy.

The initial location of the tumor gives a good indication of its behavior. Tumors of the distal penis do well after partial penectomy. Tumors at the penile root, near the peritoneum, show a more aggressive course. Visceral metastasis, including pulmonary, may occur.[46,65,98]

A number of leiomyosarcomas arising in the scrotum have been reported, predominantly in older men.[14a,15a,23a,44] In several of these there has been a history of prior irradiation[15a] or prior surgical trauma[14a] to the scrotum. The lesions are presumed to have arisen from the dartos muscle in the scrotal wall, although arrectores pilorum, vessel walls or any other smooth muscle in the vicinity would be equal candidates. The lesions have been histologically typical of leiomyosarcomas, and staining for desmin was positive in two recent cases.[15a,23a] They have tended to local recurrences, with mestastases heralding a poor outcome.

Rhabdomyosarcoma, arising from voluntary muscle, was mentioned in the British series, but the cases were quite old and poorly described.[4] More recent and better documented cases are not readily available.

FIBROUS SARCOMAS

A number of malignant tumors of fibrous tissue origin are reported, although many of the cases go back to the nineteenth century when this term was applied indiscriminately to many sarcomas of various origins.[4] Both fibrosarcoma and dermatofibrosarcoma protuberans may affect the penis. The fibrosarcoma may develop as a bundle of spindled cells, often growing in a stellate or herringbone pattern. The nuclei are often oval or cigarshaped with tapering ends, and mitotic figures may be readily demonstrable. The cells are relatively compact with only a small amount of intercellular collagen present.[5] Dermatofibrosarcoma protuberans may have features similar to those of fibrosarcoma but shows a more "cartwheel" arrangement to the fibers, with radiation about a central point.[18] The tumors recur locally and repeatedly,[5] although surgical resection may give good results in some cases.[110]

Recently, a case of epitheloid sarcoma was described in a patient originally diagnosed as having Peyronie's disease. This was a spindle cell tumor with plump cells showing considerable cytoplasm, epithelial-like in appearance. The patient eventually died of metastatic disease.[69] One similar case was subsequently identified.[81]

A single case of clear cell sarcoma, a tumor usually found on the extremities, has been reported. The lesion is composed of spindled cells with pale cytoplasm. Electron microscopy reveals melanosomelike structures, suggesting neuroectodermal origin. As is the case in extremity lesions, these are aggressive neoplasms.[91]

Metastatic Tumors

The final type of tumor that may involve the penis is the metastatic tumor. Analogous to the spleen, the penis is unusual in being an organ with a very rich vascular supply and relatively rare metastases. Only about 200 instances of metastasis to the penis had been documented as of 1984.[88]

Metastatic disease may affect the penis by a variety of mechanisms. These were described in detail by Paquin and Roland[77] in the 1950s, but even the most recent discussions still accept their concepts of mechanisms of spread.[10] The first mechanism is direct extension into the corpora cavernosa via the ischiorectal fossa into the superficial perineal space. This could explain the high relative frequency of bladder, prostate, and rectal tumors metastatic to the penis. Second is retrograde venous metastasis via collateral circulation between the dorsal penile vein and the vesical, prostatic, and pudendal venous plexuses. Reversal of flow could be due to coughing, straining, or other means of increasing intra-abdominal pressure. Paquin and Roland[77] believed this to be the major mechanism

of metastasis for bladder, rectal, and prostatic tumors. Other mechanisms described include retrograde lymphatic metastasis and spread by instrumentation.

Multiple series have confirmed that tumors of the bladder and prostate are the major source of penile metastasis, followed by rectosigmoid and renal neoplasms[1,10,26a,35,48,64,72,104] (Figs. 37-21 and 37-22). In addition, metastases from skin, lung, and testicular tumors have been reported, along with leukemic and lymphomatous infiltrates of the penis.[31,49,54]

Metastasis usually affects the vascular tissue of the corpora cavernosa. Stasis in the obstructed vasculature may lead to priapism, which is the most common symptom of penile metastasis. Hematuria, dysuria, and penile nodules may also be seen.[88] Caverosography may prove helpful in localizing the site of metastasis.[26a]

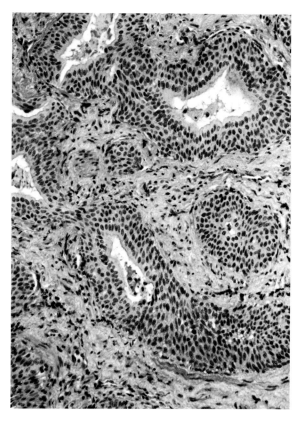

Fig. 37-21 Metastatic transitional cell carcinoma of bladder. Well-differentiated transitional cell carcinoma of the bladder metastatic to penile shaft is illustrated. The polygonal cells grow along the vascular tissue of the corpus cavernosum and mature nicely toward the centers of the vessels. ×154. (Courtesy of J. Tomaszewski.)

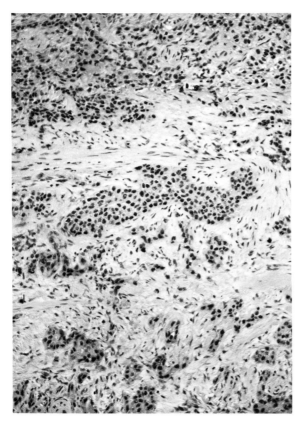

Fig. 37-22 Metastatic prostate carcinoma. The histology of the prostatic tumor is apparent as groups of cells and single cells infiltrate the connective tissue of the penis. ×116.

Penile metastasis is an ominous sign. Survival is usually less than 1 year,[103] with metastases elsewhere appearing shortly after those in the penis. A few patients have been reported with genitourinary primary tumors and no evidence of metastasis outside of the corpora cavernosa. These patients did well after surgical excision of the metastases.[88] Some patients have briefly benefitted from palliative radiation therapy.[30] However, these cases are rare, and most penile metastases are harbingers of short survival.

REFERENCES

1. Abeshouse B, Abeshouse G: Metastatic tumors of the penis: a review of the literature and a report of two cases. J Urol 86:99, 1961

2. Ackerman LV: Verrucous carcinoma of the oral cavity. Surgery 5:670, 1948

3. Andersson L, Jonsson G, Brehmer-Andersson E: Erythroplasia of Queyrat-carcinoma-in-situ. Scand J Urol Nephrol 1:303, 1967

4. Ashley DJB, Edwards EC: Sarcoma of the penis. Br J Surg 45:170, 1957

5. Ashley DJB: Evans' Histological Appearances of Tumours. 3rd Ed. Churchill Livingstone, Edinburgh, 1978

5a. Barrasso R, De Brux J, Croissant O, Orth G: High prevalence of papillomavirus-associated penile intraepithelial neoplasia in sexual partners of women with cervical intraepithelial neoplasia. N Engl J Med 317:916, 1987

6. Bernstein G, Forgaard DM, Miller JE: Carcinoma in situ of the glans penis and distal urethra. J Dermatol Surg Oncol 12:450, 1986

7. Bissada NK, Morcos RR, El-Senoussi M: Post-circumcision carcinoma of the penis. I. Clinical aspects. J Urol 135:283, 1986

8. Blau S, Hyman A: Erythroplasia of Queyrat. Acta Derm Venereol 35:341, 1955

9. Boczko S, Freed S: Penile carcinoma in circumcised males. NY J Med 79:1903, 1979

9a. Boon MD, Schneider A, Hogewoning CJA, et al: Penile studies and heterosexual partners: peniscopy, cytology, histology, and immunocytochemistry. Cancer 61:1652, 1988

10. Bosch PC, Forbes KA, Kollin J et al: Secondary carcinoma of the penis. J Urol 132:990, 1984

11. Bowen JT: Precancerous dermatoses: a study of two cases of chronic atypical epithelial proliferation. J Cutan Dis 30:241, 1912

12. Bracken RB, Diokno A: Melanoma of the penis and the urethra. J Urol 111:198, 1974

13. Bruns T, Lauvetz R, Kerr E, Ross G: Buschke-Lowenstein giant condylomas: pitfalls in management. Urology 5:773, 1975

14. Bulkley G, Wendel R, Grayhack J: Buschke-Loewenstein tumor of the penis. J Urol 97:731, 1967

14a. Collier DStJ, Pain JA, Hamilton-Dutoit SJ: Leiomyosarcoma of the scrotum. J Surg Oncol 34:176, 1987

15. Coulson WF: The male reproductive system. p. 564. In Coulson WF (ed): Surgical Pathology. Vol. 1. JB Lippincott, Philadelphia, 1978

15a. Dalton DP, Rushovich AM, Victor TA, Larson R: Leiomyosarcoma of the scrotum in a man who had received scrotal irradiation as a child. J Urol 139:136, 1988

16. Danczak-Ginalska Z: Treatment of penis carcinoma

with interstitially administered iridium. p. 127. In Grundmann E, Van Lensieck W (eds): Recent Results in Cancer Research. Vol. 60. Springer-Verlag, Berlin 1977

17. Dawson D, Duckworth J, Bernhardt H, Young JM: Giant condyloma and verrucous carcinoma of the genital area. Arch Pathol 79:225, 1965

18. Dehner LP, Smith B: Soft tissue tumors of the penis. Cancer 25:1431, 1970

19. DeKernion J, Tynberg P, Persky L, Fegen J: Carcinoma of the penis. Cancer 32:1256, 1973

20. Derrick F, Lynch K, Kretkowski R, Yarbrough W: Epidermoid carcinoma of the penis: computer analysis of 87 cases. J Urol 110:303, 1973

21. Dodge OG, Linsell CA: Carcinoma of the penis in Uganda and Kenya Africans. Cancer 16:1255, 1963

22. Durack DT: Opportunistic infections and Kaposi's sarcoma in homosexual men. N Engl J Med 305:1465, 1981

23. Dwosh J, Mininberg DT, Schlossberg S, Peterson P: Neurofibroma involving the penis in a child. J Urol 132:988, 1984

23a. Echenique JE, Tully S, Tickman R, et al: A 37-pound scrotal leiomyosarcoma: a case report and literature review. J Urol 138:1245, 1987

24. Ekstrom T, Edsmyr F: Cancer of the penis. Acta Chir Scand 115:25, 1958

25. Elhosseiny AA, Ramaswamy G, Healy RO: Epitheloid hemangioendothelioma of penis. Urology 28:243, 1986

26. Elliott F, Eid T, Lakey W: Genitourinary neurofibromas: Clinical significance. J Urol 125:725, 1981

26a. Escribano G, Allona A, Burgos FJ, et al: Cavernosography in diagnosis of metastatic tumors of the penis: 5 new cases and a review of the literature. J Urol 138:1174, 1987

27. Ferenczy A, Mitao M, Nagai N et al: Latent papillomavirus and recurring genital warts. N Engl J Med 313:784, 1985

28. Fronstin M, Hutcheson J: Malignant melanoma of the penis. Br J Urol 41:324, 1969

29. Ghandur-Mnaymneh L, Gonzalez, M: Angiosarcoma of the penis with hepatic angiomas in a patient with low vinyl chloride exposure. Cancer 47:1318, 1981

30. Gillatt DA: Secondary carcinomatous infiltration of the penis: palliation with radiotherapy. Br J Surg 72:763, 1985

31. Gonzalez-Campora H, Nogales F, Lerma E et al: Lymphoma of the penis. J Urol 126:270, 1981

32. Graham J, Helwig E: Erythroplasia of Queyrat. Cancer 32:1296, 1973

33. Graham S, Priore R, Graham M et al: Genital cancer in wives of penile cancer patients. Cancer 44:1870, 1979

34. Grossman H, Sogani P: Basal cell carcinoma of scrotum. Urology 17:241, 1981

35. Haddad FS, Kivirand AI: Metastases to the corpora cavernosa from transitional cell carcinoma of the bladder. J Surg Oncol 32:19, 1986

36. Hall T, Britt D, Woodhead D: Basal cell carcinoma of the penis. J Urol 99:314, 1968

37. Hanash K, Furlow W, Utz D, Harrison E: Carcinoma of the penis: A clinicopathologic study. J Urol 104:291, 1970

38. Helwig E, Graham J: Anogenital (extramammary) Paget's disease. Cancer 16:387, 1963

39. Hendrickson MR, Kempson RL: Surgical Pathology of the Uterine Corpus. p. 469. WB Saunders, Philadelphia, 1980

40. Hood AF, Farmer ER, Weiss RA: Kaposi's sarcoma. Johns Hopkins Med J 15:222, 1982

41. Hoppmann H, Fraley E: Squamous cell carcinoma of the penis. J Urol 120:393, 1978

42. Huggins C, Warden J: Cancer of the scrotum. J Urol 62:250, 1949

43. Ichikawa T: Chemotherapy of penis carcinoma. p. 140. In Grundmann E, Van Lensieck W (eds): Recent Results in Cancer Research. Vol. 60. Springer-Verlag, Berlin, 1977

44. Johnson S, Rundell M, Platt W: Leiomyosarcoma of the scrotum. Cancer 41:1830, 1978

45. Kaplan C, Katoh A: Erythroplasia of Queyrat (Bowen's disease of the glans penis). J Surg Oncol 5:281, 1973

46. Kathuria S, Jablokow VB, Molnar Z: Leiomyosarcoma of penile prepuce with ultrastructural study. Urology 27:556, 1986

47. Kherzi A, Dounis A, Roberts J: Primary malignant melanoma of the penis. Br J Urol 51:147, 1979

48. Khubchandani M: Metachronous metastasis to the penis from carcinoma of the rectum. Report of a case. Dis Colon Rectum 29:52, 1986

49. Knight E, Post G, Morabito R et al: Leukemic infiltration of penis. Urology 14:83, 1979

50. Kochen M, McCurdy S: Circumcision and the risk of cancer of the penis. Am J Dis Child 134:484, 1980

51. Kossow A, Cotelingham J, MacFarland F: Bowenoid papulosis of the penis. J Urol 125:124, 1981

52. Kraus F, Perez-Mesa C: Verrucous carcinoma. Cancer 19:26, 1966

53. Lane J: Hamangioma of the glans penis. US Armed Forces Med J 4:139, 1953

54. Lanesky J, Law D, Roth S, Wadle R: Burkitt's lymphoma metastatic to penis. Urology 15:610, 1980

55. Leiter E, Lefkovits A: Circumcision and penile carcinoma. NY J Med 75:1520, 1975

56. Lichtenauer P, Scheer H, Louton T: On the classification of penis carcinoma and its 10-year survival. p. 110. In Grundmann E, Van Lensieck W (eds): Recent Results in Cancer Research. Vol. 60. Springer-Verlag, Berlin, 1977

57. Licklider S: Jewish penile carcinoma. J Urol 86:98, 1961

58. Loewenstein L: Carcinoma-like condylomata acuminata of the penis. Med Clin North Am 23:789, 1939

59. Lowe FC: Squamous cell carcinoma of the scrotum. J Urol 130:423, 1983

60. Mabogunje O: Kaposi sarcoma of the glans penis. Urology 17:476, 1981

61. Manglani K, Manaligod J, Ray B: Spindle cell carcinoma of the glans penis. Cancer 46:2266, 1980

62. Margolis S: Genital warts and molluscum contagiosum. Urol Clin North Am 11:163, 1984

63. McCance DJ, Kalache A, Ashdown K et al: Human papillomavirus types 16 and 18 in carcinomas of the penis from Brazil. Int J Cancer 37:55, 1986

64. McCrea L, Tobias G: Metastatic disease of the penis. J Urol 80:489, 1958

65. McDonald MW, O'Connell JR, Manning JT, Benjamin RS: Leiomyosarcoma of the penis. J Urol 130:788, 1983

66. Merino M, Livolsi V, Lytton B: Penile Paget's disease and prostatic carcinoma. J Urol 120:121, 1978

67. Merrin C: Cancer of the penis. Cancer 45:1973, 1980

68. Millstein D, Tang C, Campbell E: Angiosarcoma developing in a patient with neurofibromatosis (von Recklinghausen's disease). Cancer 47:950, 1981

69. Moore S, Wheeler J, Hefter L: Epithelioid sarcoma masquerading as Peyronie's disease. Cancer 35:1706, 1975

70. Mortensen H, Murphy L: Angiomatous malformations of the glans penis. J Urol 64:396, 1950

71. Mostofi FK, Price E: Tumors of the Male Genital System. Armed Forces Institute of Pathology, Bethesda, 1973

72. Narayana A, Olney L, Howard D, Culp D: Metastatic tumors of the penis. Eur Urol 5:262, 1979

73. Narayana A, Olney LE, Loening SA et al: Carcinoma of the penis. Cancer, 49:2185, 1980

74. Obalek S, Jablonska S, Beaudenon S et al: Bowenoid papulosis of the male and female genitalia: risk of cervical neoplasia. J Am Acad Dermatol 14:433, 1986

75. Ogawa A, Watanabe K: Genitourinary neurofibromatosis in a child presenting with an enlarged penis and scrotum. J Urol 135:755, 1986

76. Panda K, Nayak C: Clinicopathological studies on cancer penis. J Indian Med Assoc 75:25, 1980

77. Paquin AJ, Roland SI: Secondary carcinoma of the penis. Cancer 9:626, 1956

78. Persky L, deKernion J: Carcinoma of the penis. CA 36:258, 1986

79. Persky L: Epidemiology of cancer of the penis. p. 97. In Grundmann E, Van Lensieck W (eds): Recent Results in Cancer Research. Vol. 60. Springer-Verlag, Berlin, 1977

80. Peters MS, Perry HO: Bowenoid papules of the penis. J Urol 126:482, 1981

81. Pueblitz S, Mora-Tiscareno A, Meneses-Garcia AA et al: Epithelioid sarcoma of penis. Urology 28:246, 1986

82. Queyrat L: Erythroplasie du gland. Bull Soc Fr Dermatol Syphil 22:378, 1911

83. Ray B, Whitmore W: Experience with carcinoma of the scrotum. J Urol 117:741, 1977

84. Ray B: Condyloma accuminatum of the scrotum. J Urol 117:739, 1977

85. Reddy C, Devendranath V, Pratap S: Carcinoma of the penis — role of phimosis. Urology 24:85, 1984

86. Rege P, Evans A: Erythroplasia of Queyrat. J Urol 111:784, 1974

87. Riveros M, Lebron R: Geographic pathology of cancer of the penis. Cancer 16:798, 1963

88. Robey EL, Schellhammer PF: Four cases of metastases to the penis and a review of the literature. J Urol 132:992, 1984

89. Roman A, Fife K: Human papillomavirus DNA associated with foreskins of normal newborns. J Infect Dis 153:855, 1986

89a. Rogus BJ: Squamous cell carcinoma in a young circumcised man. J Urol 138:861, 1987

90. Rosai J: Ackerman's Surgical Pathology. CV Mosby, St. Louis, 1981

91. Saw D, Chan J, Watt CY, Poon YF: Clear cell sarcoma of the penis. Hum Pathol 17:423, 1986

92. Scappini P, Piscioli F, Pusiol T et al: Penile cancer. Aspiration biopsy cytology for staging. Cancer 58:1526, 1986

93. Schellhammer P, Grabstald H: Tumors of the penis and urethra. p. 1171. In Harrison JH (ed): Campbell's Urology. 4th Ed. Vol. 2. WB Saunders, Philadelphia, 1978

94. Seftel AD, Sadick NS, Waldbaum RS: Kaposi's sarcoma of the penis in a patient with the acquired immune deficiency syndrome. J Urol 136:673, 1986

95. Senoh K, Miyasaki T, Kikuchi I et al: Angiomatous lesions of glans penis. Urology 17:194, 1981

96. Shabad A: Some aspects of etiology and prevention of penile cancer. J Urol 92:696, 1964

97. Shah P, Abrams P, Gaches C et al: Verrucous carcinoma of the penis or Buschke-Lowenstein tumor. Eur Urol 7:78, 1981

98. Smart RH: Leiomyosarcoma of the penis. J Urol 132:356, 1984

99. Smith R, Young H, Chaffey B: Verrucous carcinoma of the penis. Br J Surg 41:327, 1969

99a. Srinivas V, Morse MJ, Herr HW, et al: Penile cancer: relation of extent of nodal metastasis to survival. J Urol 137:880, 1987

100. Stone NN, Sun CC, Brutscher S, Sein T: Granular cell tumor of the penis. J Urol 130:575, 1983

101. Suarez GM, Lewis RW: Granular cell tumor of the glans penis. J Urol 135:1252, 1986

102. Thomas J: Pathology of carcinoma of the penis. J Indian Med Assoc 52:461, 1969

103. Trulock T, Wheatley J, Walton K: Secondary tumors of penis. Urology 17:563, 1981

104. van den Berg GM, Menke HE, Stolz E: Nodules on the glans penis, an unusual metastatic pattern of prostate carcinoma: case report. Genitourin Med 62:126, 1986

105. Villa LL, Lopes A: Human papillomavirus DNA sequences in penile carcinomas in Brazil. Int J Cancer 37:853, 1986

106. Wade T, Kopf A, Ackerman A: Bowenoid papulosis of the genitalia. Arch Dermatol 115:306, 1979

107. Wajsman Z, Moore R, Merrin C, Murphy G: Surgical treatment of penile cancer. Cancer 40:1697, 1977

108. Weiss JP, November S, Curtin CT: Recurrent penile condylomata acuminata in a 17-month-old boy. J Urol 136:468, 1986

109. Wespes E, Simon J, Schulman CC: Cabanas approach: is sentinel node biopsy reliable for staging penile carcinoma? Urology 28:278, 1986

110. Wilson LS, Lockhart JI, Bergman H, Politano V: Fibrosarcoma of the penis. J Urol 129:606, 1983

38

Tumors and Tumorlike Conditions of the Male Urethra

Robert S. Katz

Tumors of the male urethra are quite rare and comprise less than 1 percent of all male genitourinary neoplasms. In general, they are histologically similar to tumors seen elsewhere in this region.

BENIGN TUMORS

Condyloma Acuminata

Condyloma acuminata are virus-induced growths that are common on the external penile surface. Although primary urethral neoplasms are rare, perhaps nearly one-third are condylomata.[33] Intraurethral condylomata are generally found in young men and are spread by sexual contact. Papillomavirus has been identified as the etiologic agent.[33] As with other penile condylomas, HPV types 6 and 11 are most common, with type 18 also seen.[9a] In general, the condylomas are located within the first portion of the urethra near the meatus. However, the lesions may extend into the remainder of the urethra and into the bladder.[9] The virus enters the urethra at the anterior portion by direct implantation and may then grow in a retrograde manner. Patients usually report symptoms of bloody urethral discharge, dysuria, difficulty in in-

itiating voiding, or change in the caliber of the urinary stream.

Grossly, the condyloma of the urethra has the typical warty appearance seen elsewhere in the genitourinary system. The histology and behavior have been discussed previously (see Ch. 37). There is acanthosis and papillomatosis of the epithelium, with an upward growth of the cell layers. There is also hyperkeratosis and clearing of some of the more superficial nuclei. The cells mature with no significant atypicality and do not press downward into the submucosa as with the verrucous carcinoma (giant condyloma of Buschke-Loewenstein). The submucosa shows a chronic inflammatory infiltrate.[31]

A variety of therapeutic approaches have been attempted including intraurethral instillation of 5-fluorouracil, as well as surgical remedies. With patient compliance, good results seem attainable.[9]

Urethral Polyps

Urethral polyps are unusual tumors of the pediatric age group that are probably congenital in nature. The usual symptoms involve hematuria, voiding difficulties, and infection.

1369

The polyps are generally located in the posterior urethra just distal to the bladder. They are exophytic masses with a pedunculated stalk. The polyps, on microscopic examination, are composed of a connective tissue stalk with small blood vessels in the central portion. The fibrovascular core is covered with transitional epithelium that is usually histologically normal or may display some squamous metaplasia.[16] Polyps of the anterior portion of the urethra are reported but are exceedingly rare. They have the same gross and microscopic appearance.[12]

The tumors can be easily removed and the obstructive symptoms alleviated. This is generally accomplished by cystoscopy.

Hemangioma

Less than 20 cases of capillary hemangioma have been reported. The growth generally occurs in young men, although children may be affected.[37] The tumors are generally polypoid lesions involving the anterior urethra, which may protrude through the urethral meatus and produce a bloody discharge.[28,44a] Sometimes they are multiple, extending along the length of the urethra.[44a]

Microscopically, the hemangioma is similar in appearance to those elsewhere in the body. The lesions are polypoid and covered by squamous epithelium. Underneath the epithelium is an accumulation of irregular, thin-walled vascular channels, lined by a layer of flat endothelial cells in a large collagenous matrix.[28] Although these lesions are basically benign, they may recur if not adequately removed. Wide excision may be necessary.[37,44]

Leiomyoma

Two cases of leiomyoma of the male urethra have been reported. In the more recent case, bloody discharge was the presenting symptom. The tumor was

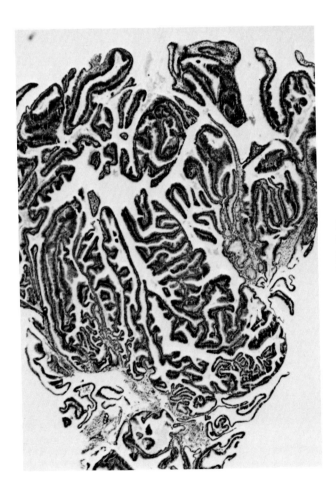

Fig. 38-1 Prostatic epithelial polyp. Benign prostatic epithelial polyp showing interdigitating channels of fibrovascular cores and overlying epithelium. ×30. (From Murad et al.,[32] with permission.)

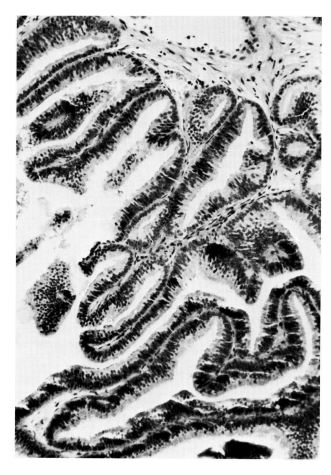

Fig. 38-2 Prostatic epithelial polyp. Higher magnification of the columnar epithelium showing basal position of the nuclei. (From Murad et al.,[32] with permission.)

resected and was histologically similar to leiomyomata in other sites. The patient did well after resection of the lesion.[34]

Benign Prostatic Epithelial Polyp

This unusual tumor apparently develops from prostatic epithelium and projects into the urethral lumen. A variety of names have been given to this neoplasm, including villous polyp and papillary adenoma of the prostatic urethra. The lesion is generally found in postpubertal men. Although rare in the United States, it is rather common in the Middle East,[4] although no explanation for this geographic difference is provided.

Immunoperoxidase techniques have demonstrated the presence of prostatic acid phosphatase and prostate-specific antigen in the epithelium of tumors, confirming their histogenesis. Ectopic prostatic tissue

in the posterior urethra is the apparent site of origin, with enlargement occurring after puberty.

This polyp appears as a papillary lesion of the prostatic urethra. Hematuria or hematospermia are the usual symptoms.[11] Microscopically, the lesions are polypoid, with a branching fibrovascular core covered by tall columnar or cuboidal cells (Fig. 38-1). Cytoplasm is abundant, clear to finely granular, and the nuclei are basally located (Fig. 38-2).[32] The epithelium is identical to that seen in the prostate.

These lesions behave in a benign fashion, with excision producing alleviation of symptoms.[11]

MALIGNANT TUMORS

Malignant tumors of the male urethra are extremely rare. In fact, they are the rarest tumors of the male genitourinary apparatus. Less than 500 cases of primary neoplasms of the male urethra have been reported in the literature.

Urethral Carcinoma

Urethral carcinoma is predominantly a disease of older men over the age of 45 years, with most cases in the 60 to 80-year age group.[30]

Tumors of the urethra may arise from the posterior (prostatic) urethra or the anterior (membranous, bulbous, penile, and glanular) urethra. Approximately 15 percent of urethral tumors develop from the transitional epithelium of the posterior urethra and are, as expected, transitional cell carcinomas. Approximately 75 percent of urethral tumors develop from the columnar and stratified squamous epithelium of the anterior urethra and are squamous cell carcinomas (Fig. 38-3). Adenocarcinoma and melanoma compose the remaining few tumors. Adenocarcinomas develop in the bulbomembranous urethra, with melanomas closer to the meatus.[23]

The clinical symptoms of transitional cell carcinoma of the posterior urethra are nonspecific. Prostatism and hematuria are reported, with some patients having a firm prostate on palpation.[15] Tumors of the posterior urethra drain to pelvic nodes.[23] The much more common tumors of anterior urethra generally arise in the bulbomembranous area. Signs and symptoms include obstruction (47 percent), mass (39 per-

cent), periurethral abscess (31 percent), fistula (20 percent), and urethral discharge (22 percent).[13] The neoplasm may invade the adjacent tissues, with involvement of the corpora, penile, and even scrotal skin.[26] When the patient attempts to void, urine may exit from a variety of urethral-cutaneous fistulae and give the impression of a spray can or "water pot perineum."[30] Anterior urethral lesions drain to inguinal lymph nodes.[23]

The etiology of urethral carcinomas in general is uncertain. The development of transitional cell carcinoma may represent extension of the "field effect" of carcinogenesis in the more proximal urothelium (see Ch. 6). A substantial number of cases of transitional cell carcinoma of the urethra have been found in patients undergoing cystectomy for bladder carcinoma.[41] In one large series, 5 percent of patients undergoing prophylactic urethrectomy with cystectomy had unsuspected carcinoma in situ. An additional 27 patients (7 percent of the total) needed urethrectomy for clinically apparent carcinoma, with 24 cases after cystectomy and 3 cases at the time of cystectomy.[41] Most of these tumors were in the distal urethra, not usually the site of transitional cell carcinoma. These lesions may reflect either the multicentricity of urothelial neoplasms or direct extension of tumor down the urethral walls.[42] A few cases of Paget's disease of the urethral meatus have been described in patients with prior cystectomies for bladder

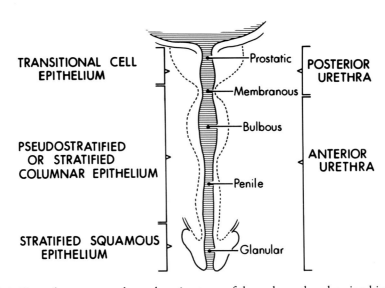

Fig. 38-3 Normal anatomy, male urethra. Anatomy of the male urethra showing histology of the mucosa and anatomic divisions. (From Levine,[23] with permission.)

carcinoma. The transitional cell bladder cancer spread to the urethral epithelium, producing the pagetoid cells described in Chapter 37.[45]

Tumors of the anterior urethra, usually squamous cell carcinoma, also have an uncertain etiology. Approximately one-third of patients with urethral carcinomas have a history of "venereal disease."[21] However, the nature and duration of these processes are not defined clearly.[30] A considerable association with stricture has also been discussed, with as many as 88 percent of patients with cancer said to have an associated stricture.[23] However, looking at the process from the opposite point of view, only about 15 percent of men with a history of stricture manifest urethral carcinoma.[23,27] A number of researchers postulate that squamous carcinoma of the urethra follows long-standing inflammation, with associated squamous metaplasia of the columnar epithelium.[15,23,30] A

few patients have documented postgonococcal strictures, and some patients have developed squamous carcinoma post-urethroplasty,[40a] but many have no history of previous urethritis.[27] Some patients have recurrent urethral strictures that respond poorly to dilatation. After episodes of bleeding, pain, and dysuria, the persistent stricture may be biopsied. By then the tumor may have penetrated so deeply that no tumor is seen in the pathologic material. Deeper biopsies may finally reveal tumor, suggesting that the tumor was present all along. In fact, one wonders whether most of the patients with a history of "stricture" who eventually developed carcinoma had tumor as the real cause of all their symptoms.

The pathology of urethral carcinomas is straightforward. Tumors of the posterior urethra may infiltrate the prostate. The transitional cell carcinoma, developing from urethral lining cells, shows large,

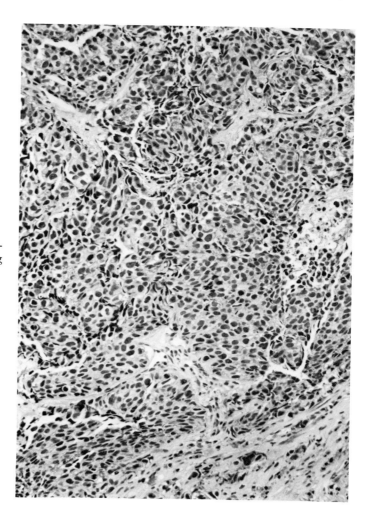

Fig. 38-4 Transitional cell carcinoma. Transitional cell carcinoma of the urethra, showing invasion of underlying tissue. ×165.

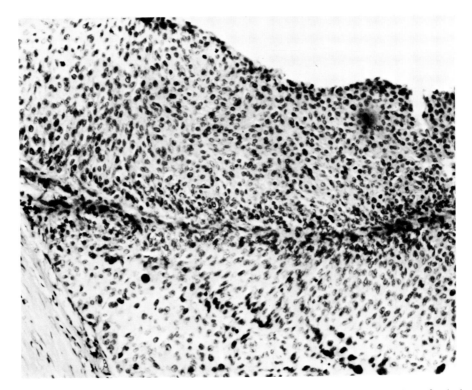

Fig. 38-5 Transitional cell carcinoma. Superficial transitional cell tumor showing loss of orderly mucosal maturation. (From Levine,[23] with permission.)

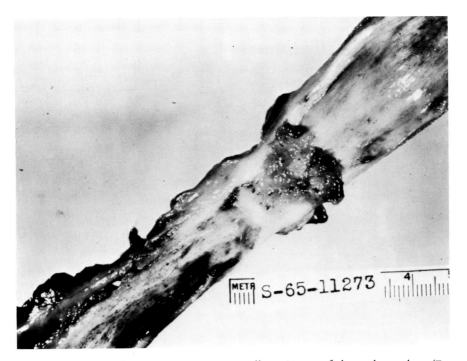

Fig. 38-6 Squamous cell carcinoma. Squamous cell carcinoma of the male urethra. (From Levine,[23] with permission.)

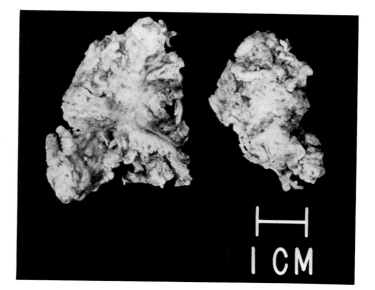

Fig. 38-7 Squamous cell carcinoma. Resection specimen of squamous cell carcinoma of the urethral orifice.

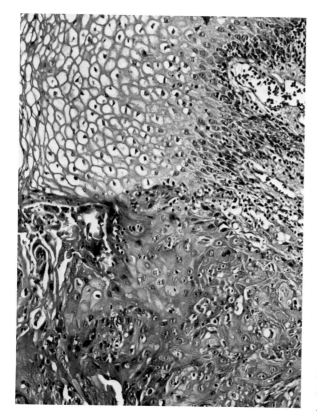

Fig. 38-8 Squamous cell carcinoma. Example of squamous cell carcinoma arising in glandular epithelium. The cellular atypicality and intercellular bridges are evident. ×138.

cuboidal transitional cells growing without normal maturation at the surface of the urethra (Figs. 38-4 and 38-5). A papillary apperance may be seen, with projections of transitional cells above the surface.[8,23] The nuclei are round and rather uniform.

The squamous cell carcinoma, most frequent in the anterior urethra, shows characteristic intercellular bridges, keratinous pearls, and intracellular keratinization (Figs. 38-6, 38-7, and 38-8). The lesions both project into the lumen and grow into surrounding tissues. Squamous carcinomas are less exophytic than transitional neoplasms.[27] The degree of differentiation of these tumors is not discussed in most series, although histologic diagnosis has not presented major difficulties.

Adenocarcinomas of the urethra are exceedingly rare. A few cases have been described in some detail. The tumors may arise in the bulbous urethra as polypoid lesions projecting into the lumen. Histologic evaluation showed papillary projections of columnar cells, with invasion of underlying corpus spongiosum. The columnar cells were pleomorphic, with large, dark nuclei. The lesions resembled adenocarcinoma of the colon and rectum, but in the reported cases, neoplasia in the prostate or bowel was not found.[24,39] Adenocarcinoma of the urethra may arise from the glands of Littre or through glandular metaplasia of the urethral epithelium.[3,24] One case showed adenosquamous carcinoma, the histogenesis of which was puzzling.[39] It was uncertain whether this tumor represented glandular metaplasia in a primary squamous carcinoma, squamous metaplasia in a primary adenocarcinoma, or another phenomenon. Urethral adenocarcinoma is so unusual that discussion of histogenesis is conjectural only.

The prognosis of primary carcinoma of the male urethra depends most on the site of origin of the tumor. In a recent series,[2] anterior urethral carcinomas, usually squamous cell carcinomas, presenting without lymph node metastasis seemed to be curable by radical surgery. However, only about 50 percent of distal (anterior) tumors present in this fashion.[2] Patients with lymph node metastasis or distant metastases have a very poor survival (dying within 2 years or less). Radiotherapy is not helpful in this process.

Patients with more posterior lesions (bulbomembranous) have a somewhat poorer prognosis.[8] Most tumors have infiltrated the prostate, bladder, or perineum at the time of presentation. Widespread metastasis is not unusual in these lesions, which include the less common transitional cell carcinomas. A variety of surgical and radiation regimens have been used, giving only a 8 percent to 10 percent 5-year survival rate, contrasted with an approximately 50 percent 5-year survival ran in anterior tumors.[18]

Flow cytometry studies have been helpful in understanding the behavior of squamous carcinoma of the urethra.[47a] A study of 30 cases revealed that among those with a normal diploid pattern of DNA only 18 percent progressed, whereas 93 percent with an aneuploid or tetraploid pattern progressed. More interestingly, among histologically low-grade lesions, none with a diploid pattern progressed versus 90 percent with an aneuploid pattern. To predict that a high-grade lesion will progress is no great feat. The real value of flow cytometry is in discerning which cases among seemingly similar low-grade lesions will progress and which will not.

Survival in patients with urethral carcinoma after cystectomy for bladder cancer appears rather dismal, with nearly all patients dying of recurrent carcinoma.[41,45]

Malignant Melanoma

Malignant melanoma of the male urethra is extremely rare. A recent review recorded a total of 24 cases.[40] The tumor may develop from almost any portion of the urethra, although those in the more ante-

rior portion are slightly more common. Most cases involve symptoms of dysuria or bleeding.[22] The melanoma has been described, anecdotally, as sometimes arising de novo and sometimes arising from a pre-existing nevus. Histogenesis of the melanoma has not been studied in a systematic fashion, owing to the rarity of cases in both the penis and the urethra.[5]

The histology of the tumor is similar to that described as a penile primary. The typical cell is a large one, with considerable eosinophilic cytoplasm. Nuclear pleomorphism is common, and considerable pigment may be evident on routine staining or special techniques may be needed to demonstrate the melanin. The tumors have been described as growing either radially in a spreading manner along the epithelium or mucosa or in a nodular, invasive fashion.[5]

Most investigators claim that good survival depends on rapid diagnosis and therapy. Only 5 of 23 patients reported in the literature were free of disease after 9 to 24 months of follow-up.[5] Melanoma of the urethra spreads by lymphatic and hematogenous routes. Penectomy, lymphadenectomy, immunotherapy, and chemotherapy have all been tried with poor results.[22]

Sarcoma

Sarcoma of the urethra is virtually unknown. However, one recent report of a leiomyosarcoma of the bladder with subsequent urethral recurrence is of some interest. The patient underwent cystectomy for this sarcomatous neoplasm and 5 months later was noted to have a mass protruding through the external meatus.[1] The tumor and the recurrence showed the spindle cells and fascicle formation typical of leiomyosarcoma (see Ch. 37).

The recurrence of the tumor in the urethra is reminiscent of the development of transitional cell carcinoma in men undergoing surgery of the bladder. The possibility of a multicentric origin of the tumor or of intraurethral metastasis must be entertained.

A single case of rhabdomyosarcoma of the male urethra was reported in a Malayan man. The patient had extensive metastatic disease and died shortly after diagnosis.[36]

Cowper's Gland Carcinoma

Adenocarcinoma supposedly arising in Cowper's gland has been infrequently described. The cases described in the literature develop mostly in the bulbous urethra. Histologically, they appear as typical adenocarcinomas.[7] While discussed as a distinct entity, it is unclear how they may be distinguished from other adenocarcinomas of the urethra. Distinction cannot be made by histologic means but may be suggested by the anatomic location of the tumor. Perhaps the Cowper's gland should be regarded as simply another possible site of origin for the rare primary adenocarcinoma of male urethra.

TUMORLIKE CONDITIONS OF THE URETHRA

A number of unusual conditions may simulate urethral carcinoma. Although these lesions are quite rare, they should be kept in the differential diagnosis of mass lesions in the urethral area.

Malakoplakia

A single case of malakoplakia of the urethra has been reported. The patient had voiding difficulty and a mass in the bulbous portion of the urethra. It was excised and showed the usual features of malakoplakia as described elsewhere (see Ch. 9). An ulcerating chronic inflammatory infiltrate was noted with lymphocytes, plasma cells, and histiocytes. The characteristic laminated calcospherules, the Michaelis-Gutmann bodies, were observed extracellularly. This disorder presumably reflects an abnormality of cellular response to urothelial infection.[43]

Balanitis Xerotica Obliterans

Balanitis xerotica obliterans has been reported to involve the anterior urethra in a single biopsy-proven case. The patient had a long history of urethral strictures that were treated by dilatation. He eventually developed balanitis xerotica obliterans on the glans, and the process involved the anterior urethra as well. The patient was of particular interest in that a squamous cell carcinoma appeared on the glans 3 years after balanitis xerotica obliterans was diagnosed.[17]

The histopathology of balanitis xerotica obliterans was described earlier (see Ch. 35). There is epidermal atrophy and the characteristic hyalinization of the dermal collagen. The relationship of this process to the eventual cancer of the penis remains uncertain.

Amyloid

Localized amyloidosis may produce a mass in the urethra that may mimic carcinoma. Amyloid of the penis was described elsewhere (see Ch. 36), and involvement of both the urethra and corpora cavernosa is possible.[46] Most patients with urethral amyloid are middle-aged, and some, but not all, have a history of gonorrhea or other infections in this region.[10]

When it is a solitary urethral mass, amyloidosis may be firm and gritty. It may appear quite similar to carcinoma, and biopsy is indicated to establish the diagnosis.[14] The lesion is submucosal and shows the typical amorphous, eosinophilic material in the connective tissue.[20] Periurethral glands may be surrounded by the amyloid, and blood vessel walls may be thickened by the deposits. Congo red stains show green birefringence of the acellular material when examined under polarized light.[35]

In general, patients have done well after resection of the localized lesions, with resolution of dysuria and hematuria. The localized forms have not been reported to progress to systemic disease, although careful follow-up is indicated because of the recognized association of amyloidosis with both chronic inflammatory and malignant diseases.[47] Although the diagnosis is not difficult to establish upon microscopic examination, it indicates the need for biopsy diagnosis of mass lesions in this area before attempting surgery.

Urethral Prolapse

Urethral prolapse is a benign process that involves the distal portion of the urethra. Although physical examination should reveal the nature of the condition without much difficulty, other lesions (urethral polyp, condylomas, caruncle, and prolapsed ureterocele) may be seen in this area.

Urethral prolapse is usually found in prepubertal girls, who usually present with vaginal spotting.[25]

As surgical repair of this problem generally produces no resected tissue, material is rarely available for pathologic evaluation. However, one recent study in autopsy material demonstrated the presence of a cleavage plane (Fig. 38-9) between the longitudinal and circular-oblique smooth muscle layers of the urethra.[25] In addition, most of the patients with urethral prolapse had a history of disorders associated with increased intra-abdominal pressure. Poor attachment between the two muscle layers and raised intra-ab-

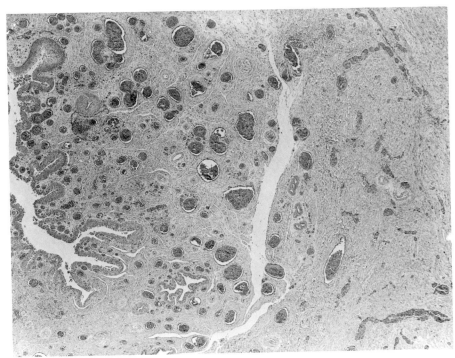

Fig. 38-9 Urethral prolapse. Note the cleavage plane between the longitudinal and circular-oblique smooth muscle layers. (From Lowe et al.,[25] with permission.)

dominal pressure (resulting from profound cough, trauma, or seizures) caused the muscle to "give way" leading to prolapse.

Surgical reduction techniques have had good results.[25]

TUMORS OF THE FEMALE URETHRA

Although this section stresses the pathology of lesions of the male external genitalia, a few comments should be made about lesions of the female urethra.

Caruncle

The most common lesion of the female urethra is the caruncle. These are polypoid masses that project from the meatus in older women. They may be asymptomatic or cause bleeding and pain. The only way to diagnose these benign growths is by excision and microscopic evaluation. It is imprudent to diag-

nose a caruncle by external inspection alone as it may, in fact, represent a primary carcinoma.[29]

Microscopically, caruncle shows large, dilated vessels surrounded by chronic inflammation, akin to a hemorrhoid.[13] Areas of granulation tissue are common (Fig. 38-10). One wonders whether these really are true neoplasms or represent inflammatory or degenerative processes in the aged.

Carcinoma

Malignant tumors of the female urethra are quite rare but are found somewhat more commonly than in men. Most (50 percent to 70 percent) of the malignancies are squamous cell carcinomas, not surprising since the anterior two-thirds of the female urethra is lined by squamous epithelium.[6,23] Adenocarcinoma is the second most frequent type, with some clear cell variants. Transitional cell carcinomas and a few malignant melanomas make up the remainder of the lesions.[6,19,38] The transitional cell carcinomas and ade-

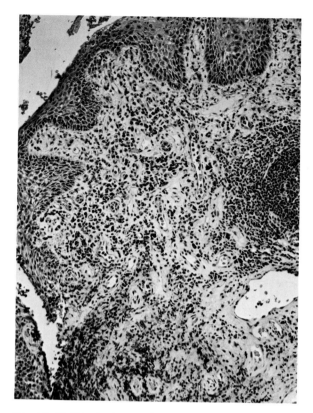

Fig. 38-10 Urethral caruncle. Large, dilated blood vessels and chronic inflammation fill the submucosa, along with numerous small blood vessels (granulation tissue). ×118.

nocarcinomas originate in the proximal one-third of the urethra.

Signs and symptoms are vague but include spotting and a variety of urinary difficulties.[23] Some patients are asymptomatic with the diagnosis established during routine examination upon the finding of a palpable mass.

The tumors have been treated by a variety of measures, including radical surgery procedures and radiation. As for male urethral carcinomas, the histology bears little relationship to prognosis. Patients with anterior tumors and tumors of limited extent have a better survival than patients with proximal lesions or lesions who have enlarged, positive pelvic lymph nodes.[19] It should be noted that most females with urethral cancer are elderly, the same age group that develops caruncles. Thus, biopsy of any mass lesion in the female urethra is mandatory.

One case of non-Hodgkin's lymphoma presenting as a urethral mass in a 63-year-old woman has been reported.[45a]

REFERENCES

1. Alabaster AM, Jordan W, Soloway M et al: Leiomyosarcoma of the bladder and subsequent urethral recurrence. J Urol 125:583,1981
2. Anderson KA, McAninch JW: Primary squamous cell carcinoma of anterior male urethra. Urology 23:134, 1984
3. Assimos D, O'Conor V: Clear cell adenocarcinoma of the urethra. J Urol 131:540, 1984
4. Baroudy AC, O'Connell JP: Papillary adenoma of the prostatic urethra. J Urol 132:120,1984
5. Begun FP, Grossman HB, Diokno AC, Sogani PG: Malignant melanoma of the penis and male urethra. J Urol 132:123, 1984
6. Bolduan J, Farah R: Primary urethral neoplasms: review of 30 cases. J Urol 125:198, 1981
7. Bourque J-L, Charghi A, Gauthier G-E et al: Primary carcinoma of Cowper's gland. J Urol 103:758, 1970
8. Bracken RB, Henry R, Ordonez N: Primary carcinoma of the male urethra. South Med J 73:1004, 1980
9. Debenedictis T, Marmar J, Prass D: Intraurethral condylomas acuminata: management and review of the literature J Urol 118:767, 1977
9a. Del Mistro A, Braunstein JD, Halwer M, Koss LG: Identification of human papillomavirus types in male urethra condylomata acuminata by in situ hybridization. Hum Pathol 18:936, 1987
10. Dounis A, Bourounis M, Mitropoulos D: Primary localized amyloidosis of the urethra. Eur Urol 11:344, 1985
11. Eglen DE, Pontius EE: Benign prostatic epithelial polyp of the urethra. J Urol 131:120, 1984
12. Foster R, Weigel J, Mantz F: Anterior urethral polyps. J Urol 124:145,1980
13. Friedrich EG, Wilkinson EJ: The vulva. p. 13. In Blaustein A (ed): Pathology of the Frmale Genital Tract. Springer-Verlag, New York, 1977
14. Fujime M, Tajima A, Minowada S et al: Localized amyloidosis of urethra. Report of two cases. Eur Urol 7:189, 1981
15. Grabstald H: Tumors of the urethra in men and women. Cancer 32:1236, 1973
16. Hanani Y, Hertz M, Jonas P: Congenital urethral polyp in children. Urology 16:162, 1980
17. Herschorn S, Colapinto V: Balanitis xerotica obliterans involving anterior urethra. Urology 14:593, 1979

18. Hopkins SC, Nag SK, Soloway MS: Primary carcinoma of male urethra. Urology 23:128, 1984

19. Johnson DE, O'Connell JR: Primary carcinoma of the female urethra. Urology 21:42, 1983

20. Kaisary AV: Primary localized amyloidosis of the urethra. Eur Urol 11:209, 1985

21. Kaplan GW, Bulkley GJ, Grayhack JT: Carcinoma of the male urethra. J Urol 96:365, 1967

22. Kokotas N, Kallis E, Fokitis P: Primary malignant melanoma of male urethra. Urology 18:392, 1981

23. Levine R: Urethral cancer. Cancer 45:1965, 1980

24. Lieber MM, Malek RS, Farrow GM, McMurtry J: Villous adenocarcinoma of the male urethra. J Urol 130:1191, 1983

25. Lowe F, Hill G, Jeffs R, Brendler C: Uretheral prolapse in children: insights into etiology and management. J Urol 135:100, 1986

26. Mahmood SA, Thomas JA: Primary penile urethral carcinoma. Br J Urol 58:333, 1986

27. Mandler JI, Pool TL: Primary carcinoma of the male urethra. J Urol 96:67, 1966

28. Manuel E, Seery W, Cole A: Capillary hemangioma of the male urethra: case report with literature review. J Urol 117:804, 1977

29. Marshall FC, Uson A, Melicow M: Neoplasms and caruncles of the female urethra. Surg Gynecol Obstet 110:723, 1960

30. Melicow M, Roberts T: Pathology and natural history of urethral tumors in males. Urology 11:83, 1978

31. Mostofi FK, Price EB: Tumors of the Male Genital System. Armed Forces Institute of Pathology, Bethesda, 1973

32. Murad T, Robinson L, Bueschen A: Villous polyps of the urethra: a report of two cases. Hum Pathol 10:478, 1979

33. Murphy WM, Fu YS, Lancaster WD, Jenson AB: Papillomavirus structural antigens in condyloma acuminatum of the male urethra. J Urol 130:84, 1983

34. Ohtani M, Yanagizawa R, Shoj F et al: Leiomyoma of the male urethra. Eur Urol 8:372, 1982

35. Ordonez N, Ayala A, Gresik M et al: Primary localized amyloidosis of male urethra (amyloidoma). Urology 14:617, 1979

36. Painter MR, O'Shaughnesy EJ, Larson PH, Ribbe RE: Rhabdomyosarcoma of the male urethra. J Urol 99:455, 1968

37. Roberts JW, Devine CJ: Urethral hemangioma: treatment by total excision and grafting. J Urol 129:1053, 1983

38. Robutti F, Betta PG, Bellingeri M, Bellingeri D: Primary malignant melanoma of the female urethral meatus. Eur Urol 12:62, 1986

39. Saito R: An adenosquamous carcinoma of the male urethra with hypercalcemia. Hum Pathol 12:383, 1981

40. Sanders TJ, Venable DD, Sanusi ID: Primary malignant melanoma of the urethra in a black man: a case report. J Urol 135:1012, 1986

40a. Sawczuk I, Acosta R, Grant D, White RD: Post urethroplasty squamous cell carcinoma. N Y State J Med 86:261, 1986

41. Schellhammer P, Whitmore W: Transitional cell carcinoma of the urethra in men having cystectomy for bladder cancer. J Urol 115:56, 1976

42. Schellhammer PF, Whitmore WF: Urethral meatal carcinoma following cystourethrectomy for bladder carcinoma. J Urol 115:61, 1976

43. Sharma T, Kagan H, Sheils J: Malacoplakia of the male urethra. J Urol 125:885, 1981

44. Sharma SK, Reddy M, Joshi V et al: Capillary hemangioma of male urethra. Br J Urol 53:277, 1981

44a. Steinhardt G, Perlmutter A: Urethral hemangioma. J Urol 137:116, 1987

45. Tomaszewski JE, Korat OC, LiVolsi VA et al: Paget's disease of the urethral meatus following transitional cell carcinoma of the bladder. J Urol 135:368, 1986

45a. Touhami H, Brahimi S, Kubisz P, Crongberg S: Nonhodgkins lymphoma of the female urethra. J Urol 137:991, 1987

46. Vasudevan P, Stein A, Pinn V et al: Primary amyloidosis of urethra. Urology 17:181, 1981

47. Walzer Y, Bear RA, Colapinto V et al: Localized amyloidosis of urethra. Urology 21:406, 1983

47a. Winkler HZ, Lieber MM: Primary squamous cell carcinoma of the male urethra: nuclear deoxyribonucleic acid ploidy studied by flow cytometry. J Urol 139:298, 1988

Index

Page numbers followed by *f* denote figures; those followed by *t* denote tables.

Abdomen
  fibrous histiocytoma of, 690
  in prune-belly syndrome, 121f, 122
Abdominal bruit, in renal artery
        stenosis, 189
ABO blood group, in urinary tract
        infection, 292
ABO blood group antigen, in
        bladder cancer, 775
Abscess
  in acute pyelonephritis, 338
  of kidney, 345, 346f
  perinephric, 347–348f
  retroperitoneal, 561–563
Acid phosphatase marker. *See also*
        Tumor marker.
  enzymatic procedures, 1265–1266
  in prostate carcinoma, 1235–1236
    bone marrow determinations,
        1266–1267
    clinical stage and, 1266
    predictive value of, 1265
    production and release of, 1265–
        1268
    therapeutic response and
        survival, 1267
    tumor grade and, 1267–1268
Acinar adenocarcinoma, of prostate,
        1211–1212
Acquired cystic disease. *See* Dialysis
Acquired immune deficiency
        syndrome, penile Kaposi's
        sarcoma in, 1361, 1362f
Acrolein, in cystitis, 437–438
Actinomyces, in epididimitis, 1122
Actinomyces israelii, in cystitis, 439
Actinomycin D, in Wilms' tumor,
        636

Actinomycosis, in cystitis, 439, 440f
Adenocarcinoma. *See also specific organ*
  in bladder exstrophy, 249–252,
        251–252f
  in ectopic ureterocele, 52, 65f
  renal cell. *See* Kidney, renal cell
        adenocarcinoma of.
Adenoma, 652–653, 653–654f
  Brunnian, 741–742f
  nephrogenic, 742–743f, 743–744
  of testis, 1080–1082, 1081f
  villous, 743
Adenomatoid polyp, 742–743f,
        743–744
Adenomatoid tumor, or epididymis,
        1139f, 1146–1150,
        1148–1149f
Adenomyoma, of epididymis, 1146
Adenosis, 742–732f, 743–744
Adenovirus infection, in acute or-
        chitis, 1035
Adhesion factors, in UTI
  bacterial, 284–287, 285–286f
  host, 290–292
Adolescent, Ask-Upmark kidney in,
        89
Adrenal gland
  in 17-hydroxylase deficiency, 981
  congenital hyperplasia of
    in female pseudohermaphrodi-
        tism, 989
    in Leydig cell tumor, 1078–1079
    sexual differentiation disorders
        and, 968t, 971–972
Adrenal hemorrhage, retroperitoneal
        bleeding in, 560
Adrenal insufficiency, 1104
Adrenal rests, intrascrotal, 1104f

Adrenal-cortical rests, paratesticular,
        961–963, 962f
Adrenalectomy, in prostate carci-
        noma, 1272–1273
Adrenocorticotropic hormone
  in Cushing's syndrome, 962–963
  in prostate carcinoma, 1232–1233
Adrenogenital syndrome, male, 968t,
        978–981, 980f, 981t
Adventitial fibroplasia, 200
Alcoholism
  in male infertility, 1027
  in renal papillary necrosis, 408
Alkylating agent. *See also specific*
  in bladder cancer, 708, 827, 828
  in hypospermatogenesis, 1018
  -induced disease, 893
  in renal cell adenocarcinoma, 651
  in Sertoli-cell-only syndrome, 1022
  in urothelial neoplasm, 708–709
Allantois, 235
Allergic granuloma, of prostate, 1185
Alpha-1-antitrypsin
  in germ cell tumor, 1055
  in malakoplakia, 448
Alpha-fetoprotein. *See also* Tumor
        marker.
  in endodermal sinus tumor, 1071,
        1072
  in germ cell tumor, mixed,
        1074–1075
  in mixed germ cell tumor,
        1074–1075
  in renal agenesis, 118
  in testicular lymphoma, 1085
  in testicular tumor, 1053, 1054,
        1055f
    metastatic, 1089

Bladder *(Continued)*
congenitally enlarged. *See* Mega-
 cystitis.
distension of, artifactual, 720f
diverticula of, 602–608
 calculi in, 605f
 carcinoma of, 823, 824f
 congenital vesical, 606–608,
  608–609f
 in hydronephrosis, 603
 in lower urinary tract obstruction, 602–608
  acquired, 602–606, 603–607f
  congenital, 606–608,
   608–609f
  malignancy in, 605–606,
   606–608f
 in prune-belly syndrome, 125
 UTI in, 300
 vesical, carcinoma of, 823, 824f
duplication of, 241f, 242
embryologic development of,
 235–237, 236f
endometriosis of, 746, 747f
eosinophilic granuloma of, 449
exstrophy of, 245–253
 adenocarcinoma in, 249–252,
  251–252f
 clinical features of, 247–248f
 embryology of, 245, 246f
 glandular metaplasia in,
  723–724f
 incidence of, 245
 inheritance in, 245
 pathology of, microscopic,
  248–250f
 squamous metaplasia in, 723
 ureterosigmoidostomy in,
  tumors in, 252–253, 253f
 urothelial neoplasm in, 711–712
exstrophy-epispadias complex, 244
extramedullary plasmacytoma of,
 868
glycocalyx, in urinary tract
 infection, 292
granular cell myoblastoma of, 862
hyperplasia of, 817
hypertrophy of, 601f
immunoblastic sarcoma of, 868
infection of. *See* Cystitis.
leiomyoma of, 861–862
lymphoma of, 867–868
lymphomatoid granulomatosis of,
 868
malakoplakia of, 401, 445f,
 446–448, 447–448f
malignant fibrous histiocytoma of,
 868
malignant melanoma of, 868
malignant mesenchymoma of, 868

megacystis of, 254–256
 isolated, 254
 -microcolon-intestinal hypoper-
  istalsis syndrome, 254–256
mucinous metaplasia of, 724–725
neck
 hypertrophy of, in posterior
  urethral valves, 256
 obstruction of, isolated, 600–602
neurofibroma of, 862–863
neurofibromatosis of, 862
neurogenic, cystitis in, 433
neuropathic, in reflux nephropathy, 358, 377
 obstruction of, 600–602
 in renal agenesis, 120
osteosarcoma of, 868
outlet obstruction of, 522–523
 in cervical carcinoma, 533–534f
papillomata of, 827
pheochromocytoma of, 868–870
 clinical presentation of, 868
 pathology of, 868–870, 869f
plasma cell granuloma of, 863
in prune-belly syndrome, 124f, 125
in renal agenesis, 115
schistosomiasis of, 440–441, 441f
squamous metaplasia of, 722
suprapubic needle aspiration of, in
 UTI, 304
surface mucous layer of, in
 interstitial cystitis, 445, 446
transitional cell papilloma of, 793
 inverted, 793
transurethral resection of, vesicoureteral reflux in, 378
trigone, embryologic development
 of, 12f
tumor of
 benign, 793, 861–863
 malignant. *See* Bladder cancer.
vesical duplication of, 241f, 242
villous adenoma of, 743
yolk sac tumor of, 868
Bladder cancer, 793–835
 adenocarcinoma
  bladder diverticula and, 605
  bladder exstrophy in, 249–252,
   251–252f, 711–712
  cecal adenocarcinoma and, 772
  clinical presentation of, 795
  colloid, 764f
  cytologic examination and, 909,
   910f
  distribution of, 798
  gland-forming, 763f
  grade of, 803
  incidence of, 794
  lymphatic invasion in, 815
  mucinous, 764f

number of, 799
papillary, 763f
prognosis of, 800, 811
vs. prostatic adenocarcinoma, 770
staging of, 811t
urachal origin in, 825
urethral stricture in, 616
vascular invasion in, 815
advanced, 831–832
age factors in, 794
alkylating agents in, 708, 827, 828
analgesic abuse in, 707–708
aromatic amines in, 703
 smoking and, 705
artificial sweeteners in, 706–707
Bacillus Calmette Guerin in,
 826–827
bilharziasis in, 709, 710
biopsy abnormalities in, frequency
 of, 816
Brunn's nests in, 724f
carcinosarcoma, 767
chemotherapy in
 in advanced disease, 831–832
 in superficial disease, 827–828
chondrosarcoma, 767–768, 768f
cisplatin in, 827–828, 831
clinical presentation of, 794–795
coffee drinking in, 705–706
cyclamate in, 706, 707
cyclohexylamine in, 706, 707
cyclophosphamide in, 438,
 831–832
cystectomy in, 828
 radical, 830–831
 salvage, 829–830, 892
cystoscopy in, 796, 797t
cytologic examination in, 796,
 917–918t
distal ureters in, 818–819,
 819–821f
doxorubicin in, 828, 831–832
epodyl in, 828
grade of, 801–802f
granuloma, plasma cell, 863
hematoporphyrin derivative photodynamic therapy in, 829
hematuria in, 794–795
immunotherapy in 826–827
incidence of, 793–794
in situ
 asymptomatic, 828
 chemotherapy in, 828
 cystitis cystica in, 726f
 grading of, 803
 overt symptomatic, 828
 prior or concurrent bladder
  tumor in, 828–829
 prognosis of, 817–818
 prostate in, 819, 821–822f

transitional cell papilloma, 734,
739–741, 740f
inverted, 741–742f
tryptophan in, 711
tumor-associated antigen production in, 782–784
tumor-specific antigens in, 783
undifferentiated carcinoma, 739t,
765f
cytology of, 910–911f, 911
of upper tract. *See* urinary tract,
upper, tumors of.
ureteritis in. *See* Ureteritis.
verrucous carcinoma, 760, 762f
villous adenoma, 743
viral infection in, 710–711
Urothelium
cytoplasmic clearing in, 720–721,
721f
histologic anatomy of, 719–721,
720f
hyperplasia of, 727–729f
neoplasms of. *See* Urothelial
neoplasm.
nonneoplastic alterations of,
721–727, 722–726f
umbrella cells, 719
Uterus
atresia of, in ectopic ureter, 58
bicornuate
bladder duplications and, 242
in ectopic ureter, 57–58, 58
horseshoe kidney and, 46
in renal agenesis, 112
in renal ectopia, 35
cervix of. *See* Cervix.
didelphus of, renal agenesis and,
114
duplication of, 244
prolapse of, urinary tract obstruction in, 544, 545f
UTI. *See* Urinary tract infection

Vacuum cleaner injury, of penis, 1336
Vagina
in Behçet's syndrome, 1305
discharge of, in ectopic ureter,
55–56
duplex, in renal ectopia, 35
duplication of, 244
in ectopic ureter, single system, 58
pH of, in UTI, 293
septate
bladder duplications and, 242
horseshoe kidney and, 46
in UTI, 303
Vaginalis, meconium, 1113

Valsalva maneuver, in varicocele,
1015
Vanillylmandelic acid
in pheochromocytoma, of bladder,
868
in Wilms' tumor, 636
Varicocele, 1013–1017, 1014f
biopsy findings in, 1016
clinical and radiographic picture
in, 1015f
etiology of, 1014–1015
hormone levels in, 1015
oligospermia and, 1009
in renal cell adenocarcinoma, 671
semen analysis in, 1016
sloughing of immature cells in,
1013–1017
therapy, 1016–1017
Varicocelectomy, 1016–1017
Vas deferans
anatomy of, 936–937
artery of, 938
atresia of, 1103f
in bladder cancer, 819
calcification of, 1109, 1110f
calculi of, 1110
cyst of, 1114
duplication of, 957, 1103
in renal agenesis, 113
granuloma of, talc, 1113
infection of, acute orchitis and,
1035
syphilis of, 1122
talc granuloma of, 1113
Vasculitis
of paratesticular structures, 1129
of penis, 1328
Vasectomy
postoperative alterations in,
1007–1008
reversal of, 1007
vasitis nodosa and, 1125
Vasitis, 1123–1125
Vasitis nodosa, 1123–1125, 1124–
1125f
Vasodepressor, in hydronephrosis,
483–484
Vasoepididymostomy, in obstructive
azoospermia, 1006–1007
Vasospasm, in fibromuscular
dysplasia, 195
Vasovasotomy, in obstructive
azoospermia, 1006
VATER syndrome
in ectopic ureter, 57
megalourethra and, 267
renal agenesis and, 114
renal lesions in, 162t

Vaughan-Laragh combination
formula, in renal artery
stenosis, 192
Vena cava
duplication of, in bladder exstrophy, 245
inferior
anomalies of, hematuria in, 226
in renal cell adenocarcinoma,
656f, 673
thrombosis of, urinary tract
obstruction in, 541
Venereal disease
in acute orchitis, 1035
in prostate cancer, 1206
Reiter's syndrome following, 461
in urethral carcinoma, in males,
1373
Venous collaterals, in urinary tract
obstruction, 541
Ventriculoperitoneal shunt, urinary
tract obstruction in, 564
Verocay body
in bladder neurofibroma, 863
in penile neural tumor, 1343
Verrucous carcinoma, 760, 762f
of penis, 1349–1352, 1350–1352f
Vertebral artery stenosis, renal artery
stenosis and, 203
Verumontanum, squamous metaplasia of, 614
Vesical venous plexus, in schistosomiasis, 1233
Vesicoureteral reflux, 351–386. *See
also* Reflux nephropathy.
ascending infection in, 281
in Ask-Upmark kidney, 88,
378–379f
bladder dysfunction in, 358
classification and grading of,
352–353f
clinical aspects of, 376–379
complications of, 379–386
conditions associated with, 377–
378, 378–379f
consequences of, 359–362f
definition of, 280
diagnostic evaluation in, 379
embryologic development in,
356–357, 357t
familial incidence of, 376–377
focal segmental glomerulosclerosis
in, 380–383, 381f
grading of, 352–353f, 353
horseshoe kidney and, 46–47
hypertension in, 383–384
immunologic mechanisms in, 365
incidence and epidemiology of, 376